SIXTH EDITION

IMMUNOLOGY, IMMUNOPATHOLOGY, *and* IMMUNITY

STEWART SELL
Division of Experimental Pathology
The Albany Medical College
Albany, New York

CONTRIBUTING AUTHOR
EDWARD E. MAX
Center for Biologics Evaluation and Research
Food and Drug Administration
Bethesda, Maryland

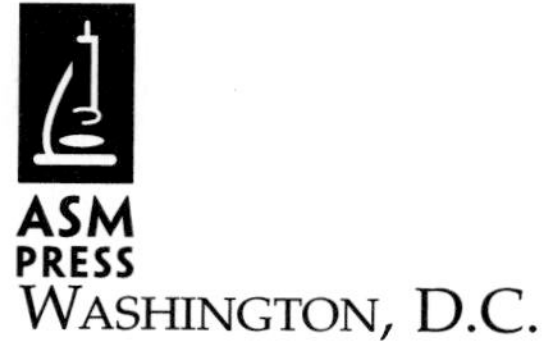

ASM PRESS
WASHINGTON, D.C.

Address editorial correspondence to ASM Press, 1752 N St. NW, Washington, DC 20036-2904, USA

Send orders to ASM Press, P.O. Box 605, Herndon, VA 20172, USA
Phone: (800) 546-2416 or (703) 661-1593
Fax: (703) 661-1501
E-mail: books@asmusa.org
Online: www.asmpress.org

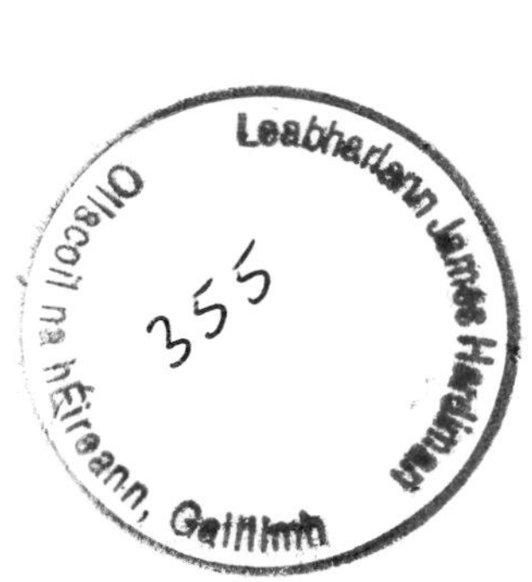

Library of Congress Cataloging-in-Publication Data

Sell, Stewart, 1935–
Immunology, immunopathology, and immunity/Stewart Sell; contributing author, Edward E. Max.—6th ed.
p.; cm.
Includes bibliographical references and index.
ISBN 1-55581-202-3
1. Immunology. 2. Immunopathology. 3. Immunity. I. Max, Edward E. II. Title.
[DNLM: 1. Immune System—physiology. 2. Immune System—physiopathology. 3. Immunity. 4. Immunologic Diseases. QW 504 S467i 2001]
QR181.S39 2001
616.07'9—dc21

00-045350

10 9 8 7 6 5 4 3 2 1

Cover photo: Scanning electron microscopic image of lymphocytes, a red blood cell, and platelets. The micrograph was taken by D. Scott Linthicum.

This book is dedicated to the graduate students and postdoctoral fellows who have made my research life interesting and rewarding: James Storey, Richard N. Baney, Teisa An, Douglas Redelman, Dorothy Hudig, Scott Linthicum, Charles Scott, Luc Bélanger, Hiro Watabe, Dennis Murayama, Kiminaro Dempo, Corey Raffel, John Brown, Daniel Keller, Sheila Lukehart, Eileen Skletsky, Stephen Norris, Harold Dunsford, Bret Steiner, Masauki Endoh, Pam Kimball, Anand Lagoo, Luoquan Wang, Zoran Ilic, Ludmilla Engele, Leonid Yavorkovsky, Masahiro Hata, Jae Hyae Lee, Nader Ghebranous, Li Yin, Thomas Shupe, Paul Yang, David Rosenberg, and Mingzen Sun. To them goes the credit for whatever scientific contributions have been made by my laboratory. In addition, I dedicate this book to the many technicians who have been with me over the years. Most, if not all, have gone on to graduate school.

Contents

Preface

The goal of this book is to emphasize what the immune system *does,* as well as *how it works.* Most immunology books focus on basic immunology or how the immune system works. The organization of *Immunology, Immunopathology, and Immunity* includes both basic immunology (how it works) and immunopathology and immunity (what it does). I have found, when teaching basic immunology, that many students raise questions about how the immune system causes diseases, such as systemic lupus erythematosus, thyroiditis, and myasthenia gravis; how the immune system may protect us against infections, such as bacterial infections and viral infections (including AIDS); and how the immune system may protect us against the development of cancer. Most immunology books have excellent coverage of basic immunology but superficial and cursory coverage of the role of immunity in disease or protection against disease. Thus, the student (or instructor) must look up in other, clinically oriented texts or search the literature to find out specific information on clinical aspects of immunology. For these questions, *Immunology, Immunopathology, and Immunity* serves as its own reference book. A teacher or student need not search for another source of information to answer clinically related questions about the role of the immune response in causing or protecting against disease. These subjects may be found in the later chapters of this text and can be easily located by looking in the index. To quote from the preface to the first edition of this book, published in 1972: "Frequently I have been asked by medical and biology students to recommend a text that covers both basic immunology and immunopathology. At best, I could recommend a basic text for immunology and individual chapters in several books for immunopathology—admitting that still, certain fundamental areas would remain uncovered. I could not identify a single text that encompasses the material that I thought important in a manner palatable to a beginner in the field."

I express my thanks and deep appreciation for the following, who have made major contributions either directly or indirectly to this effort: Phillip Gell (Oxford, England) for his original classification of and insights into immunopathologic reactions; John Fahey (University of California, Los Angeles) for his understanding of immunoglobulin structure and function; Edward Max (Food and Drug Administration) for his expertise on B cells and coauthorship of chapter 4; Ira Berkower (Food and Drug Administration) for contributions to the previous edition that have been incorporated into chapter 5; William O. Weigle (Scripps Institute, La Jolla, Calif.) for his understanding of how immune cells interact; Marion Cohen (University of Medicine and Dentistry of New Jersey) for reviewing a draft of the book; Frank Dixon (Scripps Institute) for his understanding of immune complex diseases; Frank Arnett (University of Texas, Houston) for contributions to chapter 10; William T. Shearer (Baylor College of Medicine, Houston, Tex.) for contributions to chapter 11; Byron H. Waksman (New York, N.Y.) for his many contributions to understanding delayed-type hypersensitivity and granulomatous reactions; Andrew Carlson (Albany Medical College) for his insightful information on skin diseases; Steven Baird (University of California, San Diego) for his unique understanding of immunoproliferative diseases; Rosa Ten (Mayo Clinic) for her classification of immune deficiency diseases and her review of chapter 17; Jay A. Levy (University of California, San Francisco) for reviewing chapter 19; Richard Dutton (Trudeau Institute, Saranac Lake, N.Y.), Philippa Marrack (National Jewish Hospital and Research Center, Denver, Colo.), and William T. Shearer for suggestions for the history-of-immunopathology table in appendix 1); and finally to Yale Altman (Harvard, Mass.) for his continuing enthusiastic support of this book and to Ken April (ASM Press, Washington, D.C.) for coordinating the publication process.

Immunology

Introduction to Part I

1

Immunity

The *immune system* is a collection of organs and vessels in the body involved in producing and delivering the cells and molecules that protect us from infections. *Immunology* is the study of the immune system and its products and mechanisms of defense. From the time of conception, the human organism faces attack from a wide variety of infectious agents. We must have ways to identify them and defend ourselves against their invasion, colonization, and toxic effects. This defensive ability is called *immunity.*

"Immunity" comes from the Latin word *immunitas,* which means "protection from." In legal terms, immunity means that the protected person is not subject to certain laws (e.g., diplomatic immunity) or is exempt from certain duties (e.g., not required to serve in the armed forces). In clinical terms, immunity means protection from certain diseases, particularly infectious diseases. For instance, the commonly used statement "She is immune to measles" indicates that the person referred to has had measles once (or has been vaccinated against measles) and will not get measles again. This is a form of *acquired immunity* or *adaptive immunity.*

The protective mechanisms of the body are divided into two major types: innate and adaptive (Table 1.1). Innate resistance is present in all normal individuals, does not require previous exposure to be effective, and operates on infectious agents in the same way every time the individual is exposed. The adaptive, specific immune defense system does not become active until the individual is exposed to the infectious agent; it requires stimulation or *immunization* to become activated. This system has the capacity to identify foreign agents and distinguish foreign agents from self (self and nonself discrimination). It is mediated by products that specifically recognize one agent and do not act on a different agent. In an infectious disease, such as measles, the adaptive immune system is activated during the first infection, so that upon subsequent contact with measles, no disease will occur. The immune system has learned to recognize the measles virus and react specifically to it with an accelerated protective response. This is termed *immune memory.*

Table 1.1 Comparison of innate and adaptive (acquired) immunity

Characteristic	Innate immunity	Adaptive immunity
Specificity	Nonspecific, indiscriminate	Specific, discriminate
Mechanical	Skin, mucous membrane	Immune induced reactive fibrosis (granuloma)
Humoral	pH, lysozyme, serum proteins	Immunoglobulin antibodies
Cellular	White blood cells	Specifically sensitized lymphocytes
Induction	Constitutive	Requires previous contact (immunization)

Innate Immunity

Innate defense mechanisms against foreign invaders include mechanical barriers, secreted products, and inflammatory cells (Fig. 1.1). Innate resistance is present at all times in normal individuals. Its effectiveness may be modulated by physiological conditions (e.g., nutrition, age, hormone levels). Innate resistance does not distinguish among microorganisms of different species and does not alter in intensity upon reexposure. One of the major nonspecific defense systems is the epithelial surface of the body. Externally, the skin, and internally, the mucous membrane linings of the gastrointestinal tract and the epithelium of the airways of the lungs, provide mechanical barriers to invasion. Secreted products, such as acid in the stomach, lysozyme in tears, sebaceous gland secretions, and certain proteins in the blood, are toxic to potential invaders. In addition, Paneth cells at the bottom of intestinal crypts and epithelial cells, as well as phagocytic cells, produce small antimicrobial peptides called defensins that can insert into microbial membranes and disrupt them. White blood cells are attracted to sites of infection by products of infecting organisms, necrotic tissue, and defensins and attack the invaders.

When the protective epithelial barriers are breached (as by a cut or abrasion of the skin or by penetration of invading organisms past the protective lining of the airways of the lungs), and organisms begin to grow in the tissues of the body, a more specific and more powerful backup defense system is needed. Since most infectious organisms can multiply rapidly, and the defensive reaction must be directed specifically to the infection and not to host tissues, this system must be activated quickly, be precisely directed to the infectious agent, and be very destructive.

Adaptive Immunity

The adaptive immune system is quiescent until it is stimulated by a specific infection or vaccination *(immunizing event).* Agents that stimulate the adaptive system of immunity are recognized as foreign by the immune system and are called *immunogens* or *antigens.* The adaptive system is capable of exquisitely distinguishing among different microorganisms and significantly alters its intensity and response time upon reexposure.

There are two major arms of the immune response: *humoral* and *cellular*. Humoral immunity is mediated by soluble protein molecules known as *antibodies*. Cellular immunity is mediated by specifically sensitized white blood cells known as lymphocytes. *Immunization* or *vaccination* may activate two different classes of lymphocytes. The cells responsible for antibody production are in the *B-lymphocyte* series; those responsible for cellular immunity are in the *T-lymphocyte* series (Table 1.2). *Antibodies* belong to a family of molecules termed *immunoglobulins* that are found in the

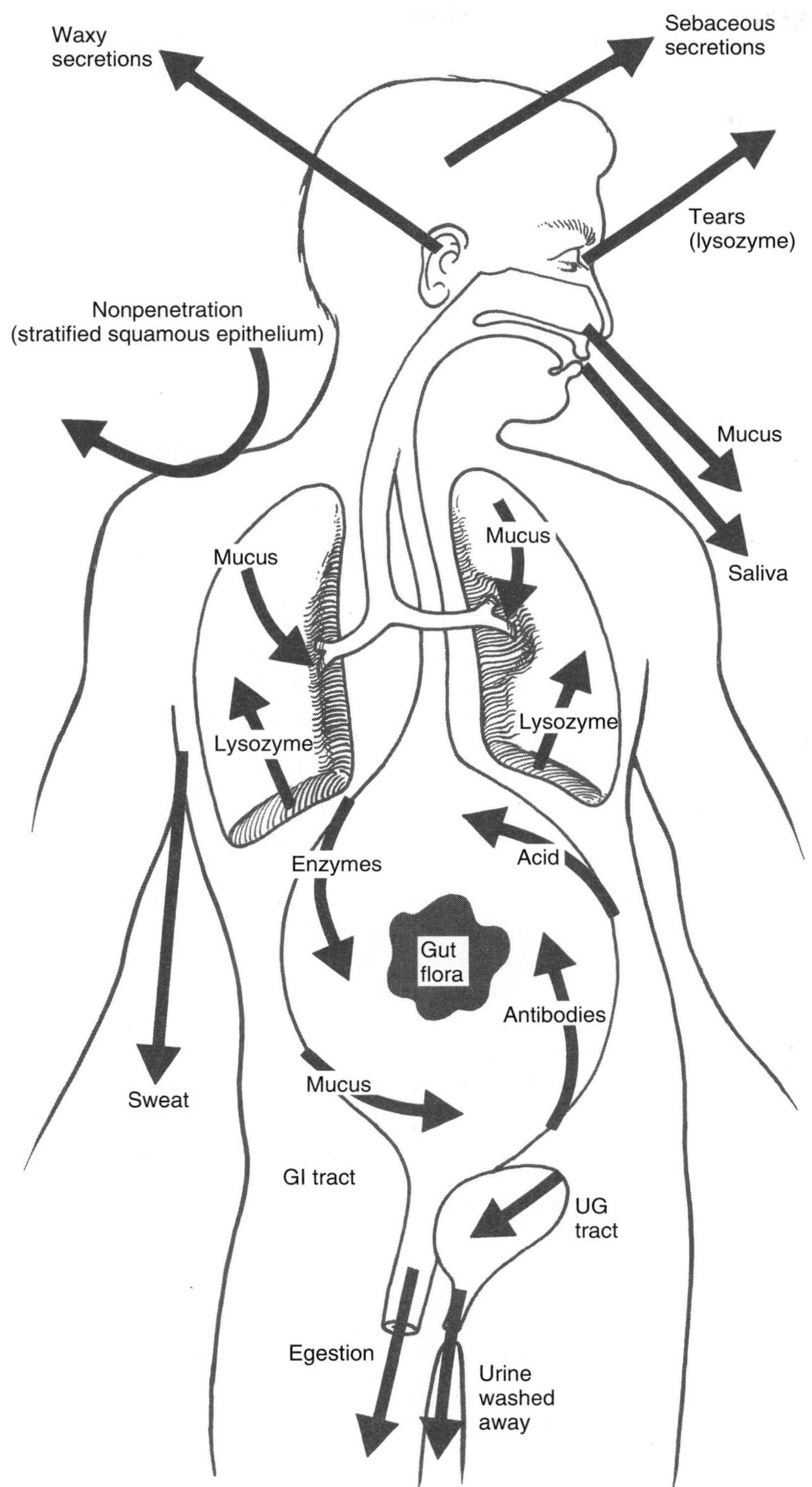

Figure 1.1 Innate immunity. Innate defenses against infectious agents include skin and mucous membrane barriers and secretions that are bacteriostatic or remove foreign agents by washing them away. GI, gastrointestinal; UG, urogenital.

Table 1.2 Two major arms of immunity

Characteristic	Humoral immunity	Cellular immunity
Cell line	B cells, plasma cells	T cells
Product	Antibody	Sensitized cells
Protection against:	Bacteria, viruses	Viruses, mycobacteria, fungi

blood or in external secretions. Antibodies are protein molecules that react specifically with structures (*epitopes*) on infecting organisms through specialized receptors (*binding sites* or *paratopes*) on the antibody molecule. *Specifically sensitized T cells* also have an antibodylike receptor (T-cell receptor), which recognizes antigens. Antigens that are capable of inducing an immune response are called *immunogens* or *complete antigens*. *Incomplete antigens* or *haptens* can elicit a reaction in an already immunized individual but cannot induce an immune reaction in an individual who is not immunized. The cells activated by immunization proliferate and differentiate in specialized organs in the body *(lymphoid organs)* and are released into the blood through specialized vessels known as lymphatics. This system allows rapid delivery to other parts of the body, where an infection may be located.

The response of the immune system to immunization has been compared to a motor neuron reflex arc, i.e., there are afferent, efferent, and central limbs. *Afferent* refers to delivery of the immunogen to cells of the immune system; *central* refers to the response of the reacting lymphoid organs resulting in production of antibody and sensitized cells; *efferent* refers to the delivery of these products to the site of antigen deposition. Once immunization has occurred, the immunized individual will respond with a more rapid and more intense response upon second exposure to the same immunogen (secondary response or immunological memory).

When an infectious agent begins to grow in our bodies, a "race of life" is started. The race is between the rate of expansion of the infection and the ability of our immune systems to combat the infection. When the antibody or sensitized cells react with antigen (infectious agent) in the tissues, very powerful immune defense mechanisms are activated. However, the infectious invaders of our bodies have many ways of evading both innate and adaptive resistance. These include such properties as the release of "toxins," the formation of protective coatings, the ability to localize in inaccessible sites, and the ability to exist within our own cells or even be incorporated into our DNA and thus evade recognition or destruction. Thus, the immune system must not only react quickly, specifically, and powerfully to an infection but must also react in a way that will overcome the evasive mechanisms of the infectious agent. Different ways in which the immune system combines specificity with the properties of inflammation are called *immune effector mechanisms*. Some of the critical characteristics of the adaptive immune system are listed in Table 1.3.

The Inflammatory Response

The response of our bodies to an infection occurs in the form of *inflammation*. The characteristics of inflammation may be modified by the presence of antibody or sensitized cells. The hallmark of an inflammatory response is the passage of proteins, fluid, and cells from the blood into focal areas in

Table 1.3 Functional abilities of the adaptive immune system

1. Specific recognition of many different foreign invaders
2. Rapid synthesis of immune products upon contact with invaders
3. Quick delivery of the immune products to the site of infection
4. Diversity of effector defensive mechanisms to combat infectious agents with different properties
5. Nonself direction of the defensive mechanisms specifically to foreign invaders rather than one's own tissue
6. Deactivation mechanisms to turn off the system when the invader has been cleared

tissues. The result is the local delivery of agents that can effectively combat infections. During an inflammatory response, components of both the innate and adaptive resistance mechanisms are often used. These include inflammatory cells, products of inflammatory cells, and certain blood proteins (inflammatory mediators).

Initiation of an inflammatory response begins with an increase in blood flow to infected tissues and with the opening of the cells lining the blood vessels or capillaries, followed by emigration of cells into the involved tissue (Fig. 1.2). Increased blood flow and vascular permeability allow fluid and/or cells to enter the tissues. The gross manifestations of

Figure 1.2 Acute inflammatory response to infection. Infectious organisms release chemicals or initiate tissue damage that produces products that are chemotactic for (attract) inflammatory cells (polymorphonuclear leukocytes) and cause constriction of vascular endothelial cells. This results in passage of fluid from the blood into the tissue (edema) and/or infiltration of tissue with inflammatory cells. Polymorphonuclear leukocytes may ingest and kill the infecting organisms or may release proteolytic enzymes into tissue, causing necrosis and formation of pus. Antibody serves to enhance this response and direct the inflammatory cells by reacting with the infecting organisms and activating bloodborne inflammatory mediators brought into the tissue during edema formation. These mediators react with cell surface receptors on the inflammatory cells and enhance the ability of the cells to ingest (phagocytose) and destroy the organisms.

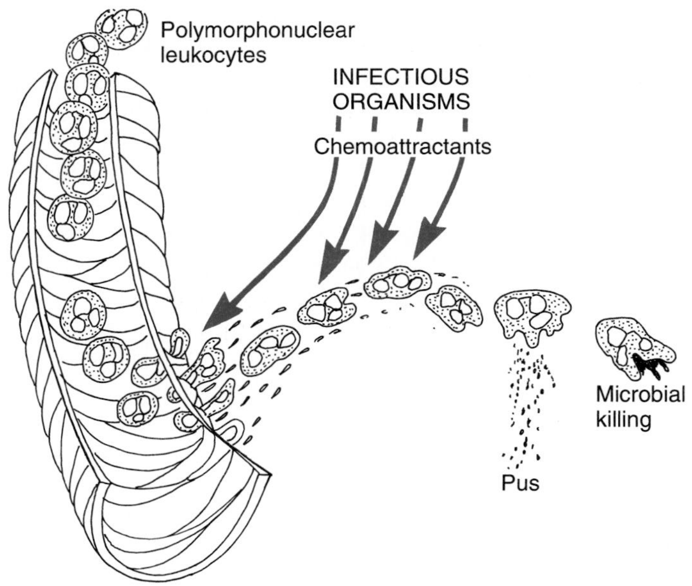

Table 1.4 Four cardinal signs of acute inflammation according to Celsus (25 B.C.)[a]

Latin	English
Rubor	Redness
Tumor	Swelling
Calor	Heat
Dolor	Pain

[a]The fifth classic sign of acute inflammation, "functio laesa" (loss of function), was added by Rudolf Virchow (1821–1902).

acute inflammation were first described by Celsus in about 25 B.C. as the *cardinal signs of acute inflammation* (Table 1.4). The signs of inflammation are manifestations of increased blood flow and infiltration of tissues by inflammatory proteins and cells. Increased blood flow causes redness and increased temperature. The presence of fluid and red blood cells in tissues is grossly recognized by swelling (edema) and redness. White blood cell (inflammatory cell) infiltrations cause a white color. If the site of inflammation is necrotic and filled with white blood cells, the inflammatory site will be seen as pus. If red blood cells are present, the pus may be yellow or bloody red, depending on the proportion of red cells. The cellular evolution of an inflammatory response eventually results in the healing or scarring of the lesion.

Immunopathology (the Double-Edged Sword)

The immune system did not evolve without ambivalence and flaws. The same system that functions so well to protect against foreign invaders may also turn against us. The term *immunopathology* is a misnomer: "immune" means protection or exemption from; "pathology" is the study of disease. Thus, immunopathology literally means the study of the protection from disease, but in usage it actually means the study of how immune mechanisms cause diseases. Immunity is a double-edged sword: on one hand, immune responses protect us from infections; on the other hand, immune mechanisms may cause disease. The most compelling evidence that immune reactions are protective is provided by the naturally occurring immune deficiency diseases. Individuals with an inability to mount an effective immune response to infectious agents invariably succumb to infections unless they are vigorously treated. However, immune reactions may also cause disease. The terms allergy and hypersensitivity are used to denote deleterious immune reactions. *Allergy* is frequently used for a particular type of rapidly developing explosive immune reaction (anaphylactic), and *hypersensitivity* is used for delayed-type or cell-mediated immune reactivity. The term immunity was once restricted to the protective effects of immune reactions, but by common usage this is no longer the case. In some diseases, immune mechanisms may actually be directed against our own tissues. This is termed *autoimmunity*.

How the immune system coordinates the process of inflammation, both in protection and in causing disease (immune effector mechanisms), is the focus of this book. Immune effector mechanisms are essentially variations of the inflammatory response influenced by specific products of the adaptive immune system. Therefore, before we can address these mechanisms and their effects, it is necessary to understand the basics of inflammation and immunology; these are covered in part I of this book.

Summary

Immunology is the study of how we protect ourselves against infection. The seemingly unlimited variations in the way that infectious agents can invade and colonize our bodies necessitates a counterbalancing system of defense that employs many different strategies. One system is constitutive and consists of mechanical barriers, pH, temperature, phagocytosis, inflammation, and so on (innate resistance). The other is induced and consists of specific products that recognize invaders as foreign (adaptive immunity). After induction (immunization), the adaptive system responds more rapidly and with greater intensity than after first exposure (immune memory). The two major arms of the adaptive immune response are humoral (antibody) and cellular (specifically sensitized cells). Specialized cells of the body known as lymphocytes are responsible for the adaptive immune response (T lymphocytes for cellular immunity and B lymphocytes for humoral immunity). In response to infection, both adaptive and innate inflammatory mechanisms may be activated. During evolution, the adaptive immune response became increasingly complex. Humans have different classes of antibody and different subsets of T cells that not only have different functions as immune effectors but also are able to direct and modify inflammatory events to provide specific direction to appropriate combinations of inflammatory events in order to combat many different infectious agents.

The immune response is not always protective; in many instances, the same immune effector mechanisms that defend us against foreign invaders may be turned against us and produce disease (the double-edged sword of immunopathology). Part I of this book (Immunology) describes the basics of the inflammatory and immune response systems. Part II (Immunopathology and Immunity) explains how the same immune mechanisms are used for both destruction and defense.

Bibliography

Abbas, A. K., A. H. Lightman, and J. S. Pober. 1997. *Cellular and Molecular Immunology*. The W. B. Saunders Co., Philadelphia, Pa.

Feron, D. T., and R. M. Locksley. 1996. The instructive role of innate immunity in the acquired immune response. *Science* **272:**50–55.

Goldsby, R. A., T. J. Kindt, and B. A. Osborne. 2000. *Kuby's Immunology,* 4th ed. W. H. Freeman & Co., New York, N.Y.

Janeway, C. (ed.). 1998. *Seminars in Immunology,* vol. 10, issue 5. *Interfaces between Innate and Adaptive Immunity.* Academic Press Ltd., London, England.

Janeway, C. A., P. Travers, M. Walport, and J. D. Capra. 1999. *Immunobiology: the Immune System in Health and Disease,* 4th ed. Elsevier Garland Publishers, New York, N.Y.

Lamont, J. T. 1992. Mucus: the front line of intestinal mucosal defense. *Ann. N. Y. Acad. Sci.* **664:**190–201.

Majno, G. 1975. *The Healing Hand.* Harvard University Press, Cambridge, Mass. (This history of inflammation and pathology is essential reading for all graduate and medical students.)

Paul, W. E. (ed.). 1999. *Fundamental Immunology,* 4th ed. Lippincott-Raven Publishers, Philadelphia, Pa.

Rich, R. R. (ed.). 1996. *Clinical Immunology: Principles and Practice.* The C. V. Mosby Co., St. Louis, Mo.

Roitt, I. J. Brostoff, and D. Male. 1998. *Immunology,* 5th ed. The C. V. Mosby Co., London, England.

Roitt, I. M., and P. J. Delves (ed.). 1992. *Encyclopedia of Immunology.* Academic Press, London, England.

Stites, D. P., A. I. Terr, and T. G. Parslow. 1997. *Medical Immunology,* 9th ed. Appleton & Lange, Stamford, Conn.

Cells of the Immune System

2

The Blood and Lymphoid Systems

To understand how the inflammatory and immune systems work, it is first necessary to know the players. The players are the cells of these systems and their products (proteins). These cells, the organs they compose, and the delivery network for the cells and their products constitute the *blood and lymphoid systems.* The blood system includes the bone marrow, where blood cells are made (hematopoiesis), and the circulating blood. The lymphoid system is a complex network of lymphatic vessels, lymphoid nodules, lymph nodes, spleen, and other organs, distributed throughout the body in places where contact is made with foreign antigens that enter the body through the skin, airways, or gastrointestinal tract. The cells of the body that react by inflammation to protect us against injury and infection are called white blood cells *(leukocytes).* The major cellular constituents of the immune system are a subgroup of white blood cells known as *lymphocytes.* However, other cells *(macrophages)* are also involved in induction of an immune response, and other white blood cell types such as macrophages and *polymorphonuclear leukocytes* take an active part in various effector inflammatory responses associated with immune reactions. The purpose of this chapter is to introduce the cellular players and the various roles they play. The effects of these players in inflammation, immunopathology, and immunity are presented in more detail in later chapters.

Blood Cells

The cells that are present in the blood represent the fully mature products of cell lineages for which the progenitors are found in other organs. There are two major cell types in the blood: *red blood cells (erythrocytes)* and *white blood cells (leukocytes)* (Fig. 2.1).

Red Blood Cells

In smears of peripheral blood stained with a special dye to bring out different cellular structures (Wright's stain), erythrocytes (red blood cells) are small, light pink, and have no nuclei. Erythrocytes are by far the most numerous cells in blood smears. The percentage of red cells in the blood is estimated from the *hematocrit* (Fig. 2.2). Red blood cells do not take part in

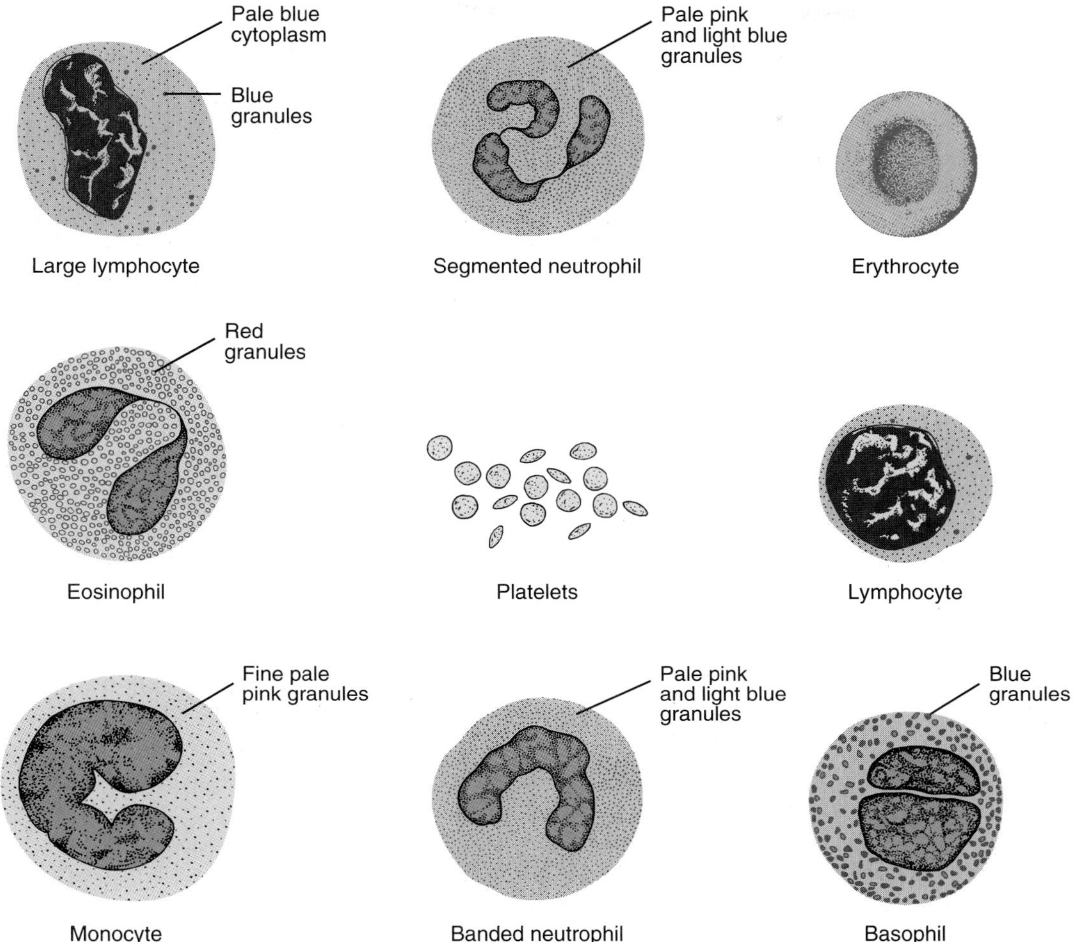

Figure 2.1 Representative cells in blood from normal individuals.

immune reactions: their major function is to carry oxygen required for metabolism of tissues throughout the body and to remove carbon dioxide produced by cellular metabolism.

White Blood Cells

White blood cells are called leukocytes *(leuko,* white; *cyte,* cell) because, when anticoagulated blood is lightly centrifuged, leukocytes sediment in a thin, white layer between the denser erythrocytes and the plasma. This layer of white cells is called the *buffy coat* (Fig. 2.2). Patients with tumors of the white blood cells often have a marked increase in this layer and blood that is more white than red: *leukemia,* or "white blood." The mature forms of these cells are most easily recognized in peripheral blood smears. The basic structure and function of white blood cells are described below; their role in immune responses and inflammation is presented in more detail in later chapters.

The various white blood cells and their normal representation in the blood are depicted in Fig. 2.3. The terms used by pathologists, immunologists, and hematologists for the various white blood cells reflect different

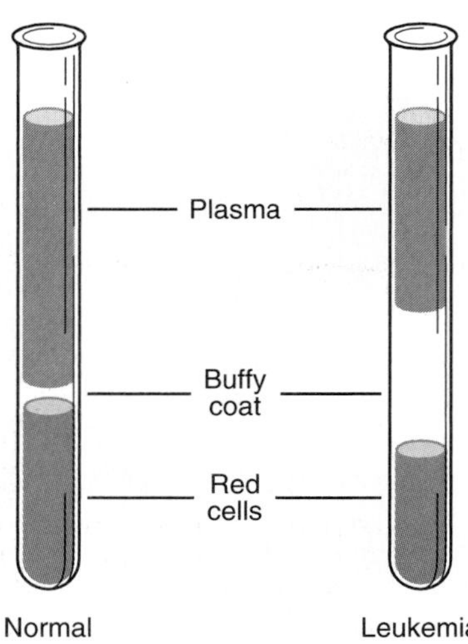

Figure 2.2 Separation of blood components by centrifugation. The red blood cells are the most dense component, sediment most rapidly and make up approximately 40% of the blood volume. This percentage is known as the hematocrit. The hematocrit is used to estimate increases or decreases in the number of circulating red cells in the blood. The plasma component (protein-enriched fluid) makes up the largest percentage (approximately 55 to 60%) and is the least dense. In between the plasma and the red blood cells, the white blood cells form a thin layer called the buffy coat, which is creamy white in color.

Figure 2.3 Leukocytes. Composite drawings indicate relative size (micrometers) and morphology of cells involved in immune reactions and in nonimmune inflammatory reactions. The erythrocyte is included for size reference, since it is the most easily identified cell in blood smears and in many tissue sections.

Cell Type	% of White Blood Cells in Blood	Diameter (μm)	Nucleus	Cytoplasm and Granules	Drawings
Erythrocytes	—	7.5	None	Pink, homogeneous cytoplasm	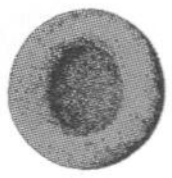
LEUKOCYTES					
Polymorphonuclear					
Neutrophils	50–70	10–12	2–5 lobules connected by thin bridges, coarse chromatin	Abundant cytoplasm/ fine pinkish granules	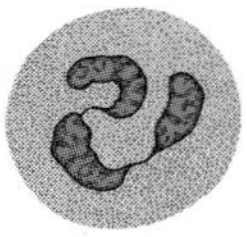
Eosinophils	1–3	10–12	Usually two oval lobes connected by bridge	Abundant cytoplasm/ coarse reflective granules stained red	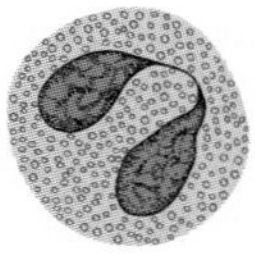
Basophils	< 1	8–10	Bent in S with two or more constrictions; obscured by cytoplasmic granules	Large and irregular granules stained deep blue	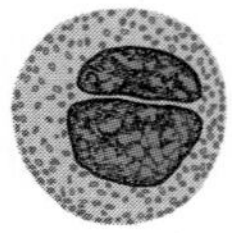
Mononuclear					
Lymphocytes	25–35	6–15	Round to oval; coarse chromatin	Bluish cytoplasm/ about 10% of cells fine azurophilic granules	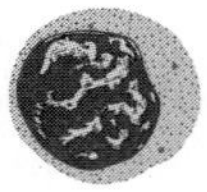
Monocytes	3–7	12–18	Kidney shaped, indented; fine chromatin	Bluish cytoplasm/ fine azurophilic granules	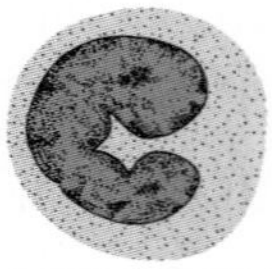

ways of looking at complex cell populations. A simplified classification of blood leukocytes is presented in Fig. 2.4.

The large mononuclear cells (macrophages) are phagocytic cells (macrophage means "large eater"). In peripheral blood, macrophages are termed monocytes; in tissues, they are called histiocytes. Particular care must be taken in understanding the terms monocyte and mononuclear. Hematologists use the term monocyte for the larger circulating mononuclear white blood cells that are found in the peripheral blood and that are in the macrophage lineage. Pathologists use the term mononuclear, or round cells, for lymphocytes and macrophages seen in tissue, to differentiate them from polymorphonuclear cells. These similar terms must be carefully distinguished to avoid confusion.

Figure 2.4 White blood cell nomenclature. White blood cells may be divided into two major populations on the basis of the form of their nuclei: single nuclei *(mononuclear* or *round cells)* or segmented nuclei *(polymorphonuclear).* Mononuclear cells are further divided into large *(macrophage* or *monocyte)* or small *(lymphocyte)* on the basis of the size of the nucleus. Lymphocytes may be further subdivided into two major populations: *T cells* and *B cells,* on the basis of function and cell surface phenotype (to be described later). B cells are the precursors of the cells that synthesize and secrete humoral antibodies. Subpopulations of T cells are responsible for a number of "cell-mediated" immune activities. T cells and B cells cannot be differentiated on the basis of morphologic appearance but do have different phenotypic markers. Some lymphocytes may "kill" certain other cell types in vitro *(natural killer* or *NK cells),* and others may become "armed" by passive absorption of antibody *(antibody-dependent cell-mediated cytotoxicity [ADCC])* or activated by lymphokines *(lymphokine-activated killer cells).* Polymorphonuclear cells play different roles in inflammation and are defined by different staining characteristics of their prominent cytoplasmic granules as eosinophils (red), basophils (blue), and neutrophils (pink) in standard blood smears.

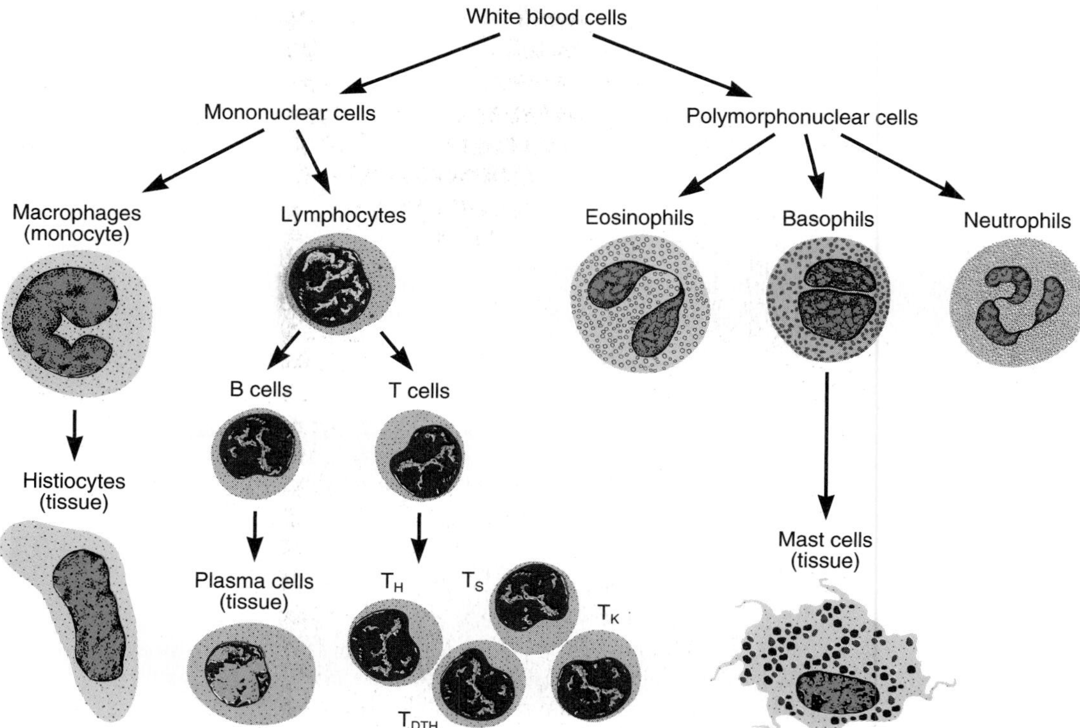

Polymorphonuclear Leukocytes/Granulocytes

Polymorphonuclear white blood cells are subdivided into three major populations on the basis of the staining properties of their cytoplasmic granules in standard hematologic blood smears or tissue preparations: neutrophil, pink; eosinophil, red; basophil, blue. Polymorphonuclear cells take part in both immune-specific and nonspecific inflammatory reactions. Because of the prominence of the granules, cells of these types are also called *granulocytes.*

Neutrophils. Neutrophils are polymorphonuclear leukocytes whose cytoplasmic granules do not take on strong acidophilic (red) or basophilic (blue) staining with the usual dyes used for staining smears of blood but show only a pale pink coloration. Such cells make up from 50 to 70% of the white blood cells of the peripheral blood and may be found scattered diffusely in many tissues, although they are most frequently found in areas of acute inflammation or acute necrosis. Like other white blood cells, neutrophils are produced from precursor cells in the bone marrow and released into the blood when mature. After entering the circulation, they last only 1 or 2 days, but their exact fate is unknown. Like its relative, the macrophage, the neutrophil is active in phagocytosis and has been called by some a microphage ("small eater"). The nucleus of the neutrophil, characteristic of polymorphonuclear leukocytes, is divided into round or oval lobes connected to one another by thin strands of nuclear material. The other outstanding feature of this type of white blood cell is the large number of membrane-delineated granules: azurophil granules, specific granules, and short rod-shaped alkaline phosphatase-containing granules (Table 2.1).

Within these granules, neutrophils carry potent microbicidal mechanisms that must be kept isolated from the cytoplasm, and they also have the ability to generate toxic oxygen species. Oxidant injury is induced by oxygen metabolites, such as superoxide anion, hydrogen peroxide, and hydroxyl radicals, that cause chemical alterations in proteins, lipids, carbohydrates, and nucleic acids. Alterations to the first three types of molecules damage membranes and protein synthesis. The azurophil granules contain *anionic granule proteins* and include myeloperoxidase, defensins, cathepsin G, azurocidin, and "lysosomal enzymes." These proteins bind to microbial cells and disrupt complex membrane functions or are released into tissues, where they may destroy host structures as well as microorganisms. For instance, in humans, defensins include four 29- to 34-amino-acid peptides (human neutrophil proteins designated HNP-1, HNP-2,

Table 2.1 Some components of neutrophil granules

Granule type	Contents
Azurophil	Microbicidal enzymes: myeloperoxidase, cathepsin G, azuroicidin, lysozyme, proteinase, elastase, protease 3
	Acid hydrolases: β-galactosidase, α-mannosidase, cathepsins A2, B, and D, α-fucosidase
	Defensins: HNP-1 to HNP-4
Specific	Cytochrome *b*, C3 receptor, β_2-integrin (CD11–CD18), lysozyme, collagenase, lactoferrin, gelatinase, plasminogen activator
Rod-shaped	Alkaline phosphatase

HNP-3, and HNP-4), which make up 30 to 50% of the azurophil granules. Defensins can insert into the membranes and kill a wide variety of bacteria, fungi, and viruses by changing the permeability of outer membranes of these organisms. Specific granules contain a specific cytochrome *b*, the complement receptor CR3, and β_2-integrin, which binds to the endothelial cells during acute inflammation. These proteins are translocated to the cell surface by certain stimuli and are important for cell activation and adhesion. Alkaline phosphatase activity is also upregulated during neutrophil activation and is located in the separate rod-shaped granule compartment.

Neutrophils are the first wave of a cellular attack on invading organisms and are the characteristic cell of acute inflammation. The appearance of neutrophils in areas of inflammation may be caused by chemicals released from bacteria or by factors produced nonspecifically from necrotic tissue or may be directed by antibody reacting with antigen. The role of neutrophils and other white blood cells in inflammation is presented in more detail in chapter 3.

Eosinophils. Eosinophils are similar in appearance to neutrophils, except that they have prominent eosinophilic (red) granules that may contain rodlike crystalloid inclusions when viewed by electron microscopy. These eosinophilic granules are membrane limited and contain large amounts of hydrolytic enzymes, including peroxidase and catalase. The chemotactic responses of eosinophils are similar to those of neutrophils, but eosinophils are found in unusually high numbers around antigen-antibody complexes and parasites in tissues. The eosinophil granule contains major basic proteins and arylsulfatase, which are toxic to parasitic worms and limit the extent of worm infestations. Eosinophils also contain histaminase and may limit or modulate mast cell-mediated inflammation. The role of eosinophil granule proteins in inflammation is covered in more detail in chapter 3. Eosinophils make up 1 to 3% of the circulating white blood cells.

Basophils and mast cells. Basophils have prominent blue-staining, finely granular cytoplasmic granules. Mast cells, related to basophils, are located in loose (areolar) connective tissue around small blood vessels. Blood basophils are round, whereas tissue mast cells may be elongated or irregularly shaped. Blood basophils make up less than 1% of the peripheral white blood cell. Basophil granules contain heparin, histamine, and serotonin (5-hydroxytryptamine); membranelike material that is metabolized to prostaglandins and leukotrienes; and a battery of hydrolytic enzymes, including a family of proteases. Heparin appears to be required for the proper formation of the basophilic granules and controls, in particular, the levels of mast cell proteases. In response to a stimulus, mast cells or basophils may spill out the contents of 60 to 70% of their granules (exocytosis). Mast cells have been nicknamed "gatekeeper cells" because they control access of blood proteins and cells to the extracellular space. The release of material from mast cell granules has a marked effect on the smooth muscles of arterioles (dilation) and the permeability of capillaries (contraction of endothelial cells). Release of these pharmacologically active agents by mast cells is the mechanism responsible for early inflammatory changes and for the unleashing of anaphylactic or atopic allergic reactions (see chapter 11). Mast cells also make many other cytokines, including interleukins 1 through 6, tumor necrosis factor, and some inflammatory cytokines, termed macrophage inflammatory proteins, that may attract macrophages, neutrophils, and eosinophils to inflammatory sites. The inflammatory cytokines of mast cells are presented in more detail in chapter 3.

Tissue mast cells have different characteristics depending on their location. This is termed *mast cell heterogeneity.* Differences in morphology, mediator content, histochemical staining, responsiveness to cytokines, and sensitivity to drugs have been described. Mast cell heterogeneity appears to be caused by microenvironmental factors. The two major subpopulations of mast cells are identified by those in the mucosa, which contain tryptase (*MC^T*), and those in the connective tissue, which contain both tryptase and chymase (*MC^{TC}*) (Table 2.2). MC^T cells predominate in lung and mucosa; MC^{TC} cells predominate in the connective tissue of bowel submucosa and skin. Each type is found about equally in nasal mucosa and ocular conjunctiva. The biological significance of these two mast cell populations is not clear, but differences in mediators suggest different functional capacities.

Lymphocytes

Lymphocytes are small, round cells found in the peripheral blood, lymph nodes, spleen, thymus, tonsils, and appendix and scattered throughout the connective tissue in many other organs. In smears of peripheral blood, lymphocytes appear slightly larger (7 to 8 μm) in diameter than red blood cells (erythrocytes) and make up about 30% of the total white blood cell count. A typical lymphocyte has very little cytoplasm and is composed mostly of a circular nucleus with prominent nuclear chromatin. The narrow rim of cytoplasm contains scattered ribosomes as well as a few ribosomal aggregates but in a resting state is virtually devoid of endoplasmic reticulum or other organelles. Once believed to be a short-lived "end" cell, some populations of lymphocytes are now known to survive for months or even years and recirculate from lymph nodes to lymph and blood. Although morphologically similar, different lymphocyte subpopulations have very different immune functions.

Lymphocytes are responsible for the primary recognition of antigen and also function as immunologically specific effector cells. Lymphocytes

Table 2.2 Characteristics of major mast cell populations[a]

Characteristic	MC^T (mucosal)	MC^{TC} (connective tissue)
Neutral protease	Tryptase	Tryptase, chymase
Tissue distribution	Mucosal (lung, bowel mucosa)	Connective tissue (skin, bowel submucosa)
Granule ultrastructure	Scrolls	Gratings/lattices
T-cell dependence	+	−
Compound 48/80 degranulation	−	+
Histamine	+	++
Leukotriene C_4/prostaglandin D_2 ratio	25:1	1:40
Cytoplasmic IgE	+	−
Fc_ϵ receptors	+++	+
Major proteoglycan	Chondroitin sulfate	Heparin

[a]Modified from L. B. Schwartz, *in* S. J. Galli and K. F. Austen, ed., *Mast Cell Differentiation and Function in Health and Disease,* Raven Press, New York, N.Y, 1989.

Table 2.3 Some basic properties of T and B lymphocytes[a]

Properties	T cells	B cells
Site of precursor	Thymus	Fetal liver, gastrointestinal tract, bone marrow
Surface markers	T antigens	Surface Ig
Rosettes	E	EAC
Tissue distribution	Interfollicular (paracortical)	Follicles (cortical)
Percentage of lymphocytes in blood	80%	20%
Radiation inactivation	+	++++
Mitogen response	Con A, PHA	PPD, LPS
Immune functions	Helper, suppressor, killer	Plasma cell precursor
Mixed lymphocyte reaction	Reactive cell	Stimulator cell

[a]E, sheep erythrocytes; EAC, sheep erythrocytes coated with antibody and complement; Con A, concanavalin A; PHA, phytohemagglutinin; PPD, purified protein derivative of *Mycobacterium tuberculosis;* LPS, *Escherichia coli* lipopolysaccharide. Subsets of T and B cells are identifed by CD markers, which are described in the text.

produce cell surface molecules that serve as receptor sites (paratopes) for reaction with antigen. The lymphocyte is the carrier of immunologically specific information. "Immunologically competent cell" and "memory cell" are functional terms for specialized cells found in immunized individuals that are not morphologically distinguishable from other lymphocytes. Two major classes of lymphocytes are T cells and B cells. Some basic differences in these cells are listed in Table 2.3; other, more sophisticated differences will become apparent later.

T cells. The term T cell is applied to the *thymus-derived lymphocyte.* T-cell precursors (prothymocytes) are produced in the bone marrow or liver during development and circulate to the thymus. Thymus-derived cells originate in the thymus from these precursor cells and, after being educated to recognize self and nonself, are re-released into the circulation; they subsequently localize in thymus-dependent areas of the other lymphoid organs (see chapter 6). Approximately 65 to 85% of lymph node cells and 30 to 50% of spleen cells are T cells.

In the human, T cells were first identified by their capacity to form rosettes with normal sheep erythrocytes (E rosette), but now many more specific markers are used. Spleen, peripheral blood, and lymph nodes contain approximately 20 to 30% B cells and 60 to 75% T cells.

T cells may be further divided into subpopulations on the basis of function and phenotypic markers. Details of the role of T cells in induction of the immune response are presented in chapter 5. Different T-cell subpopulations function to help in antibody formation (T-helper [T_H] cells), to kill target cells (T-cytotoxic [T_{CTL}] cells), to induce inflammation (T-delayed hypersensitivity [T_{DTH}] cells), and to inhibit certain immune responses (T-suppressor [T_S] cells). T_H cells are divided into two major subpopulations, Th1 and Th2. Th1 cells function primarily as helper cells for induction of B-cell proliferation and differentiation of plasma cells, which produce antibodies that activate complement, and for further development of cell-mediated immunity; Th2 cells produce factors (interleukins) that induce B cells to differentiate and produce non-complement fixing antibodies. Th1 cells may also differentiate into T_{DTH} cells, which are responsible for the inflammatory effects of T cells (e.g., delayed-type hypersensitivity) and secrete inflammatory mediators, such as lymphotoxin and gamma interferon (IFN-γ). Th2 cell products are also believed to stimulate differentiation of other white blood cells, such as eosinophils and basophils (see chapter 5).

A large number of T-cell subpopulations may now be identified by specific cell surface markers termed *clusters of differentiation (CD)*. CD markers are identified by monoclonal antibodies produced to different lymphoid cell populations. Thus, in humans, T_H cells are identified as $CD4^+$; T_{CTL} cells are identified as $CD8^+$. The expression of these markers during differentiation and in different subpopulations of lymphocytes is presented in more detail below and in chapter 6.

T lymphocytes activated by antigens produce effector molecules that activate or deactivate other lymphocytes (interleukins) or contribute to immune-mediated inflammation (lymphokines) or interact with other cell types. For instance, interleukins produced by T_H cells are required to induce activation and differentiation of B cells. These factors were first identified by their functions, as listed in Table 2.4. Many of these functions are now associated with up to 18 different interleukins, which are numbered from interleukin-1 (IL-1) to IL-18. Th1 cells produce IL-2, IFN-γ, and tumor necrosis factor in response to antigen stimulation, whereas Th2 cells synthesize IL-4, IL-5, IL-6, and IL-10. The nature and function of the interleukins are presented in later chapters.

The T cell is the maestro of the immunological orchestra. In addition to activating other cells, T cells may turn off other cells in the immune system; these are the T_S or Th3 cells. T_S cells are believed to arise in the gut-

Table 2.4 Some functional names for factors produced by activated lymphocytes[a]

Products affecting other lymphocytes (interleukins)
Helper factors
Growth-promoting factors
Differentiating factors
Suppressor factor
Transfer factor
Products affecting macrophages (lymphokines)
Migration inhibitory factor
Macrophage activation factor
Macrophage chemotactic factor
Products affecting polymorphonuclear leukocytes (lymphokines)
Chemotactic factors
Histamine-releasing factor
Leukocyte inhibitory factor
Products affecting other cell types (cytokines)
Cytotoxic factor
Growth inhibitory factors
Osteoclast activating factor
Interferon
Colony-stimulating factor

[a]These functional names have largely been replaced by specific interleukin or cytokine designations (see chapters 3 and 5).

associated lymphoid tissue and circulate to other organs, where they secrete transforming growth factor β1, which inhibits proliferation of T and B cells and increases production of immunoglobulin A (IgA) (secretory antibody). T_S cells may also be active in inhibiting production of the IgE class of antibodies, which are responsible for allergic reactions (chapter 11).

T-cell receptors and T-cell function. T-cell specificity for foreign antigens and for self (major histocompatibility complex [MHC]) is determined by the T-cell receptor (TCR). The TCR of Th1 and Th2 cells is composed of a pair of polypeptide chains termed αβ. A third type of T cell has different receptor chains, and these cells are called $T_{\gamma\delta}$ cells. $T_{\gamma\delta}$ cells appear to be part of an innate immune system and are the first to recognize infecting organisms; they are discussed further in chapter 5. The αβ TCR is specific for antigen in the form of peptide bound to a self MHC protein. MHC proteins are present on the surfaces of cells and are responsible both for the recognition of foreign cells (histocompatibility) and for "presenting" antigens to T cells. Only when presented in this form by an antigen-presenting cell does an antigen elicit a T-cell response. For a detailed description of antigen presentation by MHC, see chapter 4. Following reaction with antigen presented in the appropriate manner, T cells proliferate and differentiate into effector cells. The structure of the receptor, how different T cells are activated, and their role in immune responses are presented in detail in chapter 5.

B cells. B cells are the precursors of the cells that synthesize immunoglobulins (plasma cells). B cells express surface immunoglobulin, whereas T cells do not have surface immunoglobulin; 10 to 20% of lymph node cells, 20 to 35% of spleen cells, and 0% of thymus cells contain surface immunoglobulin. The site of B-cell differentiation may be in the fetal liver, the gastrointestinal lymphoid tissue, or peripheral lymph nodes. After antigenic stimulation, B cells differentiate into antibody-secreting plasma cells. How B cells are stimulated to proliferate and differentiate into antibody-producing cells and the nature of antibody molecules and their reactions with antigen are the subjects of chapter 4.

Plasma cells. The production of immunoglobulins (antibody) is the primary function of the plasma cell. Plasma cells differentiate from activated B cells. The plasma cell is a small round or oval cell (9 to 12 μm in diameter) with a small compact, dense nucleus located at one pole of the cell. Aggregation of the chromatin along the nuclear envelope gives rise to the characteristic "cartwheel" appearance of the plasma cell nucleus under the light microscope. The cytoplasm is dominated by rough endoplasmic reticulum organized in stocked laminae and a prominent Golgi apparatus (Fig. 2.5A). The characteristic lamellar endoplasmic reticulum and the Golgi apparatus reflect immunoglobulin synthesis and rapid secretion. These structures are also found in other cells for which protein secretion is a major function (e.g., pancreatic acinar cells). Plasma cells are prominent in the lymph nodes, spleen, and sites of chronic inflammation. Plasma cells increase in number in lymphoid organs draining the site of antigen injection during the experimental induction of antibody formation. Membrane-bound amorphous densities believed to contain stored immunoglobulins may be observed in more mature plasma cells (Russell bodies).

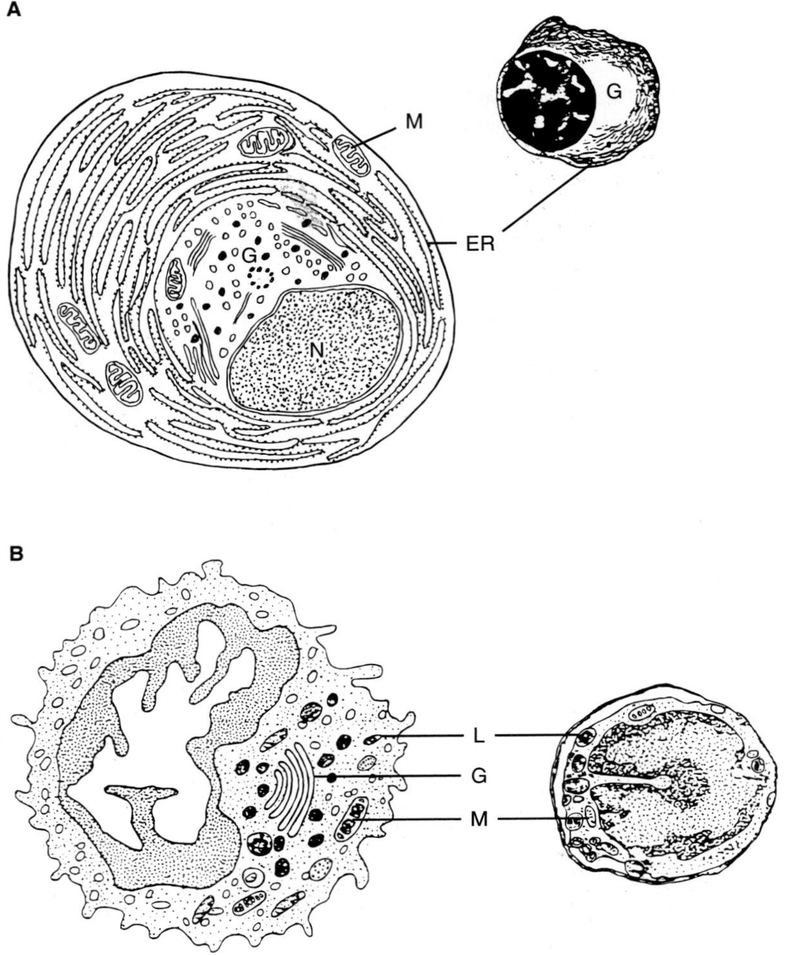

Figure 2.5 **(A)** Plasma cell. **(B)** Large granular lymphocyte (NK cell). Plasma cells contain abundant cytoplasm filled with lamellar endoplasmic reticulum and a Golgi apparatus. In tissue sections, there is polar location of the nucleus and a "cartwheel" appearance of the nucleus produced by condensation of chromatin along the nuclear membrane. Large granular lymphocytes contain mature lysosomes containing cytotoxic enzymes. ER, endoplasmic reticulum; G, Golgi apparatus; M, mitochondria; N, nucleus; L, lysosomes.

Natural killer cells. Some lymphocytes do not have detectable surface immunoglobulin or T-cell markers and are active in certain types of lymphocyte-mediated target cell killing: *natural killer (NK) cells*. The term natural is used because NK cells are present without previous immunization and act immediately on target cells; they are part of innate immunity. NK-mediated cytotoxic activity is measured by lysis of selected tumor target cells in vitro. NK activity in normal individuals was not recognized for some time because investigators considered the cytolytic activity of control (normal) cells as background in their assays for T-cell-mediated tumor cell killing. For instance, comparisons of killing activity were made by using lymphocytes from normal donors and lymphocytes from donors who had been cured of cancer (tumor regressor lymphocytes). The lytic effect of the normal NK population, determined by inhibition of tumor cell growth or lysis of tumor cells, was subtracted from the effect of regressor cells. The remaining effect was attributed to specific T_{CTL} cells. However, it was discovered that lymphocytes from many normal individuals had activity just as high as or higher than those from tumor regressors and that the tumor-killing activity was not in the T-cell population but in the T-like NK cells.

NK cells share some properties of T cells and macrophages and of B cells and granulocytes (Table 2.5). NK cells are believed to arise from a common T-cell–NK-cell progenitor before the migration of prothymocytes to the thymus (see below). NK cells have receptors belonging to three receptor families, which recognize MHC class I molecules (see chapter 4). When NK cells react with class I MHC molecules on the surface of a cell, NK activation is inhibited. Thus, cells normally expressing class I MHC are protected against NK killing, whereas cells that lack class I MHC, such as some tumor cells, are not protected. The "missing self" hypothesis proposes that NK cells detect the absence of self class I MHC. Treatment of target cells with IFN-γ increases expression of MHC class I. Whereas this increased expression of MHC class I increases the susceptibility to T_{CTL}-cell-mediated lysis, it actually protects against NK-mediated lysis. Thus, there are generally opposite requirements of T_{CTL} and NK cells for targeting cells; T_{CTL} cells require MHC class I recognition for killing (see chapter 5), and NK cells are active against targets that do not express MHC class I. T_{CTL} cells are programmed to detect foreign epitopes attached to MHC class I, whereas NK cells are directed to detect the absence of self. NK cells may be an important defense against tumor cells and some virus

Table 2.5 Comparison of NK cells with other lymphoid cells

Characteristic	NK/K cells	Similar to:		
		T cells	B cells	Macrophages
Size	16–20 nm	−	−	+
Cytoplasmic/nuclear ratio	High	−	−	+
Nuclear shape	Lobed	−	−	+
Adherence	Nonadherent	+	+	−
Phagocytosis	Nonphagocytic	+	+	−
Esterase	Absent	+	+	−
Acid phosphatase	Present	+	−	−
FcγRI receptors	Present	−	−	−[a]
Memory	None	−	−	+
ADCC	Strong	−	−	+
Markers				
Asialo-GM1	95%	+	−	−
CD2	80%	+	−	−
CD3	<5%	−	+	+
CR3 and CR4	95%	−	−	+[a]
IL-2 receptor	<5%	−	−	−[b]
NKH1	95% (NK)	−	−	−
NKH2	5% (K)	+	+	+[c]
TCR	90%	+	−[a]	−[d]

[a]Present on granulocytes.
[b]Present on activated T cells, B cells, and macrophages.
[c]Present on basophils, K cells (ADCC, antibody-dependent cell-mediated cytotoxicity).
[d]T-cell receptor gene rearranged.

infections that avoid T_{CTL}-cell killing by downregulating class I MHC expression. Cell adhesion molecules may be important, because activation of NK cells by IL-2 causes increased expression of several cell adhesion molecules (see chapter 3).

Because of the presence of large cytoplasmic granules, NK cells are also referred to as *large granule lymphocytes* (Fig. 2.5B). These cytoplasmic granules (lysosomes) contain enzymes and factors that are able to lyse target cells. Upon activation, NK cells display granule exocytosis and cytokine secretion. Killing occurs primarily by formation of "holes" in the target cell membrane by an enzyme known as perforin, as well as proteases called granzymes and other enzymes. There is evidence that this mechanism is much more efficient in vitro than in vivo. Different NK cell lines have different specificities, and not all tumor cells are susceptible to NK lysis. Targets for NK lysis include a large variety of tumor cells (leukemias, lymphomas, sarcomas, carcinomas) as well as some normal cell lines.

NK activity is increased by infections and is activated by IL-2 and IL-12. NK cells activated by IL-2 are called *lymphokine-activated killer cells.* Lymphokine-activated killer cells have been used extensively in clinical trials to treat cancer patients, with some spectacular apparent cures but with little consistency (see chapter 20). The role of NK cells in vivo is not clearly established, but they are believed to have an important role in a large number of diverse immunological functions, including defense against microbial, fungal, and parasitic infections, regulation of hematopoiesis, and natural resistance to foreign grafts, as well as in inhibiting (killing) cancer cells.

ADCC. The cells responsible for ADCC, sometimes called *K cells,* have receptors for and are able to bind antibodies. ADCC are believed to be part of the NK cell population and can be identified by the monoclonal antibody-defined surface markers NKH1 and NKH2. NK cells are $NKH1^+$; ADCC cells are $NKH2^+$. The cells responsible for ADCC have receptors for the Fc regions of IgG (FcγRIII; see chapter 4). These receptors bind IgG with low affinity but are able to direct the NK cells to antigens on target cells through the antibody-binding sites that are on the other end of the antibody molecules from the Fc region. Through these antibodies, the ADCC cells are directed to lyse target cells to which the antibody is directed. Cross-linking of the FcγRIII sends an activation signal to the NK cell (similar to T-cell activation; see chapter 5). ADCC may be an important protective mechanism against certain types of intracellular infections, such as viral infections, or against tumors.

Blast cells. A well-recognized feature of active immune responses is the presence of large blast cells. Blast cells are cells that are activated and are in the process of dividing. These cells have a large nucleus containing finely divided chromatin and prominent nucleoli. The cytoplasm of blast cells is strongly basophilic and contains dense collections of free and aggregated ribosomes. A variety of other subcellular organelles can be found in the cytoplasm, including a Golgi apparatus, various amounts of endoplasmic reticulum, and mitochondria. Blast cells are found in lymphoid organs draining sites of antigen injection and in active inflammatory lesions (particularly those of delayed-type hypersensitivity reactions) and may be induced in vitro in pure cultures of lymphocytes by certain mitogenic agents. Antigen-recognizing lymphocytes are stimulated by antigen to undergo transformation into blast cells that proliferate and differentiate into plasma cells or sensitized T cells.

Macrophages

Macrophages, the premier phagocytic cells, are the largest cells in the lymphoid system. They can range from 12 to 15 μm in diameter when in suspension but can extend cytoplasmic processes through organs for much larger distances by cytoplasmic extensions (dendritic macrophages). Macrophages in the blood are called monocytes, and those in tissue are called histiocytes. The macrophage nucleus usually has a bilobate kidney shape with considerable peripheral condensation of nuclear chromatin. The cytoplasm of the macrophage contains a great variety of organelles, including endoplasmic reticulum, a Golgi complex, mitochondria, free and aggregated ribosomes, and various membrane-limited phagocytic vacuoles (lysosomes, dense bodies, myelin figures, microbodies). The tissue macrophage, or histiocyte, is larger (15 to 18 μm) and may contain many more cytoplasmic vacuoles than blood monocytes do. Macrophages invade sites of inflammation after polymorphonuclear cells and clear the site of necrotic debris. The digestive capacity of the macrophage is more effective than that of the polymorphonuclear cell. It appears that polymorphonuclear cells (attack troops) get in quickly to act on infecting organisms, but macrophages (mop-up troops) are needed to finish the job.

Role in the immune response. The uptake of antigens by macrophages is the first step in the processing of antigen that leads to the production of circulating antibody. In such cases, the antigen is not completely degraded by the macrophage but becomes bound to macrophage RNA or membrane. The macrophage is not the cell that recognizes antigen as foreign, but the macrophage nonspecifically processes the antigen so that it can be recognized by specific antigen-reactive cells. Further definitions of antigen processing and the role of the macrophage in the induction of immunity are discussed in chapter 5.

The macrophage also plays a prominent role in the later stages of the inflammatory response and may accumulate in large numbers in sites of inflammation. The migration of macrophages (both blood and tissue) into inflammatory sites is generally believed to be non-antigen specific. Specifically sensitized lymphocytes may, upon reaction with antigen, release substances that attract and effect the migration of macrophages or products that increase the phagocytic or digestive capacity of macrophages. The role of macrophages and products of macrophages in inflammation is presented in much more detail in chapter 3.

Macrophage subpopulations. Subpopulations of cells in the macrophage family may be recognized by a combination of cell surface markers, morphologic appearance, and location in tissue (Table 2.6). Fixed histiocytes lining the sinusoids of the liver are given a special name, Kupffer cells.

Macrophages also produce factors that contribute to the induction and expression of immune responses as well as inflammation (see chapter 3). One macrophage-derived factor, IL-1, has many effects (pleiotropic) and plays a key role in the induction of immune responses, in different phases of inflammation, and on the actions of other cells.

Table 2.6 Macrophage subpopulations

Macrophage subpopulation	Organ	Presumed function
Stem cell	Bone marrow	Precursor
Monocyte	Blood	Circulating macrophage
Fixed histiocyes	Reticuloendothelial	Phagocytic cells in tissue
Dendritic histiocytes	Lymphoid organs	Process antigen for B cells
Interdigitating reticulum cells	Lymphoid organs	Process antigen for T cells
Langerhans cells	Skin, lymph nodes	Process antigen for T cells
Kupffer cells	Liver sinusoids	Clear blood of particles

Langerhans cells. Langerhans cells are a population of macrophages found within the mammalian epidermis and certain lymph nodes. They are derived from bone marrow macrophage precursors. They are able to pick up antigens encountered in the epidermis and migrate to the paracortex of the skin-draining lymph nodes, where they transform into dendritic or interdigitating reticulum cells and present antigen to T cells in a class II MHC-restricted fashion. The term veiled cells has been applied to cells believed to be Langerhans cells in the afferent lymphatics and paracortex of lymph nodes. Veiled cells have multiple long dendritic arms, as seen by electron microscopy. Langerhans cells are not usually visualized in hematoxylin-and-eosin-stained sections but can be distinguished by the presence of class II MHC markers, certain CD markers (CD1a, CD1c, CD45), and Birbeck granules. Birbeck granules, which can be seen only by electron microscopy, are rod-shaped organelles with a central zipperlike striation, occasionally having a vesicular dilation at one end, giving the structure a racketlike appearance. Adhesion molecules promote binding to T cells and provide additional activation signals that synergize through the TCR-CD3 complex (see chapter 3).

Cellular Interactions in Immune Responses

A simplified diagram of antigen processing and cellular interactions in immune responses is presented in Fig. 2.6. Two major types of antigen processing will now be discussed: exogenous and endogenous. The characteristics and mechanisms of interactions of antigen-presenting cells, T cells, and B cells in induction and expression of immune response are discussed in more detail in chapter 4. Exogenous processing can be accomplished only by cells that express class II MHC molecules (macrophages and B cells). During the induction of antibody formation, antigen is endocytosed by follicular dendritic cells and presented in association with class II MHC molecules on the surface of the antigen-presenting cell to T_H cells. T_H cells recognize class II MHC self markers and antigen and provide proliferation and differentiation signals to the precursors of plasma cells (B cells). The B cell is stimulated to divide and differentiate so that large numbers of specific antibody-producing plasma cells are produced. In some instances, B cells can present antigen to T cells and bypass the macrophage requirement, or B cells can be stimulated directly (T-independent antibody response). Interdigitating reticulum cells present exogenously processed class II MHC-associated antigen to T_H cells, which proliferate and differentiate into specifically sensitized T_{DTH} cells that mediate delayed-type hypersensitivity.

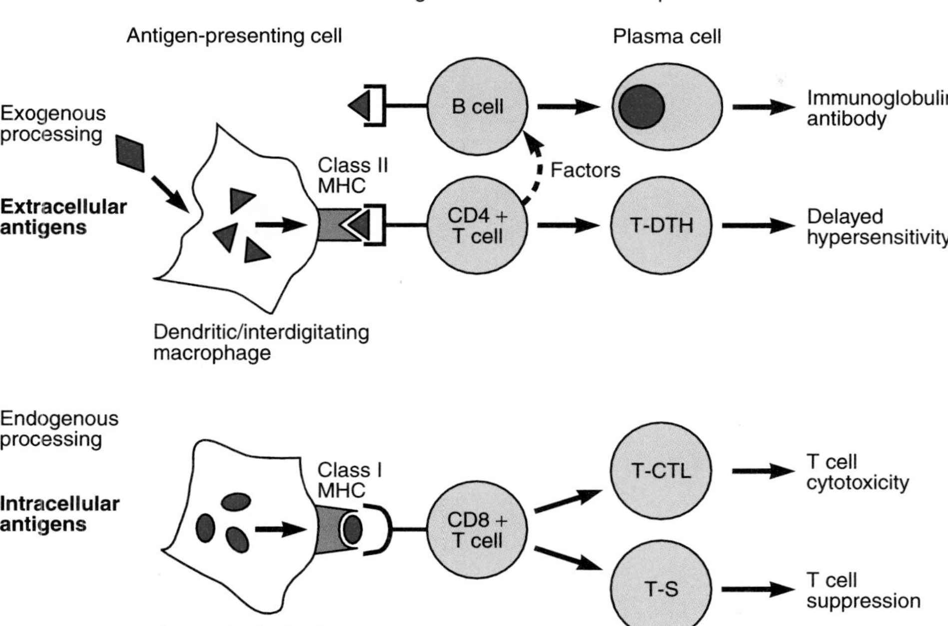

Figure 2.6 Cellular interactions in induction of antibody formation. Exogenous processing results in presentation of antigens in association with class II MHC to $CD4^+$ T_H cells. During endogenous processing, antigen is presented in association with class I MHC to $CD8^+$ $T_{CTL/S}$-cell precursors. This subject is presented here only as a preliminary introduction to antigen processing and cell-cell interactions during induction of immunity. For more details, see chapter 4.

Endogenous processing may occur in any nucleated cell that expresses class I MHC molecules. Endogenous antigens are part of the cell or are foreign antigens that have entered the antigen-processing cell by bypassing the exogenous pathway. Endogenously processed antigens are presented in association with class I MHC molecules to $CD8^+$ T cells, which proliferate and differentiate into T_{CTL} cells.

Hematopoiesis (Blood Formation)

Blood cell formation is called hematopoiesis (Greek *haemia,* blood; *poiesis,* production). A general view of hematopoiesis is presented in Fig. 2.7. The precursors of all blood cells are found normally in the bone marrow. Formation of erythrocytes is termed erythropoiesis; formation of monocytes, granulocytes, and platelets is called myelopoiesis. All blood cells arise from a common *bone marrow stem cell,* which represents less than 0.01% of bone marrow cells. This stem cell first differentiates into a stromal stem cell, which gives rise to bone marrow stroma as well as fibroblasts, adipocytes, smooth muscle, etc., and a *hematopoietic stem cell,* which gives rise to lymphoid and myeloid cell lineages. In a human survivor of the atomic bombing of Japan, a persistent clonal aberration was found in cultures of T- and B-lymphocyte colonies more than 40 years after irradiation. It is concluded that a single stem cell of an adult (containing the aberration) is capable of generating long-lived myeloid and lymphoid progeny.

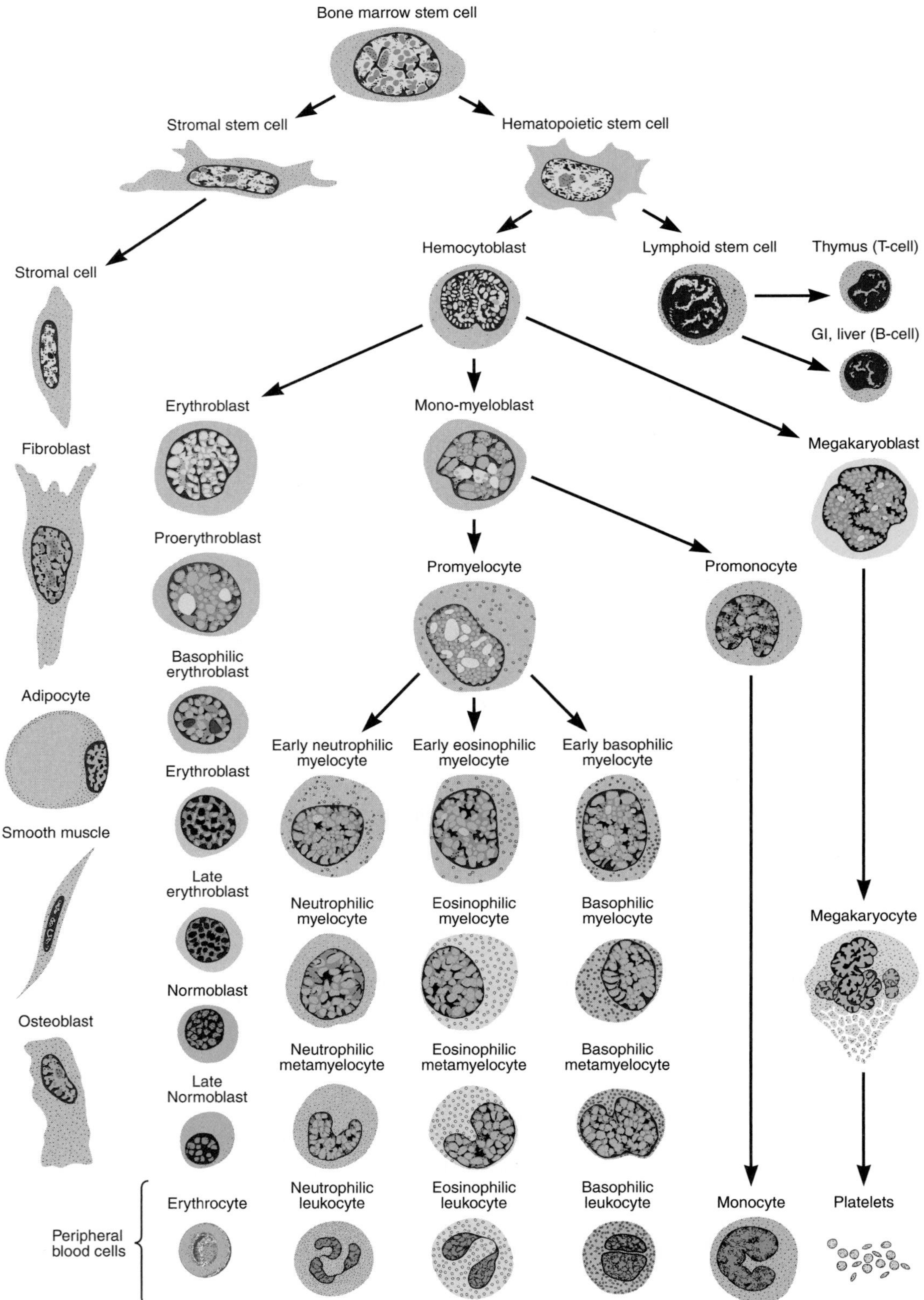

Figure 2.7 Hematopoiesis. The stroma and blood cells arise from a common bone marrow stem cell that gives rise to a stromal stem cell and a hematopoietic stem cell. The stromal stem cell differentiates into stromal cells, fibroblasts, adipocytes, smooth muscle cells, and osteoblasts, which form the supporting structure for the hematopoietic cells. The white blood cell lineages differentiate from a pluripotent hematopoietic stem cell in the bone marrow. The first differentiation step of the hematopoietic stem cell is into lymphoid and myeloid series. Lymphoid cell

In the bone marrow the stromal cells interact with the hematopoietic cells to provide a microenvironment that supports continued production and differentiation of blood cells. The myeloid stem cell then differentiates into erythrocyte (normocyte), monogranulocyte (promyelocyte), and platelet (megakaryocyte) lineages. The occurrence of leukemic cells, which share markers and properties of monocytes and polymorphonuclear cells (monomyelocytic leukemia), and the development of colonies for monocytic and granulocytic cells from a shared precursor in vitro provide evidence that monocytes and granulocytes have a common precursor. A common lymphoid stem cell differentiates into B-cell and T-cell–NK lineages. B-cell development depends on specific interactions between cell adhesion molecules on developing B cells and ligands on nonlymphoid stroma in the bone marrow, as well as the interaction of membrane-bound stem cell factor on stroma cells with its receptor, Kit, on B-cell precursors. This is followed by a reaction of IL-7 produced by the stroma cell with the IL-7 receptor, developing pro-B cells. This results in expression of primitive immunoglobulin chains in the cytoplasm of pre-B cells and eventual expression of surface IgM (see chapter 4)

Hematopoietic Factors

The ability to induce differentiation of myeloid precursors in vitro has led to a much better understanding of the role of various *colony-stimulating factors (CSF)* in controlling myeloid differentiation. Three major classes of hematopoietic factors have been identified (Table 2.7). A simplified illustration of the action of these factors is presented in Fig. 2.8. The first class is lineage specific and stimulates the final mitotic divisions and terminal differentiation (lineage-restricted CSF). The second class, pluripotent progenitor-stimulating factors, stimulates proliferation of progenitor cells, is not lineage specific, and does not support complete differentiation through mature end cells. The third class acts synergistically with other factors to augment colony development in vitro but has little or no intrinsic activity. Some of these factors also have critical roles in T- and B-cell differentiation, which are presented in later chapters.

Hematopoietic Factor Treatment of Human Diseases

Table 2.8 is a list of hematopoietic cytokines under development for treatment of human diseases. Erythropoietin has been approved by the U.S. Food and Drug Administration for use in anemia secondary to renal failure and in zidovudine therapy for AIDS. Granulocyte CSF has been approved for treatment of neutropenia in patients undergoing chemotherapy for cancer, and granulocyte-monocyte CSF has been approved for stimulation of patients receiving autologous bone marrow transplants. Other factors are being evaluated by clinical trials.

---

development takes place in other organs and is presented in chapter 6. The hemocytoblast stem cell differentiates into erythroblast, monomyeloblast, and megakaryoblast (platelets) lineages. The monogranulocyte then differentiates into monocytic and granulocytic lineages. A series of maturation stages in each lineage results in the formation of the mature cells of each lineage that leave the bone marrow and circulate in the peripheral blood. The morphologic stages of granulocytic maturation are promyelocyte, myelocyte, metamyelocyte, band, and segmented.

Table 2.7 Classes of hematopoietic growth factors[a]

Class	Factor	Cell lineage
Lineage-restricted colony-stimulating factors (CSF)	Granulocyte CSF	Granulocytes
	Macrophage CSF	Monocytes
	Erythropoietin	Red blood cells
	Interleukin-5	Eosinophils
Pluripotent colony-stimulating factors	Interleukin-3	Myeloid lineage
	Granulocyte-monocyte CSF	Granulocytes, monocytes
Recruiters	Interleukin-1	Stem cells
	Interleukin-6	Megakaryocytes
	Interleukin-9	Mast cells, erythrocytes

[a]Modified from E. M. Mazur and J. L. Cohen, *Clin. Pharmacol. Ther.* **46:**250, 1989.

Figure 2.8 Role of growth factors in hematopoiesis. Interleukins, CSFs, and erythropoietin have been shown to induce differentiation during hematopoiesis.

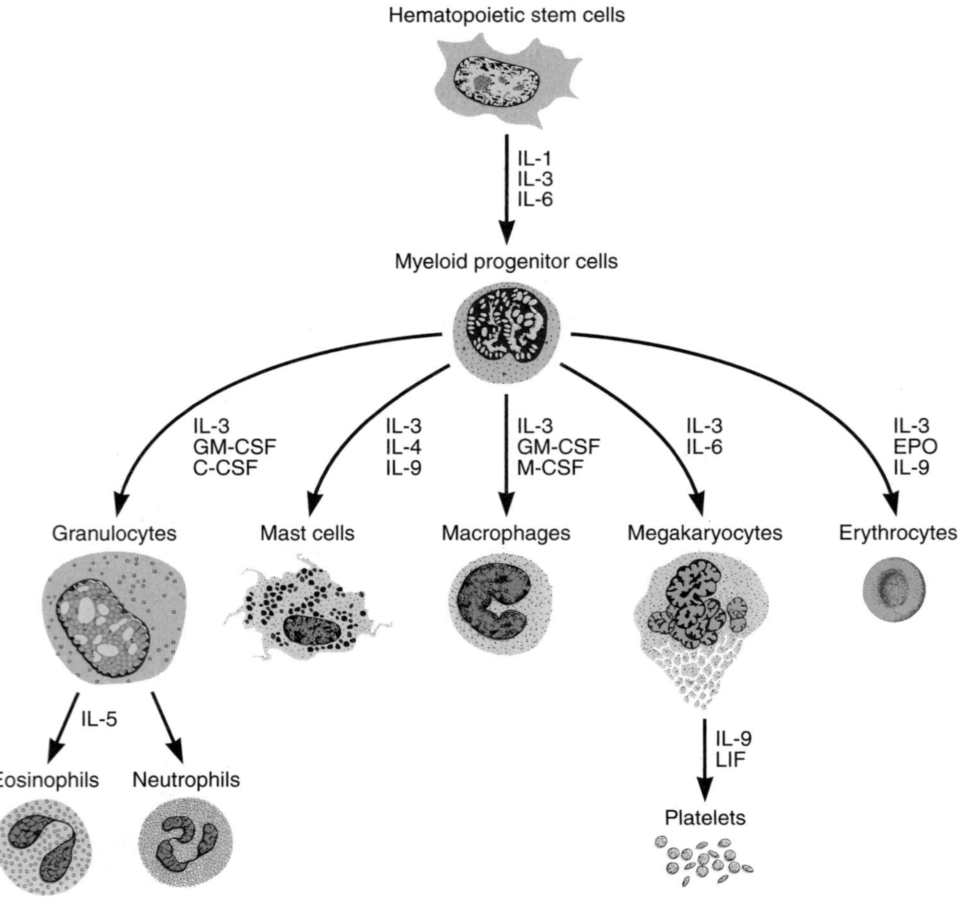

Table 2.8 Hematopoietic cytokines under development[a]

Growth factor	Site(s) of production	Effect(s)	Possible clinical use(s)	Clinical trials under way
M-CSF	Mesenchymal cells, bone marrow stromal cells	Increases production of monocytes and macrophages and phagocytic function	Stimulation of increase in macrophage antitumor activity; control of fungal infections	Yes
IL-3	T lymphocytes, mast cells	Increases production of granulocytes, macrophages, and platelets	Correction of cytopenias	Yes
PIXY321[b]		Combined features of IL-3 and GM-CSF	Correction of cytopenias	Yes
SCF	Fibroblasts, bone marrow stroma, endothelial cells, Sertoli cells, hepatocytes	Increases proliferation and differentiation of primitive hematopoietic cells	Synergy with other cytokines (e.g., erythropoietin, GM-CSF, IL-3)	Yes
IL-1	Mast cells	Increases production of other cytokines (e.g., IL-3, GM-CSF, G-CSF); synergy with other cytokines	Correction of cytopenias; radioprotection	Yes
IL-6	T and B cells, monocytes, endothelial cells, keratinocytes, bone marrow stroma	Multiple effects on T cells, mostly via other cytokines; myeloid development; regulation of acute-phase reactants; development and maturation of megakaryocytes	?	Yes
IL-2	Activated T lymphocytes	Increases growth and activation of T lymphocytes and NK cells	Stimulation of NK cell antitumor activity	Yes
IL-4	$CD4^+$ (Th2) and $CD8^+$ T lymphocytes	Increases proliferation of B and T cells, mast cells, and fibroblasts	Stimulation of antibody synthesis, inhibition of Th1 cells	Yes
IL-9	Activated T lymphocytes (especially $CD4^+$)	Increases proliferation of various progenitors, mast cells, and T cells	?	?
IL-12	B-lymphoid cell lines, mononuclear phagocytes	Increases differentiation of T_H cells and function of NK cells	Immune modulator to treat cancer	?
IL-5	Activated T lymphocytes	Activates cytotoxic T cells, increases secretion of immunoglobulins and production of eosinophils	?	?
IL-10	$CD4^+$ and $CD8^+$ T cells, mononuclear phagocytes, activated B cells	Decreases function of mononuclear phagocytes and proliferation of and cytokine production by T cells, costimulates B-lymphoid cell proliferation	Antagonist for IFN-γ, inhibitor of Th1 cells	?
IL-7	Bone marrow stroma, spleen, thymus	Increases growth of pre-T and pre-B cells and production of cytokines by monocytes	?	?
Tpo	Endothelial cells, fibroblasts, and other dividing cells	Regulates megakaryocyte development and platelet production	Correction of thrombopenia	Yes

[a]Courtesy of Stephen Baird, Department of Pathology, VA Hospital, San Diego, Calif., and Thomas Kipps, Department of Medicine, University of California, San Diego. Abbreviations: M-CSF, monocyte/macrophage colony-stimulating factor; GM-CSF, granulocyte-macrophage colony-stimulating factor; SCF, stem cell factor; G-CSF, granulocyte colony-stimulating factor; Tpo, thrombopoietin.

[b]A genetically engineered fusion of IL-3 and GM-CSF.

Table 2.9 Summary of properties of cells of the immune system

Cell type	Function	Markers
B lymphocytes	Precursor of plasma cells, antigen presentation	Surface immunoglobulin, class II MHC, complement receptors, Fc receptor, CD19, CD20, CD22, CD37, etc.
T lymphocytes		
T_H	Assists response of other lymphocytes	TCR, CD4, IL-3, IL-4, etc.
T_{DTH}	Initiates delayed-type hypersensitivity reactions	TCR, CD4, IL-2, IL-3, etc.
T_{CTL}	Kills specific target cells	TCR, CD8, perforin, granzymes
T_S (Th3)	Suppresses immune responses	TCR, CD8, suppressor factor?
Natural killer cells	Natural killers, ADCC	FcR, CD16, perforins, granzymes
Macrophages	Antigen presentation, phagocytosis, chronic inflammation	Class II MHC, CD14, CD68, FcR, and CR digestive granules (lysozyme, proteases, peroxidases), IL-1
Langerhans cells	Antigen presentation, epidermis	Class II MHC, CDI, CD45, LFA-3, ICAM-1, VLA, Birbeck granules
Neutrophils	Acute inflammation, phagocytosis, bacteriocidal	CD15, CD67, Fc and C receptors, pink granules (cationic proteins, myeloperoxidase, lysozyme, defensins)
Basophils (mast cells)	Vasodilation, vascular permeability, bronchoconstriction	Fc receptor for IgE, blue granules (heparin, serotonin, arachidonic acid), interleukins 1–6, tumor necrosis factor, etc.
Eosinophils	ADCC to parasites, anti-inflamatory	IgG, IgE, C3b receptors, red granules (major basic protein, arylsulfatase, histaminase)

Summary

A summary of the properties of white blood cells is given in Table 2.9. The cells of the lymphoid system are the white blood cells. Polymorphonuclear cells (neutrophils, eosinophils, and basophils/mast cells) have important parts to play in the inflammatory response but do not recognize antigen and are not involved in specific induction of immunity. Mononuclear cells (lymphoid cells) include macrophages, lymphocytes (T cells, B cells, and NK cells), and plasma cells. These cells are active in inflammation and in both induction and expression of immune responses. T cells, B cells, and macrophages cooperate in the induction of antibody responses to most antigens. Upon immune induction, T cells differentiate into specifically sensitized lymphocytes responsible for cellular immune reactivity, whereas B cells differentiate into antibody-secreting plasma cells. NK cells are able to lyse a variety of target cells, in particular, tumor cells that lack MHC class I antigens. Polymorphonuclear cells (granulocytes) and macrophages are active in the effector states of tissue inflammation in both a specific and a nonspecific manner.

Bibliography

Polymorphonuclear Cells

de Duve, C., and R. Wattiaux. 1966. Function of lysosomes. *Am. Rev. Physiol.* **23:**435–492. (Historical perspective.)

Dvorak, A. M. 1994. Similarities in the ultrastructural morphology and development and secretory mechanisms of human basophils and eosinophils. *J. Allergy Clin. Immunol.* **94:**1103–1134.

Hampton, M. F., and C. C. Winterbourn. 1999. Methods for quantifying phagocytosis and bacterial killing by human neutrophils. *J. Immunol. Methods* **17:**15–22.

Kaliner, M. A., and D. D. Metcalfe. 1992. *The Mast Cell in Health and Disease.* Marcel Dekker, Inc., New York, N.Y.

Lehrer, R. I., T. Ganz, and M. E. Selsted. 1991. Defensins: endogenous antibiotic peptides of animal cells. *Cell* **64:**229–230.

Spitznagel, J. K. 1999. Antibiotic proteins of human neutrophils. *J. Clin. Investig.* **86:**1381–1386.

Walsh, G. M. 1999. Advances in the immunobiology of eosinophils and their role in disease. *Crit. Rev. Clin. Lab. Sci.* **36:**453–496.

Lymphocytes

Didler, J., and A. K. So. 1998. T cells and related cytokines. *Curr. Opin. Rheumatol.* **10:**207–211.

Gowans, J. L. 1966. Life span, recirculation, and transformation of lymphocytes. *Int. Rev. Exp. Pathol.* **5:**1–24.

Kelso, A. 1999. Educating T cells: early events in the differentiation and commitment of cytokine-producing CD4+ and CD8+ T cells. *Springer Semin. Immunopathol.* **21:**231–248.

Peters, P. J., J. Borst, V. Oorschot, M. Fukuda, O. Krahenbuhl, J. Tschopp, J. W. Slot, and H. J. Geuze. 1991. Cytotoxic T lymphocyte granules are secretory lysosomes, containing both perforin and granzymes. *J. Exp. Med.* **173:**1099–1109.

Natural Killer/ADCC

Cui, J., T. Shin, T. Kawano, H. Sato, E. Kondo, I. Toura, Y. Kaneko, H. Koseki, M. Kanno, and M. Taniguchi. 1997. Requirement for Vα14 NKT cells in IL-12-mediated rejection of tumors. *Science* **278:**1623–1626.

Kos, F. J. 1998. Regulation of adaptive immunity by natural killer cells. *Immunol. Res.* **17:**303–312.

Lanier, L. L. 1998. NK cell receptors. *Annu. Rev. Immunol.* **16:**359–393.

Lee, R. K., J. Spielman, D. Y. Zhao, K. J. Olsen, and E. R. Podack. 1996. Perforin, Fas ligand, and tumor necrosis factor are the major cytotoxic molecules used by lymphokine-activated killer cells. *J. Immunol.* **157:**1919–1925.

Yokoyama, W. M. 1999. Natural killer cells, p. 575–603. *In* W. E. Paul (ed.), *Fundamental Immunology,* 4th ed. Lippincott-Raven Publishers, Philadelphia, Pa.

Macrophages

Gordon, S. 1999. Macrophages and the immune response, p. 533–545. *In* W. E. Paul (ed.), *Fundamental Immunology,* 4th ed. Lippincott-Raven Publishers, Philadelphia, Pa.

Naito, M. 1993. Macrophage heterogeneity in development and differentiation. *Arch. Histol. Cytol.* **56:**331–351.

Langerhans Cells

Steinman, R. M. 1991. The dendritic cell system and its role in immunogenicity. *Annu. Rev. Immunol.* **9:**271–296.

Teunissen, M. B. M. 1992. Dynamic nature and function of epidermal Langerhans cells in vivo and in vitro: a critical review, with emphasis on human Langerhans cells. *Histochem. J.* **24:**697–716.

Wang, B., P. Amerio, and D. N. Sauder. 1999. Role of cytokines in epidermal Langerhans cell migration. *J. Leukoc. Biol.* **66:**33–39.

Cell Interactions in Immune Responses

Braciale, T. J., and V. L. Braciale. 1991. Antigen presentation: structural themes and functional variations. *Immunol. Today* **12:**124–129.

Claman, H. N., and D. E. Mosier. 1972. Cell-cell interactions in antibody production. *Prog. Allergy* **16:**40–80.

Germain, R. N. 1999. Antigen processing and presentation, p. 287–340. *In* W. E. Paul (ed.), *Fundamental Immunology,* 4th ed. Lippincott-Raven Publishers, Philadelphia, Pa.

Mitchison, N. A. 1971. The carrier effect in the secondary response to hapten-protein conjugates. II. Cellular cooperation. *Eur. J. Immunol.* **1:**68–75.

Mosmann, T. R., and R. L. Coffman. 1989. Heterogeneity of cytokine secretion patterns and functions of helper T cells. *Adv. Immunol.* **46:**111–147.

Yewdell, J. W., and J. R. Bennink. 1992. Cell biology of antigen processing and presentation to major histocompatibility complex class I molecule-restricted T lymphocytes. *Adv. Immunol.* **52:**1–123.

Hematopoiesis

Budel, L. M., F. Dong, B. Lowenberg, and I. P. Touw. 1995. Hematopoietic growth factor receptors: structure variations and alternatives of receptor complex formation in normal hematopoiesis and in hematopoietic disorders. *Leukemia* **9:**553–561.

Kondo, M., I. L. Weissman, and K. Akashi. 1997. Identification of clonogenic common lymphoid progenitors in mouse bone marrow. *Cell* **91:**661–672.

Korbling, M. 1998. Effects of granulocyte colony-stimulating factor in healthy subjects. *Curr. Opin. Hematol.* **5:**209–214.

Kusunoki, Y., Y. Kodama, Y. Hirai, S. Kyoizumi, N. Nakamura, and M. Akiyama. 1995. Cytogenic and immunologic identification of clonal expansion of stem cells into T and B lymphocytes in one atomic-bomb survivor. *Blood* **86:**2106–2112.

Till, J. E., and E. A. McCulloch. 1980. Hematopoietic stem cell differentiation. *Biochim. Biophys. Acta* **605:**431–459.

Whetton, A. D., and G. J. Graham. 1999. Homing and mobilization in the stem cell niche. *Trends Cell Biol.* **9:**233–238.

Inflammation and Wound Healing

3

The Inflammatory Process

Inflammation is the primary process through which the body repairs tissue damage and defends itself against infection. Inflammation may be initiated by either immune or nonimmune pathways, but both pathways employ similar effector mechanisms. Nonimmune inflammation is initiated by release of bacterial products, foreign bodies, or components of dying tissue. Immune inflammation is initiated by a specific reaction of immunoglobulin antibody or sensitized T lymphocytes with antigen. The in vivo effects of immune inflammation are determined by amplification mechanisms that are also components of nonimmune inflammatory processes. These amplification mechanisms, rather than the specific immune reaction alone, are largely responsible for the tissue lesions observed. The process of inflammation is divided into acute and chronic forms.

The function of acute inflammation is to deliver plasma and cellular components of the blood to extravascular tissue spaces. The extravasation of plasma fluid into tissue (edema) causes dilution of toxic materials and increases lymphatic flow. Phagocytic blood cells infiltrate inflamed tissue, destroy infectious agents, clear the tissue of necrotic debris, and release cytokines that activate healing.

The function of chronic inflammation is to "heal" the lesion produced by the acute inflammation by clearing the site of the products of acute inflammation and replacing damaged tissue. At later stages, fibrosis serves to wall off foci of dead tissue or infection. As a physiologic response to injury, inflammation clears and restores damaged tissue; as a pathologic process, inflammation produces tissue damage and scarring. General inflammatory mechanisms are described in this chapter; their pathogenic effects in mediating immune-activated lesions are discussed in part II of this book.

The phases of inflammation are listed in Table 3.1. The following sequence of events occurs during an inflammatory response: (i) increased blood flow (vasodilation) preceded by transient vasoconstriction, (ii) increased vascular permeability leading to edema (vasopermeability), (iii) infiltration by polymorphonuclear neutrophils, (iv) infiltration by lymphocytes and macrophages (chronic inflammation), leading to (v) resolution (restoration of normal structure) or (vi) scarring (filling in of areas of tissue destruction by fibroblasts and collagen) (Fig. 3.1). The first three events are considered acute inflammation; the last three stages are chronic inflammation.

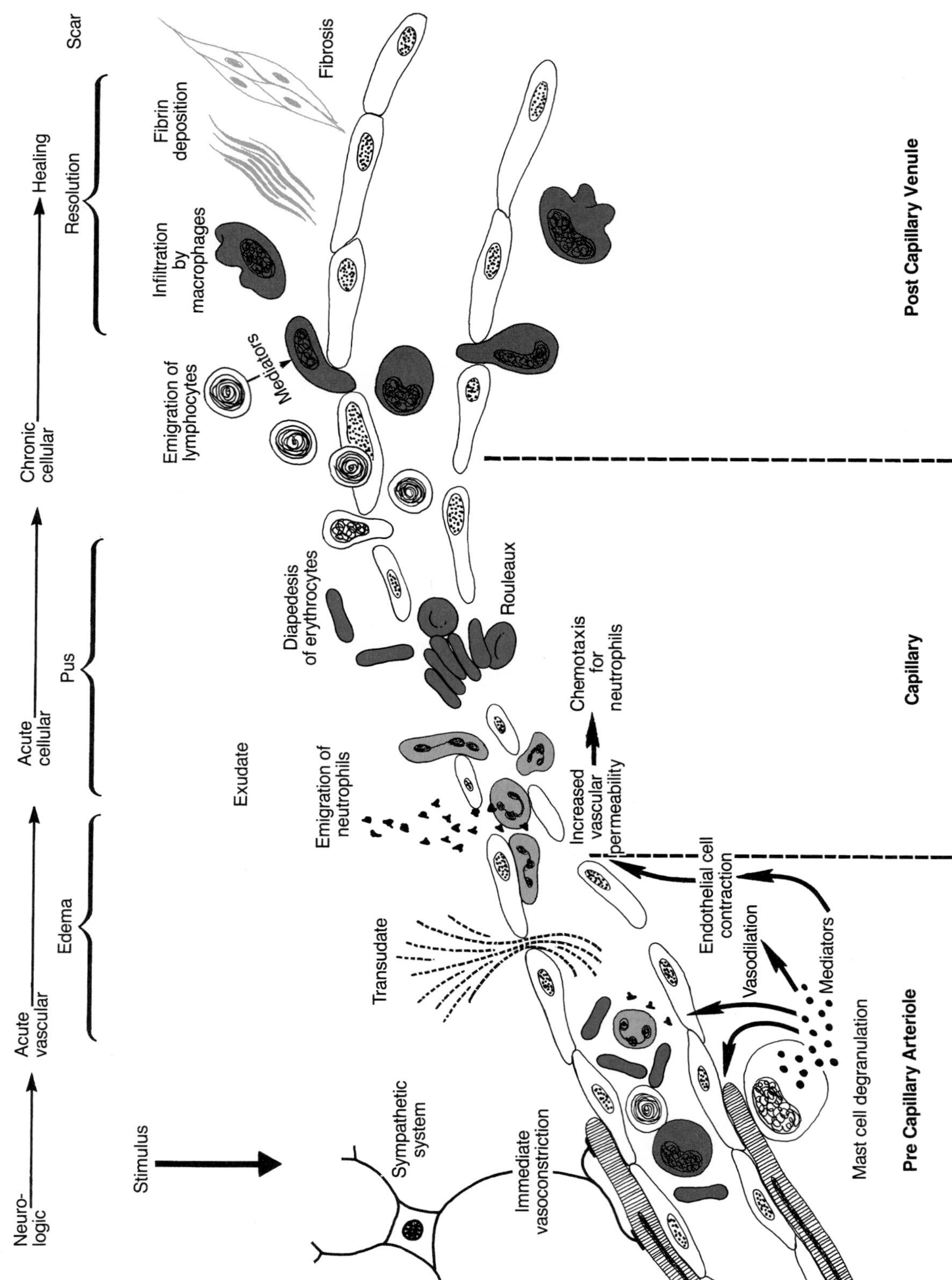

Figure 3.1 The sequence of events in the process of inflammation.

Table 3.1 Phases of the inflammatory response

Stimulus		Response		Healing and repair
	Acute	Acute	Chronic	Scarring (granulation
Initiating event ⟶	vascular ⟶	cellular ⟶	cellular ⟶	tissue) or
	response	response	response	Resolution
	(minutes)	(hours)	(days)	(week to months)
Trauma, necrosis, infection ⟶	Vasodilation, increased vasopermeability (hyperemia, edema) ⟶	Neutrophil infiltrate (pus) ⟶	Mononuclear cell infiltrate[a] ⟶	Fibrosis or clearing

[a]Lymphocytes, macrophages, and plasma cells.

Acute Inflammation

Initiation of Inflammation

Inflammation is initiated by trauma, tissue necrosis (death), infection, or immune reactions. The immediate response is a temporary vasoconstriction, causing blanching of the skin. The mechanism for this is not fully understood but is believed to be mediated by the sympathetic nervous system. This is followed within seconds by the acute vascular response, resulting in increased blood flow (hyperemia) and edema. If there has been only mild injury, such as that caused by stroking the skin, the inflammatory process may be limited to this phase. However, if there is sufficient cell death or infection, the acute cellular phase will follow. Changes in blood flow lead to adherence of neutrophils next to endothelial cells in small blood vessels or capillaries *(margination),* followed by passage of neutrophils into the adjacent tissue *(emigration).* Margination is recognized in tissues by the lining up of neutrophils along the endothelium of vessels. Emigration occurs by passage of inflammatory cells between endothelial cells. In addition, contraction of endothelial cells causes leakage (diapedesis) of red blood cells, which may progress to hemorrhage if there is necrosis of endothelial cells. Exposure of fibrinogen and fibronectin in tissues provides sites for platelet aggregation and activation with activation of fibrin (blood clot) formation, which can provide a matrix for further cellular infiltration. Alterations in the viscosity of the blood and the charge of plasma cause red cells to aggregate into stacks like pancakes (rouleau formation) as the normal negative repelling charge of the erythrocytes is lost. Depending on the degree of injury or infection, the acute cellular phase may be sufficient to clear the tissue. However, it is often necessary for the chronic cellular infiltrate of lymphocytes and macrophages to effect removal of tissue debris or dead bacteria. The macrophage is the major player in this process. If there is sufficient damage that normal tissue must be replaced, fibroblastic proliferation and scarring will occur.

Chemical Mediators

Chemical mediators are signaling molecules that act on smooth muscle cells, endothelial cells, or white blood cells to induce, maintain, or limit inflammation. The agents that act first in the sequence primarily affect smooth muscle cells of precapillary arterioles to produce dilation and increased blood flow. Increased vascular permeability occurs in two phases: early (within minutes) and late (6 to 12 h). The early phase is mediated by histamine and serotonin. Late-phase mediators of acute inflammation are derived from a variety of sources, including arachidonic acid metabolites, breakdown products of the coagulation system (fibrin split products) or peptides formed from blood or tissue proteins (bradykinin), activated complement components (C3a, C5a), as well as factors released from bacteria (formylmethionyl [fMet] tripeptides), necrotic tissue, neutrophils (inflammatory peptides), lymphocytes (lymphokines), and monocytes (monokines). The generation of these factors and their effects are presented in more detail below.

Gross Manifestations

The gross manifestations of the acute vascular response may be evoked by scratching the skin (the triple response). The triple response proceeds as follows: (i) 3 to 50 s, thin red line (vasodilation of capillaries); (ii) 30 to 60 s, flush (vasodilation of arterioles); (iii) 1 to 5 min, wheal (increased vascular permeability, edema). The term wheal refers to pale, soft, swollen areas on the skin caused by leakage of fluid from capillaries. Some individuals react to skin stroking with marked wheal formation. The areas of skin will stand out after stroking so that words can actually be written on the skin by whealing (dermatographism).

The ancient Greeks considered inflammation to be a disease. Galen, shortly after the birth of Jesus, grossly recognized the four classic cardinal signs of inflammation (Fig. 3.2). Later, the fifth sign, loss of function, was added by the great German pathologist Rudolf Virchow. Increased blood flow is manifested grossly by redness (rubor) and increased local temperature (calor). The increased blood flow delivers serum factors and blood cells to the tissue, causing an increase in tissue mass (tumor). The increase in vascular permeability permits exudation of plasma from the capillaries or postcapillary venules into the tissue, causing edema. Tissue swelling and chemical mediators act on nerve endings to produce pain (dolor). Swelling and pain lead to loss of function (functio laesa).

Histologic Features

The essential features of acute inflammation are edema (vascular response), followed by infiltration of the tissue by neutrophils (cellular response). Neutrophils pass through gaps in capillary endothelium and are attracted to sites of inflammation by chemotactic factors. Tissue necrosis is caused by release of proteolytic enzymes into the tissue from the lysosomes of the neutrophils. Neutrophil infiltration is followed by infiltration by mononuclear (round) cells, i.e., lymphocytes and macrophages. Macrophages are also attracted by chemotactic mediators and are activated to phagocytize and digest necrotic tissue or inflammatory products, including effete neutrophils that have become damaged in the inflammatory process. If tissue damage is not extensive, the inflammation will be limited by controlling factors such as enzyme inhibitors and oxygen scavengers. Macrophages will then be able to clear the inflamed area, and the tissue will return to normal (resolution). However, if tissue damage is extensive or the initiating stimulus persists, then mediators of chronic inflammation are activated. If tissue damage is significant or the organ has limited ability to regenerate, resolution cannot be achieved, and the damaged tissue will be replaced by fibroblast proliferation and collagen deposition (fibrous scar). If extensive, fibrous scarring may lead to a compromise in normal function. The fibrotic process may include proliferation of

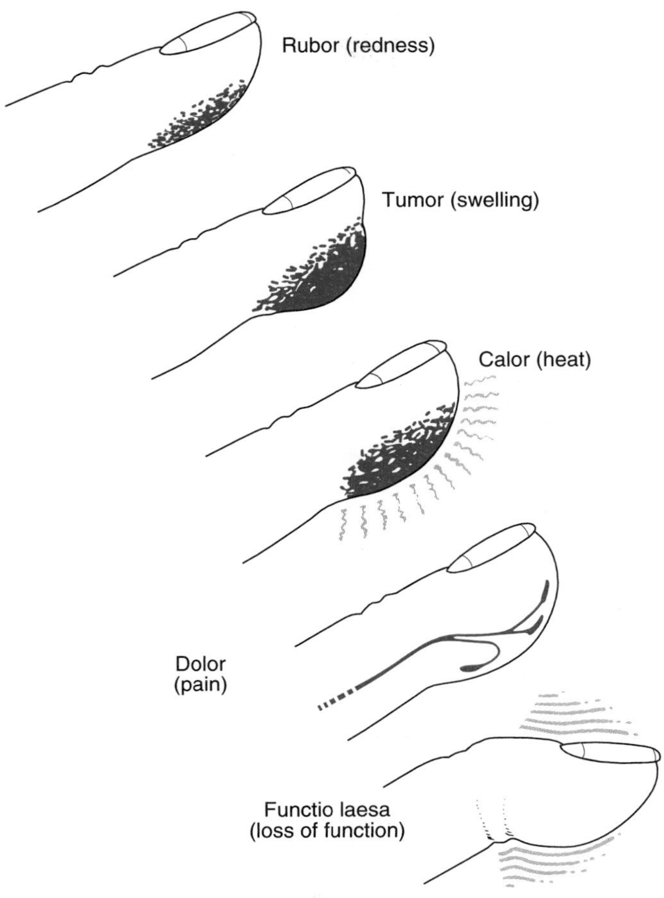

Figure 3.2 The five cardinal signs of acute inflammation.

both fibroblasts and endothelial cells (capillaries), which form a highly vascular reaction known as granulation tissue because grossly it has the appearance of small granules, like sand. If the inflamed tissue contains material that is difficult for macrophages to digest (such as silica or complex lipids), a particular form of chronic inflammation, granulomatous (like granulation tissue), may be seen (see chapter 14). The process of inflammation is modified by infection, immune products, tissue death (necrosis), and foreign bodies. Examples of the lesions of different stages of inflammation in different tissues are given below.

Classification of Inflammation

Some terms used to describe various manifestations of the inflammatory process are listed in Table 3.2. The manifestations of inflammation depend upon the severity and location of the reaction as well as the nature of the inflammatory stimulus. Systemic effects of inflammation include fever and increased numbers of white blood cells (leukocytosis). Fever is caused by an increase in the metabolic rate in muscular tissue secondary to effects of "pyrogens" released from damaged tissue that act on the hypothalamus. Leukocytosis is caused by increased production and release of white cells from the bone marrow.

Table 3.2 Definition of terms used to describe manifestations of inflammation

Hyperemia: Increased blood in tissue; caused by vasodilation

Edema: Excess fluid in tissues; caused by increased vascular permeability

Transudate: Physiologic, low-protein concentration edema fluid, containing albumin; specific gravity below 1.012; cleared by lymphatics

Exudate: Pathologic, high-protein edema fluid containing Igs and macroglobulin; specific gravity above 1.02

Pus: Exudate rich in white cells and necrotic debris; caused by emigration of neutrophils and release of enzymes

Fibrinoid necrosis: Enzymatic digestion of tissue so that it looks like fibrin, such as fibrinoid necrosis of vessels in vasculitis

Types of exudate
- Serous: Thin fluid (like transudate)
- Fibrinous: Stringy, fibrin-containing
- Suppurative: Pus (neutrophils and necrotic debris)
- Hemorrhagic: Bloody (vascular necrosis)
- Fibrous: Healed exudate, scar, adhesions

Types of lesions
- Ulcer: Surface erosion
- Abscess: Cavity filled with pus
- Cellulitis: Diffuse inflammatory infiltrate in tissue
- Pseudomembrane: Fibrous or necrotic layer on epithelial surface
- Catarrhal: Excess mucous production

The Cells of Acute Inflammation

The cellular players in the process of acute inflammation include mast cells (basophils), platelets, neutrophils, and eosinophils. These granulocytic cells are activated by a variety of chemical processes and in turn produce and release a number of chemical mediators. Most of the manifestations of the acute vascular response (vasodilation and permeability) are the result of chemical mediators released from mast cells.

Mast Cells

Mast cells have cytoplasmic granules that contain a variety of biologically active agents (Table 3.3), which, when released extracellularly (degranulation), cause dilation of the smooth muscle of arterioles (vasodilation), increased blood flow, and contraction of endothelial cells, opening up vessel walls to permit egress of antibodies, complement, or inflammatory cells into tissue spaces. Mast cells were observed by early histologists to be filled with cellular material (the granules). The term mast cell was applied to indicate that these cells appeared to be stuffed as if by overeating (mastication). The cellular granules are now known to contain biologically active agents produced by the mast cell that are released upon activation of the cells. Mast cells are usually located adjacent to small arterioles and in submucosal membranes, where released vasoactive mediators would be expected to be most active in causing dilation of smooth muscle cells of arterioles. In classic anaphylactic reactions, mast cells are degranulated by reaction of antigen with immunoglobulin E (IgE) antibody that adheres to the surface of mast cells because of a specific configuration of the Fc part of the antibody molecules.

Fcε Receptors

There are two Fc receptors for IgE: high-affinity receptors on mast cells (FcεRI) and low-affinity receptors on lymphocytes, monocytes, eosinophils,

Table 3.3 Mast cell mediators

Mediator	Structure/chemistry	Source	Effects
Histamine	β-Imidazolyethylamine	Mast cells, basophils	Vasodilation; increase vascular permeability (venules), mucus production
Serotonin	5-Hydroxytryptamine	Mast cells (rodent), platelets, cells of enterochromaffin system	Vasodilation, increase vascular permeability (venules)
Neutrophil chemotactic factor	Mol wt > 750,000	Mast cells	Chemotaxis of neutrophils
Eosinophil chemotactic factor A	Tetrapeptide	Mast cells	Chemotaxis of eosinophils
Vasoactive intestinal peptide	28-Amino-acid peptide	Mast cells, neutrophils, cutaneous nerves	Vasodilation; potentiate edema produced by bradykinin and C5a des-Arg
Thromboxane A_2	O, O, COOH, 12, OH	Arachidonic acid (cyclooxygenase pathway)	Vasoconstriction, broncho-constriction, platelet aggregation
Prostaglandin E_2 (or D_2)	O, COOH, 15, HO, OH	Arachidonic acid (cyclooxygenase pathway)	Vasodilation; potentiate permeability effects of histamine and bradykinin; increase permeability when acting with leukotactic agent; potentiate leukotriene effect; hyperalgesia
Leukotriene B_4	H OH, COOH, H OH	Arachidonic acid (lipoxygenase pathway)	Chemotaxis of neutrophils; increase vascular permeability in the presence of PGE_2
Leukotriene D_4	H OH, COOH, C_5H_{11}, $HS-CH_2$, $CHCONHCH_2COOH$, NH_2	Arachidonic acid (lipoxygenase pathway)	Increase vascular permeability
Platelet activating factor	Acetylated glycerol ether phosphocholine	Basophils, neutrophils, monocytes, macrophages	Release of mediators from platelets, neutrophil aggregation, neutrophil secretion, superoxide production by neutrophils; increase vascular permeability

and platelets (FcεRII) (Fig. 3.3A). Upon reaction of antigen with IgE antibody on the surface of the mast cells, a complex cellular activation mechanism causes the mast cells to release the pharmacologically active agents contained in cytoplasmic granules (Fig. 3.3B). The low-affinity FcεRII receptors may act to direct effector eosinophils and monocytes to parasites. The role of the FcεRII on T cells is discussed in chapter 5.

Mast Cell Mediators

Pharmacologically active agents of mast cells are the chemical mediators of atopic or anaphylactic hypersensitivity. The effects of their release are described in more detail in chapter 11. The effects of mast cell mediators are listed in Fig. 3.4. The major early events in inflammation, vasodilation

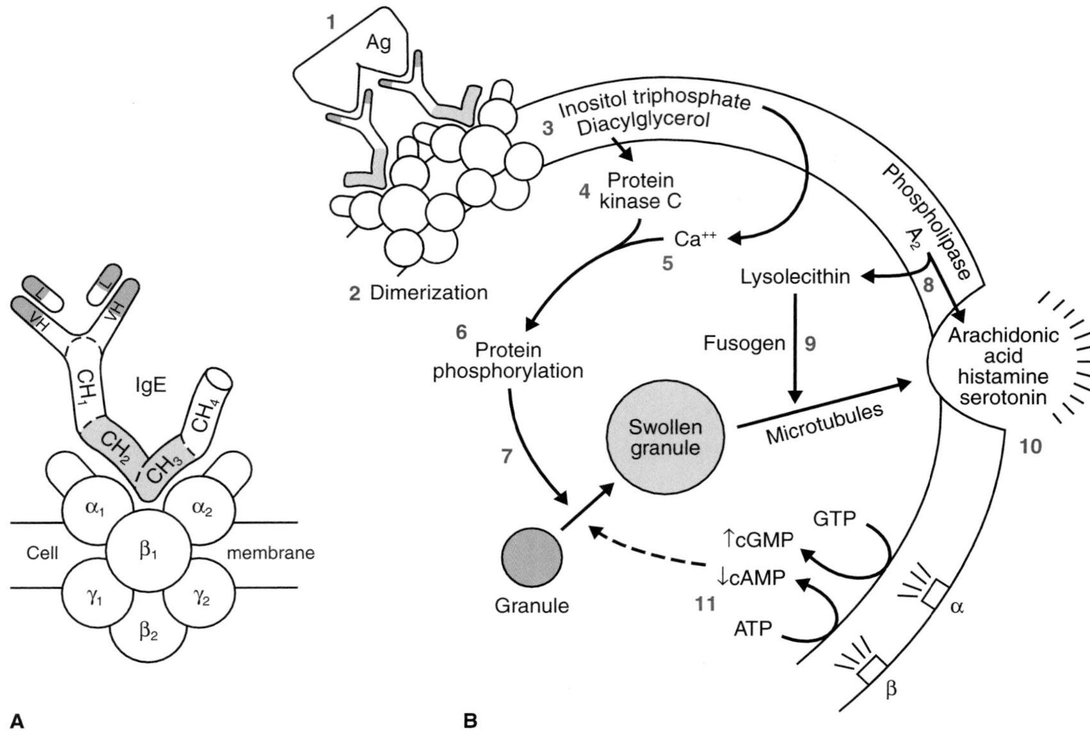

Figure 3.3 Mast cell Fc receptor and degranulation. **(A)** Diagram of the high-affinity FcεR on mast cells. The high-affinity FcεR on mast cells (FcεRI) is composed of six subunits (α1, α2, β1, β2, γ1, and γ2). The α subunits and β1 extend from the cell surface and bind to the CH2 and CH3 domains of the IgE molecule; the γ subunits (connected by a single disulfide bond) and the β2 subunit project through the cell membrane into the cytoplasm. **(B)** Postulated steps in mast cell degranulation. **(1)** Binding of antigen (allergen), cross-linking two IgE molecules on mast cell surface; **(2)** dimerization of IgE receptors; **(3)** alteration of methyltransferases; **(4)** conversion of membrane phospholipids to phosphatidylcholine; **(5)** opening of Ca^{2+} channel and influx of Ca^{2+} into cells; **(6)** activation of Ca^{2+}-dependent protein phosphorylation; **(7)** enlargement of granules by protein kinases; **(8)** activation of phospholipase A_2 with formation of lysolecithin and arachidonic acid; **(9)** lysolecithin acts as "fusogen" causing granules to fuse with cell membranes with release of contents; **(10)** activation of granules is dependent on levels of cyclic AMP and cyclic GMP, which in turn are regulated by α- and β-adrenergic receptors **(11)**.

and increased vascular permeability which occur within the first 30 min, are mediated by the immediate degranulation of mast cells and the release of histamine and serotonin. The second phase, between 1 and 2.5 h, is due to bradykinin (see "The Kinin System," later in this chapter). The third phase of persistent edema, occurring 6 to 12 h after initiation of inflammation, is mediated by prostaglandins and leukotrienes produced as a result of metabolism of phospholipids from membranelike material released from mast cell granules (see "Arachidonic Acid Metabolites," below). Chemotaxis of neutrophils and eosinophils is affected by leukotrienes as well as by platelet-activating factor. Enzymes activated by solubilization of granular material may also contribute to tissue damage and/or repair.

Histamine

Histamine is the major preformed mast cell mediator. Injection of histamine into the skin produces the typical wheal and flare reaction of the im-

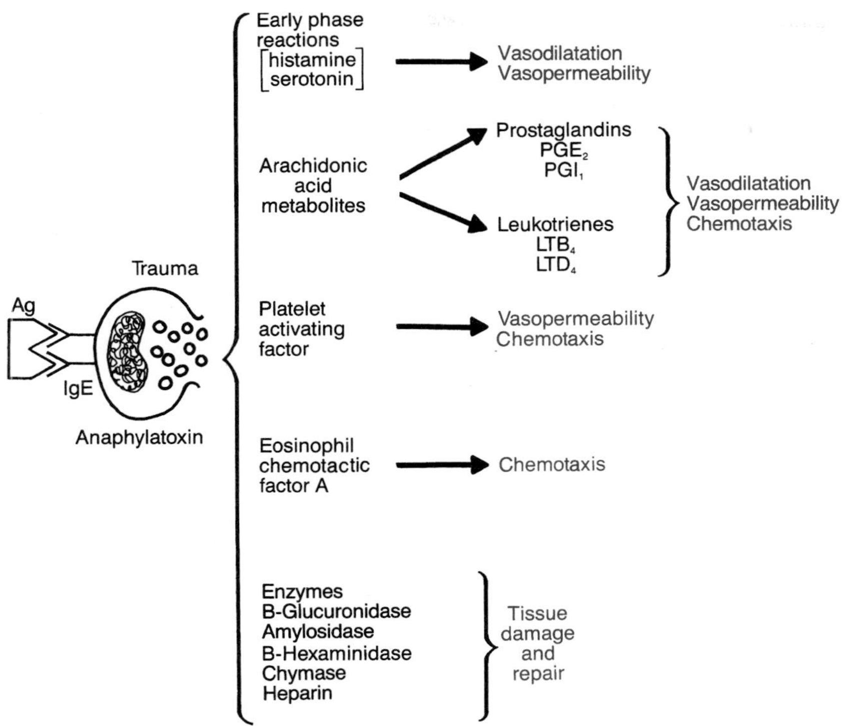

Figure 3.4 Mast cell mediators and inflammation. (Modified from S. I. Wasserman and N. A. Solter, p. 192, *in Advances in Allergy and Applied Immunology,* Pergamon Press, Inc., Elmsford, N.Y., 1980.)

mediate acute vascular response. Histamine causes endothelial cell contraction and vasodilation, leading to edema (wheal) and redness (flare). Histamine is formed from the amino acid L-histidine by the action of an enzyme called L-histidine decarboxylase found in the cytoplasm of mast cells and basophils. The biologic effects of histamine are mediated by two distinct sets of receptors, H_1 and H_2 (Table 3.4). Effects mediated through H_1 receptors are the classic acute vascular inflammatory events. Anti-inflammatory effects, as well as vasodilation, are mediated through H_2 receptors. Thus, histamine may activate acute vascular effects yet inhibit acute cellular inflammation. Acute cellular inflammation is mediated by products of arachidonic acid.

Arachidonic Acid Metabolites

Major mediators of inflammation are the metabolic derivatives of arachidonic acid. Arachidonic acid is derived from membrane phospholipids that are broken down by phospholipases. In the human, membrane phospholipids are released from mast cells during the early phase of acute inflammation but may also be derived from other cell membranes. The metabolism of arachidonic acid is believed to occur mainly in macrophages, but metabolites may also be synthesized by most, if not all, cells that take part in an inflammatory response, including mast cells. Metabolism of arachidonic acid occurs via two major pathways: the cyclooxygenase pathway, which gives rise to prostaglandins, and the lipoxygenase pathway, which gives rise to leukotrienes (Fig. 3.5).

Table 3.4 H_1- and H_2-dependent actions of histamine[a]

H_1-receptor-mediated effects	H_2-receptor-mediated effects	Shared H_1 and H_2 effects
Increased cyclic GMP	Increased cyclic AMP	Vasodilation (hypotension)
Smooth muscle constriction (bronchi)	Smooth muscle dilation (vascular)	Flush
Increased vascular permeability	Gastric acid secretion	Headache
Pruritus	Mucous secretion	
Prostaglandin generation	Inhibition of basophil histamine release	
	Inhibition of lymphokine release	
	Inhibition of neutrophil enzyme release	
	Inhibition of eosinophil migration	
	Inhibition of T-lymphocyte-mediated cytotoxicity	
Antagonized by "classical" antihistamines	Antagonized by cimetidine	

[a]Modified from D. D. Metcalfe and M. Kaliner, *in* J. J. Oppenheim, D. Rosenstreich, and M. Potter (ed.), *Cellular Functions in Immunity and Inflammation* (Elsevier Science Publishing, Inc., New York, N.Y., 1981).

Prostaglandins. The prostaglandins are derived by oxidation of prostanoic acid (cyclooxygenation).

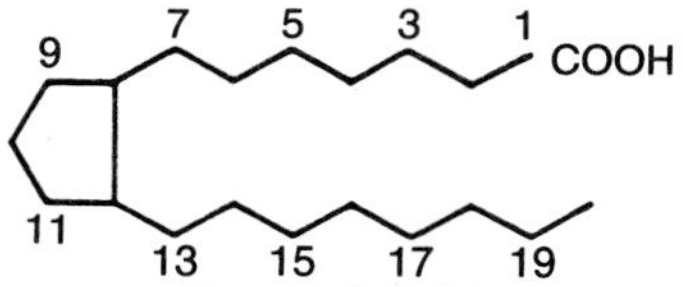

9 7 5 3 1 COOH
11 13 15 17 19
Prostanoic Acid

The numerical subscript in each prostaglandin (PG) refers to the number of unsaturated bonds. PGE_1 has one unsaturated bond at the 13–14 position; PGE_2 has two unsaturated bonds—one at the 5–6 and one at the 13–14 position. The letter designations refer to the position of bonds in the ring structure:

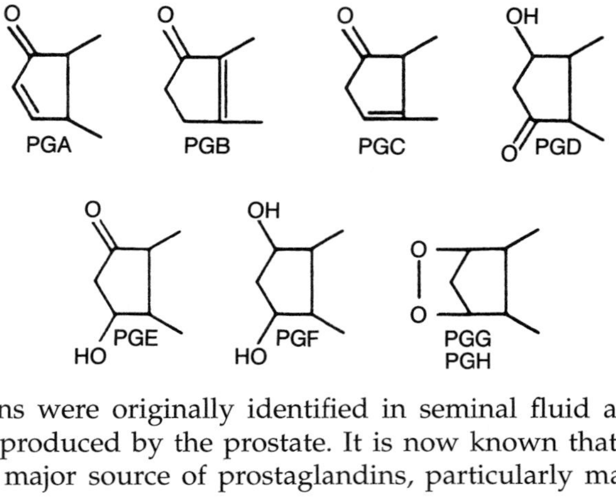

PGA PGB PGC PGD
PGE PGF PGG PGH

Prostaglandins were originally identified in seminal fluid and were believed to be produced by the prostate. It is now known that other tissue cells are the major source of prostaglandins, particularly mast cells. The

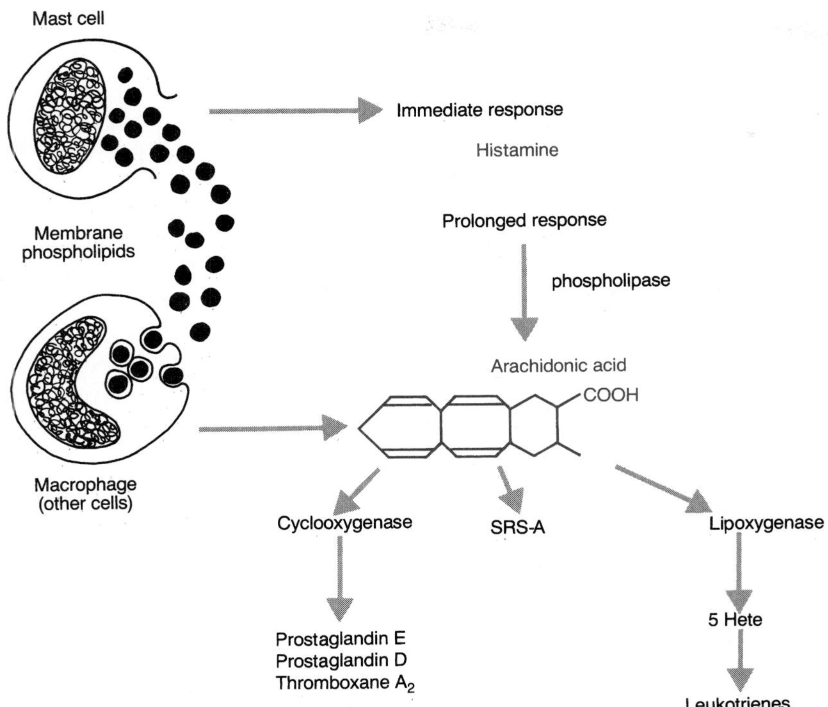

Figure 3.5 Arachidonic acid metabolism. (Modified from D. D. Metcalfe and M. Kaliner, p. 353, *in* J. J. Oppenheim, D. Rosenstreich, and M. Potter (ed.), *Cellular Functions in Immunity and Inflammation*, Elsevier Science Publishing, Inc., New York, N.Y., 1981.)

most active components are PGE_2 and PGD_2, which produce vasodilation, increase vascular permeability, and cause hyperalgesia (increased sensitivity to pain). The primary source for thromboxane A_2 is the platelet. Thromboxane A_2 is also produced by the cyclooxygenase pathway and is active in vasoconstriction, bronchoconstriction, and platelet aggregation. These metabolites are rapidly metabolized to inactive forms (PGE_1, PGD_1, and thromboxane B_2) by further oxygenation. PGE and prostacyclin (PGI_2) also act to suppress a variety of inflammatory cells, including mast cells, polymorphonuclear leukocytes (PMNs), monocytes, and macrophages, as well as natural killer (NK) cells by increasing intracellular cyclic AMP. PGE_1 also inhibits production of leukotriene B_4, suppresses lymphokine production, and inhibits increased vascular permeability and tissue injury during acute inflammation. The nonsteroidal anti-inflammatory drugs, such as aspirin, act to inhibit cyclooxygenase and block formation of these inflammatory mediators.

Leukotrienes. The products of the lipoxygenase pathway are called leukotrienes. They are generated by leukocytes and mast cells. Again, the subscript denotes the number of double bonds. The activity of leukotrienes C_4, D_4, and E_4 is believed to be responsible for a factor previously called slow-reacting substance of anaphylaxis, while that of leukotriene B_4 is chemotactic for eosinophils (eosinophilic chemotactic factor of anaphylaxis) and neutrophils. Although prostaglandins are responsible for some of the late vascular effects of anaphylaxis, they may also serve to modulate anaphylaxis by increasing cyclic nucleotide levels of mast cells and inhibiting histamine release. Leukotriene B_4 enhances adherence of PMNs to endothelial cells, a process blocked by PGE and PGI_2. In addition, leukotriene B_4 activates PMNs to migrate, degranulate, and generate superoxide anions.

Cytokines. Cytokines are small protein molecules secreted by many different kinds of cells but most prominently by activated white blood cells. Cytokines were first observed after stimulation of T cells by antigen and were identified by their biologic behavior (see Table 3.20). Mast cells produce cytokines in a pattern similar to that produced by Th2 cells and are believed to play a role in the regulation of IgE synthesis (see chapter 4). These cytokines include but are not limited to interleukin-2 (IL-2), IL-3, IL-4, IL-5, IL-6, granulocyte-macrophage colony-stimulating factor (GM-CSF), tumor necrosis factor alpha (TNF-α), and gamma interferon (IFN-γ). In particular, IL-4 drives $CD4^+$ T-helper cells to express the Th2 phenotype, and IL-4, IL-5, and IL-6 drive differentiating B cells to IgE and IgA production. The cytokine profile of mast cells helps to explain the long-standing observation of a relationship between mast cell numbers and IgE levels. The role of different cytokines in inflammation is presented in more detail below.

Platelets

Platelets are small, membrane-bound bits of cytoplasm that are pinched off from megakaryocytes in the bone marrow and circulate in the blood. The role of blood platelets in inflammation is complex. Platelets contain heparin and serotonin, so release of these mediators may contribute to the acute vascular phase of inflammation. Platelets also produce oxygen radicals, which may cause tissue damage. However, the primary role of platelets is to block damaged vessel walls and prevent hemorrhage. Platelets react with ligands in damaged vessels through a family of receptor proteins, the glycoprotein system.

Platelets react differently at sites of arterial damage (high pressure, high flow) than they do in veins (low pressure, low flow). Because of the high flow rate in arteries, platelets must first slow and stop before they can attach to the subendothelium. In arteries, platelets initially react via a single receptor on the platelet surface (glycoprotein Ib), which binds specifically to von Willebrand factor on the vessel surface. In the absence of shear forces created by high flow, these ligands will not bind to each other. Shear forces sufficient to initiate platelet-vessel binding occur when arterial blood flows over the static subendothelial surface. After initial binding, platelets are "activated," and the platelet glycoprotein IIb surface receptor undergoes a conformational change that permits it to bind to a tripeptide, arginine-glycine-asparagine (Arg-Gly-Asp, or RGD), which is present in fibrin, fibronectin, and vitronectin. At sites of vascular damage, the extracellular matrix proteins fibronectin and vitronectin are exposed, and fibrin is formed through activation of the coagulation system (see below). Platelets bind to these molecules, forming clumps of platelets that plug up leaks in the vascular system. The platelet and coagulation systems complement each other because platelet aggregation accelerates thrombin formation, and fibrin deposits strengthen platelet aggregates. Once activation and spreading of platelets are under way, the platelet becomes a nidus for binding of other platelets and for further deposition of fibrin, which strengthens the platelet aggregate by providing links between individual platelets. In the venous system, fibrin forms in the presence of red cells, and platelet deposition is less prominent.

Table 3.5 Antimicrobial systems in neutrophils

Oxygen dependent	Oxygen independent
Myeloperoxidase	Lysozyme
Superoxide anion (O_2^-)	Lactoferrin
Hydroxyl radical (OH^-)	Cationic proteins
Singlet oxygen ($^1O_2$)	Neutral proteases
Hydrogen peroxide	Acid hydrolases

Polymorphonuclear Neutrophils

Neutrophilic PMNs are the major cellular component of the acute inflammatory reaction. The vasodilation and increased permeability produced by mast cells sets the stage for tissue infiltration by neutrophils, but a number of specific signals are involved in mobilizing the neutrophils to move across the vascular wall into the tissues, and additional signals are required to activate them to destroy. Neutrophils are characterized by numerous cytoplasmic granules that contain highly destructive hydrolytic enzymes (Table 3.5). At least three cytoplasmic granules are identifiable: specific granules (e.g., lactoferrin), azurophilic granules (lysosomes containing acid hydrolases and other enzymes), and a third granule compartment containing gelatinase (see Table 2.1 for more details).

Chemotactic Factors

Neutrophils may be attracted to sites of inflammation by a number of chemotactic factors (Table 3.6). Neutrophils have cell surface receptors for some of these factors, such as activated fragments of complement (see below) and fMet tripeptides. Many chemoattractants, including *N*-formyl tripeptides, C5a, leukotriene B_4, and IL-8, bind to a heptahelical G-protein cell surface receptor on the inflammatory cell. Neutrophils are stimulated by chemotaxis to move, to adhere and de-adhere, to rearrange their cytoskeleton, and to phagocytose infectious microorganisms, secrete granule contents, and activate the NADPH oxidase system to generate toxic metabolites of oxygen. The adherence of neutrophils to cells and surfaces is mediated by cell adhesion molecules known as integrins (see below). Acute inflammatory

Table 3.6 Chemotactic and activating factors for neutrophils

Factor	Action			
	Chemoattraction	Degranulation	Adherence	NAPDH oxidase
Complement				
C5a, C5a des-Arg	X	X	X	
Kallikrein	X	X		
Fibrinopeptide B	X		X	
fMet tripeptide (Met-Leu-Phe)	X	X	X	X
Collagen peptides	X		X	
Interleukin-8	X	X		X
Platelet-activating factor	X	X		
Leukotriene B_4	X	X	X	X

reactions need not be initiated by immune mechanisms and are frequently associated with bacterial infections (such as staphylococcal and streptococcal infections) or traumatic tissue injury. In these situations, neutrophils are attracted into sites of inflammation by chemotactic factors released by the infecting organism (fMet peptides) or by products of damaged tissue, such as fibronectin, fibrin or collagen degradation products, or factors produced by other inflammatory cells. In immune complex reactions, neutrophils are attracted and activated by formation of activated complement components (see below) after antibody-antigen reaction in tissues.

The receptors for chemoattractants belong to the seven-transmembrane helix receptor family. After binding the chemoattractant ligand, these receptors become activated and transmit their signals to heterotrimeric G proteins containing α, β, and γ subunits. The G protein complex dissociates into an α subunit and a βγ subunit. The βγ subunit binds and activates target enzymes such as phospholipase C, phosphoinositide 3-kinase (PI 3-kinase), and adenylyl cyclase. These enzymes initiate a cascade of events. PI 3-kinase converts the membrane phospholipid phosphatidylinositol-4,5 biphosphate (PIP2) into phosphatidylinositol-3,4,5-triphosphate (PIP3). PIP3 in the membrane is a target for a domain on protein kinase B (the pleckstrin homology domain). Their interaction initiates migration of PIP3 to the edge of the cell reacting with the chemoattractant, producing the morphologic polarity required for directional migration. This activation mechanism appears to be involved in the chemoattraction of other cell types, such as T cells and macrophages, as well as of neutrophils.

Lysosomal Enzymes

Neutrophil granules contain a number of oxygen-independent enzymes that are able to digest foreign organisms as well as oxygen-dependent mechanisms for killing. Neutrophils engulf particles by extending pseudopodia, which surround and fuse around the particle, forming a phagosome. The phagosome then fuses with the cytoplasmic membrane granules. In some instances, such as with deposition of antigen-antibody complexes in vivo, neutrophils attempt to engulf and digest complexes as they do bacteria coated with antibody and complement but are unable to phagocytose the complexes because they are deposited in tissue structures, such as basement membranes. The neutrophils may then release their lysosomal enzymes from cells into the tissue spaces. The lysosomal acid hydrolyses cause local tissue digestion at the site of the reactions. The characteristic lesion is fibrinoid necrosis, areas of acellular digested tissue that look like fibrin but lack any fibrillar appearance.

Oxygen-Dependent Killing

Reactive oxygen metabolites (Table 3.5), primarily involved in bacterial killing, may also damage endothelial cells and adjacent tissues, resulting in the formation of pus. One of the most important components of the oxygen-dependent killing system is NADPH oxidase. Cytosolic components ras, p67, p47, and p40 translocate to cytochrome b_{558} located in the cell membrane and associate through molecular domains to form the active NADPH catalytic complex. The active complex can catalyze the conversion of molecular oxygen (O_2) by addition of one electron to form superoxide (O_2^-).

$$2O_2 + \text{NADPH} \xrightarrow{\text{NADPH oxidase}} 2O_2^- \text{ (superoxide)} + \text{NADPH}^+ + H^+$$

Superoxide can diffuse into tissue, where it is converted to other toxic metabolites active in causing tissue damage, such as in pus formation and fibrinoid necrosis. O_2^- anions serve as a substrate for superoxide dismutase to form hydrogen peroxide (H_2O_2). Additional toxic metabolites, such as hypochlorous acid (HOCl), hydroxyl radicals (HO^-), and singlet oxygen species ($^1O_2$), are formed from the action of enzymes such as myeloperoxidase, which is present in inflammatory cells and activated during inflammation. Oxygen radicals are also formed during ischemic injury (loss of blood supply) due to proteolytic conversion of xanthine dehydrogenase to xanthine oxidase, which, in the presence of O_2, catabolizes the conversion of hypoxanthine and xanthine to uric acid with the generation of O_2^- and H_2O_2. This subsequently results in generation of chemotactic mediators, neutrophil recruitment, and further tissue injury. Studies employing specific antioxidants suggest that products of O_2^- and H_2O_2 reactions and the myeloperoxidase-H_2O_2-halide systems are the most toxic mediators of acute tissue damage. In addition, O_2^- may stimulate fibroblast proliferation, and H_2O_2 activates transcription factors, such as NF-κB.

Adhesion Molecules

Adhesion molecules are responsible for inflammatory cell–endothelial cell interactions and cell-matrix interactions that take place during inflammation. The interaction of inflammatory cells with endothelial cells involves a series of interactions between cell surface ligands that are upregulated during the inflammatory process. After inflammatory cells pass through the vascular endothelium, their further reaction with extracellular matrix involves the interaction of cell receptors and matrix components. The deposition of fibrin, fibrinogen, and fibronectin from the serum during acute inflammation provides a temporary matrix into which white blood cells, fibroblasts, and endothelial cells migrate. This migration is mediated by specific cell adhesion molecules, the expression of which is upregulated during wound healing. These include *integrins, cell adhesion molecules, selectins, vascular addressins,* and *lymphocyte homing receptors* (Table 3.7).

Table 3.7 A simplified family tree of adhesion molecules[a]

Family	Subfamily	Examples	Expressed by	Receptors for:
Integrins	β1	VLAs 1–6	Activated leukocytes	Collagen, fibronectin, laminin
	β2	LFA	Lymphocytes	ICAM-1
		Mac-1	Macrophages	ICAM-1, ICAM-2, C3bi, fibrinogen
	β3	gpIIb/IIIa	Platelets	Vitronectin
Ig supergene	Adhesion molecules	ICAM-1	Activated endothelium	LFA lymphocytes
		ICAM-2	Endothelial cells	Mac-1
		VCAM-1	Endothelial cells	VLA-4 (lymphocytes)
Selectins	L-selectin	LAM-1	Granulocytes, monocytes	Activated endothelial cells
	E-selectin	ELAM-1	HEV[b] of lymph nodes	Recirculating lymphocytes
	P-selectin	GMP-140	Activated endothelium	Inflammatory cells
Vascular addressins	Peripheral lymph node	LAM-1, Leu-8	Lymph node HEV	Recirculating lymphocytes
	Mucosa	H-CAM (CD44)	Mucosal HEV	Recirculating lymphocytes
	Mucosa	VLA-4, LFA-1	Mucosal HEV (VCAM-1)	Recirculating lymphocytes

[a]Modified from S. Montefort and S. T. Holgate, *Respir. Med.* **85:**91, 1991.
[b]HEV, high endothelial veins.

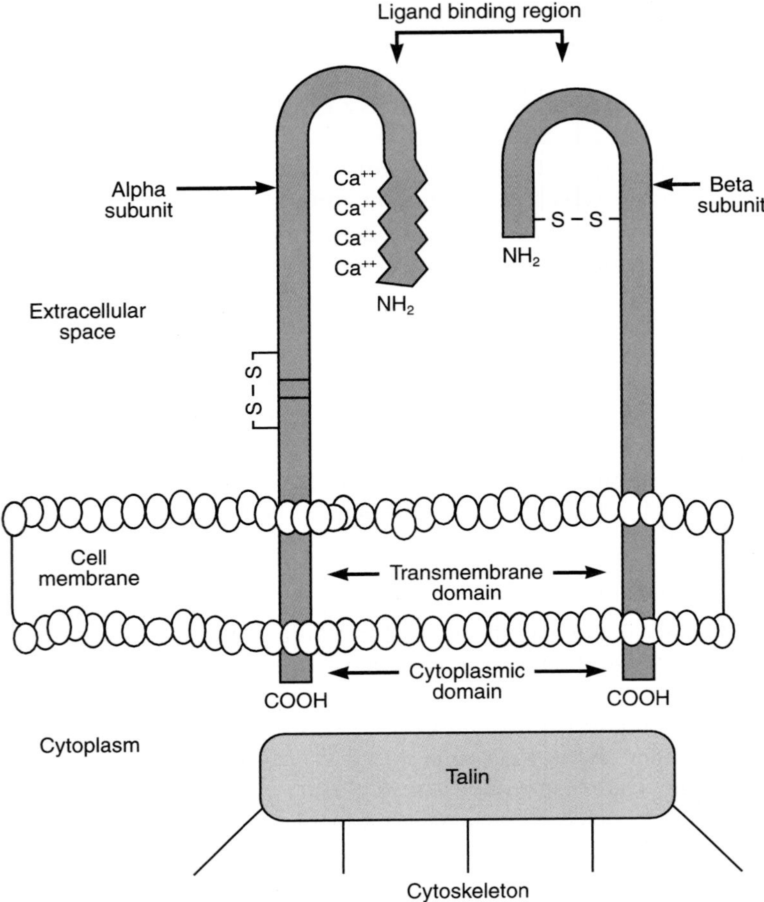

Figure 3.6 General polypeptide structure of the integrins. Integrins are composed of two similar polypeptide chains (α and β) with an extracellular receptor for matrix proteins, a membrane domain, and a cytoplasmic "tail." There is about 40 to 50% homology in amino acid sequence among the various α chains and among the three β chains but no homology between the α and β chains. The α subunit of each integrin has a matrix-binding domain, and binding to their respective ligands requires a divalent cation such as Ca^{2+} or Mg^{2+}. About one-quarter of the β subunit consists of a repeating unit with a high cysteine content. Both subunits span the cell membrane and have a cytoplasmic COOH terminal that may provide a link between the extracellular matrix and the cytoskeleton. Phosphorylation of the cytoplasmic domain may regulate the binding functions of the receptors. The integrin phenotype expressed by a particular cell imparts specificity for binding to ligands on other cells or to different extracellular matrix components. (Modified from E. Ruoslahti, *J. Clin. Investig.* **87**:1–5, 1991.)

Integrins

Integrins are cell surface molecules found on the surface of almost all cell types; they provide recognition structures for binding to other cells or to extracellular matrix (Fig. 3.6). Integrins belong to a family of heterodimeric receptors made up of α and β subunits. Each subfamily has a common β subunit, and the individual members of the subfamily each have a different α subunit. The three subfamilies are named after the common β chain, β1, β2, and β3. So far, 11 α polypeptides and 7 β polypeptides have been identified in humans (Table 3.8). The β1 subfamily consists of β1 joined to

Table 3.8 Human integrins[a]

α subunits	CD	β subunits	CD	Molecules	Designation	Receptor
α1	49a	β1	29	$\alpha_1\beta_1$	VLA-1	Collagen
α2	49b	β2	18	$\alpha_2\beta_1$	VLA-2, platelet Ia/IIa	Collagen, laminin
α3	49c	β3	61	$\alpha_3\beta_1$	VLA-3	Collagen, laminin, fibronectin
α4	49d	β4		$\alpha_4\beta_1$	VLA-4	Fibronectin, VCAM-1
				$\alpha_4\beta_7$		Fibronectin, VCAM-1
α5	49e	β5		$\alpha_5\beta_1$	VLA-5, platelet Ic/IIa	Fibronectin
α6	49f	β6		$\alpha_6\beta_1$	VLA-6	Laminin
α7	49d	β7		$\alpha_7\beta_1$		Laminin
α8				$\alpha_8\beta_1$		Laminin
αL	11a			$\alpha_L\beta_2$	LFA-1	ICAM-1, ICAM-2
αM	11b			$\alpha_M\beta_2$	iC3bR, Mac-1	iC3b, fibrinogen, LPS, ICAM-1
αX	11c			$\alpha_x\beta_2$	p150,95	iC3b
αV	51			$\alpha_V\beta_3$	Vitronectin receptor	Vitronectin, etc.
αIIb	41			$\alpha IIb\beta_3$	Platelet IIb/IIIa	Fibrinogen, vitronectin, fibronectin

[a]CD, cluster designation identified by monoclonal antibodies.

one of the eight α subunits; the β2 subfamily has αL, αM, or αx joined with β2; the β3 subfamily has αIIb or αV joined with β3.

Leukocyte integrins. The leukocyte integrins (β_2-integrins) have been identified through the use of monoclonal antibodies, including LFA-1 (lymphocyte function-associated antigen 1), Mac-1 (macrophage antigen 1), and p150,95 (named for the kilodalton molecular masses of its subunits) (Table 3.8). Monoclonal antibodies recognize the various α chains but do not distinguish among the β chains (Table 3.8). LFA-1 binds to a molecule called ICAM-1 (intercellular adhesion molecule-1), which is located on endothelial cells. The expression of ICAM-1 is upgraded during inflammation under the influence of cytokines TNF, lipopolysaccharide (LPS), IFN-γ, and IL-1 (see below). LFA-1 plays an important role in the localization of lymphocytes to tissues during inflammation as well as in the conjugation of cytotoxic T lymphocytes and NK cells to target cells and lymphocyte-lymphocyte interactions during primary induction of T-cell responses to antigens. Mac-1 is a receptor for C3bi (CR3), and p150,95 is also a receptor for C3bi (CR4). Mac-1 and p150,95 are active in phagocytosis of objects coated with C3bi (erythrocytes or organisms coated with complement), in chemotaxis of monocytes, and in the adherence of monocytes to endothelial cells.

Our understanding of the role of the leukocyte integrins in inflammation has been enhanced by the study of the naturally occurring human disease leukocyte adhesion deficiency (LAD). LAD occurs in two forms, LAD1 and LAD2. In LAD1, there is a mutation in the gene that codes for the β subunit shared by LFA-1, CR3, and CR4. In LAD2, there is an absence of neutrophil sialyl-Lewis X, a ligand of E-selectin on vascular endothelium. All cytotoxic lymphocyte functions are impaired, and patients suffer repeated infections from birth. A feature of the infectious lesions is the relative absence of granulocytes, normally a predominant feature of such lesions, in the face of elevated peripheral blood leukocyte counts (5 to 20 times normal). In vitro, neutrophils and monocytes from patients with LAD show marked defects in adhesion-related functions and deficiency in cell granule and cell surface expression of integrin molecules. Chemoattractants fail to cause upgrading of integrins on the cell surface.

Other integrins. In addition to the leukocyte integrins, there are the very late antigens of activation (VLA), the vitronectin receptor (VNR), and the platelet aggregation molecule IIbIIIa. The nonleukocyte integrins bind to extracellular matrix components such as fibronectin, collagen, and laminin. The interaction of different integrins with connective tissue molecules (Table 3.8) mediates migration of different cell types, such as fibroblasts and epithelial cells, during wound healing. One of the major binding sites is the tripeptide recognition sequence RGD. Although this tripeptide will inhibit binding of VLA-5 (fibronectin receptor), VNR, and IIbIIIa to their respective matrix structures, each is specific, indicating that amino acid substitutions adjacent to the RGD sequence determine specificity of binding. Other receptors, such as those that bind to collagen, also require the RGD sequence but have a separate specificity related to the conformation conferred on the RGD-binding tripeptide by adjacent amino acids.

Ig Supergene Family/Cell Adhesion Molecules

The Ig supergene family of cell adhesion molecules includes a pair of homologous molecules, ICAM-1 and ICAM-2, as well as vascular cell adhesion molecule 1 (VCAM-1). ICAM-1 and ICAM-2 are ligands for the β_2-integrin LFA-1 on all activated leukocytes. ICAM-1, but not ICAM-2, is also a ligand for the β_2-integrin Mac-1. VCAM-1 reacts with the β_1-integrin VLA-4. ICAM-1 and VCAM-1 expression on endothelial cells is increased by inflammatory cytokines such as IL-1, TNF, IFN-γ, and IL-4. When produced during inflammation, these cytokines will selectively increase expression of different adhesion molecules, so that induction of specific adhesion molecules can provide a means of selective recruitment of inflammatory cells.

Selectins

During normal recirculation of lymphocytes, the circulating cells bind to specialized high endothelial venules in lymphoid organs. The endothelial cell receptor belongs to another family of vascular cell adhesion molecules. These include *L-selectin* on lymphocytes, *E-selectin* on endothelial cells, and *P-selectin (granule membrane protein of 140 kDa)* on platelets (Table 3.9). L-selectin was originally identified by the monoclonal antibody Mel-14 in mice and by Leu-8 in humans. It functions as the homing receptor for lymphocytes. E-selectin mediates the interaction of cytokine-activated endothelial cells with neutrophils early in inflammation, and P-selectin serves as a site for the binding of monocytes and neutrophils to activated

Table 3.9 Properties of selectins[a]

Selectin	Molecular mass (kDa)	Cells expressing	Cells binding
L-selectin (LAM-1)	100	Granulocytes, monocytes, lymphocytes	Activated ECs
E-selectin (ELAM-1)	115	Activated ECs	HEV of lymph nodes
P-selectin (GMP-140)	140	Activated ECs, platelets	Granulocytes, monocytes

[a]ECs, endothelial cells; HEV, high endothelial veins.

platelets. These proteins share a similar domain structure, including a lectin domain, an EGF-like domain, a series of consensus repeats homologous to regulatory proteins, a transmembrane domain, and a small cytoplasmic domain (Fig. 3.7). P-selectin is located within membrane-bound granules in cells that can exocytose rapidly upon induction and appear on the cell surface. This provides a rapid mechanism of expression not requiring new protein synthesis. Expression of P-selectin may play a role in the assembly of cellular components necessary for clot formation by attachment of platelets to granulocytes and monocytes, or as a mechanism of clearance of activated platelets from the circulation by attachment of platelets to reticuloendothelial cells.

During the inflammatory process, cytokines may initially cause increased expression of E-selectin on endothelial cells, which favors the adhesion of neutrophils during acute inflammation. Over a period of 6 to 12 h, expression of E-selectin declines while expression of VCAM-1 increases, perhaps under the influence of IL-4. Now neutrophils will adhere less well, but adhesion of lymphocytes will increase. Later strong adhesion is mediated by binding of β_2-integrin (LFA-1) upregulated on activated lymphocytes to ICAM-1 and ICAM-2 upregulated on endothelial cells. Continued stimulation may result in the appearance of high endothelial venulelike postcapillary venules seen at sites of chronic inflammation, which appear to be the major sites for extravasation of lymphocytes into the lesion.

Neutrophil Adhesion and Emigration

Of critical importance in acute inflammation is the interaction of granulocytes with endothelial cells. In the process of inflammation, PMNs circulating in the blood recognize and bind to adherence molecules on endothelial cells (ECs) activated by inflammatory mediators. The strength of this initial reaction may not be sufficient to overcome the shear force of the flowing blood, resulting in the characteristic "rolling" seen as PMNs rotate along the EC surface. The adhesion of PMNs to ECs is strengthened by upregulation of other surface molecules (tethering molecules). Further

Figure 3.7 Structure of selectin. Selectins have a similar overall structure: a cytoplasmic domain, a series of C3b-C4b-like domains, an EGF domain, and a lectin domain, and a signal peptide. L-selectin has only two C3b-C4b regulatory protein repeats; E-selectin has six, and P-selectin has nine. (Modified from B. I. Johnston, G. A. Bliss, P. J. Newman, and R. P. McEver, *J. Biol. Chem.* **265**:21381, 1990.)

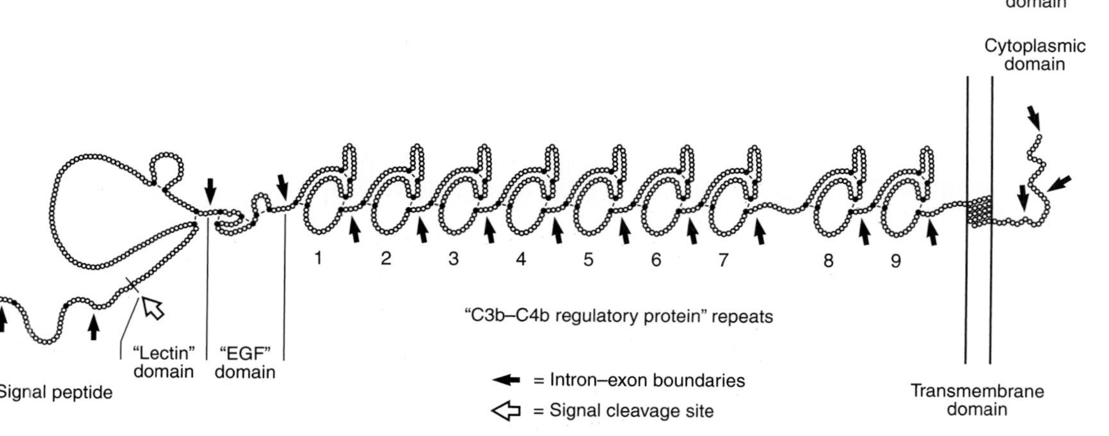

reaction of PMNs and ECs stops the rolling and is followed by transmigration of PMNs through the vascular wall.

PMN-EC interactions during acute inflammation involve an overlapping sequence of expression of signaling and binding molecules on both ECs and granulocytes (Fig. 3.8). Activated ECs produce signaling (platelet-activating factor [PAF] and IL-8) and tethering (binding) molecules (P- and E-selectins) for PMNs. There are four stages resulting in increasing binding affinity of molecules on PMNs to ligands on activated ECs: (i) reversible "rolling" mediated by L-selectin on PMNs and P-selectin on ECs, (ii) enhanced binding by G proteins on PMNs to PAF on ECs, (iii) stronger adherence mediated by β_2-integrins on PMNs and P-selectin on ECs, followed by (iv) stable binding (adhesion) and migration mediated by β_2-integrins on PMNs and E-selectin on ECs (Fig. 3.8). Immediate low-affinity binding occurs when L-selectin, which is constitutively present on PMNs, binds to the C-terminal lectin domains of P-selectin expressed on ECs within seconds after activation by thrombin, histamine, or leukotriene C_4. This is followed within minutes by synthesis and expression of PAF on the EC surface, which binds to a G protein on neutrophils. This reaction produces immediate nontranslational upregulation of expression of CD11-CD18 heterodimers (β_2-integrin) on the neutrophil, which binds to ICAMs (ICAM-1 and ICAM-2, see below) on ECs. β_2-Integrin is formed by rapid translocation of CD18 from subcellular granules to the PMN cell surface and formation of CD11-CD18 heterodimers. This is referred to as functional upregulation of the cell surface molecules and may be rapidly reversed. β_2-Integrin is also functionally upregulated after activation of PMNs with chemotactic factors or ionophores. Finally, stronger adhesion of PMNs occurs after E-selectin expression on, and IL-8 secretion by, ECs is stimulated by TNF-α, IL-1, or LPS. IL-8 (neutrophil-activating factor, or neutrophil-activating peptide 1) is released into the fluid phase and is a potent chemotactic factor for PMNs. IL-8 binds to G proteins on the neutrophils, stimulates longer-lasting translational upregulation of β_2-integrins, and enhances adhesion to ECs and to the subendothelial matrix, facilitating transendothelial migration. Clusters of differentiation (CD)

Figure 3.8 PMN-EC interactions during acute inflammation. Receptors on PMN interact with a series of cell adhesion molecules that are upregulated during the inflammatory process by mediators such as thrombin, histamine, IL-8, IL-1, and IFN.

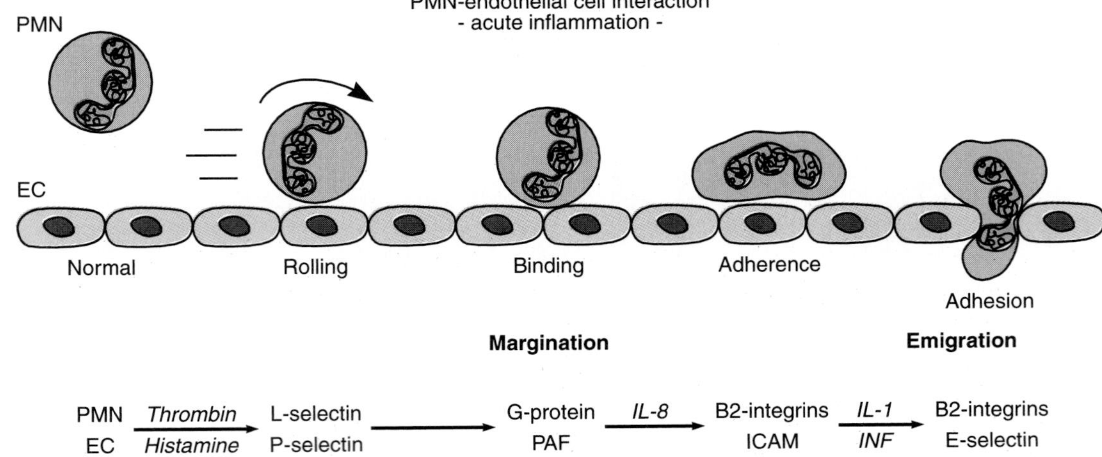

designations and other names for these molecules reflect their origin from monoclonal antibody identification.

An understanding of the role of these adhesion molecules in acute inflammation has been a major advance, but there are still many aspects of acute inflammation that are not known. This is most likely due to other combinations and interactions of recognition molecules that take place during the course of acute inflammation. Activation of ECs by cytokines such as IL-1 and TNF induces adherence of all granulocytic cell types, but there are also specific recognition molecules for eosinophils and basophils (see below).

Eosinophils

Acute Inflammation

Polymorphonuclear eosinophils, discovered by Paul Ehrlich in 1879, are distinguished from other granulocytes by the affinity of their cytoplasmic granules for acidic dyes such as eosin, resulting in an intense red staining. This staining is primarily due to the presence of a major basic protein (MBP) that binds acid dyes. Eosinophils are found predominantly in two types of inflammation: allergy and parasitic worm infections. Some chemotactic factors for eosinophils are listed in Table 3.10. These factors are derived from inflammatory cells, complement, or worm extracts. On the one hand, there is evidence that enzymes in eosinophils may serve to limit the extent of inflammation by neutralizing mediators of anaphylaxis, such as leukotriene C_4, histamine, and PAF. On the other hand, there is increasing evidence that the cationic proteins in eosinophil granules are mediators of acute inflammation. Eosinophil activation is associated with acute tissue injury. Activated eosinophils cause an initial intense vasoconstriction in lung microvasculature, followed by increased pulmonary vascular permeability and pulmonary edema. The cationic proteins that are active in this process are eosinophil peroxidase, MBP, and eosinophil-derived neurotoxin, which make up about 90% of the granule proteins. In addition, these proteins can directly injure endodermal cells, increasing the transudation of fluids into alveolar spaces as well as type II epithelial cells, leading to a decreased secretion of surfactant. This may contribute greatly to the respiratory distress syndromes (see below). Charcot Leyden crystal protein is also found in some eosinophil granules. This protein belongs to the S-type lectin family and may neutralize natural lung surfactants, causing collapse of air spaces (atelectasis).

The distribution and localization of eosinophils involves a family of adhesion molecules on endothelial cells and eosinophils similar to those for neutrophil margination and emigration. Weak binding occurs between eosinophil membrane sialyl-Lewis X to L-selectins on endothelial cells, followed by upregulation of E-selectin and PAF on the endothelial cell and binding to β_2-integrins on eosinophils. High-affinity binding specific for eosinophils or basophils occurs after activation by IL-4 of expression of VCAM-1 on endothelial cells; VCAM-1 binds to integrin ${}_{\alpha}4_{\beta}1$ (VLA-4) on eosinophils. Neutrophils do not adhere to ECs under these conditions. Expression of β_2-selectins on eosinophils is required for them to emigrate into tissues.

Eosinophils are "activated" by phosphorylation of signal-transducing proteins to release granular proteins by exocytosis. Activated eosinophils produce PAF, which acts as an autocrine to increase the activated state of

Table 3.10 Chemotactic factors for eosinophils

Factor	Origin
Histamine	Mast cells
Eosinophilic chemotactic factor A	Mast cells
Neutrophil peptides	Neutrophils
Eosinophil stimulator promoter	Lymphocytes
C5a	Complement
Worm extracts	*Ascaris* sp.

Table 3.11 Properties of eosinophil granule proteins

Name	Mol wt (10^3)	pI	Site	Activities
Major basic protein (MBP)	14	10.9	Core	Toxic to parasites, tumor cells; causes histamine release, neutralizes heparin
Eosinophil cationic proteins (ECP)	21	10.8	Matrix	Toxic to parasites, neurons; histamine release, alters fibrinolysis and coagulation, inhibits lymphocytes
Eosinophil derived neurotoxin (EDN)	18	8.9	Matrix	Potent neurotoxin, RNase activity
Eosinophil peroxidase (EPO)	71–77	>11	Matrix	Forms H_2O_2, inactivates leukotrienes, causes histamine release, kills microorganisms and tumor cells

the eosinophil, but endothelial cells are the major source of PAF for eosinophil activation. Some eosinophils have receptors for IgA and can be activated by cross-linking of these receptors by antigen.

Parasitic Diseases

Eosinophils play a major role in killing of parasites. The components of eosinophilic granules that are active against parasites and against some human tumor cells are listed in Table 3.11. Eosinophils are cytotoxic to schistosome larvae through an antibody-dependent cell-mediated mechanism. Eosinophil cationic proteins are highly toxic for schistosomes and are responsible for binding of eosinophils to worms in a way not possible for neutrophils. These proteins cause fragmentation of worms and are 10 times more toxic than MBP, although MBP makes up over 50% of the eosinophilic granule and forms the characteristic granule core seen in electron microscopy. Eosinophilic peroxidase is active in generation of H_2O_2, which is active in killing bacteria, and in degranulation of mast cells. Finally, eosinophils contain collagenase, which may function to aid in remodeling connective tissue during healing.

Serum Protein Systems

A number of serum proteins take part in acute inflammatory reactions. These include the complement, coagulation, and kinin systems as well as a number of serum proteins that regulate acute inflammation known as acute-phase reactants. The most critical player in many phases of acute antibody-mediated inflammation is the complement system.

Complement

The complement system of serum proteins is a complex set of up to 20 serum proteins that form a controlled sequence for production of activated molecules (Table 3.12). These augment inflammatory reactions mediated by classes of antibodies known as complement-fixing antibodies (see chapter 4).

Activation of the complement system may occur via two pathways: the classical and the alternate pathways. Activation via the classic sequence

Table 3.12 Complement components

Component	Function	Mol wt	No. of polypeptide chains	Concn in serum (μg/ml)	Site of synthesis
Classical pathway					
C1q	Recognition	400,000	18	200	Small intestine epithelium
C1r	Enzyme	160,000	2		Small intestine epithelium
C1s	Enzyme	80,000	1	120	Small intestine epithelium
C2	Activation	115,000	1	30	Macrophages
C3	Activation	180,000	2	1,200	Macrophages
C4	Activation	210,000	3	400	Liver epithelium
C5	Attack	180,000	2	75	Macrophages
C6	Attack	128,000	1	60	Liver
C7	Attack	150,000	3	60	
C8	Attack	150,000	3	15	
C9	Attack	75,000	1	Trace	Liver
Alternate pathway					
Properdin		190,000	4	20	Macrophages
Factor B	C3 activator	100,000	1	225	Macrophages
Factor D	C3 coactivator	25,000	4	Trace	Macrophages
C3	Activation	210,000	3	400	Macrophages

is initiated by antibody-antigen reactions, whereas the alternate pathway may be activated by certain bacterial products. The complete activation sequence occurs on the surface of cells and involves a series of molecular interactions during which molecular fragments as well as new multimolecular complexes with biologic activity are formed. The macromolecular cell-bound components serve to activate phagocytosis (opsonize) or produce "lesions" in the cell membrane that lead to lysis of the cell. This reaction is beneficial if it involves bacterial cell membranes but may be deleterious if it occurs on the surface of normal red blood cells (hemolytic anemia). In addition, complement fragments ("split products") are released into the fluid phase, where they mediate a variety of inflammatory responses, including chemotaxis of neutrophils and monocytes, enhancement of phagocytosis, and increased vascular permeability. These activated components also interact with other accessory systems, including the coagulation and fibrinolytic systems, to amplify and/or limit the acute inflammatory reaction. The major inflammatory functions of activated complement fragments are to open blood vessels and attract and activate polymorphonuclear neutrophils. Genetic defects in complement or its controlling proteins may be the cause of a variety of unusual diseases (see below).

Classical Pathway

A simplified diagrammatic representation of the classical pathway for complement activation is shown in Fig. 3.9, and the sequence is described in detail in Table 3.13. The first component of complement, C1, has the capacity to bind and be activated by antibody molecules that have been altered in their Fc region by reaction with antigen. Activation of C1 may take place in a fluid phase, such as when antibody reacts with soluble antigens in the bloodstream, or activation may occur on the surface of cells, as

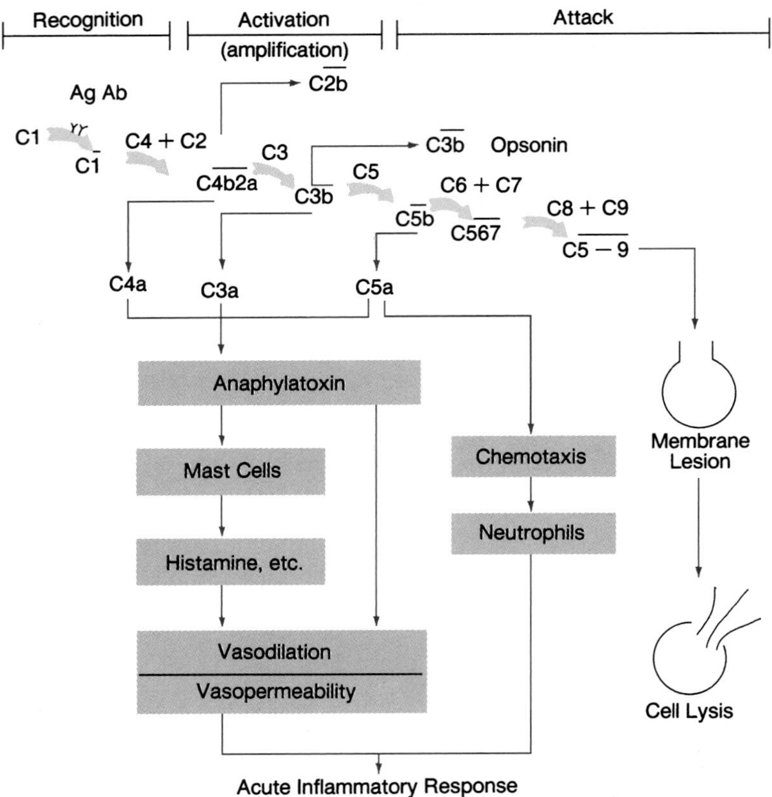

Figure 3.9 Classical pathway of complement activation. Following reaction of antibody with antigen, a cascade reaction of complement components is activated. C1 functions as a recognition unit for the altered Fc of two IgG molecules or one IgM molecule; C2 and C4 act as an activation unit leading to cleavage of C3. C3 fragments have a number of biological activities: C3a is anaphylatoxin, and C3b is recognized by receptors on macrophages (opsonin). C3b also joins with fragments of C4 and C2 to form C3 convertase, which cleaves C5. C5 then reacts with C6 through C9 to form a membrane attack unit that produces a lesion in cell membranes, through which intracellular components may escape (lysis).

when antierythrocyte antibody reacts with a red cell. The Ig classes that are active in fixing complement are IgG subclasses IgG1 and IgG3 and IgM. One molecule of IgM is capable of activating C1, whereas two molecules of IgG reacting close together are required. For two IgG molecules to achieve close enough apposition on a red cell to activate C1, approximately 600 to 1,000 molecules must bind to the cell, whereas only one IgM molecule is required. Thus, IgM antibodies are much more efficient at low concentrations in fixing complement on a cell surface.

The components of the classical pathway leading to cell lysis are C1 through C9. In the activation sequence occurring at the cell surface, C1 functions as a recognition unit, C2 to C4 function as an activation unit, and C5 to C9 function as a membrane attack unit. When C1 attaches to antibody, it becomes activated as an enzyme (C1 esterase), which cleaves C4 and C2 each into two fragments (C4a and C4b, C2a and C2b). One of the fragments of C4 (C4b) and one of the C2 fragments (C2a) join together and bind to new sites on the cell surface. The other fragments, C4a and C2b, are released into the fluid phase. C4a has weak anaphylatoxic activity,

Table 3.13 Sequence and mechanism of immune hemolysis

Reaction	Biochemical event
E + A → EA[a]	Reaction of erythrocyte and antierythrocyte antibody.
EA + C1 → EAC1q*	C1 attaches to antibody at a site on C1q and Fc portion of Ig antibody.
C1r → $\overline{C1r}$[b]	Bound C1q* converts C1r to active form by cleavage of C1r.
C1s → $\overline{C1s}$	$\overline{C1r}$ activates C1s by cleavage of C1s.
C4 → $\overline{C4a}$[c] + C4b*[d]	$\overline{C1s}$ cleaves C4 into $\overline{C4a}$ and C4b* and C2 into C2a* and
C2 → C2a* + $\overline{C2b}$	$\overline{C2b}$; plasmin acts on C2b to produce C2b kinin; $\overline{C4a}$ has weak anaphylatoxin activity.
C4b* + C2a* → $\overline{C4b2a}$	C4b* and C2a* combine to form C3 convertase.
C3 → $\overline{C3a}$ + C3b*	$\overline{C4b2a}$ cleaves C3 into $\overline{C3a}$ and C3b*; $\overline{C3a}$ (anaphylatoxin) causes smooth muscle contraction and degranulation of mast cells.
C3b* + C4b2a → $\overline{C4b2a3b}$	C3b* binds to activated bimolecular complex of $\overline{C4b2a}$ to form a trimolecular complex, C5 convertase, which is a specific enzyme for C5. Macrophages have receptors for C3b, so C3b acts as opsonin.
C5 → $\overline{C5a}$ + C5b*	C5 is cleaved into $\overline{C5a}$ and C5b* by C5 convertase; $\overline{C5a}$ has anaphylactic and strong chemotactic activity for polymorphonuclear neutrophils.
$\overline{C5b}$* + C6789 → $\overline{C5b.9}$	C5b* reacts with other complement components to produce cell membrane permeability. $\overline{C8}$ is most likely the active component, with $\overline{C9}$ increasing efficiency of $\overline{C8}$ and producing maximal cell lysis.

[a]E, erythrocyte; A, antibody to erythrocyte.
[b]$\overline{C1}$, $\overline{C4}$, etc: a line above the C number indicates the activated form of the component.
[c]C4a, C4b, etc: the lowercase letters indicate cleavage products of the parent complement molecule.
[d]C4b*, C2a*: the asterisk indicates a cleavage product that contains an active binding site for other complement components.

whereas C2b is converted by plasmin into a C2b kinin-like molecule believed to be responsible for the lesions of hereditary angioedema (see below). The complex of C4b2a on the cell surface forms an enzyme, C3 convertase, which binds and cleaves C3 into C3a and C3b. C3b binds to new sites on the cell surface. Since activated C1 can cleave many molecules of C4 and C2, and the C4b2a complex can cleave many molecules of C3, these serve as amplification steps. C3a is released into the fluid phase where it functions as anaphylatoxin. Phagocytic cells have receptors for C3b; C3b serves as an opsonin (enhances phagocytosis). In addition, C3b forms a trimolecular complex with C4b2a (C4b2a3b) that is able to cleave C5 into C5a and C5b (C5 convertase). C5a is released into the fluid phase, and C5b binds to the cell surface. C5a is a 15,000-molecular-weight polypeptide with the most potent chemotactic and anaphylatoxic activity of any chemical mediator. C4a and C3a do not have chemotactic activity. In tissues, C5a is rapidly broken down to C5a des-Arg by cleavage of the N-terminal arginine. C5 des-Arg is inactive as anaphylatoxin but retains potent chemotactic activity for neutrophils in the presence of whole serum. In addition, anaphylactic complement fragments induce the release of histamine from mast cells via receptors for C3a and C5a. C5a induces acute inflammation if activated in tissue by soluble antibody-antigen complexes (toxic complex reactions). C5b binds to the cell surface, where it reacts with the remaining complement components, C6 through C9, to produce a multimolecular complex that is capable of inserting itself into the cell membrane, forming a channel that permits release of the cytoplasm (lysis).

Alternate Pathway

The complement cascade may be activated by another set of proteins similar to C4, C2, C1, and C3; this is called the alternate pathway. A more detailed schematic representation of both the classical and alternate pathways of complement activation is shown in Fig. 3.10. The alternate pathway is activated by materials such as bacterial LPS (endotoxin), yeasts (zymosan), or IgA antibody. Three factors—initiating factor, factor B, and factor D—interact in a manner similar to that of the first three complement components of the classical pathway, producing a complex of activated B (Bb) and D that functions as a C3 convertase. A trimolecular complex of Bb, D, and C3b is then formed that is stabilized by the addition of another component, properdin. This complex functions as C5 convertase in activation of C5 and the remaining components of the membrane attack unit.

C3. C3 plays a central role in both the classical and alternate pathways of complement activation. Concealed within the C3 molecule are at least 10 binding sites for different kinds of interactions that underlie the biologic activities of C3. As the C3 molecule is processed by C3 convertase and then by I (inactivator) and its cofactors, sites appear and disappear. Some of these binding sites are to the cell membrane, to H factor, to properdin and conglutinin, as well as to complement receptors (see below), to C3d, and to the Epstein-Barr virus receptor on human B lymphocytes. Cleavage of C3 to form active fragments is illustrated in Fig. 3.11. Human C3 is a 195-kDa glycoprotein containing two polypeptide chains (α, 120,000 kDa; β, 75,000 kDa). The α chain contains an unstable thioester bond between a cysteinyl residue and a glutamic acid residue that provides a site for

Figure 3.10 Details of the classical and alternate pathways of complement activation. For description, see text.

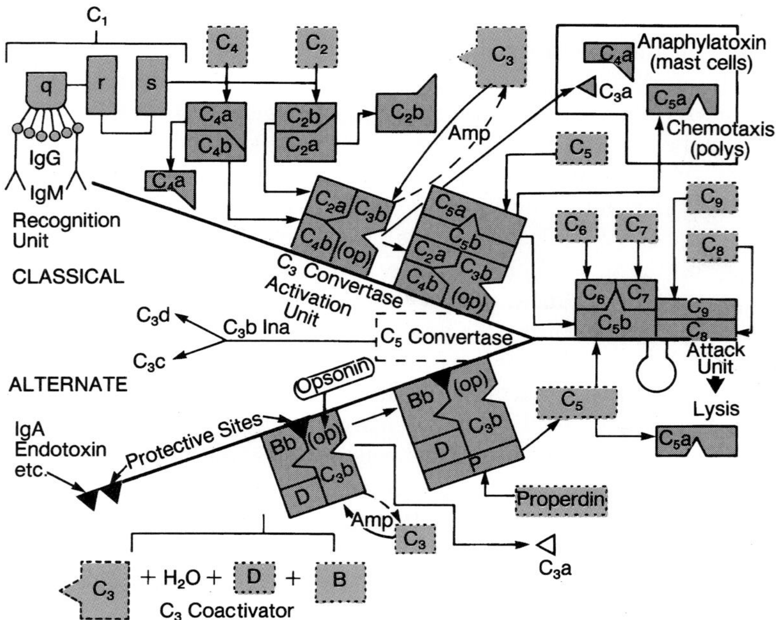

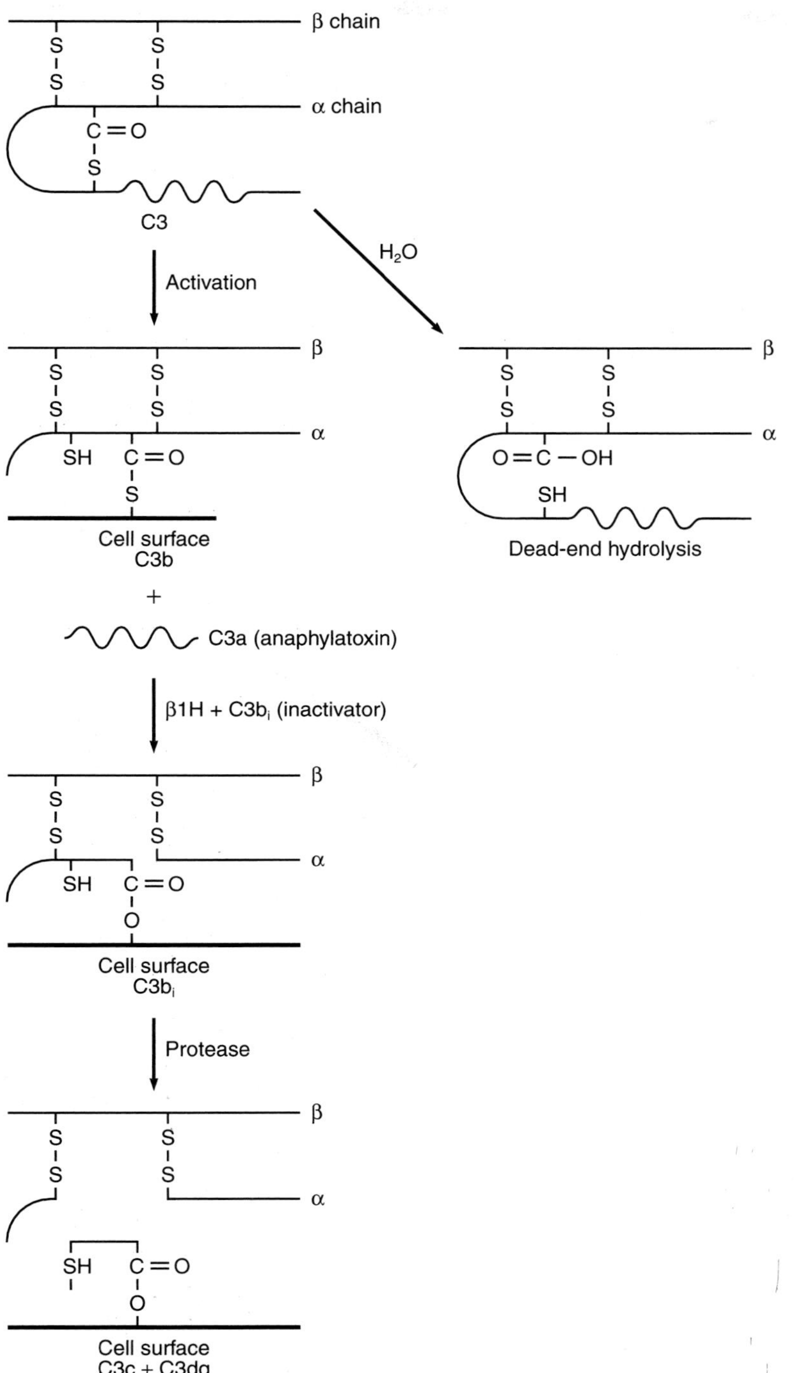

Figure 3.11 The binding and decay of C3.

covalent bonding reactions. Hydrolysis of the α-chain thioester bond causes "dead-end" inactivation. During activation, the first cleavage produces a small fragment, C3a, that has anaphylactic properties (see below). The larger fragment, C3b, has a molecular weight of 185,000 and undergoes a complex rearrangement of its tertiary structure that exposes the internal thioester bond in the α chain. This bond can be broken by aldehydes, carboxyl groups, nitrogen nucleophiles, or water, forming a new covalent bond. An ester bond between C3b and erythrocytes or bacteria is formed, whereas amide, as well as ester, bonds are formed with proteinaceous immune complexes. Since water is usually present in vast molar excess and can hydrolyze the thioester, most activated C3b does not bind to cell surfaces or immune complexes. Thus, the presence of water serves to neutralize the activated C3b and to concentrate the activity of the activated fragments to the protected sites on the cell membrane where complement activation was initiated.

C3 Receptors

There are four cellular receptors for the activated fragments of C3: CR1, CR2, CR3, and CR4. C3 receptors are instrumental in the localization of fragments of C3 that enhance phagocytosis of bacteria, yeasts, and other complement-coated particles (opsonize). Foreign organisms, such as bacteria, become coated with C3 upon reaction with antibody. Such coated bacteria will become attached to normal red blood cells because of receptors of red blood cells for the C3 fragments. This phenomenon is called immune adherence. All primate erythrocytes have such C3 receptors. C3 receptors are also found on lymphocytes, PMNs, monocytes, and podocytes of the renal glomerulus. The properties of some C3 receptors are given in Table 3.14.

Regulation and Amplification Mechanisms

Once activated, the inflammatory effects of the complement system need to be limited to the target of attack, or serious collateral tissue damage could result. Regulation of the complement system is accomplished by a set of inactivators. Complement activation occurs at low levels normally at all times and at high levels during inflammation. A number of inactivators of complement have been identified that act on different stages of complement activation (Table 3.15). Included are C1q inhibitor, C1 esterase inhibitor, the C3 esterase inhibitor system, a membrane activation complex inhibitor that competes with cell membrane sites for C5–C9, and serum carboxypeptidase N, which inactivates anaphylatoxin (C5a). A deficiency of the C1 esterase inhibitor is found in patients with hereditary angioedema (see also chapter 11). These patients exhibit massive acute tran-

Table 3.14 Complement receptors

Receptor	Ligand	Structure	Cell location	Function
CR1 (CD35)	C3b > C4b	Single chain; mol mass, 160–250 kDa	Monocytes, granulocytes, erythrocytes, lymphocytes	Cofactor for C3 inactivator, opsonization, immune adherence
CR2 (CD21)	C3 dg > C3d, Epstein-Barr virus, IFN-α	Single chain; mol mass, 140 kDa	Lymphocytes, epithelium, follicular dendritic cells (FDC)	B-cell activation, FDC activation
CR3 (CD11b/CD18)	iC3b, factor X, ICAM-1, fibronectin	Heterodimer (α and β); mol mass, 165 kDa (α), 95 kDa (β)	PMNs, monocytes, NK cells, FDC, PMNs	Opsonization, macrophage, activation, NK binding
CR4 (CD11c/CD18)	iC3b, fibronectin	Heterodimer; mol mass, 150 kDa (α), 95 kDa (β)	Monocytes, PMNs, lymphocytes, NK cells	Endothelial adhesion, causes margination of PMNs, binding of NK cells

Table 3.15 Major regulatory components of the complement system

Component	Function
C1q inhibitor	Inactivates C1q binding
C1 esterase inhibitor	Inactivates esterase activity
C3 convertase inhibitor system	Inactivates C3 convertase
Membrane activation complex inhibitor	Competes with cell surface C5–C9
Serum carboxypeptidase N	Inactivates anaphylatoxin

sient swelling of areas of the skin, the bronchi, or the gastrointestinal tract associated with depressed serum levels of C4 and C2 because of an inability to inactivate C1 esterase. This reaction results in the continued formation of C4 and C2 fragments, particularly C2b. C2b is converted by plasmin to a molecule with kininlike activity. The C2b kinin causes contraction of endothelial cells and edema. The reaction continues for approximately 24 h, which is essentially the biological life of C1 esterase in the absence of C1 esterase inhibitor.

C3 Convertase System (C3b/C4b)

C3 convertase plays a critical role in both the classical and alternate pathways of complement activation. The activity of C3 convertase is dependent upon the association of C4b and C2a in the classical pathway and C3b and Bb in the alternate pathway. C3 convertase activity is regulated by a number of regulators of complement activation (Table 3.16).

Regulators of Complement Activation

A family of proteins, termed regulators of complement activation, react with C3b or C4b and regulate their function. This family includes C2, which reacts with C4b during classical activation, and factor b, which reacts with C3b during alternate pathway activation, as well as at least six other proteins that regulate the activity of C4b/C2a and C3b/Bb (Table 3.16). The genes for these proteins are closely linked on the long arm of human chromosome 1, and each protein contains from 8 to more than 30 short homologous repeating units approximately 60 amino acids in length. The CR1, CR2, C4, Bb, and decay-activating factor (DAF) genes are very closely spaced and also show a high degree of homology, suggesting origin from a common ancestral gene.

Two proteins in the regulators of complement activation family, DAF and macrophage chemoattractant protein (MCP), protect cells from the action of C3b and C4b by inactivating these fragments on the surface of cells. DAF is a 70-kDa glycolipid protein anchored in cellular membranes. MCP is composed of two distinct but highly homologous proteins with molecular masses of 68 and 63 kDa. DAF and MCP are present on a wide variety of normal cells and provide protection from autologous tissue destruction by inactivating complement-mediated destruction. Another restriction factor, homologous restriction factor, is present on the surface of blood and endothelial cells and inhibits the terminal stage of the formation of membrane attack complexes by interfering with the binding of C8 to C5b67.

Factor H is an abundant plasma protein of 150 kDa that binds to C3b, preventing the formation of the alternate pathway convertase (C3bBb) and causing dissociation of the C3bBb complex. C4bp is a 550-kDa plasma

Table 3.16 Regulatory proteins of C3 convertase inhibitor system

Regulator	Binds to:	Properties	Function	Deficiency state
Factor I inactivator	C3b, C4b	Mol wt, 90,000; serine protease, endopeptidase	Inactivates C3b or C4b by cleavage of α chain; requires cofactors	Low C3, recurrent infections, angioedema
CR1	C3b/C4b	Mol wt, 160,000–250,000; cell membrane protein of neutrophils, macrophages, and erythrocytes	Promotes phagocytosis and degranulation; cofactor for C3b inactivator; increases decay of C4b2a and C3bBb (C3 convertases)	Hemolytic anemias, chronic granulomatous disease
CR2	C3d,g	Mol wt, 145,000; B-cell membrane	Membrane activator for B cells	Receptor for Epstein-Barr virus
Factor H	C3b	Mol wt, 150,000–160,000; serum glycoprotein	Cofactor for C3b inhibitor; binds C3b, increases decay of C3bBb in the alternate pathway	Low C3, recurrent infections, C3 detectable on erythrocytes
C4-binding protein	C4	Mol wt, 540,000–590,000; serum protein	Cofactor for C3b inhibitor; increases decay of C4b2a	
Decay-activating factor (DAF)	C3b, C4b	Mol wt, 70,000; cell membrane glycoprotein	Binds C3bBb or C4b2a; increases decay of C3 convertase of both classical and alternate pathways	Paroxysmal nocturnal hemoglobinuria (lysis of red blood cells)
JP45-70 (MCP)	C3b, C4b	Mol wt, 45,000–70,000; membrane protein	Inactivates C3 convertase (preferential for classical pathway)	

protein formed from seven identical 70-kDa subunits. It serves as a cofactor for the proteolytic digestion of C4b.

CR1 is a polymorphic 190- to 200-kDa receptor that primarily binds C3b and C4b. It is found mainly on mature blood cells. CR1 binds C3b4b complexes and processes them for clearance. Immune complexes in the circulation coated with C3bC4b bind to erythrocytes and are delivered to the reticuloendothelial system (E-IC clearance). The C3bC4 complexes are stripped from the cells and degraded.

CR2 is a 145-kDa receptor for the 40-kDa degradation fragment of C3b (C3dg) as well as for Epstein-Barr virus. CR2 is linked to surface IgM of mature B cells and plays an accessory role in the activation of B cells.

Role of Complement in Immune Reactions

Activation of complement components is an essential feature of cytotoxic and immune complex reactions and may play a role in initiating some cellular reactions. The fixation of complement to a cell surface by action of antibody or via the alternate pathway is responsible for cytolytic reactions. Opsonization is activated after coating by C3b (or C4b), and lysis of cells is activated by formation of the membrane attack complex C5–C9. The chemotactic effect of C5a attracts PMNs and is largely responsible for the participation of these cells in immune complex reactions. The anaphylatoxic effects of C3a and C5a cause separation of endothelial cells. This serves to open vascular barriers to inflammatory cells so that neutrophils, lymphocytes, and macrophages may emigrate from the blood and induce inflammation in tissues.

The Coagulation System

Any significant inflammation will result in activation of the coagulation system; several components of this system may serve as inflammatory mediators (Fig. 3.12). The coagulation system responds to various stimuli by the formation of platelet plugs and insoluble protein aggregates (fibrin) formed from soluble precursors. Fibrin forms clots that stop bleeding after injury to blood vessels. The fibrinolytic system is activated soon after clot formation in order to limit the extent of fibrin deposition and to initiate dissolution of fibrin so that circulation can be restored to injured tissues. Fibrin may also act as a scaffold for the ingrowth of fibroblasts and capillaries to initiate repair. If fibrin formed intravascularly is not cleared, multiple areas of tissue necrosis (infarcts) may occur. This is known as disseminated intravascular coagulation (see "Shwartzman Reaction" below). The kinin system increases vascular permeability in areas of inflammation and may be activated by intermediate products of the coagulation cascade.

The Shwartzman Reaction

The Shwartzman reaction is not an immune reaction but an alteration in factors affecting intravascular coagulation and reticuloendothelial clearance.

Figure 3.12 The coagulation system and inflammation. Roman numerals designate the major components of the coagulation system; a roman numeral followed by the letter "a" indicates an active fragment of that factor. Coagulation is a cascading sequence of enzyme-driven activations. Coagulation products active in inflammation are fragments of Hageman factor (XIIa), thrombin (IIa), and fibrin split products. The coagulation system consists of three major parts: the extrinsic system, the intrinsic system, and the common thrombin-fibrin pathway. The extrinsic system is activated by the action of tissue thromboplastin on factor VII. The intrinsic system involves activation of a series of components beginning with factor XII (Hageman factor). The common pathway is the activation of factors X and V on platelets with the subsequent formation of thrombin and fibrin. Kallikrein, activated factor XI, and plasmin can all act to cleave activated factor XII to produce fragments that initiate fibrinolysis and kinin release and generate a plasma factor that enhances vascular permeability. Activated factor XII converts prekallikrein to kallikrein (see "The Kinin System" in the text) so that activation of the intrinsic coagulation system also generates inflammatory mediators.

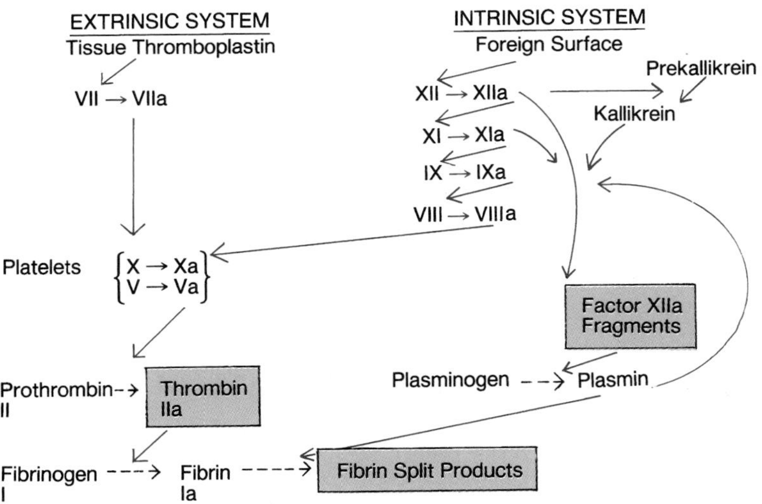

The local Shwartzman reaction. The local Shwartzman reaction is a lesion confined to a prepared tissue site (usually skin) and is a two-stage reaction (preparation and provocation). The tissue site is prepared by the local injection of an agent (gram-negative endotoxin) that causes accumulation of PMNs. The granulocytes condition the site by releasing lysosomal acid hydrolases that damage small vessels, setting up the site for reaction to a provoking agent. A relatively mild inflammatory reaction may serve as a preparative event. Provocation is accomplished by injection of agents into the prepared site that initiate intravascular coagulation (e.g., gram-negative endotoxins, antigen-antibody complexes, serum, starch). The lesion is caused by intravascular clotting with localization of platelets, granulocytes, and fibrin at the site of preparation, forming thrombi that lead to necrosis of vessel walls and hemorrhage. Although immune reactions may serve as either a preparatory or provocative event, nonimmune reactions are also effective.

The generalized Shwartzman reaction (disseminated intravascular coagulation). The classic generalized Shwartzman reaction is elicited by giving a young rabbit two intravascular injections of endotoxin 24 h apart (Fig. 3.13). The first injection serves as the preparative step; the second, the

Figure 3.13 Mechanism of the generalized Shwartzman reaction induced by endotoxin. The classic generalized Shwartzman reaction is elicited by giving rabbits two doses of endotoxin 24 h apart. The primary effect of the first (preparatory) dose of endotoxin is to cause release of platelet thromboplastin. Most of this thromboplastin is cleared by reticuloendothelial system (RES). Some thrombin triggers conversion of fibrinogen to fibrin, but again, most of this fibrin is cleared by the RES. If an animal is examined after one dose of endotoxin (preparative dose), a few fibrin thrombi are found in vessels of the liver, lungs, and spleen. These thrombi appear to be removed quickly by fibrinolysis, with no damage to the treated rabbit. However, because of the action of the RES in clearing thromboplastin and fibrin, blockade of the RES occurs. This blockade permits a second dose of endotoxin to produce severe intravascular coagulation. The second dose (provocative dose) initiates the same release of platelet thromboplastin as did the first dose, but with the RES blockaded, this thromboplastin is not cleared; most goes on to form thrombin and initiate conversion of fibrinogen to fibrin. This fibrin cannot be cleared by the blockaded RES, and most becomes lodged in capillaries, particularly capillaries of renal glomeruli. The fibrinolytic system may not be capable of overcoming large amounts of fibrin formed in a short period of time. The end result may be fatal renal cortical necrosis.

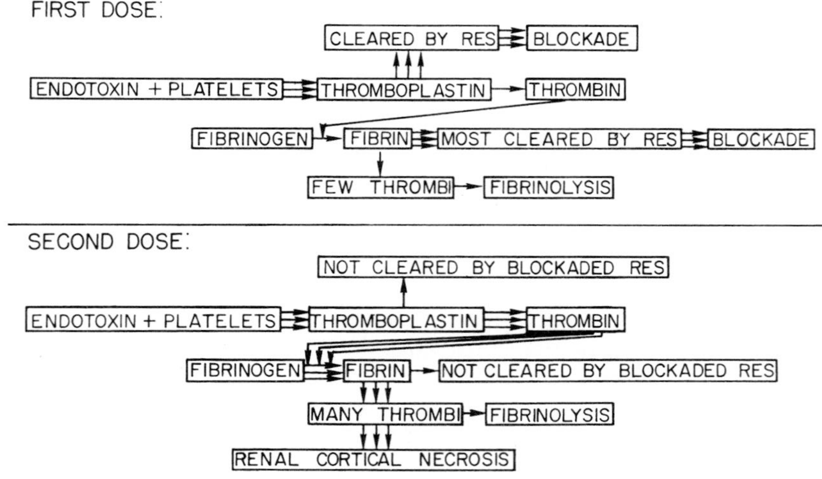

provocation step. After the first injection, a few fibrin thrombi are found in vessels of liver, lungs, kidney, and spleen capillaries. After the second injection, many more thrombi are found. Bilateral renal cortical necrosis and splenic hemorrhage and necrosis are prominent. The fibrin thrombi do not contain clumps of platelets or leukocytes. In human disease, the generalized Shwartzman reaction may develop as an acute and frequently fatal complication of an underlying disease, such as infection, and is known as disseminated intravascular coagulation. It is triggered by one or more episodes of intravascular clotting, leading to the formation of multiple fibrin or fibrinlike thrombi that lodge in small vessels. Such thrombi are prominent in the kidney or adrenal glands and cause necrosis and/or hemorrhage. Three steps appear to be necessary:

1. Intravascular clotting with fibrin formation.
2. Deposition of fibrin in small vessels. For this to happen, at least one and usually all of the following conditions must apply:

   depression of reticuloendothelial clearance of altered fibrinogen

   decrease in blood flow through affected organs

   liberation of enzymes by granulocytes, which help to precipitate fibrin

3. Once deposited, the fibrin is not removed by fibrinolysis.

Administration of agents that cause blockade of reticuloendothelial clearance (thorotrast, carbon, endotoxin, cortisone) serve as preparative agents, and agents that activate intravascular clotting (endotoxin, antigen-antibody complexes, synthetic acid polysaccharides) serve as provoking agents.

Septic shock. The release of cytokines by macrophages reacting with bacterial products produced during sepsis produces septic shock. The major bacterial factor is the LPS of the outer layer of gram-negative bacteria that is released upon lysis of the organism. This LPS is known as *endotoxin*. Other bacterial toxins, such as the peptidoglycan of gram-positive bacteria *(exotoxin)* may also cause shock. These toxins react with T cells and macrophages and activate the release of cytokines, mainly TNF, IL-1, IL-6, and IFN-γ. The cytokines, in turn, act on secondary cellular sites and produce fever or hypothermia, increased heart rate (tachycardia), increased breathing rate (tachypnea), and loss of blood pressure (shock). Endotoxin shock is produced in laboratory animals by injection of endotoxin from gram-negative organisms such as *Escherichia coli* and clinically in humans with infections with gram-negative organisms. Endotoxin shock is different from the Shwartzman reaction in the following ways: no preparative injection is necessary; shock can be induced in many species (the Shwartzman reaction occurs in only humans and rabbits); shock occurs with equal intensity at any age (young rabbits are much more sensitive to the Shwartzman reaction than old rabbits); thrombi are not prominent in endotoxin shock, which features hemorrhage and necrosis; and cortisone enhances the Shwartzman reaction but does not affect endotoxin shock. The reaction of exotoxins (superantigens) with T cells and macrophages to produce toxic shock syndrome is covered in chapter 5.

The Shwartzman reaction and pregnancy. A single injection of endotoxin in pregnant rabbits produces a generalized Shwartzman reaction. Bilateral renal cortical necrosis has been reported in septicemia following induced abortion in humans. Bilateral renal cortical necrosis in this circumstance represents a human equivalent of the generalized Shwartzman reaction due to endotoxemia during pregnancy. Pregnancy serves as the preparative step, because fibrinolytic activity and reticuloendothelial clearance are decreased during pregnancy. The occurrence of septicemia due to gram-negative organisms during delivery or abortion serves as the provocative step, leading to hypotension and intravascular clotting. In addition, intravascular dissemination of amniotic fluid during delivery may activate fibrin formation. This may be followed by thrombocytopenia and hemorrhage or a typical generalized Shwartzman reaction with bilateral renal cortical necrosis. Fibrin deposition occurs within glomerular capillary loops within 48 h of provocation. Hemorrhagic necrosis of the adrenal glands and/or renal cortical necrosis may occur 60 h to 40 days later. However, most episodes of pregnancy-associated Shwartzman reaction do not progress to fatal renal cortical necrosis.

The Kinin System

Peptides that are active as mediators of inflammation may be generated from a number of cells and tissue products. Of these, the most active is the kinin system. The components of this system are generated by the cleavage of plasma proteins into active peptides by proteolytic enzymes of the kallikrein system or by trypsin. Kallikreins are small proteolytic enzymes found in tissues (particularly glandular organs) and in plasma that act on larger molecules such as kininogens to produce active peptides. Kallikreins are activated from prekallikreins by the action of activated factor XII (Hageman factor) of the intrinsic coagulation system. Prekallikrein in plasma exists as a single polypeptide chain with an intrachain disulfide bond. There is also a tissue form that is slightly different. Activated factor XII (XIIa) cleaves polypeptide chain to form an active two-chain disulfide-linked kallikrein molecule.

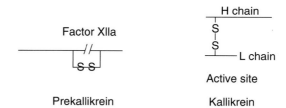

Kallikrein, factor XIIa, factor XI, or trypsin cleaves high-molecular-weight kininogen to liberate vasoactive peptides. Kallikrein in turn acts on kininogens to produce biologically active fragments (Fig. 3.14). The active peptides are kallidin and bradykinin. Kallidin is a decapeptide, and bradykinin is a nanopeptide formed by cleavage of the N-terminal lysine from kallidin. These mediators, particularly bradykinin, are highly active in stimulating vasodilation and increased vascular permeability but are rapidly catabolized by kininases into inactive peptides.

Acute-Phase Reactants

Acute-phase reactants are a heterogeneous group of serum proteins that have in common a rapid increase in concentration in the serum after acute

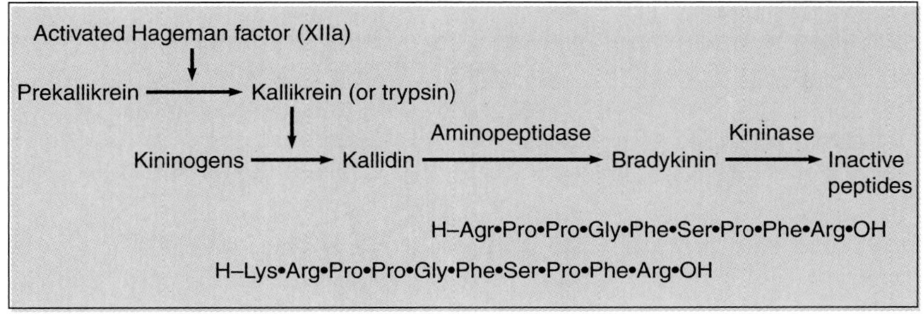

Figure 3.14 The kinin system.

tissue injury. They have varied functions in inflammation but in general serve either to increase or to limit the damage caused by inflammatory mediators such as IL-1, TNF, IFN-γ, and IFN-β2. The role of these cytokines in chronic inflammation is discussed in more detail below, but one of their actions is to stimulate production of acute-phase reactants by the liver. The major stimulators of acute-phase proteins are IL-1, IL-6, TNF-α and IFN-β2. In fact, IFN-β2 has been shown to be identical to hepatocyte-stimulating factor, which stimulates liver cell release of acute-phase reactants as well as proliferation of liver and other cells. The functions of some acute-phase proteins are listed in Table 3.17.

CRP

C-reactive protein (CRP) is the most widely used indicator of an acute-phase response in humans for the early indication of infection, inflammation, or other disease associated with tissue injury. Normally, the serum concentration of CRP is 0.1 mg/dl or less. After injury, rapid production in the liver results in concentrations as high as 100 mg/dl. CRP is synthesized only in the liver, and synthesis is stimulated by IL-6 and IL-1. CRP is composed of five identical subunits forming a unique ring-shaped molecule known as a pentraxin. A pentraxin is made up of five monomers covalently joined to form a pentamer with cyclic pentameric symmetry. Serum amyloid P component is also a pentraxin but does not increase in serum after injury. CRP got its name because it was first identified in the serum of patients with pneumonia when it precipitated with the C polysaccharide on the pneumococcal cell wall. CRP can activate both the classical and alternate pathways of complement when it binds to its ligand, the C carbohydrate of *Streptococcus pneumoniae,* and it is protective against *S. pneumoniae* infections. Cleavage of CRP by enzymes from neutrophils produces fragments that promote chemotaxis and contain the tetrapeptide Thr-Lys-Pro-Arg, known as tufsin, which is also present in the CH_2 domain of the immunoglobulin heavy chain. Thus, the biological effects of CRP are like those of immunoglobulins, including the ability to precipitate, to function as a primitive opsonin through binding to macrophages, and to fix complement. It also reacts with low affinity to other immune and inflammatory effector cells, but its immunomodifying effects are controversial.

SAA

Serum amyloid A protein (SAA) and CRP are the major human acute-phase proteins. In its denatured form, SAA is related to the amyloid A

Table 3.17 Functions of some acute-phase proteins of humans[a]

Class of function	Protein	Specific function
Mediators	C-reactive protein	Ligand binding, complement activation
	Complement components:	
	C2, C3, C4, C5, C9, Factor B	Opsonization, mast cell degranulation
	Coagulation factors	
	Factor VIII	Clotting
	Fibrinogen	Formation of fibrin matrix for repair
Inhibitors	C1 inactivator	Control of mediator pathways
	α_1-Antitrypsin	Elastase, collagenase inhibitor
	α_1-Antichymotrypsin	Cathepsin G inhibitor
	α_2-Macroglobulin	Proteinase inhibitor
Scavengers	C-reactive protein	Ligand binding (clearance of toxins)
	Serum amyloid A protein	Cholesterol binding?
	Haptoglobin	Hemoglobin binding
	Ceruloplasmin	$[O_2^-]$ inactivation
Immune regulation	C-reactive protein	Interaction with T and B cells
	α_1-Acid glycoprotein	T-cell inhibitor
Repair and resolution	C-reactive protein	Opsonization, chemotaxis
	α_1-Antitrypsin	
	α_1-Antichymotrypsin	Bound to surface of new elastic fibers
	C1 inactivator	
	α_1-Acid glycoprotein	Promotes fibroblast growth, interacts with collagen

[a]From J. T. Whicher and P. A. Dieppe, *Clin. Immunol. Allergy* **5**:425, 1985.

protein found in the tissues of patients with secondary amyloidosis. There are at least three closely related proteins in the SAA family, SAA1, SAA2, and SAA3. The function of SAA in inflammation is not clear.

α1-Proteinase Inhibitor

α_1-Proteinase inhibitor, also known as α_1-antitrypsin, inhibits the activity of proteases. It limits the effect of neutrophil-derived proteases, thus preventing systemic effects of these enzymes, and also limits the damage at the site of inflammation, so that repair can be initiated. α_1-Proteinase inhibitor is produced not only in the liver but also in macrophages. It is a single-chain glycosylated polypeptide of 394 amino acids.

α_1-Acid Glycoprotein

α_1-Acid glycoprotein, also known as orosomucoid, is a heterogeneous protein with at least seven polymorphic forms that have up to 40% carbohydrate. Its serum concentration increases up to fivefold within 24 h after acute injury. Its function is not clear.

Fibrinogen

Not only is fibrinogen a central player in coagulation, but also the fibrinopeptides produced during clotting are chemotactic for neutrophils (see below).

α_2-Macroglobulin

α_2-Macroglobulin inhibits the proteolytic activity of a wide variety of proteinases, including all classes of endopeptidases, serine, cysteinyl, aspartyl, and metallo. Most α-macroglobulins are tetramers formed from paired

180-kDa subunits. Because of its high molecular weight (720 kDa), α_2-macroglobulin does not normally pass from the blood into other tissues. Thus, it is believed to function as an acceptor of proteinases released into the blood and to prevent systemic effects of proteinase release. Although much more prominent in rats than in humans, α_2-macroglobulin was once suspected to be defective in patients with cystic fibrosis; however, this idea is not supported by clinical data.

Complement

In humans, the serum concentration of C3, the highest of any complement component, more than doubles during the acute-phase response (normal concentration is 150 to 300 mg/dl).

Adult Respiratory Distress Syndrome

An example of the inflammatory system out of control is the adult respiratory distress syndrome (ARDS). ARDS is a disorder in the regulation of acute inflammation and is manifested by diffuse damage to the alveolar epithelium and capillary endothelium of the lung (alveolar wall). This causes increased capillary permeability, interstitial and intra-alveolar edema, fibrin exudation, and hyaline membrane formation. ARDS is an all too frequent cause of death of patients with diffuse respiratory infections, burns, oxygen toxicity, narcotic overdose, and open cardiac surgery.

The etiology of ARDS is not well defined but is thought to be due to shock, oxygen toxicity, complement activation, bacterial products, or a combination of these. In oxygen toxicity associated with artificial assisted respirators, free radicals injure both endothelium and epithelium, causing increased permeability and alveolar edema. Complement activation generates C5a, which causes leukocyte aggregation and activation in the lung. Eosinophils have been shown to release cationic proteins, which also injure endothelial cells and alveolar type II pneumocytes. Alveolar cell injury leads to loss of surfactant and collapse of air spaces. Surfactant is a complex mixture of lipids, proteins, and carbohydrates that lowers alveolar surface tension and greatly reduces the work of breathing. A deficiency in surfactant is responsible for neonatal respiratory distress syndrome. Surfactant is produced by type II alveolar epithelial cells that are sensitive to various toxic agents. A loss of surfactant is believed to play a major role in both neonatal and adult respiratory distress syndromes. The role of the various acute inflammatory mechanisms in ARDS is not clear at this time but most likely involves multiple mediators and may be potentiated by a failure of inactivation mechanisms.

Interrelationships of Inflammatory Cells and Protein Systems in Acute Inflammation

A composite of inflammatory mechanisms and interrelationships is illustrated in Fig. 3.15. The complement, kinin, coagulation, and mast cell systems as well as bacterial products contribute to vasodilation, increased vascular permeability, and chemotaxis of the primary cellular mediator of acute inflammation, the neutrophil. The neutrophil and its lysosomal enzymes are responsible for killing microorganisms on the one hand and

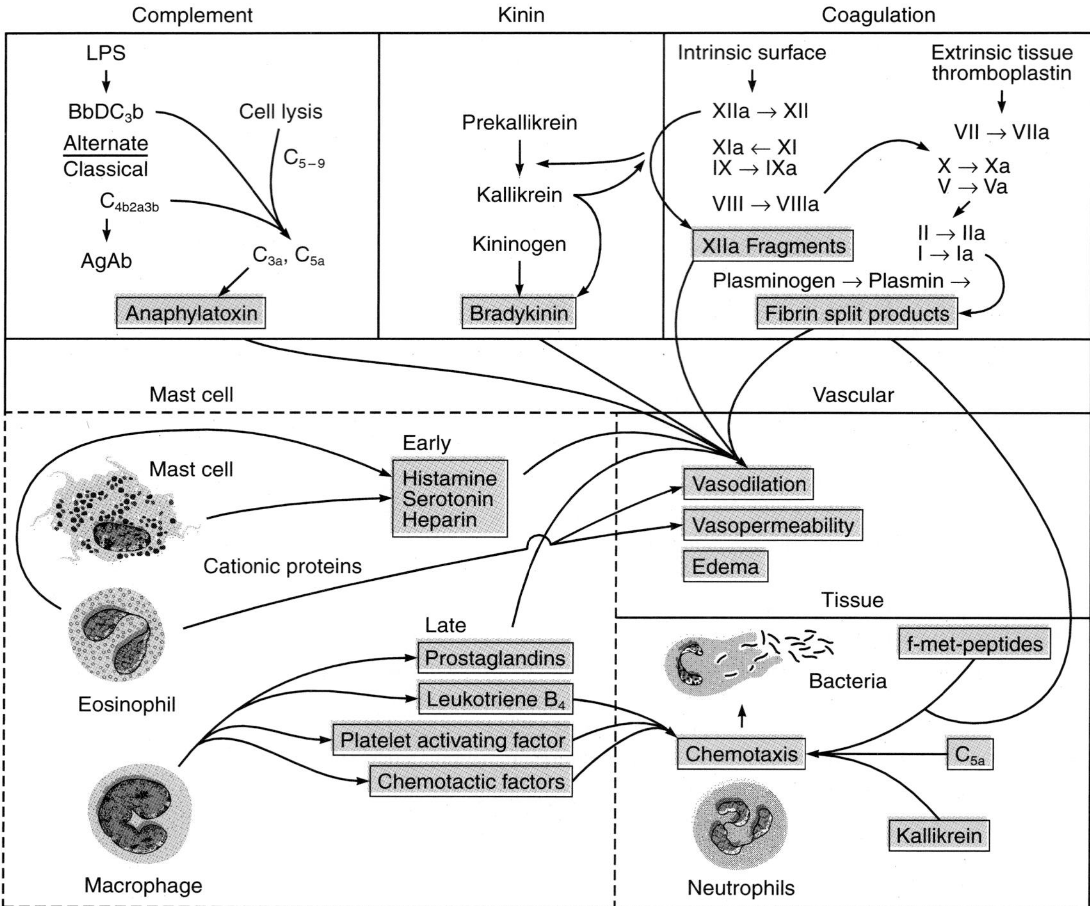

Figure 3.15 Interrelationships of inflammatory cells and systems in acute inflammation. Products of the complement, kinin, coagulation, and mast cell systems produce vasoactive and chemotactic mediators of acute inflammation. The major mediators are highlighted by boxes.

causing tissue necrosis on the other. The anaphylactic peptides C3a and C5a are the major inflammatory mediators derived from complement. Cells destroyed by the activation of complement may contribute indirectly through the release of intracellular contents that may cause further tissue destruction (enzymes) or activate the extrinsic coagulation system. Activation of the intrinsic coagulation system produces a series of active fragments. Activated factor XII (Hageman factor) contributes to generation of three inflammatory mediators, bradykinin, Hageman factor fragments, and fibrin split products. Mast cells contribute directly by release of mediators such as histamine and serotonin and indirectly by providing arachidonic acid precursors for generation of leukotrienes, prostaglandins, and other factors. These systems act to increase blood flow and vascular permeability, which leads to edema as well as attracting PMNs and eosinophils to sites of inflammation. Neutrophils destroy infecting organisms by phagocytosis and digestion but also release lysosomal enzymes that may produce tissue damage. Eosinophils are believed to modulate inflammatory reactions by deactivating mast cell mediators.

Chronic Inflammation

Chronic inflammation follows acute inflammation if the acute response is not adequate to clear the tissue. The function of chronic inflammation is to clear the tissue of necrotic debris produced by acute necrosis, provide more powerful defensive weapons against persistent infections, and complete the process of wound healing. If the tissue can be cleared with little or no damage, the structure will be returned to normal *(resolution)*; if some of the normal tissue architecture is destroyed, it may be necessary to fill in the zones of destruction with connective tissue *(scarring)*.

The Cells of Chronic Inflammation

The cells of chronic inflammation are lymphocytes, macrophages, and plasma cells. To contrast these to the PMNs that are the hallmark of acute inflammation, the cells of chronic inflammation are collectively termed mononuclear cells. Plasma cells are present in many forms of chronic inflammation and represent antibody-producing cells that migrate from lymph nodes to inflammatory sites.

Lymphocytes

Lymphocytes are prominent in chronic inflammation and are the immune specific effector cells of T-cell cytotoxicity ($CD8^+$ T_{CTL}) and of delayed-type hypersensitivity ($CD4^+$ T_{DTH}). The immune-specific effects of T_{CTL} and T_{DTH} lymphocytes in cell-mediated immunity are presented in detail in chapters 12 and 13. In nonimmune chronic inflammation, cytokines produced during acute inflammation and adhesion molecules (see below) attract and activate lymphocytes. Lymphocytes respond to specific signals and generally do not respond chemotactically to factors that attract other white blood cells. In addition to the interleukins that act on other cells during induction of immunity (see chapter 5), activated lymphocytes secrete a number of biologically active inflammatory mediators. These were originally named through identification of a functional activity found in the supernatants of cultures of activated T cells (Table 3.18). The major inflammatory function of these mediators (lymphokines) appears to be the attraction and activation of macrophages (especially by IFN-γ), but they also have other functions such as increasing vascular permeability, killing target cells, and controlling lymphocyte proliferation.

Lymphocyte-Endothelial Cell Interactions

Lymphocytes involved in chronic inflammation go through a process similar to that of neutrophils in acute inflammation, by binding to endothelial cells and emigrating across the endothelial lining to enter tissue. A schematic drawing of the sequence of events leading to lymphocyte adhesion and emigration during chronic inflammation is presented in Fig. 3.16. As a result of the interaction of lymphocytes with endothelial cells, endothelial cells may be able to present antigens to circulating memory T cells during their interaction, and endothelial cells may be injured during the process of adherence.

After arriving at sites of inflammation, lymphocytes may exert direct attacks on target cells or organisms (T_{CTL} or NK cells) or, more critical for the process of chronic inflammation, they are activated (see chapter 5) to release cytokines that attract and activate macrophages. The mechanisms

Table 3.18 Classic inflammatory lymphokines

Factor	Mol wt	Produced by	Effect
Migration inhibitory factor	15,000–70,000	Activated T_{DTH} cells	Inhibits migration of macrophages
Macrophage-activating factor (IFN-γ)	35,000–55,000	Activated T_{DTH} cells	Increases lysosomes in macrophages; increases phagocytic activity
Macrophage chemotactic factor	12,500	Activated T_{DTH} cells, lysates of PMNs, Ag-Ab complexes (complement)	Attracts macrophages; gradient chemotaxis
Lymphotoxin (cachexin)	Multiple (10,000–200,000)	Activated T-killer or NK cells	Causes lysis of target cells
Lymphocyte-stimulating factor	85,000	Activated T_{DTH} cells	Stimulates proliferation of lymphocytes
Proliferation inhibitory factor	70,000	Activated T_{DTH} cells	Inhibits proliferation of lymphocytes
Aggregation factor		Activated T_{DTH} cells	Causes lymphocytes and macrophages to adhere together
Interferon	20,000–25,000	Activated T_{DTH} cells	Inhibits growth of viruses; activates NK cells
Lymphocyte-permeability factor	12,000	Lymph node cells	Increases vascular permeability
Transfer factor	10,000	Activated T_{DTH} cells	Induces antigen-specific delayed-type hypersensitivity after passive transfer
Skin reactive factor	10,000	Activated T_{DTH} cells	Induces inflammation upon injection into skin
Cytophilic antibody	160,000	Plasma cells	Binds to macrophages; stimulates phagocytosis of specific antigen
Leukocyte inhibitory factor	68,000	Activated T cells	Inhibits neutrophil mobility
Osteoclast-activating factor	17,000	T and B cells	Stimulates osteoclasts to absorb bone

and effects of lymphocytes in immune-mediated inflammation are presented in more detail in part II of this book.

Macrophages

Macrophages play the leading roles in chronic inflammation in general and in delayed-type hypersensitivity reactions in particular. Macrophages usually infiltrate sites of inflammation several hours after lymphocytes do. The main function of macrophages is to phagocytize damaged tissue com-

Figure 3.16 Adhesion and emigration cascade of lymphocytes during the early stages of chronic inflammation. The sequence includes four stages: (i) weak binding to endothelial cells through selectin molecules, (ii) an activation signal to upregulate integrin expression, (iii) strong integrin-mediated adhesion, and (iv) migration through the vessel wall. MIP-1β, a member of the intercrine family, increases the adhesiveness of the $\alpha_4\beta_1$-integrin VLA-4 on $CD8^+$ T_{CTL} cells to VCAM-1. HA, hyaluronate. (Modified from Y. Shimizu, W. Newman, Y. Tanaka, and S. Shaw, *Immunol. Today* **13:**106, 1992.)

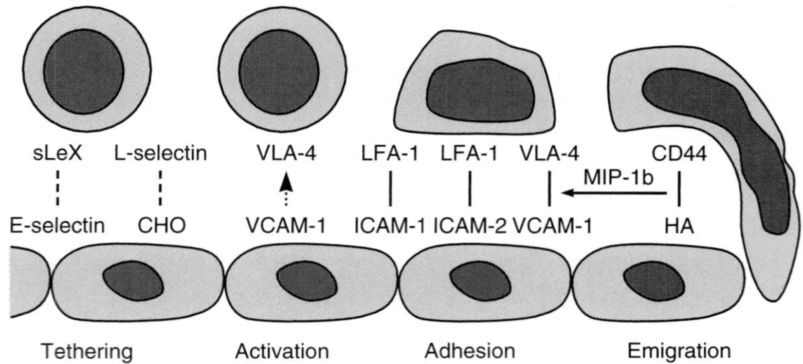

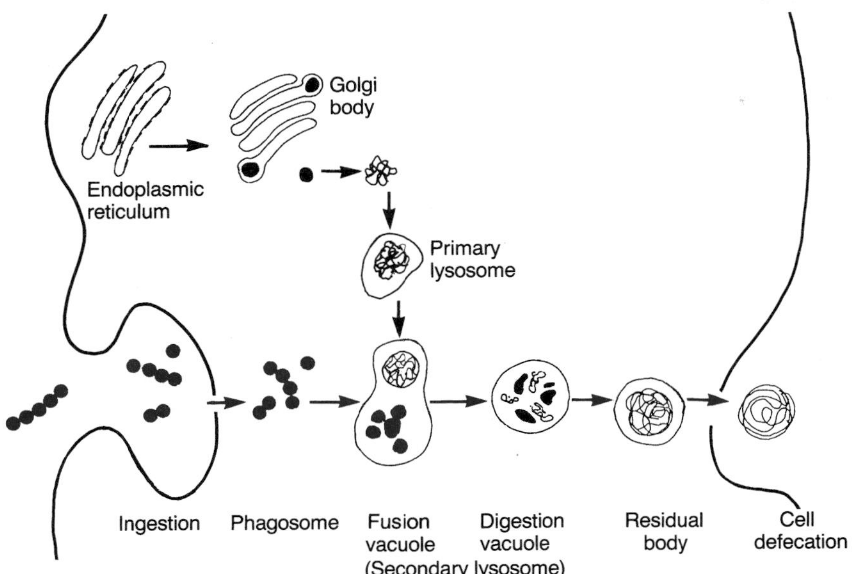

Figure 3.17 Phagocytosis. Foreign material is ingested into a phagosome. The phagosome fuses with a primary lysosome (formed by a Golgi body), which contains enzymes to digest ingested material. The resulting fusion vacuole is termed a secondary lysosome. When digestion is ended, some material may remain in the residual body or be eliminated from the cell by cell defecation. (Modified from C. de Duve, *Sci. Am.* **208:**64, 1963.)

ponents, microorganisms, or other cells (Fig. 3.17). Macrophages clear the tissue of the products of inflammation by the action of potent macrophage lysosomal enzymes and set the stage for resolution of the inflammatory process. In delayed-type hypersensitivity reactions, macrophages are attracted and activated by lymphokines produced by reaction of antigen with specifically sensitized lymphocytes (T_{DTH} cells) (see chapter 5). Activated macrophages also secrete cytokines (monokines) that are largely responsible for later events in wound healing (see below).

Phagocytosis

The stages of phagocytosis are illustrated in Fig. 3.18. Coating of bacteria by complement or antibody enhances phagocytosis, although phagocytosis certainly occurs in the absence of antibody and complement. Cell surface aggregation of receptors precedes pseudopod formation and invagination of the cell membrane. Engulfment and ingestion of material is accompanied by ion fluxes (positive ions entering cell) and superoxide formation. After formation of a phagocytic vacuole, fusion with enzyme-containing lysosomes (phagolysosomes) and digestion of phagocytosed material occurs. Macrophages have receptors for the aggregated Fc or Ig molecules and for complement fragments C3b and iC3b. Cross-linking of these receptors leads to signal transduction mediated by Syk tyrosine kinases and to mobilization of the actin cytoskeleton in intermediary steps that are still unclear.

Products of Macrophages

The products of macrophages that are important for consideration in inflammation are (i) the cytoplasmic constituents responsible for cellular metabolism and the degradation of phagocytosed material, (ii) the cell surface receptors that contribute to phagocytosis, and (iii) the secreted

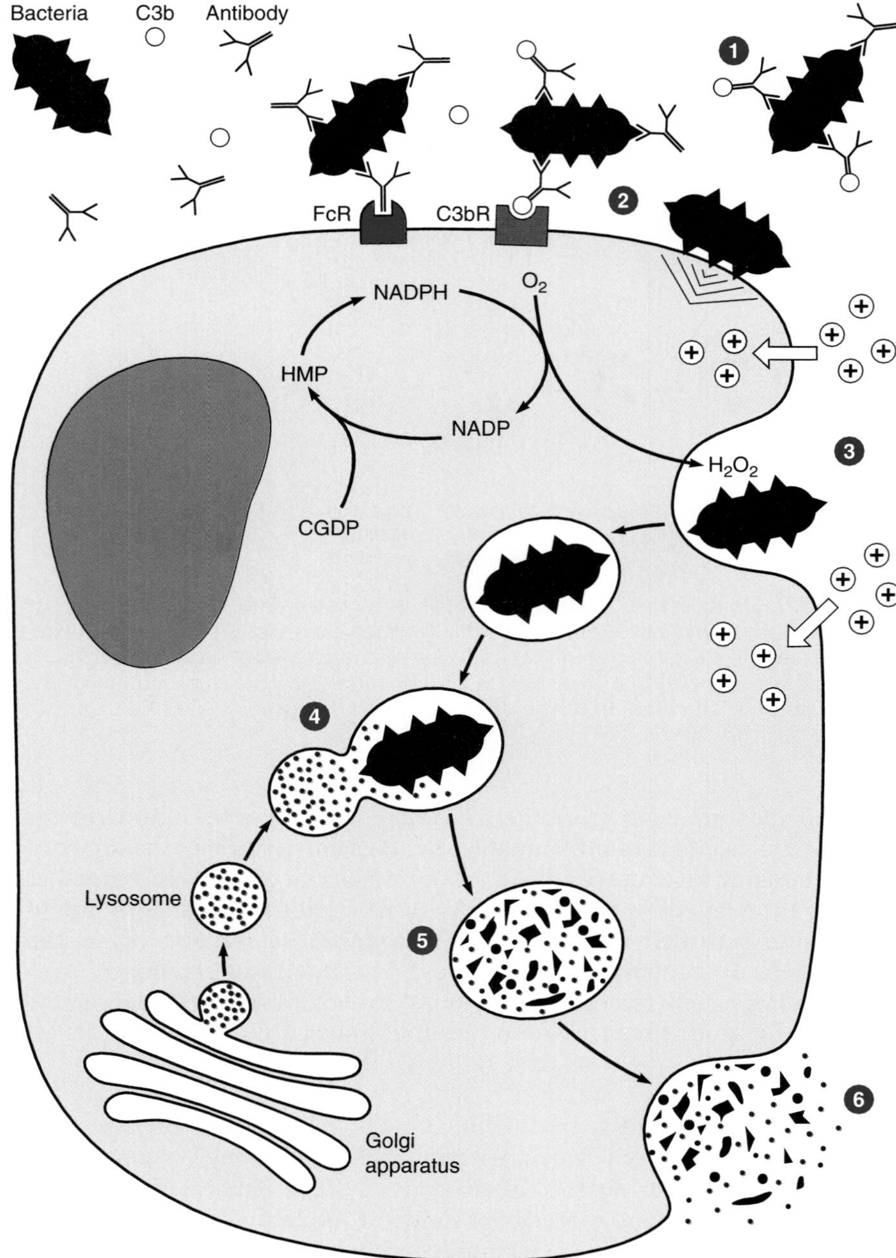

Figure 3.18 Schematic drawing of steps in phagocytosis. **(1)** Opsonization: aggregated Fc of antibody, activation of C3b. **(2)** Recognition through receptors and patching of receptors. **(3)** Ingestion: cation influx stimulates transduction of hexosemonophosphate shunt and conversion of O_2 to H_2O_2. **(4)** Fusion of lysosome and phagosome to form phagolysosome involving microtubules. **(5)** Digestion of bacteria in phagolysosome. **(6)** Exocytosis of remnants.

products (monokines) that may cause tissue damage or stimulate wound healing (Table 3.19). Depending on the nature of the inflammatory stimulus, the macrophage functions to clear necrotic tissue and to eradicate invading organisms, leading to resolution of the acute inflammatory re-

Table 3.19 Cellular, cell surface, and secreted products of macrophages

Type of product	Examples
Cellular enzymes	Peroxidase (RER), 5′ nucleotidase, aminopeptidase, alkaline phosphatase
Cell surface receptors	Fc receptor I (IgG2a), Fc receptor II (IgG2b), IgM, C3b, lymphokines, protein aggregates (nonspecific), fibronectin, high-density lipoprotein, lactoferrin, insulin, fibrinogen, asialoglycoprotein, fMet-Leu-Phe
Secreted biologically active products of macrophages	
Hydrolytic enzymes	Lysosomal hydrolases, neutral proteases, collagenase, plasminogen activator, elastase, lysozyme, arginase
Cell stimulatory proteins	Colony stimulating factor, interleukin-1, interferon, tumor necrosis factor, osteoclast activating factor
Others	Complement components (C2, C3, C4, C5, factor B), oxygen intermediates, α_2 macroglobulin, prostaglandins

sponse, or, if the organism persists, to initiate a chronic or prolonged defensive reaction, granulomatous inflammation (discussed in chapter 14).

Macrophages are attracted to sites of inflammation by a number of chemotactic factors that were originally named for their functional activity, such as migration inhibitory factor, lymphocyte-derived chemotactic factor, macrophage-activating factor, and macrophage stimulatory protein (Table 3.18). With further characterization, it is clear that the major chemoattractant and activator for macrophages is IFN-γ produced by activated $CD4^+$ T cells and NK cells. Mice deficient in IFN-γ rapidly succumb to infections with intracellular pathogens. Migration inhibitory factor (MIF), the first lymphokine shown to affect macrophage migration, has been cloned and is clearly different from IFN-γ. MIF is active in inhibiting macrophage migration in vitro. In vivo, MIF serves to hold activated macrophages in sites of inflammation, thus focusing their activity at the site of infection. In addition, macrophages are attracted by C5a, IL-8, and fMet peptides. Thus, macrophages are attracted to sites of acute inflammation both by products of immune-specific activation of lymphocytes and by products of nonimmune cells.

Activated Macrophages

Activated macrophages have an increased capacity for phagocytosis and an increased capacity to digest phagocytosed objects, and, in addition, they secrete factors (monokines) active in inflammation and immune reactions (Table 3.19). Activated macrophages have changes in lysosomal enzyme content: a decrease in 5′ nucleotidase and an increase in aminopeptidase and alkaline phosphatase as well as an increase in adenosine triphosphate and production of superoxide anion and hydrogen peroxide. There is also an increase in the activity of cell surface receptors on macrophages, in particular, for Fc of immunoglobulin and C3b.

An acquired cellular resistance to microbial infection may be observed in an infected host whose activated macrophages have an increased capacity for destroying infected organisms. Macrophage activation may occur by increasing the number of lysosomes per cell, by increasing the amount of hydrolytic enzymes in each lysosome, or by increasing the number of phagocytes available. Once such an increased capacity has been established, it is active against infections caused by unrelated organisms. A

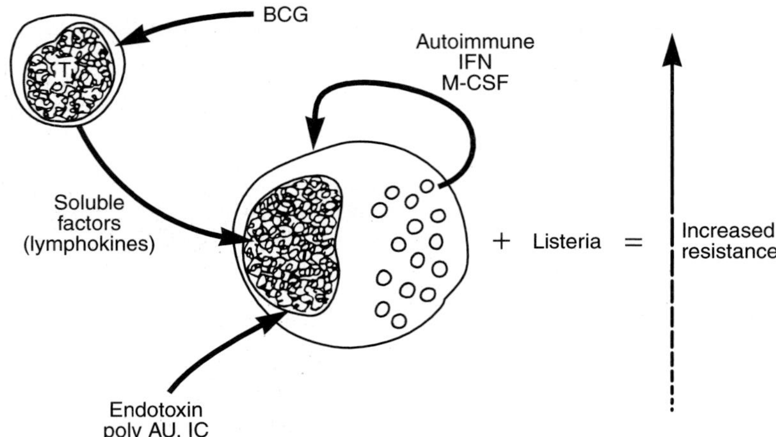

Figure 3.19 Nonspecific macrophage activation. Macrophages may acquire an increased capacity to destroy infective organisms or target cells after treatment with a variety of agents. BCG acts upon a T_{DTH} cell, which produces soluble factors that affect macrophages. Endotoxins and polynucleotides act directly on macrophages. The mechanism of action of these agents is not understood, but as a result of macrophage activation, a laboratory animal will resist a normally infectious challenge dose of an infectious agent.

number of agents have been found that cause activation of macrophages. These include bacillus Calmette-Guérin (*Mycobacterium bovis* BCG), *Listeria monocytogenes, Toxoplasma,* endotoxin, levamisole, and polynucleotides (Fig. 3.19). Activation may occur by release of macrophage-activating factors from lymphocytes or through an "autocrine" production of IFN-α/β, TNF, or monocyte/macrophage colony-stimulating factor (M-CSF). A considerable interest in the role of this phenomenon in enhancing tumor immunity has developed because of the possibility of limiting tumor growth with activated macrophages. This type of cellular immunity has been termed *immune phagocytosis,* even though this "immunity" is nonspecific.

Phagocytic Deficiencies

In some cases, because of either the nature or amount of the phagocytized material or because of an insufficiency in lysosomal hydrolases, ingested particles or organisms are not killed and digested. Some organisms *(Histoplasma capsulatum)* have the ability to survive phagocytosis and reproduce within phagocytes. Infection with such an agent may result in the presence of large numbers of viable organisms in the cytoplasm of phagocytic cells. Some inorganic particles (silica) cannot be digested, remain in phagocytic cells, and eventually cause destruction of the phagocyte (phagocytic suicide), tissue damage and fibrosis, and increased susceptibility to certain infections. Certain human diseases are characterized by abnormalities in phagocytosis (phagocytic dysfunction). Such phagocytic deficiencies are usually associated with susceptibility to infections. These diseases are presented in more detail in chapter 18. In addition, macrophages may not be able to clear tissues of some proteins that are produced in excess or abnormal proteins that are difficult to catabolize.

Accumulation of these proteins in tissues leads to a condition known as amyloidosis (see below).

Cytokines in Chronic Inflammation

The process of inflammation is mediated by a variety of proteins that are secreted by the cells involved and act on the cells involved. Cytokine is a term used for a large group of proteins that are produced by a variety of cells in the body and act to stimulate or inhibit the functions of the same cells that produce them (autocrine) or of other cell types (paracrine). Cytokines include hematopoietic growth factors, interferons, lymphokines, monokines, chemokines, and other cytokines (see appendix 4). Lymphokines are a subgroup of cytokines produced by lymphocytes; monokines are produced by macrophages. Interleukins are cytokines that are produced by white cells and act on other white cells. In general, cytokines have the following characteristics in common.

1. Low molecular weight
2. Secreted from cells, often glycosylated
3. Regulate immunity and inflammation
4. Produced transiently and act locally
5. React with high-affinity receptors on target cells
6. After reaction activate cytoplasmic tyrosine kinases through the stepwise formation of a receptor complex
7. Alter metabolism and behavior of the target cell through phosphorylation of cellular kinases
8. Have multiple and overlapping functions
9. Act in a network, either inducing or inhibiting the effect of other cytokines

The response of a cell to a cytokine depends on the local concentration of the cytokine, the simultaneous presence of other cytokines or regulators present, and the state of activation of the cell. The role of cytokines in the induction of immunity and in control of hematopoiesis is presented in chapters 2, 4, and 5. The cytokines interact in a network: one cytokine may have many actions (pleiotropy), and different cytokines may produce very similar effects (redundancy). The overlapping and varied effects of the cytokines may seem inefficient, but because there are different ways to accomplish the same thing, inflammation or other processes dependent on cytokine action may be effected successfully under many different circumstances. Thus, the cytokines provide a network of backup systems for vital functions. If one cytokine is deficient, another may accomplish the task. The major cytokines that are active in the chronic inflammatory response are IL-1, IFN-γ, TNF-β, transforming growth factor β (TGF-β), and IL-2 (Table 3.20).

IL-1

IL-1 consists of three structurally related molecules: IL-1α, IL-1β, and IL-1Ra (receptor agonist). The biologic activities of IL-1α and IL-1β overlap with those of TNF-α and IL-6. IL-1 is the epitome of a *pleotypic* cytokine with many different sources and actions. It is produced by macrophages, dendritic cells, T cells, B cells, and endothelial cells. IL-1 production is stimulated by a variety of activation signals. It was originally called lymphocyte activation factor because of its ability to stimulate

Table 3.20 Major cytokines involved in inflammation and wound healing

Name	Source(s)	Activities
IL-1	Activated macrophages, T and B cells, endothelial cells, dendritic cells, etc. (different forms)	Activates T and B cells; stimulates production of IL-2, IFN-γ, IL-3, IL-4, TGF-β, and acute-phase proteins; mobilizes PMNs, produces fever; induces adhesion molecules; stimulates hematopoiesis
IL-2	Activated T cells, B cells	Stimulates proliferation of T and B cells, production of IL-1 and IFN-γ, augments NK activity, and activates macrophages
IFN-γ	Activated T cells, large granular lymphocytes, and lymphokine-activated killer cells	Upgrades MHC class I and II expression; enhances T_{CTL}, NK and macrophage activity; margination of lymphocytes; increases TNF and IL-1 production
TGF-β	Platelets, macrophages, $CD4^+$ T cells	Stimulates wound healing; controls inflammation; inhibits IL-2, IL-4, IFN-γ, and TNF; inhibits B-cell proliferation
MIF	Activated T_{DTH} cells ($CD4^+$ T cells)	Attracts and holds macrophages in tissue
TNF-α (cachectin)	Activated macrophages, T_{DTH} cells, some T_{CTL} cells	Increases MHC class I and class II expression; activates macrophages; promotes angiogenesis; induces tumor necrosis, fever, cachexia
TNF-β (lymphotoxin)	T_{DTH} cells, NK cells, lymphokine-activated killer cells	Activates angiogenesis; increases oxygen radical production

proliferation of lymphocytes (T cells). IL-1 is critical not only for activation of T cells but also for B cells during induction of a specific immune response and as a cofactor for stimulation of proliferation of hematopoietic cells by CSFs. The precise effect of IL-1 in inflammation is not easily explained, since it has so many different direct and indirect functions. It stimulates production of other lymphokines, such as IL-2, IL-3, IL-4, IFN-γ, and TGF-β, as well as G-CSF and GM-CSF. It promotes generation of cytotoxic effector cells and synergizes with CSFs to increase production of inflammatory cells in the bone marrow. It induces fever, lethargy, and shock, stimulates the release of prostaglandins, and is found in high levels in the joint fluid of patients with rheumatoid arthritis. Thus, IL-1 affects different stages of induction of the specific immune response as well as acting at many stages of the process of inflammation and healing. Because of the wide powers of IL-1, having a way to turn off its activity is critical. Among the inhibitors of IL-1 are glucocorticoids, IL-4, IL-10, IL-13, TGF-β, and PGE_2. In general, these inhibitors act by downregulating the expression of IL-1 and upregulating the expression of IL-1Ra. IL-1Ra is the only natural competitive regulator for the action of a cytokine.

IL-2

IL-2 acts primarily during induction of immunity but also has effects in inflammation. It is produced mainly by activated T cells but also in smaller amounts by activated B cells. Its main action is as an autocrine or paracrine stimulator of proliferation of T or B cells. IL-2 also enhances the expression of other lymphokines by activated lymphocytes, especially IFN-γ and IL-1, and it synergizes with other interleukins to induce differentiation of B cells to become immunoglobulin-secreting cells. IL-2 augments NK cell activity and increases the cytotoxicity of macrophages. The major effect of IL-2 in inflammation appears to be indirect, through stimulation of production of IFN-γ and IL-1. IL-2 has been reported to have some beneficial effect on patients with solid tumor metastases, through increasing the cytotoxicity of NK cells or macrophages.

IFN-γ

IFN-γ (formerly, type II interferon) is a major mediator of inflammation. It is produced by activated T cells, large granular lymphocytes, and activated NK cells. It is the foremost attractor and activator of macrophages and plays a major role in delayed-type hypersensitivity reactions. (One of the earlier names for IFN-γ was macrophage activation factor.) IFN-γ upgrades expression of HLA class I markers on most cell types and class II markers on immune cells and vascular endothelium. The action of IFN-γ on endothelial cells may be critical in the attraction of inflammatory cells to vessel walls during inflammation (margination). It also markedly increases the expression of integrin receptors on endothelial cells. It directly enhances the cytotoxic effect of cytotoxic T cells and NK cells. IFN-γ also affects the expression of a number of other cytokines. It enhances the transcription of TNF and IL-1 but inhibits production of GM-CSF. It synergizes with other cytokines in a variety of different effects. IFN-γ has been used effectively in the treatment of leprosy and chronic granulomatous disease but is contraindicated in patients with rheumatoid arthritis, in whom it appears to increase inflammation.

MIF

MIF is the first lymphocyte-derived cytokine, defined by its ability to inhibit migration of macrophages in vitro. The gene for MIF has been cloned, and MIF is clearly different from IFN-γ, with which it shares biological effects. Although discovered in the supernatants of activated lymphocytes, MIF is present in high amounts in the granules of anterior pituitary cells and is released during stress. MIF induces TNF-α secretion by macrophages, and TNF-α in turn stimulates secretion of MIF. MIF potentiates the activation of macrophages by IFN-γ.

TGF-β1

TGF-β is named for the original function described for TGF-β, the ability to stimulate growth of some cultured cells in vitro, but actually TGF-β has much broader and more significant effects. TGF-β is a multifunctional cytokine playing an important role in embryonal development as well as in regulating repair and regeneration following tissue injury. In mammals, TGF-β exists in three closely related isoforms: β1, β2, and β3. TGF-β2 and -β3 are important in development as well as in inflammation, whereas TGF-β1 does not appear to have a developmental function. Platelets contain high concentrations of TGF-β1, and upon degranulation they release TGF-β1 at sites of tissue injury. In addition, TGF-β1 is produced by activated macrophages, T and B cells, fibroblasts, endothelial cells, osteoclasts and osteoblasts, astrocytes, and microglial cells. TGF-β1 is chemoattractive for white blood cells, induces angiogenesis, controls cytokine production, and causes increased deposition of extracellular matrix as well as decreased matrix degradation by lowering the synthesis of proteases and increasing the levels of protease inhibitors. Thus, TGF-β1 plays a key role as the "chief executive officer" of wound healing. However, like many CEOs, TGF-β1 sometimes has a vested interest in increasing its influence at the expense of the organization. In chronic progressive inflammatory diseases, TGF-β1 may act as an autocrine to increase its own production, autoactivating overproduction of extracellular matrix and producing scarring and fibrosis. This has been termed the "dark side" of tissue repair. Controlling TGF-β1 production may be the key to preventing scarring and fibrosis in diseases such as glomerulonephritis and progressive pulmonary fibrosis.

Table 3.21 Some members of the tumor necrosis family

Family member	Receptor	Function
TNF, LT-α	TNF-RI (p55)	Enhances inflammation, causes cell death (apoptosis)
TNF, LT-α	TNF-RII (p75)	Enhances inflammation
LT-α/β complex	LT-βR	Apoptosis, lymph node development
CD40 ligand	CD40R	Ig class switching costimulation of T cells
CD27 ligand	CD27	Costimulation of T cells
CD30 ligand	CD30R	Costimulation of T and B cells
CX40 ligand	CS40R	Costimulation of T cells
4-1BB ligand	4-1BB	Costimulation of T cells
Fas/Apo-1 ligands	FAS.ApoR	Apoptosis of autoreactive T cells, activation of NF-κB
TRAIL/Apo-2L	DR4	Apoptosis
Apo3 ligand	Apo3/DR3TRAMP	Apoptosis, activation of NF-κB
OCDF[a]	OPG	Regulation of bone mass

[a]OCDF, osteoclast differentiation factor; OPG, osteoprotegerin.

TNF

TNF-α, a product of activated macrophages, was discovered because of its ability to cause necrosis of tumors in laboratory animals after treatment with endotoxin (LPS) and was called *cachectin*. It is structurally related to another factor produced by activated T cells, TNF-β, also called *lymphotoxin* because of its ability to kill certain tumor target cells in vitro. Other effects, including costimulation of T cells, were also found for TNF-like proteins. These other effects (pleiotropy, again) are due to the fact that TNF actually is a family of proteins (e.g., TNF, lymphotoxin, CD40) that react with a family of related receptors (Table 3.21). The receptors have three to six cysteine-rich domains in the extracellular regions. Some (Fas/Apo1, TNF-RI, and DR4) contain a "death domain" in the cytosolic tail. Reaction of ligand with these receptors leads to cell death through activation of death domain proteins (Fas-associated death domain-containing protein [FADD/MORT] or TNF receptor-associated death 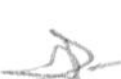 domain-containing protein [TRADD]), which results in processing of cytosolic caspases and apoptosis (see below). Other TNF receptors do not have the death domain, and reaction of their ligands may result in stimulation, such as enhancement of class I major histocompatibility complex (MHC) expression by fibroblasts and vascular endothelium, synergizing with IFN-γ to enhance class II MHC expression on many cell types, facilitation of macrophage activation and IL-1 release, and promotion of angiogenesis during wound healing (see below). In addition to producing hemorrhagic necrosis and/or apoptosis of tumors, TNF family members cause fever, hypotension, and profound weight loss (cachexia). TNF may produce dramatic regression of some tumors, but its effects are not consistent (depending on the immunocompetence of the patient) and are limited by severe systemic toxicity (see chapter 20).

Chemokines

Recently, a new cast of characters, called chemokines, have been shown to be active as chemoattractants and activators of a number of events in inflammation and wound healing, mostly through attraction and activation of macrophages but also by other effects on PMNs, angiogenesis, and fi-

Table 3.22 Some members of the chemokine family[a]

Chemokine	Cell source	Target cells	In vivo activity
CC family			
MCP-1	Many, not lymphocytes	Macrophages, T cells, basophils	Attracts monocytes, activates macrophages and Th2 cells, histamine release
MCP-2	Monocytes	T cells	Like MCP-1, blocks HIV-1 binding to CCR5
MCP-3	Monocytes, epithelial cells	Macrophage, T cells, eosinophils	Like MCP-1, also attracts eosinophils
MCP-4	Monocytes, epithelial cells	Monocytes, basophils, eosinophils	Activates monocytes, basophils, and eosinophils
MCP-5	Monocytes, smooth muscle cells	Monocytes, T cells, basophils	Like MCP-1
MIP-1α	T cells, monocytes, mast cells, fibroblasts	T cells	Enhances cell-mediated immunity
MIP-1β	T cells, monocytes, fibroblasts	T cells	Blocks HIV-1 uptake
RANTES	T cells, endothelial cells, platelets	Macrophages	Attracts macrophages
I-309	T cells, mast cells	T cells	Attracts T cells, induces tumor immunity
CXC family			
IL-8	Macrophages, lymphocytes	Neutrophils, T cells, endothelial cells	Mobilizes PMNs from bone marrow
	Fibroblasts, endothelial cells	NK cells, basophils, endothelial cells	Attracts PMNs and monocytes, angiogenesis
Gro (α, β, γ MSGA)	Macrophages, fibroblasts	PMNs, endothelial cells, fibroblasts	Attracts PMNs, fibroplasia, angiogenesis
NAP-2	Platelets, macrophages	PMNs, endothelial cells	Attracts PMNs, clot resorption
ENA-78	Keratinocytes, fibroblasts, macrophages, others	PMNs, endothelial cells	Attracts PMNs, angiogenesis, mobilizes PMNs
GCP-2	Osteosarcoma cells	PMNs, endothelial cells	Attracts PMNs
PF-4	Platelets	Endothelial cells, fibroblasts	Angiogenesis, fibrosis
IP-10	Macrophages, lymphocytes, fibroblasts, etc.	T cells, NK cells, monocytes, endothelial cells	Enhances immune response, angiostatic
MIG	Macrophages, hepatocytes	Endothelial cells, T cells	Angiostatic, attracts T cells
I-TAC	Astrocytes, macrophages, lymphocytes	T cells	Attracts T cells
SDF-1	Bone marrow stroma	T cells, B cells	Blocks HIV-1 binding, attracts lymphocytes,stimulates B-cell development in bone marrow
Lymphotactin	CD8 T cells, NK cells	T cells, dendritic cells, NK cells	Attracts lymphocytes
CX_3C			
Fractalkine (neurotactin)	Endothelial cells, microglia, macrophages	T cells, monocytes, PMNs	Attracts T cells, monocytes, and PMNs, causes inflammation in brain

[a]Abbreviations: MCP, macrophage chemoattractant protein; MIP, macrophage inflammatory protein; RANTES, regulated on activation, normal T-cell expressed and secreted; Gro, growth-related peptide; NAP, neutrophil-activating peptide; PF, platelet factor; ENA, epithelial-derived neutrophil attractant; GCP, granulocyte chemotactic protein; IP, IFN-γ-inducible protein; MIG, macrophage inflammatory globulin; TAC, T-cell attractant chemokine; SDF, stromal-derived factor.

brogenesis. At this writing, the chemokine family contains more than 50 members and is still growing. Four subgroups can be distinguished on the basis of conserved cysteine motifs: CC (β-chemokines), with two unseparated terminal cysteine residues; CXC (α-chemokines), with a nonconserved amino acid separating the two terminal cysteine residues; C (γ-chemokines), with only one terminal cysteine; and CX_3C (fractalkine or neurotactin) which has three amino acids between the amino terminal cysteines. More than 25 CC and 11 CXC chemokines have been identified (see Table 3.22 for some examples).

Table 3.23 Chemokine receptors

Receptor	Expressing cells	Reactive ligands[a]
CXCR1	Neutrophils (N), resting T cells (RT)	IL-8>GCP-2>NAP
CXCR2	N, RT	Gro, NAP-2, IL-8, ENA-78
CXCR3	Monocytes (M), activated T cells (AT)	IP-10, MIG, I-TAC
CXCR4	RT, M	SDF-1
CCR1	M, AT, eosinophils (E)	MIP-1α, RANTES, MCP-2, -3, -4
CCR2	M, AT, basophils (B)	MCP-1, -2, -3, -4, -5
CCR3	M, B, E	RANTES, eotaxin-1, -2, MCP-2, -3, -4, MIP-1α
CCR4	M, AT	TARC
CCR5	M, AT	MIP-1α, MIP-1β, RANTES
CCR6	AT	MIP-3α
CCR7	AT	ELC
CCR8	M, AT	I-309

[a]For characteristics of chemokines and definitions of abbreviations, see Table 3.22.

These chemokines have high affinity for transmembrane G-protein-coupled receptors and activate signal transduction through binding their receptors and activating the phospholipase C and Ras pathways (see T-cell activation pathways in chapter 5). Four receptors have been identified for the α family (CXCR1 through CXCR4) and eight for the β-chemokine family (CCR1 through CCR8). The various chemokines preferentially react with one or more of these receptors (Table 3.23). Other proinflammatory chemoattractants, such as PAF, leukotriene B_4, C5a, and fMet-Leu-Phe, also react with these receptors. The receptors consist of an extracellular N terminus, seven hydrophilic transmembrane domains with three extracellular and three intracellular loops, and an intracellular terminus rich in serine and threonine residues. The G protein is coupled to one of the intracellular loops.

Increased levels of chemokines have been found in a number of chronic inflammatory reactions, including a variety of human diseases, such as atherosclerosis, acute respiratory distress syndrome, and glomerulonephritis. In contrast to other proinflammatory cytokines, such as IL-1 and TNF, chemokines do not stimulate production of other cytokines or acute-phase reactants but do induce other effector molecules, such as histamine and defensins. Chemokines attract T cells and monocytes but, with the exception of reactions with CXCR1 and CXCR2, not neutrophils. A subgroup of chemokines appear to be active in allergic reactions by attracting basophils and activating histamine release (eotaxin-1, MCP-4, and, to a lesser extent, RANTES, MCP-2, MCP-3, and MIP-1α). Some chemokines also inhibit generation of new blood cells in the bone marrow (MIP-1α, IL-10, platelet factor 4, IL-8, MCP-1, MRP-1, and MPR-2), whereas eotaxin-1 and IL-8 enhance early hematopoiesis.

Some infectious agents also react with these receptors and use them for binding and entry into the cells they will infect (Fig. 3.20). For example, *Plasmodium vivax* (malaria) binds to the Duffy red cell antigen, which is also a receptor for many CC and CXC chemokines. Monotrophic human immunodeficiency virus type 1 (HIV-1) binds to CCR5; lymphotrophic HIV-1 binds to CXCR4; cytomegalovirus binds to a CCR-like receptor; human herpesvirus 8 (which causes Kaposi's sarcoma) binds to CCR1, -3 and -5. Since

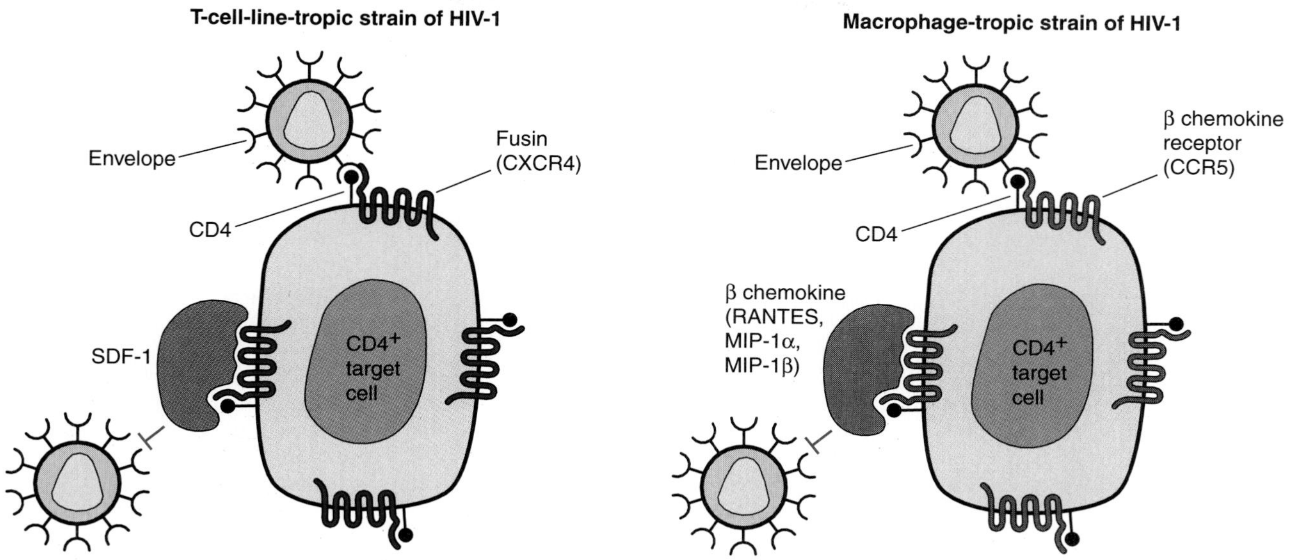

T-cell-line-tropic strain of HIV-1

Macrophage-tropic strain of HIV-1

Figure 3.20 Models of coreceptor (CCR5 and CXCR4) usage and inhibition of HIV binding by coreceptor ligands. Entry of M-tropic strains of HIV is blocked by CCR5 ligands MIP-1α, MIP-1β, and RANTES. Entry of T-tropic strains is blocked by the CXCR4 ligand SDF-1. (From A. S. Fauci, *Nature* **384:**529, 1996.)

this area of investigation is still new, it is likely that receptors for other viruses will be found in the chemokine families.

Apoptosis

The term apoptosis ("dropping out") is applied to the process of cell death that occurs during normal tissue development and renewal, so-called programmed cell death. This same process has been adapted for use by the immune system to eliminate cells, not only as part of a defense against infected or cancerous cells but also as a way of limiting proliferation of immune cells after induction of an immune response. Apoptosis is a form of cell suicide activated by metabolic alterations in the cell, DNA damage (such as by irradiation), withdrawal of growth factors, or specific interaction of ligands, such as TNF or FasL, with "death receptors" on the cell. Apoptosis employs an internally encoded death sequence involving activation of endogenous proteases known as caspases (Fig. 3.21). The activated caspases disrupt the integrity of the cytoskeleton, and the cell shrinks up, the nuclear DNA becomes fragmented, and the dying cell is usually phagocytosed by another cell without an inflammatory reaction. Apoptosis can be contrasted to necrotic or traumatic cell death, such as complement-mediated lysis, by which the cells swell up and membrane integrity is lost, resulting in leakage of cytoplasm and inflammation.

Death Receptors

Apoptosis through death receptors may be mediated by members of the TNF family, including TNF, Apo3 ligand, or Fas ligand (FasL), a product of T-killer cells or T_{CTL} cells. TNF family members react with their receptors to produce ligand-induced trimerization of the receptor in the cell membrane. Trimerization of the cytoplasmic tails of the Fas receptors leads to

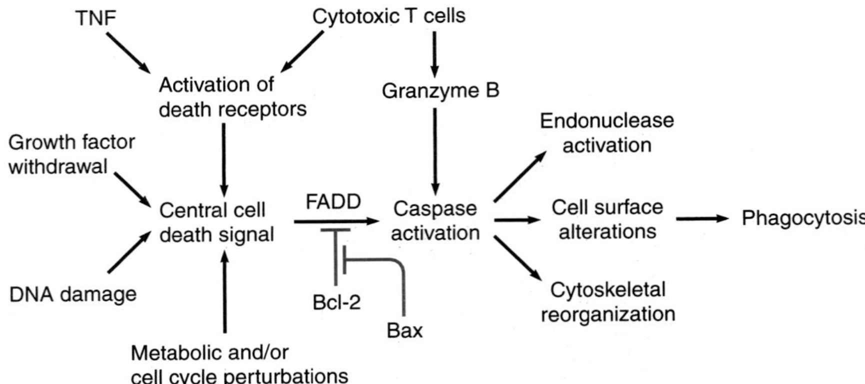

Figure 3.21 Apoptosis. Activation of the death signal may be mediated by growth factor withdrawal (reduction of Bcl-2 expression), DNA damage (p53 activation), metabolic alterations (lack of oxygen), or activation of specific death receptors by TNF or Fas ligand. Binding of the death receptor by ligand leads to trimerization of the receptor and binding of FADD. The FADD-receptor complex is internalized, and in the cytosol FADD binds and activates caspase 8, initiating the caspase activation cascade. Caspase activation is amplified by granzyme B if the cell is targeted by T_{CTL} cells. The threshold of caspase activation is controlled by Bcl-2, which blocks activation and promotes cell survival. The activity of Bcl-2, in turn, is blocked by Bax, which forms inactive heterodimers with Bcl-2. Caspases cause DNA fragmentation (endonucleases), cell surface alterations (blebbing), and cytoskeletal reorganization (shrinking), leading to cell death and phagocytosis. (Modified from C. B. Thompson, p. 813–829, *in* W. E. Paul, ed., *Fundamental Immunology*, 4th ed., Lippincott-Raven, Philadelphia, Pa., 1999.)

recruitment of an adaptor protein, FADD or TRADD. Recruitment of FADD or TRADD is followed by dimerization with caspase 8, which contains a death effector domain. Caspase 8 is cleaved, releasing active protease subunits, which then act on additional caspases. These caspases begin degradation of intracellular structures.

Caspases

Caspases are intracellular cysteine proteases that cleave after aspartic acid residues. At least 10 different caspases are known. In the cascade of activation, cleavage by one caspase results in removal of the amino-terminal prodomain and the processing of the remaining polypeptide into two subunits of the active enzyme. Once activated, most caspases catalyze the activation of several other members of the caspase family, resulting in amplification of the caspase system. Caspases act on DNA to cause fragmentation characteristic of apoptotic cells as well as reorganization of the cytoskeleton and cell surface blebbing culminating in phagocytosis, usually by macrophages, but often by other cells in the same tissue (hepatocytes can phagocytose apoptotic hepatocytes).

Table 3.24 The Bcl family

Antiapoptotic proteins
Bcl-2
Bcl-x_L
Bcl-w
Mcl-1
NR-13
Proapoptotic proteins
Bax
Bak
Bcl-x_S

The Bcl Family

B-cell lymphoma gene 2 (Bcl-2) is a member of a family of proteins that determine the threshold of the cellular apoptotic response. Bcl-2 was originally found to be upregulated in B-cell lymphomas, where it prevents apoptosis and provides "immortality" to the leukemic cells (see chapter 17). A number of Bcl family proteins have opposing effects (Table 3.24).

Five homologs of Bcl-2 inhibit apoptosis, and three enhance it by antagonizing antiapoptotic effects. This is done by forming heterodimers. For example, Bcl-2 is antiapoptotic as a homodimer in blocking caspase activity but is a heterodimer of Bcl-2, and Bax is not. The ratio of Bcl-2 to Bax in a cell determines the apoptotic threshold. An excess of Bcl-2 promotes cell survival, whereas an excess of Bax promotes apoptosis. Control of lymphocyte populations may be mediated by the Bcl family. For example, some growth factors for lymphocytes, such as IL-3, act by upregulating Bcl-2, allowing survival of lymphocytes and expansion of the population. Withdrawal of the growth factor leads to upregulation of Bax, allowing the apoptosis signals to proceed, resulting in cell death and reduction of the population. In such a way, the effect of growth signals mediated by interleukins or adhesion receptors and death signals mediated by the TNF family is modulated by the balancing cytoplasmic levels of Bcl family members.

Wound Healing

The process of wound healing can be considered to begin during the earliest phase of injury or inflammation. Wound healing involves complex interactions among various cell types as well as the extracellular matrix, inflammatory mediators, and growth factors. The time of onset of healing depends on the extent of damage and whether or not the inflammatory process has been enhanced by infection, immune mechanisms, or chronic injury. Chemotactic and growth factors present in the area of injury promote cell migration and proliferation. The cell types involved in healing include platelets, lymphocytes, endothelial cells, macrophages, and fibroblasts. In uncomplicated sterile wounds, platelets limit hemorrhage and are a source for platelet-derived growth factor (PDGF), which is most likely the first growth factor to take part in the healing process. PMNs and macrophages clear necrotic tissue by phagocytosis. Once lymphocytes and macrophages enter the wound, the healing process is controlled not only by cytokines but also by various growth factors as well as by cell matrix interactions mediated by integrins and cell adhesion molecules.

Growth Factors

Various growth factors originally recognized for their effects on tissue culture cells have been found to be critical pharmacologic agents for wound healing, and some are being successfully used to treat previously incurable wounds. Growth factor therapy is being tested on burns, ulcers, surgical incisions, dental extractions, skin grafts, and in other situations. The most important growth factors for wound healing are listed in Table 3.25. The names of the growth factors used in Table 3.25 are based on the original studies that identified the factor and do not necessarily reflect what is now known about them. For instance, PDGF is also produced by macrophages, endothelial cells, and smooth muscle cells. Transforming growth factors, originally isolated from tumor cells, are also produced by normal cells and mediate many normal functions. TGF-β, originally described as a growth factor, is a potent stimulator of extracellular matrix formation and serves to limit the proliferation and stimulate differentiation of many cell types.

The precise role of these and other growth factors in wound healing is not yet well understood. The sequence of release of various factors and activation at the site of injury controls cell proliferation, chemotaxis, cell

Table 3.25 Growth factors active in wound healing[a]

Factor	Source	Responding cells[b]
Platelet-derived growth factor	Pl, endo, macrophages	Fibroblasts, SM, glia
Acidic fibroblast growth factor	B, R, F, C	Endothelium
Basic fibroblast growth factor	Pl, B	Endothelium
Epidermal growth factor	SG, epi	Mesenchyme, epithelium
Transforming growth factor alpha	Tumor, epi	Mesenchyme, epithelium
Transforming growth factor beta	Pl, bone, other	Many
Insulinlike growth factor 1	Liver	Mesenchyme, epithelium
Insulinlike growth factor 2	Liver	Mesenchyme, epithelium

[a]Pl, platelets; endo, endothelium; F, fibroblasts; SM, smooth muscle; B, brain; R, retina; C, chondrocytes; SG, salivary gland; epi, epithelium.
[b]React with tyrosine kinase receptors.

adhesion, and interactions as well as differentiation and extracellular matrix formation. Thrombin, formed during clotting, stimulates the release of alpha granules from aggregated platelets. The alpha granules contain growth factors such as TGF-β, PDGF, and fibroblast growth factor (FGF). Thus, platelet-derived factors initiate wound healing very early after injury. The influx of macrophages into the wound sets the stage for tissue repair. Macrophages release a variety of biologically active substances, including at least six growth factors—IL-1, TNF-α (cachectin), IL-6, FGF, TGF-β, and PDGF—that alter fibroblast growth and metabolism (Table 3.26). Two of these factors, TGF-β and PDGF, stimulate the production of connective tissue. TGF-β stimulates the expression of collagen and fibronectin genes as well as protein production by fibroblasts. It increases the rate of healing, enhances angiogenesis, and stimulates the release of other growth factors.

Macrophages play a central role in wound healing. Macrophages clear the wound of necrotic tissue and initiate granulation tissue formation. TGF-β may limit the effects of activated macrophages and prevent continuing damage to normal tissue by deactivating superoxide production. FGFs stimulate proliferation of endothelial cells, cells surrounding nerves (Schwann cells), and chondrocytes as well as fibroblasts, so they are likely to be very important for initiating the proliferative phase of healing and

Table 3.26 Effect of macrophage-derived cytokines on fibroblast growth and metabolism

Cytokine	Source	Fibroblast proliferation	Connective tissue production
IL-1	Monocytes, macrophage (alveolar and peritoneal)	+	+
IL-6	Alveolar macrophages	+	+
TNF-α	Monocytes, alveolar macrophages	±[a]	±
FGF	Peritoneal macrophages	+	?
TGF-β	Monocytes	−	++
PDGF	Monocytes, macrophages (alveolar and peritoneal)	+	+

[a]±, weakly positive.

the formation of granulation tissue. Acidic FGF stimulates endothelial cells and thus could be critical for the proliferation of capillaries during healing. TGF-β and PDGF most likely act later in healing to stimulate connective tissue differentiation and extracellular matrix formation. Epidermal growth factor is chemotactic and mitogenic for epithelial cells and thus may stimulate reepithelialization of a damaged surface. TGF-β and PDGF may remodel connective tissue by stimulating collagen production by fibroblasts as well as proteinase inhibitors and collagenases. The final outcome of matrix formation and collagen remodeling is scarring or resolution.

Adhesion Molecules

(See also "The Cells of Acute Inflammation" above.) Binding of the cell surface adhesion molecules with extracellular matrix structures initiates differentiation of the cells and apparently is vital for the process of wound healing. Binding of fibroblasts to extracellular matrix fibers initiates organization and eventual reepithelialization of wound surfaces. This process depends on reaction of basic amino acid sequences on epithelial cells with matrix components and eventual formation of basement membranes. Exactly how this process takes place and the role of various cellular adhesion reactions remain to be elucidated. The participation of tissue proteoglycans in this process is under active investigation.

Proteoglycans

Proteoglycans are macromolecules composed of a protein backbone and one or more glycosaminoglycan side chains. There are four major types of glycosaminoglycans: heparan/heparan sulfate, chondroitin sulfate/dermatan sulfate, keratan sulfate, and hyaluronic acid. Many different kinds of proteins have sites for noncovalent binding of sulfated glycosaminoglycans. These binding sites are characterized by sequences of basic amino acids such as BBXB and BBBXXB. The capacity of glycosaminoglycans for many different interactions confers on them the function to serve as the "glue" to bind together extracellular matrix components, to bind cells to the matrix, and to concentrate soluble biologically active proteins such as growth factors. In addition to the glycosaminoglycan binding, many of these macromolecules can bind through domains in the core protein, such as the lectinlike domain found in the large cartilage proteoglycan. A model of adhesion molecules in a cell membrane binding to extracellular matrix is shown in Fig. 3.22.

The roles of cell-proteoglycan and growth factor-proteoglycan interactions during inflammation and healing are becoming increasingly clear. Each of the glycosaminoglycans has a strong negative charge, making it possible for them to bind many substances, including some growth factors. Binding of FGFs to heparan or heparan sulfate protects the FGF from degradation. FGF and other factors are normally tightly bound to collagens, fibronectin, and heparan sulfate in the extracellular matrix. After wounding, active FGF-glycosamine complexes can then be generated by proteolysis of the proteoglycans, such as occurs during inflammation. Other growth factors, such as GM-CSF and IL-3, as well as platelet factor-4, the prototype of a number of growth factors and cytokines, also bind to heparan and heparan sulfate. In addition, TGF-β binds to proteoglycan through the core protein. The inflammatory mediators of neutrophil granules are able to break down the extracellular matrix leading to the formation of pus, thus destroying the normal tissue organization.

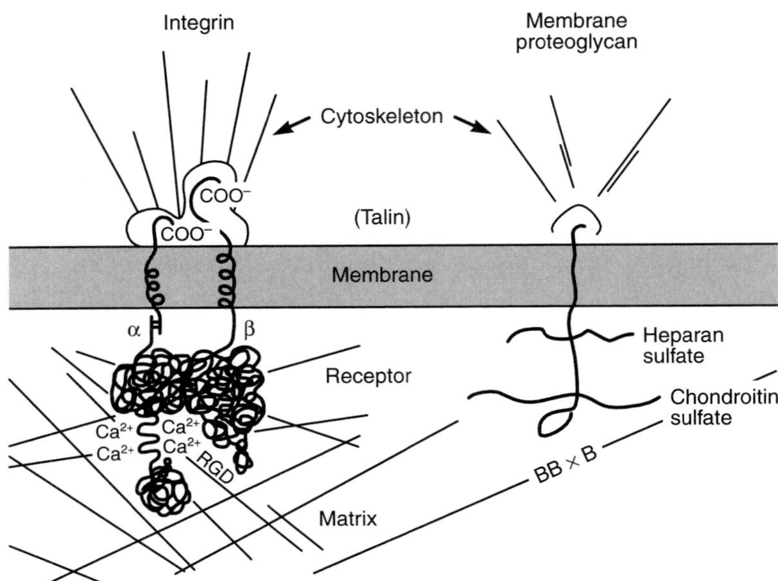

Figure 3.22 Schematic model of binding of a cellular integrin and cell surface proteoglycan to the extracellular matrix. Both the α and β chains of the cell adhesion molecule integrin bind to the cytoskeleton and extend through the cell membrane to attach to proteoglycans in the extracellular matrix, involving Ca^{2+} and the RGD sequence. Cell surface proteoglycans, such as heparan sulfate/chrondroitin sulfate proteoglycan, bind to basic amino acid sequences in fibronectin through the heparan sulfate side chains. (Modified from E. Ruoslahti, *J. Biol. Chem.* **264:**13369, 1989.)

Reestablishment of tissue during the healing process involves the reorganization of the extracellular matrix and reepithelialization of the surface of the wound. Reformation of the extracellular matrix requires synthesis of connective tissue fibers, mainly type I collagen, by fibroblasts and reattachment of extracellular matrix structures to cell surface receptors and proteoglycans. Fibroblasts responding to growth factors released from the damaged matrix, such as FGF, migrate to the wound area, proliferate, and lay down extracellular matrix. During reepithelialization, keratinocytes break free and migrate to the site of injury, attracted by a variety of chemical signals. The activated keratinocytes also display increased expression of integrins, influenced by TGF-β1, which enable them to recognize and attach to matrix molecules.

Review of Mediators of Inflammation

A summary of the roles of various mediators at different stages of the inflammatory process is given in Fig. 3.23. The early vascular stages are largely caused by mast cell mediators. In some instances, products of the coagulation, kinin, and complement systems may be active. The acute cellular stage is mediated by complement, leukotrienes, or bacterial or tissue products. The chronic cellular stage is influenced mainly by cytokines. The outcome of the inflammatory process depends largely on the degree of injury and is effected mainly by macrophages, which either clear the inflamed tissue or set the stage for fibroblast proliferation and scarring. Because of the difficulty in studying this complex process, which can really

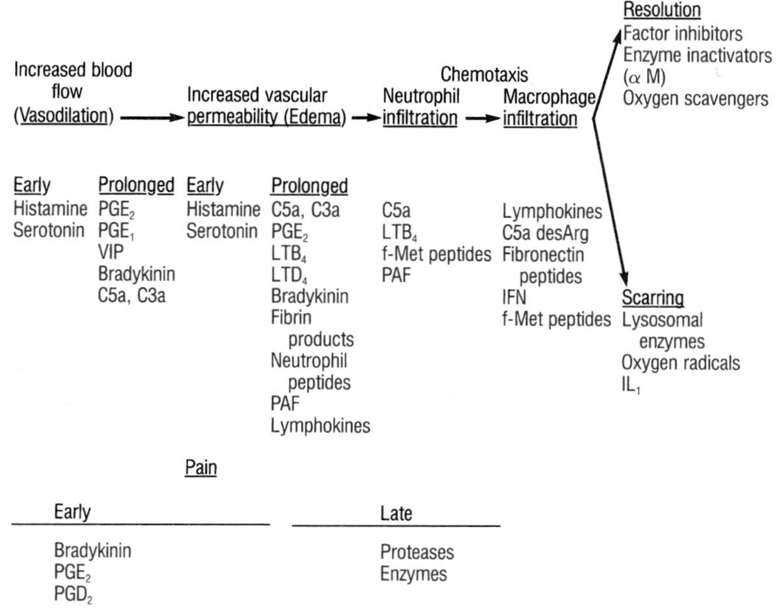

Figure 3.23 Summary of the roles of mediators in the process of inflammation. PGE, prostaglandin E; PGD, prostaglandin D; VIP, vasoactive intestinal polypeptide; LTB, leukotriene B; LTD, leukotriene D; PAF, platelet-activating factor; IFN, interferon; IL-1, interleukin-1.

only be duplicated in vivo, the precise action of the various mediators is not well understood.

Manifestations of Inflammation in Tissues

The examples of morphologic manifestations of different stages of inflammation in tissues to be discussed include four different organs in which inflammation is initiated by different etiologies: (i) vessels: vasculitis induced by antigen-antibody reaction or inflammatory mediators; (ii) lung: pneumonia induced by infection; (iii) heart: myocardial infarction induced by blockage of blood flow (coronary thrombus); and (iv) kidney: glomerulonephritis induced by antibody-antigen reaction and activation of complement (Table 3.27).

The initiating event is different, but the subsequent sequence of events is similar. Acute inflammation is first manifested in vessels by increased blood flow (congestion) and increased vascular permeability (edema). Chemotactic factors attract and activate PMNs. If enzyme release occurs in the vessel walls, fibrinoid (looks like fibrin) necrosis is seen. This will be followed by lymphocyte and macrophage infiltration. If resolution does not occur, subendothelial fibroblastic proliferation leads to narrowing of the vessel wall (endarteritis) and eventually to infarction of tissue. In the lung, congestion and edema due to increased blood flow and vascular permeability are followed by polymorphonuclear infiltration and then by macrophage infiltration, fibroblast proliferation, and scarring (organizing pneumonia). In myocardial infarction, necrosis of myocardial cells is seen first. Release of cytoplasm from necrotic cells produces vasodilation, endothelial cell contraction (increased vascular permeability, edema), and

Table 3.27 Manifestations of inflammation in tissue

Organ	Etiology	Inciting event	Stages of inflammation: Acute	Subacute	Chronic
Vessel (vasculitis)	Multiple	Multiple; cell injury, infection	Increased blood flow and vasopermeability (edema) → Resolution; PMN infiltrate (pus)—Mononuclear cells → Resolution / Scarring; *Necrosis*[a]—Hemorrhage → Scarring		Resolution; Scarring
Lung (pneumonia)	Infection	Release of bacterial products	Edema, congestion → Resolution; PMN infiltrate—Macrophages → Resolution / Scarring; Hemorrhage—*Necrosis*—Fibroblast proliferation → Scarring		Resolution; Scarring
Heart (infarct)	Disturbance of flow	Necrosis of myocardial cells	Edema, congestion; PMN infiltrate—Macrophage—Fibroblast proliferation → Scarring		Scarring
Kidney (glomerulonephritis)	Immune inflammation	Deposition of antigen-antibody complexes, activation of complement	Increased glomerular permeability (proteinuria) → Resolution; PMN infiltrate—mononuclear infiltrate; *Necrosis*—Hematuria → Scarring (uremia); Epithelial proliferation		Resolution; Scarring (uremia)

[a]Necrosis is key to chronic damage and scarring.

chemotaxis for PMNs. This is followed by macrophage infiltration, fibroblast and capillary proliferation (granulation tissue), and scarring. In the renal glomerulus, the sequence of events is initiated by activation of complement following deposition of antibody-antigen complexes in the basement membrane. This produces changes in the endothelial cells and basement membrane that result in leakage of protein in the urine (proteinuria, the equivalent of edema in other organs) and chemotaxis of PMNs. Enzymes released by PMNs cause destruction of the basement membrane, and red blood cells pass into the urine (hematuria, the equivalent of hemorrhage in other tissues). Subacute glomerular inflammation is manifested by proliferation of epithelial cells and continued thickening of the basement membrane (membranoproliferative glomerulonephritis). The major consequence of the inflammatory process changes from increased glomerular permeability (proteinuria, hematuria) to decreased filtration as the basement membrane becomes thickened (uremia). As in other organs, chronic inflammation is manifested by fibrosis and scarring. Thus, in each organ the process of inflammation is essentially the same, leading to resolution or scarring through similar stages.

Cytokines, Adhesion Molecules, and Growth Factors in Atherosclerosis

The interplay of cytokines, adhesion molecules, and growth factors in chronic inflammation is critical to the development of atherosclerotic plaques in blood vessels. The endothelial cells of blood vessels constitute a critical interface with the blood and the underlying tissues, in particular the smooth muscle cells of the vascular media. In hyperplastic arterial disease, the endothelial cells lose their anticoagulant properties and become "sticky" because of increased expression of adhesion molecules. Smooth muscle cells begin to produce increased extracellular matrix. Mononuclear cells from the blood penetrate the arterial wall, infiltrate the smooth muscle layer, and begin to accumulate oxidized low-density lipoproteins (LDL). The proliferation of smooth muscle cells and accumulation of lipid-laden macrophages leads to the formation of "fatty streaks" in the subendothelium and, eventually, atherosclerotic plaques.

This progressive tissue lesion is mediated by a hypothesized series of changes in growth factors, cell adhesion molecules, and cytokines. First, hypercholesteremia promotes lipid uptake by vascular walls. These lipids initiate a cycle of local cytokine production and lipid modification (oxidation of LDL). Adhesion of blood monocytes (macrophages) to vascular endothelial cells is mediated by ICAM-1 and VCAM-1 on endothelial cells binding to LFA-1 and VLA-4 on the monocytes. Emigration and activation of monocytes is enhanced by production of MCP-1, an adhesion molecule for monocytes, by endothelial cells. Activated macrophages in the vessel wall produce M-CSF, a ubiquitous growth factor that autoupregulates production of the cytokines IL-1, TNF, and IFN-γ. As activators of endothelial cells, both IL-1 and TNF induce syntheses of specific glycoproteins that further increase leukocyte adherence, induce rearrangements of the endothelial wall cytoskeleton, and augment synthesis of PAF and prostacyclin, which serve to increase vascular permeability and cause vasodilation. IL-1 and TNF also stimulate production of IL-8, which activates neutrophils. In addition to mediating permeability and emigration, IL-1 and TNF induce endothelium to produce PDGF, which recruits smooth muscle cells to the subendothelium and stimulates their proliferation. Within the intima, the accumulating macrophages express an acetyl-LDL receptor for oxidized LDL, and the macrophages take up and accumulate modified LDL, thus becoming lipid-laden "foam" cells in fatty streaks. Fatty streaks along the endothelium are the first grossly recognizable changes in atherosclerosis and progress by smooth muscle proliferation, lipid and matrix accumulation, remodeling, calcification, ulceration, hemorrhage, and thrombosis to lesions characteristic of atherosclerotic arterial disease.

Amyloidosis

Amyloidosis refers to a heterogeneous group of diseases in which there is an extracellular tissue deposit of a hyaline, microscopically amorphous material with a filamentous ultrastructure that gives green birefringence under polarized light after Congo red staining. This property was first associated with staining of linear polysaccharides (i.e., starch), and the name amyloid (starchlike) was applied by Rudolph Virchow in 1851. Amyloid deposits are actually made up of protein and not cellulose (amyloid), as originally proposed. The proteinaceous deposits are very difficult to solubilize, so chemical analysis has been difficult. Tissue deposits build up because the reticuloendothelial and macrophage systems, as well as other cells, are unable to effect removal of the poorly degradable materials. In some cases, amyloid deposition is caused by the overproduction of precursor molecules of plasma proteins, which accumulate because of incomplete catabolism. In other cases, an altered form of a protein is produced that is more difficult to "turn over" than the normal protein. The major protein constituents of amyloid have three common features: (i) there is a serum precursor, (ii) the protein has a high degree of antiparallel beta-sheet conformation, and (iii) there is a distinctive ultrastructural appearance. The growing mass of amyloid fibrils associates with plasma and extracellular matrix proteins and proteoglycans to form amyloid deposits, which infiltrate the extracellular species of organs, destroying normal tissue architecture and function. Amyloidosis is a group of complex diseases, caused by pathologic conformational changes and polymerization, in which normally soluble precursors are converted into insoluble fibrils.

Classification

Amyloid deposition may affect different organs and give rise to many pathologic conditions (Table 3.28). The deposits may be generalized or localized. Generalized nonhereditary amyloidosis is caused by the deposition of precursors of serum proteins and is associated with overproduction. Generalized hereditary amyloidoses result from the production of variants of prealbumin. Neuron-related proteins are found in localized cerebral amyloidoses, and hormone-related proteins are found in endocrine amyloidosis. Disease is caused when there are enough deposits to interfere with the normal function of an organ. In systemic amyloidosis, deposits in the liver, heart, or kidney may lead to failure of these organs. In cerebral amyloidoses such as Alzheimer's disease (AD), deposits in neurons lead to dementia. In hereditary cerebral hemorrhage with amyloidosis, deposits in cerebral vessels may cause recurrent cerebral hemorrhages. What chemical analysis has been possible has provided considerable insight into the pathogenesis of the different types of amyloidosis.

Amyloidogenic Proteins

Systemic Amyloidosis

The four forms of amyloidogenic proteins found in systemic amyloidosis have been classified as AL, AA, AF, and AH. AL deposits include immunoglobulin light chains; AA deposits, protein AA; AF deposits (F, familial), primarily prealbumin variants; and AH deposits (H, hemodialysis), β_2-microglobulin.

Table 3.28 Classification of systemic and local amyloidoses[a]

Type	Protein
Systemic nonhereditary	
Primary and myeloma-associated	Immunoglobulin light-chain dimers
Secondary	High-density lipoprotein–serum amyloid A protein (HDL-SAA)
Hemodialysis	β_2-Microglobulin
Systemic hereditary	
Familial Mediterranean fever[b]	HDL-SAA
Familial amyloid polyneuropathy	Prealbumin variants
Systemic senile amyloidosis	Prealbumin variant (ILE 122)
Local cerebral	
Hereditary cerebral hemorrhage with amyloidosis	
Icelandic type	Cystatin c
Dutch type	β-protein
Alzheimer's disease and Down's syndrome	β-protein
Transmissible spongioform encephalopathies	Protease-resistant protein
Local endocrine	
Medullary carcinoma of the thyroid	Procalcitonin
Pancreatic	Calcitonin gene-related peptide

[a]Modified from E. M. Castano and B. Frangione, *Lab. Investig.* **58:**122–132, 1988.
[b]Also found in nonhereditary form.

AL: immunoglobulin light chains. Deposits of immunoglobulin light chains are found in primary amyloidosis and amyloid associated with multiple myeloma (a tumor of plasma cells that may make large amounts of immunoglobulin molecules). The immunoglobulin deposits usually consist of dimers of two variable halves of the light chain, a variable half and a complete light chain, or two complete light chains. Mixing variable regions of some light chains (Bence Jones proteins) in vitro results in the formation of the β-pleated sheet structures characteristic of amyloid. Such structures are difficult to catabolize and may have an affinity to deposit in certain tissues, producing amyloidosis.

AA: protein AA. Protein AA is related to the acute-phase serum protein SAA. AA protein production by hepatocytes is stimulated by IL-1. Protein AA in tissue deposits of amyloid has a molecular weight of 8,500; that of SAA is 14,000. A proteolytic enzyme in macrophages clips off 30 to 40 amino acid residues from the carboxyl end of SAA to produce protein AA. Protein AA then deposits in tissue, forming filamentous, poorly degradable amyloid. This form of amyloidosis is most likely caused by the increased production of SAA secondary to chronic inflammatory conditions such as rheumatoid arthritis, tuberculosis, bronchiectasis, and leprosy or malignancies such as Hodgkin's lymphoma or renal cell carcinoma.

AH: β_2-microglobulin. β_2-Microglobulin is an 11.8-kDa part of the class I MHC. High serum levels of β_2-microglobulin are found during renal failure and are not removed from the circulation by conventional dialysis membranes. Up to 70% of patients receiving chronic renal dialysis may develop deposits of amyloid in bone and synovium composed of intact normal β_2-microglobulin.

AF: prealbumin variants. Genetically determined amino acid substitutions in prealbumin are found in the group of familial amyloid polyneuropathies (FAP) and in systemic senile amyloidosis. FAP is recognized in various nationality groups. In the Jewish kindred, there is a substitution of methionine for valine at position 39 and isoleucine for phenylalanine at position 33. In patients of Swiss-German origin, there is a substitution of serine for isoleucine at position 84. In Portuguese, Japanese, and Swedish families, there is a substitution of methionine for valine at position 30. In systemic senile amyloidosis, there is isoleucine at position 122. It is possible that these genetic variants of prealbumin may aggregate abnormally in tissue or be resistant to proteolytic cleavage, leading to deposition in vessel walls and peripheral nerves, areas where normal mechanisms of tissue turnover may be limited.

Protein P. Protein P is a minor component (<10%) of most amyloid deposits and is related to the acute-phase protein CRP. Protein P is made up of a double pentamer composed of 23,000-molecular-weight subunits. CRP is a single pentamer. Protein P forms from the aggregation of two CRP pentamers and can be seen by electron microscopy as an 80-Å doughnutlike structure. Protein P binds to many different ligands, including amyloid fibrils, fibronectin, and C4-binding protein. This binding may be the reason protein P is found in amyloid deposits.

HSPG. Heparan sulfate proteoglycan (HSPG) is a component of basement membrane that was first shown to be associated with protein AA deposition but now has been found in four other forms of amyloid deposits: AD, prion amyloids such as Creutzfeldt-Jakob disease, amyloid in type II diabetes, and familial amyloidotic polyneuropathy. It is not clear if this is related to a disturbance in the synthesis of basement membrane, a passive absorption of HSPG by amyloid deposits, or a response provoked by amyloid deposition. Unlike other components of amyloid, HSPG is not found in the serum and does not appear to have a serum precursor.

Local Amyloidosis

Cystatin C. Cystatin C is a 12-kDa basic protein that is an inhibitor of cysteine proteases and is related to kininogens. The variant that is found in amyloid fibrils in the walls of small arteries and arterioles in the cerebral cortex and leptomeninges starts at position 11 of the normal protein and has glutamine instead of leucine at position 68. It has been identified in amyloid deposits in an autosomal dominant form of cerebral amyloidosis in Iceland.

β-Protein. β-Protein (β-amyloid protein) is a 4-kDa protein fragment of 42 amino acids with a highly hydrophobic tail of 14 residues that is found in the senile plaques of patients with AD or Down's syndrome and in the vessel walls of patients with Dutch-type hereditary cerebral hemorrhage with amyloidosis. β-Amyloid protein deposition thus identifies a group of diseases with varied sites of deposition, from primarily neuronal (dementia) to primarily vascular (cerebral hemorrhage). Deposits of β-protein undergo fibrillogenesis, resulting in highly stable 5- to 10-nm filaments characteristic of amyloid. The precursor of β-protein is a 56-amino-acid polypeptide that spans the cell membrane of many cell types (amyloid precursor protein). It has a large extramembranous portion and a small cytoplasmic domain. The 42 amino acids of the β-protein include 28 extracellular amino acids and the first 11 to 14 amino acids of the hydrophobic transmembrane domain. The complete 56-amino-acid precursor of β-protein may be a growth factor, but the abbreviated 42-amino-acid form is inactive, suggesting that the 42-amino-acid fragment may function to block the activity of the 56-amino-acid molecule.

PrP. Protease-resistant protein (PrP) is a poorly defined 27- to 30-kDa protein that is found in amyloid deposits in the human transmissible spongioform encephalopathies (Creutzfeldt-Jakob disease, Gerstmann-Sträussler syndrome, and kuru) as well as in the sheep disease scrapie. It has been suggested that this protein is a component of an infectious agent (a prion), although it is expressed in both normal and infected brains.

Pathogenesis

The complete understanding of the pathogenesis of systemic amyloidosis remains elusive. Some common factors leading to the various forms of systemic amyloidosis include the following.

1. A circulating soluble precursor that includes an amyloidogenic primary structure that forms a proteolytic fragment. The proteolytic fragment folds into a β-pleated sheet secondary structure that assembles into a fibrillary structure in tissue and is resistant to re-

moval. In some cases, there are increased amounts of an amyloidogenic material (β_2-microglobulin) or aggregation of a precursor (P protein).
2. Increased serum levels of the precursor due to increased synthesis or decreased clearance or both.
3. Abnormal processing of the protein, such as prealbumin variants or immunoglobulin light chains, or incomplete degradation, such as for the formation of protein AA from SAA.

There appears to be a diversity of etiologic factors leading to amyloid deposition. The stimulus for the overproduction or abnormal production of some amyloid precursors may be the stimulation of liver and other tissues by cytokines (IL-1 and IL-6) from macrophages. Deposition may result from a complication of inflammatory disease or malignancy, genetic defects, chromosomal abnormalities, or environmental factors. At this time, there is an effective treatment for only one form of amyloidosis, the autosomal recessive disease familial Mediterranean fever. Long-term treatment with colchicine can prevent the deposition of protein AA that otherwise causes early death due to renal failure.

Alzheimer's Disease

AD is a progressive senile dementia of immense clinical importance. The pathologic hallmark of the lesions of AD is the deposition of amyloid fibrils in senile plaques and in blood vessels in specific regions of the cerebral cortex. The plaques contain a mixture of proteins, but the most obvious feature is that the core of AD plaques contains insoluble β-protein. The AD β-amyloid or A4 protein is derived from β-protein precursor (see above).

The gene for β-protein precursor is on chromosome 21, the same chromosome that is trisomic in Down's syndrome, in which there is premature development of the neurologic lesions of AD. Down's syndrome patients with trisomy 21 are believed to produce larger amounts of β-protein because of gene dosage—the gene for the protein precursor is located in or near 21q21. Point mutations in the β-protein precursor gene have been detected in two Swedish families with early-onset AD and in a different location in a patient with hereditary cerebral hemorrhage of the Dutch type of amyloidosis. In Dutch-type amyloidosis, deposition of β-protein is seen primarily in the walls of cerebral blood vessels, whereas in AD it is more prominent in neural plaques. The mutation in the Dutch disease occurs within the β-protein itself, whereas the mutation in the families with early-onset AD is in the precursor molecule, two amino acid residues from the end of the β-protein. However, in the nonhereditary forms of AD, there is no evidence that the β-protein gene is abnormal.

AD may be due to a genetically controlled increase in the amount of β-protein precursor that accumulates with aging because of an insidiously failing catabolic system or to aberrant function or metabolism of the β-protein precursor, most likely secondary to abnormalities in enzymes that process the precursor protein for secretion. Thus, research is now directed to the transcriptional, translational, and posttranslational events that might account for the progressive deposition of β-amyloid protein in AD. As a result, evidence has been obtained that accumulation of the β-protein may be derived from the precursor protein following uptake by neuronal lysosomes. Lysosomes in neurons are small intracellular vesicles where protein degradation normally occurs. In vitro, neurons release β-protein by cleavage of the extramembranous portion of the larger precursor molecule. This is accomplished by an enzyme called β-secretase, which cleaves one end of β-protein from its precursor. The β-protein is then taken back into the cell by endocytosis, where it is normally degraded. However, if there is increased production, such as in the Swedish families, with early-onset AD, or an inability to break down the β-protein, either because of an abnormal β-protein or defects in catabolism, gradual accumulation of the protein with aging and intracellular accumulation may occur, eventually leading to loss of the neuron. Inhibition of the activity or production of β-secretase is being investigated as a possible mode of prevention of AD.

Summary

Inflammation is the process of delivery of proteins and cells to sites of tissue damage or infection and their activation at these sites. The process moves from acute to subacute and chronic stages and to resolution or scarring. The extent of tissue lesions produced by the inflammatory process is determined by mechanisms mediated by activated serum proteins or blood cells, as well as by extracellular matrix and endothelial cells. The serum protein systems involved in acute inflammation include complement, coagulation, fibrinolysis, kinin, and acute-phase reactants. The cellular systems include PMNs, eosinophils, mast cells (or basophils), and platelets in acute inflammation and lymphocytes and macrophages, as well as fibroblasts, in chronic inflammation. Cellular infiltration involves an interactive set of receptors on the inflammatory cells (e.g., neutrophils, lymphocytes, or macrophages) that react in sequence with ligands on vascular endothelial cells. Each of these systems has a homeostatic function and is controlled by interrelated feedback systems. Manifestations of inflammation in different tissues are similar even though the process is initiated by different events (infections, tissue necrosis, antibody-antigen reactions). Excessive or prolonged activation, as well as inadequate activation, of these systems may have serious effects, leading to chronic inflammation and scarring. Inability to remove proteins related to inflammation may result in their accumulation in cells, resulting in amyloidosis or AD.

Bibliography

General

Rosenberg, H. F., and J. I. Gallin. 1999. Inflammation, p. 1051–1066. *In* W. E. Paul (ed.), *Fundamental Immunology,* 4th ed. Lippincott-Raven Publishers, Philadelphia, Pa.

Mast Cells

Costa, J. J., and S. J. Galli. 1996. Mast cells and basophils, p. 408–430. *In* R. Rich, T. A. Fleisher, B. D. Schwartz, W. T. Shearer, and W. Strober (ed.), *Clinical Immunology: Principles and Practice,* vol. 1. The C. V. Mosby Co., St. Louis, Mo.

Galli, S. J. 1993. New concepts about the mast cell. *N. Engl. J. Med.* **328:**257–263.

Lantz, C. S., J. Boesiger, C. H. Song, N. Mach, T. Kobayashi, R. C. Mulligan, Y. Nawa, G. Dranoff, and S. J. Galli. 1998. Role for interleukin-3 in mast-cell and basophil development and in immunity to parasites. *Nature* **392:**90–93.

Platelets

Malik, A. B., and S. K. Lo. 1996. Vascular endothelial adhesion molecules and tissue inflammation. *Pharmacol. Rev.* **48:**213–229.

Neutrophils

Ding, Z.-M., J. E. Babensee, S. I. Simon, H. Lu, J. L. Perrard, D. C. Bullard, X. Y. Dai, S. K. Bromley, M. L. Dustin, M. L. Entman, C. W. Smith, and C. M. Ballantyne. 1999. Relative contribution of LFA-1 and Mac-1 to neutrophil adhesion and migration. *J. Immunol.* **163:**5029–5038.

Henderson, L. M., and J. B. Chappel. 1996. NADPH oxidase of neutrophils. *Biochim. Biophys. Acta* **1273:**87–107.

Kishmoto, T. K., and R. Rothlein. 1994. Integrins, ICAMs and selectins: role and regulation of adhesion molecules in neutrophil recruitment to inflammatory sites. *Adv. Pharmacol.* **25:**117–169.

Servant, G., O. D. Weiner, P. Herzmark, T. Balla, J. W. Sedat, and H. R. Bourne. 2000. Polarization of chemoattractant receptor signaling during neutrophil chemotaxis. *Science* **287:**1037–1040.

Smith, J. A. 1994. Neutrophils, host defense, and inflammation: a double-edged sword. *J. Leukoc. Biol.* **56:**672–686.

Varani, J., and P. A. Ward. 1994. Mechanisms of neutrophil-dependent and neutrophil-independent endothelial cell injury. *Biol. Signals* **3:**1–14.

Eosinophils

Makino, S., and T. Tukuda. 1993. *Eosinophils: Biological and Clinical Aspects.* CRC Press, Inc., Boca Raton, Fla.

Martin, L. B., H. Kita, and K. M. Leiferman. 1996. Eosinophils in allergy; role in disease, degranulation and cytokines. *Int. Arch. Allergy Immunol.* **109:**207–215.

Adhesion Molecules

Albelda, S. M., C. W. Smith, and P. A. Ward. 1994. Adhesion molecules and inflammatory injury. *FASEB J.* **8:**504–512.

Butcher, E. C. 1991. Leukocyte-endothelial cell recognition: three (or more) steps to specificity and diversity. *Cell* **67:**1033–1036.

Giancotti, F. G., and E. Ruoslahti. 1999. Integrin signalling. *Science* **285:**1028–1031.

Gille, J., and R. A. Swerlick. 1996. Integrins: role in cell adhesion and communication. *Ann. N. Y. Acad. Sci.* **797:**93–106.

Kansas, G. S. 1996. Selectins and their ligands—current concepts and controversies. *Blood* **88:**3259–3287.

Ruoslahti, E., and M. D. Pierschbacher. 1987. New perspectives in cell adhesion RGD and integrins. *Science* **238:**491–497.

Strausbaugh, H. J., P. G. Green, E. Lo, K. Tangemann, D. B. Reichling, S. D. Rosen, and J. D. Levine. 1999. Painful stimulation suppresses joint inflammation by inducing shedding of L-selectin from neutrophils. *Nat. Med.* **5:**1057–1061.

Complement

Kirschfink, M. 1997. Controlling the complement system in inflammation. *Immunopharmacology* **38:**57–62.

Lae, S. K. A., and A. W. Dodds. 1997. The internal thioester and the covalent binding properties of the complement proteins C3 and C4. *Protein Sci.* **6:**263–274.

Muller-Eberhard, H. J. 1992. Complement. Chemistry and pathways, p. 33–61. *In* J. I. Gallin, I. M. Goldstein, and R. Snyderman (ed.), *Inflammation: Basic Principles and Clinical Correlates,* 2nd ed. Raven Press, New York, N.Y.

Coagulation

Altieri, D. C. 1995. Inflammatory cell participation in coagulation. *Semin. Cell Biol.* **6:**269–274.

Salgado, A., J. L. Boveda, J. Monasterio, R. M. Segura, M. Mourelle, J. Gomez-Jimenez, and R. Peracaula. 1994. Inflammatory mediators and their influence on haemostasis. *Haemostasis* **24:**132–138.

Shwartzman Reaction

Colman, R., S. J. Robboy, and J. D. Minna. 1979. Disseminated intravascular coagulation: a reappraisal. *Annu. Rev. Med.* **30:**359–374.

Septic Shock

Cerami, A. 1992. Inflammatory cytokines. *Clin. Immunol. Immunopathol.* **62:**S3–S10.

Herman, A., J. W. Kappler, P. Marrack, and A. M. Pullen. 1991. Superantigens: mechanism of T-cell stimulation and role in immune responses. *Annu. Rev. Immunol.* **9:**745–772.

Möller, G. (ed.). 1993. Superantigens. *Immunol. Rev.* **131.**

Kinin

Busse, R., and J. Fleming. 1996. Molecular responses of endothelial tissue to kinins. *Diabetes* **45**(Suppl. 1)**:**S8–S13.

Margolius, H. S. 1996. Kallikreins and kinins. Molecular characteristics and cellular and tissue responses. *Diabetes* **45**(Suppl. 1)**:**S14–S19.

Acute-Phase Proteins

Dowton, S. B., and H. R. Colten. 1988. Acute-phase reactants in inflammation and infection. *Semin. Hematol.* **25:**84–90.

Kolb-Bachofen, V. 1991. A review of the biological properties of C-reactive protein. *Immunobiology* **183:**133–145.

Kushner, I. 1993. Regulation of the acute phase response by cytokines. *Perspect. Biol. Med.* **36:**611–622.

Xia, D., and D. Samols. 1997. Transgenic mice expressing rabbit C-reactive protein are resistant to endotoxemia. *Proc. Natl. Acad. Sci. USA* **94:**2572–2580.

ARDS

Kollef, M. H., and D. P. Schuster. 1995. The acute respiratory distress syndrome. *N. Engl. J. Med.* **332:**27–32.

Ward, P. A. 1996. Role of complement, chemokines and regulatory cytokines in acute lung injury. *Ann. N. Y. Acad. Sci.* **796:**104–112.

Lymphocytes

Butcher, E. C., and L. J. Picker. 1996. Lymphocyte circulation and homeostasis. *Science* **272:**60–66.

Dunon, D., L. Piali, and B. A. Imhof. 1996. To stick or not to stick: the new leukocyte homing paradigm. *Curr. Opin. Cell Biol.* **8:**714–723.

Dustin, M. L., and T. A. Springer. 1991. Role of lymphocyte adhesion receptors in transient interactions and cell locomotion. *Annu. Rev. Immunol.* **9:**27–66.

Pober, J. S. 1999. Immunology of human vascular endothelium. *Immunol Res.* **19:**225–232.

Springer, T. A. 1994. Traffic signals for lymphocyte recirculation and leukocyte emigration: the multistep paradigm. *Cell* **76:**301–314.

Macrophages

Allen, L. A., and A. Aderem. 1996. Mechanisms of phagocytosis. *Curr. Opin. Immunol.* **8:**36–40.

Cavaillon, J. M. 1994. Cytokines and macrophages. *Biomed. Pharmacother.* **48:**445–453.

Laskin, D. L., and K. J. Pendino. 1995. Macrophages and inflammatory mediators in tissue injury. *Annu. Rev. Pharmacol. Toxicol.* **35:**655–677.

Nelson, D. S. 1976. *Immunobiology of the Macrophage.* Academic Press, New York, N.Y.

Nielsen, B. W., N. Mukaida, K. Matsushima, and T. Kasahara. 1994. Macrophages as producers of chemotactic proinflammatory cytokines. *Immunol. Ser.* **60:**131–142.

Cytokines

Baker, S. J., and E. P. Reddy. 1996. Transducers of life and death: TNF receptor superfamily and associated proteins. *Oncogene* **12:**1–9.

Bassoni, F., and B. Beutler. 1996. The tumor necrosis factor ligand and receptor families. *N. Engl. J. Med.* **334:**1717–1725.

Beutler, B., and A. Cerami. 1988. The history, properties and biological effects of cachectin. *Biochemistry* **27:**7575–7582.

Boehm, U., T. Klamp, M. Groot, and J. C. Howard. 1997. Cellular responses to interferon-gamma. *Annu. Rev. Immunol.* **15:**749–795.

Border, W. A., and E. Ruoslahti. 1992. Transforming growth factor-β in disease: the dark side of tissue repair. *J. Clin. Investig.* **90:**1–7.

Dinarello, C. A. 1994. The interleukin-1 family: 10 years of discovery. *FASEB J.* **8:**1314–1325.

Stahl, N., and G. D. Yancopoulos. 1993. The alphas, betas and kinases of cytokine receptor complexes. *Cell* **74:**587–590.

Chemokines

Baggiolini, M., B. Dewald, and B. Moser. 1997. Human chemokines: an update. *Annu. Rev. Immunol.* **15:**675–705.

Murphy, P. M. 1996. Chemokine receptors: structure, function and role in microbial pathogenesis. *Cytokine Growth Factor Rev.* **7:**47–64.

Pleskoff, O., C. Treboute, A. Brelot, N. Heveker, M. Seman, and M. Alizon. 1997. Identification of a chemokine receptor encoded by human cytomegalovirus as a cofactor for HIV-1 entry. *Science* **276:**1874–1878.

Taub, D. D. 1996. Chemokine-leukocyte interactions. *Cytokine Growth Factor Rev.* **7:**355–376.

Apoptosis

Chinnaiyan, A. M., and V. M. Dixit. 1996. The cell-death machine. *Curr. Biol.* **6:**555–562.

Goldstein, P. 1997. Controlling cell death. *Science* **275:**1081–1082.

Majno, G., and I. Joris. 1995. Apoptosis, oncosis, and necrosis. An overview of cell death. *Am. J. Pathol.* **146:**3–15.

Wound Healing

Aota, S., T. Nagai, K. Olden, S. K. Akiyama, and K. M. Yamada. 1991. Fibronectin and integrins in cell adhesion and migration. *Biochem. Soc. Trans.* **19:**830–835.

Ben-Baruch, A., D. F. Michiel, and J. J. Oppenheim. 1995. Signals and receptors involved in recruitment of inflammatory cells. *J. Biol. Chem.* **270:**11703–11706.

Martin, P. 1997. Wound healing—aiming for perfect skin regeneration. *Science* **276:**75–81.

Ruoslahti, E., and Y. Yamaguchi. 1991. Proteoglycans as modulators of growth factor activities. *Cell* **64:**867–869.

Chronic Inflammation and Atherosclerosis

Brody, J. I., N. J. Pickering, D. M. Capuzzi, G. B. Fink, C. A. Can, and F. Gomez. 1992. Interleukin-1 α as a factor in occlusive vascular disease. *Am. J. Clin. Pathol.* **97:**8–13.

Libby, P. 1992. Do vascular wall cytokines promote atherogenesis? *Hosp. Pract.* **27:**51–58.

Ross, R. 1993. The pathogenesis of atherosclerosis: a perspective for the 1990's. *Nature* **362:**801–809.

Amyloidosis

Kyle, R. A., and M. A. Certz. 1990. Systemic amyloidosis. *Crit. Rev. Oncol. Hematol.* **10:**49–87.

Sipe, J. D. 1992. Amyloidosis. *Annu. Rev. Biochem.* **61:**947–975.

Alzheimer's Disease

Selkoe, D. J. 1991. The molecular pathology of Alzheimer's disease. *Neuron* **6:**487–498.

Vassar, R., B. D. Bennett, S. Babu-Khan, S. Kahn, E. A. Mendiaz, P. Denis, D. B. Teplow, S. Ross, P. Amarante, R. Loeloff, Y. Luo, S. Fisher, J. Fuller, S. Edenson, J. Lile, M. A. Jarosinski, A. L. Biere, E. Curran, T. Burgess, J. C. Louis, F. Collins, J. Treanor, G. Rogers, and M. Citron. 1999. β-Secretase cleavage of Alzheimer's amyloid precursor protein by the transmembrane aspartic protease BACE. *Science* **286:**735–741.

All about B Cells

STEWART SELL AND EDWARD E. MAX

4

B Cells and Antibodies

B cells are lymphocytes that express cell surface antibodies. B cells are activated by interaction of antigens with these cell surface antibodies (receptors) along with costimulatory signals provided by antigen-presenting cells and T cells. B cells thus activated proliferate and differentiate into plasma cells, which provide "humoral immunity" via the secretion of circulating antibodies also known as immunoglobulins. An individual must be able to make thousands of different antibody molecules in order to identify and react with many potential infectious agents by initiating antibody-mediated immune effector mechanisms. Yet each plasma cell makes only one type of antibody that recognizes a single antigen determinant (epitope). Antibody diversity resides in the vast number of different individual B cells that express immunoglobulin targeted to different specific antigens. After an antigen binds to and activates B cells displaying specific membrane immunoglobulins, these particular B cells are activated. Activation leads to clonal proliferation of these B-cell lines, and the progeny of the specifically activated B cells differentiate into plasma cells that synthesize and secrete antibody specific for the initiating antigen. Through the activation of many different clones of B cells, a large number of antibodies that react with different infectious agents are produced in a very short period of time. This chapter describes the nature of antibodies, their reaction with antigens, how antibodies are produced, and how B cells are activated and differentiate to express different immunoglobulin classes (isotypes).

Antibodies

Antibodies were the first components of immune specificity to be recognized. For example, about a century ago, it was shown that after an animal was exposed to the bacterium *Vibrio cholerae,* protein components of serum from that animal—but not from a "naive" animal—were capable of killing live cholera organisms. Other early experiments documented other manifestations of antibodies, including their ability to neutralize and precipitate toxins and other bacterial proteins, to agglutinate bacteria, and to confer immunity when injected into a naive animal challenged with the specific organism. All of these manifestations have been shown to result from tight and specific binding between an antibody and a microbial component *(antigen)*. Although all antibodies are proteins, a variety of macromolecules act as antigens, including proteins, polysaccharides, nucleic acids, and proteolipids. The first identification of the fraction of serum proteins containing antibodies was accomplished by electrophoresis in 1938 (Fig. 4.1). When animals produced high levels of antibody, there was a marked increase in the serum gamma globulins; when immune serum was absorbed with the specific antigen, the level of gamma globulins decreased.

At this point in the history of immunology, it could have been assumed that vertebrates are endowed through evolution with a repertoire of antibodies designed to interact with the microbial molecules to which they are commonly exposed. However, it was soon demonstrated that antibodies could be induced against many nonbiological chemicals if these were injected into laboratory animals after being coupled to proteins, e.g., dinitrophenol coupled to serum albumin. The resulting antibodies could bind with specificity to small molecules like dinitrophenol, known as *haptens;* yet the administration of haptens alone failed to elicit antibodies (i.e., the haptens were not *immunogenic*) unless they were attached to a macromolecule (a *carrier*). The ability of the immune system to generate specific antibodies against a variety of nonbiological haptenic chemicals that were presumably never encountered in the evolutionary history of vertebrates suggested that antibody repertoire was not limited to any particular set of commonly encountered antigens but could potentially include specificities against a much larger universe of antigens. This raised the question of how such vast diversity might be encoded in the organism's genome; the answer could not be clarified until the development of the techniques of molecular genetics, as discussed below. A related mystery was the mechanism by which an antigen could act as an *immunogen,* i.e., induce an organism to produce a set of highly specific antibodies directed against itself, while not inducing antibodies against other antigens.

Figure 4.1 Demonstration of antibodies in the gamma globulin fraction of serum. If serum is placed under an electric field, the proteins will migrate in the charged gradient. The black line indicates the levels of proteins in the migration pattern after absorption with antigen. The blue-green line indicates the levels before absorption. By this method, the serum antibodies were shown to be the least negatively charged (gamma globulin).

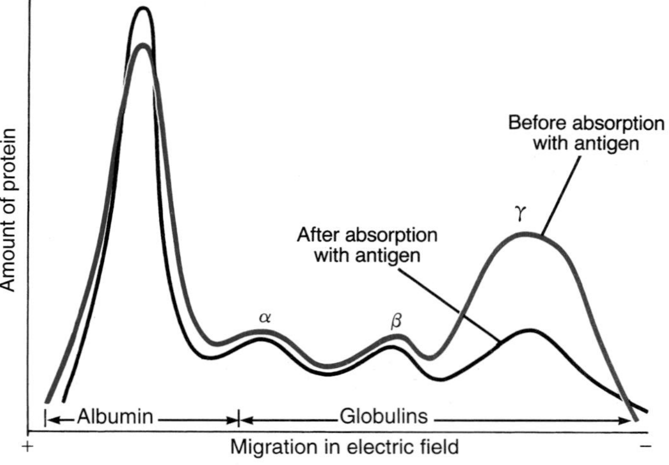

Antigen Binding

One parameter that bears importantly on the function of an antibody is its affinity for antigen, i.e., how tightly it binds the antigen molecule. As a simple paradigm for quantitating affinity, consider the binding reaction between a hapten H and antibody molecule A, a reversible reaction:

$$H + A \underset{K_d}{\overset{K_b}{\rightleftarrows}} HA$$

where K_b is the rate constant for binding, and K_d is the rate constant for dissociation. If antigen is introduced into an antibody-containing solution, the above reaction will proceed to the right until at equilibrium the rate of binding equals the rate of dissociation: $[H][A]K_b = [AH]K_d$ or $K = K_b/K_d = [HA]/[H][A]$, where K is known as the association constant, a measure of affinity.

This association constant can be measured by equilibrium dialysis (Fig. 4.2). For this determination, a known amount of antibody is placed inside of a dialysis bag, and variable amounts of radioactively labeled hapten are added to the solution outside the bag. The large size of the antibody molecule prevents efflux across the dialysis membrane, but the smaller hapten can readily diffuse through the membrane into the bag and then bind to the antibody. At equilibrium, the concentration of hapten outside the bag must equal the concentration of free (unbound) hapten inside the bag, so any excess of radioactivity/volume measured inside the dialysis bag is due to hapten bound to antibody. For a pure antibody that binds monovalently to antigen and shows no cooperativity effects, the same association constant will be calculated from the experimental data determined at every concentration of hapten. If similar experiments are performed with an antiserum containing a mixture of many antibodies with a range of affinities, the calculated association constant at low hapten concentration will reflect the antibodies of highest affinity, whereas at higher concentrations of hapten the calculated association constant will be lower. In this situation, an average association constant can be estimated

Figure 4.2 Equilibrium dialysis. A solution of antibody is placed inside a dialysis bag, and the bag is placed in a solution of free hapten. The dialysis bag is chosen to be permeable to the hapten but not to the antibody. Free hapten will dialyze into the bag, where it will be bound by larger antibody molecules. When the system reaches equilibrium, the concentration of hapten inside the bag will be equal to the concentration of free hapten outside the bag, plus the concentration of the hapten bound to the antibody inside the bag.

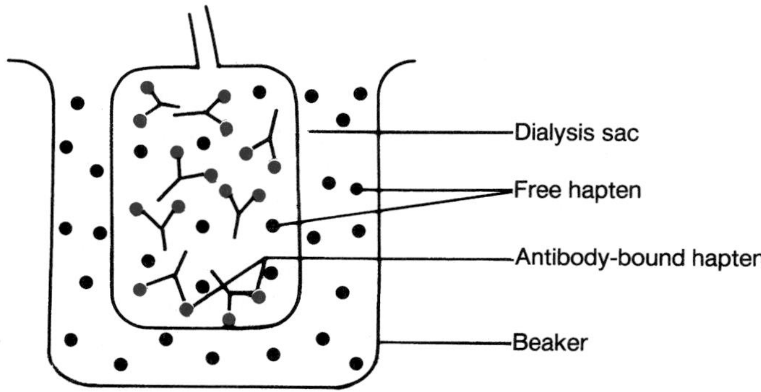

from the K measured when the antibody is 50% saturated with hapten. When such average association constants are measured at various times after immunization, it is generally observed that this average association constant increases during the course of an experimentally induced immune reaction *(affinity maturation)*. The mechanism of affinity maturation is addressed later in this chapter.

Clonal Selection

Early in the study of antibodies, it was recognized that an understanding of how these proteins recognize antigens would require knowledge of their primary structure, i.e., amino acid sequence. However, attempts at determining amino acid sequences of antibodies were hampered by the fact that any antibody response in a laboratory animal includes the products of a large number of different antigen-specific clones producing antibodies with heterogeneous structures; from such mixtures, little useful sequence information could be obtained. A logical solution to this technical problem derives from an understanding of the answer to a question posed above: how does a particular antigen elicit a narrow antibody response specifically targeted against that antigen?

The *clonal selection* theory championed by Sir Macfarlane Burnet in the 1950s, and subsequently proved correct, was based on the concept that any one B lymphocyte can make only a single species of antibody. Early in the development of an antibody-producing cell, at the B-cell stage, very little of this antibody is secreted; instead, the antibody is expressed on the outside surface of the cell membrane. This form of membrane immunoglobulin serves as an antigen-specific receptor that—on binding antigen—can trigger the B cell to proliferate and to mature to an antibody-secreting stage. Many millions of resting B cells circulate in the unimmunized animal, each displaying on its surface an antibody of a different structure and specificity. When a foreign antigen is administered, only the small population of B cells expressing a membrane antibody capable of binding the antigen will be triggered. These antigen-specific B cells then proliferate and subsequently mature into cells capable of secreting antibody of the same specificity originally displayed on the surface of the clonal progenitors. This hypothesis provided a satisfactory explanation for the selective elicitation of antibodies specific for an injected antigen, though it raised several additional questions addressed later in this chapter: (i) What is the difference in antibody structure between that expressed on the surface and the secreted form? (ii) What mechanism explains the shift between these two forms? (iii) Why does each B cell express only a single antibody, given the fact that it should have many genes for antibodies in each antibody gene locus and, as a diploid cell, two copies of each gene locus?

The clonal selection hypothesis provides a theoretical solution to the technical problem of obtaining a pure homogeneous antibody preparation for amino acid sequence analysis: homogeneous immunoglobulin can be obtained from a clonal population of lymphocytes derived from a single progenitor cell. Initially, such *monoclonal antibodies* were derived from *myelomas,* which represent clonal expansions of a single malignantly transformed B lymphoid cell; myelomas occur in humans and can be induced experimentally at high frequency in several inbred mouse strains. Generally, such myelomas are not targeted against a known antigen. To generate monoclonal antibodies against specific antigens, *hybridoma* technology was developed, originally by Milstein and Kohler. In this technique, a mouse is immunized with antigen and, after variable lengths of time, individual mice are sacrificed to obtain splenic B cells. These B cells are fused to a nonsecreting myeloma to yield hybrid cells: hybridomas. The antigen-specific splenic B cells contribute the antigen specificity of antibody production, whereas the myeloma cells contribute the transformed phenotype, allowing sustained proliferation. Cells secreting antibodies of desired properties can then be cloned from the fusion population and propagated, providing an immortal source of homogeneous antibody suitable for amino acid sequence determination.

Immunoglobulin Structure

Isotypes

A comparison of protein structural analyses of various myeloma proteins showed that human antibodies can be classified into five major classes, or *isotypes:* immunoglobulin G (IgG), IgA, IgD, IgE, and IgM, which are defined by "effector" properties that are independent of antigen specificity. In addition, IgG has four subclasses and IgA has two. The most abundant isotype in normal human serum is IgG, which exists in four subclasses designated IgG1 to IgG4 (in decreasing order of abundance in normal serum [Table 4.1]). All IgG antibodies have about the same molecular mass (about 150 kDa) and are composed of four disulfide-linked chains that can be separated by reduction in mercaptoethanol: two identical heavy (H) chains (about 50 kDa) and two identical light (L) chains (about 25 kDa). The antibody thus has a chain structure designated H_2L_2. The isotype of an antibody is defined by that of its heavy chain, which confers the biologic properties. The same two light-chain classes—κ and λ—can occur with any of the nine heavy-chain isotypes. The heavy chain contributing to IgG is known as γ, whereas the heavy chains of the other major isotype classes—IgA, IgD, IgM, and IgE—are known by the corresponding Greek letters α, δ, μ, and ϵ, respectively (see below for more details). Each heavy-chain isotype has a characteristic component of carbohydrate covalently bound at specific amino acid residues.

Prototype Molecule

Because of the high abundance of IgG (about 14 mg/ml in normal human serum) and its frequent representation in tumors of plasma cells (myelomas), it was the first isotype whose structure was determined, and it

Table 4.1 Biological properties of IgG subclasses

Property	IgG1	IgG2	IgG3	IgG4
Percentage of total IgG in serum	65	23	8	4
Complement fixation	++	+	+++	0
Placental transfer	+++	++	+++	+++
Passive cutaneous anaphylaxis[a]	+++	0	+++	+++
Receptor for macrophage	+++	0	+++	0
Reaction with staph protein A	+++	+++	0	+++
Prominent antibody activity	Anti-Rh	Anti-levan, anti-dextran	Anti-Rh	Anti-factor VIII

[a]Heterocytophilic antibody (see chapter 11).

remains a conceptual prototype for antibodies. The analysis of IgG structure was facilitated by the observation that the proteases papain and pepsin could clip the H_2L_2 IgG molecule in two different ways, defined by the position of the cleavage sites relative to the disulfide bonds linking the heavy chains (Fig. 4.3). Papain cleaves on the N-terminal side of these disulfide bonds, producing three fragments. Two identical fragments are known as Fab because they are capable of monovalent antigen binding. The third fragment is known as Fc because (in rare instances) it can be crystallized even when obtained from polyvalent antiserum (because Fc pieces lack the diversity of the antigen-binding fragments). In contrast to papain, pepsin cleaves on the C-terminal side of the disulfide linkages, yielding a fragment—$F(ab')_2$—that is divalent but lacks the effector properties characteristic of intact antibody. Apart from the importance of these protease fragments in the early protein structural analysis of IgG, they have also become useful laboratory tools because of their distinct functional properties.

Amino acid sequence analysis of purified fragments of heavy and light chains from IgG reveal repeated internal sequence similarities that reflect the domain structure of these polypeptide chains (Fig. 4.4). Each domain contains 100 to 110 amino acids (representing about 12 kDa) containing an internal disulfide loop and certain other characteristic amino acids.

Figure 4.3 Protease fragments of IgG. IgG molecules are cleaved by proteases to generate fragments that were used to determine the structure of IgG. The intact IgG molecule is indicated in the center. The heavy chain is indicated as a blue-green bar, and the light chain is indicated as a shorter white bar; in each case the N-terminal V domain is stippled, and the C domains are not. The thin black bars represent the disulfide bonds that link the heavy and light chains. Cleavage by papain produces three fragments: two identical fragments, the Fab fragments, can bind antigen but cannot cross-link the antigen (are univalent); and one, the Fc fragment, contains the C regions of the heavy chain. Cleavage by pepsin produces one fragment and many small fragments. The one large fragment consists of two Fab fragments linked by disulfide bonds because the pepsin cleaves the heavy chains on the C-terminal side of the disulfide bonds linking the two heavy chains. The Fc region is cleaved into small pieces.

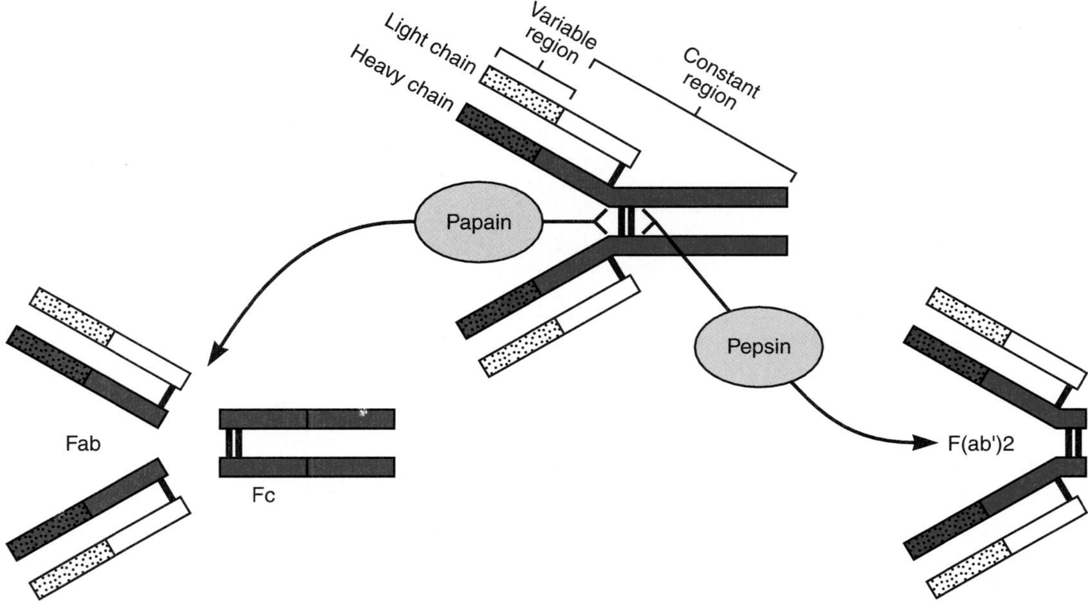

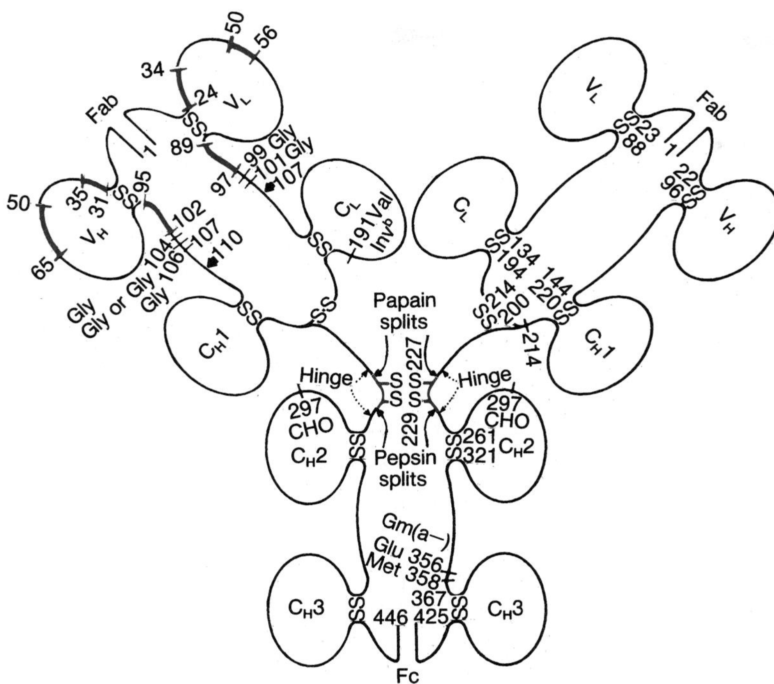

Figure 4.4 Schematic view of the four-chain structure of a human IgG molecule. Numbers on the right side indicate actual residues of a myeloma protein EU. Numbers of Fab fragments on the left side are aligned for maximum homology: light chains numbered according to E. A. Kabat (*J. Immunol.* **125:**961, 1980). Immunoglobulin domains are shown by the four "loops" formed by intrachain disulfide bonds (SS). V_L and V_H, light- and heavy-chain V domains. CH_1, CH_2, and CH_3, domains of the C region of the heavy chain. C_L, C region of the light chain. Hinge region in which two heavy chains are linked by disulfide bonds is indicated by the thin colored lines. Hypervariable regions (complementarity-determining regions) are indicated by thicker colored lines. Attachment of carbohydrate is at residue 297. Arrows at residues 107 and 110 denote the transition from V to C regions. Sites of action of papain before the hinge region and of pepsin after the hinge region show why papain produces Fab monomer and pepsin produces $F(ab)_2$ dimers. Locations of heritable allotypic differences (Gm on the heavy chain and Inv on the light chain) are shown.

Similar "immunoglobulin domains" have been found in a large number of surface proteins, probably reflecting a primitive and very ancient gene that underwent extensive duplication and diversification during evolution. These related proteins form a group known as the immunoglobulin superfamily, which includes T-cell receptors (the closest relatives of the immunoglobulins), major histocompatibility antigens, numerous cell adhesion molecules, and a number of other surface proteins with important function in the immune system (including CD4 and CD8).

Variable and Constant Domains

Sequence comparison among monoclonal antibody chains revealed a remarkable dichotomy between the N-terminal domain, which is highly variable, and all the remaining domains, which show essentially identical sequence when the corresponding domains are compared with different monoclonal chains of the same class. The diversity of the variable (V) domain reflects the function of this part of the molecule in binding diverse antigens, whereas the constant (C) domains confer the isotype-specific properties or "effector" functions of the immunoglobulin. The number of C region domains in heavy chains (C_H domains) depends on the isotype: μ and ϵ heavy chains have four C_H domains, while δ, γ, and α heavy chains each have three C_H domains, plus a "hinge" region between C_H1 and C_H2 that may be the evolutionary remnant of a primordial fourth domain. Three-dimensional structure analyses by X-ray crystallography have defined a common general structure in all immunoglobulin domains, which is conserved even in the nonimmunoglobulin members of the immunoglobulin superfamily. In this structure, the polypeptide backbone is folded into seven more or less parallel strands in the configuration known as β-pleated sheet (Fig. 4.5). In the intact H_2L_2 molecule, the V_H and V_L domains contact each other, as do the C_L and C_H1 domains; each remaining C_H domain contacts the corresponding domain of the other heavy-chain partner. These interactions lead to an H_2L_2 structure whose "Y" shape has been visualized by electron microscopy and, in greater detail, by X-ray crystallography (Fig. 4.6).

Effector Functions

The structural differences among the various heavy-chain isotypes are responsible for differences in effector functions of antibodies, i.e., their ability to act in certain locations or engage secondary protective mechanisms. These effector functions include the following:

1. *Opsonization* is the ability of an antibody to bind to a microorganism or particle to facilitate its phagocytosis or killing by cellular phagocytes (e.g., neutrophils, macrophages).
2. *Complement fixation* involves the activation of a complex cascade of serum proteins—known collectively as complement—that can lyse

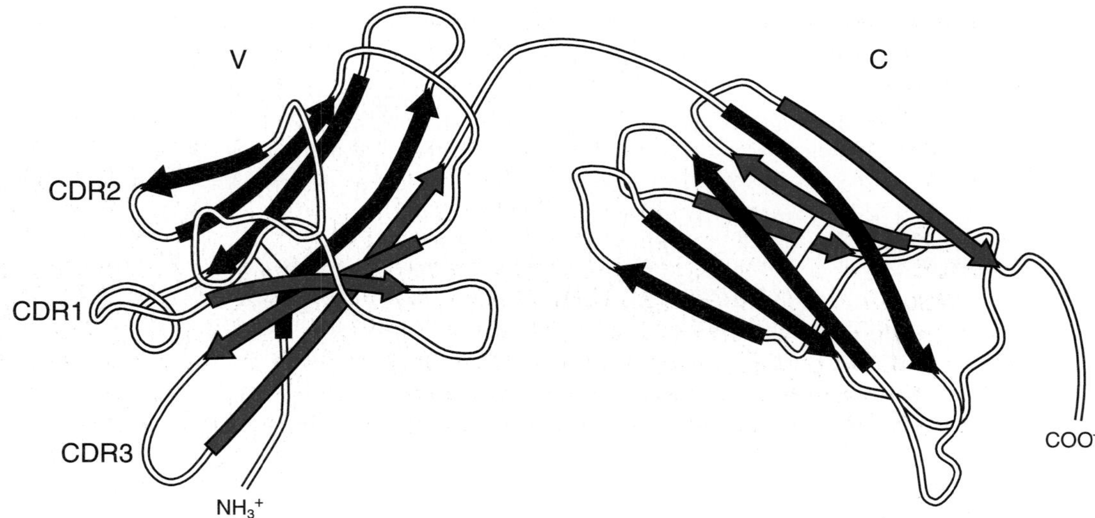

Figure 4.5 Ribbon diagram of a light chain. This three-dimensional view of the folding of the α carbon chain backbone is a visualization based on X-ray diffraction of immunoglobulin crystals. The V and C domains are rotated 160° with respect to each other. The broad arrows ("ribbons") show the seven segments of β-pleated sheet structure in each domain, with one face of three strands (blue-green) roughly parallel to another face of four strands. The loops projecting out at the left represent the three complementarity-determining regions (CDR1, CDR2, and CDR3), which, together with three similar loops from the heavy-chain V region, form the antigen-combining site.

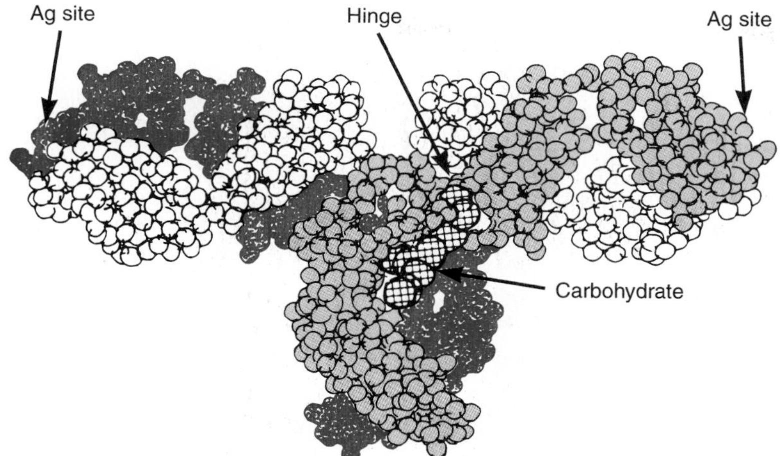

Figure 4.6 X-ray crystallographic space-filling three-dimensional model of an IgG molecule. One complete heavy chain is light blue-green, and the other is blue-green; each light chain is white, and carbohydrate is cross-hatched. The positions of the heavy-chain hinge and the two antigen (Ag) binding sites are labeled.

bacteria by chemically punching holes in them. Other functions of complement include chemotaxis (the attraction of phagocytes to an inflammatory site), enhancement of opsonization, and increasing the permeability of blood vessels (see chapter 3). Complement can be activated as a result of binding of antibody to antigen (the classical pathway) or directly by certain bacterial products (the alternate, probably more evolutionarily primitive, pathway).

3. *Neutralization* of viruses or toxins may result from binding of antibodies that produce alterations in the tertiary structure of the toxin. An antibody that neutralizes a toxin is known as an antitoxin.
4. *Antigen clearance* refers to the ability of the reticuloendothelial system to remove antigen from the serum; the presence of antigen-specific antibody can speed up antigen clearance.
5. The *release of chemical mediators* can be induced by binding of antigen to "cytophilic" antibody, i.e., antibody noncovalently bound to cell surface immunoglobulin receptors that bind via the Fc portion of the immunoglobulin molecule (Fc receptors); the classic example is IgE, discussed below.
6. *Isotypes* can be distinguished by their time of appearance after antigen administration or their ability to appear in certain locations, e.g., to cross the placenta or to appear in secretions.

Fc Receptors

The effector functions of antibodies are mediated by the Fc regions of their heavy chains. Apart from toxin neutralization and complement-mediated lysis of bacteria, most effector functions of antibodies depend on interactions of antigen-antibody complexes with cells of the immune system. These interactions are mediated by cell surface proteins known as Fc receptors (FcRs), which bind to specific isotypes of heavy-chain Fc regions: FcαR binds IgA, FcγR subtypes bind IgG, etc. FcRs generally have extracellular sections made of two—or in the case of FcγRI, three—immunoglobulinlike domains; FcϵRII, which is exceptional in several respects, has an extracellular region unrelated to immunoglobulin. On cross-linking to other FcRs or

Table 4.2 Properties of Fc receptors

	FcγRI	FcγRIIA	FcγRIIB	FcγRIIIA	FcγRIIIB	FcεRI	FcεγRII	FcαRI
Size (kDa)	70	40	40	50–70	50–70	8, 33, 45	45	60
Affinity	High	Low	Low	Medium	Low	High	Low	Medium
CD	64	32	32	16	16	NA	23	89
Distribution	Monocytes, IFN-γ-treated neutrophils	Monocytes, neutrophils, eosinophils,	Monocytes, granulocytes, B cells, platelets	Monocytes, natural killer cells	Neutrophils	Mast cells, basophils, eosinophils	B cells, monocytes, eosinophils platelets	Monocytes, neutrophils, eosinophils
Associated molecules	FcRγ dimer	γ-Like domain	γ-Like domain	β, FcRγ dimer	GP1	β, FcRγ dimer		FcRγ dimer
Activity	Antibody-dependent cell-mediated cytotoxicity, phagocytosis	Phagocytosis, granule release	Downregulate B-cell receptor activation decrease IR	Phagocytosis, antigen presentation	Clearance of immune complexes	Degranulation, phagocytosis	Antigen presentation IgE	Degranulation, phagocytosis

to other surface molecules, most FcRs transmit either of two kinds of signal. FcγRI, FcγRIII, FcϵRI, and FcαRI signal through an associated dimer of a γ-transduction protein highly similar to the ζ chain of the T-cell receptor transduction machinery (see chapter 5); FcγRIIA includes at its C terminus a similar γ-cytoplasmic domain. Like the ζ chain associated with the T-cell receptor, the FcRγ chain mediates signal transduction through phosphorylation of immunoreceptor tyrosine-based activation motifs (ITAMs). In contrast, FcγRIIB, the major FcR on B cells, signals through a cytoplasmic domain bearing an immunoreceptor tyrosine-based inhibitory motif (ITIM). A summary of some characterized FcRs is presented in Table 4.2.

Human Heavy-Chain Isotypes

A simplified comparison of the structure of the five major immunoglobulin classes is shown in Fig. 4.7. Many of their effector functions are discussed in the brief description of the human immunoglobulin isotypes below and are listed in Table 4.3.

IgM, at a concentration of about 1.5 mg/ml in normal serum, contributes about 10% of serum immunoglobulin and is present mostly as a pentamer with five H_2L_2 units covalently linked by disulfide bonds. IgM pentamers can be visualized by electron microscopy and appear to be joined at their C-terminal tips. Pentamer formation is facilitated by the presence of a 15-kDa protein known as the J chain, one molecule of which is linked by disulfide bonds to the $(IgM)_5$, creating a complex of about 950,000 kDa (with a sedimentation constant of 19S). This immunoglobulin was designated IgM because it is larger than the other immunoglobulins (macroglobulin). IgM is the first isotype expressed during fetal development and is also the first expressed during the development of each B lymphocyte. As a lymphocyte matures, it generally switches to expression of other isotypes, but, remarkably, the heavy-chain V region is not altered during this process, so the antigen-binding specificity does not change; the mechanism of the switch at the genetic level is discussed later in this chapter. The multivalency of serum IgM allows this isotype to bind efficiently to polyvalent antigen particles (such as microbes) even when the intrinsic affinity of each monomeric V_H-V_L pair for antigen may be relatively low. The Fc regions of the pentameric structure also provide very efficient complement fixation. Since aggregated Fc regions are required to fix complement, one IgM pentamer on the surface of a bacterium or cell is able to activate complement, whereas two IgG molecules must bind close together to accomplish complement activation. It is estimated that IgM is 600 times more efficient than IgG in fixing complement on reaction with a cell surface. The IgM isotype thus plays a particularly important role early in infections before affinity maturation has occurred. Because of its large size, IgM does not cross the placenta; thus, the presence in cord blood of IgM antibodies against a particular virus is presumptive evidence of fetal infection.

IgD is present in only low concentrations in serum (about 0.04 mg/ml), where it has no known function. It is present, along with IgM of the same antigen specificity, on the surface of immature B cells, where it is capable of triggering cell activation in response to antigen exposure. It is possible that IgD has its primary function in this membrane form, although extensive investigation has not fully clarified its role. Mice from a strain genetically engineered to lack IgD are competent to generate an antibody response to antigen challenge but take longer than normal to develop high-affinity antibodies through affinity maturation. When B cells are activated by antigen, cell surface IgD disappears as another isotype is expressed.

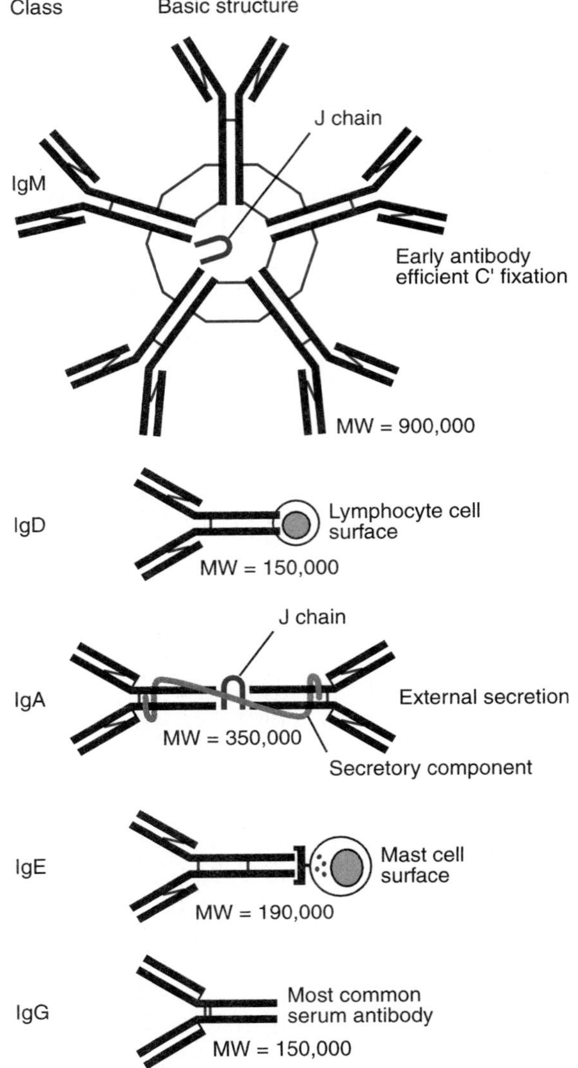

Figure 4.7 Comparison of immunoglobulin classes in humans. The five isotype classes (IgM, IgD, IgA, IgE, and IgG) contain similar basic subunits composed of two identical heavy chains (known as μ, δ, α, ϵ, and λ) and two identical light chains (either κ or λ) attached to each of the heavy chains. There are four human λ subtypes. Disulfide bonds link heavy and light chains, as shown by the thin blue-green lines, and also link IgA into dimers and IgM into pentamers. IgM pentamers and IgA dimers also contain a 15-kDa J (joining)-chain polypeptide. Two of the five Ig isotypes exert their major function bound to cells through the Fc region of their heavy chains—IgD as a lymphocyte receptor and IgE as an effector molecule on mast cells to which it is bound by the Fcϵ receptor on the mast cell.

IgA contributes only about 10 to 15% of serum immunoglobulin (normal range, about 2 to 3 mg/ml). However, since it is the predominant isotype in secretions (saliva, milk, tears, and secretions of lung, nasal, and intestinal mucosa), it is actually the predominant immunoglobulin in terms of daily production by the whole animal, playing a key role in defense against environmental pathogens. In secretions, it is generally present as a dimer of H_2L_2 units linked by a molecule of J-chain protein and covalently associated with a protein known as secretory component. The secretory

Table 4.3 Some properties of human immunoglobulins[a]

Property	Immunoglobulin class				
	IgG	IgA	IgM	IgD	IgE
Concn in serum (g/100 ml)	1.2	0.4	0.12	0.003	$<$0.00005
Sedimentation coefficient (S)	7	7 (9, 11, 13)[b]	19 (24, 32)[b]	7	8
Molecular weight	140,000	160,000[c]	900,000	180,000	200,000
Electrophoretic mobility	γ	Slow β	Between γ and β	Between γ and β	Slow β
Heavy chain	γ	α	μ	δ	ϵ
Light chain	λ or κ	λ or κ	λ or κ	λ or κ	λ or κ
Complement fixation	Yes	No	Yes	No	No
Placental transfer	Yes	No	No	No	No
Percent intravascular	40	40	70		
Half-life (days)	23	6	5	3	2.5
Percent carbohydrate	3	10	10	13	10
Antibody activity	Most antibody infections; major part of secondary response; Rh isoagglutinins; LE factor	Present in external secretions	First antibody formed; ABO isoagglutinins; rheumatoid factor	Antibody activity rarely demonstrated, found on lymphocyte surface	Reagin sensitizes mast cells for anaphylaxis

[a]Modified from J. L. Fahey, *JAMA* **194:**183, 1966.
[b]Figures in parentheses indicate the existence of other molecular forms, such as polymers.
[c]Serum IgA, 160,000; secretory IgA, 350,000; may activate alternate pathway (see chapter 10).

protein is not made by B lymphocytes but represents a fragment of the poly-Ig receptor on the surface of epithelial cells, a protein that mediates transepithelial transport of the IgA dimer into lumenal secretions. In humans, there are two IgA subclasses: IgA1, which predominates in serum, and IgA2, which is the (slightly) more abundant form in secretions.

IgE is by far the least abundant isotype in the serum of normal individuals (normal concentration, about 0.00005 mg/ml), but it is the isotype whose manifestations are perhaps most apparent to the average person because it accounts for all allergic reactions. IgE binds extremely tightly to receptors on the surface of mast cells and basophils. These receptors are known as FcϵRI to distinguish them from lower-affinity FcϵRII receptors found on some lymphocytes. When contact between antigen and surface-bound IgE causes cross-linking of the associated FcϵRI molecules, the latter can trigger the release of granules containing allergic mediators such as histamine, causing swelling, itching, rhinitis, bronchoconstriction, and so on (see chapter 11). This isotype is thought to play a beneficial role in defense against parasites, since helminth infestations are associated with striking increases in IgE concentrations.

IgG is by far the most abundant isotype in serum, contributing about 75 to 85% of total immunoglobulin. The four human IgG subclasses all have a similar monomeric H_2L_2 structure as described above, although the $\gamma 3$ subclass is distinguished by a very long hinge region containing 15 disulfide cross-links. All four subclasses cross the placenta, consistent with a major role for maternal IgG in fetal and neonatal immunity, but the subclasses do appear to have distinct functional roles. For example, IgG1 and IgG3 are able fix complement well (see chapter 3), whereas IgG2 is much weaker in this regard, and IgG4 does not fix complement at all. IgG2 is the major subtype of anticarbohydrate antibodies, for reasons unknown. Several forms of Fcγ receptor exist on macrophages, granulocytes, and natural killer cells (Table 4.2). Cross-linking of these receptors by interaction of bound antibody with polyvalent antigen particles leads to activation of cellular attack mechanisms (phagocytosis or antibody-dependent cell-mediated cytotoxicity [ADCC]). This mechanism explains the role of antibodies in promoting the killing of bacteria (opsonization), one of the earliest effects of antibodies to be described.

Light-Chain Isotypes

Each immunoglobulin molecule contains two light chains of the same isotype, κ or λ. The two light-chain classes in humans, κ and λ, are present in serum in a ratio of about 60% κ to 40% λ (in mice, the ratio is about 95% κ to 5% γ). Although one or the other light-chain class may predominate in certain immune responses, this ratio is thought to result from chance differences in the V region repertoire for these two classes; no important functional distinction between κ and λ is known.

Diversity of Antibody Specificity

The most remarkable feature of immunoglobulins is the striking diversity of the V regions. With few exceptions, all myelomas have distinct V regions, and even hybridoma antibodies specific for a particular antigen are gener-

Figure 4.8 Variability plot of the V domain of a heavy chain. A parameter reflecting sequence variability at each codon position in the heavy-chain V region shows three clusters of hypervariability. These are known as CDR1, CDR2, and CDR3. The V region of the heavy chain is folded so that the CDRs contact antigen and determine the specificity and, to some extent, the avidity of the binding reaction.

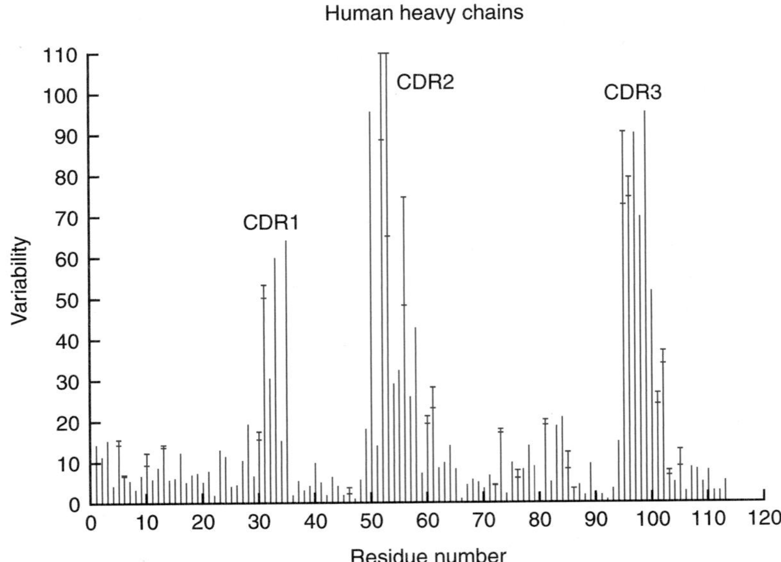

ally distinct. When this immense diversity was discovered, it was unprecedented in biology, and even now it is unmatched except for the related diversity of T-cell receptors. The puzzle of how such diversity might be encoded in the genome of an organism was complicated by the fact that the variability ended precisely at the boundary between the V and C regions of the protein; the molecular explanation for immunoglobulin diversity is discussed later. A plot of the amount of sequence variability at each of the approximately 110 positions in the V region (a "variability plot" [Fig. 4.8]) shows that the variability is not evenly distributed but rather is clustered into three "hypervariable" regions. These three hypervariable clusters were hypothesized to represent the complementarity-determining regions (CDRs), i.e., the amino acid residues that actually contact the diverse world of foreign antigens. This hypothesis was substantiated by the three-dimensional structures of antibody molecules determined by X-ray crystallography. The three hypervariable regions of the V_L and V_H domains form six loops that together constitute a surface capable of interacting with antigen (Fig. 4.4). The remaining residues of the V region domain create a framework (FR) that holds the CDR loops in proper position to contact antigen. Crystallographic analysis of several antigen-antibody complexes has characterized features of the interface between these two molecules, which generally conform to early models of a lock-and-key fit, as shown by the example in Fig. 4.9. A "bump" projecting from the antigen surface fits into a

Figure 4.9 Formation of an antigen-binding site (paratope) by folding of the V_H regions of the light and heavy chains of an antibody molecule so that the hypervariable regions responsible for binding the epitope are brought together. The numbers refer to amino acid residues. Glycine residues, which are usually present at the positions indicated, are important in chain folding. The hypervariable amino acid regions occur at specific positions in the peptide chain of the V_H regions. These "hot spots" lie relatively close together in the antigen-binding site and form a continuous surface capable of providing complementarity with a specific epitope. For a given antibody, not all the hypervariable regions need to be involved with binding of a given antigen.

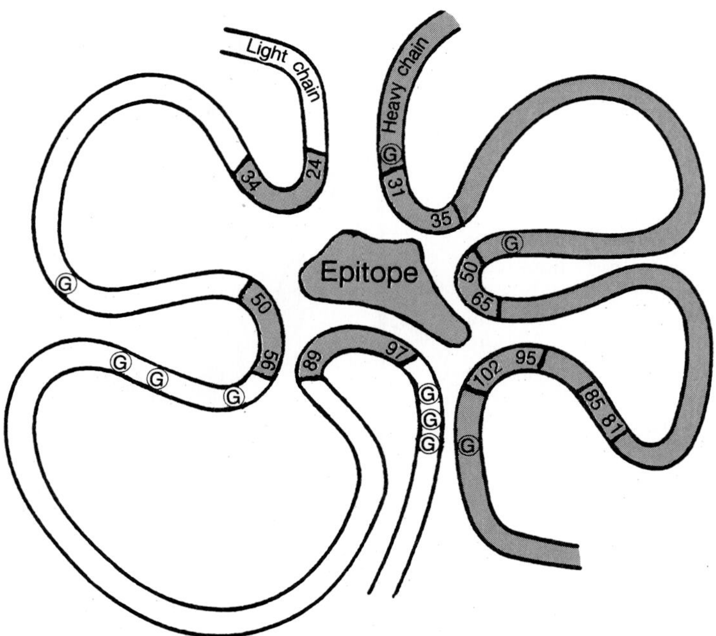

cavity on the antibody, and vice versa. The forces that bind protein antigens to antibodies are essentially the same as those that hold together the subunits of multimeric proteins: van der Waals forces, hydrophobic interactions, hydrogen bonds, and salt bridges (i.e., electrostatic forces between a positive charge on one surface and a negative charge on the other).

Antigenic Determinants (Epitopes)

The specific region on a macromolecular antigen that contacts the antibody is known as an *epitope* or *antigenic determinant* (Fig. 4.10). Most protein antigens have several epitopes. An epitope may be a linear sequence of amino acids or a protein surface composed of several loops that are not contiguous on the linear amino acid sequence of the antigen *(conformational epitopes)*. Because antibodies themselves are proteins, they can also serve as antigens (see below). The antibodies produced in a given animal are part of that individual's "self" and thus are not usually recognized as foreign by the immune system. The mechanism of this crucial discrimination, known as *tolerance,* is not fully understood, but there is evidence that during the fetal and early neonatal development of the immune system, lymphocytes making antibodies that are capable of recognizing self antigens are either eliminated or disabled from producing antibody to self antigens. B-cell tolerance is addressed later in this chapter. Failures of development of self tolerance are responsible for autoimmune diseases.

Idiotypes

In contrast to the tolerance-producing effects of potential antigens during the neonatal period, when a new foreign antigen is encountered later in life, it generally provokes an antibody response. Some V regions—either from

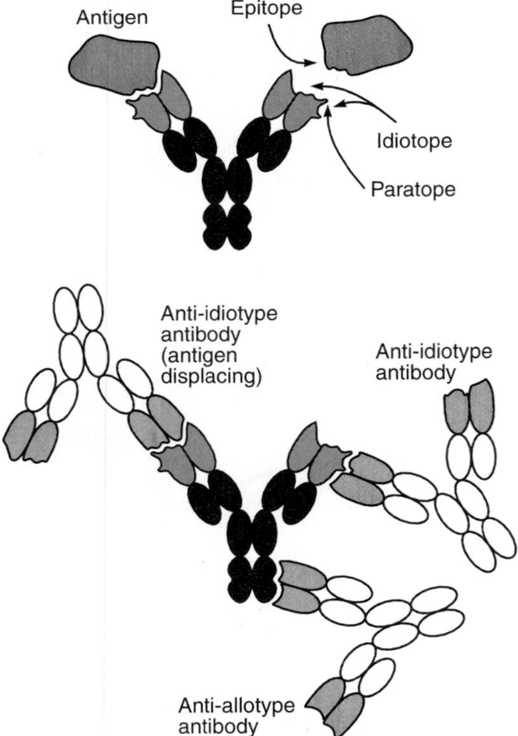

Figure 4.10 Paratopes, epitopes, idiotypes, and allotypes. The two contact surfaces between antibody and antigen (upper panel) are known as paratope (antigen-binding site) on the antibody and epitope on the antigen. An antibody may be recognized as an antigen by another antibody, and, depending on the part recognized, these are known as anti-idiotypes or antiallotypes. Anti-idiotypes are unique to each antibody and may react with the paratope, with sites adjacent to the paratope or both. Antiallotypes are genetically inherited determinants that are present in different antibodies in the same individual (see below).

antibodies newly synthesized in vivo or from antibodies injected into syngeneic animals—may look sufficiently foreign to the immune system that these antibody V regions induce their own second level of immune response. The resulting antibodies are known as *anti-idiotypic* and are said to recognize an *idiotype* in the V region of the injected antibody. An anti-idiotypic antibody may interfere with the binding of the injected antibody to its antigen if is directed against an epitope in the region of the antibody that binds antigen (paratope). Other anti-idiotype antibodies may recognize FR residues in the V region and thus fail to interfere with antigen binding (Fig. 4.9). It has been speculated that the immune response might be regulated by an idiotype/anti-idiotype network of interactions, but there is little solid evidence for a significant physiological role of such regulation.

Xenotypes and Allotypes

Another way that an antibody may act as an antigen is if it is injected into a recipient whose own antibodies differ in structure from the injected antibody. This may occur if the injected antibody derives from a different species (a *xenogeneic* antibody). Even within the same species, genetic polymorphisms between individuals—allelic genes—can create differences in immunoglobulin structure sufficient to induce an antibody response in a recipient. Such differences within a species are known as *allotypic,* and the resulting anti-allotypic antibodies can be useful laboratory reagents. For example, if B cells from a mouse of allotype 1 are injected into a recipient mouse of allotype 2, the production of antibody by the donor cells can be monitored by measuring the production of allotype 1 antibody. The allotypic variations most commonly studied are in the C regions, but V region allotypes are also known. In human immunoglobulins, about 30 different allotypic specificities have been described.

Antibody-Antigen Reactions

The laboratory techniques used to detect and measure antigen-antibody reactions have been critical tools in the development of immunological knowledge; because of the extreme specificity and sensitivity of antibodies, these techniques have also been widely used in other fields including protein chemistry, molecular biology, forensics, and clinical medicine. The first laboratory methods developed employed natural (unmarked) antigens and antibodies; in these methods, detection of antigen-antibody complex formation depended on a resulting visible change (precipitation or agglutination) or a physiological consequence of such formation (complement fixation). More modern techniques (described later) use antibodies bound to solid supports or tagged with enzymes, fluorescent dyes, or radioactivity.

Precipitin Reaction

Many techniques for detecting antigen-antibody complexes using unlabeled antibodies depend on formation of insoluble particles (precipitation). The insolubility of antigen-antibody complexes results from the fact that each H_2L_2 antibody molecule is divalent (has two antigen-combining sites), while most natural antigens are multivalent (have multiple copies of an epitope). Thus, under appropriate conditions, a complex lattice containing large numbers of antibody and antigens forms, leading to an insoluble particle (Fig. 4.11); such particles accumulate as a visible precipi-

Figure 4.11 The quantitative precipitin reaction. If increasing amounts of antigen are added in separate tubes to constant amounts of antiserum, the amount of precipitate increases to a maximum point and then decreases. This phenomenon results from the nature of the precipitate: a large network of multivalent antigen and divalent antibody forming a lattice structure that becomes insoluble as the mass of the lattice displaces surface ions required to maintain solubility. When either antibody or antigen is in excess, the amount of cross-linking is insufficient to form an insoluble lattice. The concentration ratio of antigen and antibody yielding maximum precipitation is called the "equivalence point." Determination of the equivalence point by this type of titration can be used to measure the amount of antibody if the antigen concentration is known or to measure the amount of antigen if the antibody concentration is known.

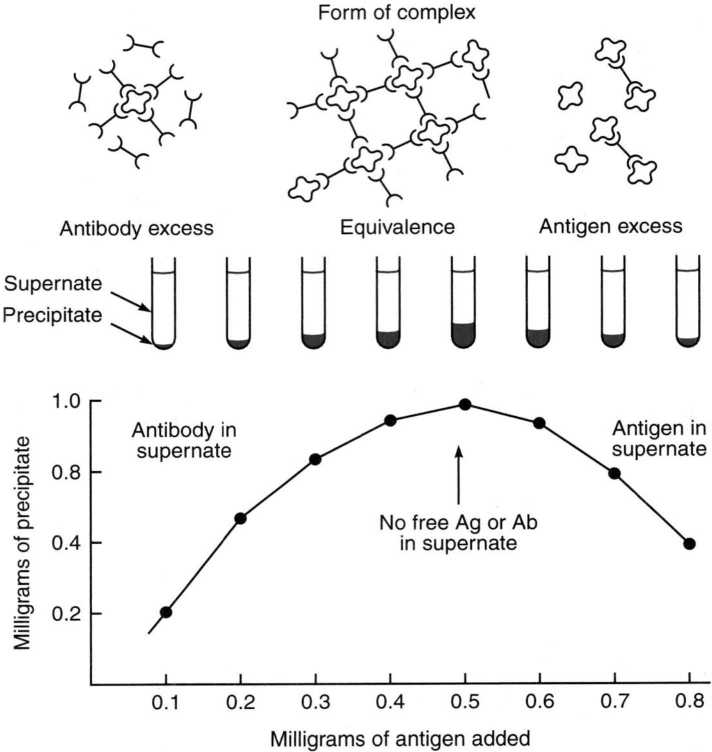

tate (precipitin reaction). Precipitates do not form if either antigen or antibody is present in too high a concentration. The sensitivity of the precipitin reaction to both antigen and antibody concentrations means that if antibody concentration is held constant, a measure of the antigen concentration can be obtained by determining the dilution of antigen that produces optimal precipitation, i.e., the "equivalence" concentration; conversely, if antigen concentration is held constant, the precipitin reaction can be used to estimate antibody concentrations.

Immunodiffusion

Several laboratory techniques are based on the fact that precipitin reactions can occur in aqueous gels like agar, which can support a concentration gradient because convection is prevented. For *single diffusion in agar,* developed by Jacques Oudin, a solution of antigen is placed over agar containing antibody in a tube (Fig. 4.12). The antigen diffuses into the agar until the equivalence point is reached. The distance that the antigen migrates can be used to measure the antigen.

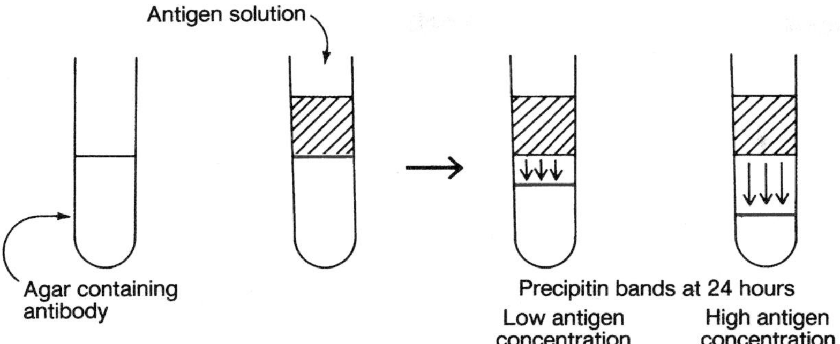

Figure 4.12 Simple gel diffusion, or Oudin, tube. A solution of antigen is placed over agar containing antibody in a tube. A precipitin band will form where the antigen meets the antibody. The precipitin band will move into the agar as more antigen from the solution diffuses into the agar. The distance that the band moves into the agar at any point in time is a function of concentration of the antigen added (higher concentration of antigen results in further diffusion into the agar). By comparison of the distance of migration of bands formed by known concentrations of an antigen with the distance of migration of band produced by solutions containing unknown amounts of the same antigen, an accurate measure of the antigen concentration in the unknown solution can be made.

In a simple *radial diffusion assay* (Fig. 4.13), antibody is incorporated into a flat gel matrix at a uniform concentration. Cylindrical holes, or wells, are cut in the gel. Then a solution of antigen—whose concentration is to be determined—is pipetted into one well, while a series of known concentrations of antigen is distributed into the other wells. A diffusion gradient of antigen concentration forms around each well, and a precipitin ring forms at a position where the diffusing antigen and the constant concentration of antibody reach the equivalence point. This will occur far

Figure 4.13 Radial immunodiffusion, a simple method for quantitation using the principle of the equivalence point between antibody and antigen. Antigen is placed in a well in an agar gel containing a known concentration of antibody. As antigen diffuses into the agar, it forms a precipitin ring at the equivalence point. The higher the concentration of the antigen, the larger the precipitin ring will be.

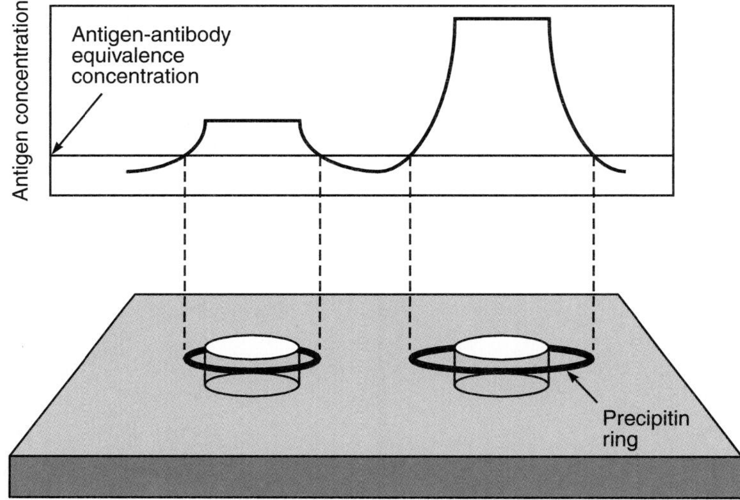

from a well containing abundant antigen, producing a large ring, while a smaller ring will form around a well containing less antigen. The concentration of the unknown solution can be determined from the diameter of the precipitin ring it produces, based on the diameters of the rings formed by the standards. The assay can be reversed to measure antibody concentration against a standard of antibody dilutions in a gel containing a constant concentration of antigen.

An elegant variation of the radial diffusion assay is the *double diffusion* or *Ouchterlony* technique. Antigen and antibody solutions are placed separately in two adjacent wells cut in a gel. As both molecules diffuse out from the wells, they form a precipitin line at a position reflecting the equivalence point. If one well containing an antiserum is placed near two wells containing two antigen preparations (Fig. 4.14), the pattern of precipitin lines can indicate whether more than one different antigen, or epitopes on the same antigen, are recognized by the antiserum.

Immunoelectrophoresis

If an antiserum recognizes many different antigens, precipitin lines in Ouchterlony plates may be too complex to be interpreted. In that case, immunoelectrophoresis may be useful (Fig. 4.15). In this method, the antigen mixture, typically serum proteins, is placed in a well and subjected to a voltage gradient that partially separates the proteins from one another electrophoretically. Antiserum is then placed in a linear well parallel to the

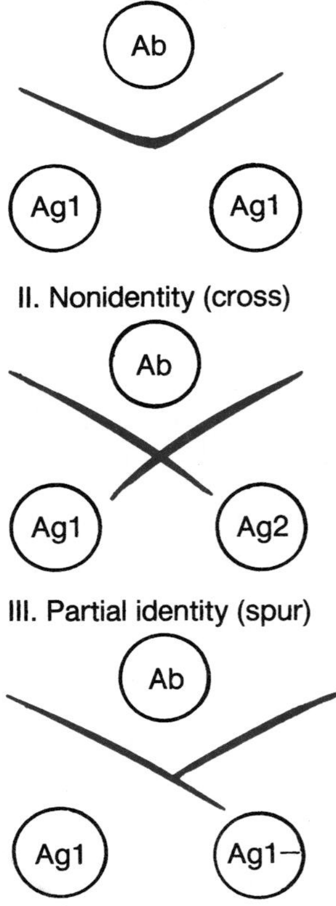

Figure 4.14 Double diffusion in agar (Ouchterlony) technique. If two identical antigen solutions (Ag1) are placed in adjacent agar wells, and an appropriate antiserum (Ab) is placed in an equidistant well, two precipitin bands will form and will fuse (reaction of identity) because the antigen is the same. If two different antigens (Ag1 and Ag2) are placed in adjacent wells, and antibody to both antigens is placed in an equidistant well, the two precipitin lines will cross since the two antigen-antibody precipitations occur independently (reaction of nonidentity). If an antigen with multiple epitopes is placed in one well (Ag1), and a related antigen sharing some, but not all, epitopes is placed in the second well ($Ag1^-$), the antibodies directed against the shared epitopes will form a fused precipitation pattern (identity reaction); but antibodies against epitopes of Ag1 missing in $Ag1^-$ will not interact with that molecule and will form a "spur," extending the precipitin line between Ab and Ag1.

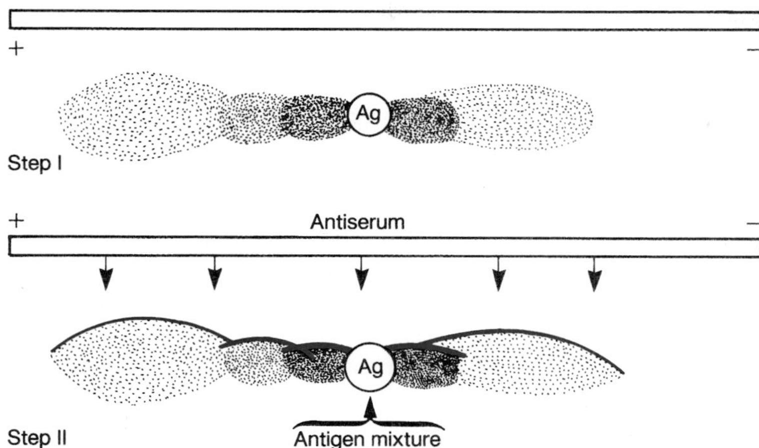

Figure 4.15 Immunoelectrophoresis. To visualize the precipitin lines formed between multiple protein antigens and a mixture of antibodies, the antigens are placed in a well cut into an agar gel (Ag) and subjected to a voltage gradient (electrophoresis), which causes the proteins to move into the gel (step I); the final position of each protein (shaded areas) depends on its charge and size. After electrophoresis, the antibody mixture is placed in a linear trough and allowed to diffuse toward the separated protein antigens (step II). An arc-shaped precipitin line is formed at the equivalence point of each antibody-antigen combination.

row of separated antigens and allowed to diffuse toward the antigens, creating precipitin lines that allow visualization of multiple antigens.

Agglutination

Antibodies may be detected by *hemagglutination* when present in concentrations too low to form a visible precipitate. This method depends on the formation of a link between two red blood cells (or bacteria or antigen-coated latex particles) by a single divalent antibody recognizing an antigen on the surface of the particles (Fig. 4.16). The complexed particles form a diffuse mat coating the round-bottomed well of a microtiter plate, whereas in the absence of agglutinating antibody, the free particles roll to the bottom in a tight grouping. The highest antibody dilution showing agglutination can be used as a measure of antibody concentration. Soluble antigen can inhibit agglutination by competing for antibody molecules, providing a sensitive assay for soluble antigen.

Complement Fixation

(See chapter 3.) Antibodies that fix complement can be detected by the consumption of complement activity. In such a *complement fixation assay,* a test antiserum is mixed with antigen, and then a small amount of complement is added. After an incubation to allow for immune complexes to consume complement, red blood cells (RBCs) and an anti-RBC antibody are added. The amounts of reagents are adjusted so that the complement added is just enough to lyse the RBCs coated with antibody; then the persistence of unlysed RBCs can be used as a measure of complement consumed by the initial antigen-antibody reaction. Some antisera may contain preexisting complement-consuming immune complexes, and some sera or

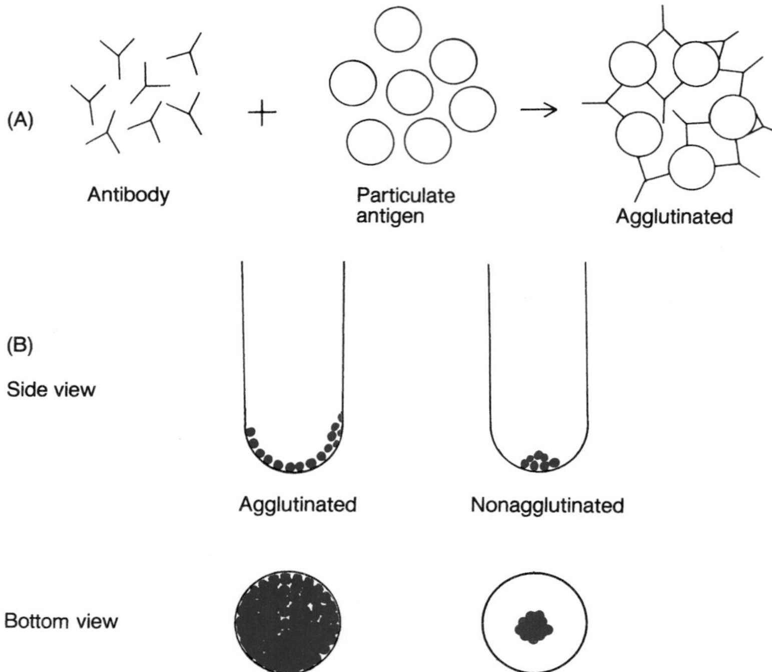

Figure 4.16 Agglutination of particulate antigens. **(A)** Divalent antibody forms a lattice with multivalent particulate antigen. **(B)** Agglutinated particles settle to the bottom of a round-bottomed tube in a diffuse layer, whereas nonagglutinated particles roll down the sides of the tube to form a tight "button" at the bottom. The difference between these patterns is easily seen from below the tube.

antigen preparations contain complement inhibitors; these possibilities require careful controls for complement fixation assays.

Radioimmunoassay

The detection of binding between antigen and antibody has in recent years benefited from a variety of technologies that allow one or the other reactant to be bound to solid supports or to be tagged with dyes, enzymes, or radioactive markers. A diverse repertoire of assay techniques has resulted. In the *radioimmunoassay,* antibodies have been used to quantitate the amount of a specific antigen (Fig. 4.17).

A standard amount of radioactively labeled antigen is incubated with an antigen-specific antibody in amounts that bind to about 60 to 70% of the antibody. The antibody is removed from solution (by ammonium sulfate precipitation or adsorption to a solid support), taking with it any bound radioactive antigen, which can be measured by quantitating the radioactivity. If unlabeled antigen is added in the initial incubation, some radioactive antigen will be displaced from the antibody. By measuring the displacement caused by standard amounts of unlabeled antigen, a standard curve can be prepared that allows one to deduce the amount of antigen in an unknown sample by the amount of radioactivity it displaces.

Immunolabeling

Antibodies can be tagged with fluorescent dyes or enzymes using chemical techniques that leave antigen binding intact. Tagged antibodies specific for cell components or surface markers can be used to stain tissue sections

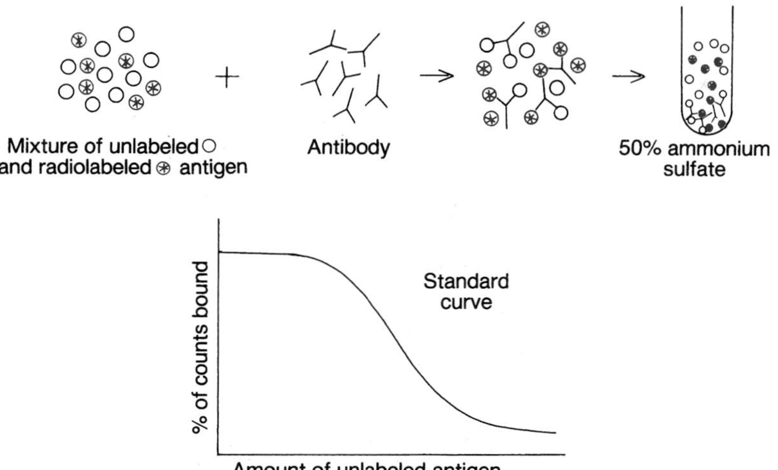

Figure 4.17 Radioimmunoassay. Very small amounts of antigen may be accurately measured by the ability of the antigen to compete with radiolabeled antigen binding to antibody. If a mixture of unlabeled and radiolabeled antigen is added to an antibody solution in slight antigen excess, the amount of labeled antigen bound to the antibody is a function of the amount of unlabeled antigen present. On the basis of this competition, a standard curve can be constructed by adding increasing amounts of unlabeled antigen to constant amounts of labeled antigen and antibody. When relatively small amounts of unlabeled antigen are present, all of the radiolabeled antigens will be precipitated. As the amount of unlabeled antigen is increased, less radiolabeled antigen is bound to the antibody. When a standard curve using increasing amounts of known unlabeled antigen has been constructed, the amount of antigen in an unknown solution can be determined by comparing the degree of inhibition of binding of labeled antigen by the unknown antigen solution to that produced by known amounts of the same antigen.

or live cells. An indirect staining strategy relieves investigators of the necessity to individually tag multiple antibodies: nontagged murine monoclonal antibodies against various cell components can be incubated with tissue sections, and then the location of bound antibodies is determined by staining with a single fluorescence-tagged xenogeneic antibody directed against murine immunoglobulin (Fig. 4.18). In these techniques, it is important to control for natural fluorescence of the cells and for nonspecific binding of the fluorescence-tagged antibody. One variation of fluorescent antibody staining with clinical importance is a test used to detect antibodies against *Treponema pallidum,* the infectious agent of syphilis. A patient's serum is incubated with a slide on which *T. pallidum* bacteria have been fixed, and the slide is treated with fluorescence-tagged anti-human antibody; the presence of fluorescent-labeled bacteria indicates that the patient was exposed to this agent.

Fluorescent antibody tagging has been extensively exploited in a technique widely used in immunology to characterize different cell populations in the immune system by the surface markers exposed on their cell membranes. In *flow cytometry,* a population of cells is stained with a fluorescent antibody against a specific membrane antigen. The solution with suspended cells is then passed in a thin stream through a laser fluorometer, which measures the fluorescence of each cell as it passes the detector and stores the information on a computer. Antibodies with different colored fluorescent dyes can be used to stain simultaneously for more than

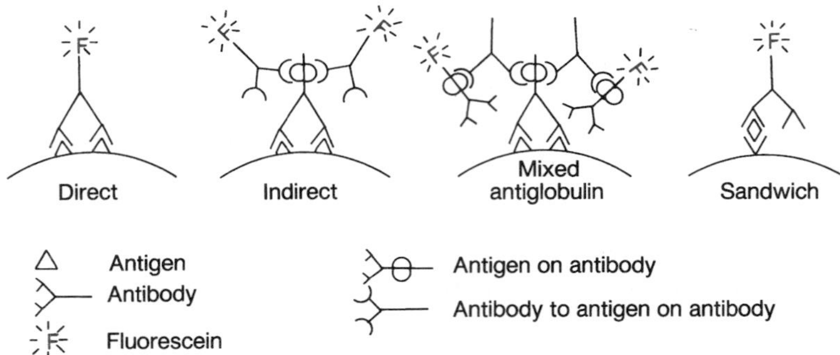

Figure 4.18 Fluorescent antibody techniques for detecting antigens in tissues. In the direct technique, specific antibody is labeled with fluorescent compound and added to tissue sections. The reaction of specific antibody to antigenic sites in the tissue sections is detected by exposing the labeled tissue sections to UV light and visualizing areas that "light up" under a fluorescence microscope. In the indirect technique, unlabeled antibody is incubated with tissue antigen. Fluorescein-labeled antibody to the first antibody is then added. The first antibody provides more antigenic sites for the second antibody to bind than was provided by the tissue antigen, increasing the technique's sensitivity. In the mixed antiglobulin technique, antigens on the first antibody are used to react to binding sites of the second antibody. The second antibody is then labeled by adding fluorescently labeled immunoglobulin of the same species as that of the first antibody. This variation of the technique is especially useful in labeling surface immunoglobulin molecules when the tissue antigen is an immunoglobulin. To identify antibody rather than antigen in tissue sections, a "sandwich" technique is used. Antigen is added to tissue and is bound by the specific antibody in the tissue. Specific fluorescein-labeled antibody to antigen is added and reacts with antigen now bound to the antibody in the tissue.

Figure 4.19 Identification of different cell types in the blood by flow cytometry. **(A)** In the first passage, preparations of white blood cells that have had red cells removed by lysis are "gated" by forward and side light scattering. Light is scattered by cytoplasmic granules. This identifies those white cells that contain granules (polymorphonuclear leukocytes and monocytes) and separates them from lymphocytes. Each dot represents a cell. The large groups of cells to the right with high side scatter are granulocytes; the group of cells at the top to the left with high forward scatter are monocytes. The cells in the area outlined in blue-green are lymphocytes. **(B)** The fraction containing the lymphocytes (which do not scatter light) is stained for CD3 (T-cell receptor) and CD4 (T-helper cells). Four quadrants are identified: $CD3^-$ $CD4^-$, $CD3^-CD4^+$, $CD3^+$ $CD4^-$, and $CD3^+$ $CD4^+$. The first quadrant identifies null cells; the second identifies residual monocytes that are weakly $CD4^+$; the third identifies non-$CD4^+$ T cells, most likely $CD8^+$ T-suppressor cells; and the fourth identifies $CD4^+$ T-helper cells.

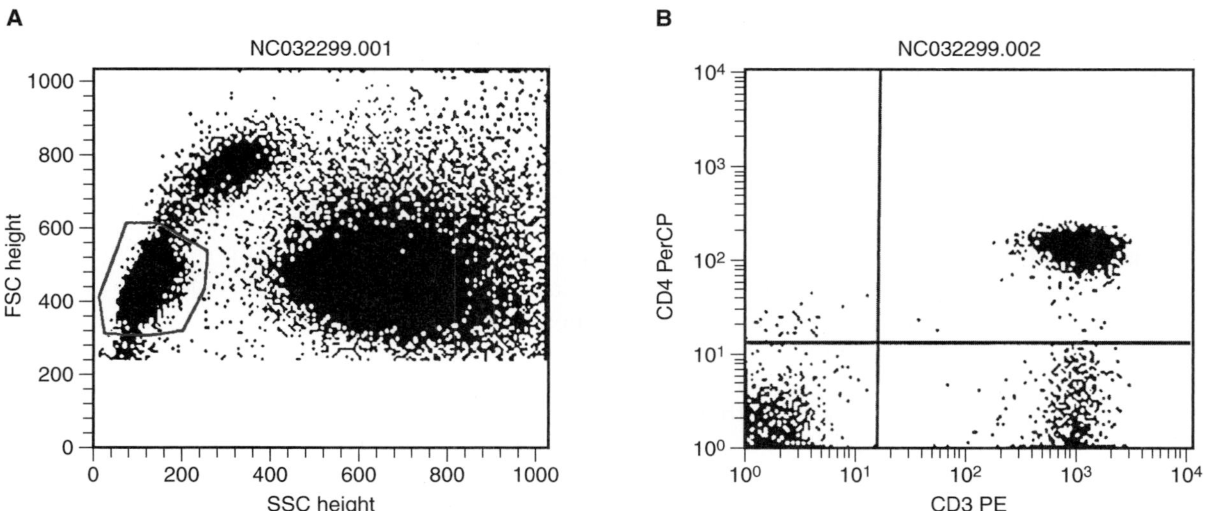

one antigen. The fluorometer can also be adjusted to detect the size of the cells and the presence of granules in the cells by properties of the scattered light. Thus, as shown in Fig. 4.19, it is possible to identify the phenotypes of different cell populations in a mixture of cells.

In a powerful preparative variation of this technique known as *fluorescence-activated cell sorting (FACS),* cells with particular staining characteristics can be sorted into separate tubes; this is done by converting the stream into droplets containing single cells, giving each droplet a measured charge according to its staining characteristics, and then deflecting the charged droplets into the appropriate tube by a controlled electric field (Fig. 4.20). Cell populations expressing certain surface markers can also be purified by antibodies coupled to microscopic magnetic beads; the bound cells are then separated from unbound cells by subjecting the cell suspension to a strong magnetic field.

As an alternative to fluorescence, antibodies can be labeled with enzymes, whose catalytic activity can be used to amplify the signal of an antigen-antibody complex by causing the deposition of an insoluble product or the release of a colored or fluorescent product. Such labeled antibodies can be used to stain tissue sections *(immunohistochemistry)* or

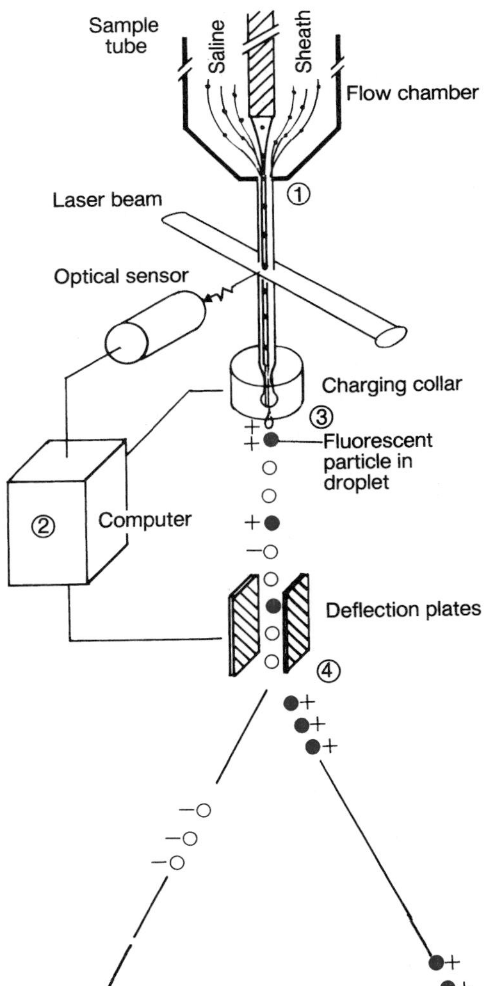

Figure 4.20 Fluorescence-activated cell sorting. **(1)** Fluorescently stained cells are forced out of a small nozzle, forming a stream in which they pass through a laser beam one cell at a time. **(2)** An optical sensor linked to a computer detects fluorescent characteristics and classifies each cell according to conditions set by the investigator (e.g., light scattering, different fluorescent wave lengths, size). **(3)** As the stream forms droplets—containing no more than one cell—the computer imparts a positive, negative, or zero charge to each droplet based on the fluorescence wave length emitted by each labeled cell. **(4)** The charged droplets pass between charged plates, which deflect the droplets into appropriate collection tubes.

proteins that have been separated by electrophoresis and then blotted onto a membrane support *(Western blotting)* (Fig. 4.21). One of the most versatile and widely used techniques involving enzyme tagging is the *enzyme-linked immunosorbent assay (ELISA)* (Fig. 4.22). In a simple ELISA method for assaying antigen, varying amounts of the antigen—a standard curve and unknown solutions to be assayed—are adsorbed to the wells of a 96-well plastic microtiter plate; after "blocking" nonspecific protein absorption by treatment with a protein mixture and washing steps, an enzyme-linked antibody is pipetted into the wells and allowed to react with the antigen; unbound antibody is then washed out, and a chromogenic substrate of the enzyme is pipetted into the wells. The amount of colored dye released by the bound enzyme can then be determined by an automated plate reader and used to quantitate antigen based on the standard curve of known antigen concentrations. Numerous variations of this technique have been devised to take advantage of the convenience of a solid support that can be used to process multiple samples in automated machines.

Antibody Affinity Chromatography

Many of the methods discussed above require purified antibody for their operation. An antibody may be purified by column chromatography through a support on which antigen is displayed. The antigen-specific antibody is bound tightly while contaminating proteins are washed away; then the antibody can be released by altering the salt concentration or pH. Conversely, columns made with purified antibodies bound to a solid sup-

Figure 4.21 Immunodetection of proteins on one-dimensional (1D) and two-dimensional (2D) gels. The left panel shows three lanes from a Western blot. The first two lanes show protein bands as detected by a nonspecific protein stain. Lane 3 shows the result of transferring the same set of proteins in lane 2 onto a solid support and then immunostaining with a labeled antibody; a subset of the total proteins is detected (blue-green bands). The right panel shows a similar comparison between proteins detected by nonspecific protein staining after sodium dodecyl sulfate-polyacrylamide gel electrophoresis (SDS-PAGE) (upper panel) and the subset of proteins detected after blotting to a solid support and immunostaining (blue-green spots in lower panel).

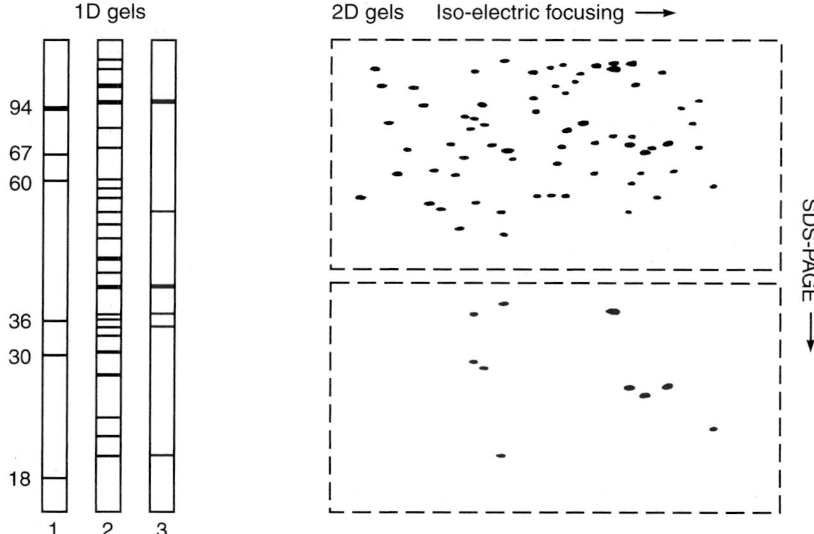

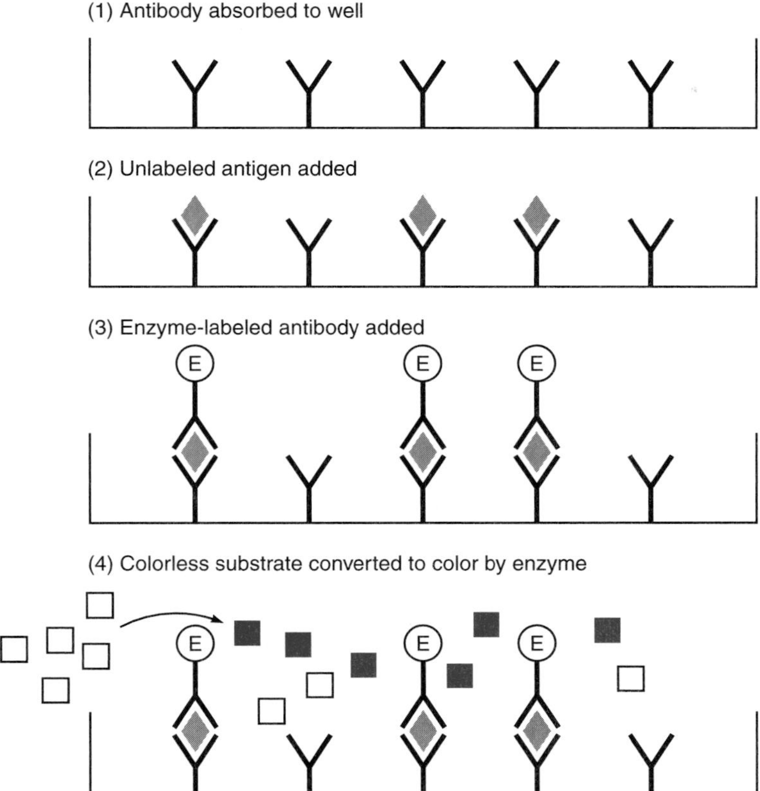

Figure 4.22 Variation of ELISA technology known as a "sandwich" assay, because the antigen is detected sandwiched between two antibody molecules—unlabeled antibody bound to the plate and an enzyme-labeled antibody added after the antigen has reacted with the antibody bound to the plate. After the wells of a microtiter plate are coated with a constant amount of antibody and then "blocked" by absorption of nonspecific proteins, varying known amounts of antigen are added to different wells and allowed to bind to antibody on the plate. An enzyme-linked antibody against the antigen is then added in excess, and unbound antibody is removed by washing. Finally, a solution containing chromogenic substrate is added, and the rate of color production is measured in an automated plate reader; fluorogenic substrates may also be used with fluorescence-detecting plate readers.

port have been widely used to purify the corresponding antigen. Recent genetic technologies have made it easier to clone genes than to purify low-abundance proteins. In many cases, it has been possible to generate antisera reactive against a protein whose structure is known only from its gene; such antisera can be obtained by immunizing with peptides synthesized according to the amino acid translation of the cloned gene. C-terminal peptides are frequently useful for this strategy.

Neutralization Tests

(See also chapter 8.) The activity of antisera to bacteria or viruses may be tested by the ability of such sera to reduce the viability of suspensions of these organisms when cultured in vitro. The effect is usually measured by the rate of loss of viability of the target organism upon addition of dilutions of the antisera. The ability to elicit "neutralizing" antibodies is crucial for determining the effectiveness of some vaccines. In experimental studies, the effect of dilutions of antisera on infectivity is titered using mixtures of infective organisms and antisera, which are then injected into test animals.

Antigen-Antibody Reaction In Vivo

Antigen-antibody reactions may occur in the blood or other tissues of living individuals. Such reactions may elicit a number of inflammatory reactions that are discussed in detail in later chapters on antibody-mediated immunopathologic reactions.

Immune Elimination

The presence of antibody in the circulation leads to rapid clearance of antigens (Fig. 4.23). Reaction of antibody with antigen results in formation of aggregated Ig components and activation of complement, which *opsonizes* the complexes and results in clearance of the antigen-antibody complexes

Figure 4.23 Immune elimination. A three-stage elimination of diffusible antigen from the bloodstream of previously nonimmunized animals has been observed. Upon intravascular injection of antigen, the blood level of antigen drops rapidly until only about 40% of injected antigen remains in blood. This is due to equilibration of diffusible antigen between intravascular and extravascular fluid compartments (equilibration phase). After this rapid equilibration, antigen is slowly removed by normal metabolic processes (nonimmune catabolism phase) until the onset of antibody production between 7 and 10 days after antigen injection. Appearance of antibody results in rapid elimination of antigen (immune elimination phase) due to formation of antigen-antibody complexes and their removal by the reticuloendothelial system. During the first part of the immune elimination phase, soluble antigen-antibody complexes (formed in antigen excess) may be demonstrated in the blood until there is enough antibody to form insoluble or antibody excess complexes. These soluble complexes are responsible for the lesions of serum sickness (see chapter 10). After antigen is completely removed, free antibody appears in the blood. If antigen is injected into an animal that already has circulating antibody, antigen is removed in one rapid immune elimination phase.

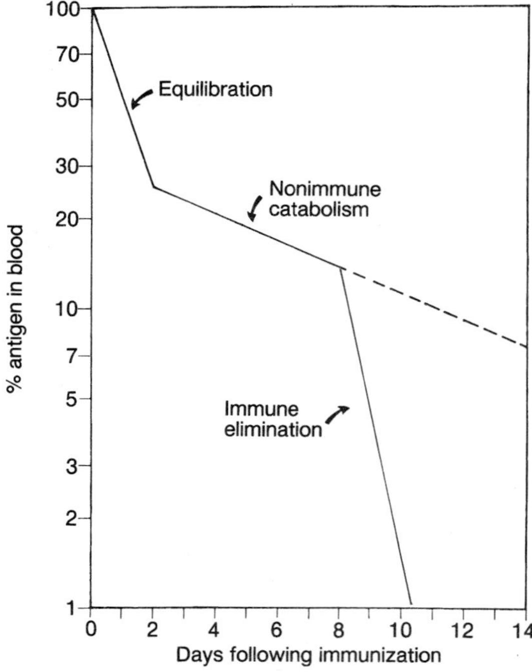

by the reticuloendothelial system. During the induction phase of antibody formation, antigen will be catabolized at a slow "nonimmune" rate. However, when antibodies are formed, catabolism occurs much more rapidly. During the early phase of immune elimination, soluble antigen-antibody complexes in antigen excess are formed in the circulation. Soluble complexes in antigen excess are not opsonized and may lodge in tissue and cause the lesions of serum sickness (see chapter 10).

Antibody-Mediated Inflammatory Reactions

The activity of antibodies in vivo in an actively immunized animal, or an animal that has received antibody by passive transfer of an antiserum prepared in another animal, may result in a reaction involving accessory inflammatory mechanisms. Intravenous injection of antigen into actively or passively sensitized animals may cause an acute systemic reaction because of the presence of IgE antibodies (anaphylaxis). If the antigen is injected into the skin of sensitized animals, erythema (redness) and swelling may be observed. These reactions depend upon tissue inflammatory responses initiated by reactions of antibody or sensitized cells with antigen and are discussed in detail in part II.

Sensitivity of Antigen-Antibody Reactions

The sensitivities of some methods for detection of antigen-antibody reactions are given in Table 4.4. For further information on how to detect and measure both primary and secondary antibody-antigen reactions, the American Society for Microbiology's *Manual of Clinical Laboratory Immunology* (5th ed., 1997) is recommended.

The B-Cell Receptor (BCR)

The BCR as a Signal Transducer

B cells express membrane immunoglobulin molecules that can bind to antigen and generate activation signals for B-cell proliferation and differentiation. The structure of antibody expressed on the surface membrane of a B lymphocyte differs from that of secreted antibody in that additional

Table 4.4 Sensitivity of some methods for measuring antibody-antigen reactions[a]

Method	Sensitivity (μg of antibody/ml)
Quantitative precipitin	4–10
Simple agar diffusion	5–10
Bacterial agglutination	0.01
Bactericidal	0.0001–0.001
Hemagglutination	0.003–0.006
Hemolysis	0.001–0.03
Complement fixation	0.1
Toxin neutralization	0.01
Passive systemic anaphylaxis (guinea pig)	30
Uterine muscle in vitro	0.01
Passive cutaneous anaphylaxis	0.003
Radioimmunoassay	<0.001

[a]Adapted from J. H. Humphrey and R. G. White, p. 201, *Immunology for Students of Medicine*, 2nd ed., Blackwell Scientific Publications Ltd., Oxford, England, 1963.

amino acids are present on the C terminus. The membrane form includes a 25-amino-acid lipophilic transmembrane segment that anchors the immunoglobulin to the membrane lipids and several additional C-terminal amino acids that extend into the cytoplasm of the cell, forming a cytoplasmic "tail." The cytoplasmic tail varies in length between 3 amino acids (μ and δ) and 28 amino acids (ε and γ).

Signal transduction mechanisms triggered by various receptor-ligand interactions in nonlymphoid cells are known to depend on enzymatic reactions carried out by cytoplasmic domains of receptor proteins, but the cytoplasmic tails of membrane immunoglobulins are too small to support such reactions. Membrane immunoglobulins mediate signal transduction through the disulfide-linked heterodimer, Igα-Igβ (CD79a-CD79b), products of the *mb-1* and *B29* genes, respectively. This heterodimer binds noncovalently to membrane immunoglobulins of all isotypes and is required for the appearance of immunoglobulin on the cell surface. Igα and Igβ each have a single extracellular Ig-like domain, a transmembrane region, and a cytoplasmic domain containing an ITAM similar to those on Fc receptors described above. Antigen-induced oligomerization of the BCRs leads to phosphorylation of ITAM tyrosine sites on Igα and Igβ by Src family tyrosine kinases. The phosphorylated ITAMs provide a binding site to recruit Syk to the receptor, whereupon Syk becomes activated by phosphorylation of two adjacent tyrosines in its kinase domain. The critical role of Syk in activation of B cells is indicated by the profound defect in B-cell development and signaling in mice lacking Syk. The activated tyrosine kinases trigger a complex cascade of early signaling events leading to the nuclear transposition and activation of transcription factors. After activation of B cells, interaction with interleukin-2 (IL-2) appears to be critical for progression of B-cell activation and completion of the cell cycle. This cytokine is probably provided by T-helper cells.

BCR signaling can be modulated by other cell surface receptors. Two of these are the CR2 receptor for complement, which promotes B-cell activation, and the Fc receptor FcγRIIb, which inhibits signaling. Antigens with fragments of C3 on them can bind both to the BCR and to the CR2 receptor complex, including CD19 and TAPA-1. This promotes phosphorylation of cytoplasmic tyrosines of CD19, which act to enhance the B-cell activation signal. If antigen is bound to antibody when it contacts the BCR, it may cross-link the BCR to FcγRIIb. This results in phosphorylation of an ITIM in the cytoplasmic domain of FcγRIIb and subsequent blocking of downstream signaling events of the BCR.

The BCR in Antigen Presentation

Apart from the function of the BCR in activating its B cell to proliferate and secrete antibody, the BCR can also mediate antigen binding that results in antigen internalization, antigen proteolysis, and presentation of antigen peptides to T cells in the context of surface major histocompatibility complex class II proteins (see chapter 5). The activated T cells in turn provide activation signals, collectively known as T-cell help, to the B cell, facilitating B-cell proliferation, isotype switching, and immunoglobulin secretion. T-cell activation is more commonly mediated by "professional" antigen-presenting cells (APCs), such as dendritic cells (see chapter 5), but the unique property of B cells as APCs is that they can efficiently present an antigen at more than 1,000-fold lower concentration than nonspecific APCs, as long as the antigen is specifically recognized by membrane immunoglobulin of the BCR. The mediation of T-cell help includes T-cell-derived lymphokines, such as IL-2, IL-4, IL-5, and IL-10, as well as signals generated by contact between the B cell and T cell. One example of such a contact signal is the interaction between the B-cell protein CD40 and its ligand CD154 on the T cell; this signal is required for isotype switching, as discussed later in this chapter.

Although most B-cell responses require T-cell help, certain antigens elicit T-cell-independent responses. These include TI1 antigens associated with intrinsic B-cell mitogens like lipopolysaccharide that are recognized by specific receptors considered to be components of the "innate" immune system, and TI2 antigens, nonprotein polymers such as polysaccharide with internally repeated epitopes.

Immunoglobulin Genes

Generation of Diversity

The most unusual feature of immunoglobulin structure is the vast diversity of antibody molecules with different antigen-binding specificities. Unique genetic mechanisms for generating antibody diversity were discovered when the genes encoding homogeneous myeloma proteins were compared with the corresponding sequences in germ line DNA. The nucleotide sequences encoding different V regions of immunoglobulins are assembled in each B lymphocyte from precursor gene segments that are not present in contiguous germ line DNA. Each B cell rearranges the DNA for one functional heavy-chain gene and one functional light-chain gene; variability in the way these genes can be assembled means that the two functional immunoglobulin V genes in a B cell are almost never assembled in exactly the same way as in another B cell. Therefore, the collective pool of millions of mature circulating B cells includes a repertoire of BCR antibody sequences so huge that when antigen is administered, some B cells with a membrane antibody capable of binding to that antigen will be available. After reacting with specific antigen, these antigen-binding B cells are triggered to proliferate and mature into secreting plasma cells, as discussed above, leading to the synthesis and secretion of antigen-specific antibodies.

An additional process accounts for affinity maturation, the progressive increase in average affinity of antibodies observed during the course of an immune response. A unique somatic mutation mechanism recognizes the functional immunoglobulin V region genes in antigen-activated B lymphocytes and somehow targets these DNA segments for random mutations. Although most mutations in antibody structure probably impair antigen binding or leave it unchanged, rare mutations that increase binding affinity are selected by their improved capacity to bind antigen and thereby respond to the antigen-dependent signal for proliferation and secretion. Successive rounds of mutation and selection lead to progressive increases in antibody affinity. How the processes of gene assembly and somatic mutation accomplish this will now be examined in more detail.

Light-Chain V Gene Assembly

The human genome contains three independent immunoglobulin gene loci capable of assembling functional immunoglobulin genes: the κ locus on chromosome 2, the λ locus on chromosome 22, and the heavy-chain locus on chromosome 14. During maturation of a B lymphocyte, heavy-chain gene assembly occurs first, followed by light-chain assembly. However, because the light-chain genes are simpler, they will be considered first.

The κ Locus

The V regions of functional κ light-chain genes encode about 108 amino acids in a contiguous DNA segment. At the 5′ end of the gene—corresponding to the N-terminal direction—additional codons specify the sequence of a "signal peptide." Signal peptides, found in all nascent proteins destined for secretion or membrane expression, are typically the first amino acid residues to be translated by the ribosome and serve as tags to attach the ribosome to the endoplasmic reticulum. As the ribosome continues the translation process, the signal peptide is cleaved by a peptidase, and the remainder of the protein is formed inside the endoplasmic reticulum, en route to ultimate secretion or membrane expression. If the V gene from a B cell is compared with the corresponding DNA in a nonlymphoid cell (loosely described as germ line DNA), it is found that the germ line V gene lacks the C-terminal 13 or so codons found in the assembled V region gene cloned from lymphocytes. These 13 residues have become known as J region residues, because they "join" the V region to the C region. The J region amino acids are encoded in the human κ locus in five Jκ region gene segments that lie 5′ of the single Cκ region gene (Fig. 4.24). A particular B cell assembles an intact Vκ gene by a DNA rearrangement that joins one of the Jκ region gene segments to one of approximately 76 germ line Vκ sequences that lie 5′ of the J-C cluster. The DNA rearrangement deletes the intervening V regions. A germ line complement of 76 Vκ sequences and five J gene segments could theoretically lead to almost 4,000 different Vκ-Jκ pairings. However, the number of potentially functional Vκ-Jκ genes is different from the number of theoretical Vκ-Jκ pairs for two reasons. First, of the 76 Vκ sequences, only about 50 are functional; the remainder are "pseudogenes," that is, these sequences contain mutations that introduce termination codons or other alterations that would preclude their translation to functional κ light-chain proteins. On the other hand, a particular pair of functional Vκ-Jκ gene segments can actually give rise to several different κ light-chain sequences. This is because the DNA recombination mechanism that joins these two segments by deleting the intervening DNA is somewhat imprecise, so the position of the crossover between V and J is somewhat flexible (Fig. 4.25).

Figure 4.24 V-J rearrangements of κ light-chain genes. In nonlymphoid tissue (germ line) DNA, there are no functional, complete immunoglobulin genes. The two segments that can form a complete κ gene lie in two clusters: the V gene segments and the much smaller cluster of J region segments. A complete functional κ gene is expressed in a lymphocyte after one of the V segments (shown in black) recombines with one of the J regions.

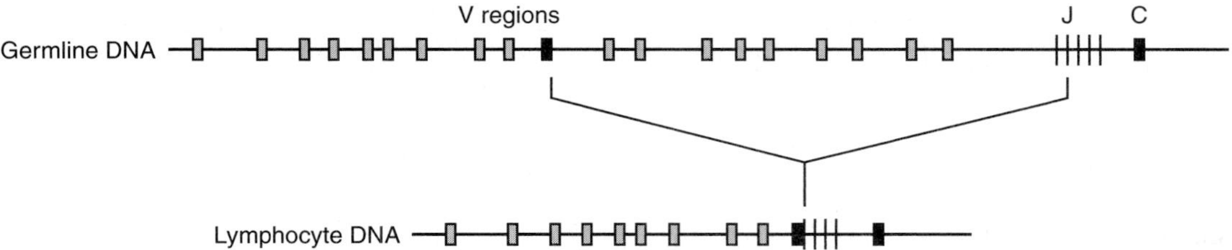

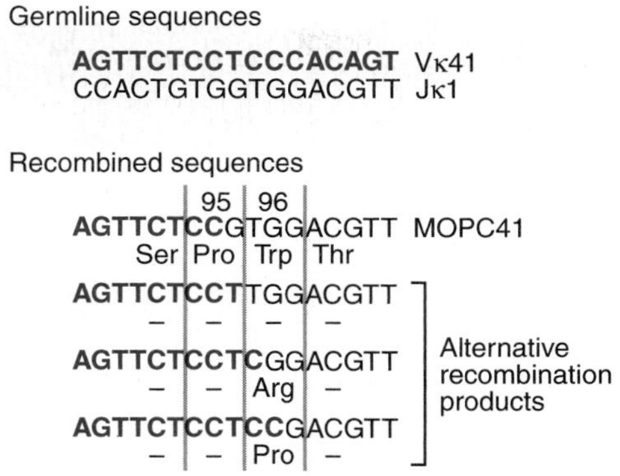

Germline sequences

AGTTCTCCTCCCACAGT Vκ41
CCACTGTGGTGGACGTT Jκ1

Recombined sequences

95 | 96
AGTTCTCCGTGGACGTT MOPC41
Ser | Pro | Trp | Thr

AGTTCTCCTTGGACGTT
– | – | – | –

AGTTCTCCTCGGACGTT
– | – | Arg | –

AGTTCTCCTCCGACGTT
– | – | Pro | –

Alternative recombination products

Figure 4.25 Junctional diversity in V gene assembly. The figure shows the DNA sequence of two germ line murine κ elements in the region involved in recombination during V gene assembly: the germ line Vκ41 segment (highlighted in blue-green) and Jκ1. The next four lines show possible recombination junctions. The first, which was found in the myeloma MOPC41, includes the Vκ41 sequence up to the second nucleotide of codon 95 and then switches to Jκ1 sequence. The next shows the consequences of a recombination junction one nucleotide further downstream; the G→T change in the last nucleotide of codon 95 does not change any encoded amino acids. The last two lines, illustrating two other possible recombination products, are associated with amino acid changes that have been observed in actual murine κ chains. The examples shown maintain the triplet reading frame between V and J, which is required for a functional gene but occurs in only about one-third of recombination events. If the triplet reading frame is not maintained, the rearranged gene will not be expressed, and recombination at the allelic gene will be attempted. If neither allele of the κ-chain gene has a productive rearrangement, rearrangement of λ light-chain gene may be attempted.

This flexibility furnishes the Vκ-Jκ junction with additional diversity that is functionally important for antigen binding since the Vκ-Jκ junction forms part of CDR3 that is generally at, or at least near, the antigen-binding site. After the assembly of a complete κ V region gene, the entire κ gene is transcribed into RNA, and the two introns—one within a signal peptide coding region near the 5′ end of the RNA and the other between J and C—are spliced out before the RNA is translated.

The V Gene Assembly Mechanism

A single common DNA recombination mechanism is thought to assemble V genes of κ, λ, and heavy-chain loci, as well as those of the four T-cell receptor gene loci (see chapter 5). Two conserved sequences (signal elements) identify the position where the DNA should rearrange (Fig. 4.25). The first is a 7-mer CACTGTG that occurs as a consensus sequence 5′ to the Jκ coding sequences, with its reverse complementary sequence CACAGTG appearing 3′ to the Vκ coding sequences. The second element is a 9-mer GGTTTTTGT spaced about 23 nucleotides 5′ to the Jκ 7-mer with its complementary sequence ACAAAAACC about 12 nucleotides 3′ to the Vκ 7-mer. Recombination occurs only between one coding sequence with a 12-bp spacer separating 7-mer and 9-mer sequences and another coding sequence with a 23-bp spacer, a requirement known as the 12/23 rule. A benefit of this rule may be that futile recombinations, such as that between two Vκ or two Jκ gene segments, are prevented. As shown in Fig. 4.26, the spacing of the 7-mer and 9-mer signal segments of the V and J regions is reversed in the λ locus compared with the κ.

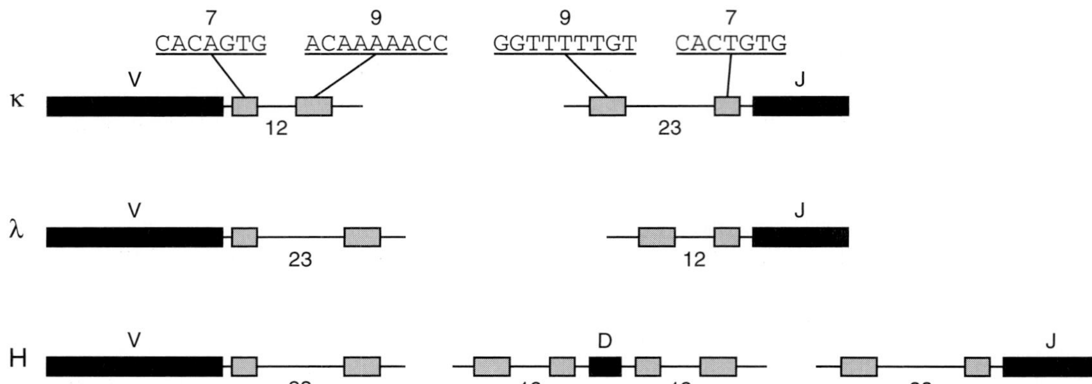

Figure 4.26 Recombination signal sequences (RSSs). The conserved 7-mer and 9-mer sequences that target V assembly recombination are shown flanking the elements involved in these rearrangements. The V, J, and D coding regions are depicted as black rectangles. The spacing between the 7-mer and 9-mer is either 12 or 23 bp as indicated. Recombination occurs almost exclusively between pairs of elements with different RSS spacing.

The earliest model for Vκ-Jκ rearrangement assumed that V segments and J segments were oriented in the same direction of transcription and that the intervening DNA was simply excised and lost from the cell, as shown in Fig. 4.25. However, it is now clear that some Vκ genes are oriented in the opposite direction from the Jκ-Cκ region. For these Vκ genes, the recombinase machinery joins V to J by inverting the DNA between the 7-mer Vκ junction and the 7-mer Jκ junction.

The conserved 7-mer and 9-mer signal sequences are recognized by two components of the "recombinase" machinery, the products of the *recombination-activating genes RAG1* and *RAG2*. These lymphoid-specific proteins cleave DNA at the end of V or J coding sequences just at the beginning of the 7-mer and catalyze the formation of hairpin loops connecting the two DNA strands of each of these coding regions. Each hairpin loop is then opened as the DNA is "nicked" by an unknown endonuclease. The resulting ends are then "nibbled" to varying extents by an unknown exonuclease, a process that contributes to the "flexibility" at the V-J junction described earlier. A variable number of nucleotides may then be added to the coding ends by the enzyme terminal deoxynucleotide transferase (TdT), producing untemplated "N regions." The enzyme is active primarily in pre-B cells undergoing heavy-chain V assembly recombination. Thus, N region nucleotides are more common in heavy-chain V genes than in light-chain genes, which rearrange later, when TdT is less active. After cleavage, exonuclease trimming, and addition of any N region nucleotides, the DNA ends are then ligated, probably by a complex involving the Ku proteins (which bind specifically to DNA ends), a Ku-associated DNA-dependent protein kinase, ligase IV, and the product of the *XRCC4* gene. The components of this complex are all ubiquitous proteins that participate in the repair of double-stranded DNA breaks that occur occasionally in all cells. V assembly recombination is thus accomplished through B-cell-specific, site-specific cleavage by the RAG proteins, followed by DNA break repair accomplished by ubiquitous enzymes. Mice with targeted deletions in either the *RAG1* or *RAG2* gene make no B cells or T cells because they cannot undergo V assembly recombination to make either immunoglobulin or T-cell receptor, but they show no defect in the repair of DNA breaks. A rare human genetic immunodeficiency, the Omenn syndrome (see chapter 18), is caused by defects in either RAG gene. Mice with targeted deletions of the nonspecific DNA end-joining complex show absence of B and T cells but also demonstrate other consequences of their inability to repair DNA breaks, including hypersensitivity to agents that cause such breaks, such as ionizing radiation.

The λ Locus

The assembly of a human Vλ gene occurs between V and J gene segments similar to those of the κ system. However, the germ line organization of the λ C region locus is significantly different from that of the κ locus. There are four nonallelic functional Cλ genes, whose protein products were identified by specific antibodies long before the genes were cloned; these are known by their serological designations $Kern^-Oz^-$, $Kern^-Oz^+$, $Kern^+Oz^-$, and Mcg. The amino acid sequences of these four C regions differ from each other in only five positions. In the human Cλ locus, the genes for these four forms are present in a cluster that also contains three Cλ-related pseudogenes. Each Cλ sequence is associated with a single Jλ gene segment located 5′ to the C sequence. The overall organization of the Jλ-Cλ locus is shown in Fig. 4.27. The λ genes also differ from κ in having the opposite distribution of recombination signal sequence (RSS) spacer lengths; that is, Vλ genes are flanked by signal sequences with 23-bp spacers, while those upstream of Jλ have 12-bp spacers. Upstream of the Jλ-Cλ cluster lie the Vλ sequences, which have been completely characterized by nucleotide sequence analysis. Of the 69 Vλ-like sequences in the locus, about 36 appear potentially active, and 30 of these have been found actively expressed in complementary DNAs. In contrast to the Vκ locus, all the Vλ-Jλ recombination occurs exclusively through deletion, with no inversion events.

Heavy-Chain Diversity

Heavy-Chain V Gene Assembly

Expression of the heavy-chain locus is more complex than either the κ or λ locus owing to (i) additional mechanisms for diversity generation in V_H gene assembly; (ii) alternative RNA splicing pathways accounting for

Figure 4.27 Structure of the human λ light-chain locus. Four of the seven Jλ-Cλ regions in the most frequent haplotype are functional (black rectangles), whereas three regions (4, 5, and 6) are pseudogenes (gray rectangles) in almost all individuals. Variant loci containing extra duplications between the second and third λ genes are indicated by the dashed lines. Flanking regions containing λ-related sequences are shown.

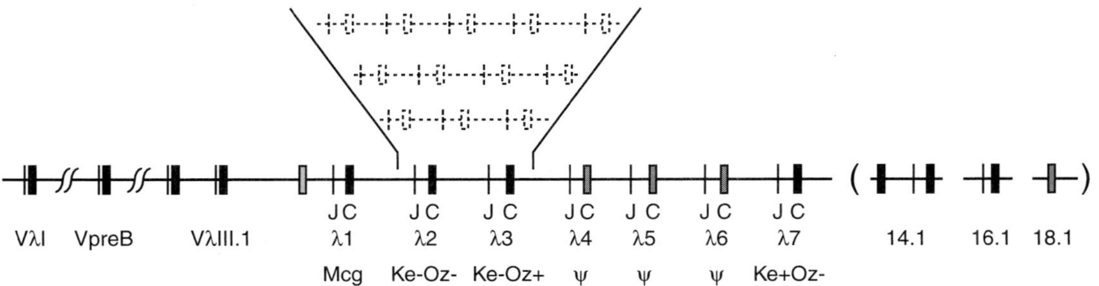

production of a membrane-bound versus secreted protein from the same gene; and (iii) the heavy-chain isotype switch. The additional complexity of V_H gene assembly is revealed by comparing the sequence of an assembled gene (isolated from a B cell or myeloma) with that of its germ line precursors. Between the DNA derived from a germ line V_H region gene and that derived from a J_H region gene segment, one typically finds a variable length of sequence derived from neither. Part of this DNA derives from an additional germ line element known as the D (diversity) segment. In human germ line DNA, the heavy-chain locus has about 30 D region genes located between six J_H regions and the upstream V_H regions. These D elements contain coding sequences of 11 to 31 bp in length that are flanked by 7-mer and 9-mer signal sequences generally having 12-bp spacers (complementing 23-bp spacing of RSSs associated with both V_H and J_H regions). In the course of B cell development, an initial recombination event joins one D region to one of the J_H regions. A second V assembly recombination then joins a V_H region to the already assembled DJ_H segment. The human V_H sequences have been completely characterized by nucleotide sequence analysis. Of 123 V_H sequences, 44 appear potentially functional, and about 40 of these have been documented as expressed in messenger RNA (mRNA) or protein. All the V_H regions lie in the same orientation, and the V gene assembly occurs exclusively by deletional recombination.

As in the case of light-chain genes, considerable diversity can occur even within V regions assembled from a particular set of germ line elements (that is, a particular V, D, and J segment) because of variations at the V-D and D-J junctions. The exonuclease trimming of coding ends in the heavy-chain locus is apparently considerably more extensive than that in light-chain genes. Furthermore, assembled heavy-chain V region genes have variable numbers of "extra" bases between V and D and between D and J. Most of these extra bases are added to coding ends of DNA by the enzyme terminal deoxynucleotide transferase without a template, as discussed earlier with reference to Vκ-Jκ recombination; but N region addition is much more extensive in the V_H gene assembly recombination than in V_L. For a productive VDJ recombination, the V and J regions must be in the same reading frame, but the D region sequence can be read in all three reading frames. Thus, several mechanisms contribute to enormous heavy-chain CDR3 diversity of expressed heavy chains: the combinatorial joining of three separate classes of sequence elements (V, D, and J), the extensive variation in trimming of these elements before joining, the three reading frames of the D regions, and the addition of untemplated "N" nucleotides.

Membrane and Secreted Immunoglobulin

The mechanism by which a single heavy-chain gene can encode either the membrane or secreted form of immunoglobulin has been explained by the analysis of the C genes and their expressed transcripts. A typical example is the Cμ gene, which lies about 3 kb downstream of the human J_H regions. Each of the four domains of internal sequence similarity observed in Cμ at the amino acid sequence level is encoded in a separate exon. The exon encoding the fourth C domain, C_H4, includes the C-terminal codons of the μ heavy-chain form found in secreted antibody. The alternative C-terminal amino acid residues of μ chain expressed on the membrane of B lymphocytes are encoded in two exons lying downstream of C_H4 (Fig. 4.28). The primary transcription product of the μ gene can be spliced to encode the

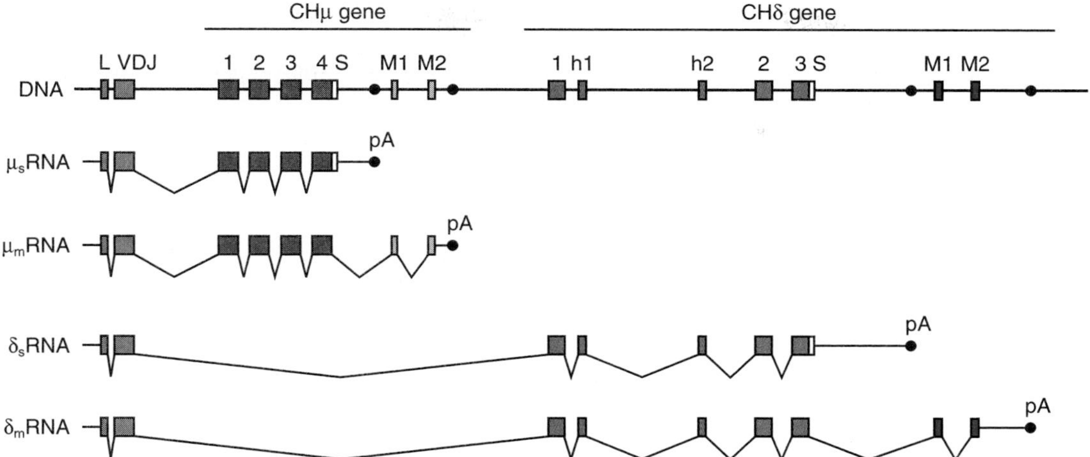

Figure 4.28 Splicing of heavy-chain exons in the formation of membrane and secreted immunoglobulin and μ and δ heavy chains. The exons of a rearranged heavy-chain gene are shown, including both μ and δ loci. Sequences that are spliced out at the RNA level are shown as V-shaped lines. In the case of μ heavy chain, all mature mRNAs show removal of the intron separating most of the signal peptide sequence from the V region, the J_H-Cμ intron, and the three intra-Cμ domain introns. In μ_s mRNA, the transcript includes the last two codons of the secreted heavy chain and terminates at a poly(A) addition site (black dot) close downstream.

last residues of C_H4 characteristic of the secreted form or may be alternatively spliced so as to exclude these residues and join the remainder of the Cμ transcript to the "membrane exons" encoding the hydrophobic transmembrane region and cytoplasmic tail characteristic of surface IgM. Analogous splice patterns account for the membrane and secreted forms of the other isotype heavy chains.

Immunoglobulin Class Switching

The isotype initially expressed in the development of all B lymphocytes is IgM. Most B cells also express surface IgD along with IgM. The simultaneous expression of μ and δ heavy chains appears to result from a long RNA transcript that begins at VDJ, reads through Cμ, and continues through the Cδ gene, which lies about 5 kb downstream of Cμ (Fig. 4.29). Such a transcript can be alternatively spliced to yield mature transcripts including either VDJCμ (encoding the μ heavy chain) or VDJCδ (encoding δ); both RNAs are produced in most early B cells. After a B cell is triggered for activation by an encounter with antigen, the cell may mature to express another isotype, such as IgE, IgA, or one of the IgG subtypes. This isotype switch is the result of a unique class of DNA rearrangements in which the C region gene of the new isotype moves to lie downstream of VDJ in the position formerly occupied by the Cμ gene. The nature of this rearrangement has been clarified by cloning of the complete set of C_H regions and the compilation of a map that orients them with respect to each other. In germ line DNA, the C region genes encoding the γ, ϵ, and α chains are arrayed downstream of Cμ and Cδ, as shown in Fig. 4.29. Thus, in the example illustrated in Fig. 4.29, the isotype switch to ϵ is associated with a DNA deletion that removes all the C regions from Cμ through Cγ4, leaving VDJ near the Cϵ gene. The recombination junctions typically occur

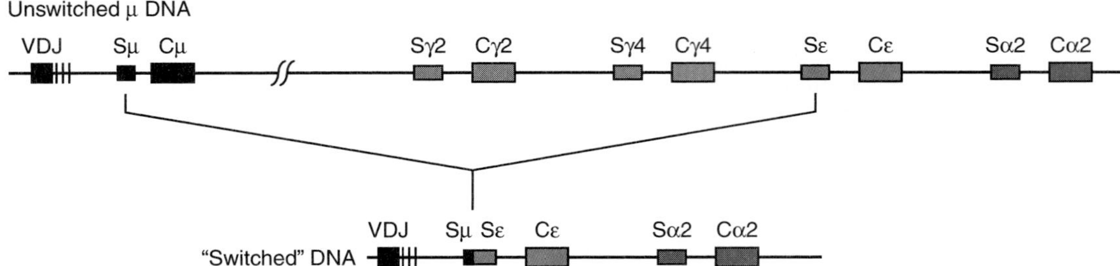

Figure 4.29 Isotype (Ig class) switch recombination. The human heavy-chain gene locus is spread out over roughly 300 kb and includes two duplication units of γ-γ-ϵ-α genes, of which only the more downstream γ2-γ4-ϵ-α2 unit is shown here. Isotype switching involves DNA deletion events whose endpoints usually fall within the repetitive switch (S) regions that lie 5′ of each C region. In the isotype switch deletion illustrated here, a composite Sμ-Sϵ region is formed by the recombination; as a consequence, the Cϵ gene is moved downstream of VDJ to the position formerly occupied by Cμ. The resulting DNA is a template for transcription of VDJ-Cϵ mRNA that encodes the ϵ heavy chain.

within internally repetitive segments of DNA known as "switch regions," which lie 5′ of all the C region genes (except Cδ, which is rarely involved in a switch rearrangement). In the example of μ to ϵ switching, the 5′ part of the μ switch region (Sμ) becomes joined to the 3′ part of Sϵ, forming a composite Sμ-Sϵ switch region. The exact position of the switch junction is irrelevant to the final structure of the expressed protein, since the recombination occurs within an intron sequence that is spliced out of the RNA transcript before it is translated into protein.

Certain types of antigen exposure are known to promote responses dominated by specific isotypes. For example, IgE is most prominent after the exposure of respiratory mucosa to inhaled allergens and in helminth infestations, whereas the B cells of Peyer's patches in the intestinal mucosa respond predominantly with IgA. The detailed mechanism of isotype selection by specific immunogen exposure is not known, but both T cells and the cytokine milieu of the B cell appear to play important roles in the isotype switch. The role of T cells is illustrated by a rare genetic immunodeficiency in which serum IgM is elevated and all other isotypes are essentially absent (hyper-IgM immunodeficiency [see chapter 18]). Incubation of B cells from affected patients with T cells from normal individuals restores isotype switching by the B cells, whereas the patients' T cells are unable to accomplish this. The effect of this specific B-cell–T-cell interaction has been traced to the binding of a B-cell membrane protein known as CD40 to a T-cell membrane protein known as the CD40 ligand (CD40L, also known as CD154); it is the gene for the latter protein that is abnormal in most cases of hyper-IgM immunodeficiency. One consequence of the interaction between CD40 and its ligand is B-cell proliferation, which is required for isotype switching. The importance of cytokines is exemplified by switching to IgE. For this switch, it is clear that IL-4 is necessary, while gamma interferon is inhibitory. Since these cytokines are characteristic of two different classes of $CD4^+$ helper cells—Th2 and Th1, respectively—it is apparent that selective isotype switching can depend on T cells in several different ways.

Despite the observation that specific isotypes play unique roles in specific immune responses, several human pedigrees are known with individuals who are homozygous for extensive deletions in the C_H locus (Fig. 4.30). These individuals generally do not present with serious clinical immunodeficiency, suggesting that there is considerable potential for compensation by the remaining available isotypes.

Allelic Exclusion and the Regulation of V Assembly

Most autosomal genes are expressed in roughly equal amounts from the two homologous loci on the maternal and paternal chromosomes. In contrast, each B lymphocyte expresses only a single light-chain gene and a single heavy-chain gene; the allelic light-chain and heavy-chain locus in each cell is excluded from expression ("allelic exclusion"). If both alleles were expressed, each cell might be capable of producing four different V_HV_L pairs, some of which might react with self antigens, and individual H_2L_2 molecules with two different V_HV_L pairs might be produced. Allelic exclusion is apparently important for efficient clonal selection of immunoglobulin targeted against a specific foreign antigen and not against other molecules. But how is allelic exclusion maintained? Two general mechanisms have been proposed. First, the stochastic model suggests that a single allele is expressed simply because of the extremely low probability of more than one functional rearrangement in a single developing B cell. The regulation model suggests that allelic exclusion results from the tight developmental control of V gene assembly recombination, such that expression from one allele prevents V assembly at the other alleles, as described in the following scenario.

The initial recombination in the B lymphocyte is D-J_H joining, which commonly occurs on both heavy-chain alleles before V_H genes become activated for recombination and before any recombinations have occurred in the light-chain genes. When V_H genes do become activated, and a VDJ rearrangement first occurs in a cell, a μ heavy chain can be produced only if the VDJ recombination is "in frame" (or "productive"), which happens in roughly one-third of recombinations. If the initial VDJ recombination is productive, a μ heavy chain is made, a step defining the developmental stage of a pre-B cell. The heavy chain appears on the surface of the cell and

Figure 4.30 Human immunoglobulin heavy-chain gene locus deletions. This map shows the J_H regions and the entire C region gene locus. Black rectangles represent C region genes for the nine expressed isotypes (Ig classes): gray rectangles represent two pseudogenes in the locus. The numbers indicate the approximate distances between the C region genes in kilobases. This map order has been deduced from overlapping clones and Southern blotting of large fragments and is confirmed by analysis of natural germ line deletion mutations in humans (shown by the lines underlying the locus).

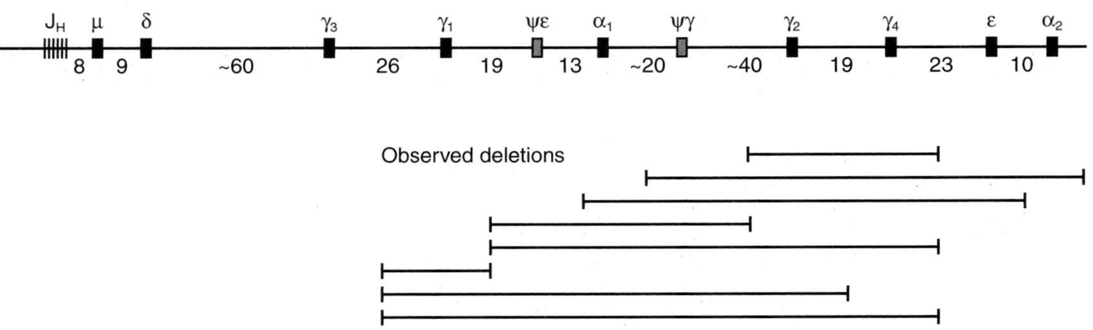

transmits a signal that shuts off further heavy-chain recombination, thus preventing expression of the allelic heavy-chain locus. Because heavy chains are apparently unable to be expressed on the cell membrane in the absence of a light chain, and at this stage no light-chain gene has yet been assembled, the μ protein of the pre-B cell is expressed on the membrane with a "surrogate" light chain composed of a V-like and a C-like protein known respectively as VpreB and λ5 (mouse) or 14.1 (human). These proteins are encoded near the λ locus and show sequence similarity to that chain. If the initial VDJ_H recombination is out of frame ("nonproductive"), then no μ protein is made to generate a shutoff signal, so recombination can proceed on the other allelic locus. Some cells undoubtedly recombine both alleles nonproductively; these cells may be lost to the immune system as functional participants.

In addition to shutting off VDJ_H recombination, the production of a μ heavy chain in the pre-B cell has a second regulatory effect: it activates the κ locus for rearrangement. A feedback mechanism similar to that described for heavy chains prevents the production of two different κ chains; in this case, the signal that shuts off further κ rearrangement is the appearance of functional IgM antibody ($\mu_{H2}\kappa_2$) on the surface of the cell, an event that defines the cell as developmentally at the B-cell stage.

The λ locus is apparently not usually activated for recombination in human B cells unless κ recombination is nonproductive on both chromosomal κ loci. The evidence for this is that B-cell leukemias and lymphomas expressing κ chains usually have their λ-chain genes in germ line (i.e., unrecombined) organization. Surprisingly, if B-cell malignancies expressing λ light chain are examined, not only are their λ genes in recombined organization (as expected), but their Cκ genes are generally deleted from both allelic κ loci. This deletion represents a programmed step in B-lymphocyte maturation and occurs at specific sites in the DNA.

Exactly how the feedback mechanisms described above activate or shut off recombination at specific loci is not known in detail. According to the current model, the enzymatic machinery for each V assembly recombination is essentially identical for κ, λ, and heavy-chain genes, but the recombination reactions can occur at a particular locus only after that locus becomes "accessible" to the recombination machinery. Accessibility appears to be associated with gene transcription, since a cell capable of recombination at a particular immunoglobulin locus generally transcribes the germ line elements that are targets for the recombination. The resulting transcripts of isolated V regions and C regions are known as germ line or "sterile" transcripts, because they cannot encode a functional immunoglobulin chain. The regulation of recombinational accessibility may thus be achieved by transcriptional regulatory mechanisms, which are actively being investigated.

Somatic Mutation

The mechanism responsible for affinity maturation of antibodies during the course of an immune response is somatic mutation. This process can lead to increases of over 100-fold in affinity binding to antigen. The process has been most fruitfully investigated in mice, in which the availability of inbred strains—with identical complements of germ line V region genes—facilitates recognition of individual mutations. Thus, the extensive published sequence data on germ line V region genes cloned from the BALB/c mouse generally mean that if the V_H and V_L gene sequences of any BALB/c myeloma or hybridoma protein are known, the germ line V region precursors can be identified; therefore, any V region sequence differences between the expressed gene and its germ line precursor can be attributed to somatic mutation. (By contrast, the genetic polymorphisms of germ line V genes in humans may complicate the identification of somatic mutations.)

The time course of somatic mutation during an immune response has been studied by immunizing mice and analyzing the V region sequences of hybridomas made at various times after immunization. In the first week after immunization, antigen-specific antibodies are generally unmutated. After this time, mutations begin to appear and increase over the next week or so. Late booster immunizations can induce additional mutations. The mutations are clustered around the rearranged V_HDJ_H or V_LJ_L gene, extending from the transcriptional initiation site through a domain of about 2 kb; homologous unrearranged sequences on the other chromosome remain essentially unmutated. Apparently, a specific "hypermutation" mechanism is able to recognize an assembled and expressed immunoglobulin V region as a target for mutation. The mutations are not specifically targeted to CDRs to create higher-affinity antibodies but occur in FR codons as well as in intron and flanking regions. In accordance with the evolutionlike model discussed earlier in this chapter, mutated V regions may encode an antibody with an affinity for antigen that is higher, lower, or unchanged in comparison with the unmutated antibody. However, cells making high-affinity antibody have a proliferative advantage as antigen concentration falls, since they are better able to receive antigen-dependent activation signals than are lower-affinity cells that bind antigen less efficiently. The beneficial mutations tend to cluster in the CDRs, since these are the regions most critical for antigen affinity. The proliferative advantage of high affinity cells—which acts like evolutionary selection pressure—was demonstrated by experiments in which antigen concentration was maintained at a high level by repeated injections; this protocol abolished the development of affinity maturation, as would be expected from the reduced selection pressure for efficient antigen binding.

Somatic mutation occurs in the germinal center (see chapter 6), as shown by experiments in which polymerase chain reaction was used to clone immunoglobulin genes from selected regions of thin sections of lymphoid tissue. Each precursor area to a germinal center is apparently colonized by very few B cells before the onset of somatic mutation, since the cells in a particular germinal center appear to be clonal progeny derived from very few founder cells. In several cases, it has been possible to analyze multiple mutated sequences from a single germinal center and to derive a genealogic tree that traces how early mutations were retained in later progeny sequences that have additional mutations. Some evidence suggests that the germinal center B cells undergoing somatic mutation represent a separate B-cell lineage, different from the population that responds in the first few days after antigen administration. The population susceptible to mutation appears to require T-cell help to initiate the hypermutation process; the antibody response to T-cell-independent antigens like polysaccharides does not show affinity maturation.

The combination of the diversity resulting from joining of multiple gene elements (V_L, J_L, V_H, D, and J_H) and the amplification of that diversity by somatic mutation provides powerful and flexible mechanisms capable of creating antigen-combining sites of extremely high affinity, exquisitely tailored to the specific foreign antigen under immunologic attack.

B-Cell Development

Ig Gene Expression

A model for B-cell maturation and immunoglobulin expression is illustrated in Fig. 4.31. There are two major phases of B-cell development: antigen independent and antigen dependent. Differentiation of B cell precursors to B cells expressing cell surface IgM and IgD is antigen independent. By assembling a specific pair of heavy- and light-chain genes, the B cell determines its antigen-recognizing specificity before antigen enters the system. The first identifiable cell in the B-cell lineage is the pro-B cell, in which D-JH recombination is occurring in cells expressing the surface markers CD19 and B220. The pro-B cell expresses neither cytoplasmic nor cell surface immunoglobulin. In the next cell in the lineage, the pre-B cell, rearrangement of immunoglobulin heavy-chain genes occurs, but the light-chain genes have not rearranged. Pre-B cells express cytoplasmic μ chains but not cell surface immunoglobulin. Immature B cells have rearranged heavy- and light-chain genes and express both. These cells exist in two forms, those that express cell surface IgM only and those that express cell surface IgM and IgD. Upon antigen stimulation and given appropriate second signals from T-helper cells, B cells proliferate to expand the clone and often switch to express a different isotype (IgG, IgA, or IgE). The differentiated progeny of B cells—plasma cells—express little, if any, surface immunoglobulin but rapidly synthesize and secrete antibody of a single immunoglobulin isotype.

CD Markers of B-Cell Differentiation

The differentiation of B and T cells may also be characterized phenotypically by the expression of markers detected by monoclonal antibodies known as *clusters of differentiation,* or CD. The markers were analyzed on different cell populations in the 1970s and 1980s and were found to identify different stages of development. A short list of some of these markers for B and T cells is presented in Table 4.5; a more extensive listing is given in Appendix 3. The expression of CD markers during B-cell differentiation is presented in Table 4.6. These markers have been helpful in defining the stage of differentiation of B-cell lymphomas (see chapter 17).

B-Cell Tolerance

As discussed earlier, tolerance mechanisms must exist to prevent B cells from reacting with self antigens (self tolerance). B cells may become inactivated by antigen contact at two critical stages. (i) If the BCR of the immature B cell contacts antigen in the bone marrow, the cell is arrested in development and the receptor is edited by re-expression of recombinases (RAG1 and RAG2) to form a new BCR. (ii) B cells that mature and enter the long-lived circulating pool become activated by contact with antigen, depending on the presence of second signals, usually in the form of IL-2 from T-helper cells. B cells that contact antigen in the absence of second signals are either inactivated (anergy) or deleted by apoptosis.

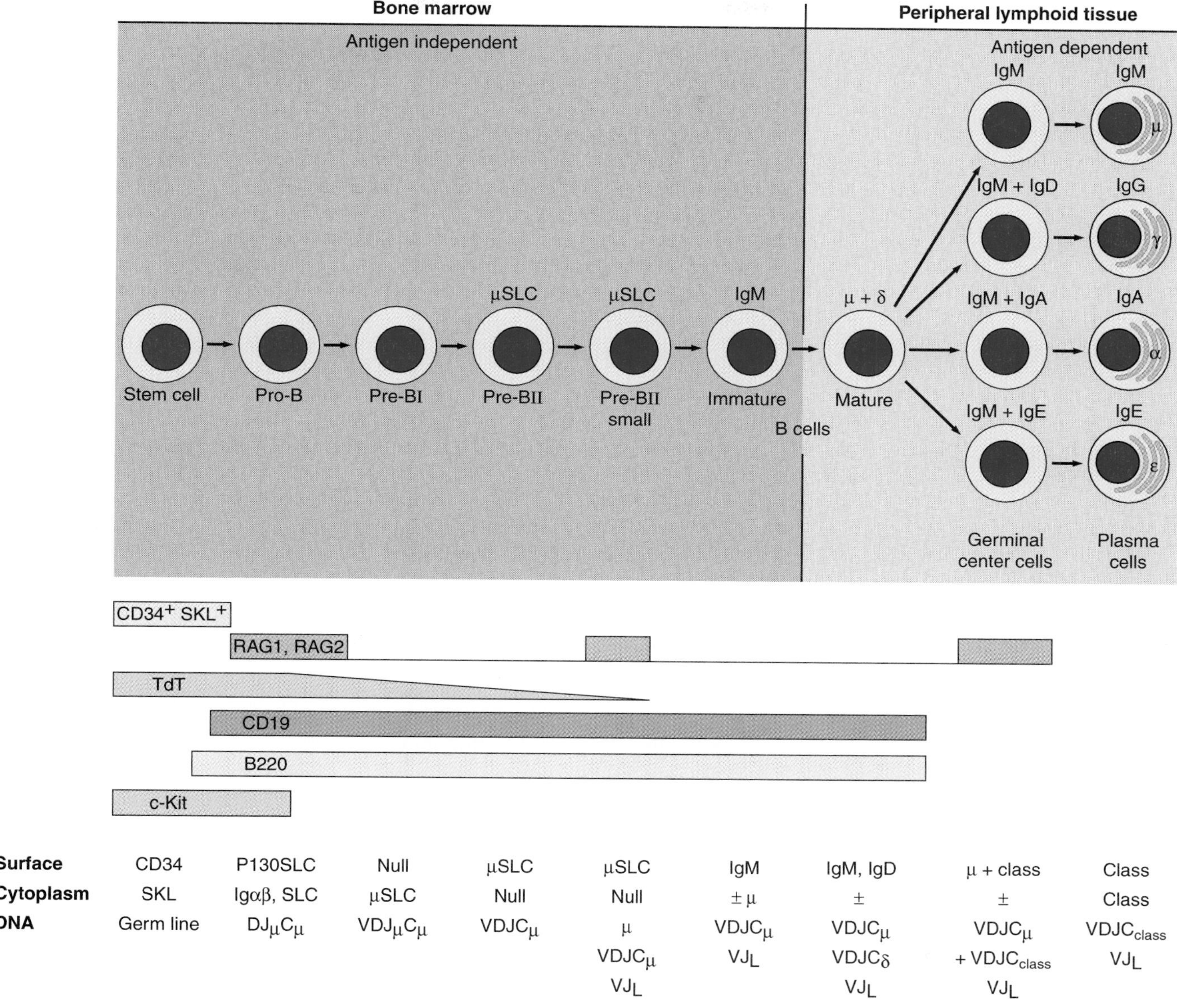

Figure 4.31 B-cell differentiation. Shown is the sequence of marker and Ig gene rearrangements during stages of B-cell differentiation. Cells of the B-cell lineage arise from a multipotent hematopoietic stem cell and are first identified by the presence of RAG1,2 and rearrangement of the DJ regions of the μ-chain gene, as well as the early B-cell markers CD19 and B220, and the nonimmunoglobulin components of surface Ig, Igα and Igβ. The pro-B cells share c-Kit, the receptor for stem cell factor, and TdT with more primitive stem cells. In the absence of heavy-chain expression, the pro-B cell expresses segments of the J and C regions of λ surrogate light chains (SLC), which are later expressed on pre-B cells associated with a μ heavy chain (μSLC). In pre-B cells, rearrangement of the VDJC of the μ-chain gene occurs, and later the VJ segments of the light-chain genes are rearranged. B cells are recognized by the presence of IgM chain on the cell surface, and in the more mature stage in the periphery, by the presence of IgM and IgD. T-cell stimuli (CD40L and cytokines) lead to immunoglobulin class (isotype) switching in germinal centers of peripheral lymphoid tissue (mostly in lymph nodes) and differentiation to plasma cells secreting antibody of only one immunoglobulin class.

Table 4.5 A beginner's CD subclassification of lymphoid cells

Marker	Property	Tissue distribution
CD1	Cell surface glycoprotein	Cortical thymocytes, Langerhans cells, dendritic cells, Reed-Sternberg cells
CD2	Sheep RBC receptor	All T cells and thymocytes, T-cell leukemias and lymphomas
CD3	T-cell receptor chain	Medullary thymocytes, peripheral T cells, T-cell leukemias and lymphomas
CD4	Receptor for human immunodeficiency virus	T-helper cells, T-delayed-type hypersensitivity cells
CD7	Glycoprotein	T cells and bone marrow prothymocytes
CD8	Glycoprotein	T-cytotoxic cells (suppressor cells)
CD5	Glycoprotein	All T cells, some B-cell tumors (chronic lymphocytic leukemias, CLL)
CD10	Glycoprotein	B cells early in differentiation (acute leukemias, ALL)
CD19	Glycoprotein	All B cells (ALL, CLL, and large cell lymphoma, LCL)
CD22	Glycoprotein	All B cells except late in differentiation (ALL and CLL, not LCL)
CD34.	Glycoprotein	T and B cells as well as bone marrow precursors of T and B cells
CD45	Membrane protein tyrosine phosphatase	Most white blood cells, differentiates lymphomas from other small cell tumors

Gene Rearrangements in Lymphomas and Leukemias

Because the V assembly recombinations that occur in any one B lymphocyte are generally unique, these recombinations provide genetic markers that are clinically useful in the diagnosis and management of B-cell malignancies. Most B-cell tumors are made up of cells that have a unique clonal set of immunoglobulin gene rearrangements. A V(D)J recombination can be readily detected in DNA from a clonal source by Southern blotting (Fig. 4.32). In a nonclonal population such as peripheral blood lymphocytes or bone marrow biopsy, rearranged immunoglobulin genes resulting from diverse recombination events produce a faint smear on a Southern blot because of multiple rearrangements characteristic of nonclonal populations. However, DNA from a clonal population constituting as few as 5% of the lymphocytes will generate discrete bands by Southern blot, which can be

Table 4.6 Expression of some CD markers during B-cell differentiation[a]

	Antigen independent					Antigen dependent		
Antigen	Pro-B	Pre-pre-B	Pre-B	Immature B	Mature B	Activated B	Memory B	Plasma cell
CD10	X	X	X					
CD19	X	X	X	X	X	X		
CD22/24		X	X	X	X	X		
CD21			X	X	X	X		
CD23			X	X	X	X		
CD38		X	X					X
CD39				X	X	X		
PAC1								X

[a]Modified from F. M. Uckun, *Blood* **76:**1908, 1990.

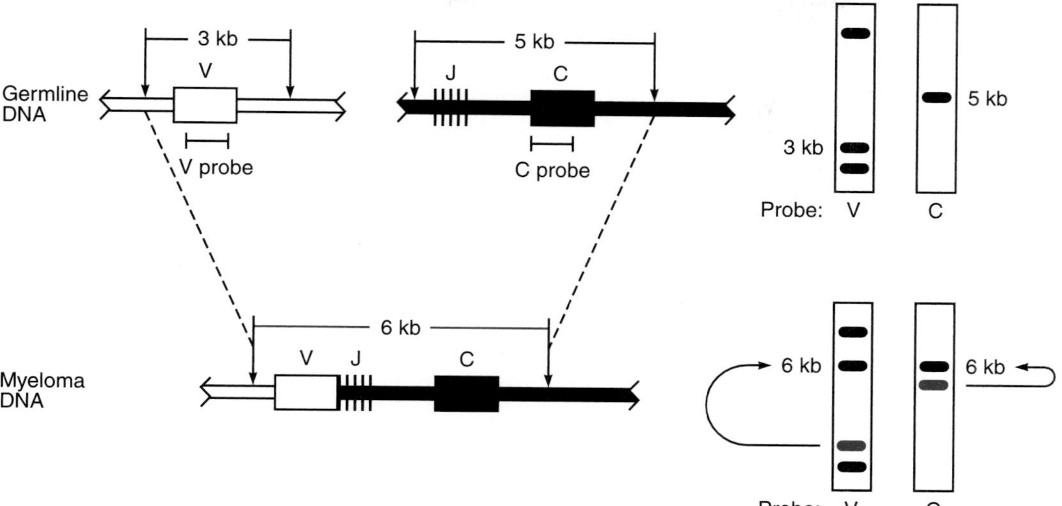

Figure 4.32 Detection of a V-J rearrangement in a B-cell tumor by Southern blotting. The upper part of the figure shows nonlymphoid (germ line) DNA (left) and resulting Southern blots (right); the lower part of the figure shows the corresponding features of DNA from a myeloma containing a Vκ-Jκ rearrangement. When germ line DNA is digested with a restriction endonuclease (having sites indicated by the arrows), and blots of the resulting DNA fragments are probed for V and C regions, the bands for the V and C regions will be different. After V-J recombination, both V and J lie on a single restriction fragment, here illustrated as 6 kb. With appropriate choice of endonuclease, a given myeloma should always show at least one rearranged band representing the rearranged gene expressed by the myeloma. If the κ allele on the other homologous chromosome has not rearranged, a germ line band may also be visible (blue-green band); alternatively, a second rearranged band may be seen, or there may be no second band at all if the other allele has been deleted.

distinguished from the diffuse smear. Thus, the intensity of a rearranged band in DNA from a blood sample or bone marrow biopsy of a leukemia patient can be used to assess the extent of clonal cells representing residual disease after treatment. An even more sensitive method for detecting clonal rearrangements is the polymerase chain reaction, which can detect an immunoglobulin rearrangement characteristic of a leukemic cell when such cells are as rare as 1 leukemic cell in 10,000 normal cells.

Application of Antibody Technology to Therapy

The recognition that immunity to a disease could be conferred by administration of serum fractions to laboratory animals *(passive immunity)* led to numerous applications in clinical medicine, including the use of animal antibodies (now largely abandoned because of the risks of serum sickness), immunoglobulin-containing human serum fractions *(gamma globulins)* from normal donors, and immunoglobulins from humans known to have recovered from a specific disease. More recently, monoclonal antibodies have been proposed for the diagnosis and treatment of cancer. In diagnostic applications, antibodies against tumor antigens have been tagged with radioactive elements and administered to patients so that cancers, including metastases, can be visualized by nuclear medicine imaging. Therapeutic approaches involve both antibodies tagged with radioactivity to provide localized radiotherapy and antibodies tagged with various toxins.

The antibodies that have been used to target these poisons specifically to tumor cells have frequently been murine monoclonal antibodies, since in comparison with human hybridomas, murine hybridomas are easier to make, more productive of antibody, and more stable. Some murine antibodies have shown some promise in clinical situations in humans, but a major drawback is that the murine proteins are frequently recognized as foreign by the patient's immune system, leading to the development of a human anti-mouse antibody *(HAMA)* response. Such a response can diminish the effectiveness of the murine antibody and carries the risk of serum sickness.

The availability of immunoglobulin genes of mice and humans has led to several strategies aimed at avoiding the HAMA response. An initial idea was to fuse murine V genes—carrying the specificity for the tumor antigen—to human C genes and to express the encoded chimeric antibody by transfecting the genes into a nonexpressing myeloma; the resulting *transfectoma* expresses an antibody that carries murine determinants only on the V_H and V_L regions. An even more elegant approach has exploited our understanding of the three-dimensional structure of immunoglobulin V region protein domains. As discussed earlier, it is the three CDR loops of each chain that contact antigen, while the remaining FR residues serve primarily to hold the CDR loops in the correct position. Therefore, it was reasoned that it should be possible to use genetic engineering to graft the CDR sequences from a murine antitumor antibody onto human V region FR codons to produce an antibody that is human except for murine sequences at the antigen-binding site. Such "humanized" antibodies have in fact been found to carry the antigen specificity of the original murine monoclonal antibody but to evoke almost no HAMA response. Antibody genes have been altered in various ways to construct novel proteins with the desired properties of immunoglobulins. One interesting engineered structure is the *Fv chain,* which contains a V_H domain directly linked to a V_L domain through a spacer polypeptide of about 15 residues.

Several other strategies may also prove useful for generating human monoclonal antibodies. Large segments of the human germ line immunoglobulin locus can be introduced into murine strains, creating *transgenic mice* that can synthesize human antibodies. Alternatively, immunodeficient mice engrafted with human B-cell precursors may be immunized and then used to generate human hybridomas (though it is not clear whether the murine advantages of stability and high antibody production would be achieved). A completely different strategy avoids hybridoma technology completely. A "library" of human V_H and V_L genes is constructed so that Fv proteins are expressed on the surface of bacteriophages; the resulting *phage display library* is then selected for the desired antigen specificity by affinity chromatography on a solid support containing antigen. The bound bacteriophage are then eluted, and the resulting V_H-V_L gene pair can be used for further constructions.

Antigen-binding domains from antibodies have also been fused (via bioengineering) to other effector proteins. For example, protein toxins can be delivered to cancer cells via tumor-specific antibodies. In another example, tissue plasminogen activator (an enzyme used to dissolve clots after coronary thrombosis) was targeted to clots by linking it to an antifibrin antibody. These approaches illustrate the potential of biotechnology for providing new therapeutic strategies based on antibodies to specific molecules on tumor cells, microbial invaders, or pathogenic structures.

Summary

Antibodies are proteins that show vast diversity in the antigens that they can bind, yet fall into subclasses showing common effector functions. The basic structure of an antibody is the L_2H_2 unit, composed of two identical heavy chains and two identical light chains. The vast diversity of antibodies resides in the N-terminal V regions of both light and heavy chain, whereas the common effector functions are determined by structures in the heavy-chain C regions. Antibodies are important both for their protective functions (e.g., their roles in virus neutralization, bacterial opsonization, complement activation) as well as their disease-producing actions (autoimmunity, allergy, etc.), and an impressive technology has been developed for analyzing their presence in body fluids. Specific antibodies developed against antigens of interest can also be used in the laboratory to purify or assay those antigens. The great mystery of how the enormous binding diversity of antibodies could be encoded in the genome has been explained by the finding that unique antibody V region genes are assembled in each B lymphocyte from a common germ line endowment of V_H, D, J_H, V_L, and J_L sequences. In addition to this combinatorial diversity, the precise junctions between any two germ line elements may vary depending on how many nucleotides are "nibbled" from the coding sequence ends and the nature of the "N" nucleotides added before the elements are joined. A final measure of diversity results from V gene somatic mutation, which occurs within cells residing in germinal centers of lymphoid tissues; rare mutations that increase antibody affinity are selected for expression by a signaling mechanism acting through the form of antibody that is displayed on the cell membrane of B lymphocytes. After a B lymphocyte has been committed to a particular antigen specificity, the effector functions of the expressed antibody may be altered by isotype switch recombination, a process regulated by the immunologic milieu, including the mix of locally expressed cytokines. The potential importance of specific antibodies as reagents for diagnosis and therapy has motivated scientists to engineer new genes encoding immunoglobulin segments in novel contexts, a technology offering exciting prospects for the future.

Bibliography

Antibodies and Immunoglobulins

Burnet, F. M. 1959. *The Clonal Selection Theory of Acquired Immunity.* Vanderbilt University Press, Nashville, Tenn.

Fahey, J. L. 1966. Antibodies and immunoglobulins. *JAMA* **194:**71–74, 255–258.

Frazer, J. K., and J. D. Capra. 1999. Immunoglobulins: structure and function, p. 37-74. *In* W. E. Paul (ed.), *Fundamental Immunology,* 4th ed. Lippincott-Raven Publishers, Philadelphia, Pa.

Kabat, E. A. 1980. Origins of antibody complementarity and specificity—hypervariable regions and the minigene hypothesis. *J. Immunol.* **125:**961–969.

Kennett, R. H., T. J. McKearn, and K. B. Bechtol. 1980. *Monoclonal Antibodies: Hybridomas: a New Dimension in Biological Analysis.* Plenum Press, New York, N.Y.

Kohler, G., and C. Milstein. 1975. Continuous cultures of fused cells secreting antibody of predefined specificity. *Nature* **256:**495–497.

Porter, R. R. 1958. Separation and isolation of fractions of rabbit λ-globulin containing the antibody and antigenic combining sites. *Nature* **182:**607–671.

Pressman, D., and A. L. Grossberg. 1968. *The Structural Basis of Antibody Specificity.* Benjamin, New York, N.Y.

Silverton, E. W., M. A. Navia, and D. R. Davies. 1977. Three dimensional structure of an intact human immunoglobulin. *Proc. Natl. Acad. Sci. USA* **74:**5140–5144.

Antibody-Antigen Reactions

Bullock, G. (ed.). 1982. *Techniques in Immunochemistry,* vol. 1. Academic Press, Inc., Orlando, Fla.

Bullock, G. (ed.). 1983. *Techniques in Immunochemistry,* vol. 2. Academic Press, Inc., Orlando, Fla.

Coons, A. H. 1956. Histochemistry with labeled antibody. *Int. Rev. Cytol.* **5:**1.

Crowle, A. J. 1961. *Immunodiffusion.* Academic Press, Inc., New York, N.Y.

Engvall, E., and P. Perlmann. 1971. Enzyme linked immunoabsorbent assay (ELISA). Quantitative assay of immunoglobulin G. *Immunochemistry* **8:**871–874.

Farr, R. S. 1958. A quantitative immunochemical measure of the primary interaction between I*BSA and antibody. *J. Infect. Dis.* **103:**239–262.

Gill, T. J., III. 1970. Methods for detecting antibody. *Immunochemistry* **7:**997–1000.

Loken, M. R., and A. M. Stall. 1982. Flow cytometry as an analytical and preparative tool in immunology. *J. Immunol. Methods* **50:**R85–112.

Mancini, G., A. O. Carbonara, and J. F. Heremans. 1965. Immunochemical quantitation of antigens by single radial immunodiffusion. *Immunochemistry* **2:**235–254.

Mariuzza, R. A., R. H. Poljak, and F. P. Schwarz. 1994. The energetics of antigen-antibody binding. *Res. Immunol.* **145:**70–72.

Ouchterlony, O. 1962. Diffusion-in-gel methods for immunological analysis. *Prog. Allergy* **6:**30–154.

Oudin, J. 1946. Method of immunochemic analysis by specific precipitation in gel medium. *C. R. Acad. Sci. Ser. D* **222:**115.

Rodbard, D., and G. H. Weiss. 1973. Mathematical theory of immunoradiometric (labeled antibody) assays. *Anal. Biochem.* **52:**10–44.

Weigle, W. O., and F. J. Dixon. 1957. The elimination of heterologous serum proteins and associated antibody response to guinea pigs and rats. *J. Immunol.* **79:**24.

Yalow, R. S. 1978. Radioimmunoassay: a probe for the fine structure of biologic systems. *Science* **200:**1236–1245.

Cell Membrane Immunoglobulin, B-Cell Activation, and Antigen Presentation

Allen, R. C., R. J. Armitage, M. E. Conley, H. Rosenblatt, N. A. Jenkins, et al. 1993. CD40 ligand gene defects responsible for X-linked hyper-IgM syndrome. *Science* **259:**990–993.

DeFranco, A. L. 1999. B-lymphocyte activation, p. 225–261. *In* W. E. Paul (ed.), *Fundamental Immunology,* 4th ed. Lippincott-Raven Publishers, Philadelphia, Pa.

Neel, B. G. 1997. Role of phosphatases in lymphocyte activation. *Curr. Opin. Immunol.* **9:**405–420.

Sandor, M., and R. Lynch. 1993. The biology and pathology of Fc receptors. *J. Clin. Immunol.* **13:**237–246.

Zoller, K. E., I. A. MacNeil, and J. S. Brugge. 1997. Protein tyrosine kinases Syk and ZAP-70 display distinct requirements for Src family kinases in immune response receptor signal transduction. *J. Immunol.* **158:**1650–1659.

Immunoglobulin Genes

Agarwal, A., and D. G. Schatz. 1997. RAG1 and RAG2 form a stable postcleavage synaptic complex with DNA containing signal ends in V(D)J recombination. *Cell* **89:**43–53.

Han, S., S. R. Dillon, B. Zheng, M. Shimoda, et al. 1997. V(D)J recombinase activity in a subset of germinal center B lymphocytes. *Science* **278:**301–305.

Matsuda, F., K. Ishii, P. Bourvagnet, et al. 1998. The complete nucleotide sequence of the human immunoglobulin heavy chain variable region locus. *J. Exp. Med.* **188:**2151–2162.

Max, E. E. 1999. Immunoglobulins: molecular genetics, p. 111–182. *In* W. E. Paul (ed.), *Fundamental Immunology,* 4th ed. Lippincott-Raven Publishers, Philadelphia, Pa.

McBlane, J. F., D. C. van Gent, D. A. Ramsden, C. Romeo, C. A. Cuomo, M. Gellert, and M. A. Oettinger. 1995. Cleavage at a V(D)J recombination signal requires only RAG1 and RAG2 proteins and occurs in two steps. *Cell* **83:**387–395.

Schwarz, K., G. H. Gauss, L. Ludwig, U. Pannicke, Z. Li, et al. 1996. RAG mutations in human B cell-negative SCID. *Science* **274:**97–99.

Storb, U. 1996. The molecular basis of somatic hypermutation of immunoglobulin genes. *Curr. Opin. Immunol.* **24:**206–214.

Biotechnology Application of Antibody Genes

Boulianne, G. L., N. Hozumi, and M. J. Shulman. 1984. Production of functional chimaeric mouse/human antibody. *Nature* **312:**643–646.

Persic, L., A. Roberts, J. Wilton, A. Cattaneo, A. Bradbury, and H. R. Hoogenboom. 1997. An integrated vector system for the eukaryotic expression of antibodies or their fragments after selection from phage display libraries. *Gene* **187:**9–18.

Thrush, G. R., L. R. Lark, B. E. Clinchy, and E. S. Vitetta. 1996. Immunotoxins: an update. *Annu. Rev. Immunol.* **14:**49–71.

All about T Cells and Induction of Immunity

5

T Cells and the Immune Response

T cells are lymphocytes that do not express surface immunoglobulin but do express a different cell surface receptor for antigen, the T-cell receptor. T cells serve as the director or "maestro" of the immune response, controlling both the extent and the manner of the response. The immune system is organized to solve the problem of rapid specific recognition of an enormous number of potential antigens by efficient cell-to-cell collaboration and clonal expansion of specifically selected cells, which depend on T cells acting at each step. This collaboration occurs at three steps: (i) between antigen-presenting cells (macrophages and B cells) and T cells, (ii) between T-helper cells and antibody-producing B cells, and (iii) between T-helper cells and other T cells. In each step, the ability of T cells to respond in an antigen-specific manner is central to the strategy of the immune system. In addition to recognizing foreign proteins, T cells also retain a functional memory of virtually all self proteins, which enables them to distinguish between self and nonself antigens. How T cells become educated to recognize self and nonself is described in the section on the thymus in chapter 6.

T-Cell Recognition of Antigens

Although potential invaders contain a variety of proteins, nucleic acids, carbohydrates, and lipids, T cells respond almost exclusively to proteins of the pathogen. In the case of viruses, this focuses the immune response on structural and nonstructural proteins coded by viral genes. To recognize these protein antigens, T cells depend on the function of accessory cells, called antigen-presenting cells (APCs), and on the major histocompatibility complex (MHC) molecules of the APCs. T cells also depend on their own T-cell receptor (TCR) for antigen, as well as additional accessory molecules expressed on the T-cell surface, including CD4 and CD8.

T cells respond to antigen by cell activation and proliferation, with release of factors called cytokines, lymphokines, or interleukins. Activated T cells can then act as T-helper cells by providing essential signals needed for the clonal expansion of other antigen-specific cells, including B cells and T-cytolytic cells (T_{CTL} cells), as well as the cells that mediate delayed-type hypersensitivity (T_{DTH} cells), which are effector cells derived from T-helper cells. T_{CTL} cells recognize "target" cells after infection and destroy them before they can release new virus and infect other cells. T_{DTH} cells activate macrophages to phagocytose and kill organisms. The coordinated response of different cellular players follows prearranged scripts, and these are controlled and directed via signals from the T cell.

The immune response starts when foreign proteins are ingested by macrophages or when endogenous antigens in macrophages are "processed" (Fig. 5.1). These APCs do not have specific receptors for antigen but "present" antigen, which consists of processing the antigen into fragments and presenting the antigenic fragments to T-helper cells in a form that is recognized specifically by the T cells. APCs take up the antigen by endocytosis, and the early endosomes become acidified, which activates proteases. Partial enzymatic degradation of proteins occurs, yielding peptides. The most antigenic peptides bind to MHC molecules, which transport them to the cell surface of the APC for T-cell stimulation. Antigen presentation gets the immune response going by triggering the response of antigen-specific T-helper cells.

Clonal Expansion of T Cells

The T-cell response to antigen may be measured by mimicking clonal expansion in culture. In this method, T cells are cultured with antigen plus APCs. As the responding T cells start to grow, they actively synthesize new DNA. By adding radiolabeled thymidine, a building block of DNA, to the culture, the T-cell response can be measured as the incorporation of radioactive counts into newly synthesized DNA. This assay, which has revealed many properties of antigen recognition by T cells, exploits the

Figure 5.1 General scheme of antigen processing and presentation. Exogenous antigen is taken up in endosomes (lower pathway), where it is partially degraded to peptide fragments. Those peptides that bind MHC class II will be transported to the cell surface for presentation to $CD4^+$ T-helper cells. Alternatively, endogenously expressed antigen is processed by cytoplasmic proteases, and the peptide fragments that bind MHC class I are transported to the cell surface and presented to the precursor of $CD8^+$ T_{CTL} cells.

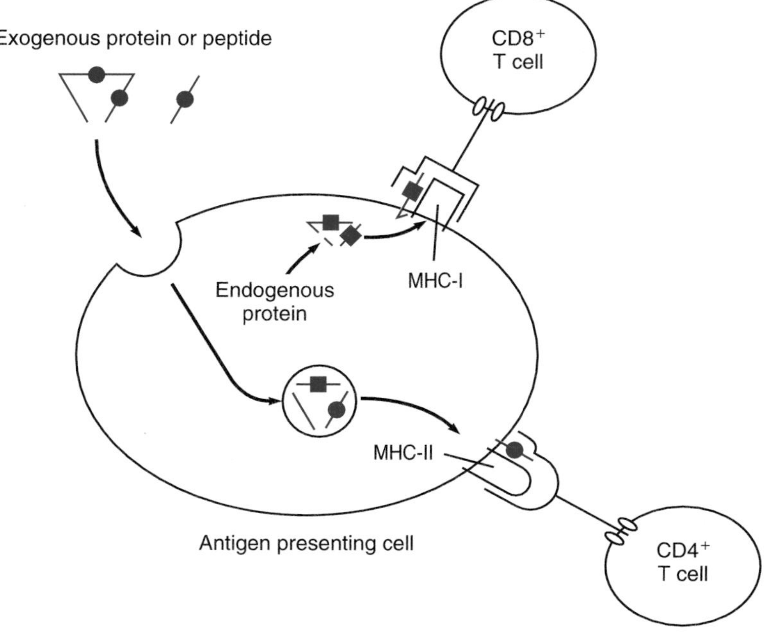

basic strategy of the immune system, namely, clonal selection by exponential growth of antigen-specific T cells. Through several lines of evidence, the proliferation assay revealed that T cells cannot respond directly to protein antigens but can only respond to antigen after processing.

Using repeated doses of antigen stimulation, T-cell proliferation may be driven to obtain a line of antigen-specific T cells. Consecutive rounds of antigen stimulation must be separated by a resting culture in the absence of antigen. This is necessary because antigen stimulation leads to temporary nonresponsiveness, but responsiveness can be recovered during resting periods without antigen. A second useful trick is to add T-cell growth factor, now called interleukin-2 (IL-2), to the cultures. This cytokine, found in the culture medium of stimulated T cells, is able to keep T-cell lines growing even in the absence of other signals and is particularly useful in maintaining T cells in resting cultures. Viability and expansion of responding T cells is enhanced by IL-2 because antigen stimulation induces expression of the receptor for IL-2 during the resting culture. As shown in Fig. 5.2, during the early rounds of antigen stimulation, the total number of cells in culture (mostly not antigen specific) falls rapidly, while the number of antigen-specific cells increases from nearly undetectable to the point where they exceed the number of nonspecific cells. By the third or fourth round of stimulation and rest, nearly all the cells of the line are antigen specific, as shown by exponential growth of the total cell number with subsequent rounds of antigen stimulation.

Figure 5.2 Theoretical growth curve for an antigen-specific T-cell line. Initially rare, these cells increase exponentially through successive rounds of antigen stimulation. In contrast, the nonspecific cells decline over time, due to lack of stimulation. The total cell number declines initially, then increases as antigen-specific T cells become the majority of the population. At this point, cloning by limiting dilution will give a high yield of antigen-specific T cells.

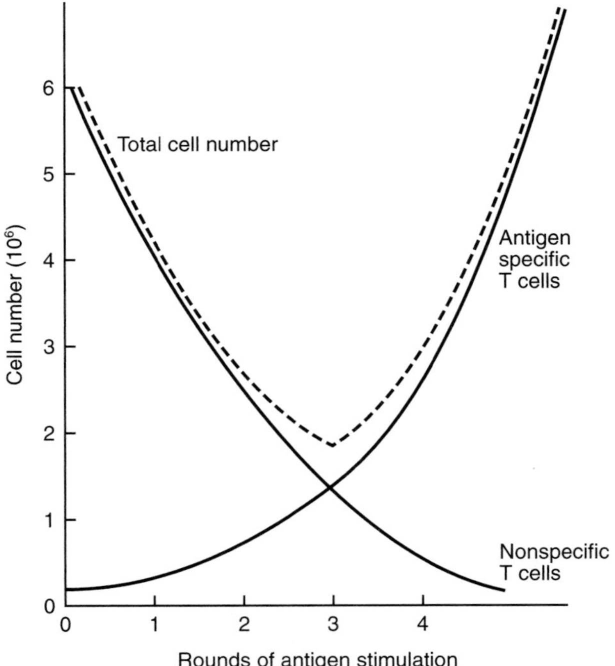

T-Cell Cloning

At this point, T-cell "lines" may be "cloned" by limiting dilution. In this method, the cells are spread among hundreds of microtiter wells at a low cell density so that, on average, there is less than one cell per well. In the presence of IL-2 and feeder cells, a line of T cells can be grown from a single cell. After 2 or 3 weeks in culture, some of the wells contain clumps of growing T cells. After further expansion, many of these growing colonies are found to be antigen-specific T cells. Since the original cloning was done, on average, at less than one cell per well, each of the cells in a well should be derived from the same parental cell, and they all should have the same specificity for antigen and MHC. Cloned T cells have been very useful in defining antigenic determinants (epitopes) recognized by T cells, as well as the MHC restriction and antigen-processing pathways, as described below.

T-Cell Hybridomas

Another highly successful technique is to fuse the antigen-specific T cells, after a single step of antigen stimulation, with a drug-sensitive T-cell tumor. The normal cells provide antigen specificity and the ability to survive drug selection, whereas the tumor cells confer unlimited growth potential on the product of cell fusion. After a few days in culture, the selecting drug is added to the culture, so only the fused cells can grow out. Thanks to the insight of John Kappler, the antigen-specific cells are detected by their production of IL-2 in response to antigen in combination with APCs, providing a way to measure the response to antigen, independent of T-cell growth. These T-cell hybridomas have become the best way to establish long-term T-cell lines in sufficient quantity to study the TCR for antigen.

T-Cell Epitope Mapping

Because a cloned T-cell line reacts to a single peptide antigen, the T-cell line responds to the same antigenic site, regardless of whether it occurs in a protein, polypeptide, or short peptide. Thus, the antigenic determinant (epitope) recognized by the T cell can be determined by replacing the native protein with large fragments or short peptides and measuring the T-cell proliferative response to each. This is called epitope mapping.

T-Helper-Cell Epitope Mapping

For example, for a specific T-helper-cell line, the peptide epitope hepatitis B antigen (HBsAg) was mapped, starting with large polypeptide fragments of the antigen and proceeding to a set of overlapping peptides (Fig. 5.3). Since native HBsAg protein exists in two forms, pre-S + S and S, the first step was to determine which form stimulated the T-cell line. As shown at the bottom of Fig. 5.3, the T-cell line responded to pre-S + S but not to S alone, indicating that it was specific for a site contained in the pre-S sequence. Similarly, large fragments of pre-S, called pre-S1 and pre-S2, were tested, and the response was mapped to pre-S1. Then a series of synthetic peptides corresponding to the pre-S1 sequence were tested, and three peptides, corresponding to amino acids 1 to 28 and 21 to 40, as well as amino acids 12 to 32, were found to stimulate the line. Since these three peptides overlap at just eight residues, the results map the site to amino acids 21 to 28 of the pre-S region. They clearly show that peptides, large or small, can replace a native protein for stimulation of T cells, provided that

T Cell Response to Synthetic Peptides of HBsAg

Antigen	Site	^{3}H – TdR Incorporation (Δcpm) Expt I	Expt II
Pre S_1	1–120	31,521	54,321
Pre S_2	121–174	– 1401	ND
1 – 21		4937	ND
1 – 28		29,866	65,432
12 – 32		23,601	ND
21 – 47		25,475	39,921
32 – 53		1567	ND
53 – 73		– 197	ND
94 – 117		1801	1715
120 – 145		1336	ND
Pre S + S Antigen		ND	62,944
S Antigen		ND	174
Medium Control		5374	1,731

Figure 5.3 Mapping the epitope specificity of a human T-cell line. The response to large recombinant fragments of HBsAG showed specificity for the pre-S1 region. A series of synthetic peptides were tested, and three overlapping peptides stimulated the line, mapping the epitope to the 8-amino-acid sequence shared by all three peptides.

they contain the antigenic sequence. By repeating this process for a number of T-cell clones, the predominant epitopes of HBsAg were identified. An alternative approach to mapping the epitopes recognized by T cells is to synthesize a series of synthetic peptides covering the entire protein sequence. Each peptide is tested individually to identify the most important sites for T-cell recognition.

T-Cytolytic-Cell Epitope Mapping

A similar approach has been used to find the epitopes recognized by T_{CTL} cells. These cells are capable of recognizing a virally infected cell at an early stage in the viral life cycle, before infectious virus has assembled. By lysing the cells at this time, it is possible to kill the infected cell without releasing infectious virions (Fig. 5.4A). The lytic activity of the T_{CTL} cells is measured by release of the radioisotope ^{51}Cr from radiolabeled target cells. The infected target cells are first allowed to take up ^{51}Cr, which binds covalently to intracellular proteins. The labeled target cells are then mixed with T_{CTL} cells at various ratios of T_{CTL} effectors to infected targets (E:T ratio). As the target cells are broken open, or lysed, by the action of T_{CTL} cells, ^{51}Cr-labeled proteins will be released. These can be detected by measuring ^{51}Cr radioactivity released into the culture supernatant. Using this assay, the ability of T_{CTL} cells to destroy infected target cells was shown to depend on the MHC class I antigens of the host, as well as the viral proteins synthesized inside the target cell. Uninfected cells could become targets of T_{CTL} cells by uptake of viral peptides, suggesting antigen processing within target cells. Since viral proteins were processed inside the cell (endogenous processing), T_{CTL}-cell specificity was not limited to proteins naturally expressed on the cell surface. Rather, viral proteins localized inside the target cell were also perfectly good target antigens for T_{CTL} cells.

For example (Fig. 5.4B), when a T_{CTL} line specific for influenza virus-infected cells is tested on target cells expressing individual viral proteins, lysis is specific for influenza nucleoprotein. Although this protein does not normally localize to the cell surface, it is a good target for T_{CTL} cells, because it can be processed to antigenic fragments and presented on the cell

Figure 5.4 **(A)** T_{CTL} cells (CTL) lyse the infected cell before assembly and release of new infectious virus, terminating the infection. **(B)** Epitope mapping with a series of peptides from influenza nucleoprotein. Target cells were labeled with ^{51}Cr and either infected (A), uninfected (0), or pulsed with nucleoprotein peptides. They were then incubated with influenza-specific T_{CTL} cells from the same donor. Cell lysis was detected as the release of ^{51}Cr from the target cells. (Modified from A. R. M. Townsend, J. Rothbard, F. M. Gotch, G. Bahadur, D. Wraith, and A. J. McMichael, *Cell* **44**:959–968, 1986.)

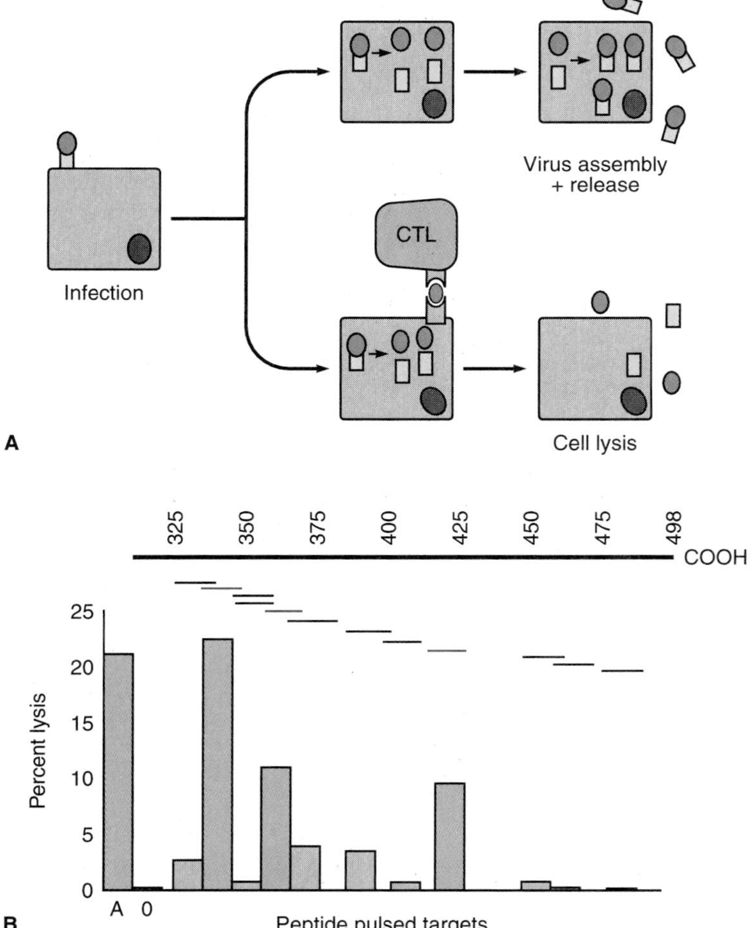

surface during infection. Using a series of synthetic peptides of the nucleoprotein sequence, the major antigenic epitopes recognized by T_{CTL} cells was localized to just a few sites on nucleoprotein. Thus, epitope mapping indicates that both stimulation of antigen-specific T-cell proliferation and T-cell cytotoxicity requires recognition of MHC molecules on the APCs.

The T-Cell Receptor

Structure

T-cell specificity for antigen and MHC is determined by the TCR. The TCR is specific for antigen in the form of peptide bound to an MHC protein (see below). Only when presented in this form by an APC does an antigen elicit a T-cell response. The TCR forms a complex of six proteins (Table 5.1 and Fig. 5.5), two of which, the α and β chains, have variable regions coding for the antigen plus MHC specificity and are responsible for antigen and MHC recognition. The TCR γ, δ, and ϵ chains, known as the CD3 complex, and the ζ chain assemble first, and then the α and β chains are added to form the complete receptor complex (Ti). The transmembrane and nearby segments of the CD3 proteins hold the complex together, whereas the cytoplasmic tails of CD3 and ζ are important for receptor signaling. Once the TCR binds antigen in association with the appropriate MHC structure, the intracellular segments of the CD3 and ζ chains become phosphorylated as an important early step in T-cell activation (discussed below).

The TCR α and β chains are like surface immunoglobulin on B cells and recognize each foreign antigen with a high degree of specificity. As with surface immunoglobulin, the TCR is present on the T-cell surface before antigen enters the system, and antigen recognition leads to rapid clonal expansion of antigen-specific T cells. The general scheme for generating diversity of the TCR α and β chains is remarkably similar to that for heavy and light chains of antibodies. There are two types of receptors on the T-cell surface. About 95% of mature T cells express TCRs with an α and a β chain ($T_{\alpha\beta}$ cells), whereas 5% bear γ and δ chain receptors ($T_{\gamma\delta}$ cells). These two groups of T cells are derived from distinct T-cell lineages. The $T_{\gamma\delta}$ cells are found more often in specialized locations, such as

Table 5.1 Properties of the protein chains of the TCR

Chains	Mol wt		Function
	Nonreduced	Reduced	
Ti			
α and β	90,000	41,000–43,000	Dual recognition of antigen and MHC
Cd3 complex: δ	25,000	25,000	Phosphorylated during cell activation
γ	26,000	26,000	Unknown
ϵ	21,000	21,000	Phosphorylated during cell activation
ζ	32,000	16,000	Phosphorylated during cell activation
CD4	51,000	51,000	Class II MHC recognition
CD8	76,000	76,000	Class I MHC recognition
Protein tyrosine kinases			
Lck	56,000		CD4 and CD8-associated signal transduc tion
ZAP-70	70,000		TCR-associated signal transduction
CD45	Isoforms 180,000–220,000		Stabilizes activated LcK kinase

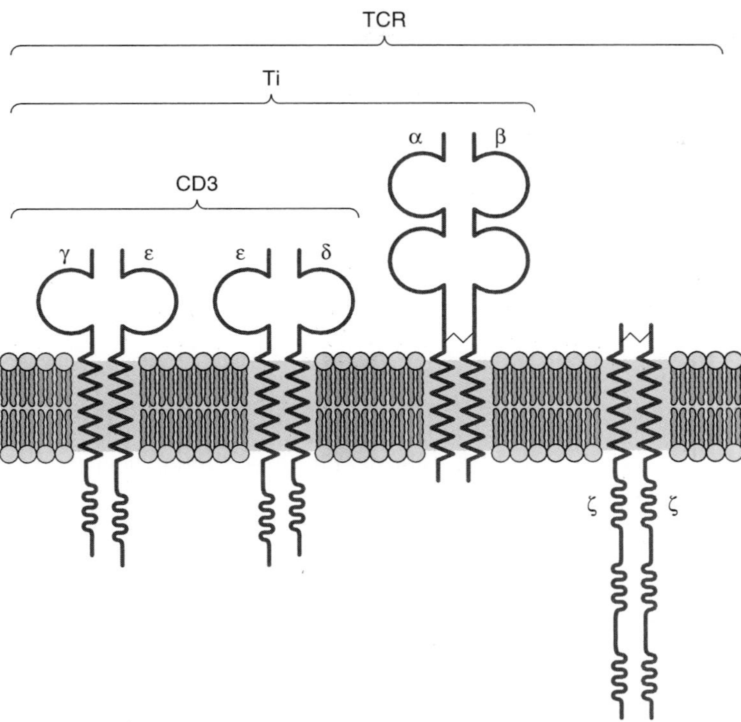

Figure 5.5 The TCR. Shown is the α- and β-chain heterodimer in association with the γ, δ, and ϵ chains of CD3 and the homodimer of the ζ chain. Within the TCR complexes are two copies of the CD3 ϵ chain forming dimers with either γ or δ chains. These chains interact with the enzymatic machinery on the cytoplasmic side of the membrane to generate intracellular activation signals (see below). The TCR chains have cytoplasmic tails of various lengths, which contain immunoreceptor tyrosine-based activation motifs (ITAM) that become phosphorylated at specific sites during T-cell activation through the action of receptor-associated protein tyrosine kinases. These phosphorylations initiate the process of T-cell activation.

the gastrointestinal tract and skin, and are thought to play a role in early immunosurveillance of infections. $T_{\alpha\beta}$ cells are more generally disbursed in lymphoid tissues and are the cells that provide help for induction of acquired immunity. As shown in Fig. 5.6, the diversity of TCR V_β chains is generated by recombination between separate variable, diversity, joining, and constant regions.

Unlike the surface immunoglobulin on B cells, once the TCR genes have recombined, there is no further somatic mutation. While this may prevent affinity maturation (higher binding to antigen with time), it may have the important advantage of preventing changes in receptor specificity that could lead to autoimmunity after thymic selection has occurred. As with immunoglobulins expressed by B cells, T cells show allelic exclusion of V_β chains, so each T cell can express only one V_β chain and has a single antigen specificity. Of the 70 germ line V_β genes, each is expressed on between 1 and 10% of all T cells. An extreme example of allelic exclusion occurs in transgenic mice, which have had transcriptionally active TCR V_α and V_β genes inserted into their germ line. Since these mice express the TCR transgenes early in T-cell development, other V_α and V_β genes are not expressed, owing to allelic exclusion. Thus, virtually every T cell in these mice expresses the V_α and V_β chains of the transgene.

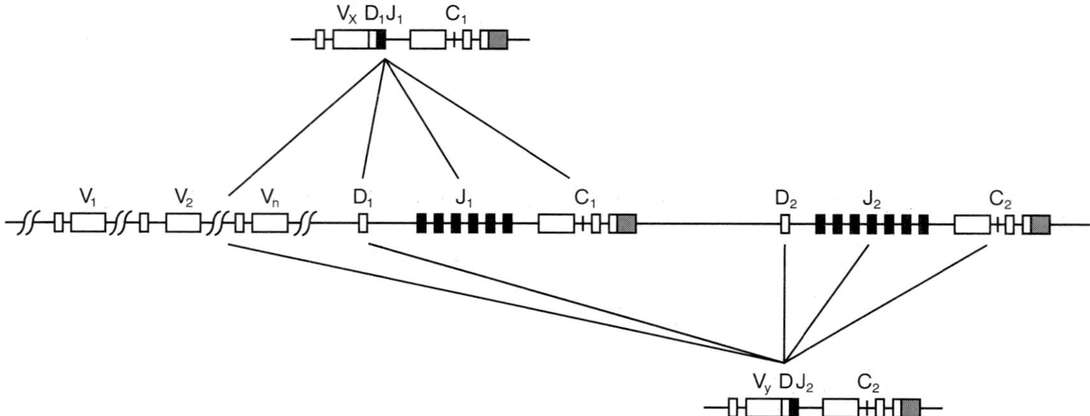

Figure 5.6 Combinatorial rearrangement of the variable (V), diversity (D), joining (J), and constant (C) gene segments of the germ line TCR β chain to form two possible TCR genes, one above and one below the germ line gene. The germ line V regions are arranged in tandem. In the process of forming an expressed TCR gene, one of them recombines with a D region, which then recombines with one of the J_β regions to form a transcriptionally active unit. In general, besides forming a contiguous gene, recombination also brings a promoter upstream of the V region into proximity of an enhancer region located near the C region, causing active transcription of the rearranged gene. Given the 70 V regions times 2 D regions times 6 J regions for each D region, recombination can generate over a thousand distinct TCR α and β chains with different specificities. This number is further greatly increased by junctional diversity, in which new sequences are filled in at the junctions between the V, D, and J regions, in locations that produce new contact residues for antigen binding. Altogether, over 10^5 combinations of α and β chains are possible, and the product of these (10^{10}) is an upper estimate of the possible number of different receptor specificities.

Chromosomal Location

The chromosomal locations of genes coding for all four variable and constant regions (αβ or γδ chains) have been identified (Table 5.2). Interestingly, the δ chain locus is contained completely within the variable and constant genes coding for the α chain. One might imagine that prior rearrangement of δ could occur in a precursor T cell, followed by rearrangement of α, with deletion of δ. However, there is no evidence for gene switching between these two subsets. Instead, they appear to represent distinct T-cell lineages, starting in the thymus.

Superantigens

TCR V_β chains can be stimulated by a special type of antigen called a superantigen. To trigger T cells, these superantigens must first bind to MHC class II of the APC, but they do not require antigen processing. Then they bind the TCR V_β chain, regardless of the antigen specificity of the V_β chain. By binding all T cells bearing a particular V_β chain, superantigens can activate an entire T-cell subset at once. Certain bacterial toxins, such as staphylococcal enterotoxin A, act by stimulating all murine T cells bearing $V_\beta1$, 3, 10, 11, and 17. Others, such as toxic shock syndrome toxin 1 (TSST-1), induce massive release of cytokines by stimulating all T cells with $V_\beta2$, resulting in the toxic shock syndrome. (For more details on how this works, see chapter 13). The hallmarks of superantigen-induced T-cell stimulation are (i) lack of antigen processing; (ii) flexible MHC requirements,

Table 5.2 Chromosomal location of TCR genes in humans and mice

Gene	Chromosomal location	
	Humans	Mice
TCR-α	14q11	14C-D
TCR-β	7q32-35	6B
TCR-γ	7q15	13A2-3
TCR-δ	14q11	14C-D

(iii) stimulation of all mature T cells with a particular V_β chain, regardless of antigen specificity, and (iv) ability to delete all immature thymocytes of the same V_β type.

T-Cell Activation

Antigen Signaling

Upon reaction of the TCR for antigen peptide-MHC complexes, T cells are activated to synthesize and secrete lymphokines and to proliferate. As defined above, the TCR consists of six different proteins. The Ti αβ or Ti λδ heterodimer extends from the surface of the cells. The αβ-, and γδ-chain pairs have both variable and constant regions, and, like antibodies, the variable regions determine specificity for recognizing antigen and MHC complexes. However, the α and β chains and γ and δ chains have short cytoplasmic tails, so they are not capable, by themselves, of triggering the cellular response to antigen. Instead, they rely on the CD3 chains (γ, δ, and ε) and the ζ chains to transmit a signal across the plasma membrane. These chains interact with the enzymatic machinery on the cytoplasmic side of the membrane to generate intracellular activation signals. Stimulation of the T cell by reaction of the TCR with peptide antigen-MHC molecules is accomplished by linkage of the TCR immunoreceptor tyrosine-based activation motifs (ITAMs) to intracellular activation pathways. These ITAMs interact with protein tyrosine kinases, resulting in a cascade of phosphorylations, activation of transcription factors, and production of lymphokines (Fig. 5.7).

Tyrosine Kinases

Two tyrosine kinases, Lck and ZAP-70, are directly involved in the CD3 and ζ-chain phosphorylation and the generation of the intracellular activation signal. Lck is a member of the Src family of protein tyrosine kinases. The amino half of Lck contains two Src homology sequences, called SH2 and SH3, while the carboxyl half contains the catalytic site. SH2 domains play a critical role during signal transduction. They recruit signal transduction molecules to activate protein tyrosine kinases (PTKs) and they protect tyrosine-phosphorylated sites from the action of protein tyrosine phosphatases, thereby prolonging the effects of tyrosine phosphorylation. In addition, they may allow the recruitment of kinases or phosphatases to potential substrates and regulate other enzymatic functions. Other sequences near the amino terminus of Lck code for binding to CD4 or CD8. Up to 90% of the Lck molecules are bound to CD4 in a $CD4^+$ T cell. The complex of CD4 plus Lck forms a receptor for MHC class II, with CD4 providing the ligand-binding function and Lck serving as the signal

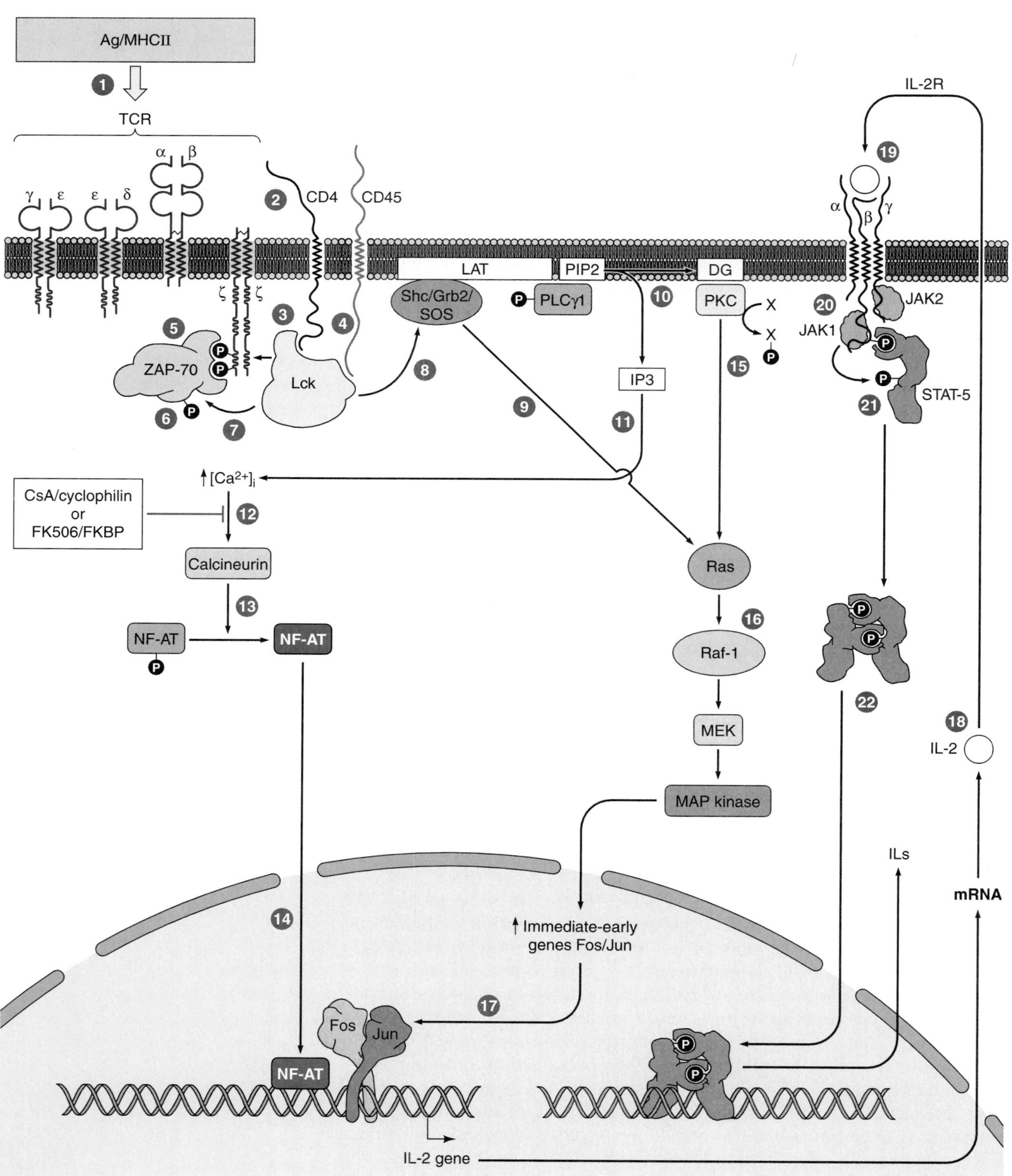

Ag/MHCII
1
TCR
γ ε ε δ
α β
2 CD4 CD45
ζ ζ
3 4
5
ZAP-70
P
P
Lck
6 P
7
8
LAT
PIP2
DG
Shc/Grb2/SOS
P PLCγ1
10
PKC
X
X
P
15
IP3
9
11
$\uparrow[Ca^{2+}]_i$
CsA/cyclophilin
or
FK506/FKBP
12
Calcineurin
13
NF-AT
P
NF-AT
Ras
16
Raf-1
MEK
MAP kinase
14
↑ Immediate-early genes Fos/Jun
17
Fos
Jun
NF-AT
IL-2 gene
IL-2R
19
α β γ
20
JAK2
JAK1
P
P
STAT-5
21
P
P
22
18
IL-2
ILs
mRNA
P
P

generator once ligand has bound. Similarly, CD8 and Lck form a combined receptor for MHC class I in $CD8^+$ T cells. In each case, the associated Lck kinase phosphorylates other proteins that are brought near CD4 or CD8 during antigen recognition. Mice deficient in Lck have a marked deficiency in protein tyrosine phosphorylation and markedly impaired T-cell function, including a profound arrest in thymic development at the $CD4^-/CD8^-$ to $CD4^+/CD8^+$ transition.

A second Src kinase, Fyn, with structural similarities to Lck, may play a role in activation of mature T cells. This protein tyrosine kinase also has two Src homology-2 domains and a catalytic domain, and it binds ζ chains as well as the CD3 chains. This binding increases in activated T cells, apparently because Fyn has greater affinity for the phosphorylated chains. Together, these two protein kinases make it possible to hypothesize an integrated model of TCR-mediated cell activation.

As the peptide plus MHC of the APC approaches the T-cell surface, it is bound by both the TCR α and β chains and by CD4. By binding the same antigen plus MHC ligand, the CD4-Lck receptor is brought close to the CD3 plus ζ complex, providing a substrate for the Lck protein kinase.

Figure 5.7 The TCR and activation of $CD4^+$ T cells. At the upper left is depicted the TCR. The sequence of events during T-cell activation upon reaction of the TCR with antigen/MHC complex is as follows. **(1)** Binding of extracellular domains of α and β chains of Ti to antigen in association with class II MHC. **(2)** Engagement of CD4/Lck with the TCR and MHC-antigen complex. **(3)** Activation of Lck protein-tyrosine kinase. **(4)** CD45 stabilizes active Lck. **(5)** Phosphorylation of ITAMs on γ and ζ chains of TCR. **(6)** Binding of ZAP-70 SH regions to PO4 on γ and ζ chains of TCR and phosphorylation of ZAP-70 by activated Lck. **(7)** ZAP-70 interacts with LCK SH2 domain to form a stable complex and activate LAT in the cell membrane. **(8)** LAT recruits the Grb2-Sos complex and PLC to the plasma membrane with phosphorylation and activation of PLCγ1 as well as adaptor proteins Grb2 and Shc, which bind to protein-rich regions in Sos, a guanine nucleotide exchange protein. **(9)** The Shc-Grb2-Sos complex activates Ras by nucleotide exchange (PKC-independent pathway). **(10)** PLCγ1, activated by Tec kinase, cleaves phosphatidylinositol 4,5-biphosphate into diglycerol (DG) and inositol phosphate (IP3). **(11)** IP3 mobilizes intracellular Ca^{2+} and increases transmembrane flux of extracellular Ca^{2+}. **(12)** Elevated cytoplasmic Ca^{2+} activates calcineurin. **(13)** Calcineurin acts to dephosphorylate and activate nuclear factor of activated T cells (NF-AT). **(14)** NF-AT relocates to the nucleus, where it binds to DNA and assists in transcriptional activation of the IL-2 gene. **(15)** Increased PKC activity of membrane DG leads to phosphorylation of a number of cellular proteins and activation of Ras (PKC-dependent pathway). **(16)** Ras activation leads to a cascade of protein kinase activities culminating in expression of immediate early genes Fos and Jun. **(17)** Fos/Jun bind to regulatory sequences in DNA along with NF-AT and act to upregulate IL-2 gene expression. **(18)** IL-2 is secreted and acts as an autocrine factor for stimulating the cell to transit G_1 after reaction with the IL-2 receptor (IL-2R). **(19)** After reaction with IL-2, there is rearrangement of the receptor chains allowing juxtaposition of the Jak kinases (Jak1 with the β chain and Jak3 with the γ chain) and phosphorylation of the β chain. **(20)** One phosphorylation site on the β chain leads to phosphorylation of Shc and activation of Ras. **(21)** A second dual phosphorylation site further into the cytoplasmic tail of the β chain allows docking of signal transducer and activator of transcription 5 (STAT-5) through its SH2 domain. **(22)** STAT-5 is phosphorylated, dimerizes, and translocates to the nucleus, where it activates genes for a variety of interleukins and cytokines involved in proliferation of T cells and other cell types. Different STAT molecules may be involved in activation of genes for different cytokines, including but not limited to IL-3, -4, -5, -7, -12, and granulocyte-monocyte colony-stimulating factor as well as IFN-γ. (Modified from A. Weiss, p. 411–447, *in* W. E. Paul, ed., *Fundamental Immunology,* 4th ed., Lippincott-Raven, Philadelphia, Pa., 1999.)

In the second step, the phosphorylated CD3 and ζ chains induce binding of Fyn and its activation by Lck. Fyn then phosphorylates downstream effectors, which activate the entire cell. Presumably, this process occurs each time the T cell encounters its antigen plus MHC, as during antigen priming and T-helper cell activation of B cells. Lck activation also occurs during thymic maturation, whereas Fyn appears mainly to be involved in activation of mature T cells. Mice lacking Fyn develop normally but have deficiencies in activation of single-positive $CD4^+$ or $CD8^+$ T cells. Fyn may cooperate with Lck during development, because a complete developmental block in development of $CD4^+/CD8^+$ thymocytes is seen in double-negative mice.

The Syk family of PTKs includes Syk and ZAP-70. Syk is found in immature thymic cells and in $T_{\gamma\delta}$ cells. ZAP-70 is expressed in mature T cells and natural killer cells. These molecules each have two SH2 N-terminal domains and a C-terminal catalytic domain. ZAP-70 binds with high affinity to doubly phosphorylated ITAMs to the more C-terminal SH2 domain. The Src and Syk kinases interact with the TCR in a highly coordinated and sequential manner during T-cell activation. When the TCR and CD4 engage an MHC class II molecule, Lck is brought into close proximity with the TCR cytoplasmic domain and phosphorylates CD3 and ζ chains. ZAP-70 is recruited to the tyrosine-phosphorylated CD3 and ζ chains by its SH2 domains, which allows Lck to transphosphorylate and activate ZAP-70.

The role of ZAP-70 is revealed further by a genetic defect in humans. Homozygous patients have a form of severe combined immunodeficiency that causes a defect in T cells and in antibody formation. In these patients, the mutations produce an unstable form of ZAP-70, depriving the T cells of detectable ZAP-70 protein or function. As expected, the peripheral T cells lack the ability to signal via the TCR, measured as loss of response to either mitogens or antibodies that cross-link the TCR. In contrast, receptor-independent cell activation, via phorbol ester and calcium ionophore, is normal. Thymic maturation of $CD8^+$ T cells is blocked. Surprisingly, however, normal numbers of mature $CD4^+$ T cells are produced, suggesting the possibility that other kinases, such as Syk or Fyn, may supply this function during thymic development of $CD4^+$ cells. However, once they mature, none of these T cells is able to function without ZAP-70, and the result is a profound T-cell-deficiency syndrome, despite normal numbers of $CD4^+$ T cells.

Tec Kinases

Tec kinases are a distinct family of PTKs that are expressed in lymphoid cell lineages and involved in T-cell activation. Loss of Tec kinases does not affect events immediately downstream for TCR activation, but loss of Tec is associated with impaired IP3 production, calcium mobilization, and mitogen-activated kinase activation. Thus, Tec kinases appear to be a link between the ZAP-70 and Src families and phospholipase $C\gamma$ activation.

CD45

CD45 (leukocyte common antigen) is a transmembrane protein tyrosine phosphatase found in all cells of the hematopoietic lineage except mature red blood cells. Different isoforms are expressed differently. CD45 exists in isoforms with molecular masses of 180, 190, 205, and 220 kDa that identify cells that die or develop further in the thymus. Thymocytes that express CD45 p180 are designated CD45RA and are destined to die in the thymus;

those with CD45 205/220 are called CD45RO and are in the lineage that will become functional T cells. In the periphery, 60% of T cells are CD45RA and 40% are CD45RO. On peripheral T cells, CD45 p180 (RA) identifies resting memory T cells. Activation of these cells in the periphery is associated with conversion to reexpression of CD45 p205/220 (RO). It is concluded that inappropriate rearrangement or specificity of the TCR in the thymus activates expression of CD45 p180 and cell death. Loss of CD45 in engineered cell lines is associated with a loss in TCR signal transduction. CD45 can dephosphorylate the negative regulatory site of Lck, resulting in activation of Lck. Thus, CD45 acts to remove the negative regulation of Lck and allow the Lck to become activated.

Phospholipase Cγ1

TCR induction of PTK activity results in the phosphorylation of a large number of cellular proteins, in addition to the chains of the TCR, Src, and Syk kinases. One of the most important is membrane-associated phospholipase Cγ1 (PLCγ1). Although normally PLCγ1 is a cytoplasmic enzyme, some is translocated to the membrane through interaction with phosphorylated SH2 domains on Syk or ZAP-70, where it is in a position to be phosphorylated by any of the TCR-regulated kinases, most likely a Tec kinase. Activation of PLCγ1 by tyrosine phosphorylation leads to generation of second messengers of the phosphoinositol pathway. Hydrolysis of the membrane-associated phosphatidylinositol 4,5-biphosphate results in formation of inositol 1,4,5-triphosphate (1,4,5-IP3) and 1*m*2-diacylglycerol (DG). These act as second messenger to induce an increase in concentration of calcium ions ([Ca^{2+}]) and activation of protein kinase C (PKC). This occurs within seconds of the binding of the TCR by antigen and will last as long as the TCR is occupied. The intracellular calcium ion levels are raised first by mobilization of Ca^{2+} from the endoplasmic reticulum (ER) and then from transmembrane flux from extracellular sources of Ca^{2+}. Elevated calcium activates calmodulin-dependent events through the activation of calcineurin and Ca^{2+}/calmodulin-dependent kinase. The immunosuppressive agents cyclosporine and FK506, which have played a spectacular clinical role in prolonging human allograft survival, act by inhibiting calcineurin. Calcineurin dephosphorylates nuclear factor of activated T cells (NF-AT), revealing a binding site of NF-AT for the IL-2 gene promoter. NF-AT passes into the nucleus and combines with the immediate early genes Fos and Jun to activate the transcription of many lymphokine genes, including IL-2. Nuclear transport of NF-AT by itself is not sufficient to activate transcription of NF-AT target genes, as NF-AT becomes engaged with a nuclear export protein Crm1 and undergoes futile cycling across the nuclear envelope. Calcineurin masks the nuclear export signals on NF-AT and blocks Crm1-mediated export, allowing NF-AT to bind to DNA and other transcription proteins.

The Ras Pathway

One of the other effects of PKC activation is activation of Ras. Ras is active in the GTP-bound state and inactive in the GDP-bound state. Ras is also activated through PKC-independent pathways through guanine nucleotide exchange proteins, such as Shc-Grb2-SOS complexes. Grb2 is an adaptor protein containing SH2 and SH3 domains. In activated cells, Grb2 binds to another adaptor protein called Shc and then, through its SH3 domain, to proline-rich regions in SOS. The GTPase activity of Ras is regulated by interaction with SOS. With formation of this complex, there is inactivation of Ras triphosphatase activity and activation of Ras. Activation of Ras leads to a sequence of activation of kinases, including Raf, MEK, and mitogen-activated protein kinase, followed by upregulation of the immediate early genes Fos and Jun, which interact with NF-AT to upregulate lymphokine synthesis, including IL-2.

IL-2 and IL-2 Receptors

IL-2 can function as an autocrine stimulator, interacting with IL-2 receptors (IL-2Rs) on the same cell that produced the IL-2, which is also upregulated during T-cell activation. Three IL-2Rs have been detected on T cells with high, intermediate, and low affinity for IL-2. These are composed of different transmembrane chains: α, β, and γ. The low-affinity receptor has only α chain, the intermediate affinity receptor has β and γ, and the high-affinity receptor has α, β, and γ. Each chain appears to have a separate receptor for IL-2, but the β and γ chains will bind IL-2 only when present as a dimer. The low-affinity receptor is found on activated T cells and is identified as CD25. Only the high-affinity receptor binds IL-2 at physiologic conditions, internalizes it, and initiates T-cell proliferation. Mutations in the IL-2R γ chain are responsible for most cases of X-linked severe combined immunodeficiency syndrome. The cytoplasmic chain of the β and γ do not encode enzymatic activity and are not involved in the initial activation signal of T cells but interact with cytoplasmic proteins to initiate signals required for proliferation and differentiation.

The Jak/STAT Pathway

The cytoplasmic chains of the IL-2R react with the cytoplasmic Jak family of PTK and signal transducers and activators of transcription (STAT). Conserved cytoplasmic domains of β and γ chains react with Jak1 and Jak3 PTKs, respectively. Dimerization of the β and γ chains leads to activation of the associated Jak1 and Jak3 PTKs and phosphorylation of STAT-5 proteins. Activated STAT proteins dimerize and translocate to the nucleus where they bind to specific DNA sequences and contribute to transcription of immediate early genes, as well as B-cell lymphoma gene 2. The IL-2R may also activate T cells through other mechanisms, such as by Src, Shc, and P13 kinases. Although IL-2 is the major molecule driving T-cell proliferation, other lymphokines, such as IL-4 and IL-15, may function as T-cell growth factors in the absence of IL-2.

The complexity and subtlety of TCR signaling may reflect the varied responses of activated T cells. In addition, certain signals may be responsible for a specific step in T-cell maturation, such as thymic maturation or peripheral tolerance, whereas others may be used for a variety of responses of mature peripheral T cells, including T-cell help and release of cytokines involved in inflammatory reactions.

Antigen Processing and Presentation

T cells cannot respond to protein antigens unless they have been processed and presented by the MHC of an APC. T cells do not respond to protein antigens directly. Instead, they require partial proteolytic degradation to antigenic peptides. As indicated in Fig. 5.1, two processing pathways have been identified: (i) endosomal or exogenous and (ii) nonendosomal or endogenous. The endosomal pathway produces peptides for association with MHC class II in endosomes. The proteasomal pathway produces peptides for association with MHC class I in the ER. The peptide-MHC complex is transported to the cell surface for presentation to T cells. Immunogenicity reflects high-affinity binding between a peptide and the peptide-binding groove of MHC. In this way, T cells may look at either their own proteins or "foreign" proteins produced by intracellular infectious agents by endogenous processing through MHC-I or "foreign" proteins ingested from the extracellular environment through MHC-II. In using these pathways, the immune system appears to have adapted well-established pathways of intracellular protein trafficking in order to process antigens for immune recognition.

The alleles of the MHC were first identified as responsible for tissue graft rejection. If donor and recipient share the same MHC markers, then grafts are generally accepted (although other genetic differences may lead to rejection, the minor histocompatibility antigens), whereas if the donor contains MHC antigen not present in the recipient, the graft will be rapidly rejected (see below). It was later found that the same cell surface molecules of the MHC also were responsible for antigen recognition by T cells.

Endosomal or Exogenous Processing

In the endosomal or exogenous pathway, extracellular or exogenous antigens are taken up by endocytosis into early endosomes of APCs (Fig. 5.8). Acidification of endosomes activates resident proteases, such as cathepsin D, which partially degrade the foreign proteins into antigenic fragments. As the proteins are cut to smaller fragments, they are also unfolded, exposing the anchor residues for MHC binding. Meanwhile, MHC class II proteins, following their synthesis on polyribosomes and assembly in the ER, travel through the Golgi and enter endosomes. When first assembled, they consist of three chains, called the alpha, beta, and invariant chains. The invariant chain apparently binds the other chains and blocks the peptide-binding groove on the MHC. When invariant chain is removed in the endosomes, the peptide-binding groove is exposed for peptide binding. MHC will acquire any available peptides, and, if the peptide binds stably, the peptide-MHC complex will be transported to the cell surface for presentation to T cells. Thus, the affinity of peptide binding to MHC class II determines which peptides will be immunogenic and which will not. Since the endosomal proteases are activated by the acid pH of endosomes, they can be inhibited by weak bases that prevent acidification, such as chloroquine and ammonium chloride. They are also sensitive to the protease inhibitors leupeptin and E-64. Inhibition by these agents is evidence that the protein was processed via the endosomal pathway.

Nonendosomal or Endogenous Processing

Nonendosomal or endogenous processing usually begins when a virus takes over the cell and directs the cell's transcription and translation machinery to synthesize viral proteins (Fig. 5.9). A small percentage of these "endogenously" synthesized proteins are diverted for processing by a proteolytic particle, called the proteasome. Proteasomes are assembled from 15 to 20 low-molecular-weight proteins, and they normally function to remove defective or senescent proteins from the cell. During infection, they also degrade viral proteins that have reached the cytoplasm, producing viral peptides for MHC binding and presentation to T cells. However, before they can bind MHC, the peptides must get into the same intracellular

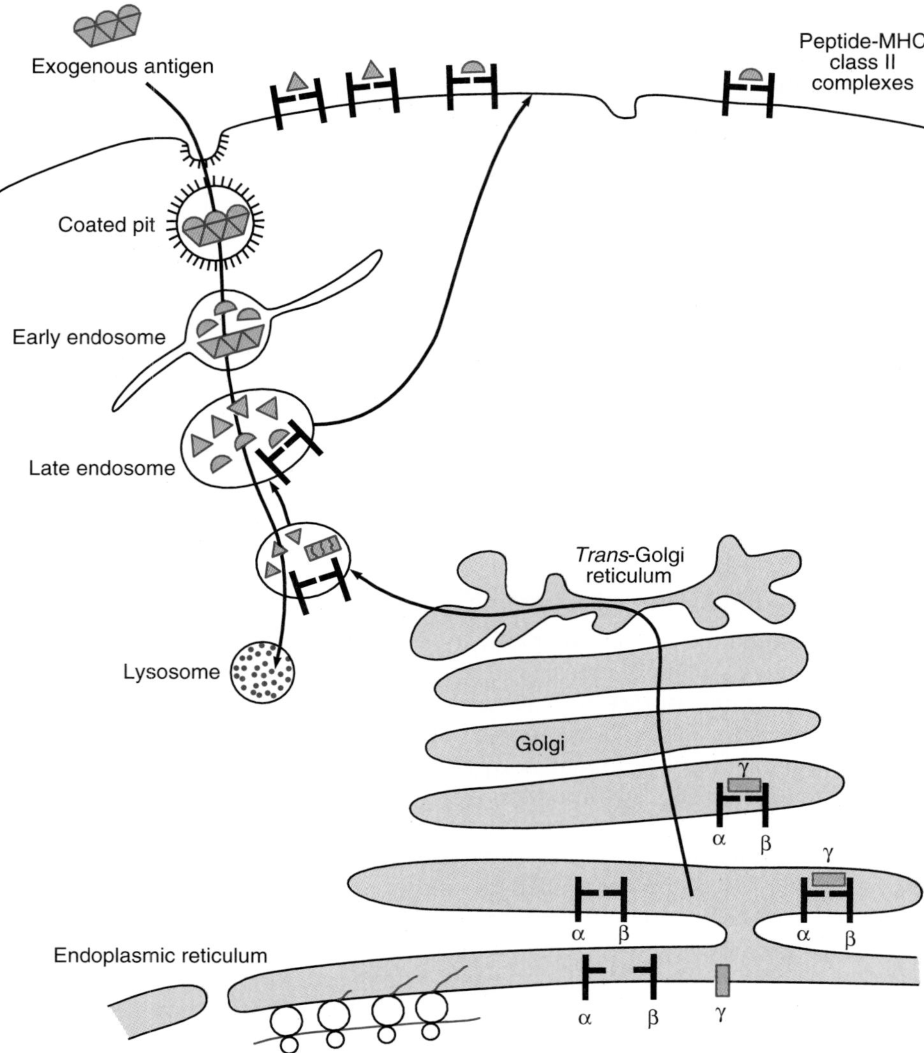

Figure 5.8 Endosomal processing pathway leading to antigen presentation with MHC class II. Class II alpha and beta chains assemble with invariant chain (γ chain) in the ER. They are transported to endosomes, where the invariant chain comes off so peptide can bind. They are then transported to the surface with peptide in the binding groove.

compartment as MHC. Newly synthesized MHC class I molecules are held in the ER and wait there until they either bind peptides or are degraded. Thus, it is essential for peptides to be transported from the proteasome to the ER, which requires the activity of a peptide transporter.

At least four proteins are implicated in the supply of peptides for antigen presentation. Two of these, called TAP-1 and -2, are members of the ATP-binding cassette transporter family. Together, they form a heterodimer that transports peptides from the proteasome to the ER for MHC class I binding. Mutant cells, which lack the normal supply of peptide transport proteins, fail to transport MHC class I to the cell surface. Mutations in another two genes, RMA-S and CEM.174, result in deletion of two additional proteins, LMP-2 and -7 (for low-molecular-weight proteins), associated

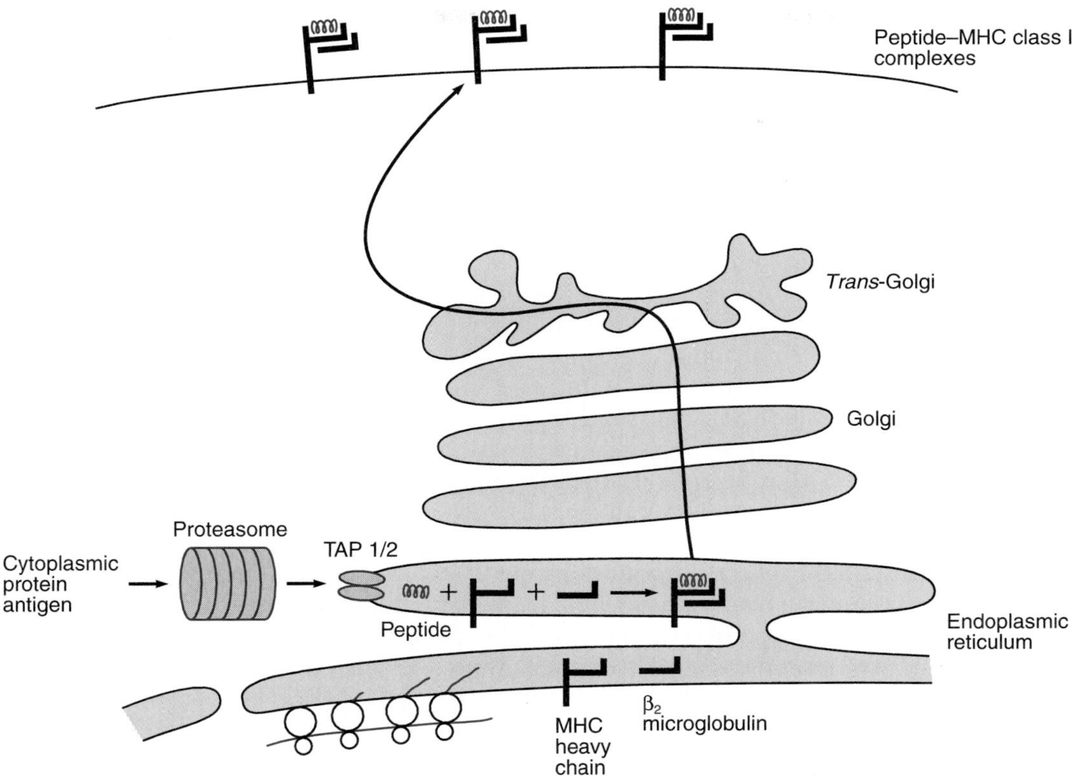

Figure 5.9 Nonendosomal (proteasomal) processing pathway leading to antigen presentation with MHC class I. Class I heavy-chain and β_2-microglobulin must wait in the ER until peptide is supplied by the TAP-1/2 peptide transporter. MHC class I needs peptide to form a stable complex that can be transported through the Golgi apparatus and on to the cell surface.

with the proteasome, which play a role in the specificity of proteasomal degradation and production of peptide fragments. During infection, the MHC-encoded proteins function as an elaborate peptide production and transport system, starting with peptide generation in the proteasome (LMP-2 and -7), followed by peptide transport into the ER (TAP-1 and -2) and out to the cell surface (MHC class I heavy and light chains).

The difference between the two processing pathways may be blurred in certain cases. What distinguishes them is the intracellular compartments for peptide binding to MHC. Exogenous proteins are usually degraded to peptides in the endosomal compartment, where they are acquired by MHC class II molecules. Endogenous proteins are usually degraded in cytoplasmic proteasomes and transported into the ER by TAP-1 and -2 for MHC class I binding. However, exceptions to this simple rule are well known, particularly for endogenous proteins presented with MHC class II. This could occur if endogenous proteins were processed endosomally or if proteasomal peptides could escape the TAP-1 and -2 transporter and reach endosomes instead.

Because of the large number of self peptides, it might be difficult for viral peptides to compete for the available binding sites on MHC class I molecules. Recent studies have shown that viral peptides need to bind only a small fraction of MHC class I molecules, as few as 200 per cell, to trigger a T-cell response. This suggests that the immune system may be tuned to respond to virus-sized aggregates of foreign proteins, while ignoring smaller units of self proteins. This may be important for vaccine design, since particulate antigens such as HBsAg, which contain about 200 copies of HBsAg protein per particle, are 1,000 times more immunogenic than the same amount of HBsAg monomers.

Peptide-MHC Binding

The basis for T-cell recognition of antigen in association with MHC is that antigenic peptides bind directly to MHC molecules. To demonstrate this binding, an antigenic peptide fragment of ovalbumin (egg albumin) corresponding to amino acids 323 to 339 was radiolabeled and incubated with MHC class II molecules purified from mouse APCs. Bound peptides were separated from free peptides by passing the mixture over a Sephadex column, which separates molecules by size. Since the complex of peptide plus MHC is quite large, it comes through the column first, whereas the unbound peptide comes through later. The extent of peptide binding was estimated by comparing the area under the two peaks. These experiments demonstrated several important properties of peptide binding to MHC class II. First, the binding sites on MHC are saturable, since excess unlabeled peptide could compete off the radiolabeled peptide. Second, two different peptides can bind the same site on MHC, since they also compete for binding. Third, those peptides capable of binding a particular MHC type correspond closely to those known to be immunogenic in mice of the same MHC type. These results suggested that MHC proteins should have a peptide-binding site.

The Peptide-Binding Groove of MHC

The three-dimensional structure of MHC (Fig. 5.10) showed that MHC class I molecules have a lower part anchored in the cell membrane and an

Figure 5.10 Structure of the peptide-binding groove of class II HLA-A2. The black areas at the base of the receptor groove indicate the polymorphic residues of the class II MHC molecule, which are reflected in genetic variations in the ability of different alleles of the class II MHC to present immunogenic peptides. Peptides fit into the groove and interact with the floor and walls. The strength of binding in the groove determines immunogenicity. (Modified from P. J. Bjorkman, M. A. Saper, B. Samraoui, W. S. Bennett, J. L. Strominger, and D. C. Wiley, *Nature* **329**:512–518, 1987.)

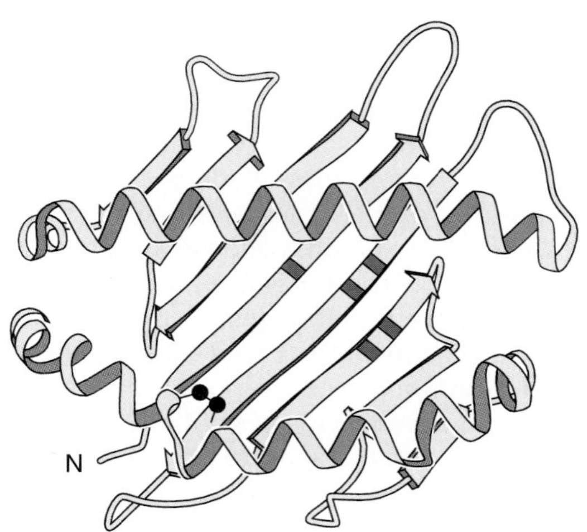

upper part with a binding groove large enough to bind antigenic peptides. The sides of the groove consist of alpha-helical structures of the HLA heavy chain, and the floor consists of β-pleated sheet. The walls and floor provide numerous contact sites for bound peptides. Those peptides that form noncovalent bonds to the amino acid side chains of the binding groove will bind stably. Other peptides, lacking "goodness of fit," will come out of the groove as fast as they go in and will not survive long enough for antigen presentation to T cells.

Since the walls and floor of the peptide-binding groove are lined with residues that vary from one MHC type to another, this structure explains why different peptides will bind to different MHC types. Since a given peptide could bind stably to the MHC of one type and not another, different peptides will be immunogenic in different people, depending on their MHC types. This could present a major obstacle to developing a vaccine based on synthetic peptides, since a number of different peptides might be needed to immunize a population of diverse MHC types.

Anchor Residues

Binding of peptides to MHC is through shared amino acids in the peptide known as "anchor residues." Analysis of peptides eluted after binding to MHC revealed that different MHC molecules generally bind different peptides, but the peptides bound by a given MHC molecule share amino acid residues (anchor residues) and correspond to the binding motif for the MHC groove. For example, peptides eluted from the mouse class I molecule H-2 Kd gave more than 10 well-resolved peaks, plus many additional minor peaks. Most of these peptides were nanomers, with variable sequences at seven positions but fairly strict conservation of amino acids Tyr or Phe at position 2 and Ile or Leu at position 9. This motif was also found in the sequences of individual peptides from viruses, tumors, and parasites that were known to be presented by H-2 Kd.

The shared anchor residues have been determined for other MHC class I binding molecules, including H-2 Kd, Kb, and Db in mice and HLA-A2.1 and B27 in humans. In general, all peptides binding MHC class I are eight or nine amino acids long. The second or fifth position and the eighth or ninth position are conserved among all the peptides binding a given MHC molecule, but they are unique for each MHC type. Although these anchor residues are conserved, the rest of the peptide sequence can vary widely, allowing many different peptides to bind the same MHC groove, provided they conform to the binding motif. Once an MHC binding motif is known, it can be used to search for as yet unidentified antigenic sites on foreign proteins.

HLA-B27

Another interesting example is provided by the peptides binding to the class II HLA-B27 molecule. The anchor residues are Arg at position 2 and Lys or Arg at position 9. These anchor residues, spaced seven amino acids apart, can be used to scan amino acid sequences in search of new antigenic sites likely to bind HLA-B27. Some of these were found on foreign proteins, such as human immunodeficiency virus type 1 (HIV-1) envelope glycoprotein gp120 and influenza virus nucleoprotein. But other peptides were derived from self cellular proteins. The significance of this will be discussed further below.

The Major Histocompatibility Complex

The organization of MHC genes in mice and humans is shown in Fig. 5.11. The MHC occupies 4 million base pairs on the short arm of chromosome 6 in humans and a similar length on chromosome 17 of mice. These regions contain a number of genes related to MHC class I and class II proteins as well as some with other immunologic functions.

New alleles of MHC are constantly being identified. An update is maintained by Steven Marsh at The Anthony Nolan Bone Marrow Trust in

Figure 5.11 Genetic maps of the MHC of humans and mice. Three markers, Ke3, Bat I, and Mog, serve to define the relative positions of the other genes in the two species. The human MHC region contains clusters of genes in three designated regions: *Mhc* class II, *Mhc* class III, and *Mhc* class I. The *Mhc* class II region includes the seven genes encoding the class II MHC molecules, as well as the LMP (processing) and TAP (transporter-associated proteins) involved in antigen processing and presentation. HLA-DR proteins are the major antigen-presenting molecules for exogenous processing and are highly represented on professional APCs, such as memory B cells, macrophages, and tissue resident macrophages. However, they can also be induced on activated T cells and in other tissues when stimulated by inflammatory cytokines such as IFN. The *Mhc* class III region contains genes for complement components (C4, Bf, and C2) and tumor necrosis factor (TNF-α and -β). The *Mhc* class I region encodes HLA-A, B, C, E, F, G, and H. HLA-A, B and C are the major class I *Mhc* antigen-presenting molecules for endogenous antigen processing. The class I antigens are largely responsible for tissue graft rejection and are found on virtually every nucleated cell in the body but are not found on red blood cells. This is why blood transfusions must match for the blood group antigens A, B, and O but not for tissue type, whereas other transplants must match for both or be rejected. Since each person inherits two copies of HLA genes, their tissue type may include up to six different class I alleles. Comparison of the mouse MHC with the human MHC shows that the order of the regions is not the same, with the proximal segment of the mouse region encoding MHC-I. The mouse MHC class I gene *H-2K* is separated from the other class I genes, *H-2D* and *H-2L*, by the MHC-II and MHC-III regions, including the class II genes coding for 1-A and 1-E, and the class III genes for complement components (C2 and C4), enzymes (21-hydroxylase, 21-OH, and glyoxalase [GLO]), and cytokines (TNF). (Modified from D. H. Margulis, p. 263–285, *in* W. E. Paul, ed., *Fundamental Immunology*, 4th ed., Lippincott-Raven Publishers, Philadelphia, Pa., 1999.)

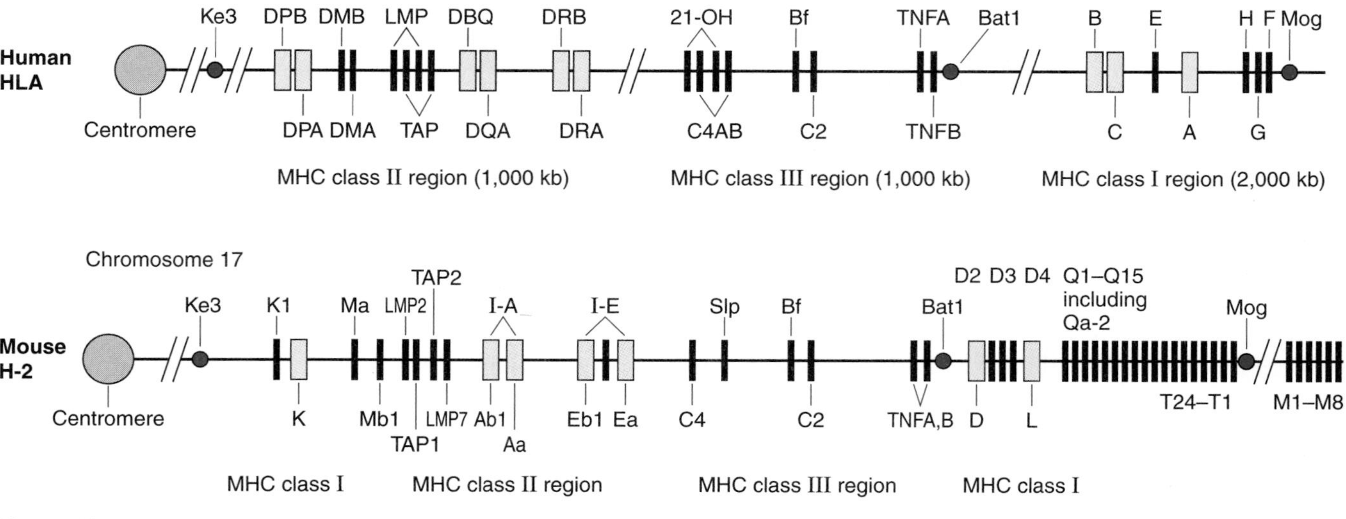

England and can be searched through the website http://www.anthonynolan.com/HIG/index.html. As of January 1998, 298 HLA-DRB, 20 HLA-DQA1, 44 HLA-DQB1, 19 HLA-DPA1, 86 HLA-DPB1, 4 HLA-DMA, and 6 HLA-DMB class II alleles and 165 HLA-A, 327 HLA-B, 88 HLA-C, 5 HLA-E, and 14 HLA-G class I alleles had been identified. Within the human population, the number of possible combinations on each chromosome for HLA class I, largely responsible for tissue graft recognition, would be the product of 165 HLA-A alleles × 327 HLA-B × 88 HLA-C × 5 HLA-E × 14 HLA-G = 332,362,800 combinations. This number is increased further, since each person has two copies of chromosome 6, but is reduced slightly by the fact that certain alleles tend to occur together, a phenomenon called linkage disequilibrium.

Structure

When expressed on the cell surface, class I MHC antigens consist of two subunits of 45 and 12 kDa. Only the larger subunit is encoded in the MHC; the smaller is the cell surface form of β_2-microglobulin and does not vary with MHC type. The MHC class II proteins also have two subunits, an alpha chain of 34 kDa and a beta chain of 29 kDa. The human class II genes encode seven proteins, and both subunits of the cell surface dimer are polymorphic. Some have one alpha chain and one beta chain, whereas others have two beta chains. Each person has two copies of the seven class II genes, giving up to 14 MHC class II tissue types. These provoke a strong T-cell response between lymphocytes from mismatched individuals, and the mixed lymphocyte reaction was the earliest way that MHC class II differences in humans were detected. The large number of possible combinations of class I and II tissue types produces the marked HLA diversity observed in human populations and explains the low probability of finding a perfect HLA match between unrelated organ donors and those in need of a transplant.

Inheritance

Within a family, all of the HLA alleles on each parental chromosome 6 are inherited together in a block, called a haplotype. Thus, for purposes of tissue transplantation, all seven of the class I MHC genes on one chromosome are inherited together, unless there is a crossover. The pedigree of a typical family, with parental haplotypes AB and CD, is shown in Fig. 5.12A. According to Mendelian genetics, the children will inherit one haplotype from each parent, giving just four possible combinations: AC, AD, BC, and BD. For each child, the likelihood of matching another sibling for HLA is 25% for a perfect match at both haplotypes and 50% for matching at just one haplotype. Neither parent will match perfectly, since the children must inherit one haplotype from the other parent. For transplantation purposes, it makes an enormous difference whether both haplotypes are shared between donor and recipient, in which case most transplanted organs will be accepted. This is reflected in the 90% 1-year survival of renal allografts from a perfectly matched sibling donor (Fig. 5.12B). In contrast, haplotype mismatched organs are rejected, and renal graft survival decreases in proportion to the number of HLA mismatches.

HLA Matching

For unrelated donors, matching of HLA type of donor and recipient increases the survival time of the grafted organ (Fig. 5.13). The methods of

A

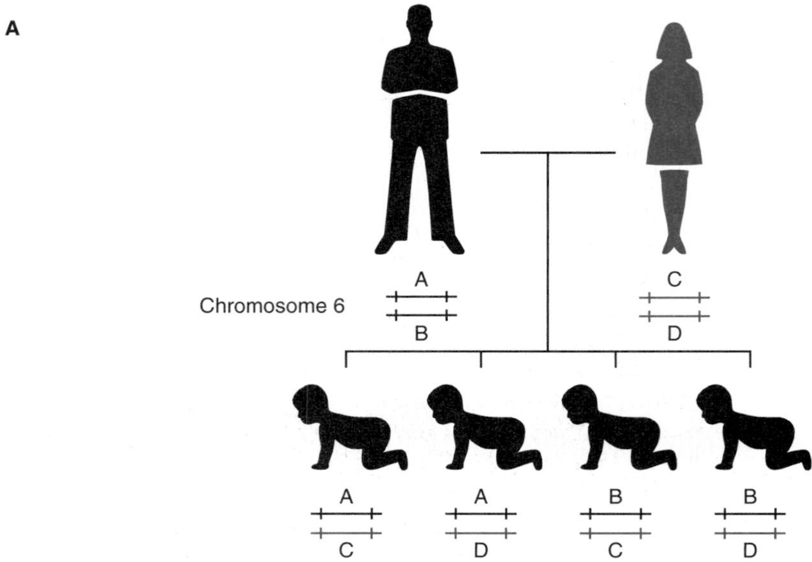

B

	Donor	Recipient	Skin graft (mean survival) days	Kidney graft (1-year graft survival), %	Bone marrow graft
Siblings	*a/c* →	*a/c*	20.0	90	Often successful
	a/d →	*a/c*	13.8	70	Failure
	b/d →	*a/c*	12.5	60	Failure
Unrelated	*x/y* →	*a/c*	12.1	50	Failure

Figure 5.12 **(A)** HLA inheritance within a family, where the probability of a perfect match between two siblings is 0.25. **(B)** Effect of HLA mismatches on the survival or graft rejection of a transplanted origin.

typing include the selectivity of antibodies to lyse lymphocytes (serologic) and dot blot hybridization of polymerase chain reaction-amplified DNA using known sequence-specific oligonucleotide probes (molecular). Of the 906 possible alleles, approximately 24 HLA-A, 53 HLA-B, 14 HLA-DR1, and 9 HLA-DQ1 alleles are identified in order to attempt to find the closest match between donor and recipient.

In the special case of transplanted bone marrow, the donor lymphocytes may recognize the tissues of the recipient as foreign. The ensuing rejection episode can be severe, involving the skin, gastrointestinal tract, and liver of the recipient in a process known as graft-versus-host disease. At the present time, graft-versus-host disease is the major impediment to the use of bone marrow transplantation in a variety of conditions, and only HLA-matched donors are used. Precise matching may be less important if the mature T cells responsible for graft-versus-host reaction are removed. To do this, small mononuclear cells are fractionated by reaction to CD34, a marker for immature hematopoietic stem cells. By transplanting only stem cells, it is thought that the progeny will be influenced by the developmental environment of the host so that donor cells reactive to the host will be eliminated. In many cases, a graft-versus-host reaction is seen, but if the patient survives, the cells responsible for the reaction appear to develop

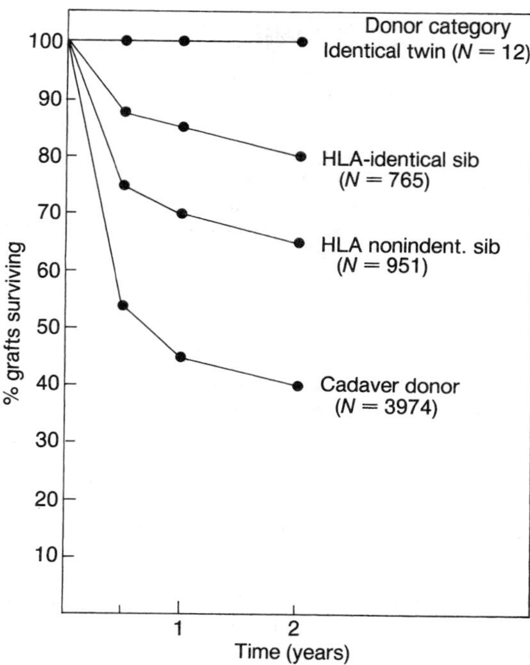

Figure 5.13 Survival times of kidney allografts among people of different genetic relationships ranging from identical twins to unrelated individuals (cadaver donors). (From W. H. Hildemann, *Tissue Antigens* **22:**1–6, 1983.) Because of better matching and more controlled immunosuppressive regimens, the survival of renal grafts has improved since the time these data were available, but these earlier data show more clearly the effect of tissue matching. At the present time, the 10-year expected survival rates for kidneys from HLA-matched siblings, one haplotype-matched related donors, and cadaver donors are 74, 51, and 40%, respectively. The effects of matching have been largely superseded by controlled immunosuppression.

mutual tolerance with the host, resulting in survival of both host, and donor hematopoietic cells.

Self Recognition

Continuous presentation of self peptides by normal cells may be important for maintaining tolerance to self antigens. But during an infection, processing and presentation of viral proteins activates the immune response. One particular HLA type, HLA-B27, is closely associated with certain autoimmune diseases, including ankylosing spondylitis (arthritis of the spine) and Reiter's syndrome (arthritis with uveitis of the eye). The relative risk of these two syndromes is increased 87- and 37-fold, respectively, for people with HLA-B27, compared with those lacking HLA-B27. Perhaps the disease could be triggered when foreign peptides bind to HLA-B27 and initiate a T-cell response. Then it may be perpetuated by self peptides, which could even direct the response to target organs. According to this hypothesis, the cause and pathogenesis may be found among the self and foreign peptides that bind HLA-B27. Other HLA types are less strongly associated with insulin-dependent diabetes (HLA-B8, B15, DR3, DR4, etc.), rheumatoid arthritis (HLA-DR4), Hodgkin's disease (HLA-A1), and so on. In these cases, something may go wrong with this process of distinguishing self from foreign antigens, related to properties of these particular HLA molecules.

T-Cell–B-Cell Interactions, the MHC, and the Immune Response

The first definitive evidence that two different cell types played different roles during induction of antibody formation was obtained by Avrion Mitchison using analysis of antibody production after adoptive transfer of T cells and B cells to irradiated recipients. As shown in Fig. 5.14, if T cells were from a donor immunized with bovine gamma globulin (BGG), and B cells were from a second donor immunized with dinitrophenol (DNP) bound to a different protein, then both cell types were required for the recipient animal to produce anti-DNP antibodies in response to the combined antigen DNP-BGG. Without the addition of immune T cells, the transferred B cells could not respond by themselves, and no anti-DNP antibodies were made. In this system, T-helper cells recognize the BGG, whereas the B-cell precursors of the antibody-producing plasma cells recognize the DNP-BGG immunogen.

Even though the T cells and B cells recognized different parts of the combined antigen, they could still cooperate to produce antibodies. The part of the combined antigen recognized by B cells is called the hapten (DNP), and the part recognized by T cells is the carrier protein (BGG). Both parts must be covalently attached, not simply mixed together, in order to elicit T-cell help. The first plausible interpretation of these results was that the combined antigen held together the T and B cells by forming an "antigen bridge" (Fig. 5.15A), so that "helper" factors secreted by the T cell could activate and maintain the B-cell response.

Figure 5.14 Adoptive transfer of carrier BGG-primed T cells and hapten DNP-primed B cells into an MHC-compatible host. Subsequent immunization with the conjugate DNP-BGG results in antibodies due to T-cell–B-cell collaboration. However, T-cell help requires MHC matching with the B cell (inset).

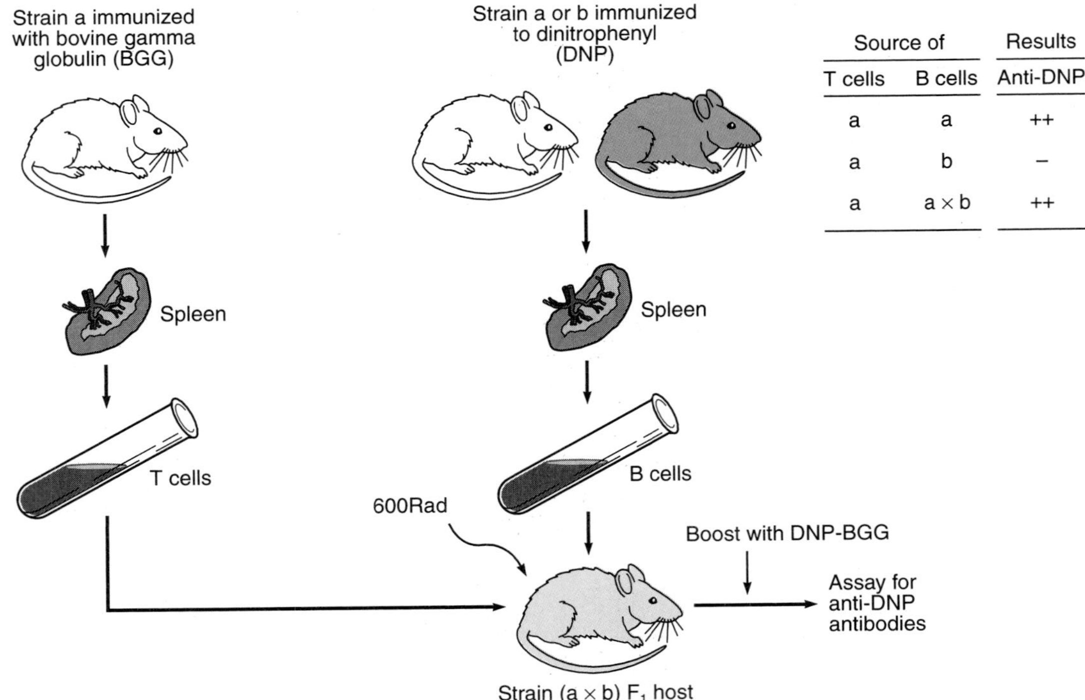

Source of		Results
T cells	B cells	Anti-DNP
a	a	++
a	b	–
a	a × b	++

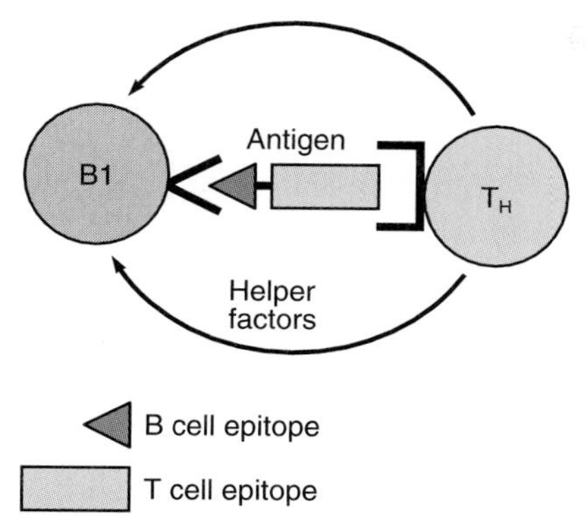

A. 'Traditional' antigen bridge model of T cell help

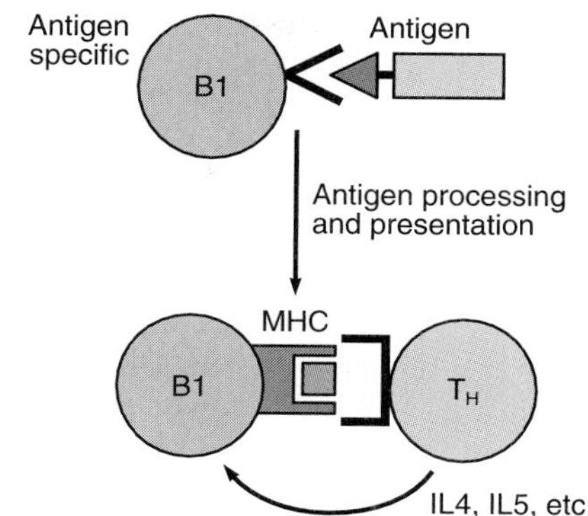

B. Antigen presentation model of T cell help

Figure 5.15 **(A)** Traditional antigen bridge model of T-cell help. Explains why hapten and carrier must be covalently attached. **(B)** Antigen presentation model of T-cell help. B cell takes up the antigen via hapten-specific surface immunoglobulin. B cell then processes and presents peptide fragments plus MHC to the T cell.

MHC Recognition by T Cells

Besides allowing the antigen to be varied, adoptive transfer could be used to mix T and B cells from different strains of mice with different MHC types. As shown in the inset of Fig. 5.14, the B cells only made antibodies when they matched the MHC type of the T-helper cells. This indicates direct contact between the two cells and could be explained as dual recognition of both antigen and MHC by T cells. As we now know, the TCR can respond to antigen only after it is processed to antigenic fragments and presented by the MHC of the APC, which is the B cell or dendritic macrophage. The need for MHC compatibility is explained by the TCR's specificity for self MHC.

The results can be explained by the antigen presentation model of T-cell–B-cell help (Fig. 5.15B). In this model, surface immunoglobulin serves as a high-affinity receptor for antigen binding to specific B cells. Antigen is internalized by endocytosis, followed by dissociation and partial degradation in endosomes. Those peptides that bind MHC class II are transported to the B-cell surface for presentation to T-helper cells. When the TCR binds this antigen-MHC complex, the T cell is triggered to produce a variety of cytokines needed for B-cell activation and differentiation. This model is supported by the observation that B cells (usually memory B cells) function as efficient APCs and can stimulate T-cell proliferation and cytokine secretion, even at low antigen concentrations. Only those B cells with antigen-specific surface immunoglobulin would take up sufficient amounts of antigen to elicit T-cell help.

According to the model, covalent linkage between hapten and carrier is not needed to hold the two cells together via an antigen bridge (Fig. 5.15A) but simply allows both hapten and carrier determinants to enter the B cell together (Fig. 5.15B). In the experiment shown in Fig. 5.14, DNP-BGG would be taken up by a DNP-specific memory B cell via its surface immunoglobulin. Partial degradation would produce BGG peptides for presentation on the surface of the B cell. T-helper cells specific for these BGG peptides could then respond by releasing helper factors as well as contact-mediated help. Since antigen recognition by the two cells is sequential, the B cell can respond to native antigen before processing, whereas the T cell responds to denatured fragments after processing. In this way, the antigen receptors of both cells contribute to the specificity of the response.

Activation Signals

B-cell activation signals can be divided into three types. The first signal is generated by surface immunoglobulin binding to antigen-MHC complex. This signal is particularly important for T-independent antigens, such as bacterial polysaccharides. These antigens can activate B cells directly by cross-linking surface immunoglobulin without antigen processing or presentation to T cells. Antigen valency is important for cross-linking, so polymers are more likely to activate B cells in this way.

For most protein antigens, however, the B cells must rely on T-cell help. Signal 2 is contact-mediated help from T cells, whereas signal 3 is mediated over a short distance by soluble cytokines, such as IL-2 and IL-4 secreted by T-helper cells.

Contact-Mediated Help

Direct contact between the T-helper cell and the B cell permits a number of molecular interactions to occur at the cell surface (Fig. 5.16). Some of these simply hold the two cells together, whereas others confer antigen specificity or transmit activation signals. As described earlier, each cell contributes to specificity via its antigen receptor. The B cell internalizes and processes antigen based on specific binding to surface immunoglobulin. Then, after antigen processing and presentation, the TCR binds antigenic peptide plus MHC of the B cell, resulting in activation of the T cell.

Figure 5.16 Interactions at the T-cell–B-cell interface. Some are antigen specific, such as TCR binding MHC plus peptide. Others are MHC specific, such as CD4 binding MHC class II. Other interactions are stimulatory, such as CD40L binding CD40 and B7 binding CD28. Finally, some simply help hold the two cells together, such as ICAM-1 and LFA-1 or LFA-3 and CD2.

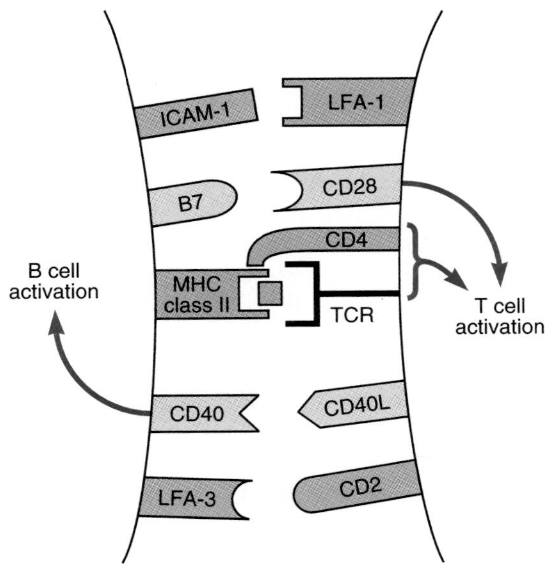

Cell adhesion molecules (see chapter 3), such as LFA-1 on the T-cell surface and ICAM-1 on the B cell, hold the two cells together without contributing to antigen specificity. Similarly, CD2 on the T cell binds LFA-3 on the B cell and stabilizes the pair. But the interaction between CD40 on the B cell and a T-cell surface molecule called CD40 ligand (CD40L) provides an essential activation signal for resting B cells (Table 5.3).

CD40L is a 33-kDa molecule that is induced on activated T cells but absent from resting T cells. Once expressed, CD40L is quite stable, surviving cell fixation with paraformaldehyde or even cell fractionation, when it is found on membranes prepared from activated T cells. The CD40L gene sequence shares homology with secreted cytokines, such as tumor necrosis factor alpha (TNF-α). Thus, CD40L is a T-cell membrane-bound cytokinelike molecule with potent B-cell-activating properties.

The B-cell receptor CD40 has a molecular mass of 45 to 50 kDa and resembles the receptor for TNF-α. When bound to CD40L, and in cooperation with IL-4 (see below), it activates resting B cells for clonal expansion and triggers immunoglobulin class switching. By rearranging the immunoglobulin variable genes on a different constant region, this allows the cell to switch from producing IgM to producing IgG or IgA while retaining its original antigen specificity, coded by the variable region.

A second activation signal results when CD28 protein on the T-cell surface (a 44-kDa homodimer) binds B7 protein on the surface of activated B cells. But in this case, the direction of activation is reversed, as the B cell activates the T cell to proliferate and release cytokines. This stimulatory effect could also be produced artificially by cross-linking CD28 with monoclonal antibodies, combined with other costimulatory signals, such as cross-linking the TCR with antibodies to CD3. Thus, in each T-helper-cell–B-cell pair, activation signals flow in both directions.

The result is a positive feedback loop between the two cells (Fig. 5.17). Cellular activation could start when the TCR binds antigen plus MHC

Table 5.3 T and B-cell activation signals

Signal 1: Antigen plus MHC binds to B-cell receptor
Signal 2: Contact-mediated help

Surface protein	Mol wt (10^3)	Found on	Effect
B7	44–54	B cells	Binds CD28
CD28	44	T cells	Activates T cell
CD	40–50	B cells	Activates B cell
CD40L	39	T cells	Binds CD40

Signal 3: Cytokines

Factor	Mol wt (10^3)	Produced by	Receptor (kDa)	Effect
IL-2	15	Th1 cells	55, 70, 64	Growth factor
IL-4	20	Th2 cells	140, 64	Growth factor, IgG2, IgG4, IgA, IgE class switch
IL-5	30	Th2 cells	140, 70	IgA production
IL-13		Th2 cells		IgE class switch

Regulatory cytokines

Factor	Mol wt (10^3)	Produced by	Receptor	Effect
IL-4, IL-13, IL-10	35–40	Th2/B cells	On APCs	Inhibit IL-12 (APC) and IFN-γ production
IL-12		APCs	On Th1	Activates Th1 cells, stimulates IFN-γ production

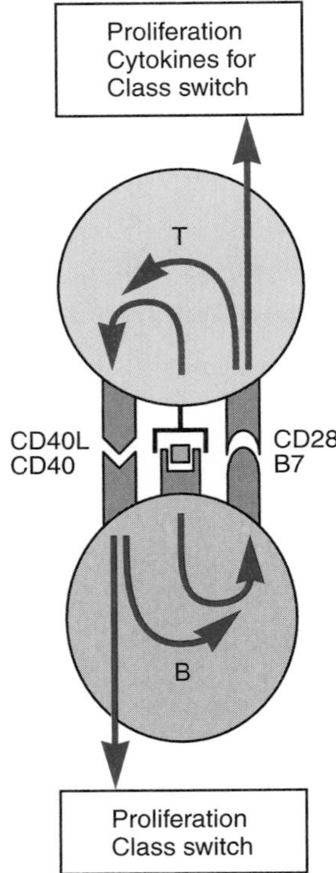

Figure 5.17 Feedback stimulation between activated T-helper cell expressing CD40L and activated B cell expressing B7. Stimulatory signals flow in both directions, resulting in T-cell production of cytokines. The B cell responds to CD40L plus cytokines by proliferating and by activating class switching. (Modified from E. A. Clark and J. A. Ledbetter, *Nature* **367**:425–428, 1994.)

presented by the B cell. This partial activation signal, combined with B7 binding CD28 on the T cell, results in a complete activation signal. Activation induces CD40L expression by the T cell. When the induced CD40L binds CD40 on the B cell, a positive feedback loop is created between the B cell and the T-helper cell. These signals are important both for the initial activation of resting B cells and, later on, as B cells pass through germinal centers and undergo class switching and affinity maturation. Activated T cells also release cytokines, which provide additional important activation signals for the B cell.

Soluble Helper Factors

Activated T cells release cytokines that play an important role in B-cell proliferation and differentiation to antibody-secreting cells (Table 5.3). The first to be discovered was B-cell stimulatory factor 1, now known as IL-4. This 20-kDa protein diffuses from T-helper cells to the IL-4 receptor found on resting and activated B cells. IL-4 has multiple effects on B cells, including increased expression of MHC class II and costimulation of B-cell proliferation. But the most striking effect of IL-4 is to induce class switching. In this process, the variable region of surface immunoglobulin is retained, while the constant region is changed from IgM to other immunoglobulin classes. This preserves the antigen specificity, while changing from membrane-bound IgM to secreted antibodies with different biological activities. Class switching can be demonstrated in cell culture, where B cells stimulated by the mitogen lipopolysaccharide can be switched from making IgM exclusively to IgG2 or IgE by adding IL-4. Under these conditions, the IL-4 effect can be directly antagonized by gamma interferon (IFN-γ). In turn, IFN-γ elicits its own signal for class switching but directs the B cells to produce IgG1 or IgG3 instead. The physiological importance of IL-4 in class switching can be demonstrated in vivo, since mice pretreated with monoclonal anti-IL-4 fail to make an IgE antibody response to parasites. The influence of soluble helper factors on B-cell class switching and induction of cell-mediated immunity is largely determined by different populations of T-helper cells.

T-Cell Populations and Control of the Immune Response

Most $\alpha\beta$ T-helper cells fall into two subpopulations, either the CD4 (helper) or CD8 (suppressor/cytotoxic) populations. The CD8 population mediates specific T-cell toxicity, and the activities of these cells are presented in chapter 12. The CD4 population not only is the effector cell for delayed-type hypersensitivity (DTH) (see chapter 13) but also is the major helper cell for induction of immune responses. The CD4 population is further divided into Th1 and Th2 helper cells. The differential effects of Th1 and Th2 populations are mediated through their characteristic cytokines (Fig. 5.18). Th1 cells are active in three inductive responses: (i) production of IL-2 and IFN-γ, which stimulate immunoglobulin class switching of B cells to produce complement-fixing antibodies of the IgG1 and IgG3 complement-fixing antibody subclasses, (ii) secretion of the proinflammatory TNF, which acts in cooperation with IFN-γ to activate macrophages and initiate DTH reactions, and (iii) secretion of IL-2 and IFN-γ, which activate resting CD8 cells to become active cytotoxic cells. Each of these functions activates an arm of cell-mediated inflammatory reactions. In contrast, the second type of CD4 helper cells (Th2) secretes IL-4, IL-5, IL-10, and IL-13 but not IL-2 or IFN-γ. IL-4 and IL-13 stimulate immunoglobulin class

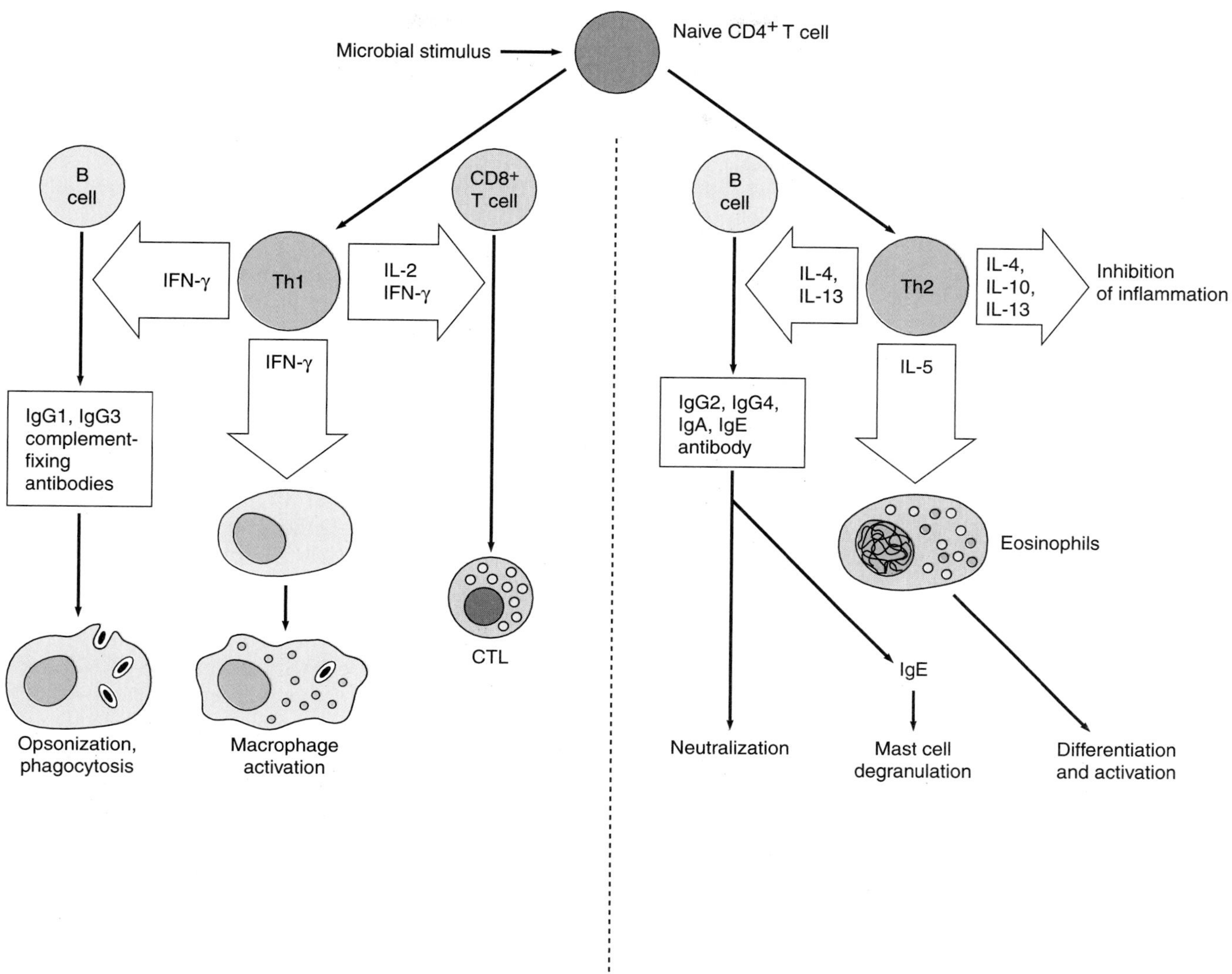

Figure 5.18 Differential induction of immune response by Th1 and Th2 helper cells. The activities of Th1 and Th2 cells are characterized by the cytokines they produce. Th1 cytokines IL-2, IFN-γ, and TNF-β activate cell-mediated reactions, including immunoglobulin class switching for production of complement-fixing antibodies (opsonins), macrophage activation, and differentiation of CD8 cytotoxic cells. Th2 cytokines IL-3, IL-4, IL-5, and IL-10 are responsible for immunoglobulin class switching for non-complement-fixing antibodies IgG2, IgG4, IgA, and IgE, responsible mainly for mucosal immunity. In addition, IFN-γ secreted by Th1 cells inhibits Th2 effector functions, and IL-4, IL-10, and IL-13 secreted by Th2 cells inhibit Th1 functions. (Modified from A. K. Abbas, K. M. Murphy, and A. Sher, *Nature* **383:**787–793, 1996.)

switching of B cells to IgG2, IgG4, and IgA. These plus IL-5 stimulate switching to IgE antibody and IL-5-activated eosinophil differentiation. In addition, activation of one Th population results in inhibition of the other population. For example, IL-4, IL-10, and IL-13 inhibit Th1 cells and inflammation, whereas IFN-γ inhibits Th2 cells. Both Th1 and Th2 secrete IL-3 and granulocyte-monocyte colony-stimulating factor.

The ability to direct the immune response to one or the other of the Th populations may provide powerful new ways to control the immune response. For example, allergic individuals may have increased numbers of IL-4 producing Th2 cells as compared with Th1 cells and thus may be more likely to develop allergies owing to IL-4-mediated class switching and production of IgE antibodies in response to antigen. Alternatively, a relative lack of Th1 cells could also account for this, since Th1 cells secrete IFN-γ, which has a direct antagonist effect against IL-4 and reduces class switching. In addition, direction of the immune response to cell-mediated immunity by preferential activation of Th1 cells is critical in determining the outcome of some infections. For example, the major protective mechanism against a variety of infections, including tuberculosis, syphilis, leprosy, and fungal infections, is cell-mediated immunity through activation of macrophages. Individuals who exhibit a high degree of resistance to these infections most likely preferentially respond to infection by activation of Th1 cells, whereas those individuals who have poor resistance and progressive infections most likely respond to infection by activation of Th2 cells.

Vaccines for induction of protective immunity must be designed to induce the appropriate immune response, cell mediated (Th1) or antibody mediated (Th2). Unfortunately, even if the Th1/Th2 paradigm is correct, it does not separate cell-mediated immunity from most IgG antibody responses. Humoral antibodies are effective against most bacterial infections; DTH (initiated by T_{DTH} cells) is the mechanism of protection against organisms, such as mycobacteria, that infect macrophages; T-cell cytotoxicity (mediated by T_{CTL} cells) is the most effective response to viruses, such as smallpox, that infect epithelial cells. For other viruses, such as poliomyelitis virus or influenza virus (see below), circulating antibodies that "neutralize" the virus are most effective. Thus, to design a successful vaccine, it is critical to select an immunization strategy that will induce the type of immunity best suited to defend against a specific infection.

Prophylactic Immunization (Vaccination)

History: Smallpox

The term vaccine is derived from the cowpox virus known as vaccinia, which is used in the process of vaccination against smallpox (variola). This was accomplished before the immunologic principles behind the induction of T_{CTL} cells were known, and it represents one of the most spectacular successes in the control of an infectious disease. Smallpox was once one of the most lethal and disfiguring human diseases. In ancient China, names were not given to infants until they had survived smallpox, because so many children died from smallpox that families would run out of favorite names. The Chinese noted that milder forms of smallpox could be induced by using infected tissue from people with a relatively benign course of the disease. From this observation, they developed the first method of artificial active immunization. A powder from smallpox crusts was made into a snuff that was inhaled into the nose. Although this practice produced fatal smallpox in up to 1 in 50 exposed individuals, the course of the disease induced in most individuals was generally much milder than that in the naturally acquired disease. Although this would be an unacceptable result by present-day standards, it was a great improvement over the fatality rate of the natural infection. In the Western world, the use of mild forms of smallpox became known as *variolation*.

The introduction of variolation is largely attributed to the efforts of Lady Mary Wortley Montagu, who was the wife of the British ambassador to Turkey. She learned of the practice of variolation in Constantinople. Infected tissue from individuals with mild forms of smallpox was injected into young uninfected people. The inoculated individuals developed mild disease and recovered. She returned to England and persuaded King George I to conduct clinical trials on prisoners at Newgate Prison. The trials were successful, and variolation become a regular practice in England. In the United States, variolation was introduced by Zabdiel Boylston in Boston in 1721 through the urging of Cotton Mather. During the Revolutionary War, smallpox broke out among the American army late in 1775. However, the disease was controlled by variolation, and by September 1776, the army was again prepared to take the field free of smallpox.

In 1770 Edward Jenner noted that milkmaids who contracted cowpox had a mild smallpoxlike disease but never developed any of the serious manifestations of smallpox. In 1796 he inoculated a healthy young boy with cowpox (vaccinia) from the sore of a dairymaid. The boy developed cowpox, which healed and was subsequently found to be resistant to challenge with smallpox. In 1807 a National Vaccine Establishment was set up in London to evaluate and compare the results of vaccination with those of variolation. By 1840 compulsory vaccination was established by law, and variolation was made illegal.

Vaccinia virus has low pathogenicity for humans and contains antigens that cross-react with smallpox virus. Dermal inoculation induces cell-mediated immunity, which results in a cytotoxic delayed skin reaction at the site of inoculation approximately 8 days after application (see chapter 12). This long-lasting T_{CTL}-cell-mediated immunity protects the vaccinated person against smallpox. The term vaccination, now used to cover all kinds of protective immunization, is derived from the use of the vaccinia virus.

Through the application of worldwide vaccination programs monitored by the World Health Organization (WHO), the once great killer disease of smallpox has been eliminated. A few cases of smallpox were reported in Somalia in 1976, and the last known case was diagnosed in October 1977. In December 1979, an independent scientific commission certified the global eradication of smallpox. WHO continues to monitor rumors and coordinate the investigation of suspected cases, but during the last 12 years all suspected cases turned out to be chicken pox, a skin disease other than smallpox, or a mistake in reporting. Inoculation with vaccinia virus sometimes leads to complications such as postvaccinial encephalitis or disseminated vaccinia in a small but significant number of vaccinated individuals. Because the untoward consequences of vaccination are now more significant than the naturally occurring disease, vaccination against smallpox has been discontinued. By 1984 all countries had ceased smallpox vaccination of the general public. Until 1987, WHO maintained a stock of vaccine sufficient to immunize 300 million people, but this reserve is no longer maintained. Since the virus gene pool has been cloned in bacterial plasmids, which provide sufficient material to solve future research and diagnostic problems, it was decided that there is no need to maintain stocks of viable virus. Vaccinia virus is available for experimental use and for production of vaccinia vectors for carrying the DNA of other organisms (recombinant vaccines). Smallpox virus is now maintained in only two WHO-supervised laboratories under high security. However, the possibility that smallpox could be used for biological warfare has led to recommendations that military personnel continue to be vaccinated. There is an ongoing debate on whether or not all remaining repositories of smallpox virus should be destroyed.

Vaccination for Antibody Production

For most successful vaccines that induce antibody, collaboration between the T-helper cell and the B cell is a crucial step in generating protective levels of antibodies. Historically, vaccines using killed organisms or modified toxins (Table 5.4) were effective in stimulating antibody production. To induce high antibody levels, it is often necessary to prime and boost one or more times with vaccine antigen. A typical response to primary immunization and boosting is shown in Fig. 5.19. Primary immunization elicits antibodies after a lag of 10 to 14 days. These are mostly of the IgM class and have low titer and affinity. After a rest period of 4 or more weeks, secondary immunization gives a much more rapid "memory" antibody response within 7 to 10 days, and the antibody titer generally increases greatly, by as much as two logs. These antibodies differ qualitatively as well as quantitatively. They are of the IgG class and have greater affinity for the antigen than in the primary response. Subsequently, an infectious challenge will elicit a rapid increase in antibodies resembling the secondary response in titer, immunoglobulin class, and affinity.

The observed serologic effects of immunization can be explained in terms of fundamental cellular responses to antigen. During the primary immunization, the few antigen-specific T cells and B cells must quickly expand their numbers through clonal selection. Since antigen-specific T-helper cells are scarce at this time, T-helper function is limiting. Without

Table 5.4 Types of vaccines[a]

Type of vaccine	Infectious diseases		
	Viral	**Bacterial**	**Parasitic**
Live, attenuated organism	Polio, measles, mumps, rubella, varicella, yellow fever, rotavirus (e) dengue (e), hepatitis A (e)	Tuberculosis, typhoid, cholera (e), shigellosis (e), leprosy (e)	
Killed organism	Polio, influenza, rabies, Japanese B encephalitis, hepatitis A	Pertussis, typhoid, cholera, leprosy (e), *Helicobacter* (e)	Malaria (e)
Toxoid		Diphtheria, tetanus, shigellosis (e), enterotoxigenic *Escherichia coli* (e)	
Vectored	HIV (e), measles (e), rabies (e)	Typhoid (e), cholera (e), tuberculosis (e), shigellosis (e)	Malaria (e)
DNA (all e)	HIV, influenza, herpes simplex type 2, rabies, HBV, HCV, HDV, papillomavirus, HTLV-1, CMV, St. Louis encephalitis	Typhoid, tuberculosis	Malaria, leishmaniasis, schistosomiasis

[a]Abbreviations: HBV, hepatitis B virus; HCV, hepatitis C virus; HDV, hepatitis D virus; HTLV-1, human T-cell leukemia virus type 1; CMV, cytomegalovirus; e, experimental.

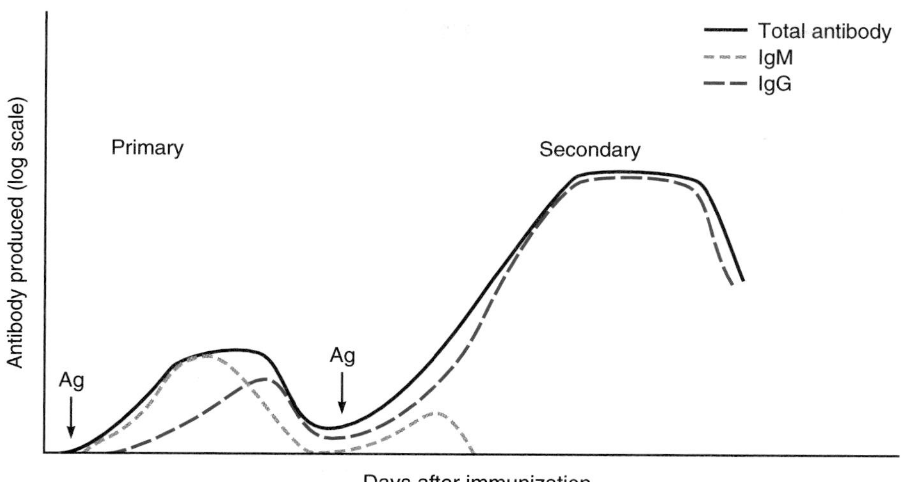

Figure 5.19 Antibody class switching during primary and secondary immunizations. Priming elicits IgM antibodies of low affinity. During the secondary immunization, B cells receive abundant T-cell help under optimal conditions for class switching from IgM to IgG production and maturation to high-affinity antibodies.

contact help or IL-4, B cells fail to form germinal centers, so little class switching or affinity maturation occurs. Thus, primary immunization elicits mainly IgM antibodies of low to moderate affinity.

After the primary immunization, the number of antigen-specific T-helper cells increases rapidly. By the secondary immunization, primed B cells respond to antigen in the presence of excess T-cell help. These B cells increase rapidly and produce a corresponding rise in the level of specific antibodies. Under the influence of T-cell help—both contact help and cytokines such as IL-4—antigen-specific B cells mature in germinal centers, where they switch from IgM to IgG or IgA. Somatic mutation of V-region genes, followed by selective growth, yields B cells producing antibodies with progressively greater affinity for the antigen. At the same time, a subset of B cells become memory B cells and enter a resting phase that can last for decades. Upon subsequent infection, these memory B cells are quickly activated to produce high titers of IgG antibodies with high affinity for the antigen.

Vaccine Design: Influenza Virus

For many pathogens, the first infection elicits prolonged immunity against subsequent infections. In such cases, it should be possible for vaccines to elicit protective immunity by eliciting neutralizing antibodies comparable to those found after infection. In designing such a vaccine, the two most important issues are (i) identifying the major neutralizing sites (the target of neutralizing antibodies) and (ii) achieving sufficient vaccine potency to elicit protective levels of neutralizing antibodies in virtually all vaccine recipients. While the first issue depends primarily on the virus or pathogen, the second depends on the ability of the vaccine antigens to mobilize T cells and B cells to collaborate in producing a vigorous immune response.

Most antiviral antibodies bind without neutralizing the virus. In part, this is because relatively few sites on the virus are neutralizing sites, which perform essential viral functions that can be blocked by antibodies binding nearby. For example, if located on a viral envelope protein, each of these sites may correspond to a particular envelope function, such as binding to a receptor on the host cell, fusing with the host cell membrane to allow viral penetration, or uncoating inside the cell. By binding these sites, antibodies can neutralize the virus either by blocking an essential viral function or by triggering the function, but at the wrong time or place. For example, if antibodies triggered viral uncoating, it could be a lethal event if it occurred outside the host cell. A variety of approaches have been used to locate and characterize the major neutralizing sites of a virus.

A particularly illustrative case is influenza virus. Neutralizing sites were found by combining epidemiologic data with data from research laboratories. Influenza is highly mutable. Its hemagglutinin protein, a predominant target of neutralizing antibodies, accumulates mutations from one year to the next, a process called antigenic drift. In some years, this random process yields a virus variant that escapes from the antibodies that neutralized earlier influenza strains. This results in a new influenza epidemic among previously infected populations, whose antibodies no longer protect them. Epidemiologic studies of these variants indicate that a limited number of point mutations can account for these epidemics, because of escape from neutralizing antibodies directed at these sites.

Figure 5.20 Neutralizing sites on influenza virus hemagglutinin are indicated by solid symbols. Residues forming each conformational site share the same symbol. Hemagglutinin structure is based on X-ray crystallography. (Modified from D. C. Wiley, I. A. Wilson, and J. J. Skehel, *Nature* **289**:373–378, 1981.).

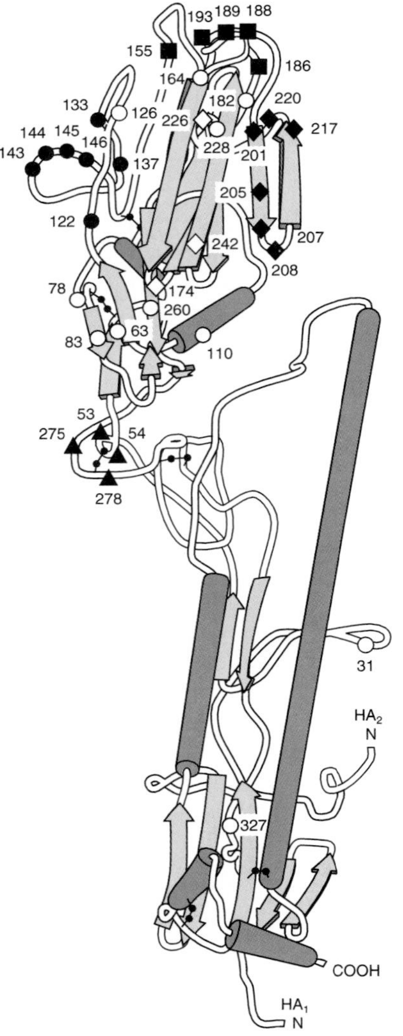

As shown in Fig. 5.20, the accumulated mutations accounting for the decade 1977 to 1986 can be mapped to a few nearby sites on the three-dimensional structure of hemagglutinin. These sites are generally close to the receptor-binding site of the hemagglutinin, but distinct. This allows the virus to mutate at the neutralizing sites without affecting its ability to bind its receptor on the cell surface. Quite often, these sites consist of residues that are far apart in the primary sequence but are brought together by the three-dimensional folding of the protein, and these are called "conformational sites." For a vaccine antigen to elicit neutralizing antibodies to these sites, the correct protein folding is just as important as the correct sequence.

A second approach is to generate "escape mutants" in the laboratory, using a panel of neutralizing monoclonal antibodies specific for hemagglutinin. Virus is grown in the presence of a lethal amount of antibody. Since each antibody binds a single neutralizing site, it applies selective pressure on the virus and favors the outgrowth of a rare mutant within the virus stock that could escape neutralization by mutating this site. The surviving virus is analyzed for mutations in the hemagglutinin gene. The neutralizing sites identified by "artificial selection" agree closely with those observed among the naturally selected strains causing influenza epidemics. These sites are important to vaccine design, because just as the virus changes from year to year, so must the vaccine. Changes affecting neutralizing sites are the most important, since they may herald the appearance of a new epidemic of influenza.

Other viruses, such as HIV-1, mutate even more quickly than influenza, varying from one isolate to another. However, variation per se is not proof of natural selection by neutralizing antibodies. Ever since Darwin, it has been clear that random variation is necessary but not sufficient for evolution. Without selection and escape from neutralizing antibodies, as occurs when a previously infected patient is reinfected, it is premature to conclude that variation in HIV-1 is anything more than random variation produced by a promiscuous reverse transcriptase. Conversely, we cannot be sure that those neutralizing sites that are relatively conserved would remain stable if infection occurred in a previously immune population.

Vaccine Potency: *Haemophilus influenzae*

The second major issue for induction of a successful antibody-based immune response is immunogenicity, or vaccine potency. This can be particularly important when the group at risk of serious infection is unable to respond to the vaccine antigen. For example (Fig. 5.21A), meningitis due to *H. influenzae* occurs most often in children between 2 months and 2 years of age. Younger babies are protected by maternal antibodies, and older children develop natural immunity. As with other bacteria, the neutralizing

Figure 5.21 **(A)** Incidence of *H. influenzae* meningitis (in blue) during the first 5 years of life and the corresponding level of anticapsular antibodies (in black). Most disease occurs in the first 2 years of life, after maternal antibodies have waned but before natural exposure has elicited antibodies in the baby. **(B)** Response to *H. influenzae* type b (HIB) conjugate vaccine. Unlike the free polysaccharide, the conjugate elicits high-titered anticapsular antibodies at an early age, when protection is needed. (Modified from H. Peltola, H. Kayhty, A. Sivonen, and H. Makela, *Pediatrics* **60**:730–737, 1977, and V. I. Ahonkhai, L. J. Lukacs, L. C. Jonas, H. Matthews, P. P. Vella, R. W. Ellis, J. M. Staub, K. T. Dolan, C. M. Rusk, G. B. Calandra, et al., *Pediatrics* **85**:676–681, 1990.)

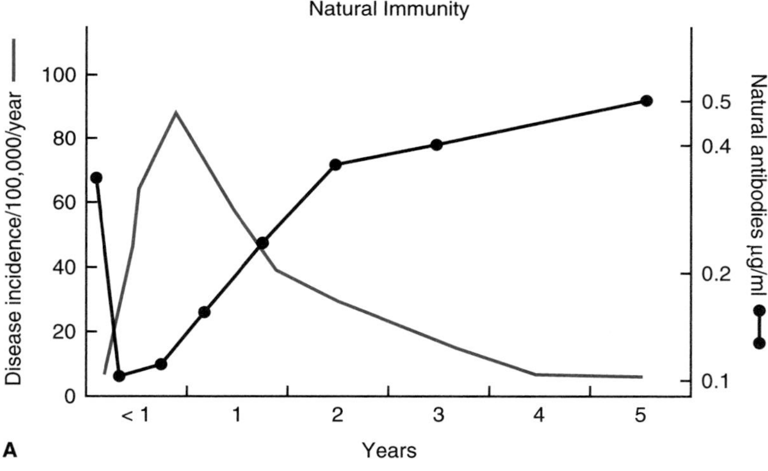

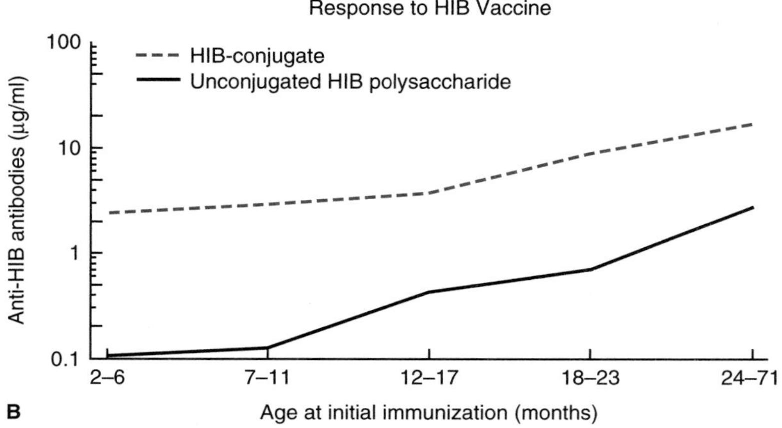

antibodies are directed at the polysaccharide capsule surrounding the bacteria. But young children are unable to respond directly to the polysaccharide. Because the antigen is multivalent, B cells should respond without T-cell help. Since the T-independent response is weak in young children, another way had to be found to elicit antibodies to the bacterial polysaccharide.

The solution to increasing the antipolysaccharide response in these children is to enlist T-cell help. Although the capsular polysaccharide is not a T-dependent antigen, it may be converted to a T-dependent antigen by covalently coupling it to a protein carrier. As explained above (Fig. 5.15B), during immunization, the conjugate would be taken up by B cells specific for the polysaccharide, processed, and presented to T-helper cells specific for the carrier protein. These T cells would then provide contact help and release cytokines needed by B cells to make antibodies to the polysaccharide. Normally, T cells respond to an antigen after processing, whereas B cells recognize the unprocessed antigen, and they often respond to different parts of the same antigen. In this case, this is taken one step further, since each cell responds to a different component of the conjugate, with the polysaccharide acting as a hapten.

The advantages of conjugate vaccines include the ability to choose a highly immunogenic carrier protein (Fig. 5.21B), which makes it possible for babies as young as 2 to 6 months to respond to the polysaccharide in the conjugate, although they are unable to respond to the polysaccharide by itself. A potential disadvantage of conjugate vaccines is the lack of boosting through natural exposure, since the carrier protein is lacking. This is not a problem for *H. influenzae* type b vaccine, but it could be more serious when persistent high titers must be maintained over many years through natural exposure, as in the case of malaria.

Other types of vaccines under consideration include synthetic peptides corresponding to the sequence of neutralizing sites on viral proteins. These may have problems with both issues in vaccine design. Since many viral neutralizing sites depend on protein conformation, the peptides would be unable to elicit antibodies to these sites, since they lack the native conformation. In addition, a peptide vaccine may fail to immunize a number of people, since it is unlikely to bind all MHC types, and MHC binding is an essential step in eliciting T-cell help.

Control of the Type of Immune Response

Immune deviation is defined as the selection of one type of immune response over another. The classic example is the dichotomy of the immune response in infectious diseases. Thus, in some diseases, such as leprosy and tuberculosis, antibody production is not protective and is associated with progressive disease, whereas DTH is protective and associated with arrested disease. Thus, a vaccine designed for producing high antibody titers may not be protective against these diseases. How does one selectively control immune deviation to induce protective DTH rather than nonprotective antibody formation? As stated above, when presenting the differential effects of Th1 and Th2 cells, it is not possible to separate the induction of delayed-type hypersensitivity from circulating antibody production on the basis of the different effects of Th1 and Th2 cells. A hypothetical scheme for the role of antigen processing in determination of the type of immune response is presented in Fig. 5.22. According to this scheme, the immunoglobulin class of antibody and type of T cell (T_{CTL} or

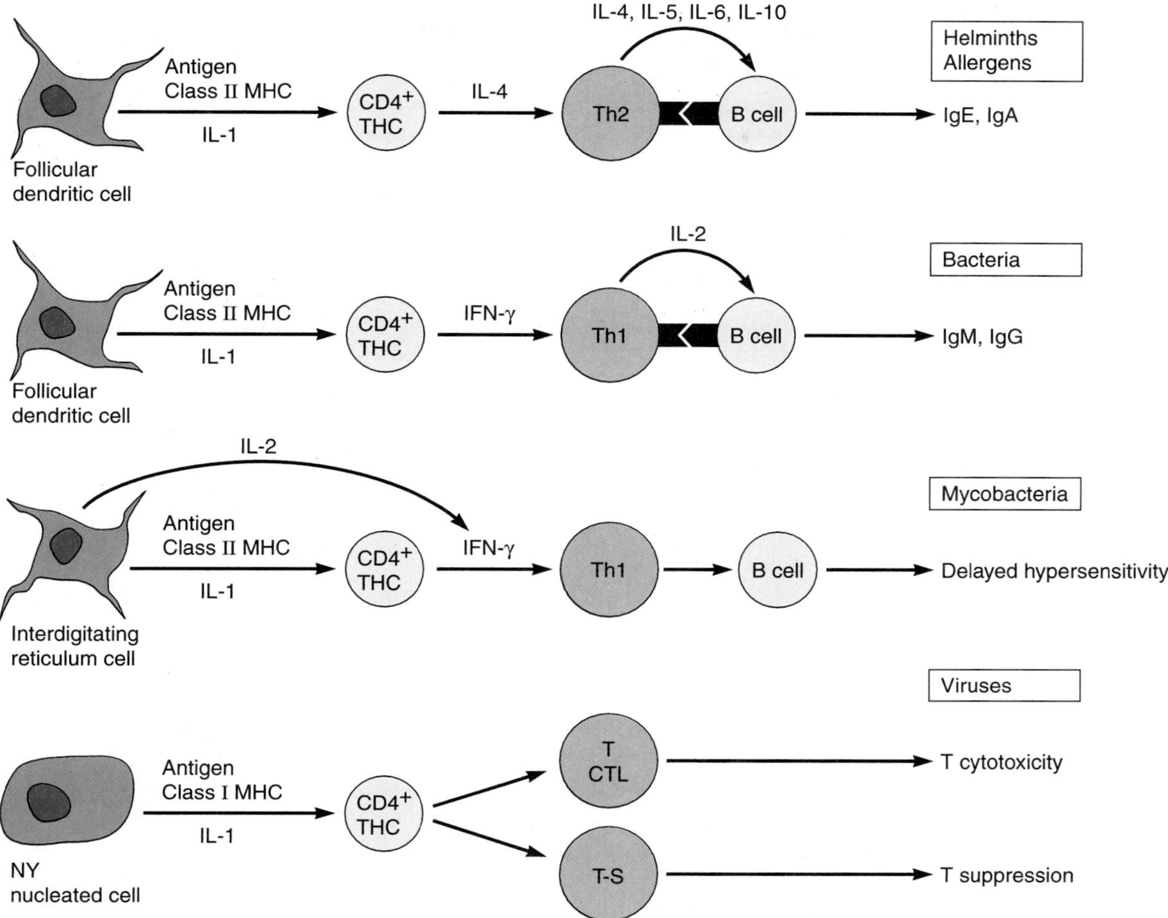

Figure 5.22 Diagram depicting the presumptive role of antigen processing and T-helper-cell subsets in different types of immune responses. IgE, IgA, and some IgG subclasses of antibodies result from antigen processing by class II MHC$^+$ dendritic cells that are located in follicles, presentation of antigen to CD4$^+$ T-helper cells, activation of Th2 cells, and differentiation of B cells to produce IgE and IgA. IgG antibodies are produced by B cells if this process involves the Th1 subset of helper cells instead of Th2. DTH also results from activation of Th1 cells, but DTH may result from antigen processing by interdigitating dendritic cells in the T-cell zones of lymph nodes and the action of IL-12. Cytotoxic CD8$^+$ T cells are produced after antigen processing by class I MHC$^+$ cells to CD$^+$ helper cells. DTH cells are CD4$^+$; CTL cells are CD8$^+$. Differentiation of CD8$^+$ cells to T_{CTL} cells is encouraged by IFN-γ and IL-12.

T_{DTH}) that is produced after immunogen recognition depends upon the type of immunogen processing and the nature of the T-helper cell involved. In the classic model of antigen presentation for antibody responses, antigen is processed by follicular dendritic cells or B cells that present the antigen to T-helper cells, which produce interleukins or lymphokines that activate antigen-reactive B cells to proliferate and synthesize antibody. The current paradigm holds that different types of immune responses can be explained on the basis of two different T-helper cells (Fig. 5.18). Th2 cells secrete lymphokines that drive B cells to IgE and IgA antibody production; Th1 cells secrete lymphokines that drive B cells to produce IgG1 and IgG3 antibodies and cell-mediated reactions. Thus, as originally presented, this model is useful for separating IgE and IgA from some IgG classes. The model has also been interpreted to separate antibody responses from cell-mediated immunity (T_{DTH} or T_{CTL} cell mediated). However, Th1 cells are implicated in induction of both cell-mediated immunity and IgG antibody (IgG1 and IgG3). If induction of both IgG antibodies as well as T_{DTH} and T_{CTL} cells employs Th1 cells, then another level of immune induction must be required to separate these responses. Separation of antibody from DTH most likely results from different antigen processing. Antibody responses occur in follicular zones of lymphoid organs after processing of antigen by dendritic cells or B cells around which follicles form; DTH responses occur in the diffuse cortex of T-cell zones after processing of antigens by interdigitating dendritic (reticulum) cells. T_{CTL} cells are produced after activation of $CD8^+$ T-helper cells following antigen processing by any nucleated MHC class I-positive cell. Effective immunization for T_{CTL} cells was accomplished historically by intentional infection with living viruses, such as vaccination for smallpox, measles, mumps, and chicken pox.

How To Select the Type of Immune Effector Mechanism

The form of delivery of the immunogen can determine the type of immune response. In the late 1950s it was shown that immunization with very low doses of protein antigens could direct the immune response to DTH rather than antibody formation, which occurred when higher doses were used. This phenomenon became known as immune deviation. Direction of immune responses to T_{DTH} cells may be encouraged by the use of complete Freund's adjuvant (a water in oil emulsion containing killed *Mycobacterium tuberculosis*), very low doses of antigen, injection of IL-12 along with the antigen, or insertion of the DNA for the antigen into a living strain of *M. tuberculosis*, BCG (bacillus Calmette-Guérin), which may direct immunogens to processing by interdigitating reticulum cells and preferentially induce DTH. Direction to $CD8^+$ T cells may be accomplished by selecting peptides that are recognized by class I-restricted T cells, through the use of antigen forms or complexes that direct antigens to class I-restricted (endogenous) processing (see below), or by inserting the DNA for the antigen into a vector (such as vaccinia virus) that preferentially infects class I MHC-positive epithelial cells and induces T_{CTL} cells.

Adjuvant stimulation of $CD4^+$ T_{DTH} cells. An effective way to increase the specific immune response to a given antigen is to administer the antigen (immunogen) along with an agent that will enhance the reactivity of the reacting cells. Such agents are termed adjuvants. The mechanism of action of adjuvants is not well understood, but they are believed to attract macrophages and reactive lymphocytes to the sites of antigen deposition, to localize antigens in an inflammatory site (depot effect), to delay antigen catabolism, to activate the metabolism of APCs, and to stimulate lymphoid cell interactions. Adjuvants will also produce a nonspecific increase in immune reactivity; much of the immunoglobulin produced by adjuvant-antigen stimulation is not specific antibody. Injection of adjuvant with or without antigen can produce a sustained hyperglobulinemia. Effective adjuvants include oils, mineral salts, double-stranded nucleic acids, products of microorganisms, and a variety of other agents.

Freund's adjuvant. The most widely used adjuvant for induction of DTH in laboratory animals is complete Freund's adjuvant. This adjuvant consists of a water- or saline-in-oil emulsion. Emulsions without mycobacteria are called incomplete (incomplete Freund's adjuvant), and emulsions containing mycobacteria are termed complete (complete Freund's adjuvant). The glycolipid and peptidoglycolipid portions (wax D) of the mycobacteria are responsible for the increased effect of complete Freund's adjuvant. In producing antisera in animals, it is common to use complete Freund's adjuvant for the initial immunization and incomplete Freund's adjuvant for booster immunizations. Repeated immunization with complete Freund's adjuvant can lead to severe necrotic reactions at the site of the injection because of extreme potency of hypersensitivity to the mycobacterial component. To be fully effective, adjuvants must be injected intradermally or subcutaneously. Unfortunately, because of the severity of the inflammatory reaction induced by complete Freund's adjuvant, its use in humans is limited to investigative studies when no alternative is available.

Cell wall extracts. Killed organisms such as *Listeria monocytogenes* or the cell walls of certain bacteria (mycobacteria) and fungi also serve to enhance immune reactivity. In general, the effect is less than but similar to that of complete Freund's adjuvant. These agents also produce a marked nonspecific activation of the effector arm of immune responses that involve macrophages. They attract and activate macrophages, thus increasing phagocytosis at the site of antigen-induced inflammation.

Synthetic immunostimulants derived from bacterial cell walls are exemplified by peptidoglycan derivatives such as muramyl dipeptide (MDP) (Fig. 5.23). MDP is a simple dipeptide derivative of muraminic acid and is the minimal molecule capable of replacing mycobacterial cell walls in complete Freund's adjuvant for increasing antibody production and for inducing DTH. However, this compound is toxic and produces fever, leukopenia, and platelet lysis in animals. Muramyl dipeptide has been combined with liposomes to stimulate the immune system of patients with cancer nonspecifically. Synthetic disaccharide peptides, such as disaccharides from lactobacilli coupled to the dipeptide L-alanyl-D-isoglutamine, may be even more active than MDP and less toxic. Other artificial saccharides, lipids, and peptidolipids structurally related to MDP are also being tested for possible clinical use. The primary action of adjuvants is on macrophage activation resulting in increased T- and B-cell proliferation, presumably through IL-1 production and induction of DTH by production of IL-12.

IL-12. IL-12 is produced by macrophages and is a potent inducer of IFN-γ by Th1 cells and natural killer cells. IL-12 in concert with presentation of antigen by dendritic APC is believed to amplify the induction of $CD4^+$ T_{DTH} cells and T_{CTL} cells, thus directing the immune response to cell-mediated immunity. Although the effect on induction of immunity has not been analyzed extensively, it is possible that incorporation of IL-12 into immunization protocols may select for DTH. By insertion of the gene for IL-12 and for the specific antigen into a plasmid, it is possible to induce production of both IL-12 and the antigen in a single immunizing plasmid.

Figure 5.23 Structure of muramyl dipeptide.

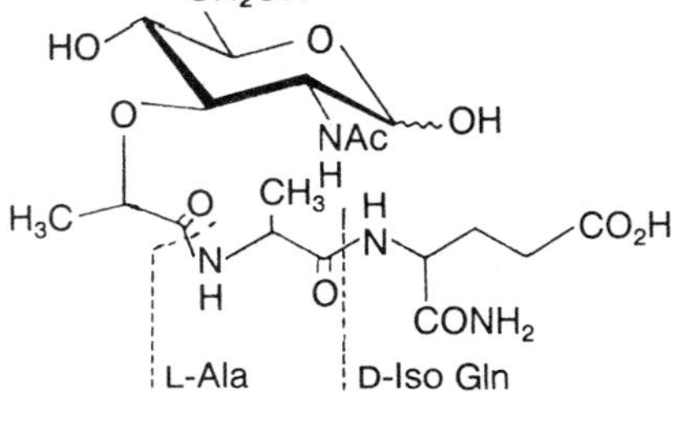

Stimulation of $CD8^+$ T_{CTL} cells. *Peptide selection.* By analysis of the primary amino acid sequence of a potential immunogen, it is possible to predict peptides that will be recognized by $CD8^+$ T cells. Such peptides are made up of 7 to 12 amino acids that form amphipathic helixes. Amphipathicity refers to alternating hydrophobic and hydrophilic residues in an alpha helix arranged so that hydrophobic and hydrophilic residues alternate about every three to four residues. Since there are about 3.6 residues per turn, this sequence aligns the hydrophobic residues on one side of the helix and hydrophilic residues on the other. The hydrophobic side attaches to the cleft in the class I MHC molecule on the surface of the class I MHC^+ APC, whereas the hydrophilic side binds to the $CD8^+$ TCR (Fig. 5.24). Using this approach, a number of T-cell epitopes in antigens of infectious agents have been identified. Once the peptide having the putative T-cell epitope has been identified and synthesized, it is necessary to be able to deliver it to the endogenous processing system (see below).

ISCOMs. Delivery of antigens to the endogenous processing pathway may be accomplished by the use of immunostimulating complexes (ISCOMs) (Fig. 5.25). ISCOMs are glycosides that form micelles with the peptide and are able to penetrate cell membranes, as liposomes do, to introduce the antigen into the ER, allowing endogenous processing and presentation by the class I pathway. This approach is now being applied to retroviruses such as feline leukemia virus and HIV. Such methods give promise of being able to direct vaccination to the type of cell-mediated immunity that is effective against tumor-specific antigens. However, some T-suppressor cells also belong to the $CD8^+$ population. In view of the ability of T-suppressor cells to inhibit induction of immune effector mechanisms, it may be that the use of peptides and ISCOMs that stimulate $CD8^{++}$ cells actually enhance infection rather than inhibit it.

DNA-based vaccines. Rapid advances in vaccine development have been made though the use of sequences of DNA encoding potential antigens as immunogens. This is based on the unexpected finding that DNA injected in solution into muscular tissue could result in synthesis of the encoded gene in recipient animals. This effect is enhanced by a commercial product

Figure 5.24 Cooperative binding of a T-cell epitope with class I MHC and $CD8^+$ TCR. Peptides processed for T_{CTL}-cell recognition have hydrophilic amino acids alternating with hydrophobic amino acids in a manner that aligns the hydrophilic sites on one side of an alpha helix and hydrophobic sites on the other side. The hydrophilic side has affinity for the TCR, whereas the hydrophobic side binds to the class I MHC on the APC. Peptides that have these "amphipathic" structures are presented to reactive $CD8^+$ T cells by the endogenous antigen-processing pathway.

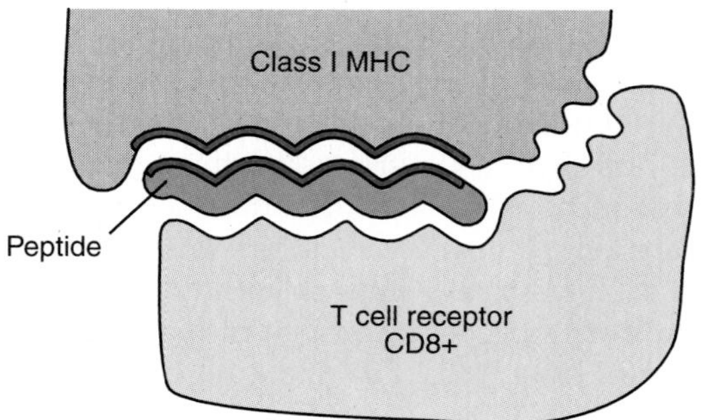

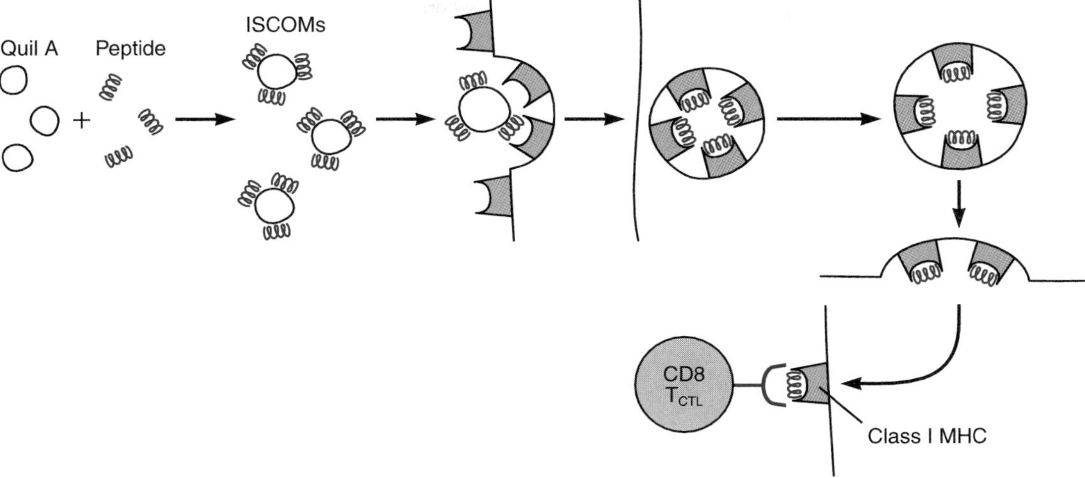

Figure 5.25 Immunostimulating complexes (ISCOMs). ISCOMs form structures with peptide antigens that direct the processing of the antigen to the endogenous pathway, presentation via class I MHC surface molecules, and induction of $CD8^+$ T_{CTL} cells.

with which very small gold particles coated with DNA are injected into superficial tissues using helium gas pressure (a "gene gun"). Mice injected with plasmids encoding an influenza A antigen developed both circulating antibodies and T_{CTL} cells and were protected against lethal challenge of the virus. The key to this approach is using a promoter, such as the cytomegalovirus promoter, to drive transcription of the plasmid DNA in the cells of the immunized individual. The antigen appears to be synthesized in muscle cells but is taken up by professional dendritic APCs, leading to stimulation of both antibody and cell-mediated immunity. This approach is now being applied for development of vaccines to a number of infectious diseases in laboratory animals, and clinical trials will most likely be under way by the time this book is published. Immunizations for human infectious diseases are listed in Table 5.5, and the recommended childhood immunization schedule is given in Fig. 5.26.

Summary

T cells occupy the center of the immune response. T cells do not respond to protein antigens directly. Instead, they have receptors for antigenic peptides generated by partial proteolytic degradation in APCs. Two processing pathways have been identified: exogenous and endogenous. The exogenous pathway involves production of peptides for association with MHC class II in endosomes and transport to the cell surface to react with CD4 T-helper cells. The endogenous pathway produces peptides for association with MHC class I in the ER of proteasomes through the function precessing and transporting molecules to present the antigen to $CD8^+$ precursors of T_{CTL} cells. In both pathways, the peptide-MHC complex is transported to the cell surface for presentation to T cells. Immunogenicity reflects high-affinity binding between a peptide and the peptide-binding groove of MHC. T-cell specificity for antigen plus MHC resides in the TCR and is augmented by CD4 affinity for MHC class II or CD8 affinity for

Table 5.5 Prophylactic immunization for human infectious diseases

Disease or organism	Antigen preparation	Indication	Immunization route	Results
Toxoids				
Diphtheria	Formaldehyde-treated toxin	All children All adults	Intramuscular	Satisfactory
Botulism	Formaldehyde-treated toxin	On exposure	Intramuscular	Needs improvement
Tetanus	Formaldehyde-treated toxin	All children All adults	Intramuscular	Satisfactory
Killed organisms				
Pertussis	Thiomersalate treated	All children	Intramuscular	Needs improvement
Typhoid[a]	Phenol inactivated	Travelers[a] on exposure	Subcutaneous, intramuscular, oral	Needs improvement
Cholera	Phenol treated	Travelers	Subcutaneous	Needs improvement
Plague	Formalin killed	High-risk groups	Intramuscular	Needs improvement
Anthrax	Phenol treated	On exposure High-risk groups	Subcutaneous	Needs improvement
Polysaccharides				
Meningococcus	Quadrivalent polysaccharide	Areas of endemicity (Africa), travelers	Subcutaneous	Needs improvement/short duration of protection in infants
Pneumococcus	Polysaccharide (23 types)	Susceptible individuals, elderly (>65 yr)	Intramuscular	Needs improvement/ antigenicity variable
H. influenzae	Polysaccharide protein conjugates (DTP-*H. influenzae* type b)	Infants and children	Intramuscular	Needs improvement
Attenuated organisms				
Poliomyelitis[b]	Monkey tissue culture (live)	All children	Oral	Satisfactory
Measles (rubeola)	Chicken tissue culture (live)	All children, adults born after 1956	Subcutaneous	Satisfactory
Mumps	Chicken tissue culture (live)	All children, adults born after 1957	Subcutaneous	Satisfactory
Rubella	Human tissue culture (live)	All children	Subcutaneous	
Yellow fever[c]	Egg tissue culture (live 7D strain)	Travelers (area of endemicity)	Subcutaneous	
Influenza	Egg tissue culture (4 strains) purified antigens	High-risk groups, elderly	Subcutaneous	Satisfactory
Varicella	Tissue culture/attenuated strain	Children with leukemia	Subcutaneous	Satisfactory
Adenovirus	Live virus/enteric capsules	Military	Oral	Satisfactory
Smallpox	Vaccinia (cowpox) virus	Laboratory markers	Intradermal or subcutaneous	Needs improvement
Tuberculosis	BCG	High-risk groups	Intradermal	Needs improvement
Killed partially attenuated organisms				
Typhus	Chick embryo culture	Travelers	Subcutaneous	Satisfactory
Rabies	Rhesus lung tissue culture/inactivated β-propiolactone	On exposure, high-risk groups	Intramuscular/ subcutaneous	Needs improvement
Cutaneous leishmaniasis	Controlled route and dose	Virulent organisms, exposed children	Intradermal	Needs improvement
Hepatitis B[d]	Recombinant protein hepatitis B virus[a] HBsAg	High-risk groups, all children	Intramuscular	Needs improvement

[a]Live attenuated oral vaccine also available.
[b]Inactivated vaccine (el PV) recommended for primary vaccination.
[c]Yellow fever vaccines must be approved by WHO.
[d]Formaldehyde-infective virus is also licensed but is no longer produced in the United States.

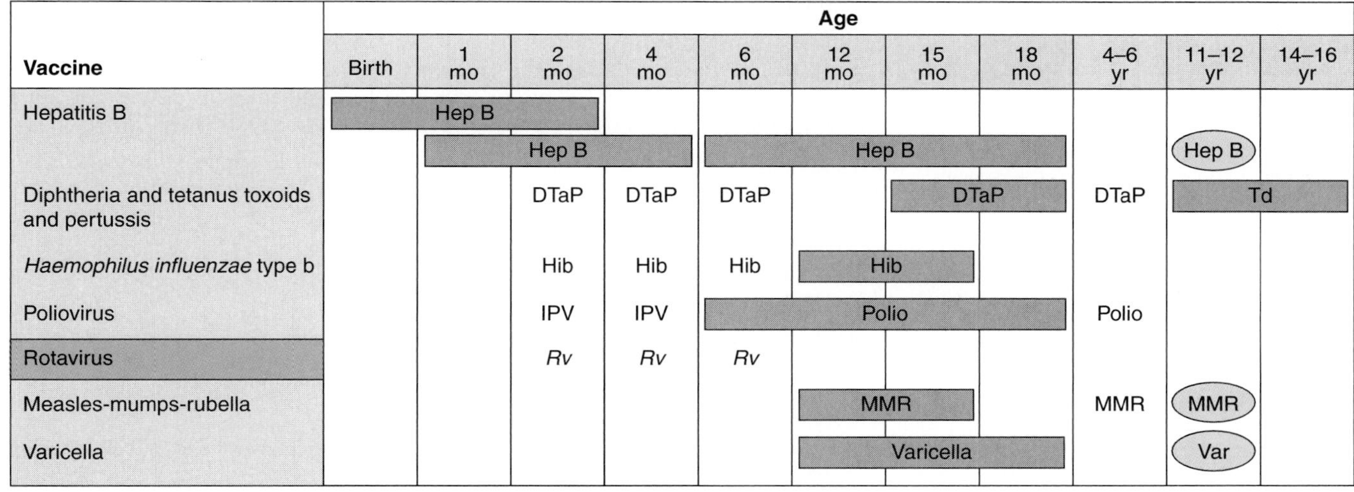

Age
Vaccine
Birth
1 mo
2 mo
4 mo
6 mo
12 mo
15 mo
18 mo
4–6 yr
11–12 yr
14–16 yr
Hepatitis B
Hep B
Hep B
Hep B
Hep B
Diphtheria and tetanus toxoids and pertussis
DTaP
DTaP
DTaP
DTaP
DTaP
Td
Haemophilus influenzae type b
Hib
Hib
Hib
Hib
Poliovirus
IPV
IPV
Polio
Polio
Rotavirus
Rv
Rv
Rv
Measles-mumps-rubella
MMR
MMR
MMR
Varicella
Varicella
Var

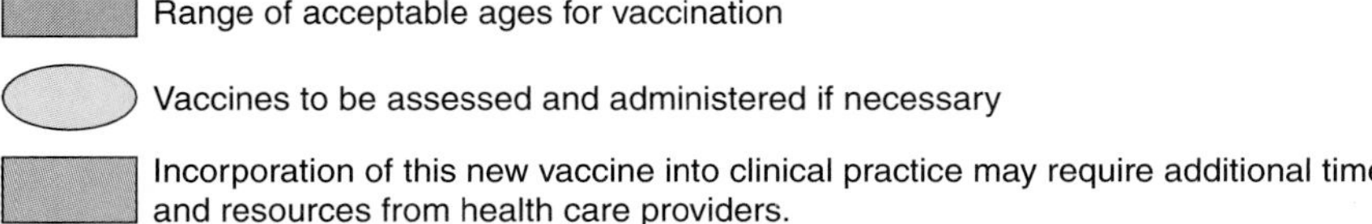

Figure 5.26 Recommended childhood immunization schedule (U.S. Public Health Service, January 1999). For details and special recommendations, see http://www.cdc.gov/epo/mmwr/preview.

class I MHC of the APC. After binding antigen plus MHC, the TCR generates a signal for T-cell activation through a cascade of protein kinase activations and protein-protein interactions that result in upregulation for cell cycle activating and differentiating proteins.

T-cell–B-cell collaboration for induction of antibody formation depends on sequential antigen recognition by both cells and an antigen presentation step. If successful, the T cell provides contact help and also secretes diffusible cytokines. Under the influence of T-cell help, the B cell undergoes activation, class switching, and affinity maturation. Two types of T-helper cells have been identified: Th1 cells on activation secrete cytokines, such as IL-2 and IFN-γ, that direct B cells to produce complement-fixing antibody (IgG1 and IgG3) and activate cell-mediated immunity (T_{DTH} and T_{CTL} cells). Th2 cells secrete cytokines IL-4, IL-5, and IL-10, which direct B cells to produce IgE, IgA, IgG2, and IgG4. Successful vaccines for antibody production use T-cell help to elicit the maximum response from B cells in making neutralizing antibodies. Direction of the immune response toward $CD4^+$-mediated T_{DTH} or $CD8^+$ T_{CTL} cells may be critical for defense against certain infections and may be accomplished through selection of specific antigenic peptides or the use of adjuvants.

Bibliography

T Cells and Induction of Immunity

Chattergoon, M. A., T. M. Robinson, J. D. Boyer, and D. B. Weiner. 1998. Specific immune induction following DNA-based immunization through *in vivo* transfection and activation of macrophages/antigen-presenting cells. *J. Immunol.* **160:**5707–5718.

Mosmann, T. R., and R. L. Coffman. 1989. Heterogeneity of cytokine secretion patterns and functions of helper T cells. *Adv. Immunol.* **46:**111–147.

Wykes, M., A. Pombe, C. Jenkins, and G. G. MacPherson. 1998. Dendritic cells interact directly with naive B lymphocytes to transfer antigen and initiate class switching in a primary T-dependent response. *J. Immunol.* **161:**1313–1319.

Zhu, J., and F. McKeon. 1999. NF-AT activation requires suppression of CRM 1-dependent export by calcineurin. *Nature* **398:**256–260.

Superantigens

Abe, R., and R. J. Hodes. 1989. T-cell recognition of minor lymphocyte stimulating (M1s) gene products. *Annu. Rev. Immunol.* **7:**683–708.

Kotzin, B. L., D. Y. Leung, J. Kappler, and P. Marrack. 1993. Superantigens and their potential role in human disease. *Adv. Immunol.* **54:**99–166.

T-Cell Receptor and T-Cell Activation

Bently, G. A., and R. A. Mariuzza. 1996. The structure of the T cell antigen receptor. *Annu. Rev. Immunol.* **14:**563–590.

Cantrell, D. 1996. T cell antigen receptor signal transduction pathways. *Annu. Rev. Immunol.* **14:**259–274.

Davis, M. M., and Y.-H. Chien. 1999. T-cell antigen receptors, p. 341–366. *In* W. E. Paul (ed.), *Fundamental Immunology,* 4th ed. Lippincott-Raven Publishers, Philadelphia, Pa.

Dong, C., D. D. Yang, M. Wysk, A. J. Whitmarsh, R. J. Davis, and R. A. Flavell. 1998. Defective T cell differentiation in the absence of Jnk1. *Science* **282:**2092–2095.

Elder, M. E., D. Lin, J. Clever, A. C. Chan, T. J. Hope, A. Weiss, and T. G. Parslow. 1994. Human severe combined immunodeficiency due to a defect in ZAP-70, a T cell tyrosine kinase. *Science* **264:**1596–1599.

Garcia, K. C., M. Degano, R. L. Stanfield, A. Brunmark, M. R. Jackson, P. A. Peterson, L. Teyton, and I. A. Wilson. 1996. An alphabeta T cell receptor structure at 2.5 A and its orientation in the TCR-MHC complex. *Science* **274:**209–219.

Healey, J. I., and C. C. Goodnow. 1998. Positive versus negative signals by lymphocyte antigen receptors. *Annu. Rev. Immunol.* **16:**645–670.

Leonard, W. J., and J. J. O'Shea. 1998. JAKS and STATS: biological implications. *Annu. Rev. Immunol.* **16:**293–322.

Oxman, N, H. Turner, S. Lucas, K. Reif, and D. A. Cantrell. 1996. The protein interactions of the immunoglobulin receptor family tyrosine-based activation motifs present in the T cell receptor ζ subunits and the CD3 γ, δ and ϵ chains. *Eur. J. Immunol.* **26:**623–633.

Schaeffer, E. M., J. Debnath, G. Yap, D. McVicar, X. C. Liao, D. R. Littman, A. Sher, H. E. Varmus, M. J. Lenardo, and P. L. Schwartzberg. 1999. Requirement for Tec kinases Rlk and Itk in T cell receptor signaling and immunity. *Science* **284:**638–641.

Weiss, A. 1999. T-lymphocyte activation, p. 411–447. *In* W. E. Paul (ed.), *Fundamental Immunology,* 4th ed. Lippincott-Raven Publishers, Philadelphia, Pa.

Antigen-Processing Pathways

Pamer, E., and P. Cresswell. 1998. Mechanisms of MHC class I-restricted antigen processing. *Annu. Rev. Immunol.* **16:**323–358.

Shen, Z., G. Reznikoff, G. Dranorr, and K. L. Rock. 1997. Cloned dendritic cells can present exogenous antigens on both MHC class I and class II molecules. *J. Immunol.* **158:**2723–2730.

Townsend, A. R. M., J. Rothbard, F. M. Gotch, G. Bahadur, D. Wraith, and A. J. McMichael. 1986. The epitopes of influenza nucleoprotein recognized by cytotoxic T lymphocytes can be defined with short synthetic peptides. *Cell* **44:**959–968.

Peptide-MHC Binding

Bjorkman, P. J., M. A. Saper, B. Samraoui, W. S. Bennett, J. L. Strominger, and D. C. Wiley. 1987. The foreign antigen binding site and T cell recognition regions of class I histocompatibility antigens. *Nature* **329:**512–518.

Cresswell, P. 1994. Antigen presentation. Getting peptides into MHC class II molecules. *Curr. Biol.* **4:**541–543.

Fremont, D. H., E. A. Stura, M. Matsumura, P. A. Peterson, and I. A. Wilson. 1995. Crystal structure of an H-2Kb-ovalbumin peptide complex reveals the interplay of primary and secondary anchor positions in the major histocompatibility complex binding groove. *Proc. Natl. Acad. Sci. USA 92:* 2479–2483.

Rudensky, A. Y., P. Preston-Hurlburt, S.-C. Hong, A. Barlow, and C. A. Janeway, Jr. 1991. Sequence analysis of peptides bound to MHC class II molecules. *Nature* **353:**622–627.

Zhang, W., A. C. Young, M. Imarai, S. G. Nathenson, and J. C. Sacchettini. 1992. Crystal structure of the major histocompatibility complex class I H-2Kb molecule containing a single viral peptide: implications for peptide binding and T-cell receptor recognition. *Proc. Natl. Acad. Sci. USA* **89:**8403–8407.

MHC

Cresswell, P. 1996. Invariant chain structure and MHC class II function. *Cell* **84:**505–507.

Gruen, J. R., and S. M. Weissman. 1997. Evolving views of the major histocompatibility complex. *Blood* **11:**4253–4265.

Jardetzky, T. S., J. H. Brown, J. C. Gorga, L. J. Stern, R. G. Urban, Y. I. Chi, C. Stauffacher, J. L. Strominger, and D. C. Wiley. 1994. Three-dimensional structure of a human class II histocompatibility molecule complexed with superantigen. *Nature* **368:**711–718.

McClusky, J. 1997. *The Human Leucocyte Antigens and Clinical Medicine,* p. 415–427. Oxford University Press, Oxford, United Kingdom.

Pelletier, R. P., C. G. Orosz, P. W. Adams, G. L. Bumgardner, E. A. Davies, E. A. Elkhammas, M. L. Henry, and R. M. Ferguson. 1997. Clinical and economic impact of flow cytometry crossmatching in primary cadaveric kidney and simultaneous pancreas-kidney transplant recipients. *Transplantation* **63:**1639–1645.

Terasaki, P. R. (ed.). 1988. *Clinical Transplants, 1988.* UCLA Tissue Typing Laboratory, Los Angeles, Calif.

T-Cell–B-Cell Interactions, MHC Recognition, and the Immune Response

Cresswell, P. 1994. Assembly transport, and function of MHC class II molecules. *Annu. Rev. Immunol.* **12:**259–293.

Elliot, T. 1997. Transporter associated with antigen processing. *Adv. Immunol.* **65:**47–109.

Gershon, R. K. 1974. T-cell control of antibody production. *Contemp. Top. Immunobiol.* **3:**1.

Mitchison, N. A. 1971. The carrier effect in the secondary response to hapten-protein conjugates. II. Cellular cooperation. *Eur. J. Immunol.* **1:**18–22.

Powis, S. J. 1997. Major histocompatibility complex class I molecules interact with both subunits of the transporter associated with antigen processing, TAP1 and TAP2. *Eur. J. Immunol.* **27:**2744–2747.

Zimmermann, V. S., P. Rovere, J. Trucy, K. Serre, P. Machy, F. Forquet, L. Leserman, and J. Davoust. 1999. Engagement of B cell receptor regulates the invariant chain-dependent MHC class II presentation pathway. *J. Immunol.* **162:**2495–2502.

Zinkernagel, R. M., and P. C. Doherty. 1974. Activity of sensitized thymus-derived lymphocytes in lymphocytic choriomeningitis reflects immunologic surveillance against altered self components. *Nature* **251:**547–548.

Contact-Mediated Help

Allen, R. C., R. J. Armitage, M. E. Conley, H. Rosenblatt, N. A. Jenkins, N. G. Copeland, M. A. Bedell, S. Edelhoff, C. M. Disteche, D. K. Simoneaux, et al. 1993. CD40 ligand gene defects responsible for X-linked hyper-IgM syndrome. *Science* **259:**990–993.

Aruffo, A., M. Farrington, D. Hollenbaugh, X. Li, A. Milatovich, S. Nonoyama, J. Bajorath, L. S. Grosmaire, R. Stenkamp, M. Neubauer, et al. 1993. The CD40 ligand, gp39, is defective in activated T cells from patients with X-linked hyper-IgM syndrome. *Cell* **72:**291–300.

Bluestone, J. A., R. Khattri, and G. A. van Seventer. 1999. Accessory molecules, p. 449–478. *In* W. E. Paul (ed.), *Fundamental Immunology,* 4th ed. Lippincott-Raven Publishers, Philadelphia, Pa.

Clark, E. A., and J. A. Ledbetter. 1994. How B and T cells talk to each other. *Nature* **367:**425–428.

Judge, T. A., A. Tang, and L. A. Turka. 1996. Immunosuppression through blockade of CD28:B7-mediated costimulatory signals. *Immunol. Res.* **15:**38–49.

Noelle, R. J. 1996. CD40 and its ligand in host defense. *Immunity* **4:**415–421.

Soluble Factors

Abbas, A. K., K. M. Murphy, and A. Sher. 1996. Functional diversity of helper T lymphocytes. *Nature* **383:**787–793.

Leonard, W. J. 1996. The molecular basis of X-linked combined immunodeficiency: defective cytokine receptor signaling. *Annu. Rev. Med.* **47:**229–239.

Leonard, W. J. 1999. Type I cytokines and interferons and their receptors, p. 741–774. *In* W. E. Paul (ed.), *Fundamental Immunology,* 4th ed. Lippincott-Raven Publishers, Philadelphia, Pa.

Lucey, D. R., M. Clerici, and G. M. Shearer. 1996. Type 1 and type 2 cytokine dysregulation in human infections, neoplastic and inflammatory diseases. *Clin. Microbiol. Rev.* **9:**532–562.

Mosmann, T. R., and R. L. Coffman. 1989. TH1 and TH2 cells: different patterns of lymphokine secretion lead to different functional properties. *Annu. Rev. Immunol.* **6***:*145–173.

Paul, W. E. 1989. Pleiotropy and redundancy: T-cell derived lymphokines in the immune response. *Cell* **57:**521–524.

Vaccination

Behbehani, A. M. 1983. The smallpox story: life and death of an old disease. *Microbiol. Rev.* **47:**455–509. See also *The Smallpox Story: In Words and Pictures,* University of Kansas Medical Center, Kansas City, 1988.

Bloch, H. 1993. Edward Jenner (1749–1823): the history and effects of smallpox, inoculation, and vaccination. *Am. J. Dis. Child.* **147:**772–774.

Jenner, E. 1798. *Inquiry into the Cause and Effects of the Variolae Vaccinae.* Low, London, England. [Republished by Cassell in 1896.]

Wilson, I. A., and N. J. Cox. 1990. Structural basis of immune recognition of influenza virus hemagglutinin. *Annu. Rev. Immunol.* **8:**737–771.

Control of the Type of Immune Response

Desmedt, M., P. Rottiers, H. Dooms, W. Fiers, and J. Grooten. 1998. Macrophages induce cellular immunity by activation Th1 cell responses and suppressing Th2 responses. *J. Immunol.* **160:**5300–5308.

Donnelly, J. J., J. B. Ulmer, J. W. Shiver, and M. A. Liw. 1997. DNA vaccines. *Annu. Rev. Immunol.* **15:**617–648.

Gabaglia, C. R., B. Pedersen, M. Hitt, N. Burdin, E. E. Sercarz, F. L. Graham, J. Gauldie, and T. A. Braciak. 1999. A single intramuscular injection with an adenovirus-expressing IL-12 protects BALB/c mice against *Leishmania major* infection, while treatment with an IL-4-expressing vector increases disease susceptibility in B10.D2 mice. *J. Immunol.* **162:**753–760.

Gately, M. K., L. M. Renzetti, J. Magram, A. S. Stern, L. Adorini, U. Gubler, and D. H. Presky. 1998. The interleukin-12/interleukin-12-receptor system: role in normal and pathologic immune responses. *Annu. Rev. Immunol.* **16:**495–521.

Kim, J. J., V. Ayyavoo, M. L. Bagarazzi, M. A. Chattergoon, K. Dang, B. Wang, J. D. Boyer, and D. B. Weiner. 1997. *In vivo* engineering of a cellular immune response by coadministration of IL-12 expression vector with a DNA immunogen. *J. Immunol.* **158:**816–826.

Sell, S., and P.-L. Hsu. 1993. Delayed hypersensitivity, immune deviation, antigen processing and T-helper cell subset selection in syphilis pathogenesis and vaccine design. *Immunol. Today* **14:**576–582.

Singh, M., and D. O'Hagan. 1999. Advances in vaccine adjuvants. *Nat. Biotechnol.* **17:**1075–1081.

Takeuchi, M., P. Alard, and J. W. Streilein. 1998. TGF-β promotes immune deviation by altering accessory signals of antigen-presenting cells. *J. Immunol.* **160:**1589–1597.

Turk, J. L., and J. Oort. 1967. Germinal center activity in relation to delayed hypersensitivity. *In* J. Cottier, N. Odortchenko, R. Schindler, and C. C. Congden (ed.), *Germinal Centers in Immune Responses.* Springer, New York, N.Y.

Yamamura, M., K. Uyema, and R. J. Deans. 1991. Defining protective responses to pathogens: cytokine profiles in leprosy lesions. *Science* **254:**277–279.

Yeung, V. P., R. S. Gieni, D. T. Umetsu, and R. H. DeKruyff. 1998. Heat-killed *Listeria monocytogenes* as an adjuvant converts established murine Th2-dominated immune responses into Th1-dominated responses. *J. Immunol.* **161:**4146–4152.

Lymphoid Organs

6

The Lymphatic System: Vessels and Organs

The lymphoid system consists of various specialized lymphoid organs and interconnecting vessels. Lymphoid organs are compartmentalized collections of specialized lymphocytes, macrophages, and supporting connective tissue that are the sites at which the cells and cell products (antibodies) responsible for the immune response are produced. Different populations of lymphocytes are preferentially located in different domains of a given lymphoid organ, where they form functional microenvironments with macrophages, dendritic cells, or epithelial cells of special types.

Lymphatic Vessels

The lymphoid organs are connected by the blood circulation as well as by a special set of lymphatic vessels (Fig. 6.1). The afferent lymphatic vessels retrieve fluid (lymph), blood proteins, and cells that escape from blood capillaries and venules and return them to the venous system after filtration through the lymph nodes. If this function of the lymphatic circulation is impaired, fluid will collect in the involved tissues (lymphedema). The lymphatic vessels also collect wandering white blood cells in tissues, including lymphocytes or dendritic cells that may have contacted antigen in the periphery, and return them to the lymphoid organs. Lymphatic vessels drain every organ of the body except parts of the central nervous system, the eye, the internal ear, cartilage, spleen, and bone marrow (Fig. 6.1).

The lymphatic circulation is different for each set of organs. Lymph nodes are located along the course of lymphatic vessels that drain from the skin, lungs, or gastrointestinal tract and are situated in the body in locations where foreign material entering the body will be filtered through the lymph nodes. Lymph nodes have both afferent and efferent lymphatics (Fig. 6.2). Specialized antigen-presenting cells in the skin (Langerhans cells) migrate to the lymph nodes after contact with antigen, thus presenting the antigen to T cells in microenvironments suitable for humoral or cellular immune responses. The products of the immune response produced in a lymph node are released into the efferent lymphatics and delivered to the bloodstream through larger lymphatic vessels. Gastrointestinal lymphoid organs are located along the absorptive areas of the gastrointestinal tract. The afferent lymphatic capillaries of the gastrointestinal tract are called lacteals. Lacteals not only deliver antigens to the

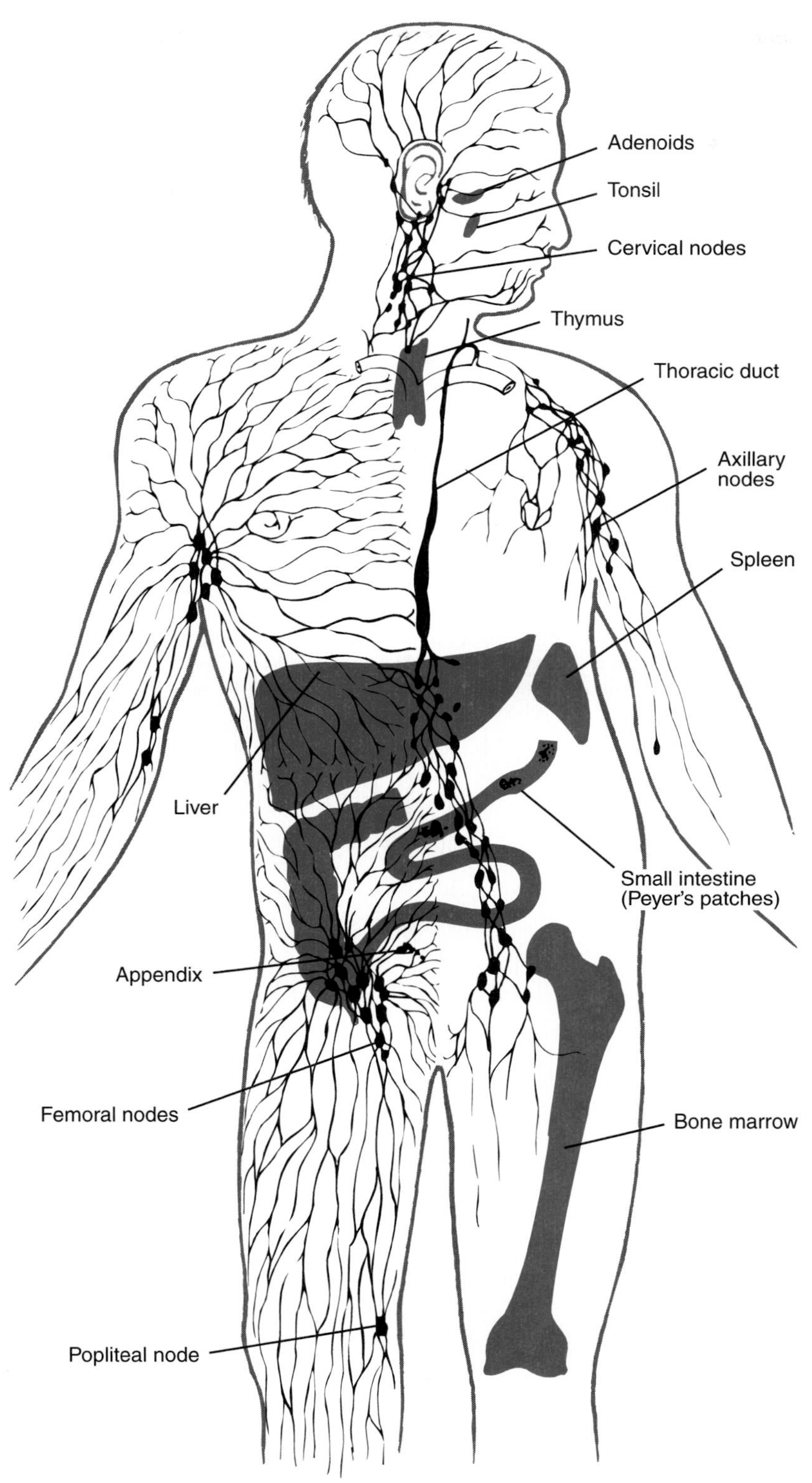

Figure 6.1 Diagram of the human lymphoid system. The system consists of circulating lymphocytes and the lymphoid organs and includes the network of lymphatic vessels and the lymph nodes stationed along the vessels, the bone marrow (in the long bones, only one of which is illustrated), the thymus, the spleen, the adenoids, the tonsils, the Peyer's patches of the small intestine (GALT), the appendix, the lung (BALT), the skin (SALT), and the mammary gland (DALT). Afferent lymphatic vessels collect the fluid and cells that escape from the blood capillaries and return them via the lymph nodes to the bloodstream at the subclavian veins. In addition, efferent lymphatics collect lymphocytes and antibody molecules from the lymph nodes and deliver them to the blood. The thoracic duct is the largest lymph vessel in the body and joins the left subclavian vein. The right lymphatic duct joins the right subclavian vein. Seventy-five percent of body tissues are drained by the thoracic duct, and 25% are drained by the right lymphatic duct. There is no pump for the lymphatic circulation, such as the heart for the systemic circulation. Lymphatic fluid is propelled by contraction of skeletal muscles or in larger vessels by smooth muscle cells that force the fluid from one level to another past valves that permit passage of fluid and cells in only one direction.

lymphoid tissue but also absorb fats in the form of chylomicra. The gastrointestinal lymphatics drain into the thoracic duct and then into the systemic circulation. The spleen does not have lymphatics and serves as a filter for the circulating blood. The bone marrow and thymus are sites of production of immature lymphoid cells (central lymphoid organs) and have no afferent lymphatics. The thymus has efferent lymphatics, whereas the bone marrow delivers maturing cells into the blood through specialized venous capillaries. The brain does not have lymphatics. Because of this and because of the blood-brain barrier, circulating lymphocytes do not enter the brain; the brain is highly susceptible to swelling, because fluid is not easily removed.

Figure 6.2 Lymph node lymphatics. Lymphatic collecting vessels are similar to veins but, except for the larger vessels, do not have muscular walls. Afferent lymphatics deliver to the lymph node lymphatic fluid-containing blood cells that have escaped through capillaries, as well as foreign material that has entered the interstitial spaces of the body. The lymph nodes act as a filter for the lymphatic fluid, which delivers antigens to the node. In response to the antigens, specific antibodies or specifically sensitized lymphocytes are produced in the lymph nodes and delivered to the systemic circulation by efferent lymphatic vessels.

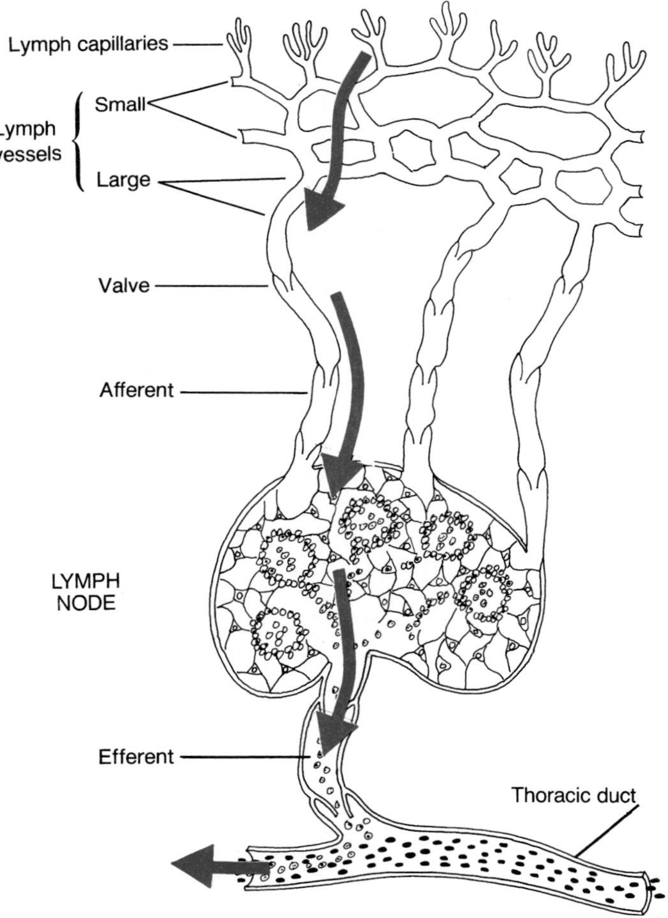

Lymphoid Organs: Structure and Function

Central Lymphoid Organs

The bone marrow, liver, and thymus are considered *central lymphoid organs* because their function is to provide precursor cells that circulate and take up residence in the *peripheral lymphoid organs.* Peripheral lymphoid organs are the lymph nodes and the spleen. Gastrointestinal tract-associated lymphoid tissue (GALT) and bronchus-associated lymphoid tissue (BALT) have both central and peripheral functions.

Bone Marrow

The bone marrow is soft tissue found within many bones of the skeleton of the body and is the site of production of new blood cells. It contains fat cells, stromal cells, and the blood-forming cells (hematopoietic tissue). The stem cells of all the blood elements, including the precursors of lymphoid cells, are located in the bone marrow. These stem cells (*multipotent hemato-lympho-myeloid stem cells*) and their progeny are organized into islands of cells within fatty tissue. There is some evidence that precursor cells in the bone marrow may also be able to differentiate into cells generally regarded as epithelial, such as hepatocytes, under stressful conditions. In the bone marrow, the cell types are admixed so that precursors of red blood cells (erythroblasts), macrophages (monoblasts), platelets (megakaryocytes), polymorphonuclear leukocytes (myeloblasts), and lymphocytes (lymphoblasts) may be seen in one microscopic field. It is impossible to differentiate stem cells for one cell line from those of another cell line by morphologic appearance alone. However, stem cells are usually surrounded by more mature cells of the same cell line, so a given cell may be identified by the company it keeps.

In normal bone marrow, the myelocytic series (polymorphonuclear cells) makes up approximately 60% of the cellular elements, and the erythrocytic series, 20 to 30%. Lymphocytes, monocytes, reticular cells, plasma cells, and megakaryocytes together constitute only 10 to 20%. Lymphocytes make up 5 to 15% of the cells of the normal adult marrow and 20 to 30% of a child's marrow. Normally, lymphocytes are mixed diffusely with the other cellular elements, but focal collections of lymphocytes may be seen in the marrow of elderly individuals. Plasma cells normally constitute fewer than 1% of the marrow cells but increase in percentage with age. Circulating blood enters via arteries that enter through the periosteum and pass through the compact bone in small canals. The marrow is drained by venous sinuses that collect mature blood elements for distribution into the peripheral blood. The mechanism whereby mature cells escape into the bloodstream while immature ones are held back is not known.

The bone marrow is not usually a site of reaction with, or response to, antigen. Marrow lymphocytes circulate from the marrow to other lymphoid organs and differentiate into lymphocytes capable of immune function. During fetal life, cells originating in the marrow populate the thymus, where they may differentiate into T cells, whereas other marrow cells differentiate into B cells (see below). In vitro studies of bone marrow after fractionation of the cells suggest that some immunologically reactive cells may be present in the bone marrow and are able to respond to antigenic stimulation. The contribution of bone marrow cells to the immune response of the whole animal remains unclear. In the human, naturally occurring tumors of plasma cells that produce immunoglobulin (multiple myeloma) are most often found in the bone marrow; extramedullary-location multiple myeloma is much less frequent. This suggests that the precursors of plasma cells with malignant potential are located in the bone marrow.

Liver

Early in ontogeny, the liver and yolk sac of mammals are the primary sites of blood cell formation and, along with the bone marrow, may be the original site of maturation or production of B cells (for more details, see "Development of Lymphoid Organs" below). The yolk sac and liver are closely related embryologically. The fetal liver is made up of immature liver cells (hepatocytes) surrounded by many islands of blood-forming cells containing essentially the same populations of hematopoietic cells as the bone marrow. Attempts to identify a tissue site for maturation of B-cell populations has largely been influenced by the finding that the *bursa of Fabricius,* a gastrointestinal lymphoid organ of birds, is required for normal avian B-cell maturation. The mammalian gastrointestinal lymphoid tissue may also be a site for B-cell development, but studies are inconclusive. Lymphocytes derived from mouse embryo liver develop surface immunoglobulin (B cells) when cultured in vitro. From this finding, it has been suggested that the fetal liver of mammals is a major tissue site of B-cell maturation. The yolk sac may also serve as a site for production of immature immune hematopoietic cells for the embryo.

Thymus

The thymus is where precursors of T cells develop and mature. T cells are, in fact, *thymus-derived cells*. Thus, cells in the thymus are technically not T cells; T cells are derived from cells that have begun maturation in the thymus and completed it in peripheral lymphoid organs (e.g., lymph node). The lymphocytes in the thymus (thymocytes) arise from precursors produced in bone marrow or liver that selectively migrate to and enter into the thymus. The structure of the thymus is shown in Fig. 6.3. The thymus differs from the lymph nodes and the spleen in three important features: (i) Normally, there are no lymphoid follicles and essentially no B cells. The cortex consists of packed small T-cell precursors and many proliferating cells in various stages of differentiation to T cells, as well as many apoptotic cells. (ii) The medulla contains remnants of epithelial islands that appear as concentric rings of eosinophilic tissue known as Hassall's corpuscles. (iii) The medulla does not contain sinusoids but is a mesenchymal-endothelial reticular network in which large numbers of lymphocytes are found. The cortex can be differentiated from the medulla because the lymphocytes are much more closely packed in the cortex. There are no afferent lymphatics in the thymus. The drainage of the thymus has not been well characterized; most drainage occurs through the vein, although significant lymphatic drainage has been claimed by some observers. The cortex is an area of active proliferation and cell death, and complete turnover of cells is believed to occur every 3 or 4 days. The primary function of the normal adult thymus is the production of thymic lymphocytes (thymocytes) that can recognize foreign antigens and the elimination or inactivation of lymphocytes that might react with self antigens (tolerance). Only a small percentage of the lymphocytes produced ever leave the thymus; most are destroyed locally by apoptosis (see

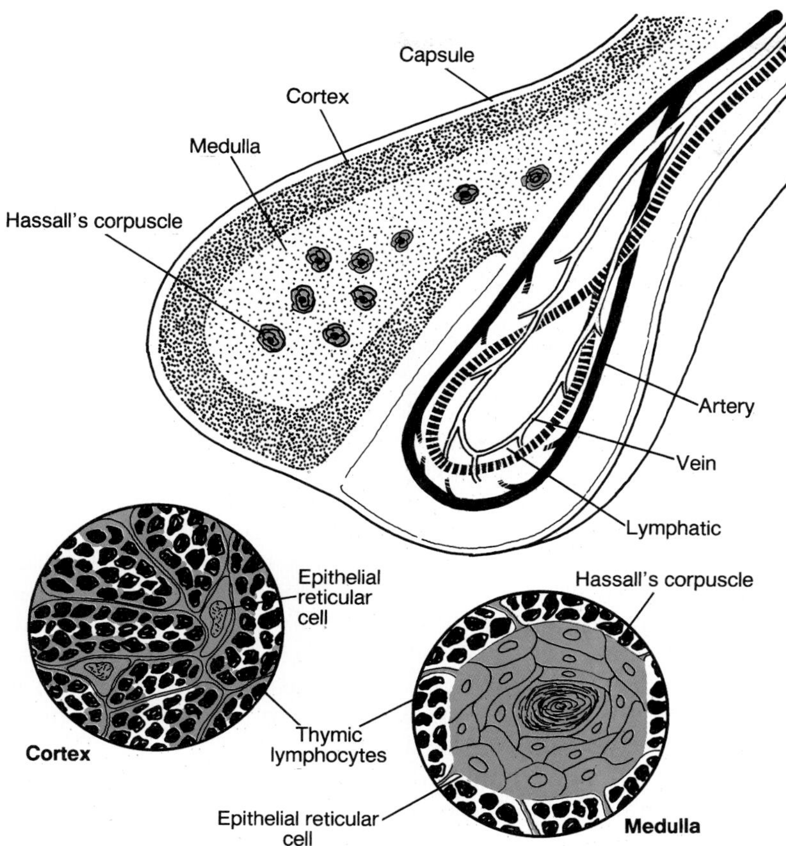

Figure 6.3 Thymus. The thymus contains an outside layer of packed lymphoid cells (cortex), an inside layer of less densely packed cells (medulla), a fibrous capsule, prominent trabeculae that divide the organ into lobules, and a hilum with entering arteries and draining veins and lymphatics. The cortex contains thymic nurse cells, which are epithelium-derived cells in the outer cortex. Each thymic nurse cell contains 5 to 20 immature thymocytes within cytoplasmic spaces, as well as thymocytes that are partially enclosed by plasma membranes on the surface of the cell. Thymic nurse cells play a critical role in the early differentiation of thymocytes.

below). The thymus is important for the development of immunity of the cellular type and for normal maturation of the paracortical areas of the lymph node and of the periarteriolar collection of lymphocytes in the white pulp of the spleen, the so-called thymus-dependent zones (see "Lymph Node" and "Spleen," below). Few B cells can be identified in the normal thymus, but B-cell zones may appear with aging or in certain diseases, such as myasthenia gravis.

Thymic stroma. Phenotypic characterization of both the thymocytes and stromal cells of the thymus reveals a complexity of cell types not apparent by conventional morphology. The cortical epithelium is derived from ectodermal branchial cleft cells, whereas the medullary epithelium is derived from the third pharyngeal pouch. The capsule is derived from mesodermal connective tissue (Table 6.1). In addition, both the cortex and the medulla

Table 6.1 Characterization of the thymic stroma

Location	Tissue type
Capsule	Mesodermal
Subcapsule	Endocrine epithelium (nurse cells)
Cortex	Nonendocrine epithelium (dendritic), dendritic cells/macrophages
Medulla	Endocrine epithelium (Hassall's corpuscles), dendritic cells/macrophages

contain macrophages and Langerhans-type dendritic cells. Maturation of thymocytes requires contact between thymocytes and thymic epithelial cells. In the cortex, many thymocytes are located within vacuolar membranes of large epithelial cells known as *thymic nurse cells*. These lymphoepithelial cell complexes provide a close association between intact, actively dividing thymocytes and large cytoplasmic vacuoles of the epithelial nurse cell. It is within the thymic nurse cells that thymocytes first learn to identify self from nonself, and presumed elimination of self-reactive cells occurs by apoptosis. Prothymocytes arriving from the bone marrow develop receptors for major histocompatibility complex (MHC) markers. If the cells do not react with these MHC markers during their residence in thymic nurse cells, they are deleted by apoptosis and phagocytosis by macrophages; many macrophages containing dying thymocytes are seen in the cortex. The process of thymic selection is described in more detail below. The thymocytes surviving selection are then ready for release into the circulation and for further maturation in the peripheral lymphoid organs.

The medullary epithelium, represented by Hassall's corpuscles, expresses different phenotypes as differentiation from medullary endocrine epithelium to mature Hassall's corpuscles occurs. This differentiation parallels that seen in skin keratinocytes (Table 6.2). The possible role of these different differentiation stages of the epithelial cells in thymic selection is not clear.

Phenotypic maturation of thymocytes. The expression of markers called *clusters of differentiation (CD)* (see appendix 3) can be used to follow maturation of thymocytes. CD34, CD7, and CD45, in the absence of other markers, identify prothymocytes (thymic precursors in the bone marrow or blood) as well as primitive cells in the thymus (Fig. 6.4 and Table 6.3). Early in thymic maturation, the cells acquire CD2 (erythrocyte receptor) and CD5 and lose CD34. CD34 is also a marker of hematopoietic stem cells. The cells then acquire CD1, CD4, and CD8, becoming $CD4^+$ $CD8^+$

Table 6.2 Comparison of differentiation stages of skin and thymic medullary epithelium

Skin						
Basal	→	Spinosum	→	Granulosum	→	Corneum
Thymus						
Medullary endocrine epithelium	→	Epithelium around Hassall's bodies	→	Outer layer of Hassall's bodies	→	Inner layer of Hassall's bodies

(called double-positive) thymocytes. The double-positive $CD4^+$ $CD8^+$ cells that recognize MHC class II molecules and survive retain CD4 and lose CD8 (helper phenotype), and those that recognize MHC class I molecules retain CD8 and lose CD4 (cytotoxic phenotype). Most thymocytes (80%) are immature double positives, whereas only 15% are mature single positives, ready to leave the thymus; the remainder are double negative. At the double-positive step, thymocytes begin to express the antigen receptor CD3, first at a low level and later at the same level as mature T cells. Since this is the T-cell receptor for antigen plus MHC, its specificity is important in determining whether the maturing thymocytes will retain $CD4^+$ and respond to antigen with MHC class II or retain CD8+ and respond to antigen plus MHC class I. In addition, now that their antigen receptor is expressed, the maturing thymocytes can be rigorously selected according to their antigen specificity, so only those maturing thymocytes with acceptable specificity will be released to the periphery as mature T cells.

Thymic selection. The critical function of the thymus is to create a population of T cells that will recognize and respond to foreign antigens through the T-cell receptor in the context of self MHC but not to self antigen alone (Fig. 6.5). This is accomplished by a systematic rescue of foreign antigen-reactive thymocytes from programmed cell death (apoptosis) based on self recognition with peptides in the groove of the MHC, most likely on thymic nurse cells. First, there is an apparent random selection of a generally diverse T-cell αβ receptor (see chapter 5) repertoire so that the thymic cells express a variety of specificities to both self and foreign antigens and with different binding affinities to self MHC. Positive selection then expands the population of cells capable of recognizing foreign peptides bound to the self MHC markers, presumably in the presence of thymic nurse cells that express both class I and class II MHC molecules—$CD4^+$ thymocytes recognizing class II and $CD8^+$ thymocytes recognizing class I antigen. Lacking positive selection, T cells unresponsive to self MHC will die in the thymus, perhaps owing to a lack of essential trophic factors or reactivity with nurse cells. Negative selection then deletes any thymocytes that respond strongly to self MHC, thereby eliminating cells that would initiate autoimmune reactions. Negative selection appears to be mediated by high-affinity reactivity with MHC on bone marrow-derived cells, such as macrophages or dendritic cells. Selection may be the result of differential avidity: low avidity on nurse cells leads to positive selection; high avidity on macrophages or dendritic cells leads to negative selection. Thymocytes with "weak" or "low" recognition of self MHC, but with the potential for high-efficiency recognition of self MHC modified by the presence of "foreign" peptide in the peptide-binding groove of the MHC, are preserved and not removed by negative selection. Negative selection occurs by clonal deletion and results in the death of T-cell precursors with potential for autoreactivity. About 50 million immature cells are produced each day in the thymus cortex, but only 2 million (4%) become mature T cells for release to the periphery; most of the loss is believed to be due to negative selection. Self antigens expressed on thymic epithelium or macrophages may simply trigger cell death. An unanswered question is why antigen binding the same T-cell receptor that normally triggers activation in mature T cells in the periphery causes the death of immature T-cell precursors in the thymus. Negative selection amounts to self tolerance through clonal deletion. Since it occurs in the

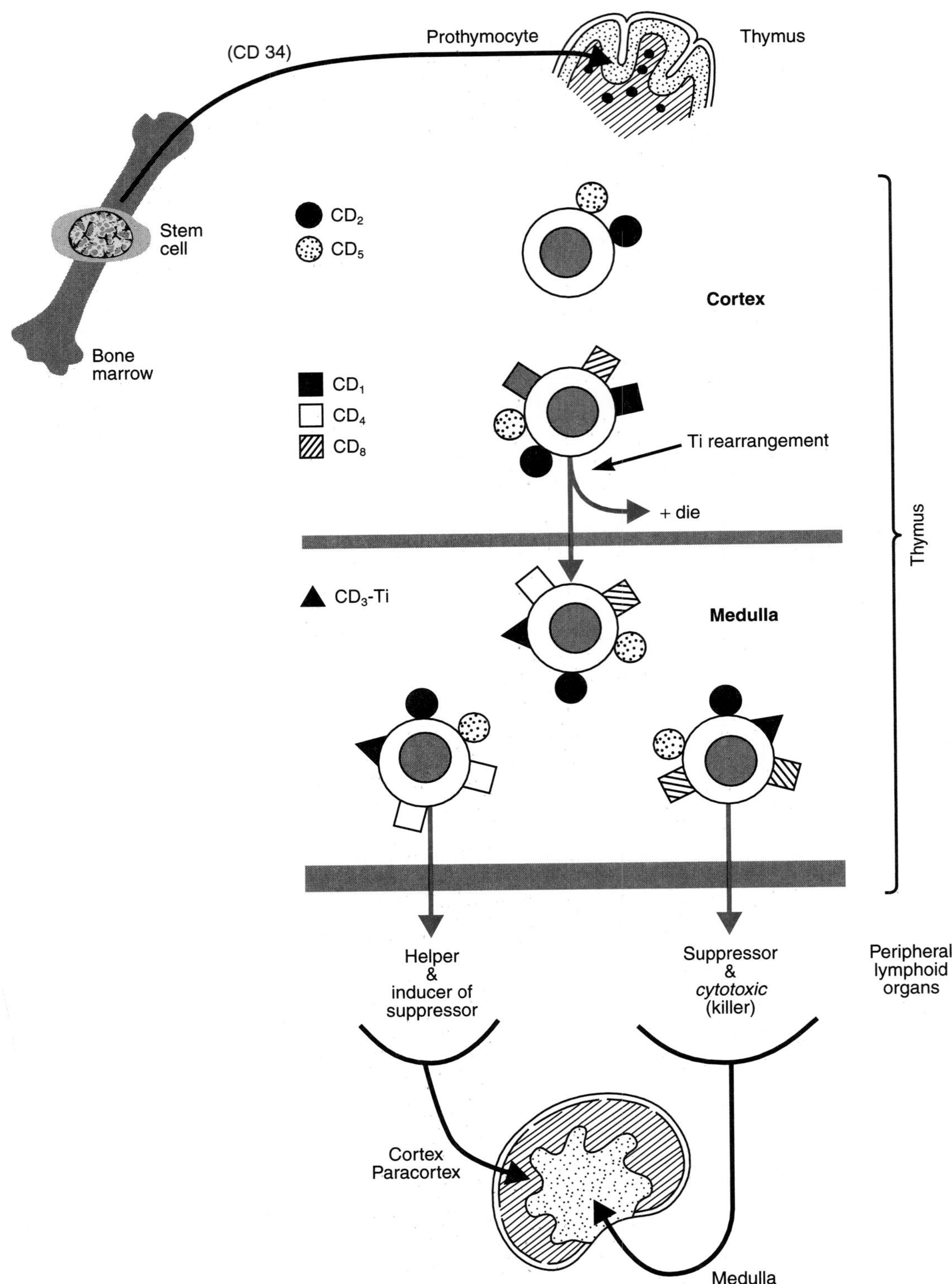

(CD 34)
Prothymocyte
Thymus
Stem cell
Bone marrow
CD_2
CD_5
Cortex
CD_1
CD_4
CD_8
Ti rearrangement
+ die
CD_3-Ti
Medulla
Thymus
Helper & inducer of suppressor
Suppressor & *cytotoxic* (killer)
Peripheral lymphoid organs
Cortex Paracortex
Medulla

Table 6.3 CD markers of T-cell differentiation in the thymus

Marker	Prothymocyte	Cortex		Medulla		Post-thymic
		Early	Late	Early	Late	
CD34	XXXXXXXXXXXXXXXXXXXXXXXXXXXXXXXXX					
CD7	XXXXXXXXXXXXXXXXXXXXXXXXXXXXXXXXXXXXXXXXXXXXXXXXXXXXXXXXXXXXXXXXXXXXXXXXXX					
CD45	XXXXXXXXXXXXXXXXXXXXXXXXXXXXXXXXXXXXXXXXXXXXXXXXXXXXXXXXXXXXXXXXXXXXXXXXXX					
CD2		XXXXXXXXXXXXXXXXXXXXXXXXXXXXXXXXXXXXXXXXXXXXXXXXXXXXXXXXXXXXX				
CD5		XXXXXXXXXXXXXXXXXXXXXXXXXXXXXXXXXXXXXXXXXXXXXXXXXXXXXXXXXXXXX				
CD1			XXXXXXX			
CD4			XXXXXXXXXXXXXXXXXXXXXXXXXXXXXXXXXXXXXXXXXXXXXXXXXX			
CD8			XXXXXXXXXXXXXXXXXXXXXXXXXXXXXXXXXXXXXXXXXXXXXXXXXX			
CD3				XXXXXXXXXXXXXXXXXXXXXXXXXXXXXXXXXXXX		

thymus, it is called "central" tolerance. Because the undesirable T cells are eliminated, it is irreversible. Negative selection is more than the lack of positive selection. Although clonal deletion is a durable form of tolerance, it is not the only mechanism to prevent a T-cell response to self antigens.

The role of the thymus in the development of other endocrine organs is not well known. Thymectomy leads to a reduction in pituitary hormone levels and atrophy of the gonads. Neonatal hypophysectomy (removal of the pituitary gland) results in thymic atrophy and wasting disease, and other evidence suggests that growth hormone may have an important effect on T-cell maturation. Much remains to be learned about thymus-pituitary interrelationships controlling T-cell development.

Peripheral Lymphoid Organs

The functionally mature cells of the immune system are located in the peripheral lymphoid organs, which include lymph nodes, spleen, and other collections of lymphoid cells throughout the body.

Lymph Nodes

Lymph nodes are located in areas of lymphatic drainage in the body and serve as filters for tissue fluid in lymphatic vessels (Fig. 6.2). Classically, the organ is divided into the inner zone, the *medulla*, surrounded by an outer zone, the *cortex*. The cortex is variable in distribution and content, depending on the state of activation (see below). The lymph node cortex contains

Figure 6.4 T-cell differentiation and acquisition of CD markers in the human thymus. Prothymocytes, bearing CD7, CD34, and CD45 markers, arise in the bone marrow and migrate to the thymus, where they mature into T cells. Thymocytes are cells in the thymus. T cells are thymus-derived cells that have matured in the thymus and have migrated to peripheral lymphoid markers. The first identifiable markers in the thymic cortex are CD2 and CD5; CD1, CD4, and CD5 are acquired as the cortical thymocytes mature. In the thymic medulla, CD1 is lost, and CD3, part of the T-cell receptor, is acquired. As a final differentiation step, $CD4^+$ cells and $CD8^+$ cells segregate into two separate populations. CD4 designates the T-helper population; CD8 designates the T-cytotoxic population. After leaving the thymus, $CD4^+$ T cells locate preferentially in the cortex of lymph nodes; $CD8^+$ T cells localize in the medulla, although there is considerable overlap.

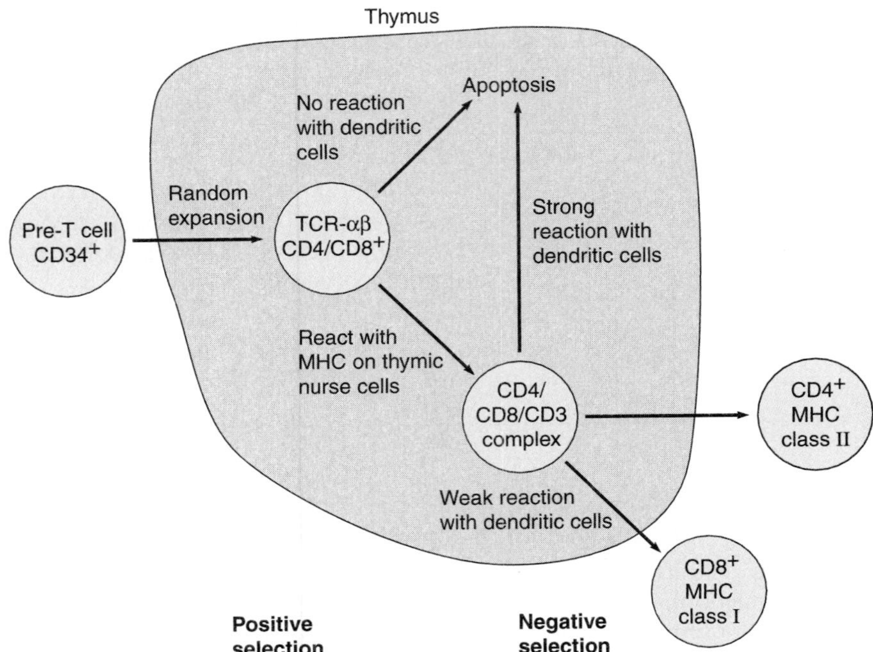

Figure 6.5 Scheme of selection of T-cell repertoire in the thymus. Pre-T cells from the bone marrow enter the thymus and develop a large variety of specificities of T-cell αβ receptor and express both CD4 and CD8. Cells at this stage of differentiation that react with MHC on thymic nurse cells are positively selected, proliferate, and express the CD3 component of the T-cell receptor. Those that do not react are eliminated by apoptosis. After this stage, $CD3^+$, $CD4^+$, and $CD8^+$ cells that react "strongly" with MHC on dendritic cells or macrophages are "negatively selected" and eliminated (clonal deletion). Those that react "weakly" with MHC (in a manner similar to that of MHC modified with foreign peptide) are allowed to survive and differentiate into $CD3^+$ $CD4^+$ or $CD3^+$ $CD8^+$ cells, which now leave the thymus for further development into T cells in the peripheral lymphoid organs.

nodules of lymphocytes (primary follicles), more loosely arranged nodules surrounded by a rim of tightly packed lymphoid cells (secondary follicles or germinal centers), and lymphocytes lying between the follicles (paracortical areas or diffuse cortex) that extend irregularly as bulges into the medulla (deep cortex) (Fig. 6.6). Thymectomy of neonatal animals leads to a depletion of lymphoid cells in the paracortical and deep cortical zones; therefore, these zones have become known as the *thymus-dependent area*. On the other hand, depletion of the primary follicles and germinal centers occurs in birds upon removal of a cloacal bursa of Fabricius (bursa-dependent zones); however, in mammals, removal of GALT does not deplete follicular zones. The medulla consists of a network of draining sinusoids alternating with a meshwork of phagocytic reticular cells. The follicles are mainly composed of B cells (B-cell domain), and the paracortical zone is mainly composed of T cells (T-cell domain). Specialized dendritic macrophages are also present in each of these domains: interdigitating reticulum cells in the T-cell domain (paracortex) and follicular dendritic reticular cells in the B-cell zones (follicles). There are also T cells within the B-cell domains, and these are highly enriched for $CD4^+$ T-helper cells.

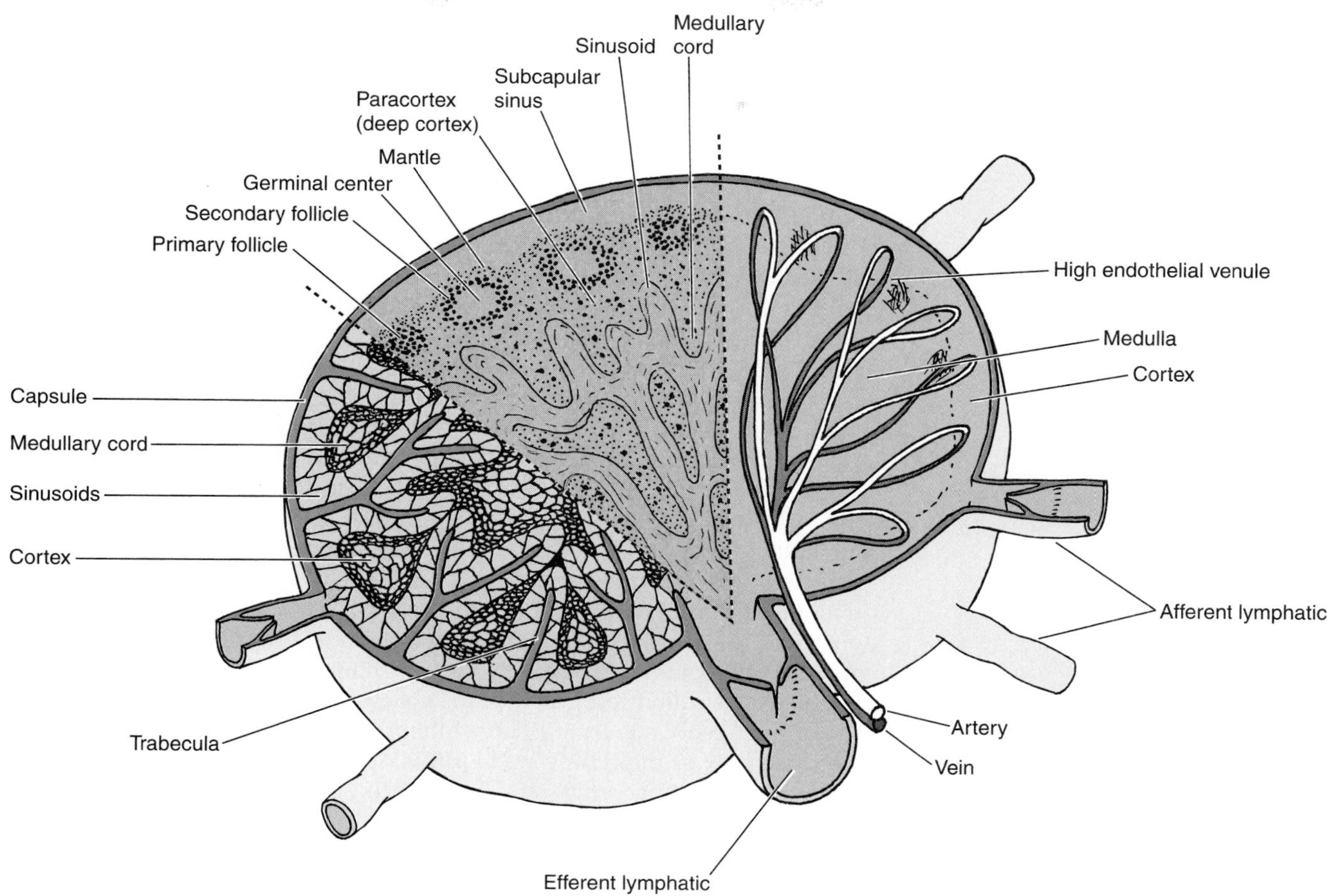

Figure 6.6 Normal lymph node. Nodes are made up of lymphoid cells contained in meshwork of reticular fibers surrounded by connective tissue capsule. Most lymph nodes are bean-shaped, with an indented area known as the hilum. The cortex (outer layer) contains densely packed lymphoid cells and includes germinal centers responsible for production of antibody-synthesizing plasma cells and paracortical areas where lymphocytes are produced. The medulla (central area) consists of sinusoidal channels maintained by reticular cells. Columns of lymphoid cells are found between sinusoids in areas containing reticular macrophages. Afferent lymphatics drain through cortex around germinal centers into medullary sinusoids. Since the medullary sinusoids contain lymphatic fluid and not blood, there are normally very few red blood cells in the medullary sinusoids. Medullary sinusoids drain into efferent lymphatics and are collected by main efferent lymphatic that drains from the hilum. The main artery divides into capillaries supplying the cortex. These capillaries drain into veins that follow the trabeculae and exit at the hilum.

Afferent lymphatic vessels drain into a subcortical sinus; lymphatic sinusoids drain through the cortex around follicles and paracortical areas into the extensive sinusoidal network of the medulla. There are also extranodal connections directly between afferent and efferent lymphatics, allowing some lymph flow to bypass the lymph node. Some efferent lymphatics arise at the junction of the paracortex and the medulla. It is here that T lymphocytes produced in the paracortex enter the medullary sinusoids. The medullary sinuses drain into efferent lymphatics, which empty into the main efferent lymphatic vessel and exit through the hilum. The arteries divide into capillaries in the cortex. These capillaries drain into veins in the cortex, so that the cortex is supplied with circulating blood in a conventional manner, whereas the medulla is mainly supplied with lymph fluid by afferent and efferent lymphatics.

Recirculating lymphocytes enter the lymph node via high endothelial postcapillary venules in the paracortex. B cells must pass through the T-cell domain and home to the B-cell domain (follicle). In reactive nodes, B- and T-cell nodular zones are located together in a *composite nodule*, which contains two clearly definable domains. The peripheral, subcapsular zone contains mainly B cells; the deeper paracortical zone contains mainly T-helper cells. These composite nodules provide anatomic structures that allow T-helper–B-cell interactions.

The Spleen

The splenic lymphoid tissue (Fig. 6.7) is analogous to that of the lymph node, but it is arranged differently. A comparison of the structure and function of the spleen to that of the lymph node is given in Table 6.4. The lymphoid follicles and surrounding lymphoid tissue are called white pulp, and the sinusoidal area, which usually contains large numbers of red blood cells, is called red pulp because of the color seen on gross examination of the freshly cut organ. The white pulp is not concentrated in an area like the cortex of the lymph node but is organized as a lumpy cylindrical sheath surrounding small arteries (central arterioles) like a bunch of grapes. T cells are located in a tight sheath around the central arteriole called the *periarteriolar lymphoid sheath (PALS)*; the B-cell domain extends as a lumpy eccentric *follicle* of white pulp. These follicles may be primary or secondary (germinal center). There is a tightly packed zone of B cells called the *mantle* that surrounds splenic germinal centers. The mantle is composed of cells of the primary follicle pushed aside by formation of the germinal center. The mantle is separated from another lymphoid zone by a venous sinus known as the *marginal sinus*. The *marginal zone* is in turn surrounded by a less dense collection of cells called the *perifollicular zone*, which separates the white pulp from the red pulp. Circulating T and B cells enter the splenic white pulp by traversing the marginal sinus, which is similar to the high endothelial venules in the lymph node. T and B cells can be found mixed in the marginal zone, which may be considered an extension of the outer layer of the PALS around the follicle. The B cells of the marginal zone appear to be in an activated state. It has been claimed that T-independent antibody responses may take place in the marginal zone. There are four types of phagocytic-macrophage cells in the spleen: (i) cells lying free in sinusoids, (ii) fixed sinusoid-lining cells, (iii) reticular cells lying between sinusoids that form a network of meshwork of reticular fibers, and (iv) cells found in areas surrounding the white pulp, the perifollicular zone.

The splenic parenchyma contains no lymphatic vessels; there are some in the connective tissue trabeculae. Blood enters through arteries running in trabeculae. The arteries branch and extend into the red pulp. The white pulp is positioned as a sleeve around the smaller arterioles. The arterioles continue out of the white pulp, where they divide

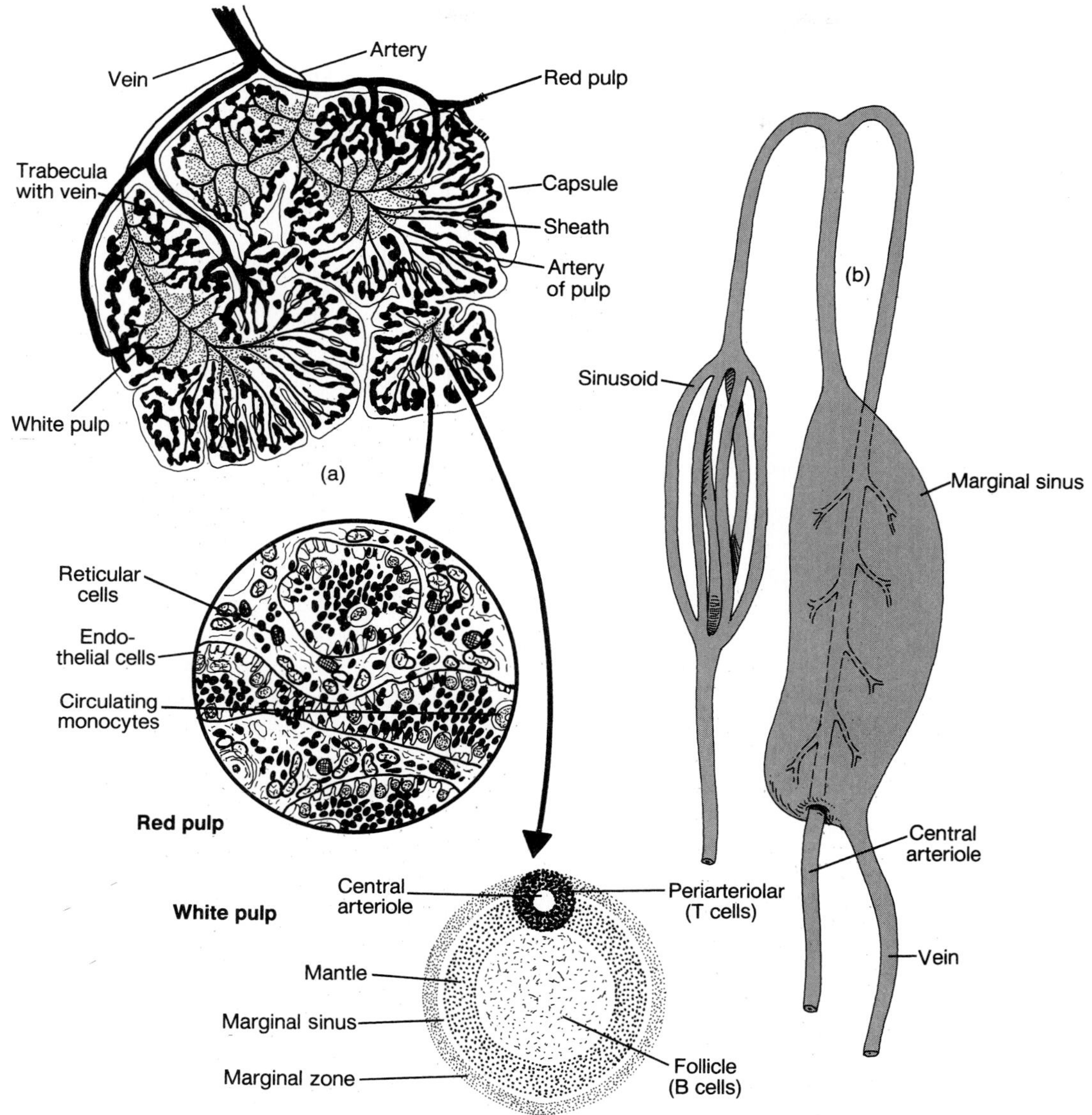

Figure 6.7 Normal splenic lobule. The spleen is composed of a network of sinusoidal channels filled mainly with red blood cells (red pulp). There are no lymphatic vessels. Blood enters through arteries that may empty directly into splenic sinusoids or into the reticular area between sinusoids. The sinusoids are drained by veins that exit via trabecular veins to a large vein that leaves the spleen at the hilus. A zone of densely packed lymphocytes surrounding the central arteriole contains T cells (thymus-dependent area), whereas B cells are found surrounding the germinal center. The mantle surrounding the germinal center is composed mainly of B cells but also T cells, which are believed to be nonactivated cells pushed aside from the B-cell zone by formation of the germinal center. Overlying the mantle is the marginal zone, containing venous capillaries that permit circulating cells to enter the white pulp. Blood flows from the central arteriole through small follicular arterioles into the marginal sinus, which drains into the red pulp. The central arteriole continues through the white pulp. Upon exiting the white pulp, the central arteriole is divided into many small branches—the penicillus arterioles—which drain into the sinusoids or the medullary cords of Billroth.

Table 6.4 Comparison of spleen to lymph node: structure and function

Structure	Description	Function or composition	Lymph node equivalent
White pulp			
T-cell zone	Periarteriolar sheath	Predominantly $CD4^+$ T cells	Paracortex
B-cell zone	Periarteriolar follicles	Production of B cells	Cortical follicle
Mantle	Rim of densely packed small lymphocytes around follicle	Small B cells not taking part in proliferation in follicle	Mantle
Marginal zone	Zone outside mantle inside perifollicular zone	Mixture of T and B cells, large activated B cells	Not known
Perifollicular zone	Zone between white and red pulp, without sinusoids	Place of retarded blood flow with interaction of circulating blood and white pulp	Medulla(?)
Red pulp			
Sinusoids/ capillaries	Meshwork of sinuses, reticulum cells, and capillaries	Clearance of particles from blood, filtering of effete red blood cells	Medullary sinuses, high endothelial venules
Nonfiltering zone	Lymphocyte zones in red pulp lacking capillaries	Site of initiation of immune reactions (?)	Primary follicle
Perivascular rim	Thin perivascular zone containing plasma cells	Connected to nonfiltering zone (?)	Medullary cords

into smaller branches, the penicillus arterioles, which supply the red pulp either by direct connection with the medullary sinusoids or by drainage into the intersinusoidal reticular tissue known as the cords of Billroth. The penicillus arterioles resemble the branches of a fine paintbrush (Latin *penicillus,* "hair pencil"). There is not complete agreement as to which arteriolar drainage is predominant, but recent evidence suggests that penicillus arterioles most likely drain into the medullary cords. Pores in the endothelial lining of the sinusoids permit easy exchange of blood from the cords to the sinusoids. In addition, small arterioles pass through the white pulp (follicular arterioles) and drain into the marginal sinus that surrounds the follicles. The medullary sinusoids have a basic structure similar to that of the lymph node but drain into branches of the splenic vein and not into efferent lymphatics. After injection of antigens, antibody-forming cells are seen in the outer layer of the PALS, from where they migrate to the coaxial sheaths of lymphoid tissue surrounding the terminal arterioles. From here, antibody-producing cells may migrate into the red pulp, where they secrete antibody into the splenic sinusoids.

It was once believed that the spleen was not an important organ for adaptive immunity. However, children who have their spleens removed surgically because of trauma, neoplastic disease, or hematologic disorders are subject to what is termed the "postsplenectomy syndrome." The postsplenectomy syndrome is caused by bacterial sepsis, usually with large numbers (approximately 100 per ml of blood) of encapsulated bacteria. Thus, the spleen does serve an important function in clearing the blood of infectious organisms!

MALT, GALT, BALT, DALT, and SALT

Local collections of lymphoid tissue underlie the submucosa of many areas of the gastrointestinal tract, airways of the lung, and the genitourinary tract. Mucosa-associated lymphoid tissue (MALT) occurs in two forms: (i) organized tissues such as the tonsils (lingual, palatine, pharyngeal, and tubal), the appendix, and Peyer's patches (Fig. 6.8) and (ii) diffuse lymphoid cells

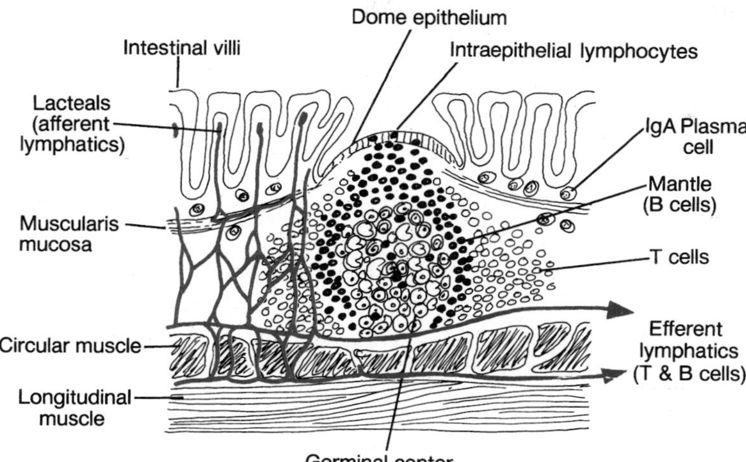

Figure 6.8 Structure of the Peyer's patch. Peyer's patches are collections of lymphoid tissue in the submucosa of the small intestine containing follicles (germinal centers) and interfollicular lymphoid tissue (thymus-dependent zones). The overlying mucosa is covered by a dome of epithelial cells, some of which (M cells) have the specialized property of transporting antigens from the lumen into the Peyer's patch. Lacteals drain filtrated from the intestinal contents into the lymphatics. In addition, both T and B cells are produced in the Peyer's patch and added to the lymphatic fluid.

in the epithelium and underlying connective tissue that is not organized into recognizable organs. Different domains of lymphoid tissues may be identified in MALT: the dome, the follicle, the thymus-dependent area, and submucosal areas. The tonsils form a ring of lymphoid tissue at the base of the tongue and pharynx, known as Waldeyer's ring, which "guards" the passageway to the esophagus and trachea. GALT is a major lymphopoietic organ in the adult and is a major site for production of T and B cells after thymic function declines with age. There is a very high rate of both cell proliferation and cell death (apoptosis) in the follicles of the GALT. Thus, the GALT may not only take over the function of the thymus in producing new T cells but also retain the function of the major B-cell-producing organ. Antigens entering through the gut or lungs may stimulate cells in the GALT or BALT, which can then circulate to other tissues. The ability of cells in the GALT to identify self from nonself may reside in the dendritic cells.

The overlying mucosa is characteristic of each location in GALT and BALT: lingual tonsil, stratified squamous; palatine tonsil, stratified squamous; pharyngeal tonsil, pseudostratified columnar; tubal tonsil, pseudostratified columnar; appendix, columnar goblet cells (crypts of Lieberkuhn); Peyer's patches, specially modified intestinal epithelium (see below); and bronchi, pseudostratified columnar. Afferent lymphatics in the form of lacteals deliver material absorbed through the intestine to the lymphatic tissue. Both immunoglobulin (antibody) and lymphoid T cells are produced by the gastrointestinal lymphoid tissue. These are delivered to the systemic circulation by draining lymphatics, but many of the proteins and cells produced are secreted into the gastrointestinal lumen. The gut and bronchial mucosae contain large numbers of immunoglobulin A (IgA)-producing plasma cells, and IgA is transported across the mucosa in large amounts by specialized processing in mucosal cells by the addition of a transport piece. Lymphocytes found in the mucosal layer of the gastrointestinal tract appear to be predominantly $CD8^+$ cytotoxic cells. $CD4^+$ helper cells are prominent in the submucosa. The intraepithelial lymphocytes of the GALT contain high numbers of $T\gamma\delta$ cells, the type of T cells that appear in the thymic cortex associated with early thymocyte maturation. It is believed that these T cells mature extrathymically and may represent discrete subsets of organ-specific lymphocytes, with unique T-cell receptor repertoires (see chapter 3).

The specialized mucosal cells overlying GALT and BALT are known as *M cells* or *follicle-associated epithelium (FAE)*. M stands for microfolds, because of the presence of ridges or folds on the surface of M cells. M cells lack the cilia of bronchial epithelium or the microvilli of intestinal mucosal cells. M cells are class II MHC^+; they take up and transport enteric antigens to the underlying lymphoid tissues. Enterocytes overlying a MALT structure can be induced to switch to an M cell by a signal from lymphocytes in the underlying lymphoid tissue. M cells do not contain a transport piece for immunoglobulin found in other mucosal cells. Antigen processing by M cells may be important in immune response to enteric pathogens such as *Vibrio cholerae, Salmonella* sp., and pathogenic *Escherichia coli*. In addition, enteric pathogens, such as poliovirus, may enter the body through M cells. M cells have abundant glycosylated surface proteins that bind to these organisms, as well as human immunodeficiency virus, through lectinlike receptors.

The mucosal lymphoid tissue produces large amounts of antibody that is secreted into the intestinal lumen. Memory B cells with a high J-chain content required for dimeric IgA and pentameric IgM secretion are produced in Peyer's patches and migrate to the lamina propria of the intestine, where they can be activated to produce IgA dimers for secretion by mucosal cells that produce a secretory piece. In addition, the lactating breast is a secretory lymphoid organ as are other glands, such as salivary glands (*duct-associated lymphoid tissue [DALT]*). Under the influence of prolactin, antibody-producing cells home to and proliferate in the breast, where they produce antibodies that are secreted into the milk. Upon suckling, these antibodies protect the newborn infant against diarrheal pathogens. IgA antibodies are also secreted in salivary glands.

GALT is believed to be a major source of new lymphocytes in the adult animal. Both T and B lymphocytes are delivered from GALT via efferent lymphatics to the thoracic duct and to the systemic circulation. These cells may then localize in any lymphoid organ of the body (except perhaps the thymus) with preferential homing to mucosal lymphoid tissue (e.g., gastrointestinal tract, lacrimal glands, mammary glands, BALT, and bladder) (Fig. 6.9).

Local immunization of the mammary gland results in the accumulation of T and B cells around ducts (DALT) with a histologic appearance similar to BALT. Lymphocytes are seen within the overlying epithelium, and local immunoglobulin production with accumulation of plasma cells follows. Normal lactating breast contains large numbers of IgA-containing plasma cells, believed to be responsible for the high levels of IgA in colostrum and milk that provide early passive immunity to newborns. In addition, transmigration of T cells through the ductal epithelium may provide passive cell-mediated immunity.

Skin-associated lymphoid tissue (SALT) includes Langerhans cells in the epidermis, recirculating T cells that pass through the epidermis and

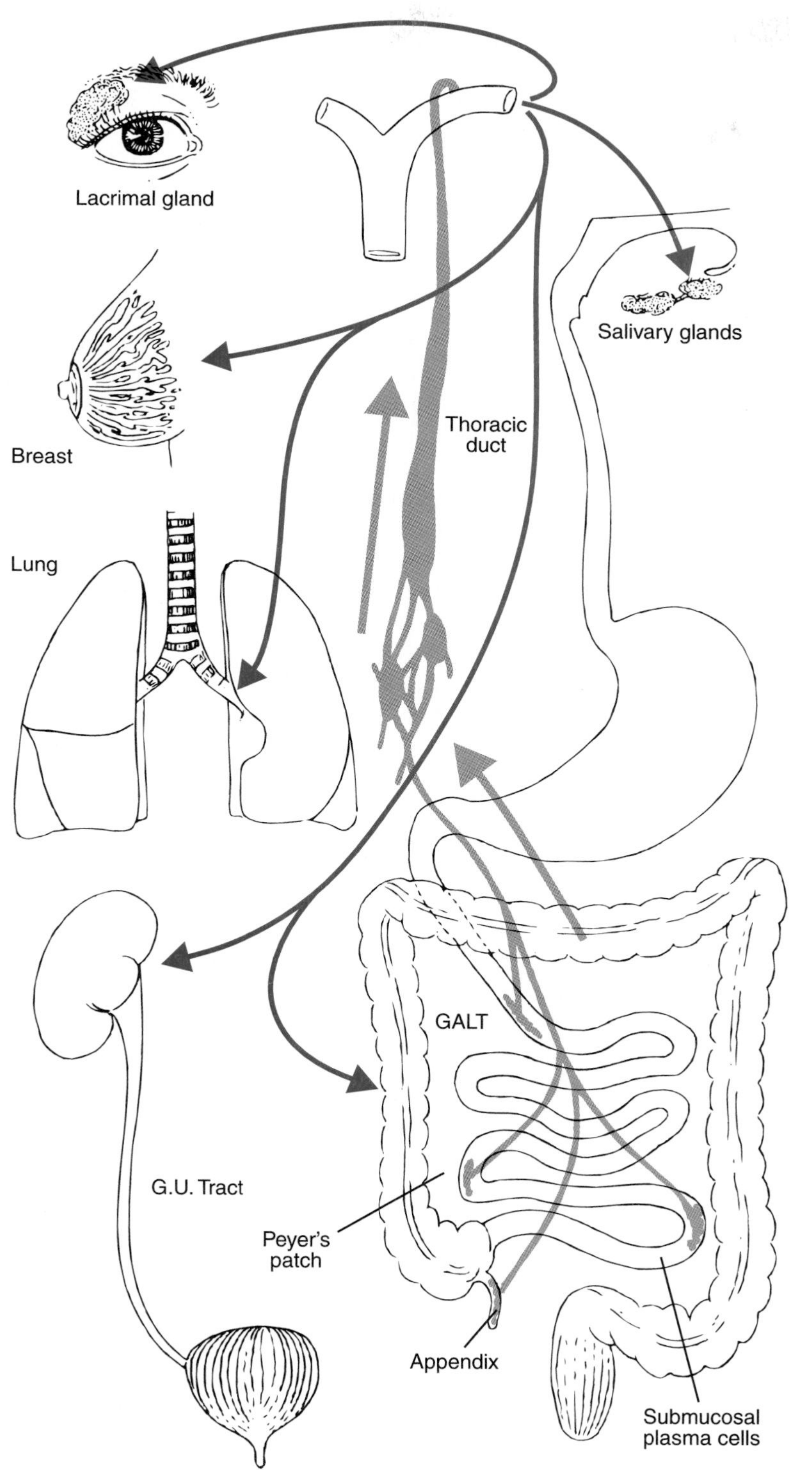

Figure 6.9 Cellular traffic in the secretory system. T and B cells produced in the GALT are delivered to the systemic circulation through the thoracic duct. These cells in the blood then may localize in other secretory lymphatic tissue, such as mammary glands, or in systemic lymph nodes. For more on the cell recognition systems involved in specific localization of lymphocytes, see the text.

dermis, keratinocytes producing epidermal T-cell-activating factors, and local draining lymph nodes (see chapter 16). The keratinized layer of the skin provides the first barrier to external organisms (antigens). Antigens that pass through the outer layers of the skin, such as the lipid soluble antigens eliciting contact dermatitis (e.g., poison ivy), will then come into contact with the MHC class II^+, Fcγ receptor$^+$ Langerhans cells. The Langerhans cells form an almost closed network of antigen-presenting cells within the spinal cell layer of the epidermis and in the form of *veiled cells* are found in afferent lymphatic vessels migrating to draining lymph nodes. Dendritic cells bearing Langerhans cell phenotypes are found in the lymph nodes draining the skin but not in mesenteric lymph nodes or spleen. It is believed that Langerhans cells are in continuous circulation, passing from the skin to the draining nodes, thus delivering processed antigens to the T cells in the paracortex of the lymph node. This system is anatomically ideally organized to react to antigens that are presented in the epidermis, such as contact sensitivity antigens. In addition, there is a subpopulation of lymphocytes that appear to home to the skin (*epidermotropic*). In the malignant form, these cells are represented by the cutaneous T-cell lymphomas, in particular, Sézary cell variant. Sézary cells have a mature T-helper cell phenotype, indicating a preference for T-helper cells to home to the epidermis. In addition, mice have an epidermal T cell not found in humans. The importance of the skin in immunopathology is recognized in this book by inclusion of a separate chapter (chapter 16) on immune reactions in the skin.

Innervation of Lymphoid Organs

The neuroendocrine system is intimately linked and involved in bidirectional communication with the immune system. There are two major linkages: the sympathetic nervous system (i.e., epinephrine) and the hypothalamic-pituitary-adrenal axis. Through these connections, one neural, the other endocrine, immune reactivity and inflammation are modulated. The immune system and its products (lymphokines and monokines) can modify neuroendocrine functions, and neuroendocrine hormones can increase or decrease immune reactions. The study of these phenomena has given rise to a variety of terms: *immunoneurology, immunoendocrinology, endocrine immunology, psychoneuroimmunology, psychoimmunology,* and so on.

There is innervation of the thymus, spleen, and bone marrow by the autonomic nervous system. The thymus is supplied by nerves derived from the vagus, phrenic, and recurrent laryngeal nerves, as well as from the stellate and other small ganglia on the thoracic sympathetic chain, but most of the innervation of the medulla of the thymus is derived from the vagus nerve, which terminates as a plexus at the corticomedullary boundary, where mid-sized and small thymocytes, believed to be partially differentiated, are located. Undifferentiated T cells occupy the outermost cortex, where nerve fibers from the phrenic and recurrent laryngeal nerve terminate. The possible role of this innervation in the development of thymocytes is poorly understood. The primary innervation of the spleen is sympathetic catecholinergic nerves from the celiac ganglion, which terminate in the central arterioles of the white pulp. It is not clear if these terminals are important for regulating blood flow, since experimental studies have shown that the spleen can contract rhythmically even after ligation of its nerves. However, ligation of the splenic nerve prevents the suppression of immunization caused by intermittent foot shock. In lymph nodes, acetylcholinergic fibers are restricted to the capsule, but catecholinergic fibers form perivascular plexuses, which are believed to regulate blood flow. The nerves that innervate bones arise from the level of the spinal cord that corresponds to the location of the bone. These nerves have medullary branches that enter the bone marrow with the nutrient arteries. The presence of both afferent and efferent nerve fibers in the marrow suggests that an autonomic reflex arc may influence marrow function, which is the production of blood cells.

Lymphocytes have been shown to have adrenergic receptors, not only for norepinephrine but also for a variety of neuropeptides, including neurotensin, vasoactive intestinal polypeptide, and so on. In addition, activated lymphocytes may be able to secrete neuropeptides. Sympathetic stimulation of lymphoid organs may increase or decrease antibody production, depending on which adrenoceptor type (alpha or beta) is activated: beta-2 adrenoceptor activation increases early antibody production but suppresses late responses; the effect of stimulation of alpha adrenoceptors is controversial.

Adrenocorticotropic hormone (ACTH) and cortisone also are active in controlling immune responses. During active immunization, cortisone levels of the blood are elevated, and immune responses to a different second antigen given during an active response are depressed (antigenic competition). It has been shown that interleukin-1 and interleukin-6 can act to increase ACTH secretion by the pituitary by increasing corticotropic releasing factor from the hypothalamus. ACTH acts on the adrenal gland to increase corticosteroid production, and corticosteroids depress lymphocyte activities. ACTH may also be increased by stress, and a number of studies have shown that immune responses may be depressed during times of psychological stress. Finally opioids may increase inflammatory effects of neutrophils, macrophages, and mast cells and natural killer activity but decrease antibody production. In conclusion, the role of neurotransmission of specific signals to cells of the immune system and the effect of hormones are not yet understood well enough to provide a clear idea of how they might influence immune responses.

Comparison of the Structures of Lymphoid Organs

A comparison of the characteristics of lymphoid organs is given in Table 6.5. The structure of each lymphoid organ is related to its functions, the most notable of which are the following.

1. The thymus, which does not normally respond to antigenic stimulus, has no afferent lymphatics and no apparent structure associated with delivery of antigen to the organ. In addition, the thymus is the site of T-cell development and does not normally contain B-cell domains.
2. The spleen, which is a filter for the blood and not the lymphatics, has no lymphatic vessels.
3. The bone marrow, which is the site of formation of blood cells, does not normally contain T- and B-cell domains.

Lymphocyte Circulation

Histologic examination of the lymphoid organs provides a static view that belies the extensive recirculation of lymphoid cells. Not only do lymphocytes and macrophages move much like maggots in infested tissue, but lymphocytes, both T and B cells, as well as macrophages leave their maturation sites, percolate through the lymphoid tissue, and enter other organs

Table 6.5 Some characteristics of lymphoid organs[a]

Organ	Cortex	Medulla	B-cell domain (follicles)	Afferent lymphatics	Efferent lymphatics	Special features
Thymus	+	+	0	0	+	Hassall's corpuscles, epithelial reticulum, no B cells
Spleen	0	0	+	0	0	White pulp and red pulp, no parenchymal lymphatics
Lymph node	+	+	+	+	+	Subcapsular sinus, prominent follicles, paracortical zones
GI tract and tonsils	+	0	+	0	+	Zones of T and B cells, no prominent medulla or draining sinusoids, active mitoses
Appendix	+	0	+	+	+	Submucosal, prominent follicles
Peyer's patches	+	0	+	+	+	M cells, active mitoses of T- and B-cell precursors
Bone marrow	0	0	0	0	0	Hematopoietic cells in fatty tissues, few mature immune cells, multipotent precursor stem cells

[a]+, present; 0, absent.

by circulation in the bloodstream. Entrance to the bloodstream occurs either via efferent lymphatics or draining veins. Mature lymphoid cells (memory cells?) as well as naive T and B lymphocytes may reenter lymphoid organs after circulating through other tissues. Lymphocytes enter the lymph node by transversing specialized cortical capillary venules known as high endothelial venules (HEV), because of the thickness of the endothelial cells. HEVs have specific surface recognition sites for different subpopulations of T and B lymphocytes. At least four functionally distinct lymphocyte-HEV recognition systems control the homing of lymphocytes separately to peripheral lymph nodes, to GALT (Peyer's patches, appendix), and to inflamed synovium. Passively transferred stem cells home specifically to the bone marrow, after bone marrow transplantation, through HEVs. Thus, there is organ selectivity for lymphocyte localization. For instance, lymph node lymphocytes preferentially localize to lymph nodes, whereas GALT lymphocytes preferentially localize to GALT, when reinfused into an animal.

Preferential homing of lymphocytes is mediated by interacting recognition molecules. Lymphocytes circulating in the blood initiate contact with HEVs in the lymph node cortex through their microvilli. This is followed by attachment and rolling, mediated by ligands on lymphocytes reacting with cell adhesion molecules (CAMs) on the HEV, and then by attachment of integrin (LFA-1) on the lymphocyte surface to intercellular adhesion molecules (ICAM-1 and ICAM-2) on the HEV. This leads to sticking and arrest of the lymphocyte to the HEV and then transendothelial migration (diapedesis).

A group of adhesion molecules, known as *vascular addressins* or *lymphocyte homing molecules,* aid lymphocytes in homing to a specific type of vascular endothelium (for an extensive presentation of this subject, see chapter 3). Endothelial cells express addressins, which are either mucosal (MAd) or peripheral lymph node (NAd) in type; expression is associated with selective homing of lymphocytes to HEVs of the mucosa or lymph node. At least four major lymphocyte surface molecules are involved in reaction with HEVs (Table 6.6). These include *L-selectin (lymphocyte adhesion molecule 1 [LAM-1]), homing-associated cell adhesion molecule (H-CAM), β_2-integrin (lymphocyte function antigen 1 [LFA-1]),* and *$\alpha_4\beta_1$-integrin (very late antigen 4 [VLA-4]).* L-selectin is a peripheral lymph node homing receptor. H-CAM is a homing receptor for all lymphocytes but is primarily reactive with a 58- to 66-kDa protein on HEVs identified as *mucosal vascular addressin (MAd).* Two integrins, VLA-4 and LFA-1, are implicated in lymphocyte homing. The ligand for VLA-4 is VCAM-1; that for LFA-1 is ICAM-1. VLA-4 directs lymphocytes to mucosal tissue; LFA-1 directs lymphocytes to both mucosa and lymph node HEVs. LFA-1 is also involved in the interaction of T-cytotoxic cells with their target cells. In the skin, preferential homing is through common leukocyte antigen (CLA) on lymphocytes and vascular E-selectin.

In the gut, slow rolling is mediated by $\alpha_4\beta_7$-integrin, and arrest and diapedesis are mediated by LFA-1. Peripheral lymph node HEVs do not express the ligand for $\alpha_4\beta_7$-integrin. Gut homing memory T cells upregulate $\alpha_4\beta_7$-integrin and so preferentially home to gut lymphoid organs. Self-reactive cells may be excluded from normal recirculation and removed by apoptosis. For more details of the cell surface molecules involved and the process during inflammation, see chapter 3.

T cells and B cells may enter at the same site but are able to go separately to their respective domains in the lymphoid organ. In the lymph node, B cells must transverse the T-cell domain (paracortical zone) to reach the B-cell domain (follicles). In the spleen, T cells and B cells first localize in the marginal zone. T cells migrate into the PALS, and B cells home to the follicle. In this way, B cells come into contact with T cells and accessory cells on their way to B-cell zones. Recirculating T and B cells enter the medullary or red pulp sinusoids before entering the efferent lymphatics. The lymphocyte fields of the lymph node thus contain slowly percolating masses of T and B cells, most of which are on their way from blood to lymph and back to blood. The ratio of the constitutive population of fixed cells to recirculating lymphocytes is not known.

The Effect of Antigens on Lymphoid Tissue

The "normal" structure of the lymphoid organs depends upon antigenic exposure. In germfree animals that have little antigenic contact, the lymphoid

Table 6.6 Lymphocyte surface molecules reacting with HEVs

Surface marker	Monoclonal antibodies	Mol mass (kDa)	Species	HEV ligand
L-Selectin	LAM-1, MEL-14, Leu-8	75–100	Mouse	Mannose-6-phosphate
H-CAM	CD44, Hermes, Pgp-1	90	Human	MAd
β_2-Integrin	LFA-1, CD11a/CD18	95/150	Human/ mouse	ICAM-I
$\alpha_4\beta_7$-Integrin	CD49d	130	Human	MADCAM-1, FBN
$\alpha_4\beta_1$-Integrin (VLA-4)	CD49d/CD29	130/150	Human/ mouse	VCAM-I

organs contain few primary or secondary follicles, sparse paracortical areas, and serum immunoglobulin levels less than one-tenth that of conventional animals. The medullary areas contain sinusoids relatively depleted of mononuclear cells or lymph fluid. If antigen is introduced, there is a marked increase in cortical follicles and paracortical tissue, and the serum immunoglobulin levels may increase to almost normal levels.

Antibody Production

The induction of antibody formation involves the interaction of four major cell types in lymphoid organs leading to formation of germinal centers. The four cell types are B cells, T cells, follicular dendritic cells (FDC), and tingible body macrophages. FDCs, B cells, and T-helper cells interact during the induction process, whereas tingible body macrophages serve to remove B cells that do not survive in the follicle (apoptotic cells). In vitro, B cells bind to dendritic cells and form clusters of cells. The B cells in these clusters are protected from apoptosis, unlike B cells not in clusters. Antigens that stimulate the production of both circulating antibody and nonantigens are taken up by the phagocytic cells (macrophages) of the medullary areas of lymph nodes and spleen (Fig. 6.10). In addition, immature dendritic cells, located at sites of antigen entry such as skin or mucosa, may capture antigen and then migrate to peripheral lymphoid organs, where they acquire the capacity to activate naive T cells carrying receptors for the antigen. In either case, a few days after exposure, antigens are found in "dendritic" macrophages in the cortex or white pulp, where germinal centers will form. Dendritic cells, when activated, both in peripheral lymphoid organs and in connective tissue of other organs, develop into elongated spindle-shaped cells with cytoplasmic extensions that envelop differentiating B cells and serve as the site for follicle development. Activated FDCs express Fc and complement receptors and will take up antibody-antigen complexes. Virgin B cells are positive for both IgM and IgD, but on stimulation the proliferating B cells in the germinal center lose their surface IgD. The nonproliferating IgD-positive B lymphocytes are pushed aside to the periphery of the nodule overlying the center of proliferation to form a *mantle* around the follicle.

The stimulated B cells either die within the follicle by apoptosis or mature into plasma cells. Decreased expression of *bcl-2* appears to prime self-reactive B cells for apoptosis. Clonal expansion, hypermutation, and affinity selection of antigen receptors all take place in the T-cell-rich FDC network. The maturing B cells form a light zone at the base of the follicle, where there are few, if any, dendritic cells. Germinal centers are dominated by a few large B-cell clones that undergo intraclonal diversity by somatic hypermutation, producing B cells with increasing affinity for the antigen. Within 5 to 7 days after immunization, plasma cells appear below the germinal center and migrate into the medullary cords, where they produce and secrete immunoglobulin antibody that is released into the medullary sinusoids. Plasma cells may be observed in large numbers in the adjacent medullary cords or red pulp for periods of at least 10 weeks after immunization. Within 1 to 2 weeks after primary immunization, memory B cells can be identified in the lymph nodes draining the site of immunization located in the mantle at the base of the follicle; later, memory B cells are present in distal lymph nodes. In addition, most of the T cells within germinal centers are specific for the immunizing antigen. After the active phase of antibody production, the germinal center involutes by apoptosis, and

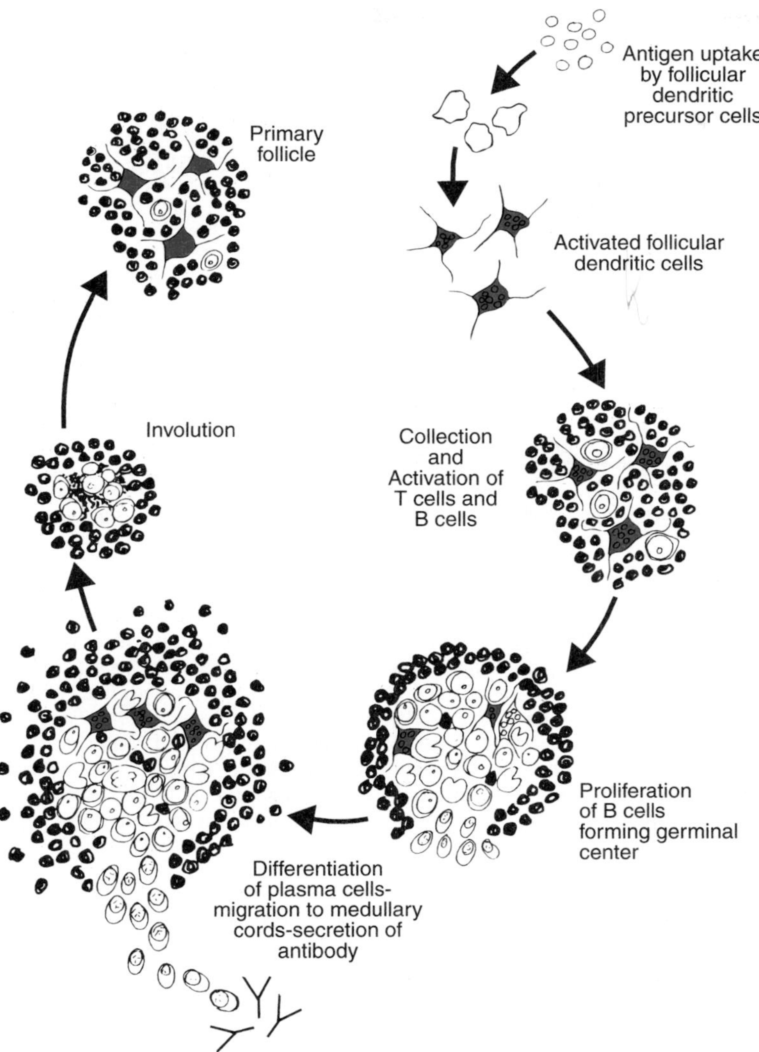

Figure 6.10 Germinal center formation. Localization of labeled antigen in lymph node following immunization demonstrates distribution in both medullary and cortical macrophages. Antigen first appears in lining cells of the subcortical sinus. On day 2, labeled macrophages are scattered through the cortex. By day 4, the label appears in cells in developing follicles (FDCs), and blast cells can be identified underlying the antigen-containing cells. Blast cells and their progeny increase in number until a typical germinal center (secondary follicle) is formed. By day 7, plasma cells and memory cells appear deep to the germinal center. Plasma cells then migrate into medullary cords and secrete antibody into medullary sinusoids. Memory B cells move to the marginal zone. During involution of the follicle, there are many tingible body macrophages that phagocytose numerous cells, even dividing cells.

tingible body macrophages become more prominent. The residual follicle may form into a collection of lymphocytes in the cortex that is recognized as the primary follicle and may be the location of memory cells. If this is the case, then the terms "primary" and "secondary" are inappropriate, because a primary follicle may derive from a secondary follicle and, if so, the primary follicle contains memory cells.

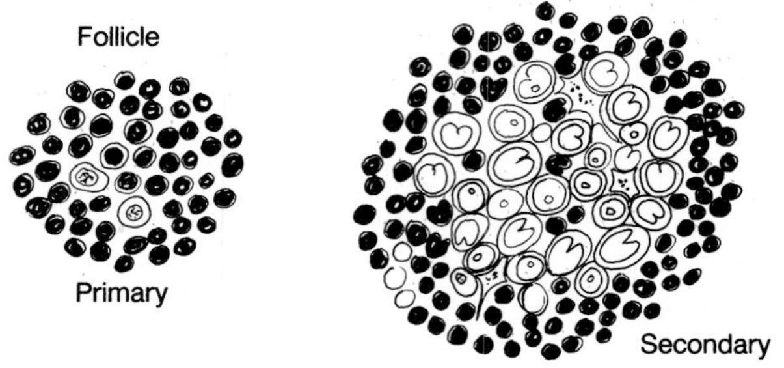

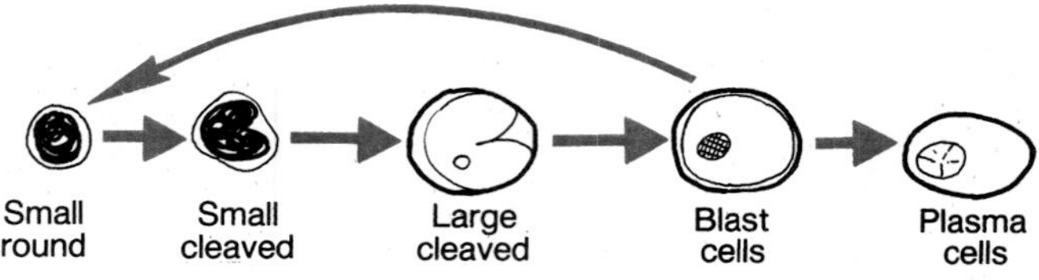

Figure 6.11 Germinal center B cells. The B cells seen in a germinal center range in size and shape from small round cells to large irregular "cleaved" cells on the basis of nuclear appearance. Primary follicles are composed of small round lymphocytes, almost all B cells. Germinal centers contain a mixture of B cells: small round, intermediate round, large round, medium cleaved, and large cleaved. Cleaved cells are believed to represent "activated" B cells; large round cells are "blast" cells that divide to produce two daughter B cells that are small and round. These morphologic cell types have been used to classify tumors arising from B cells (B-cell lymphomas). Small round B-cell tumors have a good prognosis; large round or cleaved cells have a poor prognosis; cell types in between have an intermediate prognosis.

The morphology of the B cells in an active germinal center is depicted in Fig. 6.11. The cell types in an active germinal center serve as prototypes for the changes seen in B cells that occur during proliferation and division. During the activation of B cells in the germinal center, somatic mutation is accompanied by a high rate of gene rearrangements required for isotype switching and receptor editing to produce high-affinity receptors. It is thought that this high level of genetic instability may account for the fact that most tumors of lymphocytes (lymphomas) arise in germinal centers (B-cell lymphomas). Given the principle that tumors are caricatures of the normal cells from which they arise, the cell types present in the germinal center have been used to classify tumors (lymphomas) arising from B cells (see chapter 17).

Cell-Mediated Immunity

The morphologic changes occurring in a lymph node during the development of specifically sensitized cells (T_{CTL} or T_{DTH}) are different from those occurring during the production of circulating antibody (Fig. 6.12). During the induction of cellular immunity, the proliferative changes in the lymph node do not occur in the follicles or germinal centers but in the other areas of the lymph node cortex that contain tightly packed T lymphocytes (the paracortical area). Here, there is a population of macrophages known as *interdigitating reticular cells* that process antigens in a manner similar to that of follicular dendritic macrophages but present the antigens to T cells. A few days after contact with an antigen, large "immature" blast cells and mitotic figures (dividing cells) are seen

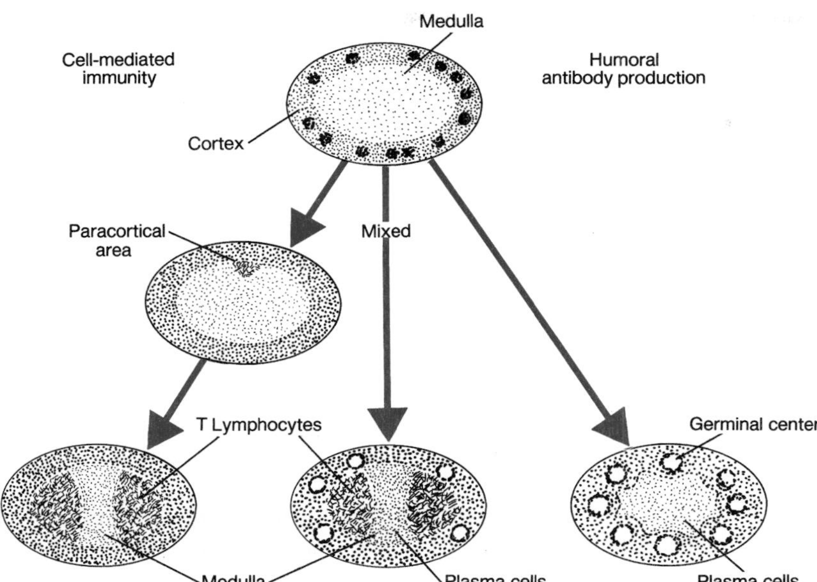

Figure 6.12 Morphologic response of lymph node to antigen stimulus. Induction of pure cell-mediated immunity leads to proliferation of lymphocytes in the paracortical zone. Induction of pure antibody formation results in germinal center formation and appearance of plasma cells in medullary cords. Immunization with most antigens produces both changes with enlargement of paracortical zones and production of germinal centers.

in the paracortex. A temporary increase in the number of small lymphocytes occurs in this area 2 to 5 days after immunization. It is likely that these are the specifically sensitized cells that are rapidly released into the draining lymph and disseminated throughout the body. It is not precisely clear where antigen is recognized during the development of delayed hypersensitivity. Lymphocytes may be able to recognize antigen at a site distant from the lymph node, where the sensitizing antigen is located, such as in the skin. The reacting lymphocyte may return to the lymph node, lodge in the paracortical area, and undergo rapid replication, resulting in the formation of large numbers of sensitized cells that now may recognize and react with the sensitizing antigen. In addition, the Langerhans cells of the skin are related to the interdigitating reticular cells of the lymph node paracortex and may carry processed antigen from contact in the skin by migration through lymphatics to the paracortical zone of the lymph node. On the other hand, antigens may be "recognized" first by reactive lymphocytes in the lymph node after delivery of the antigen to the lymph nodes by lymphatics.

Role of Cytokines, Chemokines, and Receptors in the Cellular Immune Response in the Lymph Nodes

The cellular composition of the secondary lymphoid organs is related to the interaction of cytokines and chemokines secreted by dendritic cells and receptors present on T and B cells. Activated dendritic cells upgrade expression of cell adhesion molecules ICAM-1 and VCAM-1, which interact with LFA-1 and VLA-4 on B cells and T-helper cells. In addition, chemokines produced by FDC, HEV, interdigitating reticular cells (IDC),

Table 6.7 Chemokines and receptors in lymphoid organs

Chemokine	Cells of origin	Receptor	Target cells
B-cell-attracting chemokine (BCA)	FDC	CXCR4	B cells
Secondary lymphoid chemokine (SLC)	HEV	CCR7	T cells, activated B cells
EBVI ligand chemokine (ELC)	IDC	CCR7	T cells, activated B cells
Macrophage-derived chemokine (MDC)	Activated macrophages	CCR4	T cells

and activated macrophages act to direct the structure of lymphoid organs (Table 6.7).

Normal Lymphoid Traffic

In the absence of inflammation or antigenic stimulation, macrophages and tissue dendritic cells which pass into lymph nodes provide weak attraction and localization of T cells and B cells without activation. Naive T cells and B cells enter into the cortex through HEV through reactions with SLC and CCR7 on T cells and CXCR5 on B cells. Then T cells localize in the diffuse cortex by weak reactions between CCR7 and ELC from IDC; B cells localize in the follicular cortex through weak reactions between CXCR5 and BCA from FDC. Because of the weak attraction, the cells continue to move throughout the lymph node and recirculate.

Activated Lymphoid Traffic

The key to a specific immune response is that the one in thousands of T cells and B cells that recognizes an epitope can interact in the presence of an antigen-presenting cell. The extensive dendritic extensions of the antigen-presenting dendritic cells allows them to contact many cells. The active migration of naive T and B cells in the cortical tissue allows the specifically reactive T cells and B cells to find the antigen on the dendrites of the antigen-presenting cell and to interact to consummate a T-cell-dependent B-cell response. Similarly, the dendrites of IDC in the diffuse cortex provide sites for antigen recognition of the T cells required for induction of cell-mediated immunity. This process is believed to begin when tissue macrophages or dendritic cells are activated in sites of infection or inflammation.

Tissue dendritic cells or macrophages are activated by bacterial products (such as lipopolysaccharides), tissue necrosis (fibrin breakdown products), or inflammatory cytokines (interleukin-1, tumor necrosis factor, interleukin-8, macrophage inflammatory protein, or monocyte chemotactic protein) through reactions with chemokine receptors (CXCR1, CCR1, CCR2, or CCR5). Through this action, tissue dendritic cells are activated and some reactive macrophages are activated and converted to dendritic cells. Activated dendritic cells migrate into the cortex of the lymph node and upregulate expression of their respective cytokines. IDC react with T cells to produce proliferation of T-helper cells and diffuse cortical hyperplasia. Then FDC react with activated T-helper cells and B cells to form germinal centers. Activated B cells express CCR7, and activated T cells express CXCR5 and CCR4, which increase the strength of reaction with dendritic cells as well as interaction between T-helper cells and B cells.

Development of Lymphoid Organs (Ontogeny)

Hematopoiesis

The first identifiable hematopoietic cells from which lymphoid stem cells arise appear in the ventral mesoderm and migrate extraembryonically to the yolk sac. From the yolk sac they enter the circulation to the heart and then to the liver, spleen, and bone marrow of the developing fetus. It is not clear whether the progenitor hematopoietic cells arise in the ventral mesoderm or migrate from the primitive neural crest (Fig. 6.13); there is increasing evidence of a common neuronal and hematopoietic stem cell. The first major determination stage in the differentiation of blood-forming cell lineages is the formation of oligopotent stem cells for the formation of lymphoid cells and those for the formation of myeloid cells.

Ontogeny of Lymphoid Organs

A model for the cellular development of lymphoid organs was proposed by Robert Good in the 1960s. According to this model, the precursor stem cells for all lymphoid organs arise in the bone marrow (but also could be yolk sac or liver). During fetal development, the stroma for the peripheral lymphoid organs appears first in the absence of lymphoid cells and consists of epithelial or mesenchymal supportive tissue. T and B cells are derived form bone marrow precursors and acquire immune competence by maturation in inductive microenvironments (Fig. 6.14): the thymus for T cells and the GALT for B cells.

Figure 6.13 Postulated migration of hematopoietic stem cells. Primitive hematopoietic cells may arise within the neural crest and migrate to the ventral mesenteric region or arise in the ventral mesoderm. From the ventral mesoderm, the cells migrate to the fetal yolk sac or to the primitive liver and then to fetal bone marrow and spleen. Prothymocytes arising in the dorsal mesoderm or bone marrow migrate to the thymus (T-cell development); pro-B cells in the bone marrow migrate to the gastrointestinal tract or mature in the liver to functional B cells. Maturing T and B cells migrate to the spleen or lymph nodes, where final differentiation steps occur. BM, bone marrow; GI, gastrointestinal tract; L, liver; N, neural crest; S, spleen; T, thymus; V, ventral mesoderm, YS, yolk sac.

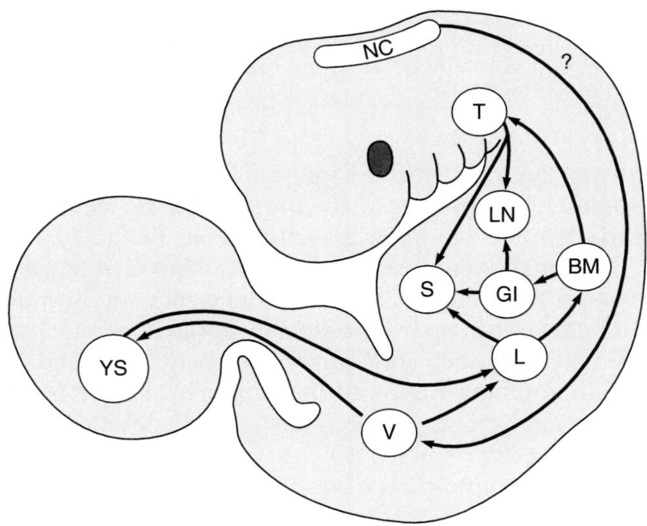

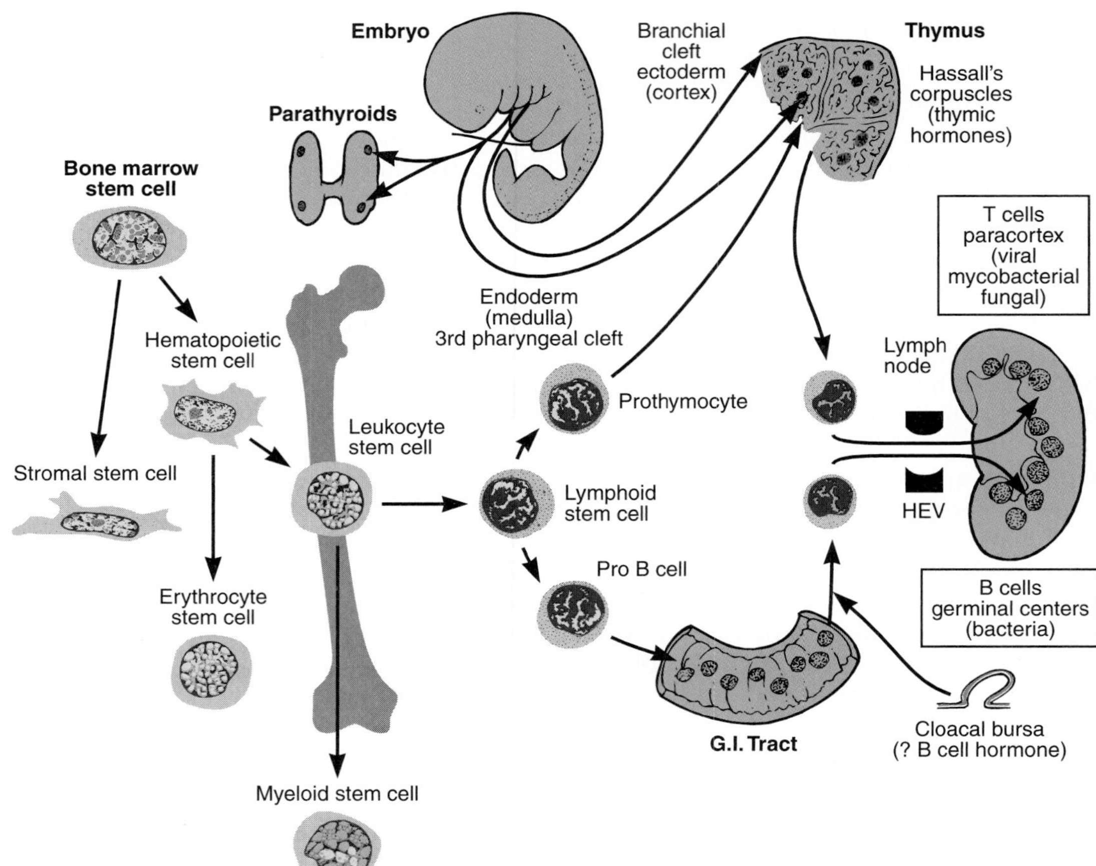

Figure 6.14 Scheme of hematopoiesis and differentiation of T and B cells. Precursors of all blood cells, as well as tissue T and B cells, arise from a common stem cell in the bone marrow. The first step in determination is between lymphoid stem cells and myeloid stem cells. Cells determined to become T cells (prothymocytes) migrate to the thymus. The interaction of these cells with thymic epithelium induces maturation of thymocytes to T cells. T cells are thymus-derived cells, which leave the thymus and migrate to thymus-dependent zones of the spleen and lymph nodes, where they undergo further maturation. B-cell maturation occurs in the bone marrow, liver, or gastrointestinal tract (cloacal bursa in fowl) and migrate to the bursa-dependent zones of peripheral organs. Myeloid differentiation occurs in the bone marrow, and normally only mature cells exit from the bone marrow and enter the blood (see chapter 2).

In mammals, the actual site of B-cell differentiation remains uncertain. In birds, a special lymphoid organ, the bursa of Fabricius, located near the anus, is clearly responsible of B-cell maturation. In the 1950s it was reported that hormonal or surgical removal of the bursa at hatching led to a loss of development of B cells and a deficiency of immunoglobulin production. There appears to be an association between follicle-epithelium in the gastrointestinal tract and bursal mesenchymal dendritic cells to form a microenvironment for B-cell development. However, it was later found that bursaless birds could produce immunoglobulins and a role for extra-bursal homing of prebursal cells had to be considered. In addition, a clear role for the gastrointestinal associated lymphoid tissue (GALT) in B-cell differentiation of mammals has not been demonstrated. Mammalian B

Table 6.8 Functional lymphoid organ microenvironments

Microenvironment	Cells present	Function
Germinal center	B cells, blasts, dendritic macrophages, T cells, tingible body macrophages	T-dependent B-cell proliferation and differentiation
Paracortex (lymph node), periarteriolar sheath (spleen)	T cells, interdigitating macrophages	T-cell proliferation and differentiation
Marginal zones	Dendritic macrophages, B cells	T-independent B-cell responses
Medulla (lymph node), red pulp (spleen)	Plasma cells, T cells, reticular cells	Rapid antibody production and release of sensitive T cells
Primary follicles	B cells, T cells, dendritic macrophages	Storage of memory cells
Mantle of germinal center	B cells	Memory B-cell differentiation

cells may arise from determined stem cells in the yolk sac, fetal liver or bone marrow and mature in the liver, bone marrow or GALT. After B cells develop, they migrate through the lymphatics to the B-cell zones of other lymphoid organs. B cells are concentrated in the lymphoid follicles of the lymph node, spleen and GALT.

Summary

The lymphoid cells responsible for specific immune responses are distributed in blood, lymphatics, and a number of tissues known as the lymphoid system. The morphologic characteristics and functional properties of the lymphoid organs that make up the lymphoid system are different. The bone marrow serves as the major source for lymphoid stem cells. T cells develop from stem cells that migrate to the thymus, learn to recognize self and nonself, and subsequently recirculate to home in thymus-dependent areas of other lymphoid organs—spleen, lymph node, and gastrointestinal tract. B cells mature in the bone marrow, liver, or gastrointestinal lymphoid tissue and migrate to B-cell areas (follicles) of the other lymphoid organs. Different immune responses take place in different lymphoid tissue microenvironments (Table 6.8). Specific T-dependent B-cell proliferation occurs in germinal centers, T-cell proliferation in the paracortex or periarteriolar sheath, T-independent B-cell proliferation in marginal zones, and antibody secretion in medullary cords. Memory B cells may differentiate in the mantle of germinal centers and be stored in primary follicles. Induction of antibody formation is associated with a hyperplasia of follicles, plasma cell production, and synthesis and secretion of immunoglobulin antibodies into the circulation by plasma cells that remain in the lymph nodes, whereas cellular sensitivity is associated with hyperplasia of thymus-dependent areas and release of sensitized T lymphocytes into the circulation.

Bibliography

Lymphatic Vessels

Yoffey, J. M., and F. C. Courtice. 1970. *Lymphatics, Lymph and the Lymphomyeloid Complex.* Academic Press, New York, N.Y.

Bone Marrow

Civin, C. I., G. Almeida-Porada, M. J. Lee, J. Olweus, L. W. Terstappen, and E. D. Zanjani. 1996. Sustained, retransplantable, multilineage engraftment of highly purified adult human bone marrow stem cells in vivo. *Blood* **88:**4102–4109.

Collins, R. J. 1994. CD 34+ selected cells in clinical transplantation. *Stem Cells* **12:**577–588.

Wu, A. M., J. E. Till, L. Siminovitch, and E. A. McCulloch. 1968. Cytological evidence for a relationship between normal hematopoietic colony-forming cells and cells of the lymphoid system. *J. Exp. Med.* **127:**455–465.

Thymus

Aguilar, L. K., E. Aguilar-Cordova, J. Cartwright, and J. W. Belmont. 1994. Thymic nurse cells are sites of thymocyte apoptosis. *J. Immunol.* **152:**2645–2651.

Crisa, L., V. Cirulli, M. H. Ellisman, J. K. Ishii, M. H. Elices, and D. R. Salomon. 1996. Cell adhesions and migration are regulated at distinct stages of thymic T cell development: the roles of fibronectin, VLA4, and VLA5. *J. Exp. Med.* **184:**215–220.

de Waal Malefijt, R., W. Leene, P. J. M. Roholl, J. Wormmeester, and K. A. Hoeben. 1986. T cell differentiation within thymic nurse cells. *Lab. Investig.* **55:**25–34.

Miller, J. F. 1994. The thymus then and now. *Immunol. Cell Biol.* **72:**361–366.

Spangelo, B. L. 1995. The thymic-endocrine connection. *J. Endocrinol.* **147:**5–10.

Waksman, B. H., B. G. Arnason, and B. D. Jankovic. 1962. Role of the thymus in immune reactions in rats. III. Changes in the lymphoid organs of thymectomized rats. *J. Exp. Med.* **116:**187–206.

Thymic Selection

Jameson, S. C., K. A. Hogquist, and M. J. Bevan. 1995. Positive selection of thymocytes. *Annu. Rev. Immunol.* **13:**93–126.

Kappler, J. W., N. Roehm, and P. Marrack. 1987. T-cell tolerance by clonal elimination in the thymus. *Cell* **49:**273–280.

Robey, E., and B. J. Fowlkes. 1994. Selective events in T cell development. *Annu. Rev. Immunol.* **12:**675–705.

Liver

Kawamoto, H., K. Ohmura, S. Fujimoto, and Y. Satsura. 1999. Emergence of T cell progenitors without B cell or myeloid differentiation potential at the earliest stage of hematopoiesis in the murine fetal liver. *J. Immunol.* **162:**2725–2731.

Owen, J. J. T., M. D. Cooper, and M. C. Raff. 1974. In vitro generation of B lymphocytes in mouse fetal liver, a mammalian "bursa equivalent." *Nature* **249:**361–363.

Lymph Nodes

Kelsoe, G. 1996. Life and death in germinal centers (redux). *Immunity* **4:**107–113.

Kowala, M. C., and G. I. Schoefl. 1986. The popliteal lymph node of the mouse: internal architecture, vascular distribution and lymphatic supply. *J. Anat.* **148:**25–46.

Leanderson, T., E. Kallberg, and D. Gray. 1992. Expansion, selection and mutation of antigen-specific B cells in germinal centers. *Immunol. Rev.* **126:**47–61.

Tsiagbe, V. K., G. Inghirami, and G. J. Thorbecke. 1996. The physiology of germinal centers. *Crit. Rev. Immunol.* **16:**381–421.

Spleen

Claasen, E., H. Kors, C. D. Dijkstra, and N. Van Rooijen. 1986. Marginal zone of the spleen and the development and localization of specific antibody forming cells against thymus-dependent and thymus-independent type-2 antigens. *Immunology* **57:**399–403.

Mebius, R. E., S. Tuijl, I. L. Weissman, and T. D. Randall. 1998. Transfer of primitive stem/progenitor bone marrow cells from LT$\alpha^{-/-}$ donors to wild-type hosts: implication for the generation of architectural events in lymphoid B cell domains. *J. Immunol.* **161:**3836–3843.

Van Krieken, J. H. J. M., and J. Te Veld. 1988. Normal histology of the human spleen. *Am. J. Surg. Pathol.* **12:**777–785.

GALT, BALT, DALT, and SALT

Bienenstock, J. 1985. Bronchus-associated lymphoid tissue. *Int. Arch. Allergy Appl. Immunol.* **76**(Suppl. 1)**:**62–69.

Boismenu, R., and W. L. Havran. 1997. An innate view of $\gamma\delta$ T cells. *Curr. Opin. Immunol.* **9:**57–63.

Bos, J. D., and M. L. Kapsenberg. 1986. The skin immune system: its cellular constituents and their interactions. *Immunol. Today* **7:**235–240.

Brandtzaeg, P., and K. Bjerke. 1990. Immunomorphological characteristics of human Peyer's patches. *Digestion* **2:**262–271.

Kraehenbuhl, J.-P., and M. R. Neutra. 1992. Molecular and cellular basis of immune protection of mucosal surfaces. *Physiol. Rev.* **72:**853–877.

Lee, C. S., E. Meeusen, and M. R. Brandon. 1992. Local immunity in the mammary gland. *Vet. Immunol. Immunopathol.* **31:**1–11.

Perry, M., and A. Whyte. 1998. Immunology of the tonsils. *Immunol. Today* **19:**414–421.

Reynolds, J. D., L. Kennedy, J. Peppard, and R. Pabst. 1991. Ileal Peyer's patch emigrants are predominantly B cell and travel to all lymphoid tissues in sheep. *Eur. J. Immunol.* **21:**283–289.

Reynolds, H. Y. 1991. Immunologic system in the respiratory tract. *Physiol. Rev.* **71:**1117–1133.

Sato, Y., and K. Wake. 1990. Lymphocyte traffic between the crypt epithelium and the subepithelial lymphoid tissue in human palatine tonsils. *Biomed. Res.* **11:**365–371.

Schuler, G. 1990. *Epidermal Langerhan's Cells.* CRC Press, Boca Raton, Fla.

Streilein, J. W. 1983. Skin associated lymphoid tissues (SALT): origins and functions. *J. Investig. Dermatol.* **80**(Suppl.)**:**12S-16S.

Waksman, B. H., and H. Ozer. 1976. Specialized amplification elements in the immune system. The role of nodular lymphoid organs in the mucous membranes. *Prog. Allergy* **21:**1–113.

Innervation

Bellinger, D. L., D. Lorton, S. Y. Felten, and D. L. Felten. 1992. Innervation of lymphoid organs and implications in development, aging, and autoimmunity. *Int. J. Immunopharmacol.* **14:**329–344.

Bulloch, K. 1985. Neuroanatomy of lymphoid tissue: a review, p. 111–141. *In* R. Guillemin et al. (ed.), *Neural Modulation of Immunity.* Raven Press, New York, N.Y.

Dunn, A. J. 1989. Psychoneuroimmunology for the psychoneuroendocrinologist: a review of animal studies of nervous system-immune system interactions. *Psychoneuroendocrinology* **14:**251–274.

Lymphocyte Circulation

Blaschke, V., B. Micheel, R. Pabst, and J. Westermann. 1995. Lymphocyte traffic through lymph nodes and Peyer's patches of the rat: B- and T-cell-specific migration patterns within the tissue, and their dependence on splenic tissue. *Cell Tissue Res.* **282:**377–386.

Butcher, E. C., and L. J. Pickler. 1996. Lymphocyte homing and homeostasis. *Science* **272:**60–66.

Cyster, J. G., S. B. Hartley, and C. C. Goodnow. 1994. Competition for follicular niches excludes self-reacting cells from the recirculating B-cell repertoire. *Nature* **371:**389–395.

Girard, J.-P., and T. A. Springer. 1995. High endothelial venules (HEVs): specialized endothelium for lymphocyte migration. *Immunol. Today* **16:**449–457.

Husband, A. 1988. *Migration and Homing of Lymphoid Cells.* CRC Press, Boca Raton, Fla.

King, N. J. C., E. L. Parr, and M. B. Parr. 1998. Migration of lymphoid cells from vaginal epithelium to iliac lymph nodes in relation to vaginal infection by herpes simplex virus type 2. *J. Immunol.* **160:**1173–1180.

Springer, T. A. 1995. Traffic signals on endothelium for lymphocyte recirculation and leukocyte emigration. *Annu. Rev. Physiol.* **57:**827–872.

Effect of Antigenic Stimulation on Lymphoid Organs

Camacho, S. A., M. H. Kosco-Vilbois, and C. Berek. 1998. The dynamic structure of the germinal center. *Immunol. Today* **19:**511–514.

Kuppers, R., M. Zhao, M.-L. Hansmann, and K. Rajewsky. 1993. Tracing B cell development in human germinal centres by molecular analysis of single cells picked from histological sections. *EMBO J.* **12:**4955–4967.

Martinez-Valdez, H., C. Guret, O. Bouteiller, I. Fugies, J. Banchereau, and Y.-J. Liu. 1996. Human germinal center B cells express the apoptosis-inducing genes Fas, c-myc, p53, and Bax but not the survival gene bcl-2. *J. Exp. Med.* **183:**971–977.

Nossal, G. J. V., G. L. Ada, and C. M. Austin. 1964. Antigens in immunity. IV. Cellular localization of 125–I and 131–I labelled flagella in lymph nodes. *Aust. J. Exp. Biol. Med. Sci.* **42:**311–330.

Sallusto, F., C. R. Mackay, and A. Lanzavecchia. 2000. The role of chemokine receptors in primary, effector, and memory immune responses. *Annu. Rev. Immunol.* **18:**593–620.

Shokat, K. M., and C. C. Goodnow. 1995. Antigen-induced B-cell death and elimination during germinal-centre immune responses. *Nature* **375:**334–338.

Spencer, J., M. E. Perry, and D. K. Dunn-Walters. 1998. Human marginal-zone B cells. *Immunol. Today* **19:**421–426.

Turk, J. L., and J. Oort. 1967. Germinal center activity in relation to delayed hypersensitivity. *In* H. Cottier, N. Odortchenko, R. Schindler, and C. C. Congdon (ed.), *Germinal Centers in Immune Responses.* Springer, New York, N.Y.

Ontogeny of Immunity

T-Cell Development

Clement, L. T. 1992. Isoforms of the CD45 common leukocyte antigen family: markers for human T-cell differentiation. *J. Clin. Immunol.* **12:**1–10.

Good, R. A., and A. E. Gabrielsen (ed.). 1985. *The Thymus in Immunobiology.* Harper and Row, New York, N.Y.

Von Boehmer, H., H. S. Teh, and P. Kisielow. 1989. The thymus selects the useful, neglects the useless and destroys the harmful. *Immunol. Today* **10:**57–61.

B-Cell Development

Burrows, P. D., and M. D. Cooper. 1993. B-cell development in man. *Curr. Biol.* **5:**201–206.

Cooper, M. D. 1987. Current concepts: B lymphocytes: normal development and functions. *N. Engl. J. Med.* **317:**1452–1456.

Glick, B. 1991. Historical perspective: the bursa of Fabricius and its influence on B-cell development, past and present. *Vet. Immunol. Immunopathol.* **30:**3–12.

Uckun, F. 1990. Regulation of human B-cell ontogeny. *Blood* **76:**1908–1923.

Embryologic Origin of Hematopoietic Cells

Anstrom, K. K., and R. P. Tucker. 1996. Tenascin-C lines the migratory pathways of avian primordial germ cells and hematopoietic progenitor cells. *Dev. Dynamics* **206:**437–446.

Bjornson, C. R. R., R. L. Rietze, B. A. Reynolds, M. C. Magli, and A. L. Vescovi. 1999. Turning brain into blood: a hematopoietic fate adopted by adult neural stem cells in vivo. *Science* **283:**534–537.

Bonifer, C., N. Faust, H. Geiger, and A. M. Muller. 1998. Developmental changes in the differentiation capacity of haematopoietic stem cells. *Immunol. Today* **19:**236–241.

Detrich, H. W. 3rd, M. W. Kieran, F. Y Chan, L. M. Barone, K. Yee, et al. 1995. Intraembryonic hematopoietic cell migration during vertebrate development. *Proc. Natl. Acad. Sci. USA* **92:**10713–10717.

Dieterlen-Lieve, F. 1998. Hematopoiesis: progenitors and their genetic program. *Curr. Biol.* **8:**R727–R730.

Kondo, M., I. L. Weissman, and K. Akashi. 1997. Identification of clonogenic common lymphoid progenitors in mouse bone marrow. *Cell* **91:**661–672.

Robb, L. 1997. Hematopoiesis: origin pinned down at last? *Curr. Biol.* **7:**R10–R12.

Selleck, M. A. J., T. Y. Scherson, and M. Bronner-Fraser. 1993. Origins of neural crest cell diversity. *Dev. Biol.* **159:**1–11.

Immunopathology and Immunity

Introduction to Part II

7

Immunity, Immunopathology, Hypersensitivity, and Allergy

The manifestations of immunity in a living animal are expressed as variations on the theme of inflammation, directed by reaction of antibody or T cells with antigen in vivo. The specificity of antibody and specifically sensitized T-effector lymphocytes provides a means of directing the defensive force of inflammation directly to infecting foreign organisms and producing *immunity*. The immune response in this way provides *immune effector mechanisms* augmented by accessory inflammatory processes that protect us against specific infections. Antibody is generally operative against bacteria or bacterial products, whereas cellular reactivity is primarily protective against viral and mycotic organisms. However, the immune reaction of the host may also produce tissue damage (disease), sometimes as a result of reaction against an infectious agent (collateral damage) or sometimes because our immune responses are directed against self antigens (autoimmunity). *Immunopathology* is the study of the destructive effects of immune effector mechanisms. The disease states produced by the destructive effect of immune reactions were classically recognized as conditions of altered reactivity as a result of previous exposure and referred to as *allergy* or *hypersensitivity*.

The terms "immunity" and "allergy" are now generally reserved for effects mediated through immune mechanisms, whereas "hypersensitivity" has a less precise meaning. Some instances of altered reactivity as a result of a previous exposure are not mediated by immune mechanisms. These phenomena include the Shwartzman reaction (alteration in the state of blood coagulation), adaptive enzyme synthesis (substrate selection of enzyme production), anaphylactoid reactions (pseudoallergic reactions resulting from liberation of pharmacologically active agents that may also be liberated by allergic reactions), reactions to drugs caused by nonallergic physiologic hyperreactivity (idiosyncrasy), and other types of environmental adaptations (heat, cold, altitude, emotion) produced by nonimmune physiologic or psychologic mechanisms. The term allergy is now generally used for reactions mediated by one type of immune mechanism (anaphylactic). "Hypersensitivity" is a more general term meaning increased reactivity to an external stimulus, usually an antigen. Thus, the term hypersensitivity, by itself, does not indicate a defined immune mechanism. However, when combined with a descriptive term such as "delayed," i.e., delayed-type hypersensitivity, a specific immune mechanism is denoted. The term "immediate hypersensitivity" is sometimes used for allergic (anaphylactic) reactivity. How immune mechanisms protect us (immunity) and attack us (immunopathology) is the subject of part II of this book. The term "immunopathology" has a double meaning: "immune" means "protection or exempt from"; "pathology" is the study of disease. Thus, immunopathology literally means the study of the protection from disease, but in accepted usage it means the study of how immune mechanisms cause diseases.

Immune Effector Mechanisms

In the systemic study of disease, pathogenic changes are classified according to their anatomic location. In the study of diseases due to immune mechanisms, however, more than one organ system may be involved with the same process. Because the alterations in different organ systems caused by the same process have pathologic similarities, the lesions caused by immunopathologic reactions are best classified by the particular type of immunopathologic effector mechanism involved.

Until the 1960s, immune reactions were not classified according to mechanism but were presented as a bewildering list of peculiar lesions or diseases. The first working classification of four major immune mechanisms was introduced by Gell and Coombs in their classic textbook in 1963 as immune mechanisms that cause disease (Table 7.1). Since then, it has been appreciated that other mechanisms are sufficiently different from the original classification in which they were included to warrant the addition of three additional mechanisms to the classification. The classification of immune effector mechanisms used in this book includes seven general categories: *inactivation* or *activation, cytotoxic, Arthus (immune complex), anaphylactic, cell-mediated cytotoxicity, delayed-type hypersensitivity,* and *granulomatous.* These effector mechanisms are activated by the reaction of antibody or sensitized cells with antigens in vivo (Fig. 7.1).

Antibody-Directed Immune Effector Mechanisms

The first four types of immunopathologic mechanisms are mediated by immunoglobulin antibodies. These reactions may be transferred by injection of antiserum from an immune animal into a nonimmune animal. The characteristics of the reactions are determined not only by the properties of the immunoglobulin molecules involved but also by the nature and tissue location of the antigen and by the accessory inflammatory systems that are called into play.

Table 7.1 Classification of immune effector mechanisms

Classification	
Gell and Coombs (1963)	**Present**
	Inactivation or activation
Type II	Cytotoxic or cytolytic
Type III	Immune complex (Arthus)
Type I	Atopic or anaphylactic
	T-cell cytotoxic
Type IV	Delayed-type hypersensitivity
	Granulomatous reactions

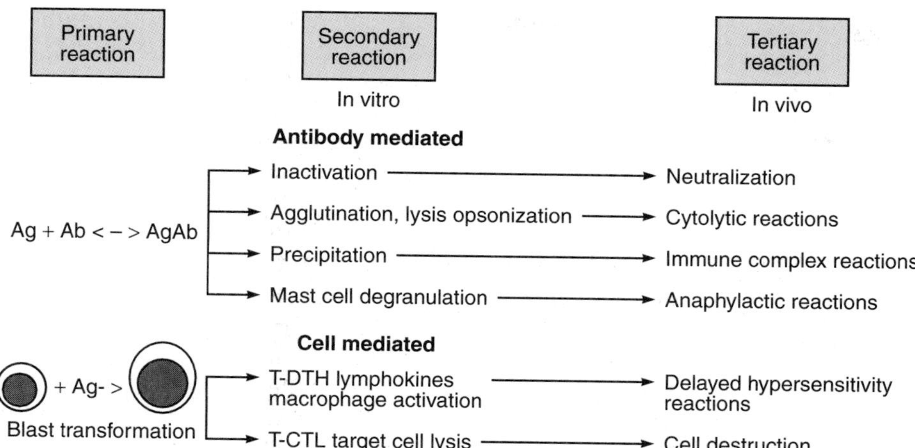

Figure 7.1 Stages of immune reactions. Primary reactions refer to binding of antigen to antibodies or cells; secondary reactions refer to various phenomena that can be measured in vitro; tertiary reactions are seen when immune effector mechanisms are activated in vivo.

Antibodies are able to inactivate biologically active molecules, such as toxins or hormones *(neutralization),* cause destruction of cells or bacteria *(cytotoxicity),* induce acute inflammatory reactions *(immune complex reactions),* and open up blood vessels to produce edema *(anaphylactic reactions).* Each of these actions has critical effects in clearing infections through activation of different stages of inflammation.

Cell-Mediated Immune Effector Mechanisms

Cell-mediated reactions are not dependent upon antibody but upon reaction of antigen with specifically sensitized cells (T_{CTL} or T_{DTH} lymphocytes). In *T-cell cytotoxic reactions,* T_{CTL} cells recognize antigen in association with class I major histocompatibility complex (MHC) markers complexed to antigens on infected cells and are usually $CD8^+$. T_{CTL} cells are effective against viral infected epithelial or solid tissue cells and kill target cells by direct transfer of cytotoxic factors or cell membrane alterations of the target cell. In *delayed-type hypersensitivity* reactions, T_{DTH} cells recognize antigen in association with class II MHC markers and are usually $CD4^+$. Activation of T_{DTH} cells leads to production and release of soluble factors (gamma interferon, interleukin-2, and other lymphokines) whose function is to attract and activate macrophages. The products of the activated T_{DTH} cells "arm" the macrophages through the production of lysosomal enzymes so that they are able to kill and digest the intracellular parasites. Delayed-type hypersensitivity is effective against intracellular parasites such as leprosy bacilli, tubercle bacilli, and viruses such as human immunodeficiency virus that infect and multiply within macrophages. The products of activated T_{DTH} cells in turn activate the infected macrophages to attack their intracellular parasites. Failure of these mechanisms leads to chronic infections. The major mechanism of tissue damage in delayed-type hypersensitivity reactions is the phagocytosis and destruction of cells by macrophages.

If macrophages are unable to eliminate the organisms completely or are unable to digest the material they phagocytose, masses of macrophages collect in the tissues and lead to space-occupying lesions (granulomas) that eventually interfere with normal tissue function. Granulomatous reactions are not separately classified in some systems but produce tissue lesions that are characteristic and clearly different from delayed-type hypersensitivity reactions or T_{CTL}-cell destruction of target organs. Granulomatous reactions may be initiated by either antibody (immune complex) or cellular reactions with antigen and may also occur to nonimmunogenic material deposited in the body (e.g., talc granulomas, urate crystals).

The "Double-Edged Sword" of Immune Defense Mechanisms

Immunity is a *double-edged sword* that cuts down our enemies with one edge and causes disease with the other. Some examples of the protective and destructive effects of immune effector mechanisms are listed in Table 7.2.

Much of what we recognize as immunopathology may result from artificial stresses put on a system that normally would not occur. The use of abnormally high doses of exogenous agents used in therapy and the delivery of these agents by unnatural routes (such as intravenously) may produce deleterious reactions such as anaphylaxis, serum sickness, transfusion reactions, and drug reactions. Tissue graft rejection is a protective response elicited by iatrogenic (physician-initiated) exposure to foreign tissue. However, there are many naturally occurring immune diseases, including autoimmune hemolytic anemia, erythroblastosis fetalis, hay fever, anaphylactic shock, polyarteritis nodosa, connective tissue diseases, and poison ivy. In many of these diseases, infectious agents are not the primary pathogenic event, although in some it is postulated that infections may initiate an "autoimmune" process that causes the disease. It may thus be said that the immune process is being used for the wrong purpose. Yet the very same processes that are responsible for the pathogenesis of these diseases are also essential for protective responses that are required for life.

In part II, immune diseases are presented according to the predominant immune effector mechanism. Although this approach emphasizes the pathologic effect of the various mechanisms, the immune response cannot

Table 7.2 The "double-edged sword" of immune reactions[a]

Immune effector type	Protective function ("immunity")	Destructive reaction ("allergy")
Neutralization	Diphtheria, tetanus, cholera, and endotoxin neutralization, blockade of virus receptors	Insulin resistance, pernicious anemia, myasthenia gravis, hyperthyroidism
Cytotoxic	Bacteriolysis, opsonization	Hemolysis, leukopenia, thrombocytopenia
Immune complex	Acute inflammation, polymorphonuclear leukocyte activation	Vasculitis, glomerulonephritis, serum sickness, rheumatoid diseases
Anaphylactic	Focal inflammation, increased vascular permeability, expulsion of intestinal parasites	Asthma, urticaria, anaphylactic shock, hay fever
T-cell cytotoxicity	Destruction of virus-infected cells: vaccinia and measles virus-infected cells, tumor cells	Contact dermatitis, viral exanthems, smallpox, graft rejection
Delayed-type hypersensitivity	Activation of macrophages against tuberculosis, leprosy, and syphilis agents	Autoallergies, multiple sclerosis, postvaccinial encephalomyelitis
Granulomatous[b]	Isolation of organisms (leprosy and tuberculosis agents, helminths) in granulomas	Beryllosis, sarcoidosis, tuberculosis, filiariasis, fungi, schistosomiasis

[a]Modified from S. Sell, *Hum. Pathol.* **9**:24–24, 1978.

[b]Granulomatous reactions, like other inflammatory lesions, may result from nonimmune stimuli as well as from an immune reaction inactivated by antibody or by sensitized cells.

be simply compartmentalized in this manner. For most diseases, more than one immune mechanism is activated, perhaps at different times, and components of one mechanism may overlap with parts of another mechanism. After presentation of the destructive effects of immune mechanisms, the protective effects are described, and specific infectious diseases are used as examples.

Bibliography

Criep, L. H. 1962. *Clinical Immunology and Allergy.* Grune and Stratton, New York, N.Y.

Gell, P. G. H., and R. R. A. Coombs. 1963. *Clinical Aspects of Immunology,* 1st ed. Blackwell Scientific Publications, Oxford, England.

Raffel, S. 1953. *Immunity, Hypersensitivity, and Serology.* Appleton-Century Crofts, New York, N.Y.

Roitt, I. M. 1971. *Essential Immunology,* 1st ed. Blackwell Scientific Publications, Oxford, England.

Sell, S. 1972. *Immunology, Immunopathology and Immunity.* Harper and Row, Hagerstown, Md.

Inactivation and Activation of Biologically Active Molecules

8

Antibody to a hormone, hormone receptor, blood clotting factor, growth factor or enzyme, or drug may inactivate, activate, protect, or have no effect on the biologic function of these molecules. The nature of the disease caused by activation or inactivation depends upon the biologic function of the biologically active molecule or cell involved.

Antibodies to biologically active molecules are produced under four circumstances:

1. Breaking of tolerance with autoantibody production
2. Immune response to a therapeutically administered hormone (insulin), enzyme, blood clotting factor, or drug that is recognized as a foreign antigen
3. Release into the body of a biologically active molecule produced by an infectious agent
4. Specific immunization with a modified toxin (toxoid) of an infectious agent

Mechanisms of Antibody-Mediated Inactivation and Activation

Inactivation

Antibody may neutralize or inactivate biologically active molecules by four major mechanisms (Fig. 8.1):

1. By direct reaction with the biologically active molecule, resulting in structural alteration of the molecule so that it is no longer active
2. By causing increased catabolism of the antibody-antigen complex, effectively lowering the concentration of the biologically active molecules
3. By reaction of antibody to cell surface receptors, causing blocking (stearic hindrance); modulation (endocytosis) or destruction of the receptor so that the cell is no longer able to respond to activating stimuli
4. By attracting inflammatory cells that destroy the surface receptors (antibody-dependent cell-mediated cytotoxicity [ADCC]). The loss of receptor function and destruction of target cells in some tissues such as insulinitis, thyroiditis, atrophic gastritis, and myasthenia gravis are often associated with a lymphocytic infiltrate. This may be due to T-cell-mediated immunity (see chapters 13 and 14), or autoantireceptors may direct ADCC.

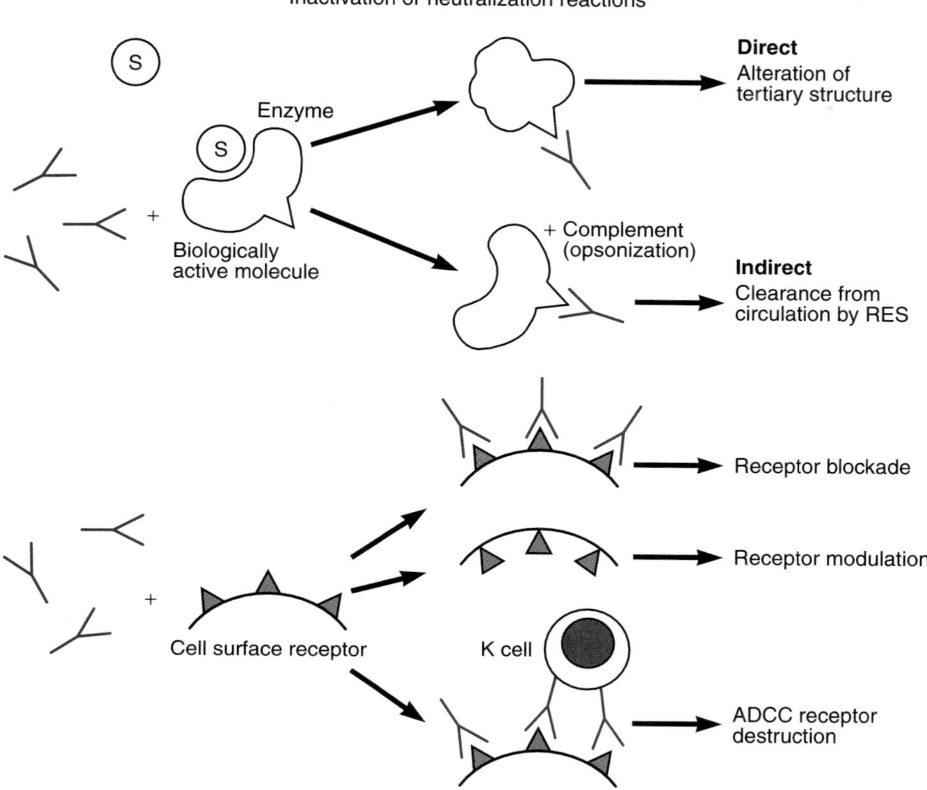

Figure 8.1 Inactivation or activation of biologically active molecules. Reaction of antibody with enzyme or other biologically active molecules may result in loss of biologic function due to stearic hindrance of binding of the activating ligand with its receptor. However, the antigenic sites (epitopes) of an enzyme are usually located on a different part of the molecule from the substrate binding site. Inactivation may occur by alteration of the tertiary structure of the enzyme following reaction with antibody. This reaction affects the structure of the substrate binding site indirectly or inactivates the enzyme molecule. In vivo, either increased or decreased catabolism of an enzyme-antibody complex may occur. The biologic effect of neutralization depends upon the molecule neutralized. Antibodies to cell surface receptors may block or stimulate the receptor or may cause receptor modulation by endocytosis or destruction of the cell by antibody-dependent cell-mediated cytotoxicity (ADCC).

5. By activating phosphorylation of biologically active molecules, such as cell surface adhesion molecules, leading to a loss of this function. The effect of this mechanism is presented in chapter 20 as the cause of blistering skin diseases.

Direct Inactivation

Antibodies may block the active site of a biologically active molecule or alter the conformation of the molecule so that it is no longer active. Biologically active molecules generally have one site that is necessary for biologic activity; a large portion of the molecule may not be directly involved. For example, an enzyme has an active site localized in a small area of the whole molecule. An antibody reacting with or near this active site may block the reaction of the enzyme with its substrate. However, most antibodies that inactivate enzymes react with an epitope (antigenic site) quite distant from the biologically active site. Inactivation occurs by alteration of the tertiary structure of the enzyme because of its reaction with antibody. Not all such reactions result in loss of substrate binding or inactivation. In fact, classic precipitin reactions with enzymes may occur with no apparent loss of activity in the precipitated enzyme. In addition, in some instances, reaction with antibody may convert an inactive form of an enzyme to an active form (see below).

Not only is the site of antibody reaction important in neutralization of a biologically active molecule, but the effect of the antibody also depends upon other characteristics of the antibody-antigen reaction, such as the ratio of antibody to antigen, the strength of antibody-antigen binding, and the biologic properties of the antibody (e.g., complement fixation, catalytic activity). Inactivation may be induced by the antibodies formed in one individual, whereas the antibodies formed in another individual may react with the same enzyme but not inactivate it.

Indirect Inactivation

In vivo, antigen-antibody complexes formed in antibody excess or at equivalence are rapidly cleared by the reticuloendothelial system due to formation of aggregated Fcs of immunoglobulin G (IgG) or fixation of complement (macrophages have receptors for aggregated Fc or C3b). An antibody that does not directly neutralize might effectively reduce the availability of an enzyme or hormone through this mechanism. However, not all antigen-antibody complexes are rapidly removed; some soluble complexes in antigen excess may continue to circulate. In some situations, binding of antibody to a hormone may actually produce a longer half-life, because bound molecules may be degraded more slowly than unbound molecules. This may lead to increased serum concentrations for the material involved but, paradoxically, a loss of biological function. On the other hand, such complexes may protect a hormone from catabolism, with later release of the active molecule (see below). The presence of such complexes may also lead to inflammatory lesions from the deposition of antibody-antigen complexes in vessels or renal glomeruli (see chapter 11).

Receptor Modulation

Antibodies may block or induce changes in cell surface receptors. Cells respond to an activating ligand through reaction with cell surface receptors for the ligand. Insulin, estrogen, and other hormones act through cell surface receptors. The ability of cells to respond to activating stimuli may be lost because of reaction of antibody with the receptor. Antibodies to cell surface receptors may occupy the receptor (stearic hindrance) or may induce endocytosis, stripping, or structural alteration of the receptor (receptor loss).

ADCC

In addition, antibodies reacting with cell surface receptors may induce the infiltration of inflammatory cells that secondarily destroy the receptors (ADCC). This is due to a reaction of K cells through Fc receptors on antibodies bound to target cells. When IgG antibodies react with a target cell, the aggregated antibodies form altered Fcs that bind to inflammatory cells.

Activation

Reaction of antibodies to a hormone, drug, or cell surface receptor may activate or enhance the biologic function of the molecule. Through the use of monoclonal antibodies that recognize distinct epitopes on hormones, it has become clear that, on the one hand, an antibody to one site may inhibit activity, whereas antibody to another site may enhance activity, depending on the effect on the hormone itself or upon the effect on the binding of the hormone to its receptors.

Conformational Stabilization

Antibodies may act with a hormone directly but away from the active binding site to stabilize the active configuration of the molecule. The enzyme β-galactosidase exists in inactive and active conformers. Some antibodies to this enzyme are able to convert the inactive conformer to the active configuration. Presumably, reaction of the antibody with the inactive form of the enzyme results in an alteration of tertiary structure so that the active site becomes available.

Increased Binding Affinity

Antibodies, through cross-linking the molecule, may increase the affinity of binding and the activity of a hormone. The activity of epidermal growth factor (EGF) on the growth of fibroblasts in vitro may be increased with Fab_2 (bivalent), but not Fab (univalent) antibody, fragments to EGF. This is believed to be caused by conversion of low- to high-affinity binding between EGF and its receptor.

Receptor Selection

Antibodies may be able to redirect hormone binding from one receptor to another. A hormone may have more than one receptor on different cells or bind to receptors in different ways. Antibodies to one epitope on the hormone may block the ability of the hormone to react with that receptor and increase the binding to another receptor. Human growth hormone has at least four distinct epitopes defined by monoclonal antibodies. A given antibody may enhance binding to one site while inhibiting binding to another site; in this way, it blocks one activity while increasing another activity or redirecting the binding to a different tissue. One monoclonal antibody to growth hormone blocks activity in vitro by inhibiting binding to the target cells yet enhances activity when injected into laboratory animals.

Buffering

Antibodies may "protect" a hormone from degradation in vivo and prolong its activity by allowing "slow release" of the bound hormone. Most hormones are degraded rapidly by enzymes. Some antibodies are able to prevent the degradation of the hormone and prolong the survival of the hormone. So-called "superactive" forms of insulin appear to be protected by binding to serum albumin, and this "carrier" function may also be provided by antibody. Anecdotal cases of patients with diabetes who show a marked decreased requirement for insulin, as well as other patients who demonstrate enhanced effects of prolactin and thyroid-stimulating hormone, may be explained by this mechanism.

Receptor Activation
Antibodies may directly bind to the receptor for a hormone and activate the cells (e.g., antithyroid receptor), because the antibody binding site mimics the structure of the activating ligand for the receptor (see below).

Examples of Antibody-Mediated Inactivation and Activation

Some specific antibodies to biologically active molecules are listed in Table 8.1.

Hormones

Diabetes Mellitus
Diabetes mellitus (*diabetes* from the Greek *dia* [through] and *bainein* [to go]; to go through; a siphon) is a general term for a heterogeneous group of diseases that have as a common denominator abnormalities in carbohydrate metabolism (Table 8.2) associated with a deficiency in the production or utilization of insulin. Insulin is an endocrine hormone produced by beta cells in the islets of Langerhans in the pancreas. Insulin specifically reacts with many other cells of the body through cell surface receptors and stimulates transport and utilization of glucose for conversion to energy or for storage as glycogen in the liver or glycosides in fat cells. Diabetes results from impaired production or decreased utilization of insulin with a resultant increase in blood glucose and related abnormalities of metabolism. Decreased insulin utilization results from impaired insulin secretion, loss of receptors or receptor response, or presence of blocking antibodies to insulin or to the insulin receptor (Fig. 8.2). About 20% of patients have "insulin-dependent" or type I diabetes (i.e., the insulin receptors or responsive cells are normal, but insulin availability is low); the remaining 80% have "insulin-independent" or type II diabetes (insulin availability is normal, but the number of receptors is low).

Table 8.1 Diseases of immune inactivation/activation

Disease	Antigen(s)
Diabetes mellitus	Insulin
	Insulin receptor
	Islet cell cytoplasm (glutamic acid decarboxylase)
	Islet cell surface
Thyroid disease	
Hyperthyroidism	Thyroid-stimulating hormone
Hypothyroidism	Triiodothyronine
Pernicious anemia	
Atrophic gastritis	Parietal cells
Megaloblastic anemia	Intrinsic factor
Infertility (induced)	Chorionic gonadotropin
	Estrogen, progesterone, prolactin
Aplastic anemia	Erythropoietin
Chronic asthma	β-Adrenergic receptor
Myasthenia gravis	Acetylcholine receptor
Polyendocrinopathy	Multiple (adrenal, thyroid, parathyroid, gonad, pancreas, melanocytes)
Hemophilia, other blood diseases	Blood clotting factors (multiple)

Table 8.2 Immunologic factors in diabetes mellitus

Type	Etiologic factor
Immune	
Type Ia juvenile onset	T-cell or ADCC-mediated destruction of beta cells; early, but not late, anti-islet cell antibody; HLA-DR3, DR4 associated
Type Ib juvenile onset	T-cell- or ADCC-mediated destruction of beta cells; both early and late islet cell antibody; associated with endocrinopathies
Insulin resistant	Anti-insulin antibodies in response to injection therapy
Insulin receptor (type II)	Autoimmune insulin receptor antibodies
Nonimmune	
Type II maturity onset	May develop insulin resistance
Secondary	Pancreatic disease (type III), hormonal (corticosteroid excess, etc.), drug-induced

Both type I and type II diabetes may have immunological origins. Of a dozen or so putative beta-cell antigens, at least five different antibodies are associated with diabetes mellitus: type I with antibodies to insulin, to islet cell cytoplasm (glutamic acid decarboxylase), to tyrosine phosphatase-like molecules, and to phogrin, and type II with antibodies to insulin receptors. In type I diabetes, there is a loss of beta cells in the pancreas as a result of immune attack early in life, or there may be neutralizing antibodies to insulin. In type II diabetes, there may be loss of receptors secondary to antibody to receptors. However, only some patients with type II diabetes have anti-receptor antibodies; most have a nonimmune pathogenesis.

Antibodies to insulin. Antibodies to insulin are often found in patients who are administered exogenous insulin, but most such patients show no increase or decrease in insulin requirements. In 1938, Banting and his group observed an antibodylike neutralizer of insulin in a schizophrenic patient who had been receiving insulin shock treatment. Insulin resistance due to antibodies to foreign insulin was then found to occur in some diabetic patients receiving exogenous (e.g., bovine or ovine) insulin for therapy. As antibodies developed, increasing doses of insulin were required. In many cases, resistance to exogenous insulin that was derived from one species (ox) did not hold for insulin derived from another species (pig). Production of human insulin by gene cloning techniques provides a less immunogenic molecule but does not completely eliminate the possibility of antibody formation, since even human insulin may be considered foreign in a diabetic who does not make insulin. Anti-insulin antibodies were first reported in 1970 in some patients who had never received exogenous insulin and who did not have islet destruction, but islet cell hyperplasia. This condition is termed spontaneous hypoglycemia.

Not all anti-insulins are neutralizing, and not all insulins are neutralizable by the same antibody, indicating that even though the insulin molecule is relatively small, it has both overlapping and distinct epitopes. The binding of insulin by anti-insulin in vivo usually causes slowing of the disappearance of insulin from the bloodstream, that is, a longer half-life. Since insulin is a small antigen available in large amounts, insulin–

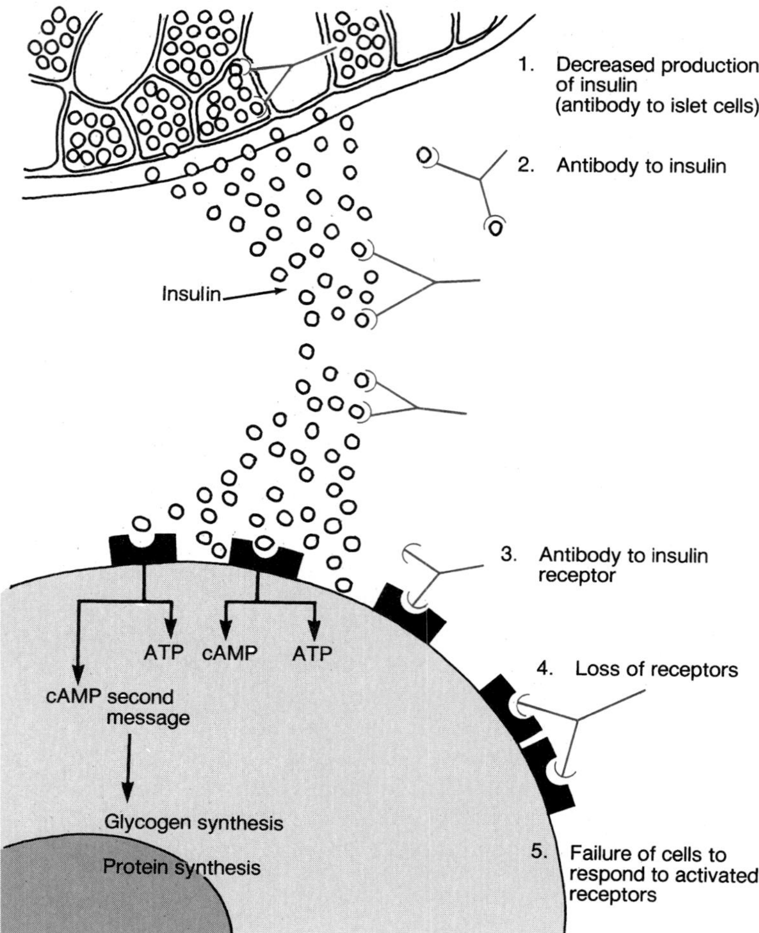

Figure 8.2 Level of abnormality in diabetes. Antibody to insulin may block insulin action, and antibodies to receptors may block or modulate receptors. However, antibody to receptors is not the only way that loss of receptors may occur. Inflammation of islet cells is associated with autoantibody to islet cells and precedes juvenile-onset insulin-dependent diabetes. The islet cell destruction is caused by immune attack by T cells.

anti-insulin complexes may not be cross-linked and are therefore not subject to clearance by the reticuloendothelial system. Reticuloendothelial system clearance is mediated by Fc or C3b receptors on macrophages, which require aggregates of IgG or complement fixation. Such complexes may not be formed with antibodies to insulin unless the epitopes involved permit cross-linking. Insulin bound to antibody is catabolized at the rate of the antibody (IgG) and not at the rate of insulin. Therefore, instead of reducing the half-life of insulin, antibody to insulin actually prolongs the half-life, because the bound insulin is protected from degradation by insulinase in the liver. Although the antibody-bound insulin is prevented from exerting its biologic activity, release of the bound insulin from the antibody may allow it to be utilized. This phenomenon may result in a decrease in the amount of insulin required for therapy because of so-called superactive forms of bound insulin. Since antibodies to insulin may either decrease or enhance insulin activity, a close correlation between antibody titers and insulin requirements is usually not seen. Acute skin reactions and systemic anaphylactic shock may also occur if insulin is injected into a sensitive individual (see below). In addition, immune complexes of various antibody-antigen proportions may be formed. These may deposit in vessel walls or in renal glomeruli and induce immune complex reactions (see chapter 11). The insulin–anti-insulin reaction has been adapted to provide a highly sensitive immunoassay for insulin.

Antibodies to islet cells. Autoantibodies to islet cell cytoplasm (beta cells) and/or islet cell surface antigens are associated with insulin-dependent (type I) juvenile onset diabetes mellitus, but the appearance of antibody in the serum *follows* the destruction of the beta cells in the islets (insulinitis). Antibodies to cow's milk albumin cross-react with beta cell surface proteins and are frequently found in patients with type I diabetes, suggesting that antibodies to beta cells may result from "molecular mimicry" between albumin and beta cell surface proteins. Eighty percent of patients with recent-onset autoimmune destruction of beta cells have antibodies to the cytoplasmic enzyme glutamic acid decarboxylase. In addition, antibodies to insulin receptors, insulin, proinsulin, glucagon, and several other peptide hormones may be found in patients with type I diabetes. The incidence of serum antibody drops markedly after onset of the disease, and after 1 year only about 20% of patients have detectable antibody.

The initial destruction of beta cells is mediated by T-cell attack, not by antibody-directed mechanisms. In laboratory animals, neonatal thymectomy can prevent diabetes in susceptible strains of mice, and the disease may be transferred with lymphocytes from animals with active disease. In humans, acute-onset juvenile diabetes begins with lymphocyte infiltration of islets (lymphocytic insulinitis), and the actual immune-mediated destruction of the beta cells is caused by cell-mediated immunity. It is not clear which T-cell subpopulation is responsible; both $CD4^+$ and $CD8^+$ cells may be found in lesions. In two cases of sudden-onset fatal type I diabetes, evidence was presented that beta cells of the islet contain a membrane-bound superantigen that stimulates a selective expansion of autoreactive clones of $CD4^+$ T cells with the β7 variable segment of the T-cell receptor. Thus, superantigen activation of these clones may produce $CD4^+$ cells that attack the islet cells. It is known that beta cells of the islet are exquisitely sensitive to the cytotoxic effects of interleukin-1, gamma interferon, and tumor necrosis factor alpha. The pathogenic significance of antibodies to islet cell surface antigens is not known. Presumably, they could play a role in the destruction of islets by an ADCC mechanism.

Treatment with immunosuppressive drugs (e.g., cyclosporine and azathioprine), anti-inflammatory agents (corticosteroids or indomethacin), monoclonal antibodies to T cells (CD3), and neutralization of gamma interferon have been shown to be effective in experimental models, and preliminary trials indicate that *immunomodulation* therapy of juvenile diabetes may be of value in preventing or limiting early destruction of the beta cells. For instance, in one study, the onset of juvenile diabetes was delayed in about one-third of patients by cyclosporine treatment if given within 6 weeks of onset. Juvenile diabetes shows a high relationship to certain histocompatibility types. It has been suggested that juvenile-onset diabetes is a genetically controlled autoimmune reaction, perhaps triggered by a viral infection.

Thyroid Hormone and Hypothyroidism

Most of the common diseases of the thyroid are immune in origin: hypothyroidism, hyperthyroidism, and thyroiditis. A number of autoantibodies to thyroid antigens are found in normal individuals (particularly with aging) and are associated with thyroid diseases (Table 8.3). Some of these autoantibodies have biologic effects, and some do not. Antibodies to thyroid hormone or thyroid-stimulating hormone (TSH) may be responsible for hypothyroidism, whereas antibodies to the thyroid receptor for TSH may produce hyperthyroidism (Graves' disease) or may block activation of the receptor (hypothyroidism). There is an associated swelling and inflammation of the orbit of the eye, Graves' ophthalmopathy. An amino acid sequence similarity between thyroglobulin and acetylcholinesterase opens the possibility that antithyroglobulin antibodies may react with epitopes common to thyroglobulin and the orbit of the eye (see below).

Antibody-dependent or cell-mediated immunity to thyroid antigens causes inflammation of the thyroid (thyroiditis) and may lead to destruction of the thyroid gland by cell-mediated immunity (see chapter 12). Autoimmune thyroiditis may be induced in animals by immunization with thyroid hormone. The major feature of this disease is infiltration of the thyroid gland with mononuclear cells. The disease is believed to be mediated by specific T_{CTL}- or T_{DTH}-cell-mediated inflammation but could be caused by ADCC. In humans with chronic lymphocytic thyroiditis, autoantibodies to thyroid hormones may be found and may be responsible for hypothyroidism by binding thyroxine or triiodothyronine. Hyperthyroidism caused by antibodies to TSH receptors (Graves' disease) is discussed below under "Receptors."

Human Chorionic Gonadotropin, Estrogen, Progesterone, and Infertility

Antibodies to the hormones required to maintain pregnancy may prevent normal pregnancy. Antibodies to human chorionic gonadotropin (hCG) have been reported in patients after hCG treatment of women with hypopituitarism as well as in apparently normal individuals. These antibodies may explain the poor results of hCG therapy in some infertile women. Antibodies to hCG are able to prevent or terminate early pregnancy. Studies of rhesus monkeys demonstrate that active immunization with hCG or

Table 8.3 Autoantibodies to thyroid antigens[a]

Antigen	Effect(s) of antibody
Thyroxine and triiodothyronine	Blocks thyroid hormone action—hypothyroidism
TSH	Blocks effect of TSH—hypothyroidism
TSH receptor	1. Stimulates receptor, hyperthyroidism (LATS)
	2. Inhibits TSH binding—hypothyroidism
Not defined (TSH related)	Stimulates growth of thyroid cells
Cell surface antigen	Cytotoxic with lymphocytes (ADCC)—lymphocytic thyroiditis
Microsomal antigen	Cytotoxic with lymphocytes—thyroiditis
Thyroglobulin	Not clear; associated with thyroiditis; cross-reacts with acetylcholinesterase, may cause Graves' ophthalmopathy
Colloid antigen	Not known; associated with thyroiditis

[a]Abbreviations: TSH, thyroid-stimulating hormone; LATS, long-acting thyroid stimulator; ADCC, antibody-dependent cell-mediated cytotoxicity.

passive transfer of antibodies to hCG can effectively reduce the number of conceptions or cause early abortions. Anti-hCG apparently blocks the luteotropic support of the corpus luteum and may affect the development of the placenta or fetus as well. Trials of hCG immunization for selected populations in which more effective birth control is considered essential have been successful, and trials using different "vaccines" incorporating the β chain of hCG, which does not share epitopes with other hormones, are now under way.

Progesterone is the major hormone required for the establishment and maintenance of pregnancy. Antibodies to progesterone are of interest as a means of interruption of pregnancy. Passive transfer of monoclonal antibodies to progesterone shortly after conception blocks pregnancy in laboratory animals. Women treated with oral contraceptive pills containing estrogenlike compounds may develop circulating antibody to ethyl estradiol, which may be detected either as free antibody or in the form of circulating immune complexes. These women have a higher incidence of thrombosis than women who do not develop antibodies. Antibodies to zona pellucida antigens can be seen in both fertile and infertile women; it is not known if there are different epitopes that could explain the apparent lack of correlation.

Prolactin

The ability to measure prolactin using immunoassays revealed a syndrome of menstrual disturbance, infertility, and galactorrhea in women and impotence and loss of libido in men associated with high levels of prolactin in the blood (hyperprolactinemia). Such patients have a form of prolactin that is larger (50 to 170 kDa) than pituitary-derived prolactin (23 kDa). The larger forms (termed "big, big") turn out to be antibody-antigen complexes. The complexing of prolactin with antibody produces soluble complexes, and the half-lives of these complexes are actually prolonged over that of the unbound prolactin. Although this may explain why the blood prolactin concentrations are higher, it is not clear why the activity is greater, as it is presumed that the antibody-bound prolactin would be inactive. However, it is possible that antibodies to prolactin may have a lower affinity for prolactin than the natural receptor. If true, the antibody-bound prolactin may serve to increase the availability of prolactin by prolonging its half-life in the blood, yet not competing well with the cellular receptor, thus making increased prolactin available for exchange with cellular receptors.

Erythropoietin

Erythropoietin is a biologically active material, produced by the kidney, that stimulates the production of erythrocytes in the bone marrow. Erythropoietic inhibitors have been identified in the plasma of patients with refractory anemia, and it is possible that these patients may have an antibody that inhibits the action of erythropoietin.

Receptors

Insulin Receptors

Antibodies to insulin receptors from different individuals recognize different antigenic determinants; some are associated with symptoms, some not. Autoantibodies to cell surface receptors for insulin may be found in patients with extreme insulin resistance. Most of these patients are female and also have a pigmented skin condition known as acanthosis nigricans. These antibodies inhibit the binding of insulin to cell surface receptors, thus interfering with the biological function of insulin. Anti-receptor antibodies are also found in patients treated with exogenous insulin, presumably because of formation of anti-idiotypes (anti-anti-insulin) that mimic part of the insulin ligand (see below). Antibodies to insulin receptors may increase basal glucose oxidation of reactive cells in vitro, thus producing insulinlike effects. Receptor cross-linking appears to be required for antibody-included insulin receptor activation, as Fab univalent fragments will not activate. Presumably, insulin activation of the receptor is different from antibody-mediated activation, since insulin is univalent and cannot cross-link receptors. However, insulin reaction with receptors does cause aggregation of receptors, presumably by perturbation of cytoskeletal elements.

TSH Receptors and Hyperthyroidism

Autoantibodies to TSH receptors that cause hyperthyroidism are termed long-acting thyroid stimulator (LATS). LATS has been shown to be an immunoglobulin antibody that can, on the one hand, inhibit the binding of TSH to human thyroid membranes and, on the other hand, stimulate thyroid cyclic AMP (cAMP) and thyroid hormone release. The levels of inhibitory and stimulating antibodies in a single patient may differ during the course of the disease. Animals that are immunized with thyroid hormones may produce not only blocking antibodies but also a thyroid-stimulating globulin. Thus, either hyperthyroidism (Graves' disease) or hypothyroidism may result from an autoimmune antibody response (Fig. 8.3). Thyroid stimulatory antibody may be measured by its ability to activate cAMP production in thymocytes in vitro; thyrotropin binding inhibitory antibody is assayed by its ability to displace radiolabeled TSH bound to the TSH receptor. There also appears to be more than one type of stimulatory antibody. A distinct population of stimulatory autoantibodies is able both to stimulate cAMP and to promote growth of thyroid cells in vitro, whereas others only stimulate cAMP. The first stimulatory antibody is associated with enlargement of the thyroid in Graves' disease and not with other thyroid diseases. Thus, some anti-TSH receptors may stimulate production of thyroid hormone and growth of thyroid cells, whereas others only stimulate hormone production. Monoclonal antibody studies indicate that the epitopes are part of the TSH receptor. Immunoglobulins from Graves' patients activate different signaling pathways, including adenyl cyclase, phospholipase C, and phospholipase A2, and different signals may correlate with different manifestations of the disease. There is a high association of hyperthyroidism with HLA-DR3 (about 60%), and those patients who are HLA-DR3 positive almost never go into remission, whereas non-HLA-DR3 patients with Graves' disease frequently have remission. A syndrome that features Graves' disease and autoantibodies to insulin (insulin autoimmune syndrome) is highly associated with HLA-DR4.

Massive swelling of the extraocular muscles and bulging of the eyes (Graves' exophthalmus or orbitopathy) are frequently associated with hyperthyroidism. The term orbitopathy is preferred, because the lesion involves the extraorbital fat and connective tissue and not the eye itself. This reaction may progress rapidly and produce blindness. The cause of the bulging eyes is not known. It has been hypothesized that there is cross-reactivity between the cell membrane of the eye muscles and some

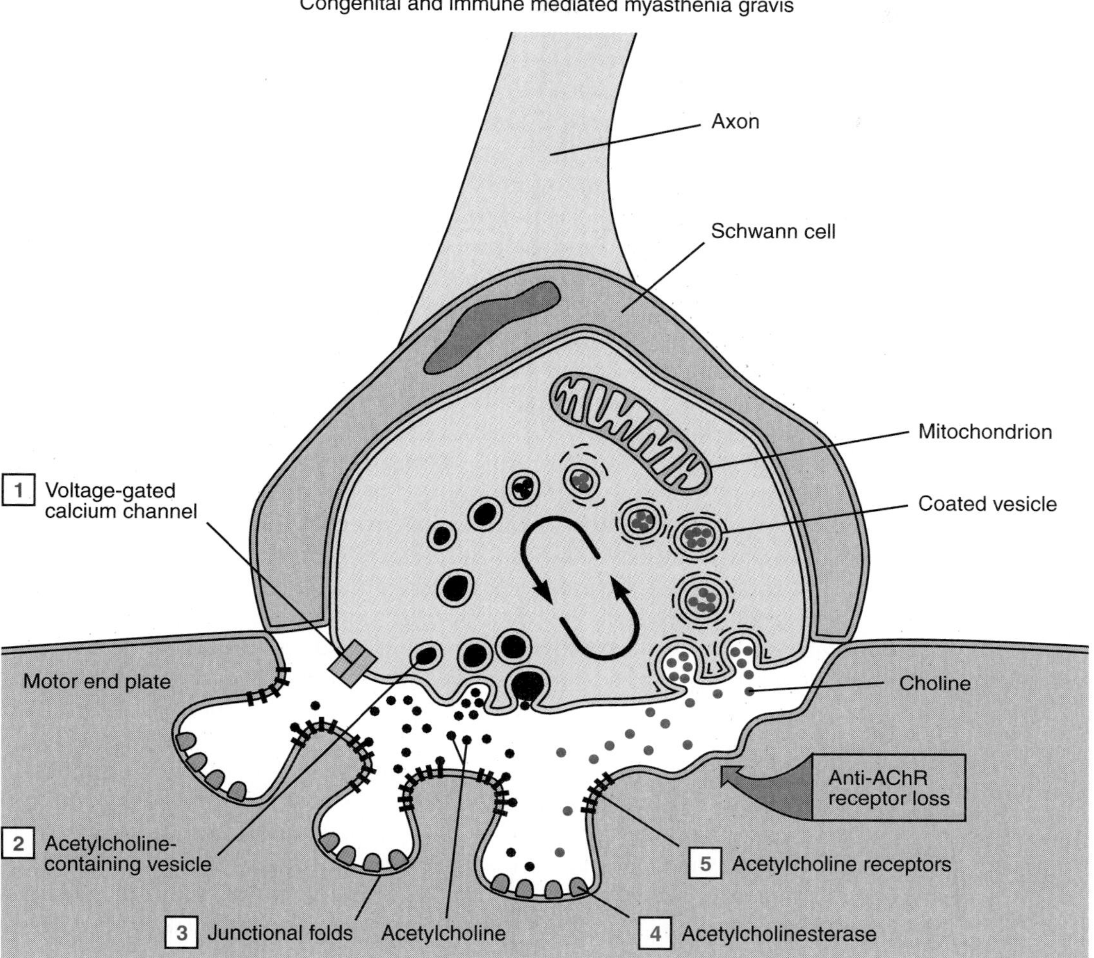

Figure 8.3 Neuromuscular transmission is mediated by acetylcholine (ACh) released from vesicles in the neuronal axon that bind to acetylcholine receptors (AChR) in the motor end plate. ACh is broken into choline and acetate by acetylcholinesterase, which inactivates ACh. Free choline reenters the neuron by endocytosis. ACh is produced in the vesicle from acetate and choline by choline acetyltransferase. ACh is released from vesicles that fuse with the cell membrane of the motor end plate. Congenital decrease in neuromuscular transmission may be impaired by **(1)** defects in voltage-gated calcium channels, **(2)** defects in ACh-containing vesicles, **(3)** defects in junctional folds, **(4)** decrease in AChR, and **(5)** acetylcholinesterase levels in the synaptic cleft. Immune-mediated myasthenia gravis is caused by action of antibodies to AChR to block or cause loss of receptors.

epitopes of the TSH receptor. IgA antibodies to eye muscles (but not to skeletal muscles) has been detected in patients with Graves' disease, but their role in the development of disease is not clear. Autoantibodies to extracellular matrix proteins and the flavoprotein subunit of succinate dehydrogenase have been implicated. Deposition of immune complexes is present on extraocular muscle membranes. These could produce cell damage and lymphocytic infiltration, perhaps by ADCC. The chronic accumulation of glycosaminoglycans in the connective tissue that is characteristic of Graves' ophthalmopathy may be caused by chronic stimulation of fibroblasts by cytokines produced by lymphocytes. Treatment with immunosuppressive drugs (cyclosporine and low-dose prednisone) may control the inflammation of Graves' ophthalmopathy, or resistant cases may be treated with orbital irradiation and steroids. Although there is no clear association with HLA typing, patients with HLA-DR4 respond better to prednisone therapy than do patients without HLA-DR4.

The Acetylcholine Receptor and Myasthenia Gravis

Myasthenia gravis (MG) is characterized by muscle weakness and easy fatigability; weakness is most prominent in the muscles of the face and throat but involves essentially all striated muscles. The disorder is the result of a functional abnormality in which the conduction of nerve impulses from the motor nerve to the muscle fiber is impaired (Fig. 8.3). Patients afflicted with this disease tire very easily; usually they awake with close to normal muscular function, but this deteriorates during the day. The clinical course is punctuated with remissions and exacerbations; total incapacitation and death from respiratory failure may occur.

MG represents more than a single disease syndrome. A partial listing of some of the recognized syndromes is given in Table 8.4. Classical MG is associated with autoantibodies to the acetylcholine receptor (AChR); some variant syndromes have defects in neuromuscular transmission at other levels. The AChR is a neurotransmitter composed of a complex transmembrane protein formed by five polypeptide chains arranged as subunits consisting of two α, one each β and δ, and one ϵ or γ chains (Fig. 8.4). An epitope located at amino acid 192 or 193 of the α chain contains a site that binds to the AChR. Most anti-AChR antibodies are directed to a major immunogenic region located between amino acids 66 and 76 of the α subunit. However, many human anti-AChRs bind to other epitopes or conformational dependent determinants and do not block binding of ACh to AChR. Impairment of neuromuscular transmission by these antibodies to AChR may be accomplished by modulation of the AChR (internalization and degradation), often associated with lymphocytic infiltration. This modulation may be blocked by Fab fragments, indicating that cross-linking is required for AChR modulation or that aggregated Fcs are required for ADCC.

In autoimmune MG, the decrease in neuromuscular transmission is associated with decreased AChRs in the postsynaptic muscle membrane. Purified radiolabeled bungarotoxin binds to AChR, and this binding may be used to estimate the number of receptors on the membrane. The number

Table 8.4 Some myasthenia syndromes

Type	Characteristic(s)	Pathogenesis
Neonatal	Transient	Placental transfer of maternal anti-AChR
Adult I	Females under 40	Auto-anti-AChR (HLA-B8, DR3 associated)
Adult II	Males over 40	Auto-anti-AChR (HLA-A2 associated)
Ocular	Eyes only	Multiple
Congenital	Permanent	Multiple
Drug-induced	Transient, drug-induced (penicillamine)	Anti-AChR (HLA-DRI associated)
Eaton-Lambert	Adults, cancer related	Autoantibody to presynaptic membrane
Engel's disease	Mild, nonprogressive	Impaired acetylcholine packaging in neural end plate

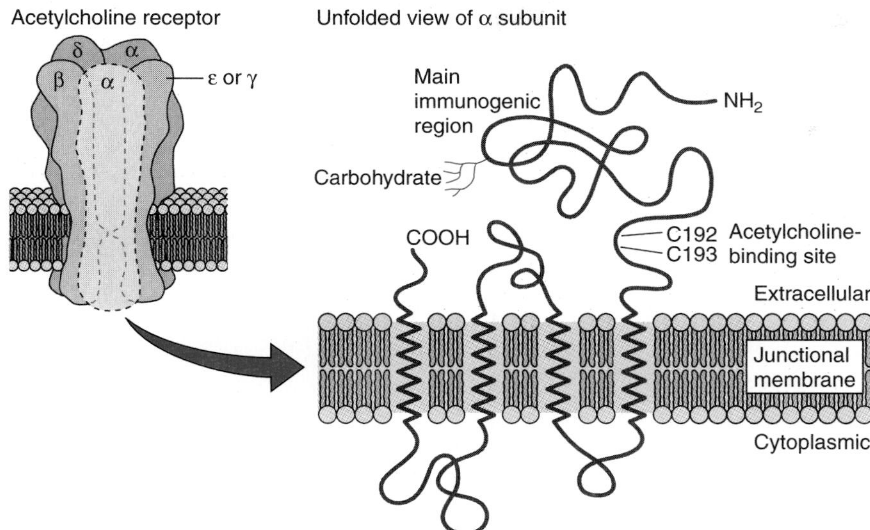

Figure 8.4 The AChR. The subunits of the receptor are arranged around a central ion pore. Each subunit has an intramembranous portion. The scheme shows the unfolded view of the α subunit. The extracellular amino-terminal end of the α subunit contains the acetylcholine binding site (C192 and C193). In autoimmune myasthenia, antibodies may bind to any of the subunits, but most bind to the major immunogenic domain of the α subunit. (From A. I. Levinson and L. M. Wheatley, p. 1354, *in* R. R. Rich [ed.], *Clinical Immunology, Principles and Practice,* The C. V. Mosby Co., St. Louis, Mo., 1996.)

of bungarotoxin binding sites is markedly decreased in muscle from MG patients, indicating a loss of AChR. The development of an experimental model of MG has provided a way to work out the autoimmune pathogenesis of MG. A syndrome with features almost identical to those of human MG has been produced by immunizing laboratory animals with AChR from the electric eel (Fig. 8.5). AChR-immunized animals develop precipitating antibody to AChR, antibody to syngeneic muscle, and a flaccid paralysis that can be reversed by neostigmine, an agent that can also temporarily reverse the muscular weakness of patients with MG. Experimental allergic MG has also been produced by immunization with syngeneic muscle AChR in complete Freund's adjuvant.

Antibody to AChR could alter neuromuscular transmission in at least three ways. It may block or inhibit AChR activity, cause modulation of AChR from muscle membranes, or fix complement and cause destruction of the postsynaptic membranes either directly or by ADCC. A simple blocking or inhibition effect seems unlikely for the human disease, because most human anti-AChRs do not affect binding of bungarotoxin by AChR and do not alter the end-plate potential of neuromuscular junctions in vitro. As mentioned above, some epitopes of the major immunogenic region of the α chain of AChR are not involved in binding ACh. A decrease in AChR activities by modulation or immune destruction appears to be more likely. The addition of immunoglobulin from myasthenic patients to mouse neuromuscular junctions leads to an accelerated degradation of the AChR receptors. Passive transfer of antibody to animals produces an acute MG syndrome associated with lymphocytic invasion of the motor end plate, suggesting ADCC.

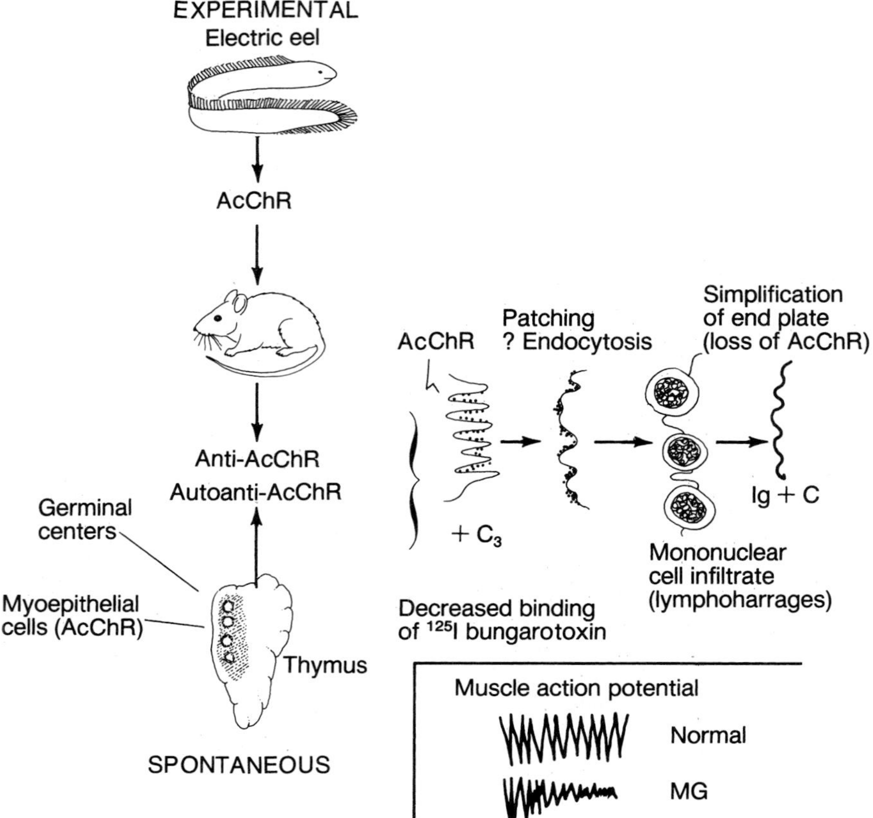

Figure 8.5 Comparison of experimental allergic and naturally occurring myasthenia gravis. Antibody to AChRs may be induced in laboratory animals by immunization with AChR from the electric eel or autologous AChR. Autoantibodies to AChR occur spontaneously in humans with myasthenia gravis. Both laboratory animals and affected humans demonstrate progressive muscle weakness, a decrease in AChR, immunoglobulin, and complement deposition, and a mononuclear infiltrate at the neuromuscular junction. On restimulation, the muscle action potential reveals a rapid decline. The thymus of affected humans may contain germinal centers not normally found in the thymus. Since the thymus contains myoepithelial cells with AChR, it is possible that autoantibody production of AChR occurs in the thymus. AcChr, acetylcholine receptor.

Anti-idiotypic antibodies have been shown to be able to cause experimental MG. Anti-idiotypic antibodies to the AChR agonist trans-3,3′-bis[α-(trimethylammonia) methyl] azo benzene bromide (Bis Q) are able to cause MG:

N=N
O
‖
$O(CH_2)_2OC(CH_2)_2COOH$
CH_2 CH_2
$N^+(CH_3)_3I^-$ $N^+(CH_3)_3I^-$

Bis Q, a potent AChR agonist that binds to AChR, was conjugated to bovine serum albumin (Bis Q acts as a hapten and the albumin as a carrier) and used to immunize rabbits. The antibodies produced to Bis Q recognize the same epitope on Bis Q as does the natural receptor for Bis Q; i.e., the paratope of anti-Bis Q mimics the binding characteristic of AChR. Immunization of rabbits with anti-Bis Q resulted in anti-anti-Bis Q, which blocked binding of ACh to AChR and reproduced experimental MG (Fig. 8.6).

Antibodies to AChR have been demonstrated in over 90% of MG patients if highly sensitive assays are employed, although lower percentages are found when other methods are used. Newborn infants of mothers with MG may be born with a temporary muscular weakness because of placental transfer of antibody from mother to fetus. Patients with other autoimmune diseases such as systemic lupus erythematosus, Graves' disease, and thymoma may also have antibody to AChR, and some of these patients develop clinical MG, suggesting that they had a latent or subclinical form of MG. Therefore, most of the evidence supports the concept that human MG and experimental allergic MG are very similar and that the major pathogenesis of the disease is an antibody-mediated modulation of AChR.

In addition to anti-AChR, many myasthenics have a variety of other immune abnormalities. They frequently have evidence of other "autoimmune" diseases. The serum of most myasthenics contains an antibody that binds to muscle fibers and epithelial reticular cells of the thymus. The level of this antibody does not always correlate to the severity of the disease. These muscle-binding antibodies could be a secondary effect of the disease or only an associated finding. Myasthenia is often associated with a peculiar thymic hyperplasia in which germinal centers are formed in the medulla of the thymus or with tumors of the thymus; thymectomy may lead to clinical improvement in these patients but may accelerate the

Figure 8.6 Production of myasthenia gravis by anti-idiotypic antibodies to anti-agonist antibody. AcChR, acetylcholine receptor.

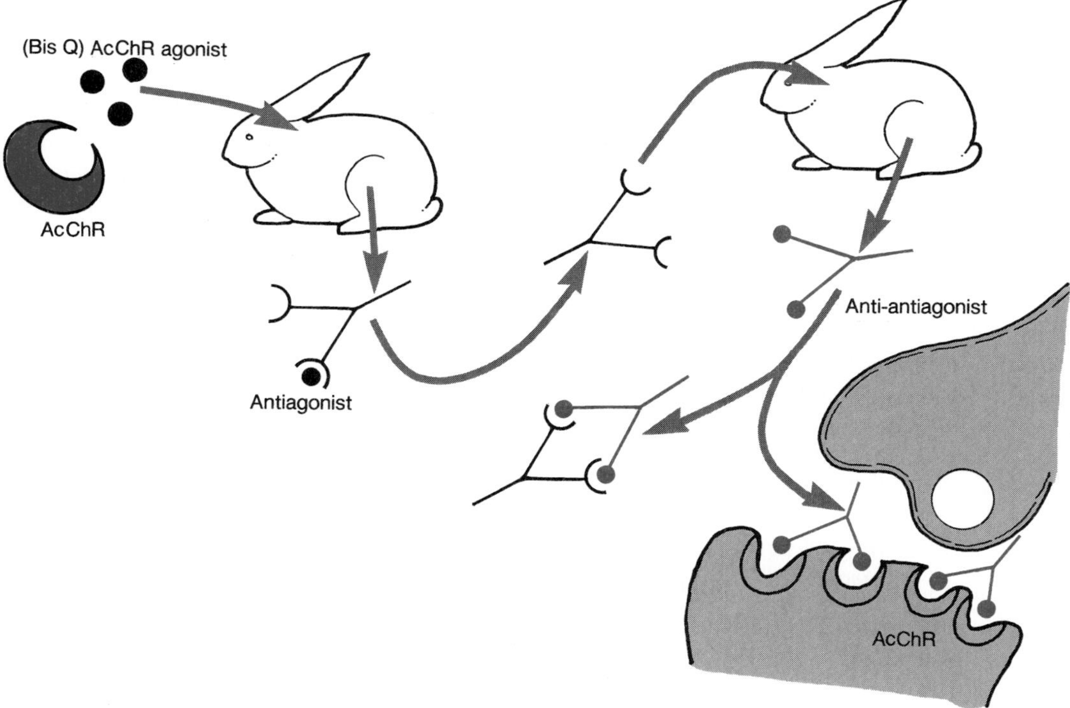

disease in others. Treatment of severely myasthenic patients by plasmapheresis (to remove anti-AChR) and immunosuppressive drugs (to suppress anti-AChR production) have produced improved muscle reactivity in some patients. This improvement is associated with a fall in anti-AChR titers in serum. Recent trials with cyclosporine indicate a more prolonged beneficial effect than other immunosuppressive drugs. In addition, specific immunoabsorption using tryptophan-linked polyvinyl alcohol gel has resulted in 50% remissions in a clinical trial.

The primary pathogenic role of antibodies to AChR does not explain all myasthenia syndromes (Table 8.4). Rare congenital disorders of neuromuscular transmission have now been recognized that mimic autoimmune MG. Five levels of defects in neuromuscular transmission are recognized: decreased function of the voltage-gated calcium channel required to initiate vesicle release (Lambert-Eaton syndrome), impaired acetylcholine packaging caused by a reduction of vesicles in the neural end plate (Engel's disease), acetylcholinesterase deficiency, congenital paucity of synaptic clefts, defects of AChR function. Extensive clinical and laboratory work-up is required to differentiate these syndromes from the autoimmune types. This is important, since therapy appropriate for immune myasthenia may be harmful to patients with congenital myasthenia.

Antibodies to a neuromuscular junction antigen may also be pathogenic for *amyotrophic lateral sclerosis.* This disease causes severe debilitating neuromuscular disease with progressive compromise of arms, legs, speech, swallowing, and eventually breathing, usually causing death within 3 to 5 years. Most patients have degeneration of corticospinal upper motor neurons. In an animal model of experimental autoimmune motor neuron disease, there is loss of motor neurons, the disease may be transferred with serum, and immunoglobulin can be demonstrated within and on the cell membranes of lower motor neurons. It has been suspected that there may be an antibody to gangliosides or motor neuron membrane proteins, but a consistent relationship has not been documented.

The *Lambert-Eaton myasthenic syndrome* occurs as a *paraneoplastic syndrome* in patients with small cell carcinoma of the lung and other cancers. Electrophysiological findings indicate that the disorder is due to reduced ACh release from the motor nerve. IgG from patients with this syndrome can passively transfer the conduction disorder to laboratory animals. Autoantibodies are directed to the presynaptic membrane and deplete the presynaptic membrane of active zones.

The *stiff-man syndrome* is a rare disease characterized by fluctuating and progressive muscle rigidity and spasms associated with autoimmune thyroiditis. Autoantibodies to the enzyme glutamic acid decarboxylase have been found that may react with cells in the gray matter of the brain. This enzyme controls the synthesis of the major inhibitory neurotransmitter γ-aminobutyric acid (GABA). It is hypothesized that these autoantibodies may cause the disorder by impairing the inhibitory function of GABA-ergic neurons.

Rasmussen's encephalitis is a unilateral cerebral dysfunction of children that presents as hemiparesis and seizures. Neuronal destruction is associated with active perivascular inflammation. A similar disease has been reproduced in animals immunized with a portion of the neuronal membrane receptor for the excitatory neurotransmitter glutamate, and increased excitability of neuronal cultures may be induced by sera from these animals or from affected patients. This disease may represent the "other side of the coin" from stiff-man syndrome. In stiff-man syndrome, there is neutralization of inhibitory functions by autoantibodies, whereas in Rasmussen's encephalitis, there is activation of stimulatory function and destruction of neurons, both resulting in muscular dysfunction.

The β-Adrenergic Receptor and Asthma

The β-adrenergic catecholamine hormone receptor-adenylate cyclase complex functions to regulate the level of cAMP in essentially all cells, but in particular those involved in anaphylactic reactions, i.e., mast cells and smooth muscle end organs (see chapter 10). The "beta-blockade" theory of asthma proposes that chronic asthma is related to a decrease in β-adrenergic sensitivity in bronchial smooth muscle, mucous glands, mucosal blood vessels, and mast cells. Autoantibodies to β_2 (lung) adrenergic receptors have been found in some patients with hay fever and/or asthma. Receptor blockade by β-receptor antibodies raises the level of excitability of the end organ cells, setting the stage for chronic asthma.

In addition, autoantibodies to β_1-receptors, muscarin-2 receptors, and angiotensin-II receptor subtype 1 and alpha-1 receptors have been found in patients with dilated cardiomyopathy. These antibodies decrease the number of binding sites for β-adrenergic agonists and selectively down-regulate the number of active binding sites on the membranes of myocardial cells, which is a characteristic of failing ventricular myocardium. Similar findings have been reported in mice with experimental Chagas' disease.

Dopamine Receptors, Schizophrenia, and Parkinson's Disease

It has been hypothesized that schizophrenia might be caused, at least in part, by autoantibodies to dopamine receptors. Dopamine receptors (D_2) are elevated in brains of schizophrenics. Antipsychotic drugs effective in the treatment of schizophrenia block dopamine receptors. Thus, it has been postulated that schizophrenia may be caused by overactivity of dopaminergic pathways. Dopamine receptor-stimulating autoantibodies have been suggested as a possible cause for overactivity. Antiserum to brain tissue evokes epileptic activity when applied topically to the cerebral cortex of animals, but a convincing role for autoantibodies in schizophrenia has not yet been demonstrated.

Associated with the pandemic of influenza between 1919 and 1926 was a variety of Parkinsonism disorders known collectively as von Economo's encephalitis. It has been postulated that certain strains of influenza virus may have had an affinity for dopamine receptors, resulting in selective destruction of extrapyramidal neurons. However, in early Parkinson's disease, the dopamine receptor density is increased, and patients respond well to dopamine mimetic medications.

Polyendocrinopathy

The autoimmune polyglandular syndromes feature circulating antibodies against multiple endocrine organs. The polyendocrinopathies, which feature two or more endocrine insufficiencies, have been divided into three types. Type I (Blizzard's syndrome) is very rare and presents almost always in childhood as Addison's disease, mucocutaneous moniliasis, and hypoparathyroidism, as well as one or more other additional endocrine abnormalities, skin lesions, and chronic active hepatitis. Type II (Schmidt's and Carpenter's syndrome) is seen in adults and features thyroiditis, Addison's disease, and insulin-dependent diabetes, often associated with pernicious anemia. Type III is the least well characterized form but the most common. It combines autoimmune thyroid disease (see chapter 12) with diabetes mellitus, with autoimmunity against gastric components (pernicious anemia), or with MG. The association of these diseases with circulating autoantibodies has stimulated the hypothesis that there is a loss of immune tolerance to endocrine hormones or receptors, perhaps through a depression of controlling suppressor T cells, resulting in autoimmune reactions to more than one endocrine system. Autoantibodies to adrenocortical cells, parathyroid cells, thyroid microsomes, pancreatic islet cells, and gastric parietal cells are often found. Shared epitopes on different endocrine organs have been demonstrated using monoclonal antibodies. It is also possible that a viral infection might stimulate such a polyspecific autoimmune reaction.

Other Biologically Active Molecules

Intrinsic Factor and Pernicious Anemia

Pernicious anemia is a disease in which there is a decrease in the intestinal absorption of vitamin B_{12} (cobalamin) associated with progressive destruction of the gastric fundic glands (atrophic gastritis) and achlorhydria. Humans acquire cobalamin solely from the diet in the form of methyl cobalamin nonspecifically bound to proteins. After ingestion and release of cobalamin by acid proteolysis in the stomach, cobalamin binds to R-protein (haptocorrin) at high-affinity sites and to intrinsic factor at lower-affinity sites. Both proteins are produced by parietal cells in the fundus of the stomach. In the duodenum, pancreatic proteases degrade the cobalamin-R complexes, but the cobalamin-IF complexes pass through to the ileum, where they bind to membrane-associated receptors on the microvilli of mucosal cells and are absorbed. Cobalamin is required for the normal maturation of all bone marrow precursors, so failure of vitamin B_{12} absorption leads to a deficit in production of mature erythrocytes and to neurologic disease. The characteristic anemia features large immature red cells (megaloblastic anemia). It is important to treat the disease by vitamin B_{12} replacement before the neurologic changes become irreversible. The diagnosis is made by demonstrating megaloblastic anemia, vitamin B_{12} deficiency, and antibodies to intrinsic factor; achlorhydria and increased serum gastrin are also found. Absorption of vitamin B_{12} requires the action of a substance known as intrinsic factor, which is secreted by some of the lining cells of the stomach (parietal cells). Pernicious anemia is associated with two distinct antibodies. One reacts specifically with the parietal cells of the gastric mucosa. The presence of this antibody is almost invariably associated with a reduction in acid secretion, atrophic gastritis, and lymphocytic infiltration. This antibody does not appear to cause gastritis. The gastritis features failure of gastrointestinal lining cells to differentiate and increased apoptosis, contributing to a depletion of end-stage cells.

The antibody to intrinsic factor was first observed because of an acquired resistance to intrinsic factor in patients being treated for pernicious anemia. Anti-intrinsic factor antibody can be demonstrated to inhibit the binding of vitamin B_{12} to intrinsic factor and is associated with abnormalities of vitamin B_{12} absorption. Two types of anti-intrinsic factor antibody have been observed: (i) blocking antibody, which prevents subsequent formation of vitamin B_{12}-intrinsic factor complexes and is associated with the presence of megaloblastic cells, and (ii) binding antibody, which can be shown to bind to intrinsic factor but does not prevent bound intrinsic factor from subsequent combination with vitamin B_{12}. Patients with pernicious anemia have an increased incidence of gastric polyps and carcinoma and should be tested for these possibilities. Pernicious anemia may also arise from nonimmune factors such as deficiency of vitamin B_{12} in the diet, gastrectomy, terminal ileal disease, or chronic infection with *Helicobacter pylori*.

Blood Clotting Factors and Hemophilia

The clotting system requires the interaction of up to 30 different factors. Antibodies that may inactivate these factors have been reported. Hemophilia A is an X-linked genetic disorder in which there is a severe deficiency of blood clotting factor VIII; hemophilia B is due to a congenital deficiency in factor IX. Antibodies to factor VIII frequently appear in hemophiliacs who genetically lack this globulin and are treated with infusions. The hemophiliac recognizes factors VIII or IX as foreign. Similarly, individuals who lack other clotting components may develop antibody to the missing component when transfused. The use of highly purified recombinant proteins has not reduced the incidence (4 to 25%) as compared with the use of plasma-derived components. Some attempts have been made to induce tolerance by high doses of factor VIII in hemophilia A. For reasons that are poorly understood, individuals with diseases such as lupus erythematosus, Sjögren's syndrome, tuberculosis, hepatitis C, or hyperglobulinemia, as well as patients treated with alpha interferon may also produce antibodies to clotting factors that complicate an already confusing clinical picture. Circulating antibodies to clotting factors have also been found in association with penicillin allergy. Finally, some individuals apparently produce circulating anticoagulants not associated with any known disease. The exact mechanism of action of antibodies to clotting factors is poorly understood. The clinical effect depends upon the particular factor or factors affected. Paradoxically, some antibodies to phospholipids may promote coagulation, perhaps by activation of platelets. In severe cases, treatment with immunosuppressive drugs such as prednisone or cyclophosphamide or extracorporeal immunoabsorption may reduce inhibitors of blood clotting factors, but care must be exercised because of possible toxicity.

Drugs

Antibodies to drugs may produce a number of different diseases, such as hemolytic anemias (chapter 9) and immune complex disease (chapter 11). Antibodies to drugs may also be used to treat drug overdoses. For instance, digoxin-specific $F(ab')_2$ antibody fragments have been used to reduce digitoxin levels rapidly in cases of digitoxin poisoning. Antibody inhibition may also affect the action of other drugs, such as steroids, chloramphenicol, morphine, oxytocin, and vasopressin.

Other Antibodies

Autoantibodies to vasopressin in rabbits produce diabetes insipidus. Antibodies to gluten may react with gluten bound to epithelial cells and damage intestinal epithelium by an ADCC mechanism causing sprue or celiac disease. Passive antibodies to gastrin have been used to induce serum gastrin levels in patients with Zollinger-Ellison syndrome (intractable peptic ulcers caused by high gastrin levels). Sheep immunized with inhibin, a nonsteroid hormone found in ovarian follicular fluid that inhibits follicle-stimulating hormone, have an increased ovulation rate. This has resulted in increased fecundity in sheep in Australia. Autoantibodies to parathyroid hormone receptors are found in patients with secondary hyperparathyroidism. These antibodies block binding of hormone to receptors.

Ligands, Receptors, and Idiotypes

Antibodies, hormone receptors, and enzymes have structural and functional similarities. Each type of molecule is organized into functional domains consisting of a specific ligand binding domain and a transmission domain. Reaction of the binding domain with ligand results in alteration of the transmission domain and activation of an effector system. Antibodies, hormone receptors, and enzymes are able to distinguish a series of ligands (antigens) with similar structures and bind the appropriate ligand with a high affinity (Fig. 8.7). Each has epitopes specific for the binding site as well as epitopes on parts of the molecule away from the binding site.

Antibodies to receptors, enzymes or other antibodies may react with ligand (antigen) binding site epitopes or with epitopes that are not part of the binding site (Fig. 8.8). Antibodies that react directly with the binding site may mimic the structure of the natural ligand and, upon reaction with the receptor, activate it. Anti-idiotype antibody is an antibody to an antibody. An anti-idiotype to the binding site (paratope) of an anti-receptor antibody may mimic exactly the structure of the ligand for the receptor. Thus, this anti-receptor antibody may actually be able to mimic the function of the ligand.

Figure 8.7 Similarities between hormone receptors, antibodies, and enzymes. **(1)** Recognition domain (paratope) that distinguishes fine structural differences. **(2)** Functional domain (constant region). Recognition domains have similar binding properties for ligands and mechanisms of activation of cells through G proteins. The black semicircles represent epitopes on the receptor for antibodies which will not block the binding of the ligand. These sites on antibody molecules are different for each antibody (non-antigen-blocking anti-idiotypes), whereas those on cell surface receptors or enzymes are shared by other receptors or enzymes of the same type.

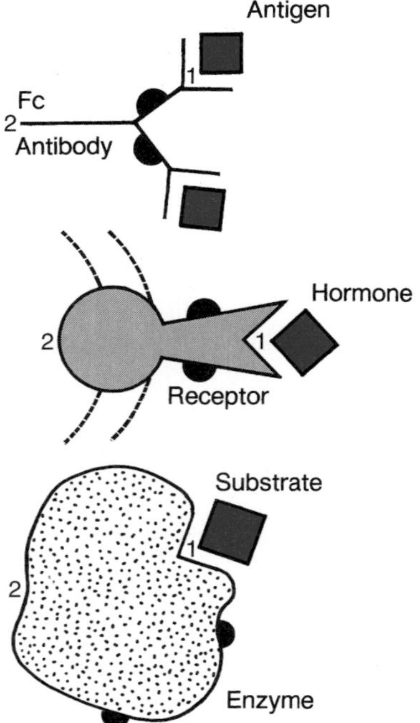

Anti-Idiotypes and Ligand Mimicry

The interrelationship of antibodies to ligands and receptors provides an idiotype network of related structures (Fig. 8.9). This relationship is difficult to explain but is essentially as follows. The structure of the paratope (antigen-binding site) of antibody to a ligand will mimic the receptor for the ligand. The anti-idiotype to the anti-ligand (anti-anti-ligand) will mimic the ligand. Similarly, antibody to the receptor may mimic the ligand, and anti-idiotype antibody to the anti-receptor (anti-anti-receptor) will mimic the receptor site for the ligand. In this way, a network of interactions may be completed (Fig. 8.10).

Anti-Idiotypes and Disease

Some examples of molecular mimicry between biologically active ligands and anti-idiotypic antibodies to anti-ligands are the following.

1. Anti-idiotypic antibodies against anti-insulin, containing the internal image of insulin, interact with the membrane-bound insulin receptor and mimic insulin action in vitro.
2. Anti-β-adrenergic ligand anti-idiotype antibodies bind to the β-adrenergic receptor and stimulate cyclase.
3. Rabbits immunized with rat anti-human TSH antibodies produce anti-antibodies that inhibit the binding of TSH to the TSH receptor (Fig. 8.11).

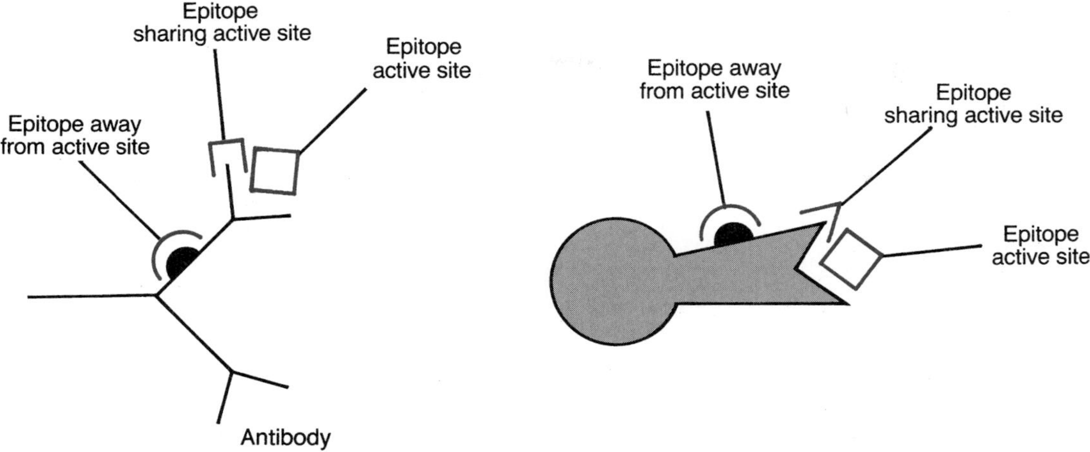

Figure 8.8 Antibodies to receptors may bind (i) the active site, (ii) epitopes away from the active site, or (iii) epitopes sharing part of the active site. Anti-idiotypes may react with (i) the active site of antibody, (ii) epitopes away from the active site, or (iii) epitopes sharing part of the active site.

4. Antibodies to an agonist of the acetylcholine receptor mimic the binding characteristics of acetylcholine receptor; i.e., the anti-agonist antibody binding site binds the same ligands as the receptor. An anti-idiotypic antibody to the anti-agonist causes MG (see above).

Neutralizing Antibodies: Cause and Effect

The presence of autoantibodies in a patient with a given disease does not necessarily mean that the antibody actually caused the disease or is even responsible for any of the symptoms of the disease. In the 1950s, Pierre Grabar postulated that most autoantibodies are part of a physiological

Figure 8.9 Relationship of ligand, anti-ligand, anti-idiotypes, receptor, anti-receptor, and anti-idiotypes. An immune response to a ligand may result in antibodies that mimic the receptor and anti-idiotypes that mimic the ligand; an immune response to the receptor may produce antibodies that mimic the ligand and anti-idiotypes that mimic the receptor.

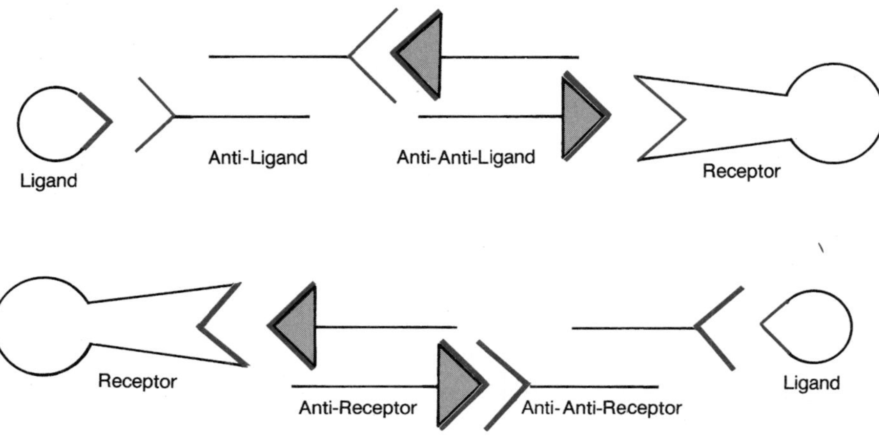

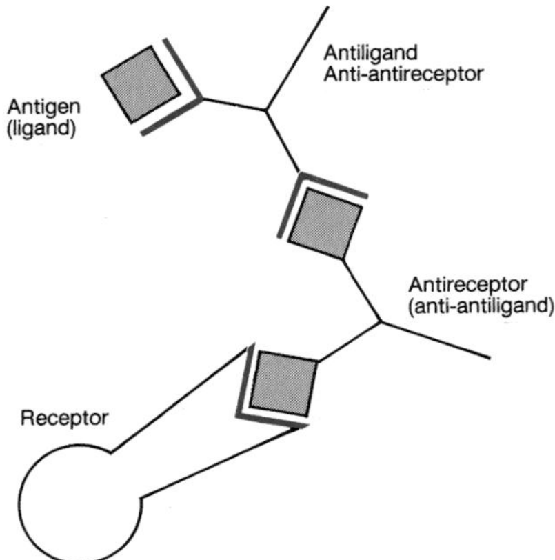

Figure 8.10 The ligand-antibody-receptor network. An immune response to a ligand may result in antibodies that mimic the receptor or the ligand (anti-anti-receptor). An immune response to a receptor may produce antibodies that mimic the ligand (anti-anti-ligand). Antibodies to the ligand may have paratopes that mimic the receptor. In this way, immune response to either ligand or receptor may produce inactivating or activating antibodies. Laboratory animals immunized with insulin develop not only antibodies to insulin but also antibodies to the insulin receptor (anti-anti-insulin).

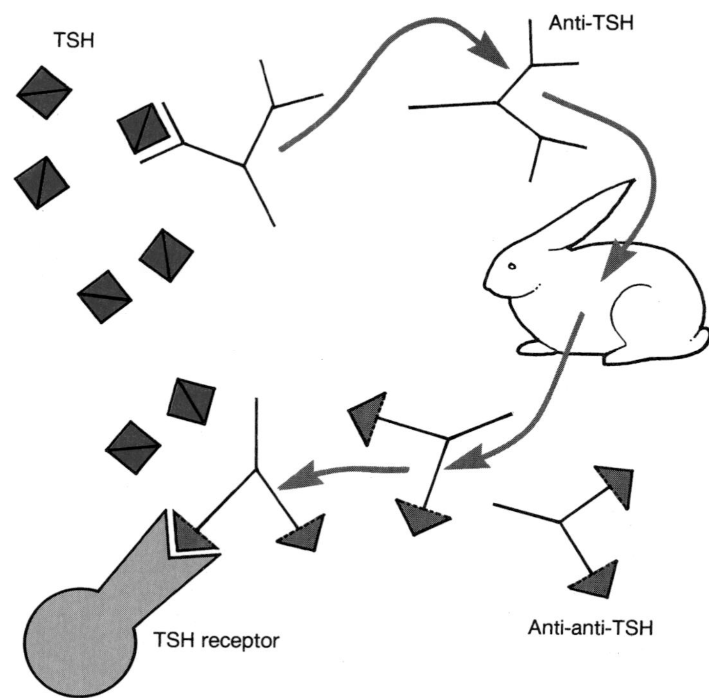

Figure 8.11 Production of TSH-blocking antibodies by immunization of rabbits with anti-TSH. Anti-idiotype to anti-TSH (anti-anti-TSH) reacts with TSH receptor and blocks TSH binding.

system of handling metabolic or catabolic products (transporters). Autoantibodies help in disposing of self materials, particularly if an unrelated event causes release of abnormally high amounts of tissue components. For example, massive tissue necrosis in an acute myocardial infarction releases intracellular antigens and triggers autoantibody formation. In this example, autoantibody formation occurs secondarily to cell necrosis and is not responsible for initiating this type of tissue damage. However, it has become increasingly apparent the autoantibodies may produce disease as a primary mechanism or may cause resistance to therapy or other secondary effects.

Protective Functions of Inactivating (Neutralizing) Antibodies

Neutralization or inactivation effector mechanisms are active in protecting us against a variety of bacterial and viral infections, both by inactivating toxins produced by bacteria and by blocking the ability of infecting organisms to react with cell surface receptors necessary for infection. Some bacteria produce disease not by direct effects of the organism but by the release of products called toxins, which may have severe destructive effects distant from the site of infection. Destructive bacterial toxins are rendered harmless by reaction with antibody (neutralization reaction). For instance, anti-toxin antibodies inactivate toxins of diphtheria or tetanus (see below). In addition, IgA antibodies in the gastrointestinal tract may be able to block the production of watery diarrhea by *Vibrio cholerae* infection of the intestinal tract by preventing the toxin from binding to gastrointestinal lining cells (neutralization). Circulating immunoglobulin antibody (usually IgG) or secretory antibody (usually IgA) also reacts with surface antigens on viruses and prevents the virus from attaching to cells (neutralizing antibody), thereby inhibiting spread of the infection. A summary of the role of various antibody-mediated mechanisms in infections is presented at the end of chapter 11.

Tetanus

Tetanus is caused by a highly fatal endoneurotoxin (tetanospasmin) released by the anaerobic gram-negative bacillus *Clostridium tetani*. Tetanus toxin is synthesized as a single polypeptide chain of 150,000 Da. Upon secretion, cleavage by a *C. tetani*-derived "nickase" results in a two-chain molecule joined by a single disulfide bond, with a heavy chain of approximately 100,000 Da and a light chain of 50,000 Da. The heavy chain is able to bind to cell surface gangliosides, and the two-chain molecule is taken into the cell. In the cell, the light chain is cleaved by cellular enzymes to produce a peptide fragment that blocks an elongation factor (EF2) required for protein synthesis. One activated light chain is able to block all EF2 activity in a cell. This effectively destroys, inhibits, or blocks protein synthesis and the function of the cell.

Viable tetanus organisms exist only in dead tissue and produce disease by release of toxin that diffuses into the adjacent living tissues. Spore forms of the organism are ubiquitous in soil and can infect a seemingly trivial wound. Natural defenses are essentially limited to local healing processes. The organisms multiply locally and produce endotoxin. The endotoxin is released when organisms are destroyed in the necrotic wound tissue and travels via the blood or by retrograde axonal transmission to the spinal cord. The toxin increases reflex excitability in motor neurons by blocking the function of inhibitory neurons. This results in rigidity and reflex spasms, with death most often due to respiratory failure. The incubation period is usually less than 14 days. The length of the incubation period is critical in determining the outcome (60% fatality if less than 9 days; 25% if greater than 9 days).

The major immune defense mechanism of the host is neutralization of the toxin by specific antibody that blocks binding of the toxin to neurons (Fig. 8.12). Unfortunately, in the natural infection, the potency of the toxin is so great that even fatal doses of tetanospasmin are not usually sufficient to stimulate antibody production. However in high-incidence countries, such as Ethiopia, up to 30% of adults have toxin-neutralizing antibody, presumably from natural exposure. Since the organism cannot survive in living tissue because it is anaerobic, *C. tetani* benefits if the infected individual dies, at which point the entire body can be colonized. Primary therapy is directed to keeping the wound clean and debrided to avoid the anaerobic conditions favoring growth of *C. tetani*. Secondary therapy is to neutralize tetanospasmin by antibody.

In 1890, von Behring and Kitasato demonstrated protective immunization using repeated small doses of tetanus toxin. Their report included the finding that the protection was due to a new factor present in the serum of immunized individuals (antitoxin). This classic report laid the foundation for subsequent development of immunoprophylaxis of infectious diseases using bacterial products. Antitoxin produced in horses was prepared and used to treat patients with tetanus or those with wounds that could accommodate *C. tetani*. Unfortunately, treated patients often developed another serious disease, serum sickness, caused by production of antibody to the horse antitoxin (see chapter 11).

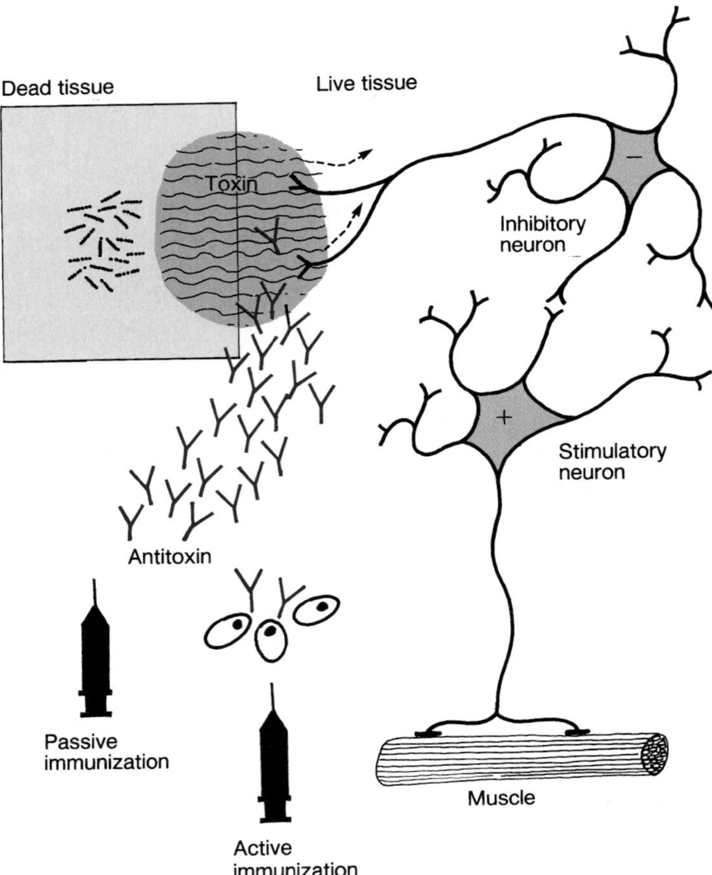

Figure 8.12 Neutralization of tetanus toxin by antitoxin. Antitoxin blocks entry of toxin into neurons. *C. tetani* releases endotoxin when the organisms die in necrotic tissue. The endotoxin is taken up by axons and delivered to nerve cells, where it inactivates protein synthesis. The loss of activity of inhibitory neurons permits hyperactivity of stimulatory neurons and muscle spasm. Antitoxin provided by active or passive immunization prevents toxin from reaching inhibitory neurons.

In 1925, Ramon introduced chemically modified toxin (toxoid) for active immunization. Active immunization with toxoid has greatly reduced the incidence of tetanus. It should be noted that antibodies directed against *C. tetani* itself would not be useful, since the organism lives only in dead tissue, and antibody cannot reach the site of infection.

For toxin to be active, it must be internalized into the neuron, presumably at the axon level. Antitoxin binding to toxin prevents entry of the toxin into the cell. This may be accomplished by alteration of the tertiary structure of the toxin molecule. Once the toxin is bound to the neuron or internalized, antitoxin is ineffective. Neutralization of tetanus toxin is a powerful specific and effective mechanism of protection. Artificial immunization with tetanus toxoid provides prolonged, but not permanent, protection. Antitoxin titers must be boosted by reimmunization if exposure to toxin is suspected. Reimmunization of an individual with a wound that may be infected with *C. tetani* induces a secondary antibody response that can effectively block the toxin. However, if reimmunization is delayed, elevation of the antibody titer may be too late to prevent clinical tetanus.

The risk for fatal tetanus is greater in people over 60 years of age who lack protective levels of antitoxin because of a failure of booster immunizations. In 1999, 32 cases of tetanus were reported in the United States, with a case fatality rate of 24%.

Diphtheria

Diphtheria is a localized infection located in the pharynx with generalized intoxication caused by release of diphtheria toxin, an extracellular protein metabolite of strains of *Corynebacterium diphtheriae* that carry the *tox*$^+$ gene. The local infection is manifested by a tightly adherent grayish plaque in the throat known as a pseudomembrane because it resembles a membrane. The bacteria multiply within the membrane and produce a toxin that is absorbed through the mucous membrane of the throat into the systemic circulation. In the late 1800s, it was deduced that the systemic effects of diphtheria infection were not caused by systemic infection by bacteria but by release of a toxin. This was finally demonstrated by Roux and Yersin in 1888, when they reproduced symptoms of diphtheria in animals by inoculation of cell-free filtrates of *C. diphtheriae* cultures. Subcutaneous injection of 25 μg of toxin into a 250-g guinea pig is lethal in 4 to 5 days. The toxin first attaches to cell surfaces at specific sites, is endocytosed and activated, and then inhibits intracellular protein synthesis. After processing in an acidic endosome, cleavage and reduction of a disulfide bond produces the enzymatically active toxin. The active toxin catalyzes the cleavage of NAD, resulting in transfer of an adenine diphosphate ribose to EF-2 (polypeptidyl transfer RNA translocase). EF-2 is then incapable of adding amino acids to peptide chains, protein synthesis stops, and the cell dies.

Diphtheria was the first disease in which passive antibody therapy was shown to be effective. The extracellular toxin may be neutralized by reaction with antibody before the toxin has a chance to bind to host cells. This is most likely due to an antibody-induced alteration of the tertiary structure of the toxin so that it cannot bind to the cellular receptor. The effectiveness of passive antibody therapy was demonstrated in 1898 by Fibiger in a controlled clinical trial. Active protective immunization was first induced by von Behring in 1913 using toxin neutralized with antibody; in 1923, Ramon used diphtheria toxin treated with 0.4% formaldehyde. Formaldehyde alters the structure of the toxin so that it can no longer bind to the target cells, yet maintains other epitopes so that a immune response results in neutralizing antibody. Neutralizing antibody most likely alters the tertiary structure of the toxin so that it cannot bind to host cells. In 1988, a conjugate vaccine consisting of type b capsular polysaccharide of *Haemophilus influenzae* (see chapter 5) linked to diphtheria toxoid was licensed for use in children younger than 18 months of age. Although the primary goal of the use of the conjugate vaccine was to prevent *H. influenzae*, it also stimulated antibody production to diphtherial toxin.

The neutralization potency of an antiserum to diphtheria toxin (antitoxin) is measured by comparison with a standard sample of antitoxin. To test a toxin preparation, increasing amounts of toxin are added to a series of tubes containing 1 unit of a standard antitoxin, and each of the mixtures is injected into a 250-g guinea pig. The amount of toxin that must be mixed with 1 unit of antitoxin to cause death in 4 days is taken as the endpoint and is called the L_+ dose. Conversely, the potency of the unknown antiserum can be determined by mixing increasing dilutions of the antitoxin with one L_+ dose of the toxin and injecting the mixture into test guinea pigs. One unit of antitoxin, when mixed with one L_+ dose of toxin, results in death in 4 days.

Schick Test

Historically, in vivo neutralization of diphtheria toxin by antibody was determined by skin testing. A small amount of diphtheria toxin injected intradermally produces a local inflammatory reaction that is maximal at 4 to 5 h and then fades. In an immunized individual, who has antibody to diphtheria toxin, no inflammatory reaction is seen; the preformed antibody neutralizes the effects of the toxin. This test was pioneered by Bela Schick between 1910 and 1930 and is known as the Schick test. A delayed-type hypersensitivity reaction to diphtheria toxin may also occur. This is known as a pseudoreaction and can usually be differentiated from the effects of the toxin, as the delayed reaction reaches a maximum at 2 to 3 days and fades by 4 to 5 days.

Viral Neutralization

Antibodies are the first line of defense against viral infections. T_{CTL} or T_{DTH} cells may be active on infected cells, but circulating antibody acts to prevent viruses from reaching target cells. Thus, for many viral diseases, vaccines that induce circulating or secreted (IgA) neutralizing antibodies are the most effective. However, for other viruses, such as smallpox or measles, which infect epithelial cells before circulating antibodies can have an effect, cell-mediated immunity is required for protection (see chapter 11).

Polio

An example of effective antibody-mediated immunization against viral infections is polio vaccination. Since the disease caused by poliovirus results from infection of anterior horn cells of the spinal cord, even if the virus establishes a foothold in the gastrointestinal tract, the presence of antibodies in the blood can prevent infection of the critical neurons. Formalin-killed (Salk) and attenuated (Sabin) vaccines are available for immunization against polio. Surprisingly few mutations in the Sabin vaccine strains are required to acquire attenuation. Although the attenuated viruses are capable of rapid variation in the vaccine that allows the virus to grow successfully, they cause almost no disease.

In evaluation of immunization to polio, factors in addition to protection of the immunized individual must be considered. Injection of formalin-killed vaccine produces good systemic immunity of the vaccinated individual. On the other hand, oral immunization by ingestion of attenuated virus induces local immunity in the gastrointestinal tract and may prevent passage of the virus through elimination of fecal contamination, whereas injection of killed virus is relatively ineffective in this regard. Polio infections are contracted naturally by swallowing of virus-contaminated materials. In an unprotected person, the virus passes into the bloodstream, leading to a systemic infection. Disease occurs when the virus attacks the anterior horn cells of the medulla and spinal cord. Antibody induced by injection prevents the systemic spread of the virus, but the gastrointestinal phase may still occur. On the other hand, oral immunization leads to local immunity in the gastrointestinal tract, presumably because of the production of secretory antibody. This reduces the gastrointestinal phase of infection and limits the spread of the virus. Persons inoculated with the killed virus may be protected from disease but can still serve as carriers to disseminate the virus during an epidemic. If a substantial portion of a population has received the oral vaccine, even the nonimmunized portion of the population is protected from epidemic disease. The incidence of paralytic poliomyelitis in the United States from 1951 to 1978 is given in Table 8.5. Although some controversy exists in regard to the efficiency of intramuscular injections of killed polio vaccine and of oral administration of attenuated poliovirus, most authorities recommend oral vaccine administered for the first time between 2 months of age and the preschool period.

Recently, largely driven by lawsuits, there has been reconsideration of the reintroduction of inactivated polio vaccine. Rare cases of polio in the United States are associated with live virus in recent vaccine recipients or with transmission to persons who were not immunized. One hundred five cases have been verified by the Centers for Disease Control in a 12-year period: 35 were vaccinees, and 50 were contacts of vaccinees. The immunization schedule now recommended is inactivated poliovirus (IPV) immunization at 2 and 4 months of age, combined with oral live virus (OPV) immunization at 6, 12, 15, and 18 months of age, and a booster combined immunization at 11 to 12 years of age.

Since 1985, through the wide surveillance of all cases of polio in the Americas, poliomyelitis is on the verge of being eradicated from the Western Hemisphere. In 1991, only nine cases of acute flaccid paralysis were confirmed to have been caused by wild-type poliovirus, and none were reported in the United States or Canada. This result may be attributed to the efforts of thousands of health workers and civil servants. However, even tighter surveillance is needed to eliminate the disease entirely.

Hepatitis

Vaccines against hepatitis viruses, if successful, would be the first vaccines for the prevention of cancer in humans. The protective effects of these vaccines are mainly mediated by the production of neutralizing antibodies. Hepatitis virus enters through the gastrointestinal tract and infects hepatocytes.

Hepatitis B. Hepatitis B virus (HBV) is acquired through the gastrointestinal tract, and the virus appears to infect hepatocytes specifically. Most infections in endemic areas occur within the first year of life, most likely from maternal-fetal transmission. After infection, HBV passes from one liver cell to another as the liver cells are killed. Thus, circulating antibodies should prevent infection of the liver by blocking reaction of the virus

Table 8.5 Correlation of paralytic poliomyelitis and vaccine use in the United States, 1951 to 1978[a]

Period	Vaccine(s)[b]	Total no. of cases	Avg no. of cases/yr	Avg no. of cases/million/yr
1951–1955	None	111,040	22,208	135
1956–1960	IPV only	22,970	4,594	26
1961–1965	IPV and OPV	2,341	468	2.4
1973–1978	OPV only	55	9	0.004

[a]Modified from A. E. Sabin, *Rev. Infect. Dis.* **3**:543–564, 1981.
[b]Abbreviations: IPV, formalin-killed polio vaccine; OPV, oral (attenuated) live polio vaccine.

with hepatocytes. In addition, IgA antibodies may block initial passage across the gastrointestinal tract.

Two types of vaccines are now available for immunization: hepatitis B surface antigen (HBsAg) subviral particles purified from the serum of asymptomatic carriers and subunit HBsAg particles produced by genetic engineering in the common baker's yeast *Saccharomyces cerevisiae* or in Chinese hamster ovary cells. The *env* gene of the virus (Fig. 8.13) was cloned, inserted into a vector, and transfected into the productive cells. Translation products of each of the small (S), medium (M), and large (L) messenger RNAs of the *env* region were identified, and subviral particles were obtained in large amounts after lysis of the yeast cells.

There is a good correlation between the presence of antibodies to the *env* gene product and protection from infection. Clinical trials have shown that there is little difference between the plasma derived or the recombinant product regarding antibody response or protection against infection. However, cell-mediated immunity to HBV protein is significantly higher after recovery from natural infection than after immunization. Thus, antibody to *env* appears to block infection. There remain a small proportion of nonresponders to the vaccines and marked individual variation in the levels of antibodies obtained. In addition, nonresponders who subsequently become infected and recover develop high titer of antibodies to the HBV *env* proteins. Thus, improvement is needed in the hepatitis B vaccines. One approach would be to produce a vaccine that includes additional epitopes of HBV, such as the core antigen or pre-S1 and pre-S2 epitopes not present in the *env* gene. Pre-S1 and pre-S2 epitopes are expressed on the surface of HBV and appear to play an important role both in immunologic recognition and in reactions with cell receptors. Originally recommended for high-risk populations (e.g., neonates born to HBsAg-carrier mothers, recently arrived immigrants from Southeast Asia or southern Africa), repeated HBsAg immunization is now included in recommended childhood immunizations, beginning as early as birth.

The high association of development of hepatocellular carcinomas in areas of the world with endemic hepatitis B has led to clinical trials with the intention of preventing hepatitis in children and thus also preventing hepatocellular carcinoma. Preliminary results indicate that best results are obtained when neonates are immunized within 1 month of birth and a booster given within 2 weeks after the first injection. Follow-up after 9 years indicates that 8% of the vaccinated children had been infected with HBV, compared with 50% of the unvaccinated children, resulting in a vaccine efficacy of 83% against infection and a 95% efficacy against chronic carriage.

Hepatitis A. During the past 15 years, the virus causing hepatitis A has been isolated and identified, and a formalin-inactivated vaccine has been produced. Hepatitis A is caused by a picornavirus that appears to have unique properties compared with other RNA viruses. As with many other infectious diseases, the incidence of the disease actually increases with improved hygienic living conditions. Thus, it is an example of an infectious agent that previously infected essentially all infants at an age when infection was asymptomatic or produced only mild symptoms indistinguishable as a specific disease. Although the incidence of hepatitis is declining in general, the majority of civilian cases in European and North American populations are acquired during travel in developing countries, and thou-

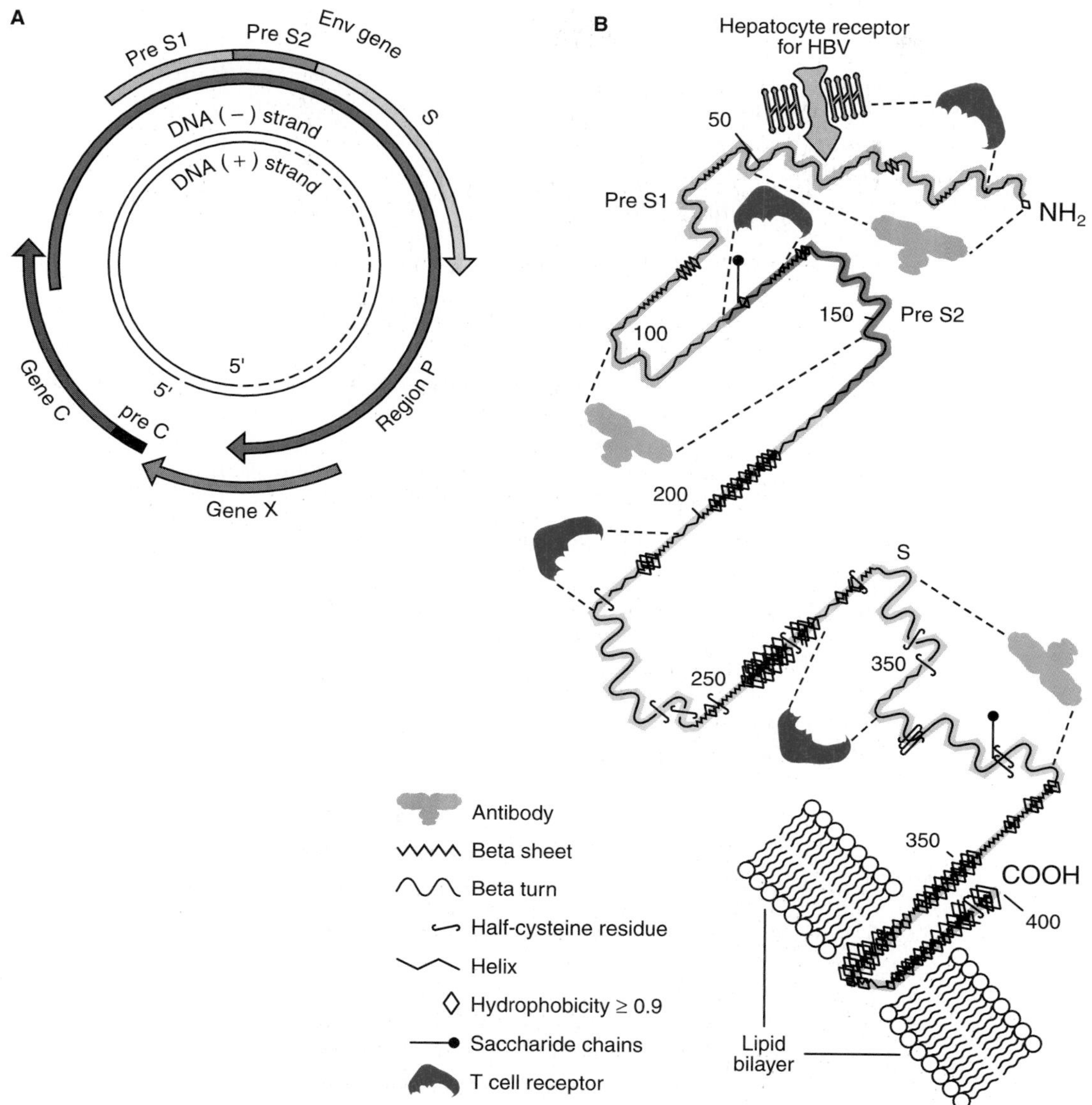

Figure 8.13 (A) Genetic map of HBV. The DNA of HBV is partially double-stranded. The two strands (+ and −) are also called large (−) and small (+) because of the different sizes. The deleted region of the + strand is indicated with a dashed line (-----). The large open reading frame for the HBsAg, the *env* region, has been cloned, and peptides representing the B- and T-cell epitopes have been identified. **(B)** Secondary structure of the HBsAg as predicted from the HBV *env* gene product. The large surface protein contains pre-S1, pre-S2, and S; the middle protein contains pre-S and S; and the small protein contains S only. The pre-S1 region contains the binding region for the hepatocyte receptor for HBV; the S region contains the hydrophobic membrane region inserted into the HBV lipid bilayer. (Modified from A. R. Neurath, B. A. Jameson, and T. Huima, *Microbiol. Sci.* **4**:45–51, 1987.)

sands of soldiers in World Wars I and II most likely had hepatitis A. Four approaches to the production of a vaccine have included production of attenuated viruses in cell culture, genetically engineered capsid vaccines, synthetic peptide vaccines, and formalin-killed cell-cultured viruses. Of these, the formalin-killed virus is now available and has been effective in inducing antibody in normal volunteers. Since licensing of hepatitis A vaccine in 1995, a program of systematic immunization of children in areas of endemicity has been recommended. However, a large change in hepatitis A incidence, mortality rates, or vaccine costs is required for intervention strategies to be cost-effective. It is not known how long immunity to hepatitis A will last after killed-virus vaccination. In developing countries, where a vaccine to hepatitis A would be most useful, it is desirable to have a vaccine that is effective in producing lifelong immunity. This objective may require an attenuated-virus vaccine.

Hepatitis C. Hepatitis C virus (HCV) infection is the major cause of post-transfusion hepatitis. Chronic HCV infection often progresses to cirrhosis and hepatocellular carcinoma. The immune response to hepatitis C infection is mediated by T_{CTL} cells (see chapter 11). Acutely infected patients who clear the infection develop a vigorous T_{CTL}-cell response, whereas those who develop progressive disease do not. The RNA genome of HCV has been cloned and consists of about 1,000 nucleotides. T_{CTL}-cell responses to HCV have been induced using DNA constructs from both nonstructural and structural regions of the HCV genome. Current therapy is not very effective, and a vaccine is not yet available. Experimental vaccines using DNA-based immunization against the HCV core are being evaluated.

Hepatitis E. Hepatitis E virus DNA has also been cloned, and a recombinant vaccine has been produced to open reading frame 2 of the Pakistani strain of the virus. Immunization trials of rhesus monkeys demonstrate protection against hepatitis caused both by the homologous and heterologous strains of the virus.

Summary

Circulating antibodies to biologically active molecules may effectively inactivate or neutralize the activity of these molecules and thus produce deficiency diseases. In some instances, autoantibodies may actually stimulate increased function. Biologically active molecules that may be affected by antibodies include hormones, enzymes, growth factors, clotting factors, and cell surface receptors. Inactivation may occur by alteration of tertiary structure, blocking of active sites, or modulation of cell surface receptors. Autoantibodies to endocrine glands, hormones, or hormone receptors are the best-understood examples of these activation or inactivation reactions. Protective immunity may be induced by immunization with altered bacterial toxins (toxoid) that will induce antibodies that inactivate the toxin or by immunization with antibodies to viruses that will block viral surface receptors.

Bibliography

Mechanisms of Inactivation and Activation

Aston, R., W. B. Cowden, and G. L. Ada. 1989. Antibody-mediated enhancement of hormone activity. *Mol. Immunol.* **26:**435–446.

Cinader, B. (ed.). 1967. *Antibodies to Biologically Active Molecules.* Pergamon Press, New York, N.Y.

Rotman, M. B., and F. Celada. 1968. Antibody-mediated activation of a defective β-D-galactosidase extracted from an *Escherichia coli* mutant. *Proc. Natl. Acad. Sci. USA* **60:**660–667.

Diabetes Mellitus

Faustman, D. 1993. Mechanisms of autoimmunity in type I diabetes. *J. Clin. Immunol.* **13:**1–7.

Marks, J. B., and J. S. Skyler. 1991. Clinical review 17: immunotherapy of type II diabetes mellitus. *J. Clin. Endocrinol. Metab.* **72:**3–9.

Roep, B. O., M. A. Atkinson, P. M. van Endert, P. A. Gottlieb, S. B. Wilson, and J. A. Sachs. 1999. Autoreactive T cell responses in insulin-dependent (type 1) diabetes mellitus. Report of the First International Workshop for Standardization of T Cell Assays. *J. Autoimmun.* **13:**267–282.

Sera, Y., E. Kawasaki, N. Abiru, M. Ozaki, T. Abe, et al. 1999. Autoantibodies to multiple islet autoantigens in patients with abrupt onset type 1 diabetes and diabetes diagnosed with urinary glucose screening. *J. Autoimmun.* **13:**257–265.

Trucco, M., and R. LaPorte. 1995. Exposure to superantigens as an immunogenetic explanation of type I diabetes mini-epidemics. *J. Pediatr. Endocrinol. Metab.* **8:**3–10.

Yoon, J. W., and H. S. Jun. 1999. Cellular and molecular roles of beta cell autoantigens, macrophages and T cells in the pathogenesis of autoimmune diabetes. *Arch. Pharm. Res.* **22:**437–447.

Thyroid Disease

Bednarczuk, T., C. Stolarski, E. Pawlik, M. Slon, M. Rowinski, et al. 1999. Autoantibodies reactive with extracellular matrix proteins in patients with thyroid-associated ophthalmopathy. *Thyroid* **9:**289–295.

DiCerbo, A., and K. Corda. 1999. Signaling pathways involved in thyroid hyperfunctions and growth in Graves' disease. *Biochimie* **81:**415–424.

Doniach, D., and I. M. Roitt. 1957. Autoimmunity in Hashimoto's disease and its implications. *J. Clin. Endocrinol. Metab.* **77:**1293–1304.

Gunji, K., A. DeBellis, S. Kubota, J. Swanson, S. Wenrowicz, et al. 1999. Serum antibodies against the flavoprotein subunit of succinate dehydrogenase are sensitive markers of eye muscle autoimmunity in patients with Graves' hyperthyroidism. *J. Clin. Endocrinol. Metab.* **84:**1255–1262.

Karlsson, F. A., L. Wibell, and L. Wide. 1977. Hypothyroidism due to thyroid-hormone-binding antibodies. *N. Engl. J. Med.* **296:**1146–1148.

Perros, P., and P. Kendall-Taylor. 1995. Thyroid-associated ophthalmopathy: pathogenesis and clinical management. *Clin. Endocrinol. Metab.* **9:**115–135.

Rasmussen, K., M. L. Hartoft-Nielsen, and U. Feldt-Rasmussen. 1999. Models to study the pathogenesis of thyroid autoimmunity. *Biochimie* **81:**511–515.

Yamano, Y., J. Takamatsu, S. Sakane, K. Hirai, K. Kuma, and N. Ohsawa. 1999. Differences between changes in serum thyrotropin-binding inhibitory antibodies and thyroid-stimulating antibodies in the course of antithyroid drug therapy for Graves' disease. *Thyroid* **9:**769–773.

hCG, Estrogen, Progesterone, and Fertility

Gupta, S. K., and V. Singh. 1988. Immunobiology of human chorionic gonadotropin. *Indian J. Exp. Biol.* **26:**243–251.

Musch, K., A. S. Wolf, and C. Lauritzen. 1981. Antibodies to chorionic gonadotropin in humans. *Clin. Chim. Acta* **113:**95–100.

Nasa, H. A., C. C. Chang, and Y. Y. Tsong. 1985. Formulation of a potential antipregnancy vaccine based on the β-subunit of human chronic gonadotropin. *J. Rep. Immunol.* **7:**151–163.

Myasthenia Gravis

Dau, P., J. M. Lindstrom, C. K. Cassel, E. H. Denys, E. E. Shev, and L. E. Spitler. 1977. Plasmapheresis and immunosuppressive drug therapy in myasthenia gravis. *N. Engl. J. Med.* **297:**1134–1140.

Engel, A. G. 1993. The investigation of congenital myasthenic syndromes. *Ann. N. Y. Acad. Sci.* **681:**425–434.

Howard, J. F., Jr. 1998. Intravenous immunoglobulin for the treatment of acquired myasthenia gravis. *Neurology* **51:**S30–S36.

Lennon, V. A., J. Lindstrom, and M. E. Seybold. 1975. Experimental autoimmune myasthenia: a model of myasthenia gravis in rats and guinea pigs. *J. Exp. Med.* **141:**1365–1375.

Lopate, G., and A. Pestronk. 1993. Autoimmune myasthenia gravis. *Hosp. Pract.* **28:**109–122.

Miyahara, T., K. Oka, and S. Nakaji. 1998. Specific immunoabsorbent for myasthenia gravis treatment: development of synthetic peptide designed to remove antiacetylcholine receptor antibody. *Ther. Apher.* **2:**246–248.

Shibuya, N., T. Sato, M. Osame, T. Takegami, S. Doi, and S. Kawanami. 1994. Immunoadsorption therapy for myasthenia gravis. *J. Neurol. Neurosurg. Psychiatry* **57:**578–581.

Solimena, M., F. Folli, S. Dennis-Domimi, G. C. Comi, G. Pozza, P. De Camili, and A. M. Vicari. 1988. Autoantibodies to glutamic acid decarboxylase in a patient with stiff-man syndrome, epilepsy and type I diabetes mellitus. *N. Engl. J. Med.* **318:**1012–1020.

Tsantili, P., S. J. Tzartos, and A. Mamalaki. 1999. High affinity single-chain Fv antibody fragments protecting the human nicotinic acetylcholine receptor. *J. Neuroimmunol.* **94:**15–27.

β-Adrenergic Receptors

Limas, C. J., and I. F. Goldenberg. 1989. Autoantibodies against beta-adrenoceptors in human dilated cardiomyopathy. *Circ. Res.* **64:**97–103.

Magnusson, Y., S. Marullo, S. Hoyer, F. Waagstein, B. Andersson, et al. 1990. Mapping of a functional autoimmune epitope on the β_1-adrenergic receptor in patients with idiopathic dilated cardiomyopathy. *J. Clin. Investig.* **86:**1658–1663.

Peukert, S., M. L. Fu, P. Eftekhari, I. Poepping, A. Voss, et al. 1999. The frequency of occurrence of anti-cardiac receptor autoantibodies and their correlation with clinical manifestation in patients with hypertrophic cardiomyopathy. *Autoimmunity* **29:**291–297.

Podlowski, S., H. P. Luther, R. Morwinski, J. Muller, and G. Wallukat. 1998. Agonistic anti-beta1–adrenergic receptor autoantibodies from cardiomyopathy patients reduce the beta1–adrenergic receptor expression in neonatal rat cardiomyocytes. *Circulation* **98:**2470–2476.

Sterin-Borda, L., G. Gorelik, M. Postan, S. Gonzalez Cappa, and E. Borda. 1999. Alterations in cardiac beta-adrenergic receptors in chagasic mice and their association with circulating beta-adrenoceptor-related autoantibodies. *Cardiovasc. Res.* **41:**116–125.

Venter, J. C., C. M. Fraser, and L. C. Harrison. 1980. Autoantibodies to β2 adrenergic receptors: a possible cause of adrenergic hyporesponsiveness in allergic rhinitis asthma. *Science* **207:**1361–1363.

Pernicious Anemia

Ingram, C. F., A. F. Fleming, M. Patel, and J. S. Galpin. 1998. The value of the intrinsic factor antibody test in diagnosing pernicious anaemia. *Cent. Afr. J. Med.* **44:**178–181.

Irvine, W. J. 1965. Immunologic aspects of pernicious anemia. *N. Engl. J. Med.* **273:**432.

Judd, L. M., P. A. Gleeson, B. H. Toh, and I. R. van Driel. 1999. Autoimmune gastritis results in disruption of gastric epithelial cell development. *Am. J. Physiol.* **277:**G209–218.

Kawashima, K. 1972. Effects of gastric antibodies on gastric secretion. II. Effects of rabbit antibodies against rat gastric mucosas and gastric juice on gastric secretion in the rat. *Jpn. J. Pharmacol.* **22:**155–165.

Prolactin

Lindstedt, G. 1994. Endogenous antibodies against prolactin—a "new" cause of hyperprolactinemia. *Eur. J. Endocrinol.* **130:**429–432.

Anticoagulants

Brackmann, H. H., H. Lenk, I. Scharrer, G. Auerswald, and W. Kreuz. 1999. German recommendations for immune tolerance therapy in type A haemophiliacs with antibodies. *Haemophilia* **5:**203–206.

Ludlam, C. A., A. E. Morrison, and C. Kessler. 1994. Treatment of acquired hemophilia. *Semin. Hematol.* **31**(2 Suppl. 4)**:**16–19.

Scandella, D., W. Mondorf, and J. Klinge. 1998. The natural history of the immune response to exogenous factor VIII in severe haemophilia A. *Haemophilia* **4:**546–551.

Scharrer, I., G. L. Bray, and O. Neutzling. 1999. Incidence of inhibitors in haemophilia A patients—a review of recent studies of recombinant and plasma-derived factor VII concentrates. *Haemophilia* **5:**145–154.

Vianello, F., T. Tison, G. Tagariello, P. Zerbinati, E. Zanon, L. Scarano, and A. Girolami. 1999. Serological markers of autoimmunity in patients with hemophilia A: the role of hepatitis C virus infection, alpha-interferon and factor VIII treatments in skewing the immune response toward autoreactivity. *Blood Coagul. Fibrinolysis* **10:**393–397.

Other References

Appel, G. B., and D. A. Holub. 1976. The syndrome of multiple endocrine gland deficiencies. *Am. J. Med.* **61:**129–133.

Butler, V. P., and J. P. Chen. 1967. Digitoxin specific autoantibodies. *Proc. Natl. Acad. Sci. USA* **57:**71–78.

Seeman, P. 1987. Dopamine receptors in human brain diseases, p. 233. *In* I. Creese and C. M. Fraser (ed.), *Dopamine Receptors.* Alan R. Liss, Inc., New York, N.Y.

Smolarz, A., E. Roesch, E. Lenz, H. Neubert, and P. Abshagen. 1985. Digoxin specific antibody (Fab) fragments in 34 cases of severe digitalis intoxication. *J. Toxicol. Clin. Toxicol.* **23:**327–340.

Volpe, R. 1977. The role of autoimmunity in hypoendocrine and hyperendocrine function. *Ann. Intern. Med.* **87:**86–99.

Idiotypes and Receptors (see chapter 4)

Courand, P. O., and A. D. Strosberg. 1991. Anti-idiotypic antibodies against hormone and neurotransmitter receptors. *Biochem. Soc. Trans.* **19:**147–151.

Strosberg, A. D. 1983. Anti-idiotype and anti-hormone receptor antibodies. *Springer Semin. Immunopathol.* **6:**67–78.

Wassermann, N. H., A. S. Penn, P. I. Freimuth, N. Treptow, S. Wentzel, W. L. Cleveland, and B. F. Erlanger. 1982. Anti-idiotypic route to anti-acetylcholine receptor antibodies and experimental myasthenia gravis. *Proc. Natl. Acad. Sci. USA* **79:**4810–4814.

Yavin, E., Z. Yavin, M. D. Schneider, and L. D. Kohn. 1981. Monoclonal antibodies to the thyrotropin receptor: implications for receptor structure and the action of autoantibodies in Graves disease. *Proc. Natl. Acad. Sci. USA* **78:**3180–3184.

Cause and Effect

Grabar, P. 1975. Hypothesis: auto-antibodies and immunological theories: an analytical review. *Clin. Immunopathol.* **4:**453–466.

Protective Effects of Neutralization Reactions

Tetanus

Blake, P. A., R. A. Feldman, T. M. Buchanan, G. F. Brooks, and J. V. Bennett. 1976. Serologic therapy of tetanus in the United States, 1965–1971. *JAMA* **235:**42–44.

Brooks, V. B., D. R. Curtis, and J. C. Eccles. 1955. Mode of action of tetanus toxin. *Nature* **175:**120.

Fraser, D. W. 1976. Preventing tetanus in patients with wounds. *Ann. Intern. Med.* **84:**95–97.

LaForce, F. M., L. S. Young, and J. V. Bennett. 1969. Tetanus in the United States: epidemiologic and clinical features. *N. Engl. J. Med.* **280:**569–574.

Prevots, R., R. W. Sutter, P. M. Strebel, S. L. Sochi, and S. Hadler. 1992. Tetanus surveillance—United States, 1989–1990. *Morb. Mortal. Wkly. Rep.* **41**(SS-8)**:**1–9.

Diphtheria

Romer, P. H. 1909. Über den Nachweis sehr kleiner Mengen des Diphtheriegiftes. *Z. Immunitaetsforsch.* **3:**208.

Schick, B. 1913. Die Diphtherietoxin-Hautreaktion des Menschen als Vorprobe der prophylaktischen Diphtherieheilserum Injection. *Munch. Med. Wochenschr.* **60:**2608.

Polio

Andrus, J. K., C. A. de Quadros, and J.-M. Olive. 1992. The surveillance challenge: final stages of eradication of poliomyelitis in the Americas. *Morb. Mortal. Wkly. Rep.* **41**(SS-1)**:**21–26.

Minor, P. D. 1992. The molecular biology of poliovaccines. *J. Gen. Virol.* **73:** 3065–3077.

Sabin, A. B. 1981. Paralytic poliomyelitis: old dogmas and new perspectives. *Rev. Infect. Dis.* **3:**543–564.

Salk, J., and D. Salk. 1977. Control of influenza and poliomyelitis with killed virus vaccines. *Science* **195:**834–847.

Hepatitis B

Chub-Uppakarn, S., P. Panichart, A. Theamboonlers, and Y. Poovorawan. 1998. Impact of the hepatitis B mass vaccination program in the southern part of Thailand. *Southeast Asian J. Trop. Med. Public Health* **29:**464–468.

Da Villa, G., M. Piazza, R. Iorio, L. Picciotto, P. Peluso, G. De Luca, and B. Basile. 1992. A pilot model of vaccination against hepatitis B virus suitable for mass vaccination campaigns in hyperendemic areas. *J. Med. Virol.* **36:**274–278.

Ellis, R. W. 1992. *Hepatitis B Vaccines in Clinical Practice.* Marcel Dekker, Inc., New York, N.Y.

Kato, H., K. Nakata, K. Hamasaki, D. Hida, H. Ishikawa, T. Aritomi, et al. 1999. Long-term efficacy of immunization against hepatitis B virus in infants at high-risk analyzed by polymerase chain reaction. *Vaccine* **18:**581–587.

Liljeqvist, S., and S. Stahl. 1999. Production of recombinant subunit vaccines: protein immunogens, live delivery systems and nucleic acid vaccines. *J. Biotechnol.* **73:**1–33.

Stephenne, J. 1988. Recombinant versus plasma-derived hepatitis B vaccines: issues of safety, immunogenicity and cost effectiveness. *Vaccine* **6:**299.

Viviani, S., A. Jack, A. J. Hall, N. Maine, M. Mendy, R. Montesano, and H. C. Whittle. 1999. Hepatitis B vaccination in infancy in The Gambia: protection against carriage at 9 years of age. *Vaccine* **17:**2946–2950.

Hepatitis A

Centers for Disease Control and Prevention. 1999. Prevention of hepatitis A through active or passive immunization; recommendation of the Advisory Committee on Immunization Practices. *Morb. Mortal. Wkly. Rep.* **48:**1–37.

Flehmig, B., U. Heinricy, and M. Pfisterer. 1990. Prospects for a hepatitis A virus vaccine. *Prog. Med. Virol.* **37:**56–71.

O'Connor, J. B., T. F. Imperiale, and M. E. Singer. 1999. Cost-effectiveness analysis of hepatitis; a vaccination strategy for adults. *Hepatology* **30:**1077–1081.

Siegl, G., and S. M. Lemon. 1990. Recent advances in hepatitis A vaccine development. *Virus Res.* **17:**75.

Hepatitis C

Hu, G. J., R. Y. Wang, D. S. Han, H. J. Alter, and J. W. Shih. 1999. Characterization of the humoral and cellular immune responses against hepatitis C virus core induced by DNA-based immunization. *Vaccine* **17:**3160–3170.

Hepatitis E

He, J., L. N. Binn, J. D. Caudill, L. V. Asher, C. F. Longer, and B. L. Inneis. 1999. Antiserum generated by DNA vaccine binds to hepatitis E virus (HEV) as determined by PCR and immune electron microscopy (IEM): application for HEV detection by affinity-capture RT-PCR. *Virus Res.* **62:**59–65.

Tsarev, S. A., T. S. Tsareva, S. U. Emerson, S. Govindarajan, M. Shapiro, J. L. Gerin, and R. H. Purcell. 1997. Recombinant vaccine against hepatitis E: dose response and protection against heterologous challenge. *Vaccine* **15:**1834–1838.

Cytotoxic and Cytolytic Reactions

9

Cytotoxic or cytolytic reactions occur when antibody reacts with either an antigenic component of a cell membrane or an antigen that has become intimately associated with a cell. The reaction of antibody with the cell activates two complement-mediated pathways of cell death or lysis: (i) activation of the complete cascade with insertion of membrane attack complexes and lysis of the target cell, or (ii) aggregated immunoglobulin Fc and/or C3b receptor binding produces "immune adherence" of antibody-coated cells to phagocytic cells and phagocytosis (Fig. 9.1). An additional method of immunoglobulin binding is by passive adsorption of antibody-antigen complexes formed in the bloodstream and subsequent activation of complement or formation of aggregated immunoglobulin. Antibody-mediated cytolytic reactions are protective when the affected cell is an invading organism but destructive when it occurs to an individual's own blood cells. Most destruction of affected blood cells occurs extravascularly by phagocytosis of antibody- or complement-coated cells in the spleen and liver, rather than by intravascular cell lysis. Blistering diseases of the skin are also mediated, in part, by cytolytic reactions (see chapter 16).

The Mechanism of Cytolytic Reactions

Cytotoxic or cytolytic reactions are initiated by immunoglobulin M (IgM) or those IgG immunoglobulin subclasses that have the capacity to activate complement. Selected IgG subclasses bind complement better than others, e.g., IgG3, IgG1. IgM is the most efficient complement-fixing antibody. One IgM antibody molecule reacting with a cell is sufficient to activate complement, whereas two IgG molecules in close apposition are required to produce an Fc aggregate that can bind complement. Antibodies of the IgM class are approximately 600 times more efficient in fixing complement than antibodies of the IgG class. IgG-coated erythrocytes are cleared predominantly in the spleen via Fc and C3b receptors, whereas IgM-coated cells are sequestered predominantly in the liver through C3b receptors. Clearance of IgM-coated cells is entirely complement dependent, whereas clearance of IgG-coated cells is not, since the clearing cells have receptors for aggregated Fc regions of immunoglobulins.

The ultimate clinical effect depends upon the type of cell involved, antibody characteristics, the number of antigen sites per cell, and the amount of antibody available. The cells usually affected are circulating blood cells:

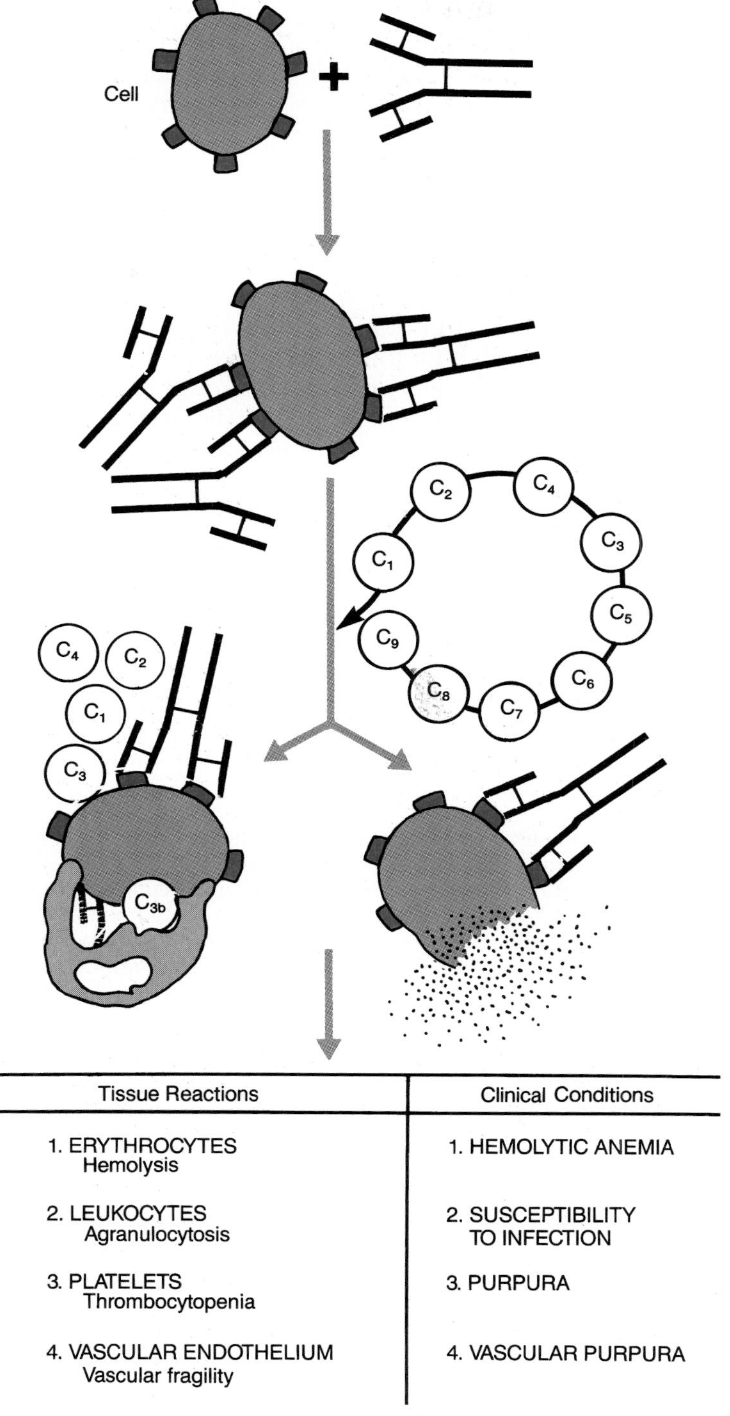

Tissue Reactions	Clinical Conditions
1. ERYTHROCYTES Hemolysis	1. HEMOLYTIC ANEMIA
2. LEUKOCYTES Agranulocytosis	2. SUSCEPTIBILITY TO INFECTION
3. PLATELETS Thrombocytopenia	3. PURPURA
4. VASCULAR ENDOTHELIUM Vascular fragility	4. VASCULAR PURPURA

Figure 9.1 Cytotoxic or cytolytic reactions. These reactions most often affect cellular elements in intimate contact with circulating plasma, such as erythrocytes, leukocytes, or platelets. Circulating humoral antibody reacts with antigens present on cell membranes. In vitro, through action of the complement system, the integrity of cell membrane is compromised and the cell is lysed. The osmotic difference in intracellular and extracellular fluids causes release of intracellular fluids. In vivo, the cells coated with immunoglobulin antibody or complement are subject to phagocytosis and sequestration in the spleen and liver.

red blood cells (RBCs, erythrocytes), white blood cells, and platelets. The resulting diseases are hemolytic anemia, agranulocytosis, and thrombocytopenia; they are grouped together as immunohematologic diseases. An experimental model of the effects of an anti-red cell antibody is illustrated in Fig. 9.2.

Immunohematologic Diseases

Erythrocytes (Anemia)

Disease conditions arising from the immune destruction of RBCs result from loss of erythrocyte function, from the damaging effects of the released cell contents, and from toxic effects due to antigen-antibody complexes formed. These disorders include transfusion reactions, erythroblastosis fetalis, acquired autoimmune hemolytic diseases (Fig. 9.3), hemolytic reactions to drugs, and some infectious diseases, such as malaria.

Transfusion Reactions

Blood group antigens are genetically controlled cell surface antigens present on blood cells. The basic structural characteristics of the ABO blood group system are presented in Fig. 9.4. An individual with blood type A has isoantibodies against type B erythrocytes. Isoantibodies are defined as antibodies to antigens within the same species. If the A individual with anti-B isoantibodies is transfused with type B blood, the anti-B antibodies coat the B erythrocytes. This coating is also called sensitization. The sensitized (antibody-coated) cells may then be lysed by complement or

Figure 9.2 Experimental model of acute hemolytic reaction. (i) Rat red blood cells (RBCs) are injected into a rabbit to produce antibodies to rat RBCs. (ii) In vitro, this antiserum will lyse rat RBCs in the presence of complement. If the antiserum is decomplemented, agglutination of the cells, but not lysis, occurs. (iii) In vivo injection of the rabbit anti-rat RBC serum into rats results in a rapid drop in the hematocrit (the percentage of the blood made up of red cells) and increasing red color in the plasma due to hemoglobin released from destroyed cells. Death of the injected rat occurs at doses sufficient to reduce the hematocrit below 20%. In the dead rat, the organs are congested with RBCs, particularly the liver and spleen.

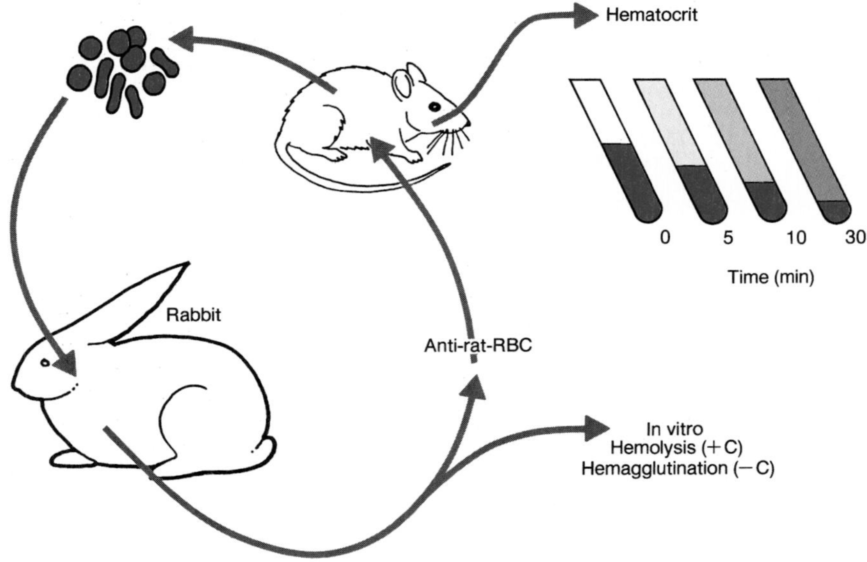

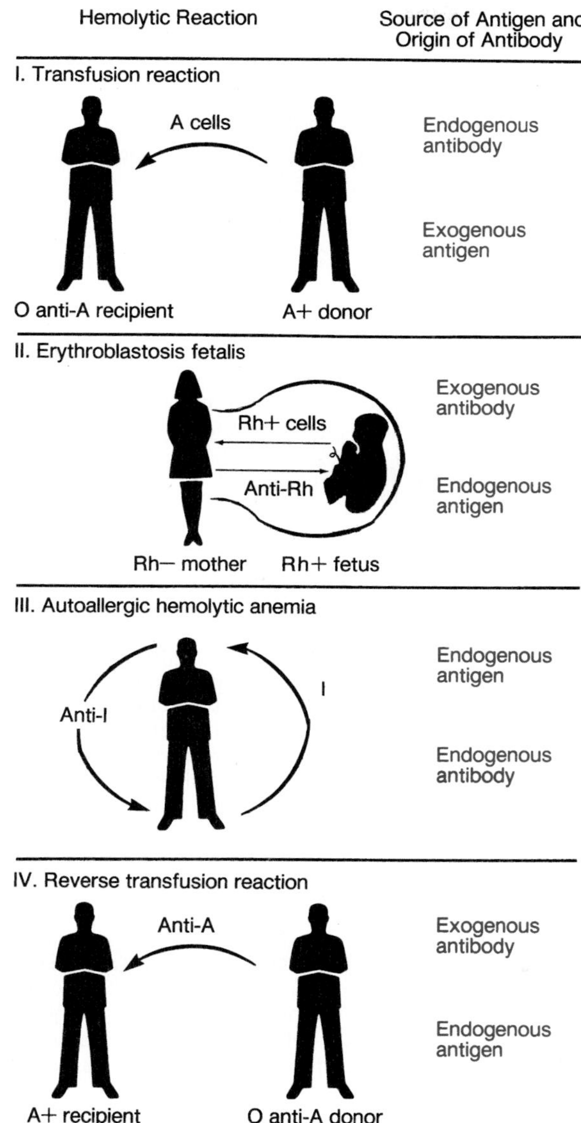

Figure 9.3 Hemolytic reactions. Shown are four types of hemolytic reactions caused by antibody-mediated complement activation in relation to the origin of the antibody and the source of the antigen. **(I)** Transfusion reactions (exogenous antigen and endogenous antibody). Erythrocytes from a donor (A+) that are antigenic for a recipient whose serum contains antibody to the donor's erythrocyte antigen (O anti-A) will be lysed upon transfusion, resulting in release of hemoglobin and a clinical syndrome known as a transfusion reaction. **(II)** Erythroblastosis fetalis (endogenous antigen and exogenous antibody). Rh^+ erythrocytes cross the placenta and stimulate the production of antibody to Rh if the mother is not Rh^+. These antibodies will cross back through the placenta to attack fetal erythrocytes. **(III)** Autoimmune hemolytic anemia (endogenous antigen and endogenous antibody). An individual becomes sensitized to the antigens of his or her own erythrocytes (autoantibody). **(IV)** Reverse transfusion reaction (endogenous antigen and exogenous antibody). Antibodies are transfused from a donor to a recipient whose red cells contain the antigen. This passively transferred antibody causes lysis of recipient red cells.

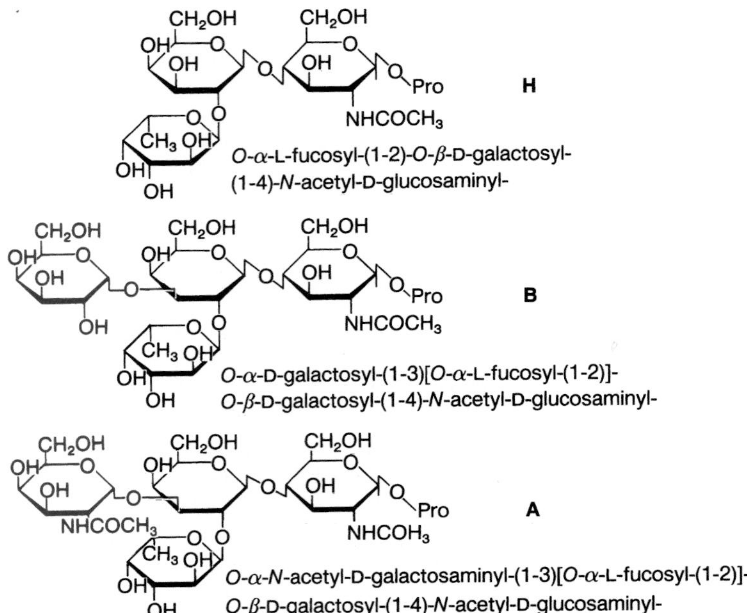

Figure 9.4 Chemistry of the ABO blood group system. ABO blood group identification depends upon the presence of carbohydrate antigenic specificities on surfaces of red cells. Blood group characteristics are inherited according to simple Mendelian laws. ABO blood group antigens have been characterized by analysis of purified blood group substances. They contain about 85% carbohydrate and 15% amino acids. The peptide component contains 15 amino acids and is the same for each blood group substance. Antigenic specificity is determined by carbohydrate structures and linkages. Individuals with type O blood who do not have A or B group specificity have a specificity now recognized as H, which consists of three sugar groups attached to a peptide. Addition of a fourth sugar group to the basic H structure produces A or B specificity. If the additional sugar is *O*-α-D-galactose, specificity is B; if it is *O*-α-*N*-acetyl-D-galactose, specificity is A. Formation of H substance is controlled by a pair of alleles, *H* and *h*. *H* gene gives rise to production of H specificity. H-active material is converted to A- or B-activate substances under the influence of galactosyl transferases determined by the *A* or *B* genes. Rare individuals lack A, B, and H reactivity, presumably because of an inability to form normal precursor for H substance. (Modified from W. M. Watkins, *Science* **152:**172, 1966.)

destroyed in the spleen. Antibodies to blood group antigens are detected in vitro by their ability to agglutinate a selected panel of red cells expressing different blood group antigens.

Immediate transfusion reactions occur when there is intravascular hemolysis due to the presence of preformed antibodies. The red cells are lysed, releasing free hemoglobin into the circulation. The free hemoglobin is bound by albumin, haptoglobin, and hemopexin or is excreted unbound into the urine. Immediate signs and symptoms are shock, fever, flushing, chest pain, difficulty breathing, hemoglobinuria, and generalized bleeding. The ABO system is responsible for about 75% of immediate fatal transfusion reactions. Death is the result of shock, disseminated intravascular coagulation, and renal failure. Extravascular hemolysis is characterized by hyperbilirubinemia from metabolized hemoglobin, elevated serum lactic acid dehydrogenase, and a falling hematocrit.

More than 14 human RBC antigen systems, which include over 60 different blood group factors, are known. The ABO and Rh systems are the most important to identify for the routine transfusion service, as these represent the majority of antibodies implicated in clinical transfusion reactions. The other antigens are less important clinically because of low antigenicity or low incompatibility frequency. Transfusion reactions are usually predictable from blood group typing, serum screening for antierythrocyte antibodies, or cross-matching. For blood typing, the red cells of an individual are tested in vitro for reaction with a panel of selected antisera that are known to react with given blood group antigens. For antibody screening, the serum of a potential recipient is tested in vitro with red cells from two or three donors who have been antigen typed and represent all of the common red cell antibodies among them. For cross-matching, the serum from a potential recipient is mixed with the cells of a potential donor. If agglutination occurs, the donor cells contain an antigen, the recipient has antibody to the antigen, and the donor cells cannot be used, even if there is no difference in ABO antigens or other detectable major blood groups. The potential for acute transfusion reactions due to the presence of preformed antibodies is easily recognized clinically and should be prevented by the appropriate cell typing, antibody screening, or cross-match testing.

In some cases, delayed transfusion reactions may occur because of induction of an immune response in the recipient to transfused cells. The transfused donor cells may survive well initially, but after 3 to 14 days, hemolysis occurs because of the production of an antibody that was not detectable at the time of the initial cross-match. This is most likely due to a secondary response in a patient previously primed but could also be due to a primary antibody response. The compatibility test relies on an agglutination end point and may, therefore, miss low concentrations of serum antibodies. Patients who receive multiple transfusions frequently develop antibodies to minor blood group antigens; the incidence of hemolytic reactions in any given individual is related to the number of previous transfusions that have been given.

Erythroblastosis Fetalis

Erythroblastosis fetalis, or hemolytic disease of the newborn, is caused by maternal antibodies that cross the placenta during the terminal stages of pregnancy and attack fetal erythrocytes. The Rh system of red cell antigens was first identified in 1939, and the first case of hemolytic disease of the newborn due to fetal-maternal Rh incompatibility was reported in 1941 by Philip Levine. The conditions for hemolytic disease exist when a pregnant woman lacks Rh antigens (Rh^-) that are present in the fetus (Rh^+) because of the contribution of paternal genes. An Rh^- mother may become sensitized to Rh^+ erythrocytes produced by the fetus. If the antibody formed by the mother crosses the placenta, it destroys the fetal erythrocytes (Fig. 9.5). Destruction of fetal erythrocytes occurs by the action of antibody and complement or by an antibody-dependent cell-mediated mechanism. Thus, RBC from infants with maternal anti-Rh may be coated with maternal antibody and killed by fetal lymphocytes or macrophages that react with the antibody on the RBC surface through Fc receptors rather than by activation of complement.

Rh antigens. The Rh antigenic system is a mosaic of genetically controlled specific antigenic determinants, which may serve as the targets for antibody from one individual to another, as in erythroblastosis fetalis or for

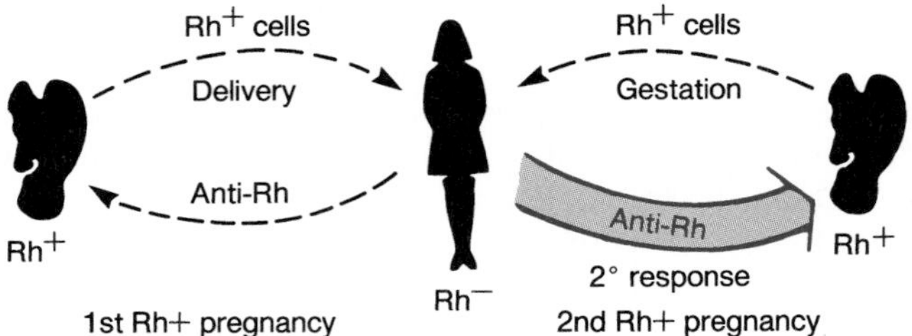

Figure 9.5 Erythroblastosis fetalis. During the first pregnancy of an Rh^- mother carrying an Rh^+ fetus, sensitization occurs during delivery when immunizing numbers of fetal RBC enter the maternal circulation. During subsequent pregnancies of a sensitized mother carrying an Rh^+ fetus, anti-Rh antibodies may cross the placenta and react with fetal RBCs. During the first pregnancy, small numbers of Rh^+ fetal erythrocytes, usually insufficient for sensitization, cross the placenta. However, at delivery, a substantial number of Rh^+ erythrocytes are released into maternal circulation. In a small percentage of Rh-incompatible pregnancies, this is sufficient to immunize the mother if the mother is not treated with passively administered anti-Rh antibody. During a second pregnancy, the small number of erythrocytes that reach the maternal circulation will induce a secondary antibody response in the mother to the Rh antigen. The maternal antibody is IgG and crosses the placenta to the fetus, where it acts on fetal erythrocytes, causing their destruction.

antibody in the same individual toward his or her own red cells (autoimmune hemolytic anemia). In the case of erythroblastosis fetalis, in which antibodies produced by the mother act on fetal red cells, the antigen is endogenous (fetal antigen) and the immune response exogenous (maternal antibody) in respect to the affected individual, the fetus. Because of the proliferation of cells by the fetus in an attempt to make up for the destruction of fetal erythrocytes in the erythrocyte series, the spleen and liver continue to contain a large number of blood-forming precursor cells (extramedullary hematopoiesis), giving rise to the name erythroblastosis fetalis. Because of the marked destruction of red cells, high concentrations of one hemoglobin breakdown product, bilirubin, during the immediate neonatal period may lead to brain damage secondary to deposition of bilirubin in the brain (kernicterus).

Prevention of Rh immunization. Hemolytic disease of the newborn is now a largely preventable disease. Prevention of immunization of Rh^- mothers carrying Rh^+ fetuses is accomplished by treating Rh^- mothers, who have just delivered an Rh^+ fetus, with passive antibody to Rh^+ antigens (Rh immune globulin). The observation that led to such a procedure was that protection against Rh immunization occurs if the fetus contains ABO blood group antigens not present in the mother (Fig. 9.6). Thus, if the blood of the fetus is A Rh^+ or B Rh^+, and the mother's blood is O Rh^-, the mother develops anti-Rh antibodies less frequently than when the blood of the fetus is O Rh^+ and that of the mother is O Rh^-, or when the blood of the fetus is A Rh^+ and the mother's is A Rh^-. The presence in the mother of antibodies to ABO group antigens on the fetal erythrocytes prevents immunization to the Rh antigens. In Rh incompatibility, fetal erythrocytes usually appear in the circulation of the mother in sufficient numbers to stimulate antibody production at the time of delivery, and this is the time most Rh^- mothers first become sensitized by Rh^+ fetal cells. Because of the possibility that such sensitization could be prevented by passive transfer of anti-Rh antisera to Rh^- mothers, trials were made on Rh^-

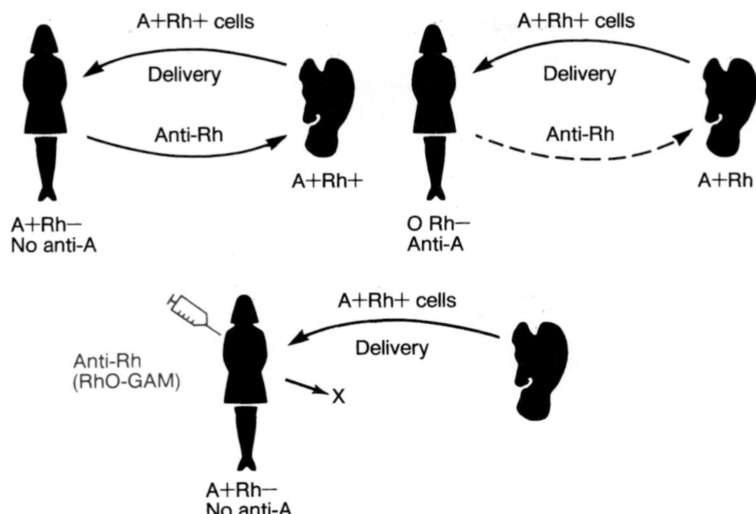

Figure 9.6 Prevention of Rh immunization by passive antibody. **(Top)** Naturally occurring situation when an ABO and Rh incompatibility are combined; sensitization of the mother to Rh^+ antigens is significantly less than when there is an Rh incompatibility but no ABO incompatibility. The presence of antibody to fetal red cell A^+ antigen in the non-A mother prevents sensitization to the Rh^+ antigen, whereas the mother with no anti-A becomes sensitized to the Rh system. This observation was used as a rationale for passively transferring antibody to Rh to mothers who were Rh^- and were carrying an Rh^+ fetus. **(Bottom)** Administration of anti-Rh at delivery significantly reduces the incidence of sensitization of the mother to the Rh system; erythroblastosis fetalis has thus become a preventable disease through the application of immunoprophylaxis.

male volunteers. Passive transfer of anti-Rh serum along with Rh^+ cells prevented immunization of these volunteers. Now adapted as a required procedure, the incidence of Rh immunization in subsequent pregnancies has been greatly reduced by the passive transfer of anti-Rh sera (or globulin) to an Rh^- mother at the time of delivery of an Rh^+ fetus. This prevention of an immune-mediated disease is considered by many to be one of the most important contributions of immunology to the prevention of human disease.

In addition, since sensitization may occur after spontaneous or therapeutic abortion of an Rh^+ fetus in an Rh^- mother, anti-Rh^+ globulin should also be administered after abortion of an Rh^+ fetus in an Rh^- mother. Rare cases of sensitization may still occur, such as by the inadvertent transfusion of Rh^+ blood to an Rh^- woman and, in a small number of instances, when sensitization occurs before delivery. Antepartum administration of anti-Rh serum can even prevent those rare cases that are due to in utero sensitization of Rh^- mothers by Rh^+ babies before delivery. An interesting relationship is that of the Rh type of the grandmother to Rh sensitization. An increased incidence of sensitization is seen when the grandmother is Rh^+, the mother is Rh^-, and the fetus is Rh^+ (about one in six mothers with this relationship will become sensitized). It appears that the Rh^- mother may be primed or sensitized by Rh^+ erythrocytes that crossed from the grandmother when the mother was a fetus, so that when she is exposed to Rh^+ cells, there is a more rapid and intense response.

Treatment of erythroblastosis fetalis. In cases where Rh sensitization has occurred, the affected fetus may be treated by intrauterine transfusion of Rh^- blood cells. Since the transfused blood does not have the Rh antigen, the erythrocytes will not be destroyed by maternal antibodies. However, this procedure has a high rate of complications and must be done only after amniocentesis and analysis of amniotic fluid by optical density to determine the severity of the hemolytic process. Fluoroscopic and ultrasound examination of the fetal position are required to place the transfusion needle in the fetal abdomen. The transfused red cells eventually transverse the peritoneum and enter the fetal circulation. In less severe cases, the patient may be followed and transfusions delayed until after birth (exchange transfusion). Exchange transfusions are usually done to remove bilirubin and prevent kernicterus. If the fetal age is sufficient, labor is induced, since the risks of prematurity are less than the risk of intrauterine transfusion.

ABO hemolytic disease of the newborn. ABO hemolytic disease of the newborn is usually mild to minimal clinically, even if the mother's blood contains high titers of anti-A or anti-B antibodies and the fetus's blood is A, B, or AB. This may be due to three reasons: (i) anti-A–anti-B antibodies are usually IgM and therefore do not cross the placenta; (ii) ABO blood group antigens are widely distributed in the fetal tissues and the placenta, so the effect upon fetal erythrocytes of any 7S anti-A or anti-B antibodies that may cross the placenta is diluted out because the antibodies react with many other tissue sites; and (iii) ABO blood group carbohydrates are not fully expressed on fetal erythrocytes. In contrast, the Rh specificity is unique for erythrocytes, and the effect of anti-Rh antibodies that cross the placenta is concentrated on the fetal erythrocytes that have fully developed Rh antigens.

Acquired Autoimmune Hemolytic Disorders

Acquired autoimmune hemolytic disorders are caused by formation of antibodies to antigens present on the affected individual's own erythrocytes. Autoimmune hemolytic anemia (AIHA) can be differentiated from congenital metabolic hemolytic disorders by careful testing. The major difference between immune and congenital hemolytic diseases is that in the latter, the erythrocytes are congenitally defective and do not survive normally in either the patient or a "normal" individual. In contrast, the erythrocytes are normal in patients with immune hemolytic disease and survive better in a "normal" recipient than in the patient. Therefore, congenital disease demonstrates an intracorpuscular defect, and immune disease demonstrates an extracorpuscular defect. The extracorpuscular defect is an autoantibody. Intravenous infusions of immunoglobulin may produce rapid reversal of acute hemolytic episodes by blocking macrophage Fc receptors, and patients maintained on long-term immunoglobulin treatment may be prevented from having additional hemolytic attacks. There are two major forms of hemolytic disease caused by autoantibodies to red cells: warm antibody mediated and cold antibody mediated, with rare patients having features of both. In a study of 1,834 patients with AIHA, 1,051 were idiopathic, and the rest were associated with a variety of other diseases, including cancer, infections, other autoimmune diseases, and other diseases.

Warm antibody disease. Warm antibody disease is almost always caused by IgG antibody that reacts with the patient's red cells. In two-thirds of the cases, the antibody reacts with Rh determinants. The antibody may appear without a known cause (idiopathic) but more frequently is associated with a collagen disease (lupus erythematosus) or with a lymphoproliferative disorder, e.g., chronic lymphocytic leukemia. The patient's erythrocytes may be coated in vivo with IgG antibody, IgG and complement, or complement alone, when tested by the Coombs' technique (see below). The action of antibody and complement leads to destruction of the erythrocytes (hemolytic anemia), mostly after phagocytosis by reticuloendothelial cells, which have receptors that bind the Fc region of IgG and C3b coating RBCs. During active anemia, the spleen or liver sinusoids may be filled with red cells. Frank intravascular hemolysis by the complete complement sequence may also be observed. Treatment with corticosteroids may abort life-threatening acute hemolytic episodes. Steroids are believed to have at least three possible effects on AIHA: (i) decreased affinity of Fc receptor binding, (ii) decreased phagocytic activity of the reticuloendothelial system, and (iii) decreased antibody production. Splenectomy is of some temporary value, but usually the anemia recurs even after the spleen is removed, indicating that the reticuloendothelial cells of other organs, e.g., liver, can cause destruction of RBCs. The reason for the production of the autoantibody is not clear.

Cold antibody disease. Cold antibody disease is usually caused by antibodies of the IgM class that may react not only with RBCs but also with other blood cells. Cold reactive antibodies are usually found in patients with a viral infection or a lymphoproliferative disease. Cold antibody hemolytic disease occurs in two forms: cold agglutinin disease and paroxysmal cold hemoglobinuria. In these disorders, the anti-erythrocytic antibody is not capable of binding to the red cell at 37°C but will do so at lower temperatures. When cells are coated by antibody in the cooler peripheral circulation and then warmed to core body temperature, complement components bind to the cell membrane, and the cells are susceptible to lysis. At warm temperatures, the antibody comes off the cell, so complement may be detected on the affected cells in the absence of antibody. Hemolytic attacks occur on exposure to cold. The cold antibody binds to cells in the exposed areas of the body (skin). These cells are coated with complement and are destroyed on entering the bloodstream of warmer parts of the body.

Paroxysmal cold hemoglobinuria. Paroxysmal cold hemoglobinuria refers to the production of dark urine after exposure to the cold because of the presence of hemoglobin from lysed red cells. The antibody responsible was first recognized in 1904 and is referred to as Donath-Landsteiner antibody. Demonstration of the antibody requires two steps: first, the patient's serum is mixed with erythrocytes at 4°C; then, the mixture is then warmed to 37°C, and lysis occurs upon warming. This type of antibody was classically found in patients with syphilis but may occur idiopathically or after a viral infection. The antibody is of the IgG class, and the specificity is usually to blood group P.

Cold agglutinin disease. Cold agglutinin disease is similar to paroxysmal cold hemoglobinuria, but intense agglutination of red cells occurs in the cold, which is not the case with Donath-Landsteiner antibody. The antibody is a monoclonal or polyclonal IgM and is directed to the blood group

I specificity. Mycoplasma infections have been associated with polyclonal anti-I formation, whereas monoclonal antibodies occur in lymphoproliferative diseases. Most patients with cold antibody hemolytic disease do well as long as they are kept warm and tolerate a chronic mild anemia with minimal disability. In fact, low titers of cold antibody are found in most normal adults and cause no apparent symptoms.

Hemolytic Reactions to Drugs

Hemolytic reactions to drugs may be activated by at least five mechanisms (Fig. 9.7).

Hapten adherence. Many drugs adhere to red cells and function as haptens. As such, the red cell-hapten complex induces an immune response, and cytotoxic reactions to the red cell or red cell-drug complex may occur. The exact mechanism of such a drug-induced hemolytic reaction depends upon the drug involved. *Penicillin* covalently binds to red cells, and the antibody formed reacts with the penicillin bound to the cell. Immunoglobulin can be demonstrated on the surface of affected cells by the direct Coombs' test. If the antibody is extracted from the red cell membrane, it will react only with cells preincubated with penicillin in an indirect Coombs' test.

Immune-complex adsorption. *Quinidine* administration can result in quinidine-antibody complexes that bind loosely to red cells. Antibody-quinidine complexes can dissociate from red cell surfaces and in complex form pass from one red cell to another. Destruction of red cells occurs as an "innocent bystander" reaction. Components of complement may be demonstrated on the affected cells in the absence of detectable antibody globulin.

Autoimmunity. *α-Methyl dopa* (aldomet) apparently induces alterations in lymphocytes so that the lymphocytes become "autoreactive." The antibody produced reacts with the patient's own red cells in the absence of bound drug. Normal erythrocytes are destroyed during a hemolytic drug reaction owing to aldomet or quinidine, because the autoantibody of the antigen-antibody complex can bind to any RBC. In cases of hemolytic reactions to penicillin or quinidine, red cell destruction ceases soon after administration of the drug is stopped; α-methyl dopa hemolytic reactions may persist for as long as a year after the drug is stopped. In hemolytic reactions to quinidine and penicillin, the source of the antigen is exogenous (or a complex of exogenous hapten and host red cell), and the origin of the allergic response is endogenous. In hemolytic anemia due to α-methyl dopa, the antigen is endogenous, and the origin of the allergic response is endogenous.

Complement transfer. During severe reactions, complement activated by reaction of antibodies to drugs on one cell may be passed into the fluid phase and bind to a second cell, leading to opsonization. Usually, activated complement components released into the fluid phase are rapidly inactivated in the blood. However, if large amounts of activated components are formed, transfer from one cell to another may occur.

Nonspecific adsorption of proteins. Cephalosporins alter the red cell membrane in a way that allows nonspecific protein absorption. Thus,

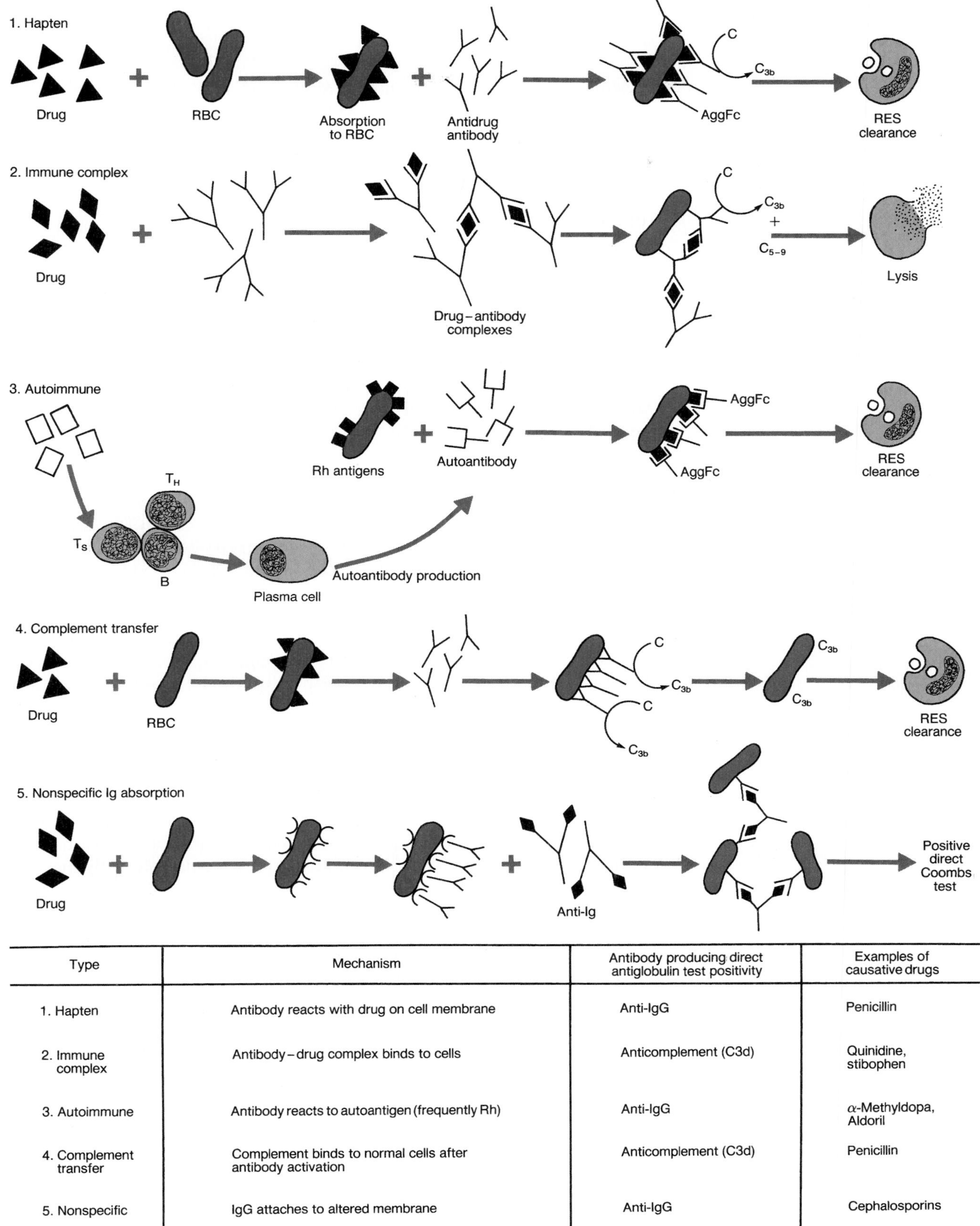

Type	Mechanism	Antibody producing direct antiglobulin test positivity	Examples of causative drugs
1. Hapten	Antibody reacts with drug on cell membrane	Anti-IgG	Penicillin
2. Immune complex	Antibody–drug complex binds to cells	Anticomplement (C3d)	Quinidine, stibophen
3. Autoimmune	Antibody reacts to autoantigen (frequently Rh)	Anti-IgG	α-Methyldopa, Aldoril
4. Complement transfer	Complement binds to normal cells after antibody activation	Anticomplement (C3d)	Penicillin
5. Nonspecific	IgG attaches to altered membrane	Anti-IgG	Cephalosporins

Figure 9.7 Mechanisms of drug-induced hemolytic drug reactions. (See text for details.)

patients receiving cephalosporins may have a positive Coombs' test without hemolytic anemia. In addition, patients on dialysis may have positive direct Coombs' tests because of anti-formaldehyde antibodies used to sterilize reusable dialysis equipment, owing to the absorption of formaldehyde to the red cells during dialysis.

Leukocytes (Agranulocytosis)

Antibody effects similar to those described above for erythrocytes may also occur with polymorphonuclear leukocytes, resulting in loss of neutrophils (neutropenia or agranulocytosis). Most cases of agranulocytosis are secondary to a lack of proliferation of granulocytes in the bone marrow on a nonimmune basis, either congenital or drug-induced. Autoimmune neutropenia (AIN) accounts for about 10% of clinically recognized neutropenia. Two major forms of AIN are primary and secondary. Primary AIN is seen in children under 3 years of age. Secondary AIN occurs with the highest frequency in adults between 40 and 60 years of age and is usually associated with autoimmune thrombocytopenia, connective tissue disease, or lymphoma. Antibodies to granulocytes in AIN are detected by immunofluorescence or agglutination. The bone marrow is usually normal or hypercellular, with a 50% reduction in mature neutrophils. The peripheral blood shows neutrophil counts around 250 cells/μl (leukopenia is defined as a reduction in the number of circulating white blood cells below 4,000/μl). At this level, patients have bacterial infections of the skin, upper respiratory tract, and middle ear. Antibiotic treatment is usually effective. Spontaneous remissions occur in most patients, and immune globulin or steroids may induce remission in prolonged cases. More recently, hematopoietic growth factors have been shown to be effective in treating leukopenia. Granulocyte colony-stimulating factor (G-CSF) is effective for autoimmune leukopenia, whereas drug-associated neutropenia responds to granulocyte-macrophage CSF (GM-CSF).

Neonatal Leukopenia (Alloimmune Neonatal Neutropenia)

Low white cell counts in a neonate may be caused by destruction of fetal white blood cells coated by antibodies that cross the placenta from the mother after immunization of the mother to fetal leukocyte antigens. The neutrophil-specific antigens are pleomorphic (at least eight have been identified) and may also be targets for AIN in infants and chronic idiopathic neutropenia in adults. Two antigens that have been identified as being associated with alloimmune neonatal neutropenia, NA1 and NA2, are located on the neutrophil Fcγ receptor III (FcγRIII). The mothers of these infants, otherwise normal, have granulocytes that lack FcγRIII.

Drug-Induced Agranulocytosis

Destruction of a patient's own white blood cells may be caused by autoantibodies or by antibodies to certain drugs that adhere to white blood cells and function as haptens. Sulfapyridine and aminopyrine are two of the drugs that have been implicated.

The consequence of leukocyte destruction is a decreased ability to defend against infection. In some situations, drugs may have a direct nonimmune cytotoxic effect (idiosyncrasy), and some cases of agranulocytosis are caused by a congenital metabolic defect (see "Immune Suppression of Blood Cell Production" below). In nonimmune agranulocytosis, more than one line of leukocyte is usually involved; for instance, in some cases, all leukocytes containing granules are destroyed or fail to develop. Antibodies to lymphocytes are found in patients with a variety of human diseases, particularly AIDS, and may be associated with lymphocyte deficiencies.

Platelets

Immune reactions to platelets may cause destruction of platelets, with resulting purpura and other hemorrhagic manifestations. The word *purpura* (purple) describes hemorrhage into the skin and is easily recognized by the red or purple spot produced by the presence of extravasated red cells. The color is first red but becomes darker (purple) and fades to a brownish yellow as the red cells are destroyed or cleared from the site of hemorrhage by macrophages. Since platelets function to prevent such hemorrhages, a loss of platelets permits purpuric lesions to develop. An anti-platelet antibody can be demonstrated in about 60% of the affected individuals. In some diseases, antigen-antibody complexes cause thrombocytopenia. Standard immunological tests such as agglutination or complement fixation usually do not detect antibodies to platelets, but antibodies are detected in many cases of thrombocytopenia by nonstandard tests, such as phagocytosis of antibody-coated platelets, lymphocyte activation by platelet-antibody complexes, competitive binding radioimmunoassays, enzyme-linked immunosorbent assays, and labeled Coombs' antiglobulin tests. Thrombocytopenia may also occur congenitally or secondarily because of increased splenic function (hypersplenism) or other nonimmune platelet consumptive disorders.

Posttransfusion Thrombocytopenic Purpura

Purpura after transfusion occurs as a result of the production of alloantibodies after transfusions of blood products containing allogeneic platelets. The cause of autologous platelet destruction is unclear. This reaction is very rare. It presents as an acute, severe thrombocytopenia occurring about 1 week after a transfusion. Antibodies to the platelet antigen Pl^{A1} are invariably found; rarely, other platelet antibody specificities have been implicated. Treatment consists of plasma exchange. This reaction is essentially seen only in women who have been pregnant, suggesting that sensitization may originally occur to platelet antigens from a fetus.

Neonatal Alloimmune Thrombocytopenia

Neonatal alloimmune thrombocytopenia (NAIT) occurs as a result of maternal IgG antibody to fetal platelet antigens contributed by the father, with thrombocytopenia occurring in the fetus when this antibody crosses the placenta. Most cases (50 to 90%) are due to antibodies to platelet antigen Pl^{A1}, but at least five other platelet antigens have been implicated. The placentally transferred antibodies affect platelets in a way analogous to the effect of anti-Rh on RBCs in hemolytic disease of the newborn. Although uncommon, bleeding may be severe, with intracranial hemorrhage and permanent neurological damage. Platelet transfusions may be very beneficial when the platelet count is very low, and at-risk pregnancies may be treated prophylactically by small weekly transfusions of antigen-negative platelets. NAIT can be distinguished from autoimmune neonatal thrombocytopenia by detection of normal levels of platelet-bound IgG on maternal platelets in NAIT.

Idiopathic Thrombocytopenic Purpura

Acute idiopathic thrombocytopenic purpura (ITP) is more common in children than in adults. Most affected individuals have a history of infection (e.g., rubella) occurring 1 to 2 weeks previously. The destruction of platelets may be due to antibodies to antigens of infectious agents adherent to platelets, to antibody-antigen complexes adsorbed to platelets (innocent bystander), or to antibodies to platelets altered by the infectious process. Platelets are destroyed rapidly when transfused into an affected individual. Chronic ITP is caused by the production of autoantibodies against altered or naturally occurring platelet antigens and is more common in adults. The chronic form is frequently associated with systemic lupus erythematosus or a lymphoproliferative disorder (leukemia, myeloma).

Quinidine (Sedormid) Purpura

Quinidine purpura is an example of a reaction to a drug acting as a hapten on the platelet surface.

Treatment with Intravenous Immunoglobulin

Children with moderate thrombocytopenia should be followed by observation only, as spontaneous remission is common. In the early 1980s, it was discovered that intravenous immunoglobulin (IVIgG) was effective in treating more severe immune thrombocytopenia. Although at least five different mechanisms have been suggested, the most important are nonspecific blockade of the Fc receptor-mediated phagocytosis of platelets and suppression of inflammatory responses. Administration of IVIgG rapidly induces FcR blockade and a reduction in immunoglobulin production, perhaps by a feedback mechanism. The mechanism of the immunosuppression is not clear. Clinically, injection of 0.4 g/kg for 3 to 5 days is effective in reversing purpura associated with transfusion, alloimmune purpura, and ITP in pregnancy. Adults tend to have more persistent symptomatic thrombocytopenia, and splenectomy is the treatment of choice for adults with refractory ITP. Patients who do not respond to splenectomy may benefit from treatment with vincristine or steroid therapy, but high-dose steroids should be avoided.

Immune Suppression of Blood Cell Production

Aplastic anemia is a general term for failure of the bone marrow to produce blood cells. This condition is associated with virus infections, drugs, or pregnancy. The cause is not known but is believed to be due to "stem cell failure." A suspected role for immunity is supported by the fact that aplastic anemia may respond to immunosuppression. However, the sera of most affected patients do not inhibit blood cell formation but actually stimulate normal colony formation. It appears that aplastic anemia is a genetically determined "premalignant" abnormality of blood-forming cells. An immune reaction does occur to the abnormal cells, but not to normal cells. If the immune reaction is strong, the abnormal cells are eliminated, and acute severe aplasia results. If the immune response is weak, abnormal blood cell formation leads to a condition known as "myelodysplasia" with chronic pancytopenia. Immunosuppression does not cure the disease but leaves the patient with a fragile hematopoietic system which is prone to malignant transformation.

On the other hand, antibody to blood cell precursors may injure proliferating cells in the bone marrow, producing an aplastic anemia or agranulocytosis. Hematopoietic stem cells may have a variety of cell surface antigens, and cells in the erythrocyte, granulocyte, or lymphocyte line may carry differentiation antigens unique for the line. Thus, immune suppression may affect all cell lines or one cell line. Antibodies to stem cells have rarely been found spontaneously in humans. Such antibodies to red or white cell precursors have been found associated with aplastic anemia, red cell aplasia, profound panleukopenia, and systemic lupus erythematosus. Thus, although rare, antibodies to blood cell precursors may produce a clinical picture similar to that of a metabolic defect in blood cell maturation (see also chapter 8). Growth factors such as G-CSF, GM-CSF, interleukin-3, and interleukin-6 may be effective treatments.

Cytolytic Skin Diseases

The pathogenic role of antibody-mediated skin diseases is described in chapter 16. The diseases include the following.

1. *Dermatitis herpetiformis and gluten-sensitive enteropathy* (sprue, or celiac disease), a blistering skin lesion with deposition of IgA and complement in microfibers in the dermal papillae. In addition, some patients have a bandlike granular deposition of IgA and complement in the dermal papillae along the epidermal basement membrane. IgA activates complement by the alternate pathway, and C3 is regularly found in areas of IgA deposition.
2. *Herpes gestationis,* a rare, blistering, skin disease associated with pregnancy and the postpartum period. C3 and properdin have been identified in the epidermal basement membrane, indicating that the alternate pathway of complement is activated.
3. *Epidermolysis bullosa acquisita,* characterized by blisters and extreme fragility of the skin due to subepidermal bullae similar in appearance to bullous pemphigoid. The autoantibody in this disease is directed to type VII procollagen (anchoring fibrils).
4. Some forms of *lupus erythematosus,* in which immunoglobulin and complement are found in the walls of blood vessels and at the dermal-epidermal junction.
5. *Vitiligo,* sharply delineated patches of depigmentation of the skin associated with autoantibodies to melanin.
6. *Alopecia,* a loss of hair found with an antibody that reacts with the capillary endothelium of the hair bulb.

Other Cytotoxic Reactions

Sperm

Autologous or allogeneic sperm is antigenic when injected into adults, and such immunization may decrease fertility in both females and males. Sperm antibodies are detected by binding assays and by their ability to agglutinate or immobilize sperm after inactivating complement in the serum by heating. The immobilizing sperm antigens are carbohydrates related to blood group antigens, having two or three repetitive Gal-Glu-NAc structures substituted with sialic acid at a terminal Gal. Sperm antibodies may prevent fertilization by decreasing motility, by inhibiting migration through female genital secretions, or by blocking fusion of the gametes. Antibodies to sperm may occur in men who have had a vasectomy because of extravasation of immunogenic sperm, and these antibodies may affect fertility after reanastamosis of the spermatic cord (vasovasostomy), despite an adequate postoperative sperm count. Anti-sperm antibodies are found more frequently in prostitutes than in normal age-matched control women. Women with sperm-immobilizing antibodies are frequently infertile and may require in vitro fertilization and embryo transfer to conceive. Intentional sperm immunization of women as a method for controlling pregnancy is possible but has not been considered practical because of possible deleterious effects of producing autoimmune reactions. Immunization of female animals with lactate dehydrogenase from testes produces highly specific antibodies and suppression of fertility.

Autoimmune Diseases

Cytotoxic antibody may produce damage in allergic thyroiditis, allergic aspermatogenesis, and other autoimmune diseases, although it is generally believed that the primary mechanism of these diseases is cell-mediated immunity. Antibody-dependent cell-mediated reactions may also be involved.

Homograft Rejection

In the 1950s, Chandler Stetson showed that specific antisera injected into a graft site may cause an acute "white" graft rejection. Although homograft rejection is usually mediated by sensitized cells (delayed sensitivity), antibody-mediated acute rejection is now recognized. Chronic graft rejection is caused by inflammation of the vessel lumen following activation of complement (see chapter 10).

Detection of Circulating Cytotoxic Antibodies

Passive Transfer (In Vivo)

The effect of the antibody may be produced by passive transfer of serum-containing antibody into a normal recipient. If this antibody is associated with cellular injury, e.g., platelet destruction in ITP, a specific cytopenia may develop.

Coombs' Test (In Vitro)

Antibody to blood cells is detected in vitro by the ability of a serum to agglutinate or lyse the target cells. In some cases, antibody does not result in agglutination unless a second antibody is added. Such nonagglutinating antibodies are termed incomplete. Incomplete antibody in serum is detected by the indirect Coombs' test; incomplete antibody already on cells is detected by the direct Coombs' test. In the *direct Coombs' test,* target cells are already coated with incomplete antibody and/or complement. The addition of an antiserum containing antibodies directed against immunoglobulin or complement components then causes agglutination of the target cells. Thus, human Rh^+ erythrocytes coated with incomplete anti-Rh antibody agglutinate when sheep anti-human immunoglobulin serum is added. For the *indirect Coombs' test,* serum containing incomplete antibody is added to uncoated target cells so that the antibody will bind to the test cells. The antibody-coated cells are then agglutinated by the addition of anti-immunoglobulin (second antibody). For detection of anti-Rh in serum, human Rh^+ cells are added to human serum containing incomplete anti-Rh antibodies. These sensitized cells are agglutinated by sheep anti-human immunoglobulin serum (Fig. 9.8). In suspected Rh hemolytic disease of the newborn, both the direct and the indirect Coombs' tests must

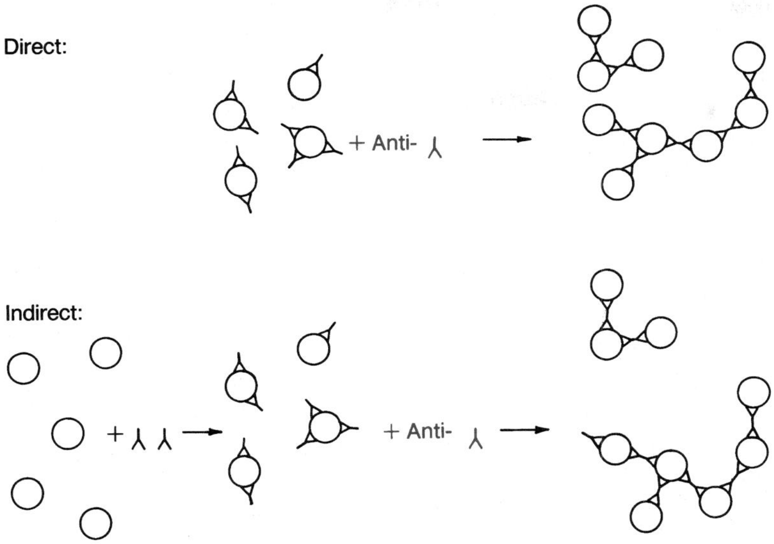

Direct:

Indirect:

Figure 9.8 Coombs' antiglobulin tests. Coombs' test for incomplete antibody to erythrocytes is carried out in two forms: direct and indirect. In the direct test, cells taken from the patient are coated with antibody in vivo and are agglutinated by the addition of anti-Ig, which reacts with the antibodies coating the cells. In the indirect test, the patient's serum contains free antibody that binds to but does not agglutinate erythrocytes added in vitro. Agglutination is accomplished by addition of a second antibody, which reacts with the first antibody (anti-Ig).

be done to rule out the presence of incomplete Rh antibodies. The direct test is usually positive for fetal erythrocytes coated with maternal anti-Rh, when free antibody is not present in the fetal serum. On the other hand, the mother's serum may contain anti-Rh antibody detectable by the indirect test; maternal serum added to fetal cells results in coating of the fetal Rh^+ cells, which are then agglutinable by antibody to human IgG. The direct Coombs' test may also be used to reveal agglutination of a patient's own cells in acquired hemolytic anemia, thus demonstrating an incomplete autoantibody.

Protective and Pathologic Effects in Infectious Diseases

The role of cytotoxic reactions in protection against bacterial infections in relation to other immune effector mechanisms is presented in more detail in chapter 15.

Malaria

During the Middle Ages, the disease malaria was named because it was attributed to bad air *(malaria)* (Torti, 1753). It is now known that malaria is caused by infection with one or more of the species of *Plasmodium* organisms. Hippocrates first recognized different types of malaria by different periods of fever. The periodic release of organisms from infected liver cells produces characteristic "cycles" of fever caused by the immune response to the released organisms. There are cyclic differences in three species of malarial parasites: *Plasmodium vivax* and *Plasmodium ovale* cause 48-h cycles; *Plasmodium malariae* causes 72-h cycles. The role of immune mechanisms in the protection against and pathogenesis of malaria is complex and includes T-cytotoxic cells (T_{CTL} cells), T-delayed-type hypersensitivity cells (T_{DTH} cells), and IgG or IgM antibodies. Both circulating antibodies and T_{CTL} cells appear to play an important role in controlling the infection through the activation of cytotoxicity directed against the infected host cells (Fig. 9.9 and 9.10).

In areas where malaria is endemic, natives develop resistance. Neonates in areas of endemicity are resistant as a result of placentally transferred maternal immunity. A peak of susceptibility occurs at about 1 year of age. However, infection at this age is less severe than in persons who first contract infection as adults. In addition, individuals of African descent lacking the Duffy blood group antigen Fy(a^-b^-) are resistant to *P. vivax* because the Duffy surface protein is required for merozoite penetration of erythrocytes. Intracellular proliferation of the *Plasmodium falciparum* malarial parasite is inhibited by sickle cell hemoglobin and is restricted in red cells with fetal hemoglobin, which persists after birth in individuals heterozygous for β-thalassemia. The red cells of the mild forms of thalassemia express higher levels of malarial antigens than do normal red cells, rendering the infected cells more susceptible to destruction by antibody, complement, and phagocytosis by neutrophils. These relationships most likely explain the genetic persistence of the lack of the Duffy blood group and the otherwise undesirable sickle cell and β-thalassemia genetic traits. The sickle cell gene and β-thalassemia are widely prevalent in areas of Africa where falciparian malaria is endemic. Even though effective innate and adaptive immunity occurs in malaria infections, it is estimated that more than 200 million people are infected worldwide and between 1 million and 2 million people per year die from complications of malarial infections.

The bite of an infected mosquito results in inoculation of hundreds to thousands of sporozoites into the bloodstream. Within minutes, the sporozoites are cleared from the bloodstream, with many going to the liver. The sporozoites invade into liver cells and develop into merozoites within a few days or a week. Thousands of merozoites are released from infected hepatocytes and begin the blood stage of the disease. The infection can be interrupted by antibody to sporozoites if present in high titer at the time of inoculation, or by antibody to merozoite antigens that present on the parasite surface or the newly infected blood cells. Protective immunity most correlates with titers of IgG antibody. However, T_{CTL} cells that recognize antigens of the sporozoites expressed on infected liver cells may destroy the infected cells before mature merozoites are released. T_{DTH} cells may also be protective, at least in some experimental models.

T_{CTL} cells are induced by endogenous presentation of sporozoite antigens in association with class I major histocompatibility complex (MHC) antigens on infected liver cells. Upon infection of liver cells, the parasites develop within a vacuole inside the hepatocyte that prevents release of malaria antigens into the cytoplasm; thus, exogenous processing of antigen cannot take place. However, the important sporozoite antigen, the circumsporate protein, is a cell surface protein that is shed into the hepatocyte during infection and appears on the surface complexed to class I MHC antigens normally expressed by the hepatocyte (Fig. 9.10). Presentation of circumsporate antigens in the form of recombinants with intracellular bacteria, such as *Salmonella,* induces $CD8^+$ T_{CTL} cells and may be a way to induce protective immunity to malaria.

After the hepatocyte phase, malaria organisms exist within erythrocytes during an established infection. Some of the major manifestations of

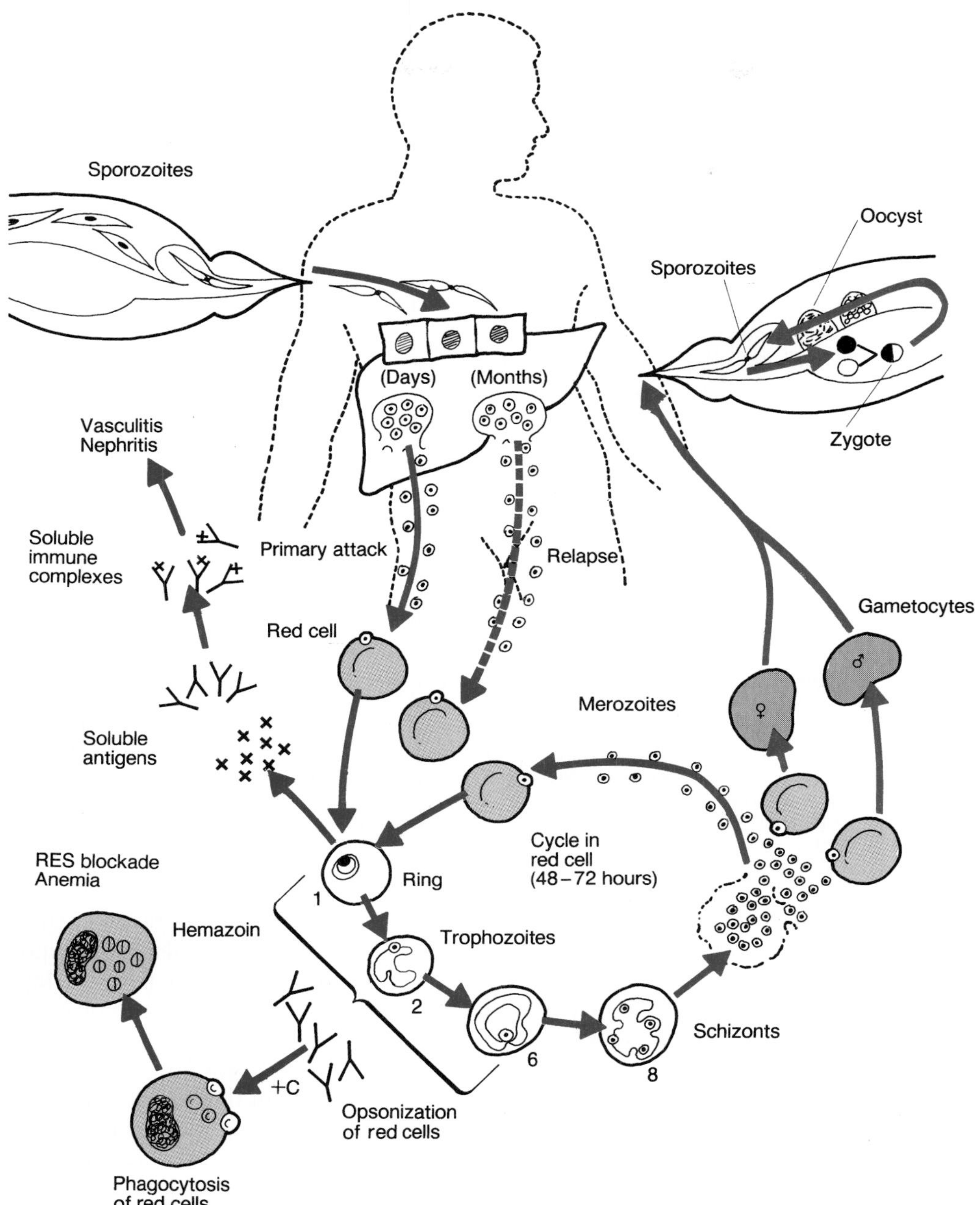

Figure 9.9 Immune mechanisms in malaria. Malaria is transmitted from the salivary glands of a mosquito to the blood of an animal by sporozoites that enter host liver cells and develop into intracellular stages. Merozoites are released into the circulation and reinfect other liver cells and RBCs. Micro- and macrogametes are produced and are taken up by mosquitoes, where they develop after fusion of micro- and macrogametes and formation of an oocyst in the stomach into sporozoites. Malaria antigens are found not only in organisms but also on the surface of infected cells. Antibodies to these antigens are able to lyse organisms or infected cells, producing anemia or liver cell necrosis. Soluble antibody-antigen complexes formed may produce immune complex lesions (glomerulonephritis). The production of large numbers of opsonized red cells and particulate antigen results in accumulation of phagocytosed material in macrophages (hemozoin pigment), reticuloendothelial blockade, and immune dysfunction. Malarial organisms are able to change antigens expressed on the cell surface, avoid destruction by antibody, and set up another cycle of infection (antigenic variation). Protective immunity may be effected by antibodies to sporozoites, which prevent infection. Protective immunity could be mediated by antibody directed to extracellular stages [(i) sporozoites, (ii) merozoites, or (iii) zygotes] or by T_{CTL} cells directed to infected hepatocytes.

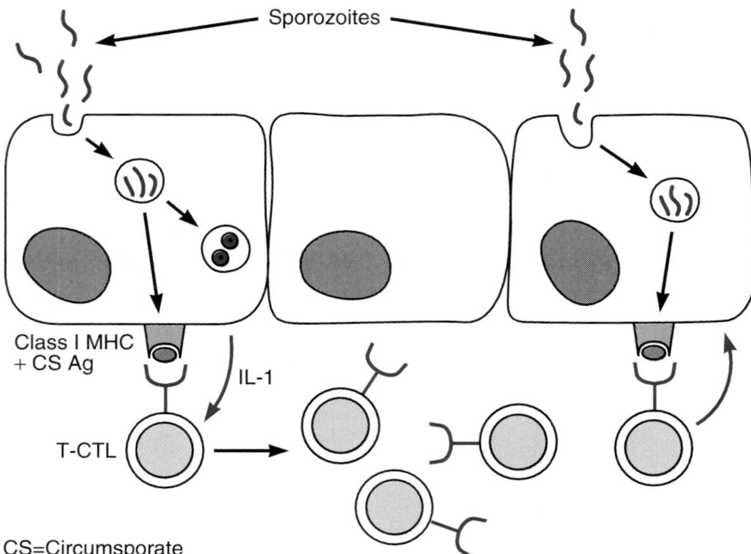

Figure 9.10 T_{CTL}-cell immunity in malaria. Sporozoite antigen is presented to T_{CTL}-cell precursors complexed to class I major histocompatibility complex cell surface markers on infected hepatocytes, leading to the proliferation of a population of T_{CTL} cells that can recognize and destroy hepatocytes expressing sporozoite antigens. Since the sporozoite antigen is expressed before infective merozoites are released, preexisting specific T_{CTL} cells may be able to destroy infected cells before systemic infection is established or prevent spread of infection from liver cells to RBCs.

malaria (anemia, fever, nephritis, and vasculitis) appear to be associated with an antibody-mediated destruction of red cells and release of hemoglobin. The erythrocytes of patients with malaria become coated with IgG or IgM and have an increased susceptibility to phagocytosis and destruction by splenic macrophages. Neutrophil killing of infected RBCs is enhanced by gamma interferon and other factors released from T_{DTH} cells. Infected red cells may be destroyed to such an extent that macrophages in the spleen and liver become loaded with malaria pigment (hemozoin) from phagocytosed and degraded RBC. Although this reaction may help to eliminate infected cells, it also contributes to the anemia. During malarial paroxysms, parasites are released from intracellular locations in large numbers, resulting in the formation of immune complexes in antigen excess. Glomerulonephritis, the nephrotic syndrome (blackwater fever), and vasculitis seen in severe cases of malaria are presumed to be consequences. Finally, the preoccupation of macrophages with erythrophagocytosis may contribute to the immunosuppression observed in association with malaria. Infected RBCs adhere to developing dendritic cells and inhibit the ability of dendritic cells to initiate immune responses. Production of tumor necrosis factor (cachexin), which is found in elevated levels in the serum of malaria patients, may contribute to the fever, chills, hypoglycemia, renal tubule necrosis, liver damage, pulmonary neutrophil accumulation, and other lesions seen in malaria.

Malaria Vaccines

The ability to produce an effective vaccine against malaria is complicated by species-specific antigens, by the stage-specific antigens that are produced during the malarial life cycle, by antigenic variation during infection, by possible genetic limitation to HLA-dependent processing of cloned peptide antigens, and by the failure of a substantial proportion of immunized individuals to develop T_{CTL} cells. Theoretically, vaccine development could be directed to prevent infection (sporozoite), to decrease the production of parasites in the infected blood (merozoite) or liver (schizont), or to the sexual stage in the mosquito (gametocyte).

Sporozoites. In the late 1960s, it was shown that vaccination with gamma-irradiated sporozoites could protect against different malaria strains. However, it was only possible to obtain enough sporozoites for limited experimental study. There is as yet no satisfactory method to cultivate the sporozoites. They must be isolated from salivary glands of infected mosquitoes. This method does not yield adequate quantities to produce a vaccine for widespread human use. Because of this, vaccine efforts then focused on isolating and cloning the gene for the circumsporate (CS) protein.

The CS protein is an antigen highly represented on the surface of the infectious sporozoite stage injected by infecting mosquitoes, and CS proteins contain repetitive amino acid sequences shared by different *Plasmodium* strains (Fig. 9.11). Since nearly all identified anti-CS antibodies react with the repeat amino acid sequences, the first vaccine tested was directed against these epitopes. Human volunteers vaccinated with the tetramer (Asn-Ala-Asn-Pro) linked to tetanus toxoid produced only low titers of antibody. To increase immunogenicity of the peptide antigen, it was complexed with epitopes that would be bound to class II MHC molecules and processed by T cells. In this way, the poorly immunogenic peptides would be provided with a "carrier" for T-cell help. This has been accomplished using "multiple-antigen peptides" (Fig. 9.11). Multiple-antigen peptides have been shown to induce higher titers of anti-CS antibody in laboratory animals and are now being tested in humans.

Merozoites and schizonts. A second approach is to suppress the effects of infection by inducing $CD8^+$ T_{CTL} cells to malaria antigens expressed on infected blood or liver cells, and by so doing decrease the production of organisms in the infected cells. Several different ways to this approach are under study. (i) A T_{CTL} epitope appears to be shared by the C-terminal CS protein and schizonts in liver cells. In mice, T-cell clones that recognize this epitope in association with class I MHC have been derived, and passive transfer of these cells protects against challenge with malarial sporozoites. Vaccination with this peptide conjugated to immunostimulating complexes or to liposomes may selectively allow presentation through class I MHC. (ii) A recombinant protein form, the p190 antigen (p190-3) of *P. falciparum* merozoites, has been found that will selectively induce $CD4^+$ and $CD8^+$ T cells when administered in Freund's adjuvant. (iii) In further studies, ampipathic analysis has been used to identify 22 putative T_{CTL} epitopes from conserved regions of 10 *P. falciparum* asexual-stage proteins that are candidates for vaccine development. Peptides containing these epitopes have been further analyzed for their ability to stimulate T cells from malaria patients. It is hoped that these approaches will result in the development of vaccines that will act to prevent relapses of malaria in infected individuals.

Gametes. The rationale for developing vaccines to the gametocytes is to produce antibodies in humans that will be ingested by the mosquitoes that are

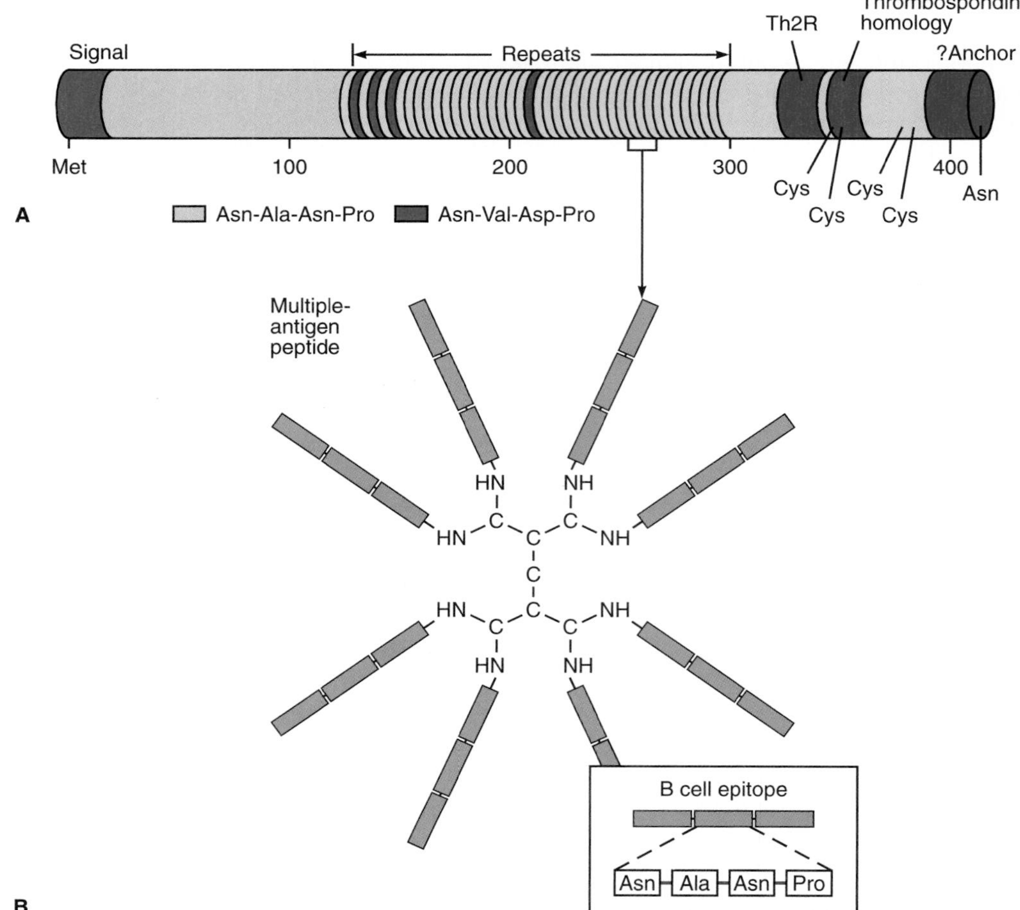

Figure 9.11 **(A)** Circumsporate protein of the malaria parasite. The middle third of the protein contains a set of repetitions of two short sequences of amino acids (Asn-Ala-Asn-Pro or Asn-Val-Asp-Pro), as well as a polymorphic region (Th2R) and two pairs of cysteine residues. Hydrophobic regions at the C terminus may anchor the protein in the plasma membrane of the sporozoite. The repetitive sequences constitute epitopes that are recognized by all known antibodies against *Plasmodium* strains. **(B)** Multiple-antigen peptide is a synthetic molecule in which a lysine core provides "mooring posts" for B-cell epitopes that can be processed by macrophages for presentation to T cells. In this example, all eight arms of the lysine core hold the same B-cell epitope (Asn-Ala-Asn-Pro). (Modified from V. Nussenzweig and R. S. Nussenzweig, *Hosp. Pract.* **25:**41, 1990.)

responsible for transmission of the infection and block or impair the sexual development of the malaria parasite in the mosquito. This approach has been attained in laboratory studies but has not yet been demonstrated in humans.

The role of cytotoxic reactions in malaria can be summarized as follows. (i) Cytotoxic mechanisms appear responsible for major immune reaction against malaria-infected erythrocytes, leading to destruction of RBCs as well as deposition of pigment in the reticuloendothelial system and formation of immune complexes during secondary lesions and immunosuppression. (ii) T_{CTL} cells play a major role in destroying infected hepatocytes. (iii) Antigenic variation of blood stages of malaria and variation in antigens in blood stages of different malarial species provide barriers to the development of an effective vaccine to these stages. (iv) Antibodies or T_{CTL} cells to sporozoites may provide protective immunity by blocking infection of liver cells but are not effective naturally (too late). Sporozoite antigen produced by cloned DNA is now being tested in clinical trials. (v) Human antibodies to micro- and macrogametes could provide passive immunity in mosquitoes and prevent the spread of malaria.

Summary

Cytotoxic or cytolytic reactions are caused by circulating antibody to cell surface structures with subsequent complement fixation. The cell surface antigens may be an integral part of the cell membrane or may be acquired by passive absorption. Reaction of antibody of the IgM or IgG class with the cell surface antigens results in activation of complement and destruction of the cell by complement-mediated lysis or by phagocytosis by macrophages with receptors for activated complement components or aggregated immunoglobulin. Cells in contact with the circulating blood are most often the target cells; these include RBCs, white blood cells, and platelets. The disease states are the result of a loss of the function of the affected cells. Examples of such diseases are hemolytic anemia, agranulocytosis, and thrombocytopenic purpura. In addition, epidermal structures may be targets of cytotoxic reactions, leading to loss of epidermal cells.

Bibliography

General

Atkinson, J. P., and M. M. Frank. 1974. Studies on the in vivo effects of antibody: interaction of IgM antibody and complement in the immune clearance and destruction of erythrocytes in man. *J. Clin. Investig.* **54:**339–348.

Boyle, M. D. P., and T. Borsos. 1980. The terminal stages of immune hemolysis: a brief review. *Mol. Immunol.* **17:**425–432.

Schreiber, A. D., and M. M. Frank. 1972. Role of antibody and complement in the immune clearance and destruction of erythrocytes. II. Molecular nature of IgG and IgM complement-fixing sites and effects of their interaction with serum. *J. Clin. Investig.* **51:**583–589.

Wintrobe, M. M. 1974. *Clinical Hematology,* 7th ed. Lea & Febiger, Philadelphia, Pa.

Transfusion Reaction

Salmon, C., J. P. Carton, and P. Rouger. 1984. *The Human Blood Groups.* Masson, New York, N.Y.

Watkins, W. M. 1978. Genetics and biochemistry of some human blood groups. *Proc. R. Soc. Lond. (Biol.)* **202:**31–53.

Erythroblastosis Fetalis

Bowman, J. M. 1986. Fetomaternal ABO incompatibility and erythroblastosis fetalis. *Vox Sang.* **50:**104–106.

Clarke, C. A., and P. L. Mollison. 1989. Deaths from Rh haemolytic disease of the fetus and newborn, 1877–1987. *J. R. Coll. Phys. Lond.* **23:**181–184.

Levine, P. 1984. The discovery of Rh hemolytic disease. *Vox Sang.* **47:**187–190.

Szulman, A. E. 1964. The histologic distribution of the blood group substances in man as determined by immunofluorescence. III. The A, B, and H antigens in embryos and fetuses from 18 mm in length. *J. Exp. Med.* **119:**503–516.

Taylor, J. F. 1967. Sensitization of Rh-negative daughters by their Rh-positive mothers. *N. Engl. J. Med.* **276:**547–551.

Voak, D. 1969. The pathogenesis of ABO hemolytic disease of the newborn. *Vox Sang.* **17:**481–513.

Autoimmune Hemolytic Anemia

Adams, J., V. K. Moore, and D. D. Issitt. 1973. Autoimmune hemolytic anemia caused by anti-D. *Transfusion* **13:**214–218.

Sokol, R. J., D. J. Booker, and R. Stamps. 1992. The pathology of autoimmune haemolytic anaemia. *J. Clin. Pathol.* **45:**1047–1052.

Drug-Associated Hemolytic Reactions

Kerr, R.-O., J. Cardamone, A. P. Dalmasso, and M. E. Kaplan. 1972. Two mechanisms of erythrocyte destruction in penicillin-induced hemolytic anemia. *N. Engl. J. Med.* **287:**1322.

Wolledge, S. M. 1973. Immune drug-induced hemolytic anemias. *Semin. Hematol.* **10:**327–343.

White Blood Cell Reactions

Bux, J., K. Kissel, K. Nowak, U. Spengel, and C. Mueller-Eckhardt. 1991. Autoimmune neutropenia: clinical and laboratory studies in 143 patients. *Ann. Hematol.* **63:**249–252.

Madyastha, P. R., and A. B. Glassman. 1989. Neutrophil antigens and antibodies in the diagnosis of immune neutropenias. *Ann. Clin. Lab. Med. Sci.* **19:**146–154.

Shastri, K. A., and G. L. Logue. 1993. Autoimmune neutropenia. *Blood* **81:** 1984–1995.

Platelets

Baldini, M. 1966. Idiopathic thrombocytopenic purpura. *N. Engl. J. Med.* **274:** 1360–1367.

Schiffer, C. A. 1991. Prevention of alloimmunization against platelets. *Blood* **77:**1–4.

Skacel, P. O., and M. Contreras. 1989. Neonatal alloimmune thrombocytopenia. *Blood Rev.* **3:**174–179.

Cytotoxic Skin Diseases

Clark, W. H., R. J. Reed and M. C. Mich. 1975. Lupus erythematosus: histopathology of cutaneous lesions. *Hum. Pathol.* **4:**157–165.

Cochran, R. E. I., J. Thompson, and R. M. N. MacSween. 1976. An autoantibody profile in alopecia totalis and diffuse alopecia. *Br. J. Dermatol.* **95:**61–65.

Hall, R. P. 1992. Dermatitis herpetiformis. *J. Investig. Dermatol.* **99:**873–881.

Jordon, R. E., K. G. Heine, G. Tappeiner, L. L. Bushkell, and T. T. Provost. 1976. The immunopathology of herpes gestationis. Immunofluorescence studies and characterization of "HG factor." *J. Clin. Investig.* **57:**1426–1431.

Ortonne, J.-P., and S. K. Bose. 1993. Vitiligo: where do we stand? *Pigment Cell Res.* **6:**61–72.

Pedro, S. D., and M. V. Dahl. 1973. Direct immunofluorescence of bullous systemic lupus erythematosus. *Arch. Dermatol.* **107:**118–120.

Other Cytolytic Reactions

Dondero, F., A. Lenzi, L. Gandini, and F. Lombardo. 1993. Immunologic infertility in humans. *Exp. Clin. Immunol.* **10:**65–72.

Stetson, C. A. 1963. The role of humoral antibody in the homograft rejection. *Adv. Immunol.* **3:**97–130.

Waksman, B. H. 1958. Cell lysis and related phenomena in hypersensitivity reactions, including immunohematologic diseases. *Prog. Allergy* **5:**349–458.

Coombs' Test

Bohnen, R. F., J. E. Ultman, J. G. Gorman, et al. 1968. The direct Coombs' test: its clinical significance. Study in a large university hospital. *Ann. Intern. Med.* **68:**19–32.

Coombs, R. R. A., A. E. Mourant, and R. R. Race. 1945. A new test for the detection of weak and "incomplete" Rh agglutinins. *Br. J. Exp. Pathol.* **26:**255–266.

Coombs, R. R. A., and F. Roberts. 1959. Antiglobulin reaction. *Br. Med. Bull.* **15:**113–118.

Malaria

Hollingdale, M. R. 1988. Biology and immunology of sporozoite invasion of liver cells and exoerythrocytic development of malaria parasites. *Prog. Allergy* **41:**15–48.

Quakyi, I. A., D. W. Taylor, A. H. Johnson, J. B. Allotey, J. A. Berzofsky, L. H. Miller, and M. F. Good. 1992. Development of a malaria T-cell vaccine for blood stage immunity. *Scand. J. Immunol.* **36**(Suppl. 11)**:**9–16.

Rodrigues, R. S., R. S. Nussenzweig, and F. Zavala. 1993. The relative contribution of antibodies, CD4+ and CD8+ T cells to sporozoite-induced protection against malaria. *Immunology* **80:**1–5.

Suss, G., and J. R. L. Pink. 1992. A recombinant malaria protein that can induce Th1 and CD8+ T-cell responses without antibody formation. *J. Immunol.* **149:** 1334–1339.

Urban, B. D., D. J. P. Ferguson, A. Pain, N. Willcox, M. Plebanski, J. M. Austyn, D. J. Roberts. 1999. Plasmodium falciparum-infected erythrocytes modulate the maturation of dendritic cells. *Nature* **400:**73–77.

Immune Complex Reactions

10

Immune Complexes In Vivo

Immune complex reactions are caused by immunoglobulin antibody reacting directly with tissue antigens (usually basement membrane antigens) or by antibody reacting with soluble antigen in the blood to form soluble antigen-antibody complexes that deposit in tissues. Although these initiating events are different, the subsequent inflammatory reaction, mainly mediated by complement, is essentially the same (Fig. 10.1). Immunoglobulin G (IgG) antibody reacting with tissue antigens accumulates to form aggregates in tissues. Soluble complexes, formed in the circulation by a single IgG molecule reacting with a soluble antigen, or antigens shed from cell membranes, form aggregates of IgG when complexes from the blood deposit closely in tissue. These aggregated antigen-antibody complexes fix complement with activation of the anaphylactic and chemotactic activities of C4a, C3a, and C5a. This results in the accumulation of neutrophilic polymorphonuclear leukocytes, which release lysosomal enzymes and reactive oxygen metabolites that, along with the membrane attack complex of complement, cause destruction of the elastic lamina of arteries (serum sickness), basement membrane of the kidney glomerulus (glomerulonephritis), walls of small vessels (Arthus reaction), articular cartilage of joints (early rheumatoid arthritis), or basement membrane of skin (cutaneous lupus erythematosus).

The alternate pathway for complement activation, entered by activation of C3 (the C3 shunt; see "Complement" in chapter 3), is active in the pathogenesis of some types of lesions that are similar to immune complex-mediated lesions. Activation of either the classical or alternate pathway results in formation of C3a and C5a, production of complement chemotactic factors (mostly C5a), accumulation of polymorphonuclear cells, and destruction of tissue. Complement mediators such as anaphylatoxin (C4a, C3a, and C5a) may induce endothelial cell contraction and open cell junctions so that soluble complexes can deposit in basement membranes or inflammatory cells can enter into tissue spaces.

The Arthus Reaction

The Arthus reaction is a dermal inflammatory response caused by the reaction of precipitating antibody with antigen placed in the skin (Fig. 10.2). It

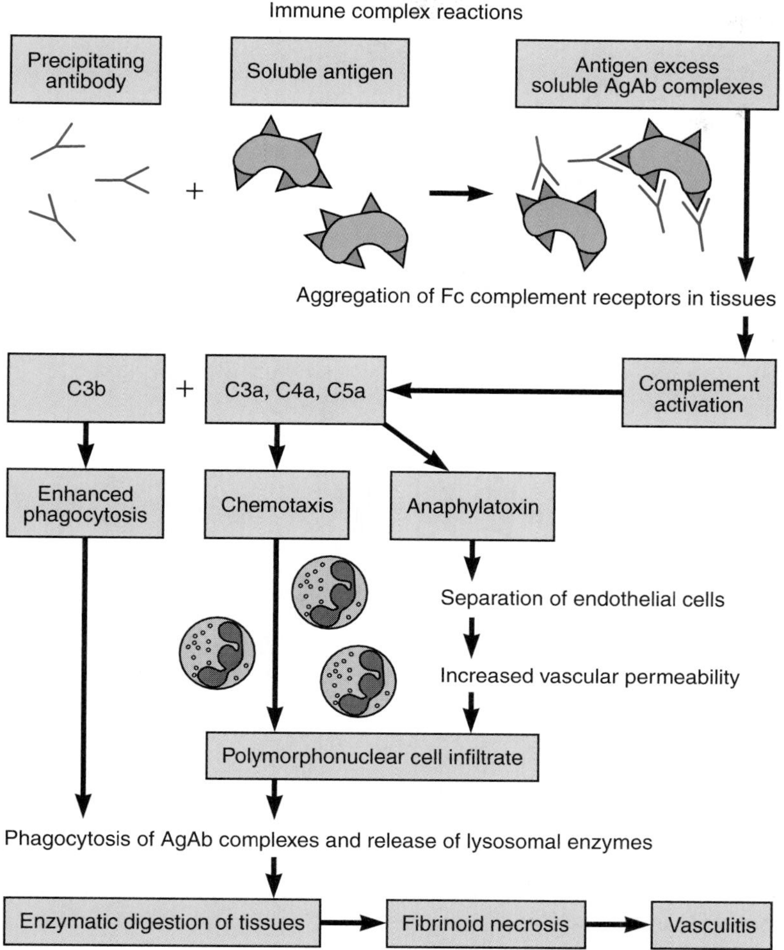

Figure 10.1 Immune complex reactions. Antibody (usually IgG) reacts with soluble antigens to produce soluble circulating immune complexes or with basement membranes (such as renal glomerular basement membrane). Antibody-antigen complexes cause activation of complement with formation of inflammatory (phlogistic) complement fragments. Fragments C3a, C4a, and C5a (anaphylatoxin) cause constriction of vascular endothelium (increased vascular permeability). C5a is also chemotactic for polymorphonuclear leukocytes, and C3b enhances phagocytosis. Released lysosomal polymorphonuclear enzymes digest tissues, producing "fibrinoid" necrosis. Fibrinoid means "fibrinlike" and refers to the histologic appearance of the acellular amorphous areas produced by "digestion" of tissue by lysosomal enzymes that resemble the appearance of fibrin in clotted blood.

is named for Marcel Arthus, who first described it in 1903. The reaction is characterized grossly by edema, erythema, and hemorrhage, all of which develop over a few hours, reaching a maximum in 3 to 5 h, or even later if the reaction is severe (Fig. 10.3). Emigration of neutrophils and eosinophils and vascular fibrinoid necrosis are seen. If the reaction is severe, there is thrombosis with resulting ischemic necrosis. This lesion is caused by the reaction of antigen with antibody, forming microprecipitates of antigen-antibody complexes in vessel walls or in adjacent tissue spaces and activation of complement. This results in vasodilation and endothelial contraction by the activated complement inflammatory peptides as well as

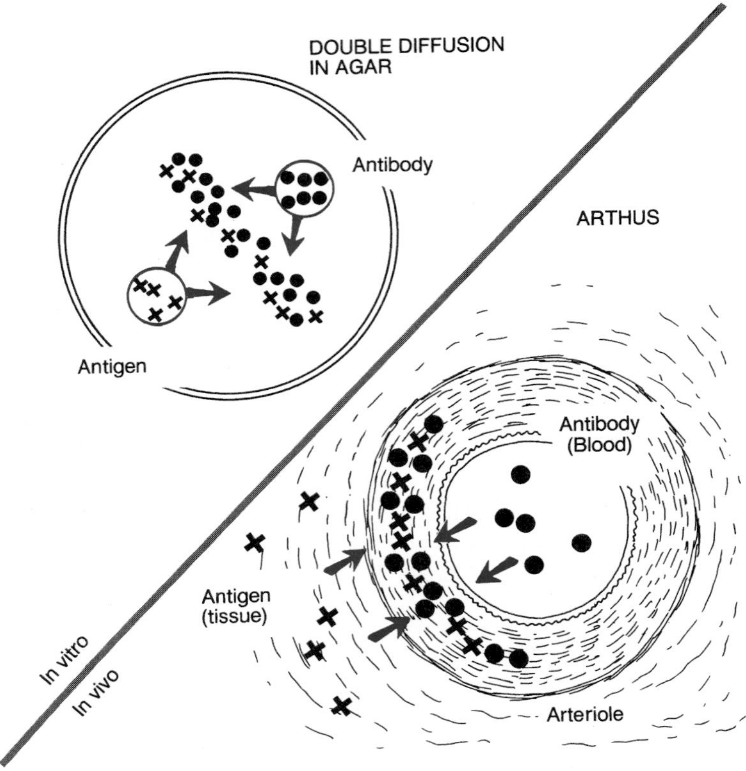

Figure 10.2 Comparison of double diffusion in agar precipitin reaction and Arthus reaction. When antibody and antigen are allowed to diffuse toward each other in agar, a precipitin band forms when the antigen and antibody concentration in the agar are in equivalence. Similarly, if antigen is injected into the skin, it will diffuse toward the vessels. The major precipitin reaction occurs in the walls of small vessels, usually arterioles, where antibody in the circulation diffuses out to meet antigen diffusing in from the tissue.

chemoattraction of polymorphonuclear neutrophils (PMNs). Platelet-activating factor-mediated release of prostaglandins and leukotrienes (see chapter 11) may also contribute to the increased blood flow and vascular permeability. PMNs infiltrate and attempt to phagocytose the complement-coated complexes. The PMNs discharge their lysosomal contents, and the resulting oxygen radicals and released lysosomal enzymes produce damage to vascular walls and surrounding tissue. Clumping of cells and activation of the clotting system may result in occlusion of small vessels and ischemic necrosis. The presence of antigen and antibody may be demonstrated in vascular wall deposits by the fluorescent antibody technique. In this reaction, complexes in different ratios of antibody to antigen (antibody excess, equivalence, or antigen excess) are present and are active in fixing complement if the Fcs of two IgG antibody molecules are juxtaposed. Reaction of macrophages with Fcγ receptor (FcγR) type I on macrophages for IgG in the immune complexes may also contribute to the inflammatory response through release of tumor necrosis factor alpha (TNF-α).

Serum Sickness

Untoward systemic effects of the administration of xenogeneic serum were noted by von Behring in 1891, when hyperimmune serum was introduced

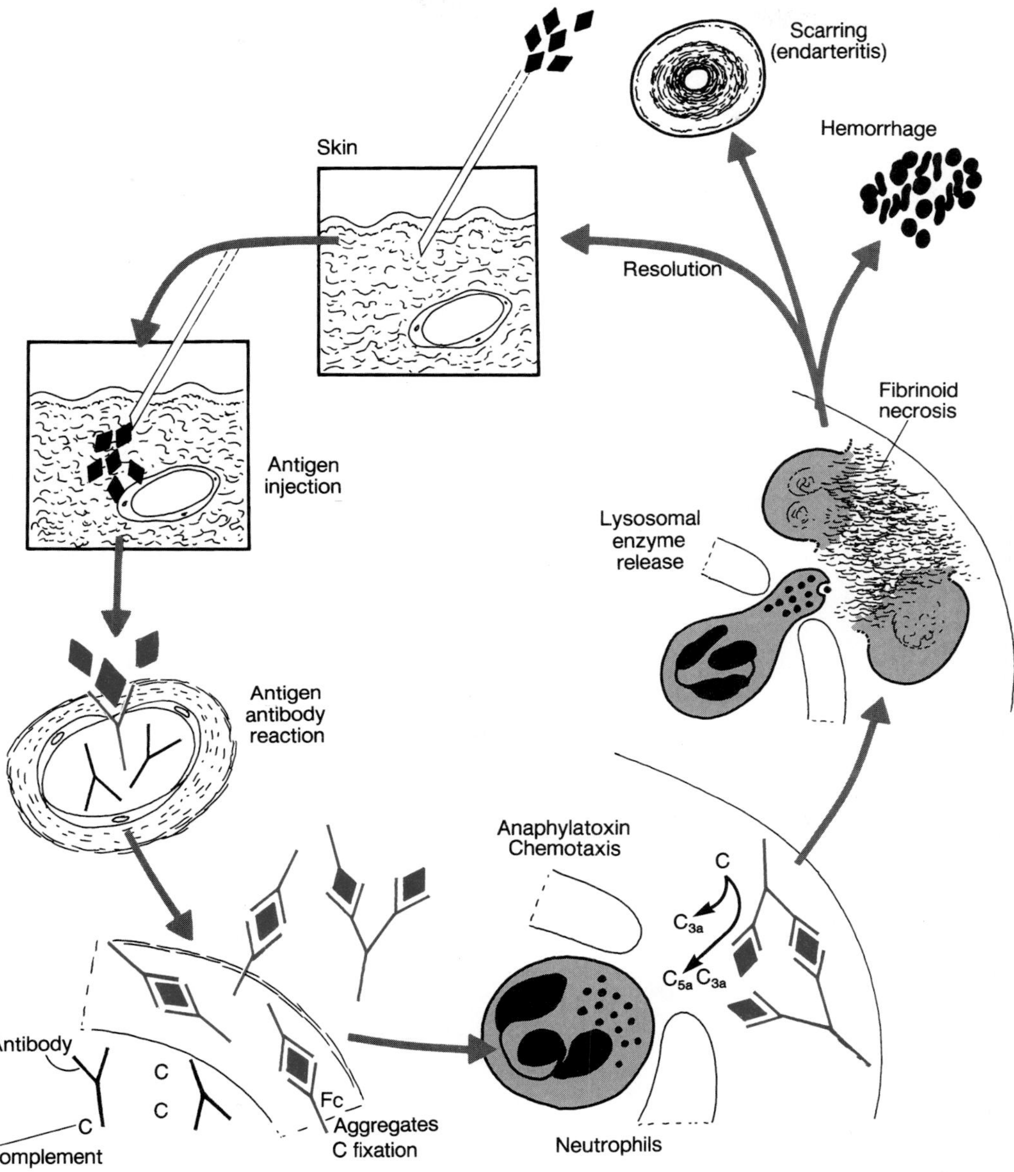

Figure 10.3 Steps in the Arthus reaction. **(1)** Injection of antigen into the dermis. **(2)** Diffusion of antigen in tissue to vessels. **(3)** Reaction of antigen with circulating antibody in the wall of small arterioles. **(4)** Formation of antibody-antigen complexes, aggregation of Fc of antibody, and activation of complement. **(5)** Contraction and separation of endothelial cells by C3a, C5a (anaphylatoxin), and attraction of neutrophils by C5a and C5a des-Arg chemotactic factors. **(6)** Activation of neutrophils in vessel wall with release of lysosomal enzymes. **(7)** Digestion of vascular wall producing fibrinoid necrosis. **(8)** Resolution or scarring, depending on severity of reaction.

for the treatment of children with diphtheria. The syndrome of serum sickness was first described in detail by von Pirquet and Schick in 1905. It consisted of fever, arthritis, glomerulonephritis, and vasculitis appearing 10 days to 2 weeks following passive immunization with horse serum (i.e., horse anti-tetanus toxin). The disease is the result of the production by the treated individual of circulating precipitating antibody to the injected horse serum (Fig. 10.4). In a recent study in Ukraine, 24 of 1,556 children to whom antidiphtheric serum was administered developed serum sickness.

The lesions of serum sickness directly correlate with the presence of soluble immune complexes. In experimental models, the lesions of serum sickness appear at the time of immune elimination or when soluble complexes in antigen excess are present in the serum (Fig. 10.5). During a continuous infusion of large amounts of a soluble antigen, such as bovine

Figure 10.4 Steps in serum sickness. **(1)** Formation of soluble antibody-antigen complexes in circulation. Such complexes do not fix complement because Fcs are not aggregated. **(2)** Soluble complexes pass through open endothelial spaces in glomeruli and deposit on the epithelial side of the basement membrane or in walls of small arteries. Accumulation of complexes results in formation of aggregates of immunoglobulin, activating complement. **(3)** Neutrophils are attracted, pass into basement membrane or vessel wall, and release lysosomal enzymes, causing destruction of basement membranes.

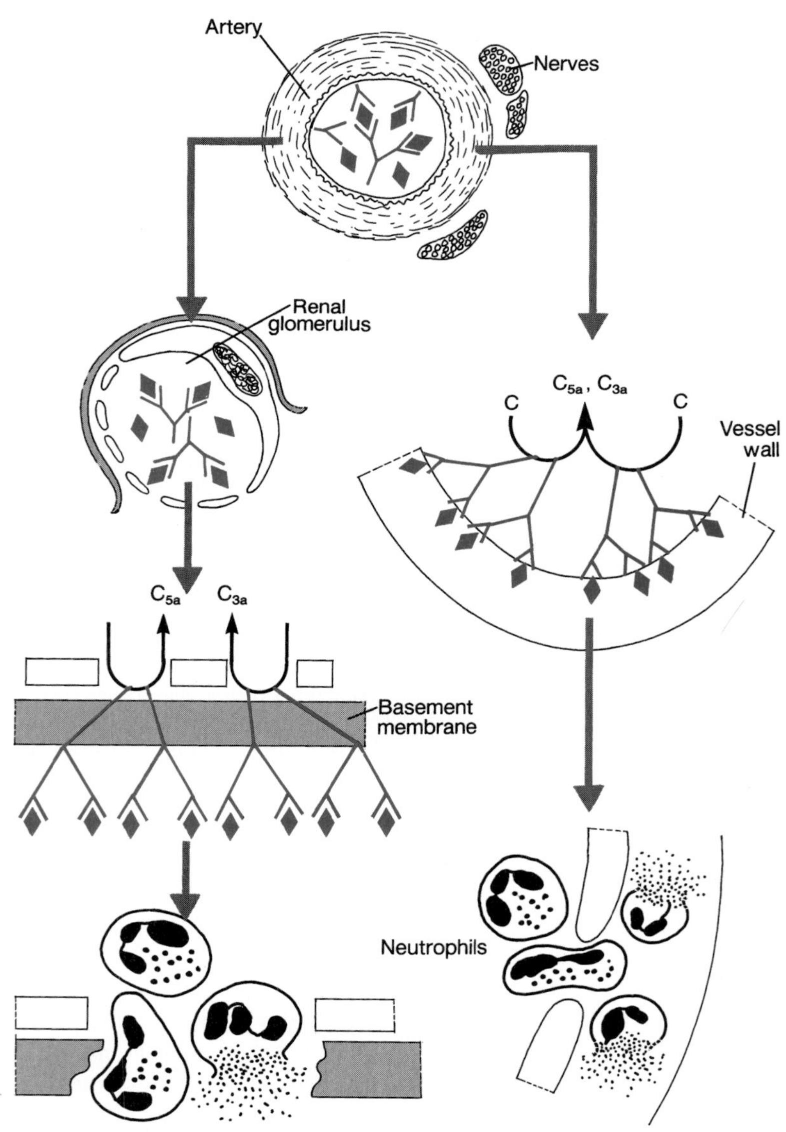

serum albumin, into rabbits, individual animals may exhibit one of three types of immune responses: (i) the production of no antibody to bovine serum albumin (high dose tolerance) or the production of antibody in such small amounts so that insufficient immune complexes are formed to produce serum sickness; (ii) the production of large amounts of antibody, which forms complexes with antigen in antibody excess that are cleared by the reticuloendothelial system (RES) and do not induce lesions; or (iii) the production of a moderate amount of antibody, with formation of soluble antigen-antibody complexes in antigen excess that deposit in tissue and induce typical lesions of serum sickness. Antibody-antigen complexes formed in vitro and injected into animals may also produce lesions, but only if the complexes are formed in antigen excess. Thus, antigen-excess immune complexes are required for the production of the lesions of serum sickness. Immune complexes in antibody excess or equivalence form aggregated Fcs or C3b and are cleared by the RES because of the presence of receptors for aggregated Fcs and C3b on the phagocytic cells of the RES. However, soluble complexes in antigen excess (toxic complexes) are not cleared efficiently by the RES and deposit in vessels and glomeruli, where accumulation of complexes results in aggregation of Fcs and complement activation.

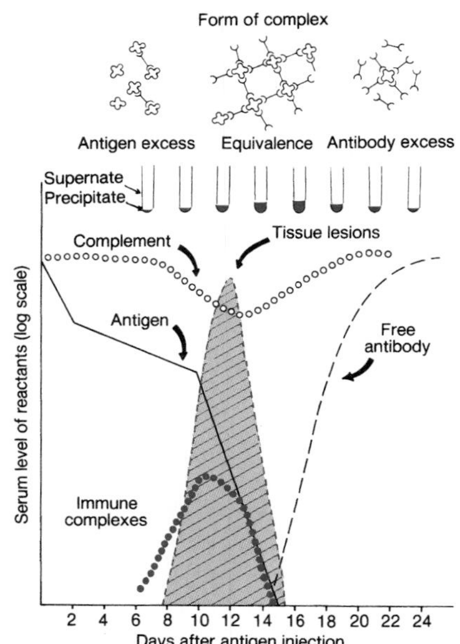

Figure 10.5 Comparison of antigen elimination, precipitin reaction, and serum complement levels during experimental serum sickness. Immune elimination of antigen follows production of antibody that binds to antigen in the circulation. When antibody first appears, there is an excess of antigen so that soluble immune complexes in antigen excess are formed. These complexes lodge in arteries and, in particular, in glomeruli, where aggregates of immunoglobulin fix complement. This results in lesions of serum sickness and a fall in serum complement. As more antibody is produced, complexes in equivalence and then antibody excess are found. Since these complexes contain aggregated Fc regions of immunoglobulin, they will be cleared from the circulation by the reticuloendothelial system because of receptors on macrophages for aggregated Fc and C3b.

Horse serum contains at least 30 different, separate antigens, so complexes of one or more of these antigens may be present in the circulation even though excess antibody or other free antigens may be present at the same time. In addition, different proportions of antibodies with different electrostatic charges may be formed. Immune complexes may activate platelets to release leukotrienes, and some individuals may produce reaginic (IgE) antibodies or a state of delayed hypersensitivity to some of the antigens in horse serum. The presence of different forms of immune complexes, as well as activation of different immune mechanisms, can result in a very complicated clinical picture. In a study of 35 patients treated with anti-thymocyte globulin for bone marrow failure, over 80% developed fever, malaise, cutaneous eruptions, arthralgias, gastrointestinal complaints, headache, blurring of vision, arthritis, and lymphadenopathy beginning 1 week after initiation of therapy and lasting for about 10 days after termination of therapy. The development by protein engineering of humanized antibodies in which antigen-combining sites of the antibodies of animals are joined with the constant regions of human immunoglobulins may eliminate the problem of immune complex serum sickness reactions.

Immune Complexes in Infectious Diseases

Transient serum sickness-like episodes are frequently associated with infections. In many instances, antibody-antigen complexes may be demonstrated, and in some cases the antigen has been identified as a component of the infectious agent. Immune complexes have been documented in glomerular or vascular deposits in animals infected with lymphocytic choriomeningitis virus, *Schistosoma mansoni,* leprosy bacilli, *Treponema pallidum,* and a number of other agents. In humans, vasculitis, glomerulonephritis, arthritis, and skin lesions may be associated with deposition of hepatitis antigen-antibody complexes in patients with hepatitis B virus or hepatitis C virus infection. Immune complexes may have a role in the inflammatory pulmonary lesions and serum sickness-like symptoms seen in cystic fibrosis patients with *Pseudomonas aeruginosa* lung infection. Chronic infectious endocarditis, during which there is continued release of organisms into the blood, features positive serum tests for immune complexes as well as a number of immune complex-associated lesions, such as vasculitis, arthritis, and glomerulonephritis. In lepromatous leprosy, antibody production to leprosy antigens is associated with circulating immune complexes, rheumatoid factor, and vasculitis (erythema nodosum leprosum), as well as renal disease. During chemotherapy, large amounts of mycobacterial antigens are released locally in the skin, and in the presence of antibodies to these antigens, a marked local acute necrotic neutrophil inflammation in the skin is often seen (type II leprosy reaction). Circulating immune complexes may also be found in high frequency in patients with recurrent infections in the absence of serum sickness-like lesions. The presence of immune complexes in the circulation does not necessarily correlate with lesions. The form of the complexes, the class of the antibody, and the properties of the antigen are all important factors, as is the ability of the RES to remove immune complexes. Continued formation of immune complexes in equivalence or antibody excess may lead to RES blockade. The role of immune complexes in rheumatic fever is presented below.

Glomerulonephritis

Acute Glomerulonephritis

Inflammation of the glomeruli of the kidney is known as glomerulonephritis. The nature of the lesion in the glomerulus reflects the stage of the process of inflammation from acute through subacute to chronic (see Table 3.27). Acute inflammation causes leakage of blood components into the urine because of damage to the glomerular basement membrane; chronic inflammation produces scarring and thickening of the glomerulus and loss of filtration (renal failure). Inflammation of the glomeruli follows the formation of immune complexes in the glomerular basement membrane. Lesions are caused by deposition of antibody-antigen complexes formed elsewhere and deposited in the glomeruli, such as that seen in serum sickness, by shedding of antibody-antigen complexes from endothelial cells into the basement membrane, or by direct reaction of antibody with glomerular basement membrane or other antigens.

To appreciate the nature of antibody-mediated glomerulonephritis, an understanding of the normal structure of the glomerulus and the form of deposition of antibody or immune complexes is necessary (Fig. 10.6). The nephron is the unit of the kidney that filters metabolites and electrolytes from the blood and produces urine. It is made up of glomerulus and tubule. An ultrafiltrate of the blood is produced by filtration through the basement membrane of the glomerulus into the epithelium-lined collecting space. The tubule collects this filtrate and resorbs electrolytes as urine passes into the collecting system. The glomerulus is made up of four principal cell types, each of which has a specific function: endothelial cells, which line the glomerular capillary network; mesangial cells, which form a stalk that supports the basement membrane of the capillaries; and two types of epithelial cells, visceral and parietal. The visceral epithelial cells cover the external surface of the capillary basement membrane and, along with the parietal epithelial cells, which cover the inside of the capsule of the glomerulus, line the space in which the glomerular filtrate is collected.

A critical feature of the glomerulus is that the capillary basement membrane is not completely covered by endothelial cells. This permits antibodies to the basement membrane or circulating immune complexes to pass into the basement membrane. Complement activation (anaphylatoxin) or

Figure 10.6 Pathogenesis of glomerulonephritis. Depicted is part of a glomerulus. The mesangial cells are located in the center and support the endothelial cells (END), which line the inside of the basement membrane. There are gaps in the cytoplasm of the endothelial cells, which expose the basement membrane to blood components. The upper left part of the figure illustrates deposition of anti-glomerular basement membrane (anti-GBM) antibody as a linear deposit of immunoglobulin on the endothelial side of the basement membrane. The upper right depicts deposition of soluble immune complexes on exposed basement membrane after contraction of endothelial cells by vasoactive amines or activation of anaphylatoxin. The lower left segment illustrates that the complexes may deposit as large clumps, distorting the foot processes of the endothelial cells. Dissolution of the basement membrane by release of lysosomal enzymes from polymorphonuclear leukocytes (POLYS) activated by complement or alterations in the electrostatic properties of the basement membrane by anti-GBM or immune complex deposition leads to leakage of proteins into the urine (proteinuria) (upper right). If more extensive destruction of the basement membranes occurs, cellular elements of the blood, as well as basement membrane fragments, may be detected in the urine. Prolonged accumulation of immune reactants leads to thickening of the basement membrane and fusion of the foot processes of epithelial cells (EPI). Clinically, this is expressed as a loss of the filtering capacity of the kidney and retention of toxic metabolites (uremia).

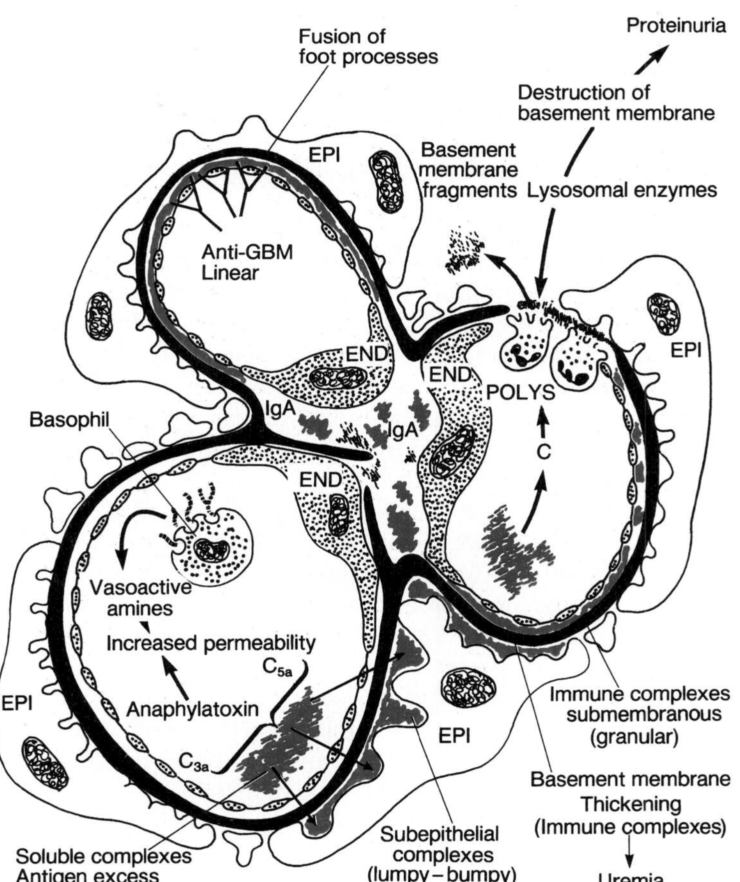

mast cell mediators may produce further separation by causing contraction of endothelial cells. In addition, the membrane attack complex of complement (MAC) may deposit in the basement membrane. If the MAC deposits are not lytically active, they are associated with a protein called clusterin. The exact pathologic role of MACs and clusterin in the glomerular basement membrane is not known, although it appears that the lytically active MACs could contribute to glomerular leakage and the MAC-clusterin deposits could contribute to membrane thickening.

Mechanisms

The lesions of immune complex glomerulonephritis are produced by alteration of the basement membrane by four mechanisms: (i) by the deposition of complexes, antibody, or complement, which cause changes in the electrostatic properties of the basement membrane and consequent leakage of serum proteins, (ii) by complement-mediated attraction of PMNs, which in turn release enzymes that digest the basement membrane, (iii) by long-term deposition of complexes that cause thickening of the basement membrane and fusion of the foot processes of the epithelial cells, leading to a loss of the filtering ability of the glomerulus (membranous glomerulonephritis), and (iv) by activation of chronic inflammatory mechanisms leading to proliferation of mononuclear and epithelial cells (proliferative glomerulonephritis). Influx of PMNs is associated with acute destruction of the basement membrane and hematuria characteristic of acute glomerulonephritis. This appears to require the involvement of TNF, because upregulation of intercellular adhesion molecule 1 (ICAM-1) and vascular cell adhesion molecule 1 (VCAM-1) and acute PMN infiltrate does not occur in TNF-deficient mice. Dissolution of the basement membrane is associated with leakage of blood components into the urine (proteinuria, hematuria, the nephrotic syndrome); whereas thickening of the basement membrane causes a loss in filtration capacity and uremia (the uremic syndrome).

Role of Electrostatic Charge

The charge of the immune complex in the glomerular basement membrane in glomerulonephritis determines to a large extent the nature and location of the deposited immune complexes. The basement membrane contains a large amount of sialic acid and is strongly negatively charged (anionic). The anionic membrane can be neutralized by deposits of cationic molecules. The charge of the complex is most important for the initial binding of complexes. In experimental immune complex glomerulonephritis models, highly cationic antigens, in the form of soluble antigen or soluble immune complexes, tend to localize within or pass though the basement membrane, whereas complexes of anionic antigens deposit on the endothelial side (Fig. 10.7). After the initial binding, the complexes condense to form large deposits, and forces other than charge retain the complexes in the membrane. Neutralization of the charge of the basement membrane causes increased permeability to smaller serum proteins, such as serum albumin, which are also strongly cationic and usually repelled from the basement membrane. This increased permeability leads to proteinuria, which may occur following immune complex deposition, without neutrophil-mediated basement membrane damage.

Size and Solubility of Immune Complexes

In addition to charge, the size and solubility of immune complexes determine the type of glomerulonephritis (Table 10.1). There are two major

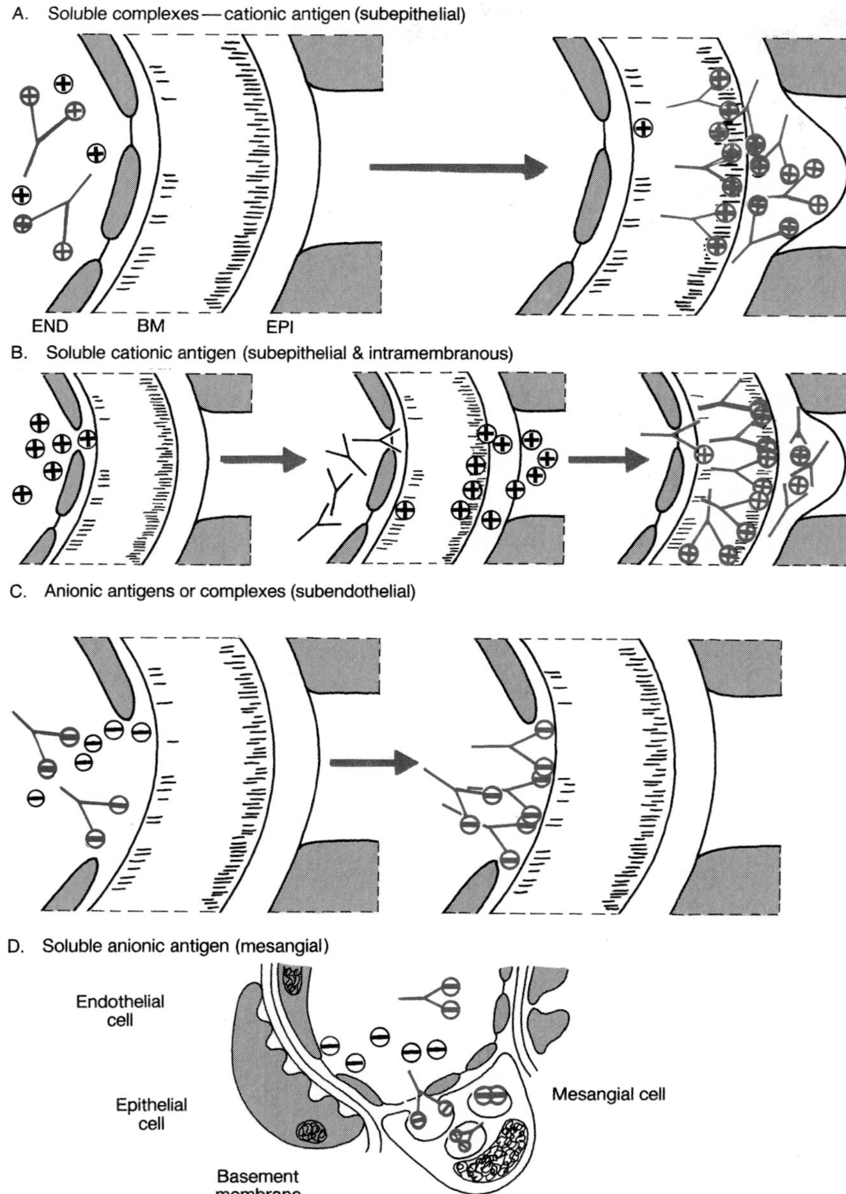

Figure 10.7 Effect of charge on immune complex localization in glomeruli. Cationic immune complexes (positively charged) preferentially localize in the glomerular basement membrane **(A)**. Subepithelial localization may be explained by a higher density of anions on the epithelial side of the basement membrane. Cationic free antigen may deposit in the basement membrane **(B)**, and subsequent reaction with antibody leads to formation of immune complexes within the basement membrane. Anionic complexes tend to be taken up by the mesangial cells **(C)** and are less pathogenic but may also localize on the endothelial side of the basement membrane **(D)**.

types of complex deposition related to glomerular injury: class I (transmembranous or diffuse) and class II (subendothelial-mesangial). Because of size, solubility, and charge, class I complexes pass into or through the basement membrane and deposit within the membrane or on the epithelial side of the membrane, whereas class II complexes deposit on the

Table 10.1 Classification of immune complex glomerular disease

Location of immune complex deposits	Proposed nomenclature
Beneath epithelium	Class I deposit disease
At epithelial slits	Transmembranous glomerulonephritis
In subepithelial space	Transmembranous glomerulopathy
Subendothelial-mesangial	Class II deposit disease
In subendothelial space	Endomembranous glomerulonephritis
At lamina densa	Laminal glomerulonephritis
In mesangium/loop	Mesangiopathic glomerulonephritis

endothelial side of the basement membrane or are phagocytosed by the mesangial system. Class I complexes are small, soluble antigen-excess complexes that usually deposit in small amounts over a long period of time, producing granular deposits of immunoglobulins or complement distributed diffusely along the epithelial side of the basement membrane or at the epithelial slit membranes. Subepithelial deposits are a common feature of idiopathic membranous glomerulonephritis (MGN) and lupus membranous glomerulopathy (LMG). In MGN, there is diffuse capping of the deposit with IgG. In contrast, the distribution of IgG is diffuse in LMG with a greater deposit of C3c. This may explain the more progressive inflammation in LMG than in MGN. In addition to deposition of complexes from the circulation, granular immune complex deposits are also formed when antibodies react with the surface antigens of the cells of the glomerular endothelial cells. The complexes containing plasma membrane antigens are shed between the endothelial cells and the glomerular basement membrane, where they form local granular deposits. Class II complexes are larger, less soluble complexes and accumulate in the subendothelial space or within the mesangium.

Chronic Glomerulonephritis

Chronic glomerulonephritis (uremic syndrome) may be produced experimentally by repeated injections of small amounts of antigen into an appropriately immunized animal or by repeated injections of soluble complexes. The prolonged deposition of class I complexes leads to variable amounts of PMN infiltration and endothelial proliferation, but the most prominent result is progression to marked thickening of the basement membrane and eventual scarring and destruction of the glomerulus. Cellular inflammation involving activation of lymphocytes, recruitment of macrophages, release of cytokines, and proliferation of epithelial cells leads to destruction of the glomerulus. The production of extracellular matrix (collagen type IV), as well as increased expression of matrix-degrading metalloproteinases, contributes to the structural remodeling process of the glomerulus. Increased expression of monocyte chemoattractant protein 1 (MCP-1) has a fibrogenic effect through the stimulation of transforming growth factor beta (TGF-β) by macrophages. In addition, release of gamma interferon (IFN-γ) from Th1 cells in the glomerulus during chronic inflammation promotes cell-mediated immune injury and contributes to crescentic (proliferative) glomerulonephritis. These mechanisms are responsible for the chronic membranoproliferative glomerulonephritis associated with various human diseases, such as lupus erythematosus (DNA–anti-DNA), diabetes mellitus (insulin–anti-insulin), and thyroiditis (thyroglobulin-antithyroglobulin). In addition, the deposition of toxic complexes of antibody and viral antigens, in particular, hepatitis B and hepatitis C, is responsible for some cases of human glomerulonephritis. Deposits of the tumor antigen carcinoembryonic antigen and antibody to carcinoembryonic antigen have been identified as being responsible for renal damage in some patients with colonic carcinoma. Rare instances of glomerulonephritis from the deposition of IgE antibody-antigen complexes may occur in atopic individuals.

Anti-Glomerular Basement Membrane Nephritis

Human and experimental glomerulonephritis may also be initiated by antibodies to glomerular basement membrane (anti-GBM) or to antigens on epithelial cells. The experimental model is known as experimental autoimmune glomerulonephritis; the human diseases caused by anti-GBM are poststreptococcal glomerulonephritis, Goodpasture's disease, and anti-GBM nephritis associated with vasculitis.

Experimental Autoimmune Glomerulonephritis

Experimental glomerulonephritis caused by anti-GBM may be induced by immunization of animals with glomerular basement membrane extracts in complete Freund's adjuvant. Anti-GBM first contacts and binds to antigens on the capillary side of the basement membrane and can be seen by immunofluorescence as a continuous thin layer along the membrane. Early in the course of anti-GBM disease, the antibodies deposit in a linear pattern, but with time, reformation of the antibody-antigen complexes by rearrangement and condensation results in the formation of dense deposits. The reaction of antibody with the basement membrane results in the binding of complement, PMN infiltration, and basement membrane destruction. A transient form of the experimental disease may be passively transferred with serum from an affected animal on injection into a normal animal, but the antiserum donor must be nephrectomized several days before transfer. Nephrectomy is necessary to allow the accumulation of the antibody, because the nephritogenic antibody is absorbed in vivo by the glomerular tissue of the serum donor. Anti-GBM is responsible for Goodpasture's disease and may by pathogenic in poststreptococcal glomerulonephritis in humans (see below).

Nephrotoxic Serum (Masugi) Nephritis

Experimental glomerulonephritis may also be produced in animals by the passive transfer of heterologous antisera to glomeruli. For example, the passive transfer of rabbit anti-rat glomerulus serum to rats causes nephrotoxic serum nephritis. The nephritis consists of a biphasic response: (i) an acute transient proteinuria is observed as a result of the formation of complexes of rabbit antibodies and antigens present in rat glomerulus; (ii) after 10 days to 2 weeks, a potentially fatal chronic proliferative glomerulonephritis may develop. This second lesion is caused by the production of host (rat) antibodies to donor (rabbit) immunoglobulin. These rat antibodies react with the rabbit antiglomerular antibodies localized on the rat glomeruli, causing the second-phase lesions. The second-phase lesions feature production of TNF and other cytokines from macrophages in involved glomeruli.

Poststreptococcal Glomerulonephritis

The occurrence of acute glomerulonephritis in humans is associated with exposure to some strains of group A beta-hemolytic streptococci. Such streptococcal strains have been termed nephritogenic. The acute infection usually presents as a sore throat and fever. There is a characteristic latent period following the onset of infection during which no significant renal symptoms are observed. Acute poststreptococcal glomerulonephritis is characterized by the onset of proteinuria and hematuria, which correspond in time with the appearance of host antibodies to streptococcal antigens. Immunofluorescence examination of affected kidneys reveals typical immune complex glomerulonephritis (described above); complement, immunoglobulins, and streptococcal antigens are found in glomeruli.

Several theories have been put forward to explain the pathogenic mechanisms for poststreptococcal glomerulonephritis:

1. Some staphylococcal products are toxic to glomeruli.
2. Antibodies to glomerular basement membranes including a GBM-deposited streptococcal antigen, a cross-reacting GBM antigen, or an altered GBM antigen.
3. Deposition of immune complexes of streptococcal antigens or autoantigens formed in the blood.

There is increasing evidence that poststreptococcal glomerulonephritis is caused by a cationic protein designated nephritic strain-associated protein (NSAP), which is a plasminogen activator. The interaction between NSAP and plasminogen splits the C3 molecule activating the alternate complement pathway, initiating inflammation in the glomerulus. Further progression of the disease might be a consequence of the deposit of antibody to the highly immunogenic NSAP trapped in the basement membrane or to basement membrane components. Antibodies to all the major basement membrane macromolecules are present in sera from patients with poststreptococcal glomerulonephritis.

Goodpasture's Disease

The combination of pulmonary hemorrhage and glomerulonephritis is known as Goodpasture's syndrome. In severe cases, there is extensive intra-alveolar hemorrhage and marked proliferative glomerulonephritis. Immunoglobulin and complement may be identified in the basement membrane of pulmonary alveoli and renal glomeruli. Antibody eluted from the kidneys of such patients binds to lung tissue, and antibody eluted from lung tissue binds to kidney. The shared antigen is α3 chain of type IV collagen in the basement membrane, shared by lung and kidney (Fig. 10.8).

Anti-GBM Nephritis Associated with Vasculitis

Rare cases of rapidly progressive glomerulonephritis with evidence of systemic disease, including myalgia, arthritis, skin rash, and vasculitis are seen in patients with anti-glomerular basement membrane antibodies and antibody to myeloperoxidase (anti-neutrophil cytoplasmic antibody, or MPO-ANCA). Pulmonary hemorrhage is seen in about half of these patients. The role of the ANCA in this disease is not clear, but patients with ANCA tend to have a better prognosis than those with rapidly progressive anti-GBM glomerulonephritis with only anti-GBM.

Other Glomerulopathies

Hypocomplementemic Glomerulonephritis

A chronic form of glomerulonephritis without evidence of immunoglobulin in the glomerulus but associated with low levels of serum complement has

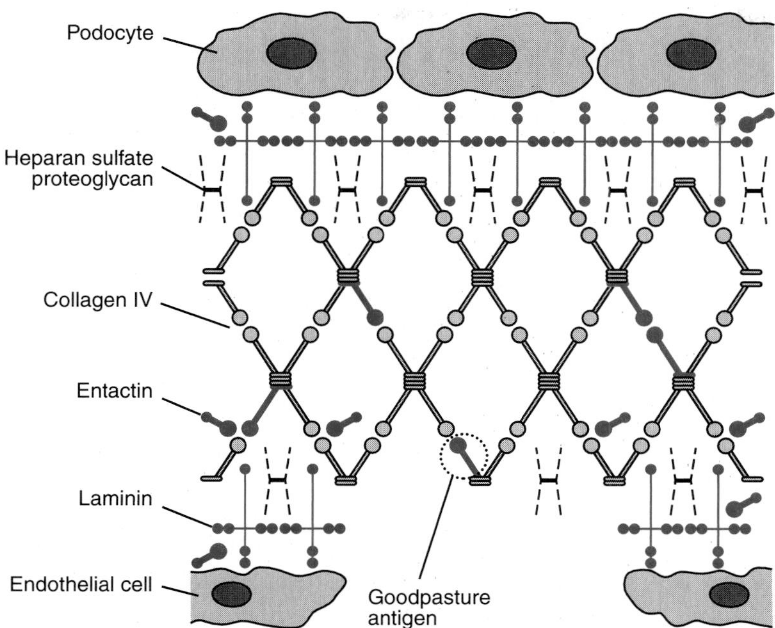

Figure 10.8 Schematic localization of Goodpasture antigen α3 chain of type IV collagen in glomerular basement membrane. The endothelial and epithelial surface of the glomerular basement membrane is lined with laminin, the membrane itself is composed of a scaffold of two subtypes of type IV collagen molecules (building blocks). Subtype A (classical) contains α1 and α2 chains; subtype B contains the α3 chain (Goodpasture antigen). The endothelial surface has a net negative charge; it repels negatively charged antibodies, but cationic antibodies pass into the membrane to react with Goodpasture antigen. Serum of patients with poststreptococcal glomerulonephritis may bind with any of the major components of the basement membrane. (Modified from B. G. Hudson, J. Wieslander, B. J. Wisdom, Jr., and M. E. Noelken, *Lab. Investig.* **61:**256–269, 1989.)

been termed hypocomplementemic glomerulonephritis. Nonimmune activation of complement via the alternate pathway may lead to deposition of complement in renal glomeruli and produce glomerulonephritis. A so-called C3 nephritic factor, which acts like an antibody to altered C3, may be responsible for chronic deposition of C3 in the glomerulus and lowered serum levels of C3. It is also possible that immune complexes may initiate the deposition of complement but be undetectable when the complement components are still active. C3 receptors may be present on glomerular endothelial cells and serve to activate C3 under some circumstances. In any case, glomerulonephritis associated with deposits of complement components without detectable immunoglobulin and lowering of the serum complement is termed hypocomplementemic glomerulonephritis.

IgA Nephritis

First identified as a mild proliferative form of glomerulonephritis associated with mesangial deposition of polymeric IgA1, IgA nephritis is now recognized to have more severe outcomes in up to 40% of patients after 5 to 25 years. In contrast to IgG complex-related tissue damage, which is primarily mediated by complement activation of neutrophils, IgA injury is predominantly mediated by macrophages. In addition, IgA antibody-antigen complexes are more negatively charged than IgG complexes, and after formation in the circulation are cleared by the glomerular mesangial cells. The reason that IgA has an affinity for mesangial cells is not clear, but there is some evidence that mesangial cells may have receptors for IgA. Many patients have IgA antibodies to gluten, the antigen responsible for celiac disease. However, there is no documented association between the presence of IgA antibodies to gluten and lesions of celiac disease, and mesangial IgA deposits occur in patients who do not have antibodies to gluten. Mesangial IgA deposits have been found in patients with Henoch-Schönlein purpura, systemic lupus erythematosus, dermatitis herpetiformis, and viral hepatitis. The etiologic implications of such associations are not clear, although the presence of shared antigens between mesangium and cutaneous capillaries might account for the IgA deposits seen in Henoch-Schönlein purpura. There are no good experimental models of IgA nephritis, most likely because other species do not have the equivalent of human IgA1.

Henoch-Schönlein Nephritis

Henoch-Schönlein purpura is a unique form of immune complex-mediated systemic vasculitis that involves the skin (purpura), kidneys (hematuria), and gastrointestinal tract (abdominal pain) and usually occurs in children below age 15. Clinically, urticarial and hemorrhagic lesions are the most prominent features and tend to occur around joints. Variations in the clinical syndrome include abdominal involvement with edema and hemorrhage into the gastrointestinal tract (Henoch's syndrome); joint involvement with effusion, swelling of the soft tissues, redness, and pain (Schönlein's syndrome); or renal lesions of focal proliferative glomerulonephritis. Granular deposits of IgA and C3 are found in the walls of small vessels in intestine and skin and in the glomerular mesangium. It is possible that an abnormal mucosal immune response to negatively charged antigens may result in IgA complexes that preferentially lodge in the mesangium. Complement may then be activated via the alternate pathway, leading to glomerular damage. Focal lesions in the glomerular basement membrane (splitting, duplications, and spikelike subepithelial protrusions) as well as immune deposits are seen. This disease is usually self-limiting and does not lead to chronic renal disease.

Renal Tubular Disease

Heymann Nephritis

Experimental immunization of rats with renal cortex extract may result in production of autoantibodies to the brush border of the proximal renal tubular cells, immune complex deposition on the epithelial side of the tubular basement membrane, and vacuolization of the proximal tubular cells. The tubular cell damage may be caused by a cytotoxic effect of the antibody. The role of this mechanism in human disease is not clear at this time.

Experimental Allergic Interstitial Nephritis

Immune injury to renal tubules may be induced by immunization of laboratory animals with whole kidney or an antigen from the basement membrane of the renal tubule. The lesion begins as a polymorphonuclear infiltrate but progresses to a chronic mononuclear infiltrate with atrophy and degeneration of the tubules. Linear deposits of IgG may be detected along the basement membrane of the proximal tubules. Immune-mediated interstitial nephritis may occur in association with collagen diseases or renal graft rejection in humans.

Clinical-Immunopathologic Correlations in Glomerulonephritis

Glomerulonephritis may be caused by deposition of immune complexes formed elsewhere, by reaction of antibody directly with glomerular basement membrane antigens, or by the activation of complement by the alternate pathway. Each of these mechanisms may produce an identical clinical picture or pathologic lesion (Fig. 10.9). Clinically, glomerulonephritis is a syndrome with markedly variable expression, but the disease can be classified generally into acute, subacute, and chronic. The acute disease may

Figure 10.9 Glomerulonephritis: clinical-pathologic correlations. The mechanisms of glomerulonephritis illustrated may produce a varied clinical and pathologic picture. **(I)** Anti-glomerular basement membrane antibody reacts with antigens on the lumenal side of the glomerular basement membrane and produces a linear deposition when examined by immunofluorescence. **(II)** Soluble immune complexes formed elsewhere pass through the glomerular basement membrane and lodge on the epithelial side, producing lumpy-bumpy deposits, or lodge within or on the endothelial side of the basement membrane as granular deposits. Granular deposit disease may also be produced from endothelial cell surface antigen-antibody complexes shed into the basement membrane. **(III)** Complement in the absence of immunoglobulin may be detected as a granular deposit. Hypocomplementemic glomerulonephritis may be caused by a preceding immunoglobulin deposit or by the action of properdin, both of which may activate complement. No single mechanism produces a particular type of clinical picture or pathologic lesion, although hypocomplementemic glomerulonephritis is usually of the chronic variety. A capillary lumen, basement membrane endothelial cell foot plates, and an epithelial cell are illustrated. (Modified from an illustration by C. Wilson, Scripps Clinic and Research Foundation, La Jolla, Calif.)

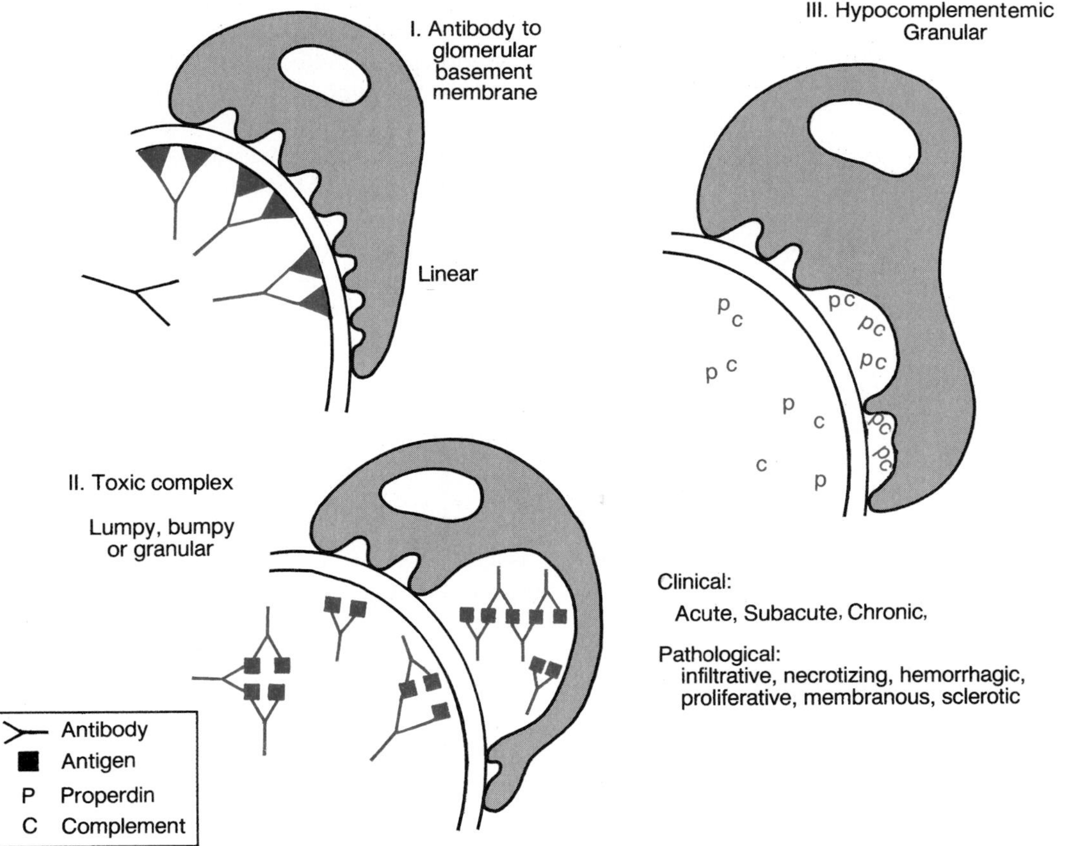

include proteinuria, gross hematuria, oliguria or anuria, edema, azotemia, and rapid death due to renal failure. However, recovery from the acute disease occurs in more than 99% of cases. Adults may develop a more persistent subacute or chronic progression to renal failure. Pathologically, a variety of lesions may be seen in the glomeruli. During the acute stage, the lesions may be minimal (proteinuria associated with fusion of epithelial foot plates), necrotic (death of glomerular cells), infiltrative or exudative (glomeruli full of PMNs), or hemorrhagic (red blood cells in glomeruli). Subacute glomerulonephritis is associated with proliferative (increased number of mononuclear cells or glomerular epithelial cells) or embolic (fibrin thrombi in glomerular capillaries) lesions. Chronic glomerulonephritis features membranous (thickening of glomerular basement membrane) or sclerotic (scarring of glomeruli) changes. Intermediate stages of the disease usually demonstrate an overlap of lesions.

Any of these lesions may be produced by one of the three basic immunopathologic mechanisms. The pathologic type of lesion depends upon the degree of injury produced in a given period of time, not upon the immunopathologic mechanism. Thus, the deposit of small amounts of immune complexes in the basement membrane may cause proteinuria. The deposit of large amounts of immune complexes or of antibodies to the basement membrane in a short period of time will lead to infiltration of the glomerulus with a large number of PMNs and extensive dissolution of the basement membrane. The dissolution permits proteins of high molecular weight to pass through the basement membrane. If larger segments of the basement membrane are destroyed, larger blood components such as erythrocytes will pass through the basement membrane, producing hematuria. The loss of protein leads to hypoproteinemia, decreased intravascular osmotic pressure, edema, and heart failure—the clinical picture of acute glomerulonephritis. The deposit of small amounts of immune complexes over long periods of time may produce some disruption of the basement membrane and leakage of serum proteins but mainly causes a buildup on or in the basement membrane leading to thickening of the basement membrane and a gradual loss of the filtering capacity of the glomeruli (membranous glomerulonephritis). This results in retention of nitrogen and waste products (azotemia) and gradual renal failure. The pathologist is not usually able to identify the immunopathologic mechanism responsible for a given case of glomerulonephritis by defining the histopathologic lesion. Identification of the mechanism requires immunofluorescent studies, serologic workup, electron microscopy, and careful clinical documentation of the course of the disease.

Human Glomerular Diseases

Human glomerulonephritis is classified by a combination of pathologic findings, clinical features, and course. A pathologic classification is given in Table 10.2.

Vasculitis

Inflammation of vessels is a primary feature of many immune complex-mediated diseases that are covered in various chapters in this book. The endothelial lining of the blood vessels usually repels white blood cells and has been called "Teflon-like." This protective barrier becomes less effective

Table 10.2 Some forms of glomerulonephritis of humans[a]

Type	Mechanism	Pathologic findings	Immunofluorescence	Clinical features	Prognosis
Postinfectious glomerulonephritis (human counterpart of acute serum sickness)	Immune complex	LM: Diffuse cellular proliferation, neutrophils EM: Subepithelial deposits ("humps")	Coarse granular or lumpy-bumpy pattern in basement membranes (IgG, C3)	Acute nephritis[b]	Good
Membranous nephropathy (human counterpart of chronic serum sickness)	Immune complex	LM: Diffuse basement membrane thickening EM: Subepithelial deposits, several small	Fine granular along basement membranes (IgC, C3)	Nephrotic syndrome[c]	Slowly progressive (renal failure)
Minimal change disease	Immunological (exact mechanism unknown)	LM: Normal glomeruli EM: Effacement of epithelial cell foot processes	Negative or nonspecific	Nephrotic syndrome	Good
IgA nephropathy (Berger's disease)	Immune complex (IgA)	LM: Increase in mesangial matrix and cells EM: Electron-dense deposits in the mesangium	Positive in the mesangium (IgA, IgG, C3)	Hematuria, proteinuria	Usually good
Goodpasture's disease	Antibasement membrane (kidney, lung)	LM: Crescentic glomerulonephritis EM: No evidence of deposits	Linear positivity along basement membranes (IgG, C3)	Acute renal failure, hemoptysis (lung hemorrhage)	Rapidly progressive (renal failure)
Membranoproliferative GN (type I)	Immune complex	LM: Mesangial proliferation, basement membrane alteration EM: Split basement membranes, subendothelial deposits	Granular irregular pattern in basement membranes (IgG, C3)	Variable (nephrotic syndrome, nephritis)	Progressive (renal failure)
Dense deposit disease (membranoproliferative GN, type II)	Alternate pathway of complement	LM: Mesangial proliferation, basement, membrane alteration EM: Very dense material of unknown nature deposited in basement membranes	Focal C3 (IgG and early-acting complement components absent)	Variable (nephrotic syndrome, nephritis hypocomplementemia)	Progressive (renal failure)

[a]Abbreviations: LM, light microscopy; EM, electron microscopy; GN, glomerulonephritis. Note: These are basic characteristic features; variations occur in pathological and clinical findings.
[b]Nephritis: hematuria, red cell casts, hypertension.
[c]Nephrotic syndrome: proteinuria >3.5 g/24 h.

when vasculitis develops, allowing the deposition of immune complexes on vascular endothelial surfaces, where they aggregate to fix complement, which, in turn, attracts and activates granulocytes. In 1990, the Diagnostic and Therapeutic Criteria Committee of the American College of Rheumatology published a classification of seven major vasculitic diseases (Table 10.3). In addition, vasculitis is associated with a large number of independent conditions, including infectious diseases, connective tissue diseases, malignancies, inflammatory diseases, such as Crohn's disease and cirrhosis, and as complications of atherosclerosis. There are definite associations between the size of the vessel and the underlying disease or syndrome. Each of these vascular lesions has a component of neutrophil infiltrate as well as lesions associated with other immune mechanisms. Often, the lesions are biopsied at a stage of development when the neutrophils have partially disintegrated. This is referred to as "leukoclastic vasculitis." Antineutrophil antibodies to proteases (C-ANCA, cytoplasmic immunofluorescence) or to myeloperoxidase (P-ANCA, perinuclear immunofluorescence) released from neutrophils may form and are used to help make the diagnosis of vasculitides such as polyarteritis nodosa (PAN), Churg-Strauss syndrome, systemic vasculitis, Wegener's granulomatosis, and idiopathic concentric glomerulonephritis.

The presence of vasculitis in the early stages of the collagen-vascular diseases (see below) implies an important role for immune complexes in the pathogenesis of these diseases. Immune complex-mediated vasculitis is often manifested in the skin. Because immune lesions in the skin may be used to compare different immunopathologic mechanisms, the skin diseases due to immune complexes are presented in a separate chapter (chapter 20). Some rare vascular diseases with peculiar features are presented here.

Behçet's Syndrome

Behçet's syndrome, rediscovered in 1937 by Hulusu Behçet, a Turkish dermatologist, was first described by Hippocrates. The disease consists of a clinical triad, which includes oral and genital aphthous ulcerations, vascular skin lesions, and arthritis and inflammation of the eye, for which an exact pathogenesis has not been determined. Involvement of infectious agents or superantigens involving overexpression of Th1 activity and interleukin-12 (IL-12) production has been suspected, but not proved. This disease is common in Japan, Korea, and China. It is believed to be an immune complex disease. About half of the patients with this disease have a correlation with their disease activity and the level of circulating immune complexes. There is an increased incidence in individuals with HLA-B51. Positive delayed-type hypersensitivity skin reactions to streptococcal antigens and exacerbations of the disease in 15 of 85 patients given a skin test suggest that an immune reactivity to streptococcal antigens is responsible. About 25% of the patients develop arterial and venous large vessel disease, including arterial aneurysms and venous thrombosis. Treatment with a variety of immunosuppressive regimes is sometimes effective.

Kawasaki Syndrome (Mucocutaneous Lymph Node Syndrome)

Kawasaki syndrome is similar to rheumatic fever involving the heart (vasculitis and pancarditis) with frequent involvement of the coronary arteries leading to thrombosis, infarction, aneurysms, and scarring. The acute dis-

Table 10.3 Pathologic overlap in selected vasculitis syndromes[a]

Syndrome	Vessels involved	Sites involved	Types of vasculitis	Special features	Other comments
Polyarteritis nodosa	Medium and small muscular arteries; sometimes arterioles	Visceral, cutaneous; infrequently cerebral and lung vessels	Necrotizing, with mixed cells and few eosinophils; rarely granulomatous	Focal segmental involvement; coexisting acute and healed lesions or normal and affected vessels; micro-aneurysms	Vascular lesion in infants is indistinguishable from fatal Kawasaki disease
Churg-Strauss syndrome	Small arteries and veins, often arterioles and venules	Upper and lower respiratory tract; viscera, heart, and skin	Necrotizing or granulomatous, with mixed cells, prominent eosinophils	Extravascular necrotizing granulomas with prominent eosinophils; may manifest as "limited form"	Most patients have asthma or history of allergy
Wegener's granulomatosis	Usually small arteries and veins; sometimes larger vessels	Upper and lower respiratory tract; often kidney; infrequently skin, heart, and viscera	Necrotizing or granulomatous, with mixed cells and occasional eosinophils	Geographic pattern of tissue necrosis and anti-neutrophil cytoplasmic antibodies; may manifest as "limited form"	Occurs in all ages, with a slight male preponderance; associated with HLA-DR2; may respond to antimicrobials
Hypersensitivity vasculitis	Arterioles and venules; often small arteries and veins	Predominantly skin; less commonly viscera, heart, and synovium	Leukocytoclastic or lymphocytic, with variable number of eosinophils; occasionally granulomatous	May be associated with myocarditis, interstitial nephritis, or hepatitis	Patients may have occult malignancy or history of drug or chemical allergy, vaccination
Henoch-Schönlein purpura	Arterioles and venules; often small arteries and veins	Predominantly skin, gastrointestinal, kidney, and synovium	Leukocytoclastic, mixed cell, or lymphocytic, with variable number of eosinophils	IgA immune deposits	Predominantly children and young adults
Giant cell (temporal) arteritis	Vessels of all sizes	Predominantly temporal arteries; less often, any other vessels	Granulomatous, with variable number of giant cells, sometimes only lymphoplas-macytic	Affected extracranial large vessels; indistinguishable from Takayasu's arteritis; may form aneurysm or cause dissection	Virtually all patients are over age 50; may be asymptomatic
Takayasu's arteritis	Elastic arteries and selected muscular arteries	Aorta, arch vessels, other major branches (coronary, renal, visceral), and pulmonary arteries	Granulomatous, few giant cells in active phase and sclerosing fibrosis in chronic stage, with scanty infiltrate	Aneurysmal in 20% may be segmental and cause rupture or dissection	Most common in women of childbearing age; more prevalent in Asia; important cause of renovascular hypertension in adolescents

[a]From E. C. LeRoy, *Hosp. Pract.* **27:**77–81, 85–86, 88, 1992.

ease features fever, conjunctivitis, erythematous skin rash, mucous membrane ulcerations, edema, and lymphadenopathy. An infectious agent is suspected but not identified. Most of the morbidity and mortality involves the development of coronary artery aneurysms.

Hypocomplementemic Vasculitic Urticarial Syndrome

This syndrome includes urticaria, leukoclastic vasculitis, arthritis, and neurologic abnormalities. Laboratory findings are a low C1q, C4, C2, and C3 with normal C1r and C1s, C5-9, and properdin. A 7S protein that precipitates C1q is found (C1q activating factor) and is believed to be responsible for complement activation.

Giant Cell Arteritis

Giant cell arteritis features a granulomatous reaction (see chapter 17) in and around the internal elastic lamina of the temporal artery. It is suspected that either there is an alteration in the elastic lamina leading to an immune response (perhaps due to solar radiation) or a congenital (perhaps HLA-D4-linked) disposition to development of an autoimmune response to elastin.

Post-Cardiac Bypass Syndrome

Patients who have been on cardiac bypass develop fever, leukocytosis, and edema believed to be secondary to nonimmune specific activation of C3 to C3a.

Aleutian Mink Disease

Aleutian mink disease is caused by the immune response to a persistent virus infection and offers an animal model for the relationship of the humoral immune response to the development of lesions found during a viral infection. The disease is characterized by a proliferation of lymphoid tissues, hypergammaglobulinemia, glomerulonephritis, hepatitis, and arteritis. There is an overproduction of IgG antibody and the formation of immune complexes because the humoral immune response is unable to control viral reproduction. This results in hyperplasia of IgG-forming cells, formation of antibody-virus complexes, and immune complex lesions of vasculitis and glomerulonephritis. The intracellular virus infection could possibly be controlled by the cellular reactivity of delayed-type hypersensitivity. However, for as yet undefined reasons, the affected mink produce a nonprotective, lesion-producing IgG antibody response. Thus, Aleutian mink disease is a prime example of the destructive effects of an immune response when the response is inappropriate (e.g., humoral rather than cellular; see also the discussion of leprosy in chapter 15). If the mink manifested a cellular rather than a humoral immune response to the virus, the disease in this form would not occur.

Dermal Vasculitis

Immune complex reactions are responsible for a variety of vascular reactions in the skin. Most lesions are secondary to deposition of immune complexes in dermal vessels. These include erythema nodosum, erythema marginatum, and erythema multiforme. These are discussed in more detail in chapter 16, where they are included as examples of immune complex-mediated skin diseases.

Cutaneous Vasculitis in Infectious Diseases

A variety of vascular skin lesions may be associated with infections such as viral hepatitis, infective endocarditis, infectious mononucleosis, and a number of bacterial infections, in particular, streptococcal and pseudomonal. In some cases, immunoglobulin and complement have been identified in cutaneous vessels, and circulating immune complexes are present. Often, these patients have glomerular or pulmonary lesions as well.

Rheumatic Fever

Acute rheumatic fever and chronic rheumatic heart disease are examples of different stages of damage caused by an immune complex mechanism activated after an immune response to an infection. Rheumatic fever is an acute systemic inflammatory sequel to group A beta-hemolytic streptococcal pharyngitis (not to streptococcal skin infections) that can lead to scarring of the valves of the heart and chronic heart disease. The heart lesions of rheumatic fever are sterile. Refinement of the diagnosis of streptococcal infection and prompt introduction of measures to eliminate the infection, usually by intensive therapy with penicillin, significantly reduce the occurrence of cardiac sequelae. The many early manifestations of this multiorgan disease often make the diagnosis difficult. To codify the diagnosis, a classification of the diagnostic criteria for rheumatic fever devised by T. Duckerr Jones in 1944 was revised in 1992 (Table 10.4). The clinical picture may be one of fleeting and transient joint pains and fever to full-blown acute rheumatic fever. Acute rheumatic fever begins with abrupt elevation of temperature, malaise, skin rash, and pain and swelling of the joints occurring within 4 to 5 weeks after a streptococcal throat infection. Myocarditis may be detected clinically using antimyosin antibody radioimaging. Subcutaneous nodules, Sydenham's chorea or St. Vitus's dance (involuntary and jerky movements of the extremities), and signs of acute left ventricular failure may also be seen at the beginning of the acute illness. The symptoms usually last for a month or two, although fatal heart failure can occur. After a symptomless period, the initial clinical pattern is repeated with subsequent infections of rheumatogenic strains of beta-hemolytic streptococci. If the first episode has prominent cardiac symptoms

Table 10.4 Revised criteria for the diagnosis of rheumatic fever (updated 1992)[a]

Major manifestations
Carditis
Polyarthritis
Chorea
Erythema marginatum
Subcutaneous nodules
Minor manifestations
Clinical findings
Fever
Arthralgias
Laboratory findings
Elevated ESR or C-reactive protein
Prolonged PR interval
Supporting evidence of previous group A streptococcal infection
Positive throat culture or rapid streptococcal antigen test
Elevated or rising streptococcal antibody titer

[a]ESR, erythrocyte sedimentation rate; PR interval, timing of signal on electrocardiogram consistent with myocarditis. Modified from A. D. Dajani, E. Ayoub, F. Z. Bierman, and the Special Writing Group of the Committee on Rheumatic Fever, *Circulation* **87**:302–307, 1992.

and little joint inflammation, the following episodes will follow the same pattern. Thus, involvement of the heart during the first episode indicates that repeated episodes will eventually lead to chronic rheumatic heart disease.

Although the incidence of acute rheumatic fever in children has decreased markedly in North America and Europe from that of 20 to 40 years ago, rheumatic heart disease still ranks as a major cause of disease in adults who contracted rheumatic fever as children. The number of admissions to the children's service at Johns Hopkins Hospital in Baltimore declined from 25 to 30 per year from 1952 to 1961 to less than 3 per year from 1976 to 1981. The decrease in the number of new cases may be due to the widespread, and often indiscriminate, use of antibiotics effective against streptococci, better general living conditions with less crowding, and a decline in the prevalence of the rheumatogenic strains of beta-hemolytic streptococci. However, the disease is still common in Third World countries, and occasional local resurgences of the disease have been reported in the United States. In Connecticut, the number of throat cultures positive for streptococci rose from less than 5,000 in 1955 to over 250,000 in 1972. The reasons for the overall decline and the local resurgences remain poorly understood, but there appears to be an increase in the prevalence of "rheumatogenic" strains of beta-hemolytic streptococci. Attempts to develop a protective vaccine using M proteins or other components of the streptococcus have not been successful. One of the problems is that immunization with streptococcal antigens may cause harmful autoimmune reactions.

The major pathologic features of rheumatic fever are widespread inflammation and scarring in connective tissue in the heart, joints, lungs, pleura, subcutaneous tissue, and skin. Vasculitis may involve many small and medium-sized arteries. The inflammation of the heart is a "pancarditis" involving the pericardium, myocardium, and endocardium. Myocardial fibers may show dissolution associated with a diffuse mixed inflammatory infiltrate. Scarring of the endocardium leads to marked thickening and shortening of the chordae tendinea and thickening of the valve leaflets. This may produce severe insufficiency and stenosis of the cardiac valves, most commonly the mitral valve. The classic myocardial lesion, the Aschoff body, begins as a loose focal mononuclear infiltrate around small arteries and evolves to a fibrous scar. The histological appearance of later valvular and myocardial lesions suggests that cell-mediated immunity may be active during the chronic stages of the inflammation. Lymphocytes from rheumatic fever patients react with streptococcal antigens in vitro by proliferation, and lymphocytes from animals immunized with streptococcal antigens kill myocardial cells in vitro. Patients with late effects of rheumatic endocarditis are a major source of candidates for corrective valvular surgery.

The lesions of rheumatic fever are caused by immune-mediated inflammation. As a protective response to infection, anti-streptococcal antibodies neutralize toxins and opsonize organisms. However, destructive lesions are caused by the formation of immune complexes and of antibodies to streptococcal antigens that cross-react with antigens present in the tissues of the host (molecular mimicry) (Fig. 10.10). Antibodies to a number of streptococcal antigens as well as to host proteins are found in postinfection serum. Antibodies to streptococcal M protein cross-react with heart muscle and are believed to be responsible for inflammation of the heart (pancarditis). Monoclonal antibodies produced to group A streptococci have identified cross-reacting antigens on cardiac myocytes, smooth muscle cells, cell surface and cytoplasm of endothelial lining cells, and valvular interstitial cells. Antibodies to group A streptococcal carbohydrate correlate with the development of valvular heart disease. The chorea of rheumatic fever has been associated with autoantibodies to basal ganglia. These antibodies can be absorbed with streptococcal cell walls. Other lesions of rheumatic fever are most likely the result of immune complex formation, in particular, erythema marginatum (vasculitis in the dermis) and glomerulonephritis. Rheumatic nodules are small, rubbery granulomas and are most likely the end result of vasculitis caused by the deposition of immune complexes containing antigens resistant to degradation, leading to accumulation of macrophages and the formation of granulomas. In addition, streptococcal M protein can act as a superantigen, activating T cells and possibly stimulating subsets of T cells that react with self antigens. Although there is no clear association of rheumatic disease with HLA phenotype, the B-cell alloantigen 833 is significantly more common in rheumatic fever patients than in control subjects.

In summary, antibodies to streptococcal products serve to inactivate streptococcal organisms and products as well as to initiate acute inflammatory reactions (immune complex mechanism). Cross-reaction of antistreptococcal antibodies with host tissues and formation of soluble complexes of antibodies and streptococcal antigens may cause immune complex-mediated inflammatory reactions distant from the site of infection.

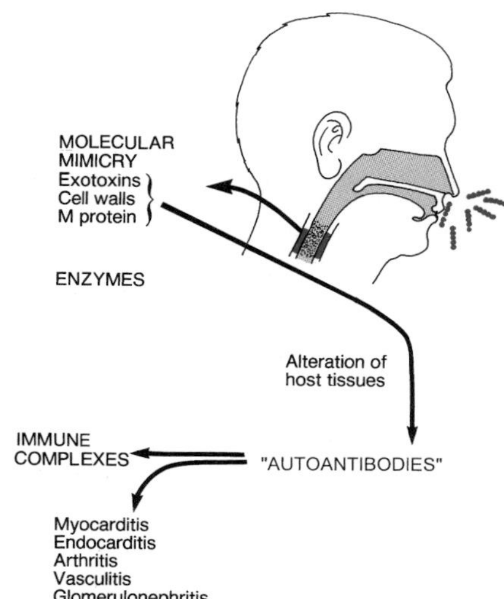

Figure 10.10 The immune response to streptococcal group A antigens and rheumatic fever. Antibodies produced to streptococcal antigens cross-react with host tissue antigens. These "autoantibodies," as well as soluble immune complexes, are responsible for the lesions of rheumatic fever (myocarditis, endocarditis, arthritis, vasculitis, and glomerulonephritis).

Diffuse Connective Tissue Diseases

The diffuse connective tissue diseases include rheumatoid arthritis, systemic lupus erythematosus, Sjögren's syndrome, polymyositis (dermatomyositis), and progressive systemic sclerosis (scleroderma). These diseases were previously termed collagen-vascular diseases or rheumatoid diseases. The term "collagen-vascular" was used because of lesions believed to be in the collagen of connective tissues and the association with vascular lesions. The term "rheumatoid" was used because of the use of the general term "rheumatism" to cover a number of diseases now known to be different, in particular, rheumatic fever and skeletal tuberculosis.

Rheumatoid diseases got their name because of the resemblance of these diseases to rheumatic fever (see above). The term *rheumatologist* in reference to physicians who diagnose and treat patients with *rheumatoid diseases* was introduced by Comroe in Philadelphia in 1940.

In 1942, Klemperer coined the term "collagen disease" for a group of diseases that had in common a morphologically similar lesion in collagen—fibrinoid necrosis, an increase in ground substance with swollen, fragmented collagen fibers and necrosis, resulting in a structureless eosinophilic area resembling fibrin in appearance. The concept that one disease could affect the function of many organs was revolutionary at the time. The discovery of rheumatoid factor and the lupus erythematosus cell in 1948 and the application of cortisone for therapy in 1949 led to major advances in understanding the connective tissue diseases. Most of the lesions of the connective tissue diseases are caused by immune complex-mediated mechanisms, but other mechanisms, in particular cell-mediated hypersensitivity, may also contribute, in particular for Sjögren's syndrome.

Each of the connective tissue diseases has its own pattern of clinical features, time course, location of lesions, autoantibody reactivities, and immunopathologic mechanisms. Rheumatoid arthritis mainly affects joints; Sjögren's syndrome, the exocrine glands; polymyositis, the skeletal muscle; and scleroderma, the dermal and submucosal connective tissue. Systemic lupus erythematosus has a multiplicity of autoantibodies and a wide spectrum of tissue involvement. As depicted in Fig. 10.11, there is considerable overlap of pathologic features within the connective tissue disease group, and a given patient may have features of several connective diseases (overlap syndromes). Many individuals with a connective tissue disease have angiitis or glomerulonephritis, immunoglobulin abnormalities, and autoantibodies with varied specificities of reactivity, including falsely positive tests for syphilis. Some of the protean manifestations of syphilis, and other chronic infectious diseases, are not unlike many of the features of the connective tissue diseases and may be the result of autoimmune reactions caused by alteration of host tissue or allergic reactions to the infecting organisms located in host tissue. Similarly, the lesions seen in the connective tissue diseases may result from immune reactions to as yet undetected infectious agents.

The variable clinical and pathologic features of the connective tissue diseases may be the result of the operation of different types of immune reactions with different degrees of severity at different times, directed to-

Figure 10.11 Pathologic features of connective tissue diseases. The relative frequency of the lesions associated with connective tissue diseases (bottom) is indicated by the thickness of the boxes (top). Serum sickness is included because its characteristic lesions (vasculitis, glomerulonephritis, myocarditis, and arthritis) are also found in the connective tissue diseases. This suggests a primary role for immune complex mechanisms in connective tissue disease.

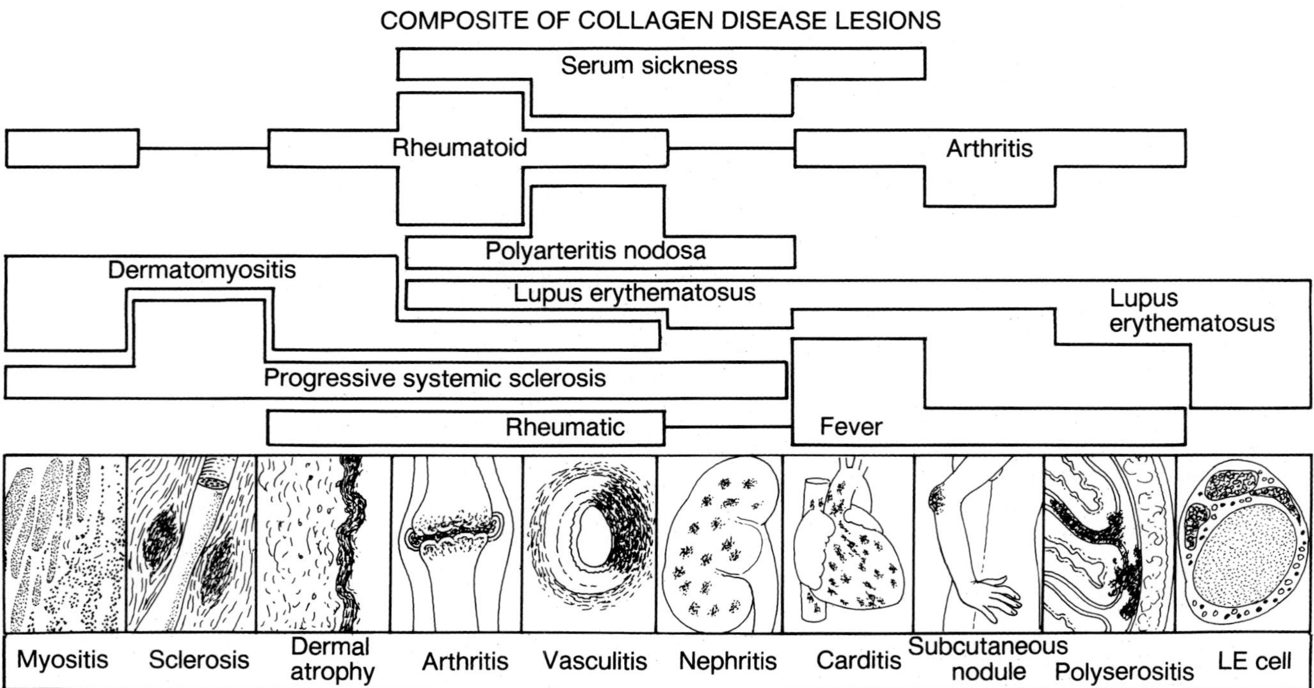

ward different antigenic specificities with different tissue locations. The interplay of these variables could produce varying clinical pictures during the course of a disease in a given individual. For further information, the reader is referred to the *Primer on the Rheumatic Disease* published by the Arthritis Foundation, Atlanta, Georgia.

Polyarteritis Nodosa

Although PAN is not officially a connective tissue disease, it is included here to illustrate the features of a multiorgan disease caused by immune complex vasculitis.

Diagnosis

The clinically apparent lesions of PAN consist of multiple foci of localized infarcts affecting almost any organ or combination of organs in the body. Inflammation of small and medium-sized arteries results in thrombosis and obstruction to blood flow, leading to many areas of necrosis and scarring. There is characteristically necrosis of a portion of the arterial wall, leading to scarring of this segment, with the rest of the wall of the vessel appearing normal. The necrotic segment may become distended owing to intra-arterial pressure, resulting in the formation of microaneurysms, giving rise to the term "nodosa," hence polyarteritis nodosa. Microaneurysms (pseudoaneurysms) may be seen in the medium-sized arteries of the liver and kidney by angiography. Initial symptoms may include malaise, fatigue, fever, myalgias, muscle weakness, and pain in various locations. Renal involvement with glomerulonephritis or vasculitis is common. Inflammation of the arteries of the heart or brain may cause myocardial or cerebral infarcts. Infarction of the pancreas may mimic the symptoms of acute pancreatitis.

The arterial lesion is similar to that seen in serum sickness arteritis, and immunoglobulin may be identified in the areas of fibrinoid necrosis. The role of this immunoglobulin in the production of the lesion is unclear. The immunoglobulin may be antibody that is reacting with antigen that is part of the vessel wall; it may be part of an antigen-antibody complex formed in the circulation and deposited in the vessel wall; or it may be nonspecifically absorbed to an arterial lesion evoked by a unrelated mechanism.

Complexes of viruses and immunoglobulin appear to be responsible for some cases of PAN. There is a high association of PAN with hepatitis B and hepatitis C, suggesting that polyarteritis occurring naturally may be due to an immune response to viral hepatitis infection with viral antigen release. The association of polyarteritis with drug administration also suggests that some cases of polyarteritis may be caused by an immune response to drugs administered for therapy of other diseases. In addition, PAN has been reported rarely in patients undergoing hyposensitization for allergic diseases (asthma), perhaps because of the production of complement-fixing IgG antibody to the desensitizing allergen.

Until the introduction of cyclophosphamide, only about half the patients with histologically proven PAN survived more than 5 years. Early and vigorous treatment with corticosteroids and cyclophosphamide or other immunosuppressive and anti-inflammatory drugs may significantly improve the prognosis of severe progressive PAN. Cyclophosphamide induces remission in cases that have been refractory to other treatments. For a more detailed comparison of PAN with other forms of vasculitis, see "Vasculitis" above.

Rheumatoid Arthritis

Rheumatoid arthritis (RA) is a systemic syndrome in which chronic inflammation of the joints is believed to be initiated by autoantibodies and maintained by cellular inflammatory mechanisms. The most clearly defined autoantibodies are directed to self immunoglobulin determinants (rheumatoid factor). The formation of immune complexes in the joint spaces leads to activation of complement and destructive inflammation (see below). The acute phase is followed by a delayed-type hypersensitivity (DTH) chronic inflammation. Chronic rheumatoid arthritis is believed to be driven by macrophages after initiation by T_{DTH} cells. T_{DTH} cells are present in large numbers in rheumatoid synovium, and cytotoxic T cells (T_{CTL} cells) may contribute to chronic articular damage. However, the major cytokines found in the joint are macrophage derived, such as IL-1, TNF-α, granulocyte-monocyte colony-stimulating factor (GM-CSF), and IL-6, whereas T_{DTH} cell factors (IL-2 and IFN-γ) are present in only very small amounts. Thus, the pathogenesis of rheumatoid arthritis involves a complex interplay of immune complex and DTH reactions. A current thought is that local dendritic cells in the synovium may play a critical role in antigen processing and development of the lesions of rheumatoid arthritis.

Diagnosis

The precise diagnosis of mild RA is difficult, as evidenced by the criteria established by a committee of the American Rheumatism Association (Table 10.5). The most common symptoms include a symmetric arthritis usually involving the small joints of the hands or feet and the knees. The arthritis is the result of an inflammatory synovitis that begins as a chronic inflammatory infiltration but usually proceeds to destructive inflammation and proliferation (pannus) eroding the articular surface. The synovia becomes hyperplastic and filled with lymphocytes and plasma cells, and prominent germinal center formation is seen as the disease progresses. Muscle wasting and the formation of subcutaneous nodules (see below) are found in about 20% of patients. Serositis, myocarditis, vasculitis, and peripheral neuropathy may also be found. Many attempts have been made to measure the progression of RA using mechanical and electrical instruments, laboratory tests, radiologic changes, and clinical measurements such as discomfort and disability. It appears that the best predictor of the prognosis for RA is loss of function as determined clinically. For the classic case of seropositive nodular erosive disease, functional disability occurs early and continues to worsen despite treatment to severe functional loss within 10 years.

Rheumatoid Factor

One of the diagnostic features of RA is rheumatoid factor (RF), a circulating autoantibody with reactivity to immunoglobulins. RF was discovered in 1940 by Waaler, who observed the agglutination of immunoglobulin-coated sheep red blood cells by factors in human sera. Historically, three general reactive specificities were recognized: (i) to xenogeneic immunoglobulins (rabbit or horse), (ii) to allogeneic immunoglobulins (denatured human IgG), and (iii) to autologous immunoglobulins (the patient's own IgG). RF is usually an IgM antibody that reacts with one or more of the above antigens, although IgG RFs are also found in some cases. The formation of RF is the result of an immune response by the host to one or more specific antigenic determinants present in his or her own

Table 10.5 The 1987 revised criteria for the classification of rheumatoid arthritis (traditional format)[a]

Criterion	Definition[b]
1. Morning stiffness	Morning stiffness in and around the joints, lasting at least 1 h before maximal improvement
2. Arthritis of 3 or more joint areas	At least 3 joint areas simultaneously have had soft tissue swelling or fluid (not bony overgrowth alone) observed by a physician. The 14 possible areas are right or left PIP, MCP, wrist, elbow, knee, ankle, and MTP joints
3. Arthritis of hand joints	At least 1 area swollen (as defined above) in a wrist, MCP, or PIP joint
4. Symmetric arthritis	Simultaneous involvement of the same joint areas (as defined in 2) on both sides of the body (bilateral involvement of PIPs, MCPs, or MTPs is acceptable without absolute symmetry)
5. Rheumatoid nodules	Subcutaneous nodules, over bony prominences or extensor surfaces or in juxtaarticular regions, observed by a physician
6. Serum rheumatoid factor	Demonstration of abnormal amounts of serum rheumatoid factor by any method for which the result has been positive in <5% of normal control subjects
7. Radiographic changes	Radiographic changes typical of rheumatoid arthritis on posteroanterior hand and wrist radiographs, which must include erosions or unequivocal bony decalcification localized in or most marked adjacent to the involved joints (osteoarthritis changes alone do not qualify)

[a]For classification purposes, a patient is said to have rheumatoid arthritis if he or she has satisfied at least four of these seven criteria. Criteria 1 through 4 must have been present for at least 6 weeks. Patients with two clinical diagnoses are not excluded. Designation as classic, definite, or probable rheumatoid arthritis is *not* to be made. From F. C. Arnett, S. M. Edworthy, D. A. Block, D. J. McShane, J. F. Fries, et al., *Arthritis Rheum.* **31:**315–324, 1988.

[b]Abbreviations: MCP, metacarpal phalangeal; MTP, metatarsal phalangeal; PIP, proximal interphalangeal.

immunoglobulins. RF is usually detected by agglutination of particles (erythrocytes, latex) coated with IgG; it also reacts with antigen-antibody complexes. RFs most often react with antigenic groupings of IgG that are buried in the native molecule and may be shared with immunoglobulins of other species. These antigenic specificities may be revealed by unfolding of the IgG molecule due to various denaturing processes or to the reaction of IgG antibody with antigen. RFs may also react with genetically controlled isoantigens (allotypes) located on immunoglobulins. The specificity of RFs produced by synovial tissue may be different from that reflected in the serum. The major antigenic determinant for synovial fluid RF appears to be in the CH3 domain of the IgG3 molecule. The significance of this is not clear.

Reaction of RF with IgG occurs in vivo and is believed to be the initiating factor for the early lesions associated with RA. Another possibility from a mouse experimental model is an autoimmune response to glucose-6-phosphate, but this has not yet been examined in human disease. Necrotizing arteritis is especially likely to evolve in patients with high titers of RF, presumably caused by deposition of immune complexes in vessels. In most cases, RF (anti-IgG) forms large complexes with IgG in vivo. These complexes are cleared from the circulation by the RES with no further tissue damage. In rare cases, the RF-immunoglobulin complexes are soluble at body temperature but can be precipitated from the patient's serum by cooling (cryoglobulins). Patients with cryoglobulins are more apt to develop secondary vascular lesions. Some cryoimmunoglobulins are not immune complexes but abnormal immunoglobulins found in the sera of patients with connective tissue diseases and patients with lymphoproliferative disorders. These "monoclonal" cryoimmunoglobulins do not cause the significant vascular and glomerular lesions found with the immune complex (mixed) cryoimmunoglobulins.

Since rheumatoid arthritis occurs in the joint, it seems reasonable that the pathogenically important RF for arthritis is in the synovium and not in the serum. The titers of RF in serum do not correlate closely with the occurrence or severity of arthritis. However, in several studies, RF in the sera predated the appearance of RA. In addition, the serum levels of RF correlate well with the appearance of subcutaneous nodules, the presence of deforming arthritis, and the incidence of systemic disease.

Pathogenesis

The role of antibody and cellular immune mechanisms in rheumatoid arthritis is depicted in Fig. 10.12. The acute inflammatory process is initiated by an immune complex reaction, but in chronic progressive RA, it resembles a chronic cell-mediated immune reaction. Although most of the serologic findings do not support an etiologic role for serum RF in the pathogenesis of RA, observations on synovial fluid (the fluid of the articular cavity) indicate an immune complex RF autoimmune mechanism for the early inflammation of RA and cell-mediated immunity for the chronic disease. The formation of immune complexes of RF and altered host immunoglobulins in the joint initiates immune complex-mediated inflammation. The synovial fluid aspirated from patients with active RA contains immune complexes, and the PMNs in such fluids may have complexes of RF and IgG in their cytoplasm (RA cells). There is also a selective lowering of complement components in the synovial fluid during active RA. The synthesis of complement components by synovial inflammatory tissue may also contribute to the severity of the early stage of arthritis. Eventually, the synovium is converted into a lymphoid organ containing germinal centers and T-cell domains mimicking the structure of a lymph node.

The chronic stage of RA is cell-mediated with involvement of T cells, macrophages, endothelial cells, cytokines, and cell adhesion molecules, as well as fibroblasts and osteoclasts. The phenotype of synovial T-cell infiltrates during active inflammation is predominately $CD3^+$ $\gamma\delta$ T cells. The function and role in pathogenesis of this particular type of T cell has not been determined. Costimulation of T cells via the CD28/B7 pathway through interaction of synovial cells may result in increased inflammatory cytokine release. There is local production of IL-2, IL-6, GM-CSF, TNF-α, and TGF-β, presumably from activated T cells; IL-1, TNF-α, IL-6, IL-8, M-CSF, platelet-derived growth factor, TGF-β, and osteoclast-activating factors from activated macrophages; as well as factors from fibroblasts, synoviocytes, and endothelial cells in the synovium, including arachidonic acid metabolites, vasoactive amines, platelet-activating factor, IL-8, and endothelin-1. TGF-β is a strong chemoattractant for granulocytes and may be a major factor in recurrent acute inflammation in the joint, whereas IL-1 mediates destruction of bone and cartilage. The production of IL-1 by activated macrophages during early synovial inflammation appears to in-

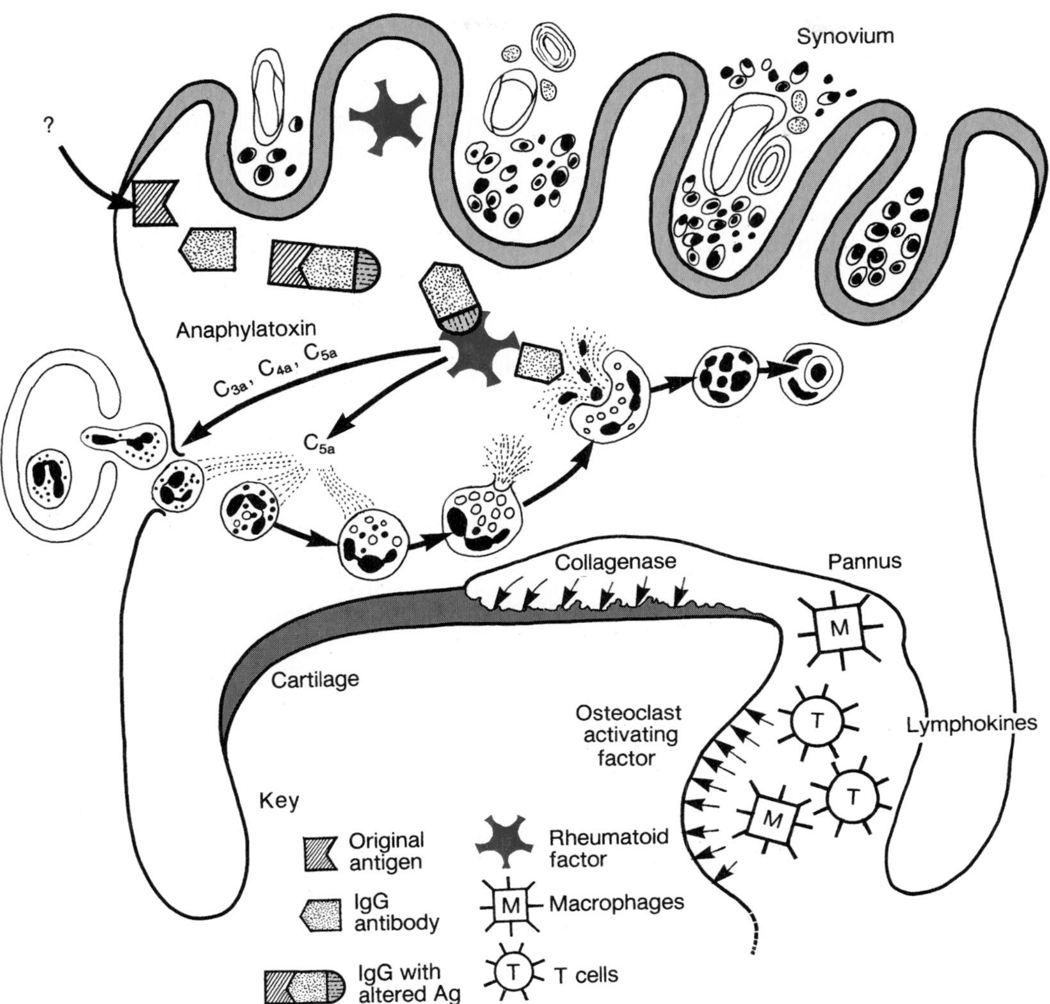

Figure 10.12 Current concepts of the pathogenesis of rheumatoid arthritis postulate that an as yet unidentified antigen (infectious agent, host autoantigen) present in the joint cavity stimulates the production of an antibody. Antigen-antibody complexes that produce an alteration in the tertiary structure of the antibody, revealing new or buried antigenic determinants, are formed. These determinants in turn stimulate the production of another antibody, RF (IgM or IgG), which can react with IgG. Complexes form in the synovial fluid and activate complement components which attract PMNs. A proliferation of lymphocytes and plasma cells in the synovial lining tissue converts the synovium into a lymphoid organ, which produces RF that is released locally into the synovial fluid. T_{DTH} lymphocytes in the synovium are activated to produce lymphokines that attract and activate macrophages. Activated macrophages and lymphocytes secrete cytokines that upregulate expression of cell adhesion molecules on endothelial cells and synovial fibroblasts. Macrophages also produce osteoclast activating factor and other activation factors that lead to destruction of adjacent bone. Hyperplasia of granulation tissue and inflammatory cells occurs and extends as a mass (pannus) over the articular cartilage. The pannus produces collagenase and elastase that destroys the joint cartilage. This pannus may progress to form a scar in the joint that leads to immobilization.

duce development of postcapillary venules with high endothelium, not found in normal synovium. The high-endothelium venules and capillaries of the synovium contain increased ELAM-1 and VCAM-1 and thus have increased adhesiveness for inflammatory cells. IL-1, TNF-α, and IFN-γ activate synovial fibroblasts and macrophages to express increased ICAM-1, which may promote lymphocyte adhesion through LFA-1 (see chapter 3). IL-1 also stimulates synovial cells to secrete collagenase, neutral proteases, plasminogen activator, and prostaglandin E_2, as well as chrondrocytes to secrete collagenase, proteoglycase, and neutral proteases. IL-1 also directly activates osteoclasts to effect bone resorption. Endothelin-1 stimulates proliferation of fibroblasts and smooth muscle cells. Thus, the process of chronic inflammation is activated, leading to production and release of lymphokines and cytokines, upregulation of cellular adhesion molecules, activation of endothelial cells and macrophages, cartilage and bone destruction, and scarring, resulting in loss of function and deformation of the involved joints. TNF may be the major factor in induction of inflammation, whereas activation of synovial cells, chrondrocytes, and osteoclasts by IL-1 may be the major pathway for cartilage destruction and bone remodeling. Transgenic mice carrying and expressing the TNF gene develop an inflammatory arthritis similar to RA, but without extensive bone destruction.

Rheumatoid nodules are granulomatous collections of mononuclear cells, primarily consisting of palisading macrophages surrounding a central area of fibrinoid necrosis. Rheumatoid nodules are prominent in the skin but may form in any tissue of the body. In the lung, rheumatoid nodules are worsened or exacerbated by tissue injury, such as that produced by silica exposure in hard-coal miners (Caplan's syndrome). Nodules are believed to form around inflamed blood vessels. The central necrotic areas contain fibrin, immunoglobulins, and complement. Thus, it is thought that nodules represent chronic destruction and scarring from a previous immune complex-mediated vasculitis.

Etiology

The relative roles of a transmissible agent and genetic factors in the etiology of RA are still open for speculation. RA was first described by Landre-Beauvais 200 years ago. Studies of remains of Native Americans for arthritic changes have led to the hypothesis that RA may have been a disease localized to certain areas of the New World, later spreading to the Old World (Europe) after European exposure to New World inhabitants with RA. A search for an infectious agent initiating RA has yielded a number of possibilities, but as yet there is no clear identification of an etiologic agent. Streptococci, diphtheroids, mycoplasma, and clostridia each have been proposed and later discarded because of lack of evidence. The presence of human T-cell leukemia virus type 1-related proteins in cells in rheumatoid synovium suggests a possible retroviral agent. There is stronger evidence that Epstein-Barr (EB) virus may be associated with RA. EB virus is believed to be the causative agent for infectious mononucleosis and lymphoid tumors in humans (Burkitt's lymphoma). The sera of patients with RA contain antibody activity to a nuclear antigen found only in B-cell lymphoid cell lines that have been transformed (immortalized) by EB virus. This antigen is not the same as the EB virus antigen found in Burkitt's lymphoma and has been termed rheumatoid arthritis-associated nuclear antigen. An EB protein shares the same five amino acids as the HLA-Dw4, four of five amino acids of DR4 (Dw14), and DR1 molecules that are implicated in genetic susceptibility to RA (see below), suggesting that molecular mimicry may be a mechanism. A direct etiologic relationship between EB virus infection and rheumatoid arthritis has not been demonstrated, but further studies on this possibility are under way. Any postulated infectious etiology must include a mechanism that leads to the stimulation of B cells to produce autoreactive rheumatoid factor.

Clinical Course

The clinical course of RA is quite variable; in some cases, there is rapid progression to severe disability, and in others there is a prolonged progressive course, leading to moderate, little, or no joint deformity. Spontaneous remissions and exacerbations occur frequently and make evaluation of therapy difficult. RA may shorten life and can lead to total disability in about 10% of cases. Inflammation of the heart, small or medium vessels, and lung (diffuse interstitial pulmonary fibrosis) is infrequent but may occur and is believed to be part of the rheumatoid process.

Therapy

Therapy is directed toward controlling pain, reducing inflammation, and preventing severe deformities by active physical therapy or orthopedic surgery. Early attempts to move through stages of therapy starting with relatively mild anti-inflammatory agents such as salicylates and other nonsteroidal anti-inflammatory agents and adding stronger agents if the disease progressed ("pyramid therapy") did not prove effective. There is growing use of multiple disease-modifying antirheumatic drugs (DMARDs) as well as the application of aggressive therapy early in the course of the disease. For example, a single injection of corticosteroids during early mild arthritis appears to produce remission in about 25% of patients, with the others showing progressive disease. DMARDs for progressive disease include various combinations of drugs. Combination therapy with sulfasalazine and prednisolone that is started at high doses and tapered over 28 weeks is more effective than sulfasalazine alone. Other combinations tested include methotrexate and cyclosporine, hydroxychloroquine, sulfasalazine, etc. A number of clinical trials are now being conducted to determine which combinations are more effective for long-term remissions. More recently, the use of monoclonal antibodies directed to $CD4^+$ T cells or to interruption of various factors believed to be important in the progression of the disease, such as IL-1, TNF-γ, CD5, IL-2R, and ICAM-1, have resulted in clinical improvement in about 25% of patients. Despite the various drugs and regimens used, therapy is still unsatisfactory. Surgical restoration is very effective in some cases, restoring much of the function of deformed hands. Physical therapy can help minimize pain and improve functional activity.

HLA Associations

Genetic susceptibility was originally demonstrated by RA clusters in families, and there is a higher concordance of RA in monozygotic than in dizygotic twins. Genetic predisposition to RA is associated with HLA-DR4 in whites and with HLA-DR1 in other ethnic groups. HLA-DR4 subtypes Dw4, Dw14, and Dw15 predispose to RA, whereas Dw10 and Dw13 do not. These subtypes contain only a few amino acid differences in the third hypervariable region of the HLA-DR4 β chain. HLA-DR1 shares the same third hypervariable region as the Dw14 subtype of DR4. The critical shared epitope of the RA subtypes appears to be on a combining site for the T-cell antigen receptor. Thus, these class II major histocompatibility complex (MHC) subtypes may present processed antigen, perhaps altered host immunoglobulin, to T-helper cells in a manner that results in the abnormal autoimmune response inherent to the etiology of RA.

Spondyloarthropathies and HLA-B27

The spondyloarthropathies include three joint diseases: ankylosing spondylitis, Reiter's syndrome (RS), and psoriatic arthritis, which involve the interarticulating joints of the spine (sacroiliitis or spondylitis). These are also called "seronegative arthritides," because there is a lack of RF or antinuclear antibodies. The occurrence of these diseases is clearly associated with HLA-B27 (Table 10.6). Ankylosing spondylitis is a chronic inflammation, fibrosis, and ossification of the articulations of the axial skeleton that occurs in young adults. More than 90% of patients with ankylosing spondylitis are HLA-B27 positive. RS, or reactive arthritis, is an acute peripheral arthritis, nongonococcal urethritis, and conjunctivitis that characteristically develops 2 to 4 weeks after an infection with *Shigella, Salmonella, Yersinia, Campy-*

Table 10.6 Spondyloarthropathies associated with HLA-B27[a]

Characteristic	Disorder				
	Ankylosing spondylitis	**Reactive arthritis**[b]	**Juvenile spondyloarthropathy**	**Psoriatic arthropathy**	**Enteropathic arthropathy**
Sacroiliitis or spondylitis[c]	100%	<50%	<50%	20%	10%
Peripheral arthritis[d]	25%	90%	90%	95%	90%
Gastrointestinal inflammation	Common, usually asymptomatic	Common, often asymptomatic	Not known	Uncommon	All
Skin and nail involvement	Rare	Most	Uncommon	All	Uncommon
Genitourinary involvement (males only)	Uncommon	Most	Uncommon	Uncommon	Rare
Eye involvement[e]	25%	Common	Common	Occasional	Occasional
Cardiac involvement	<5%	5%–10%	Not known probably rare	Rare	Rare
Usual age of onset (years)	18–40	18–45	7–18	20–50	15–50
Sex prevalence	Males 3:1	Males 3:1[f]	Males 10:1	Equal	Equal
Type of onset	Gradual	Acute	Variable	Variable	Gradual
Role of infectious agents	Unknown	Definite trigger	Unknown	Unknown	Unknown
Prevalence of HLA-B27[g]	>90%	60–80%	80%	50%[h]	50–75%

[a]From R. E. Hammer, S. D. Maika, J. A. Richardson, J. P. Tang, and J. D. Taurog, *Cell* **63:**1099–1112, 1990.
[b]Includes Reiter's syndrome, classically defined as the triad of arthritis, conjunctivitis, and urethritis.
[c]Inflammation in the spine or sacroiliac joints.
[d]Inflammation in joints of the extremities.
[e]Predominantly conjunctivitis in reactive arthritis; iritis with the other disorders.
[f]Male-to-female ratio is 10:1 if venereally acquired, 1:1 if enteropathically acquired.
[g]Whites of northern European extraction only. General prevalence in this population is 6 to 8%. Some variation is seen in other populations, but the basic associations with HLA-B27 are seen worldwide.
[h]Frequency elevated only in those with spondylitis or sacroiliitis.

lobacter, or *Chlamydia* infection. Antigens from the triggering organisms can be demonstrated in synovial fluid leukocytes and macrophages, but viable microorganisms are not present. More recently, chlamydia has emerged as the primary pathogen for RS. Antibodies against the chlamydia 57-kDa heat shock protein have been found in the sera and spinal fluid of RS patients after chlamydial infection. The significance of this observation is not clear. Seventy-five percent of cases are HLA-B27. Patients with psoriasis and inflammatory bowel disease without joint disease generally do not show a higher frequency of HLA-B27 than the normal population, but approximately 50% of those with spondylitis associated with psoriasis or inflammatory bowel disease carry HLA-B27.

Mechanisms to explain the association of spondylitis and HLA-B27 are not known at this time. Transgenic rats expressing HLA-B27 and human β_2-microglobulin spontaneously develop inflammatory lesions similar to those in human spondyloarthropathies. It has been hypothesized that there may be selective class I MHC antigen processing by HLA-B27 to $CD8^+$ T_{CTL} cells and induction of autoimmunity because of molecular mimicry between bacterial antigens and host B27 residues. Six identical residues on B27 and *Klebsiella pneumoniae* have been identified, but there is no proof that the cross-reactivity between bacteria and HLA-B27 causes the arthritis. Up to 11 subtypes of HLA-B27 based on amino acid substitutions have been identified. All but one of these, B2703, is associated with spondyloarthropathies. This finding explains why the previous lack of correspondence between spondyloarthropathies and B27 in Gambian blacks, who carry a relatively high (up to 3%) incidence of B2703. Peptides from gram-negative enteric microorganisms specifically bind to HLA-B27, and this may provide enhanced processing for immune stimulation of a subset of T-cell receptors.

Systemic Lupus Erythematosus (SLE)

SLE is a multiorgan disease caused by autoantibodies produced to a wide variety of the patient's own nuclear, cytoplasmic, and cell-membrane antigens. Most, but not all, of the lesions can be explained by the effects of formation of circulating immune complexes to altered DNA that deposit in different organs. This disease appears most frequently in women of childbearing age but can occur at any age.

Diagnosis

The classical presentation of a young woman with a history of recent sun sensitivity and development of a "butterfly rash" on the upper cheeks, pleuropericarditis, arthritis, fever, fatigue, seizures, and nephrotic syndrome occurs in only a few patients. However, these findings illustrate the major features of the disease. Untreated, the progressive form is a rapidly advancing systemic disease featuring high fever, skin rash, nephritis, polyarthritis, polyserositis (pleural, pericardial, and peritoneal effusions), and central nervous system symptoms. With more sensitive diagnostic techniques (mainly tests for antinuclear antibodies), milder forms of SLE have been recognized that may include only a remitting arthralgia, myalgia, and malaise. Degrees of severity between these extremes are common, and the clinical course is usually characterized by spontaneous remissions and exacerbations. The diagnosis and classification of SLE in a given patient is based on the results of a series of clinical findings and laboratory tests (Table 10.7).

Table 10.7 The 1982 revised criteria for classification of systemic lupus erythematosus[a]

Criterion	Definition
1. Malar rash	Fixed erythema, flat or raised, over the malar eminences, tending to spare the nasolabial folds
2. Discoid rash	Erythematous raised patches with adherent keratotic scaling and follicular plugging; atrophic scarring may occur in older lesions
3. Photosensitivity	Skin rash as a result of unusual reaction to sunlight, by patient history or physician observation
4. Oral ulcers	Oral or nasopharyngeal ulceration, usually painless, observed by a physician
5. Arthritis	Nonerosive arthritis involving two or more peripheral joints, characterized by tenderness, swelling, or effusion
6. Serositis	a) Pleuritis: convincing history of pleuritic pain or rub heard by a physician or evidence of pleural effusion *OR* b) Pericarditis: documented by electrocardiogram or rub or evidence of pericardial effusion
7. Renal disorder	a) Persistent proteinuria greater than 0.5 g per day or >3+ if quantitation not performed *OR* b) Cellular casts: may be red cell, hemoglobin, granular, tubular, or mixed
8. Neurologic disorder	a) Seizures: in the absence of offending drugs or known metabolic derangements, e.g., uremia, ketoacidosis, or electrolyte imbalance *OR* b) Psychosis: in the absence of offending drugs or known metabolic derangements, e.g., uremia, ketoacidosis, or electrolyte imbalance
9. Hematologic disorder	a) Hemolytic anemia: with reticulocytosis *OR* b) Leukopenia: $<4,000/mm^3$ total on two or more occasions *OR* c) Lymphopenia: $<1,500/mm^3$ on two or more occasions *OR* d) Thrombocytopenia: $<100,000/mm^3$ in the absence of offending drugs
10. Immunologic disorder	a) Positive lupus erythematosus cell preparation *OR* b) Anti-DNA: antibody to native DNA in abnormal titer *OR* c) Anti-Sm: presence of antibody to Sm nuclear antigen *OR* d) False-positive serologic test for syphilis known to be positive for at least 6 months and confirmed by *T. pallidum* immobilization or fluorescent treponemal antibody absorption test
11. Antinuclear antibody	An abnormal titer of antinuclear antibody by immunofluorescence or an equivalent assay at any point in time and in the absence of drugs known to be associated with "drug-induced lupus" syndrome

[a]The proposed classification is based on 11 criteria. For the purpose of identifying patients in clinical studies, a person is said to have SLE if any 4 or more of the 11 criteria are present, serially or simultaneously, during any interval of observation. From E. M. Tan, A. S. Cohen, J. F. Fries, A. T. Masi, D. J. McShane, et al., *Arthritis Rheum.* **25:**1271–1277, 1982.

Pathogenesis

Most of the lesions of SLE are related to autoantibodies, and the primary mechanism is immune complex-mediated inflammation. The heterogeneity of clinical, pathologic, and laboratory abnormalities suggests more than one simple pathogenesis, but the leading player is believed to be anti-double-stranded DNA. The major pathologic changes of SLE most frequently involve the kidney and skin, but systemic vasculitis may lead to symptoms relating to any organ of the body. The lesions reflect the progression of immune complex vasculitis and may involve arterioles, venules, and sometimes larger arteries and veins. The early lesions are characterized by granulocyte infiltration, leukoclasia, and periarteriolar edema; later lesions, by mononuclear cell infiltration and fibrinoid necrosis. The kidney lesions also reflect stages of immune complex disease and vary from mild to severe glomerular inflammation to chronic membranoproliferative glomerulonephritis. Chronic deposition of immune complexes may result in marked thickening of the basement membranes seen in histologic sections as so-called "wire loops." Hyaline thrombosis and hematoxylin bodies (nuclear debris deposited in tissue; the tissue equivalent of the lupus erythematosus [LE] cell) are also classic findings. Glomerular crescent formation and sclerosis indicate poor prognosis.

In addition to the kidney, other major organs involved are the skin, spleen, heart, and brain. The characteristic skin lesions are patchy atrophy, hyperkeratosis, and lymphocytic infiltration of the epidermis and collagen degeneration of the dermis, both of which occur more frequently in areas of the skin exposed to sunlight, as well as leukoclastic vasculitis. The spleen may have a marked periarteriolar fibrosis described as "onion skin" because of the layering of fibrous tissue around the arterioles. Scattered focal thickening, necrosis, and fibrosis of medium-sized arterioles may be found in many different organs. Nonbacterial verrucous endocarditis (Libman-Sacks endocarditis) are ovoid sterile vegetations on the undersurface of the heart valves or chordae tendineae. These are composed of fibrin- and fibrous tissue-containing platelets, lymphocytes, and plasma cells. The vegetations are usually 1 to 4 mm in diameter but can become quite large and serve as a source for emboli to the brain or even to the coronary arteries. Vasculitis in the brain may cause a variety of neurologic symptoms.

Antinuclear Antibodies

Two major diagnostic advances in SLE were, first, the recognition of LE cells by Hargraves in 1948 and, later, the identification of specific antinuclear antibodies. An LE cell is a PMN that has phagocytosed nuclear material. Its formation depends on the presence of an antibody capable of reacting with nucleoprotein. When whole anticoagulated peripheral blood from a patient with SLE is incubated in vitro, this antibody reacts with the nuclei of lymphocytes. The swollen nuclear material is then phagocytosed by PMNs in the peripheral blood, and LE cells are formed (Fig. 10.13).

A variety of antinuclear antibodies have been identified in the sera of patients with SLE, and their identification has replaced the LE cell test in the clinical laboratory. They include anti-DNA, antinucleoprotein, antinuclear membrane proteins, antihistones, antiacidic nuclear proteins, antinucleolar DNA, and antibodies to fibrous or particulate nucleoprotein (Table 10.8). The immunofluorescent staining pattern observed when serum from a patient with SLE is allowed to bind to tissue nuclei provides

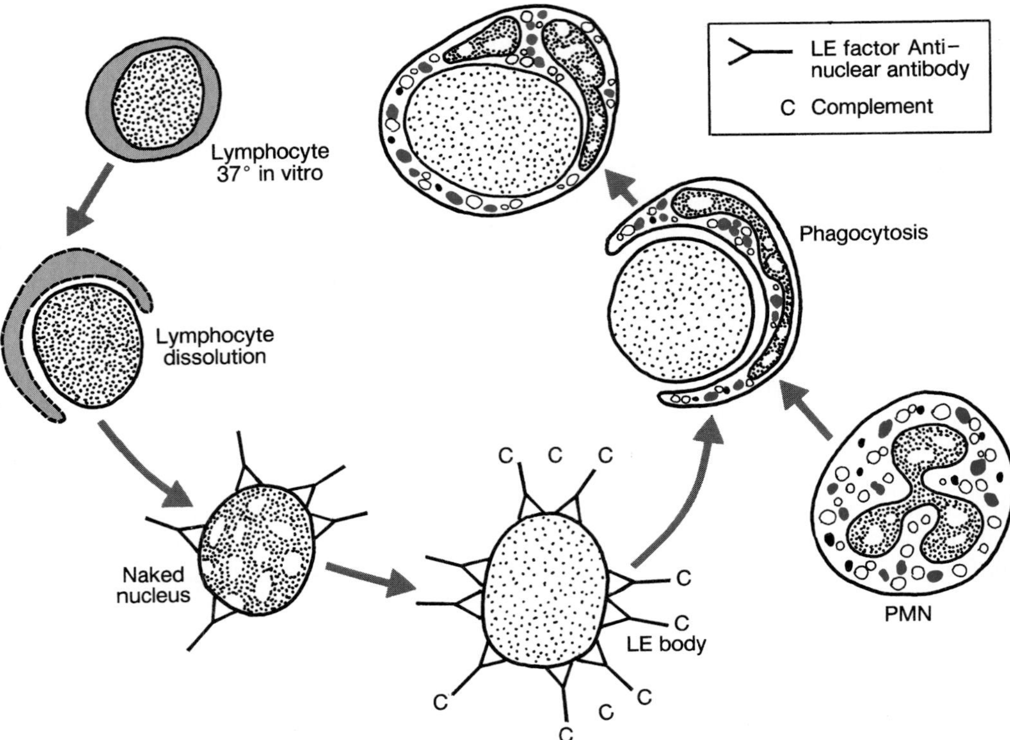

Figure 10.13 Formation of LE cells. LE cells are PMNs that have phagocytosed the nuclei of lymphocytes by coating the nuclei with antibody. This takes place at 37°C upon incubation of the whole blood of a patient with SLE who has antibody to nucleoprotein or other nuclear antigens. Lymphocytes break up, and lymphocyte nuclei become coated with antibody (LE factor), swell, and are phagocytosed by PMNs. LE cells may also be formed by phagocytosis of the nuclei of cells other than lymphocytes.

some clues to diagnosis. The localization of the bound immunoglobulin is determined by addition of fluorescent-labeled antibody to immunoglobulin (indirect fluorescent antibody test). Four major patterns are seen: nuclear rim (antimembrane proteins), speckled (antiacidic nuclear proteins), nucleolar (antinucleolar DNA), and homogeneous (not antigenically specific) (Table 10.9). The association of antibodies of different specificities with the connective tissue diseases is shown in Table 10.8.

Patients with SLE may have a number of serologic abnormalities in addition to antinuclear antibodies. These include antibodies to basement membranes of the skin, antibodies to red blood cells (positive Coombs' test), antibodies to phospholipids involved in blood clotting (lupus anticoagulant), antibodies to lymphocytes (usually to T-suppressor cells), falsely positive serologic reactions for syphilis, and antibodies to cytoplasmic antigenic components. These "autoantibodies" may be responsible for some SLE lesions and for associations of SLE with other connective tissue diseases (Table 10.10).

Antiphospholipid antibodies (APAs) (the lupus anticoagulant, cardiolipin, VDRL for syphilis) are associated with vascular thrombosis in the brain and elsewhere and deposition of fibrin and platelet thrombi in the heart valves (Libman-Sacks endocarditis; see above). Although called lupus

Table 10.8 Some reactivities of antinuclear antibodies[a]

Type of antibody[b]	Disease in which antibodies seen	Characteristic of antigenic determinants	Nuclear pattern observed by indirect immunofluorescence test
Antibody to DNA			
Reacts only with double-stranded DNA	Characteristic of SLE; correlates with nephritis	Double-strandedness of DNA essential	Rim and/or homogeneous
Reacts with both double- and single-stranded DNA	High levels in SLE; lower levels in other rheumatic diseases	Related to deoxyribose, purines, and pyrimidines but not dependent on double helix	Rim and/or homogeneous
Reacts only with single-stranded DNA	Rheumatic, nonrheumatic diseases	Related to purines and pyrimidines, with ribose or deoxyribose equally reactive	Not detected on routine screen; special treatment necessary
Deoxynucleoprotein, soluble form	LE cell antibody in SLE, drug-induced LE	DNA-histone complex necessary; dissociated components are nonreactive	Rim and/or homogeneous
Histone	SLE, drug-induced SLE	Different classes of histones may have different determinants	Homogeneous and/or rim
Sm	Highly diagnostic of SLE	U1-RNP, U2, U4-6	Speckled
Nuclear RNP (Mo)	High levels in mixed connective tissue disease; lower levels in other rheumatic diseases	U1-RNP (RNA-splicing enzymes)	Speckled
Ribosomal P	Highly diagnostic of SLE; correlates with psychosis	Ribosome P protein	Cytoplasmic
Scl-70	Highly diagnostic of scleroderma	Extractable antigen, topoisomerase I	Speckled
Ku	20% of all connective tissue diseases	DNA binding protein	Speckled
SS-A (Ro)	High prevalence in Sjögren's syndrome sicca complex (40%); lower prevalence in other rheumatic diseases (SLE 25%)	Chemical nature unknown	Negative
SS-B (La) (Ha)	High prevalence in Sjögren's syndrome sicca complex (20%); lower prevalence in other rheumatic diseases (SLE 10%)	Extractable antigen, transcription termination factor for pol III	Speckled
PM-Scl	High prevalence in myositis and scleroderma overlaps	Chemical nature unknown	Nucleolar
RNA polymerase I, II, III	Scleroderma	RNA polymerase I, II, III	Nucleolar
U3-RNP (fibrillarin)	Scleroderma	Splicing enzymes	Nucleolar
Centromere	High prevalence in mild scleroderma (CREST syndrome)	Centromere antigens (CENP-B)	Discrete centromeric staining
Jo-1	Highly specific for polymyositis	Histidyl tRNA synthetase	Cytoplasmic or nuclear
Mi-2	Specific for dermatomyositis	Chemical nature unknown	Speckled

[a]Table contributed by Frank Arnett, University of Texas Medical School, Houston.
[b]Abbreviations: RNP, ribonuclear protein; Sm, Smith; Scl, scleroderma; SS, Sjögren's syndrome.

Table 10.9 Nuclear staining patterns observed in patients with connective tissue diseases

Staining pattern	Major disease association	Specificities of antibody
Rim	SLE	Nuclear membrane protein
Speckled	SLE, scleroderma, other connective tissue diseases	Ribonucleoprotein
Nucleolar	Scleroderma, Sjögren's syndrome	U3-RNP, RNA polymerase I, Pm-Scl
Homogeneous	SLE, Sjögren's syndrome, RA	Nucleoprotein, unknown

anticoagulant, APAs may be found in individuals without SLE and produce the primary APA syndrome, which is defined by the presence of antiphospholipid and any or all of the following clinical events: recurrent thrombosis, recurrent fetal losses, thrombocytopenia, and livedo reticularis. APAs were first identified by Wassermann in 1906 when serum from patients with syphilis was mixed with saline extracts of liver. The reactive antigen was later identified as cardiolipin. The antigens in cardiolipin are negatively charged phospholipids (phosphatidyl choline, phosphatidyl serine, sphingomyelin, etc.), resulting in identification of a family of APAs with different specificities. The common feature of these antibodies is their reactivity with cell membrane phospholipids on platelets and endothelial cells, activating vasospasm (livido reticularis) and coagulation (thrombosis).

Antibody to Ro (SS-A) antigen may cause a transient annular erythematous skin rash or permanent heart block in neonates of mothers with

Table 10.10 Autoantibodies in SLE and other connective tissue diseases[a]

Disease and organ involvement	Associated autoantibodies	Proposed mechanisms
Systemic lupus erythematosus	Anti-dsDNA, anti-Ro (SS-A), other (?)	Immune complex
Glomerulonephritis		
Cerebritis (psychosis), seizures, infarction	Antineuronal, antiribosomal P, antiphosholipid	Antibody mediated; immune complex vasculitis; vascular thrombosis
Dermatitis	Anti-Ro (SS-A), anti-DNA, others (?)	Immune complex; antibody-dependent cytotoxicity (?)
Libman-Sacks endocarditis	Antiphospholipid	Endocardial thrombosis
Heart block in neonates	Anti-Ro (SS-A)	Antibody mediated
Red blood cell	Anti-RBC	Antibody mediated
Lymphocyte	Antilymphocyte	Antibody mediated
Platelet	Antiplatelet	Antibody mediated
Arthritis, serositis	DNA?	Immune complex
Sjögren's syndrome		
Exocrine glands (eyes, nose, mouth, skin, GI, lungs, GU)	Anti-salivary gland, anti-sweat gland, other auto-antibodies	Infiltration by lymphocytes and plasma cells, antibody mediated, cell mediated
Extraglandular (vasculitis)	Anti-Ro (SS-A), anti-La (SS-B)	Immune complex
Polymyositis (dermatomyositis)		
Skeletal muscle	Anti-Jo1, Mi, Pm-Scl, RNP	Antibody-dependent cell-mediated cytotoxicity
Progressive systemic sclerosis (scleroderma)		
Severe skin and visceral fibrosis	Anti-Scl-70	Immune attack of unknown kind on endothelium of arterioles and capillaries with proliferative endarteritis
Mild disease (CREST syndrome)	Anticentromere	

[a]Modified from the lecture notes of Frank Arnett, University of Texas, Houston.

antibody to Ro (SS-A) antigen owing to passive transfer of antibody from mother to fetus. This may occur when the mother is asymptomatic. Anti-Ro reactivity is also seen in subacute cutaneous lupus erythematosus, a subgroup of SLE patients with prominent photoaggravated skin rash and musculoskeletal pains, but who do not usually develop significant systemic disease.

Anti-Sm antibodies are highly specific for the diagnosis of SLE but probably do not play a critical role in the pathogenesis. Anti-Sm antibodies include antibodies to U1 small nuclear RNP (U1 snRNP) and small cytoplasmic RNP (scRNP), as well as U2, U4 to U6 small nuclear RNP (snRNP), that are ribonuclear protein particles involved in splicing of precursor messenger RNA during posttranscriptional regulation of gene expression. These antibodies, as well as anti-La and Ro, react with RNPs of infectious agents, such as human cytomegalovirus RNA. The reason that antibodies to these antigens, as well as to the nucleosome, are highly diagnostic of SLE is not known. The continuing subclassification of lupus patients according to the predominant autoantibodies promises to lead to more precise diagnosis and prognosis of the disease, as well as give clues to the pathogenesis.

The membranous glomerulonephritis of SLE may contain deposits of immunoglobulin and DNA; both granular and linear deposits of immunoglobulin have been observed. Immunoglobulin and complement may also be detected in the vascular lesions of the spleen and other organs, in the basement membrane of skin, and along the dermal-epidermal junction of grossly normal-appearing skin (positive lupus band test). These antibodies are associated with liquefaction necrosis of the basement membrane of the skin and subendothelial deposits in the basement membrane of renal glomeruli. In addition, antibodies to lymphocyte antigens that cross-react with neurons may be found in LE sera, and immune complexes are frequently found in the basement membrane of the choroid plexus (see above). The relationship of these to the central nervous system symptoms associated with lupus erythematosus remains unclear.

Etiology

The etiology of naturally occurring SLE remains unsolved. Although it is clear that the major signs and symptoms are caused by autoantibodies, the reasons why these autoantibodies are produced is not so clear. There appear to be both genetic and environmental factors.

The genetic factors (Table 10.11) include the tendency to produce high antibody responses in general, as well as to produce antibodies to particular nuclear antigens, to have reduced clearance of immune complexes, or to have impaired DNA repair. Hormonal factors are implicated, because androgens tend to protect against SLE. Bacterial or viral infections may stimulate the immune system to produce autoantibodies either nonspecifically through polyclonal B-cell activation or specifically to nuclear antigens through molecular mimicry. There may be an imbalance of humoral immunity similar to that described for NZB mice (see below). This leads to abnormal antibody formation to a variety of antigens, including host molecules. Multiple MHC and non-MHC genes appear to predispose to this imbalance. There is an increased incidence of HLA-DR2 and/or HLA-DR3, as well as inherited deficiencies of complement due to null alleles at complement C4 loci. The frequency of certain autoantibodies is related to HLA types (HLA-DQ1/DQ2 heterozygotes, anti-Ro (SS-A); HLA-B8 and DR3,

Table 10.11 Genetic features of SLE

Feature	Example(s)
Inheritance of autoimmune predisposition	Increased familial incidence of SLE (10–12%)
	Concordance in identical twins (70%)
	Family members develop other autoimmune diseases or produce autoantibodies
Androgens suppress expression; estrogens promote expression	Female/male ratio, 10:1
Multiple genes involved	Associated with complement deficiencies (C4, C2, C1r, C1s), MHC class II alleles, correlate with different autoantibodies
Independent predisposing factors	Inherited tendency to produce antibody

anti-La (SS-B); HLA-DR4, anti-nuclear RNP (Sm). There does not appear to be a linkage between SLE and polymorphisms at the heavy- and light-chain genes, because no differences in restriction endonuclease fragments in the germ line immunoglobulin heavy-chain or kappa-chain variable regions have been detected between healthy individuals and lupus patients.

The role of environmental factors in SLE has centered on photosensitivity. One theory is that exposure of females to sunlight during menstruation, when DNA is circulating, causes denaturation of DNA and results in production of antibodies to DNA. Exposure of the skin to UV radiation induces the release of proinflammatory mediators and produces photodimers, leading, for example, to production of antibodies to Ro/SS-A. However, a correlation between photosensitivity and antibodies to UV-altered DNA is not found. Some drugs (see below) have been shown to cause symptoms similar to SLE. Many infectious agents have been accused, but none have been convicted. Analysis of the antibodies to double-stranded DNA, believed to be key to the pathogenesis of SLE, indicates that they are not germ line-encoded but antigen driven, indicating that the autoantibody response in SLE is initiated by antigen exposure. Elevated levels of plasma nucleic acids are found in lupus patients, and these nucleic acids have a striking homology with the gag-pol overlap region of human immunodeficiency virus type 1, leading to the hypothesis that a retrovirus infection may lead to induction of autoantibodies to DNA. In support of this is the observation that the snRNPs that react with antibody in SLE sera have remarkable sequence homology with p30gag sequences of several oncoviruses. The most acceptable explanation at the present time is that an abnormal humoral antibody response to an infection leads to formation of antibodies that cross-react with a wide variety of human tissues in individuals who are genetically predisposed to produce autoantibodies.

Drug-Induced SLE

The features of SLE may appear in patients receiving certain drugs. The important difference between drug-induced SLE and naturally occurring SLE is that the drug-induced symptoms generally disappear upon discontinuation of the drugs. Drugs that are associated with SLE include diphenylhydantoin, isoniazid, hydralazine, and procainamide, used for the treatment of epilepsy, tuberculosis, hypertension, and cardiac arrhythmias, respectively. Other drugs produce LE-like syndromes less frequently. The mechanisms of induction of drug-associated LE-like syndromes are not yet fully understood. Patients with hydralazine-induced LE may have antibodies to hydralazine as well as antibodies to native DNA. In contrast, procainamide induces antibodies to denatured DNA, presumably because of complexes of the drug and host DNA; antibodies to native DNA or to procainamide alone are not produced. Procainamide acts by stabilization of cell membranes. It may bind to erythrocyte surfaces, alter red cell membranes, and produce immunogenic membrane fragments that lead to autoantibody formation and a Coombs'-positive hemolytic anemia. Hydralazine and isoniazid may form reactive intermediate radicals that inactivate and alter DNA, producing immunogenic DNA fragments. Thus, the induction of autoantibodies or formation of drug-antibody toxic complexes results in drug-induced LE-like syndromes; different drugs may act by different mechanisms.

Treatment

Treatment of SLE is generally designed to reduce both the inflammatory reaction of the disease and the amount of pathogenic antibodies. Treatment for mild or moderate manifestations of SLE includes avoidance of the sun, rest, and aspirin or other nonsteroidal anti-inflammatory drugs, as well as effective emotional support. Foods containing psoralens, such as celery, parsnips, figs, and parsley, as well as alfalfa sprouts, which contain L-canavanine, should be avoided. High doses of corticosteroids and/or immunosuppressive drugs may be required for life-threatening episodes. The protocol used for steroid treatment calls for high initial doses (1 mg/kg/day) with tapering after 7 to 10 days when fulminant disease manifestations are controlled. Steroid therapy not only prolongs the lives of patients with severe SLE but also significantly changes the character of the syndrome. Before the advent of steroid therapy, patients frequently died of an acute crisis; now the disease is more protracted, and chronic renal or neurologic problems cause death. Patients with acute disease who respond to steroids should have steroids withdrawn as soon as possible. The major deleterious effect of steroids is a decrease in immune defensive reactions, resulting in susceptibility to a variety of opportunistic infections (secondary immune deficiency). Extreme progressive cases may also be reversed by aggressive immunosuppression followed by transplantation of T-cell-depleted hematopoietic stem cells. Mild forms of the disease with skin lesions, but without major organ involvement, may be controlled by immunosuppressive agents. A number of agents have been evaluated and found effective in clinical trials, including methotrexate, cyclosporine, bromocriptine, and hydroxychloroquine. The optimal drug and treatment protocol has yet to be established. Two important prognostic indicators are the severity of renal disease (a creatinine level greater than 3.0 mg/dl) and the presence of antibodies to skin basement membrane (lupus band test). These indicators are associated with a poor prognosis. Lupus nephritis may be controlled effectively with monthly cyclophosphamide or intravenous passive immunoglobulin, both of which result in a decrease in anti-DNA antibodies. Although the present therapy considerably improves the prognosis and condition of patients with SLE, it is far from satisfactory. At least 90% of well-managed SLE patients have at least a 10-year survival, but more than 50% of those with renal or neurologic involvement die within 10 years of the onset of symptoms. Plasmapheresis may be used for acute severe exacerbations but does not improve the long-term clinical outcome over standard therapy.

"Lupus Mice"

New Zealand Black (NZB) mice, F_1 hybrids of NZB mice, and some other inbred mouse strains spontaneously develop lesions similar to human SLE and serve as animal models of lupus erythematosus. The NZB inbred mouse strain was developed by Marianne Bielchowsky in New Zealand in the 1950s for cancer research. These mice were found to respond immunologically quite differently from other mouse strains. After immunization with a variety of exogenous antigens, NZB mice produce abnormally high humoral antibody responses but less intense, delayed (cellular) hypersensitivity than other mice. The "lupus" strains of mice spontaneously develop a number of immunopathologic abnormalities, including a Coombs'-positive hemolytic anemia, LE and rheumatoidlike factors, hypergammaglobulinemia, circulating immune complexes, and glomerulonephritis. The thymi of NZB mice develop germinal centers with aging; germinal centers are not normally found in the thymus but sometimes occur in humans with myasthenia gravis. Other lupus mouse strains have atrophy of the thymic cortex. The development of these immunologic abnormalities occurs after about 4 to 6 months of age. Female mice develop more severe abnormalities than male mice, and at an earlier age.

The reason for development of "lupus" in these mice is not clearly understood but appears to depend on multiple factors, including genetically controlled tendencies to abnormally high antibody responses associated with virus infections. Multiple immune controlling factor abnormalities have been described, including polyclonal B-cell activation, decreased T-suppressor cell activity, increased T-helper activity, antilymphocyte antibodies, increased complement activation, and increased T-killer activity. A constellation of these incompletely understood factors appears to contribute to the lupus erythematosus disease syndrome in these mice.

Sjögren's Syndrome (Sicca Complex)

Description

Sjögren's syndrome (SS) is inflammation of the salivary glands (sialoadenitis) and lacrimal (tear) glands. This causes decreased secretions, symptoms of dry mouth and difficulty in swallowing (xerostomia), and sore eyes (keratoconjunctivitis sicca) resulting in the sensation of a sandy foreign body in the eye. The name Sjögren's syndrome pays homage to the description of 19 women with keratoconjunctivitis sicca and xerostomia by Henrik Sjögren in 1933. Earlier descriptions of xerostomia were most likely recorded by Hadden in 1888 and keratoconjunctivitis sicca by Mikulicz in 1892. Clinically, there is swelling of the lacrimal and salivary glands. If the parotid gland alone is involved, the eponym Mikulicz's syndrome has been used. The inflammation is mononuclear with features consistent with cell-mediated immune destruction of glandular tissue. Lymphocytes and plasma cells infiltrate the salivary and lacrimal glands, and fibrosis, acinar atrophy, and proliferation of the myoepithelial cells of the ducts may lead to obstruction. In small lesions, B cells predominate and germinal centers may be seen; in large lesions, T cells are found centrally and B cells peripherally. Similar findings may be observed in the mucosal glands of the pharynx and larynx and the submucosal glands of the esophagus, trachea, and bronchi.

Associations

SS may occur alone (primary SS) or be associated with other connective tissue diseases, such as RA, SLE, or scleroderma (secondary SS). It is associated with HLA-B8 and HLA-DR3 MHC types. Precipitating and complement-fixing antibody to salivary gland tissue is associated with the disease, as are other serologic abnormalities, such as antinuclear antibodies (anti-Ro [SS-A], 50%; anti-La [SS-B], 20%), RF, and antibodies to thyroglobulin. The diagnosis of SS has been reviewed by various groups. The European Cooperative Group (EEC) criteria for SS requires either a positive minor salivary gland biopsy or a positive autoantibody against Sjögren's-associated A (Ro) or B (La) antigen. There is a close relationship between the presence of anti-Ro (SS-A) antibody and the co-occurrence of SS and SLE. Patients with anti-Ro-positive SS for many years may suddenly develop SLE. On the other hand, SLE patients with anti-Ro tend to have prominent cutaneous SLE (psoriasiform cutaneous lupus) for many years and suddenly develop SS. The overlap disease tends to occur in older patients and in association with the HLA-DR3 MHC phenotype. The mechanism responsible for the clinical expression of disease in the anti-Ro (SS-A) patients with SS/SLE is not known.

Pathogenesis

SS may be initiated by immune complexes in the salivary glands, and the chronic disease may be maintained by cell-mediated immunity, similar to what occurs in the articular (joint) space in RA. The presence of antibodies to salivary ducts is associated with less cellular infiltrate in the salivary glands of patients with SS when these lesions are compared with those of patients who lack this antibody. Thus, antibody to salivary gland may block cellular-mediated tissue destruction or could contribute to inflammation through an antibody-dependent cell-mediated mechanism. It is more likely, however, that a major component of SS or sialoadenitis in humans is caused by a toxic immune complex mechanism (vasculitis is increasingly recognized in lesions). The salivary gland normally serves as a site for production of secretory antibody responsible for local defense. In experimental autoimmune sialoadenitis, as well as in the human disease, there is substantial infiltration of the glandular tissue with plasma cells and local synthesis of large amounts of immunoglobulin with RF activity. Thus, the initial inflammation may be caused by immune complexes formed from antibody produced locally, and the chronic destructive inflammation may be maintained by cell-mediated immunity. Mononuclear inflammatory lesions have been reported in laboratory animals after the injection of salivary gland tissue in complete Freund's adjuvant, but the relationship of this experimental disease to the human disease is not clear. An increase in $CD4^+$ cells that transcribe IL-2 and IFN-γ, as well as T_{CTL} cells that express perforin and dendritic cells has been reported. However, $CD8^+$, but not $CD4^+$, T_{CTL} cells are located around apoptotic acinar cells. The mononuclear infiltrate in SS may become so pronounced that the term *benign lymphoepithelial lesion* or *pseudolymphoma* has been applied. Extensive lymphoid infiltrates may also be seen in the lung, kidney, or skeletal muscle. Occasionally, these pseudolymphomas progress to frank, primarily marginal zone B-cell lymphomas. These patients also have a high incidence of systemic symptoms, such as skin vasculitis and peripheral nerve involvement. The differential diagnosis of pseudolymphoma and malignant lymphoma may be very difficult, but pseudolymphomas are polyclonal and malignant lymphomas are usually monoclonal.

Further insight into the pathogenesis of SS has come from an animal model, the nonobese diabetic (NOD) mouse. With aging, NOD mice develop histologic and clinical manifestations very similar to those of human SS. These mice have been crossed with mice lacking T and B cells (SCID). The NOD mice lacking T and B cells do develop apoptosis of acinar cells but do not progress to the inflammatory phase and do not lose secretory function. NOD mice that cannot make antibodies also do not develop progressive lesions. These results suggest a two-phase process: the initial phase is lymphocyte independent and occurs as a consequence of an innate error in exocrine tissue homeostasis; the second phase in an autoimmune attack generated in part by autoantibodies.

Etiology

Viral infection has long been suspected as a potential cause of SS, but proof of a single cause has been elusive. Recently, an association with hepatitis C infection has been identified, with about 20% of SS patients having antibodies to hepatitis C virus.

Treatment

There is no curative treatment for SS. It is usually a benign disease in which conservative treatment involving fluid replacement, such as eye drops and frequent ingestion of water, is effective. Oral pilocarpine may improve sicca symptoms in the eyes, mouth, and other sites. If pseudolymphoma lesions become large, immunosuppressive agents or corticosteroids may shrink them. The malignant lymphomas that develop require aggressive lymphoma therapy, depending on the location and extent of disease.

Inflammatory Myopathies (Dermatomyositis and Polymyositis)

The inflammatory myopathies include three major groups: polymyositis, dermatomyositis, and inclusion body myositis (Table 10.12). The first case

Table 10.12 Characteristics of inflammatory myopathies[a]

Characteristic	Dermatomyositis	Polymyositis	Inclusion body myositis
Age at onset	Children and adults	>18 yr	>50 yr
Skin rash	Yes	No	No
Pathogenic mechanism	Immune complex	T_{CTL} cells	T_{CTL} cells
Associated conditions			
Connective tissue diseases	Scleroderma and mixed connective tissue diseases	Yes	Yes, in 15% of cases
Systemic autoimmune diseases	Infrequent	Frequent	Infrequent
Malignant conditions	Sometimes	No	No
Viruses	Not clear	HIV, HTLV-1[b]	Not clear
Parasites, bacteria	No	Yes (protozoa, nematodes, etc.)	No
Drugs	Yes (penicillamine, tryptophan)	Yes	Yes
Familial	No	No	Yes, in some cases

[a]Modified from M. C. Dalakas, *N. Engl. J. Med.* **325:**1487, 1991.
[b]HIV, human immunodeficiency virus; HTLV-1, human T-cell leukemia virus type 1.

of classic dermatomyositis was reported by Wagner in 1886. The characteristic symptom of all three groups is muscle weakness of insidious onset. The major feature is diffuse muscle damage manifested by swelling, pain, and weakness associated with a perivascular and/or interstitial infiltrate of lymphocytes. Symptoms of this disease complex may also include an erythematous skin rash (in dermatomyositis), mild arthritis, and progressive muscular weakness, each of which may occur with a different degree of severity. The primary lesion is in muscle and consists of a degeneration of muscle fibers (myositis). There is a statistically increased incidence of dermatomyositis associated with specific alleles of HLA-DM A (*0103) and B (*0102).

Diagnosis

Four clinical or laboratory abnormalities are used to make the diagnosis and are found in most patients: (i) progressive symmetrical muscle weakness; (ii) electromyographic demonstration of short-duration, small polyphasic potentials, fibrillation potentials, and bizarre high-frequency repetitive discharges; (iii) muscle biopsy showing muscle degeneration, mononuclear cell infiltration, and phagocytosis of muscle fibers; and (iv) elevated muscle enzymes in the blood. The activity of the disease process may be followed by detection of enzymes (especially creatine phosphokinase) released from affected muscle tissue. In addition, the characteristic symptoms of dermatitis (erythematous, scaly rash on the face, neck, elbows, and knees; a heliotrope periorbital discoloration; and Grotton's papules, scaly erythematous flat plaques over the dorsum of the hands) are seen in dermatomyositis. In general, a poor prognosis is indicated by older age, an associated malignancy, and involvement of respiratory muscles.

Pathogenesis

The pathogenesis of dermatomyositis is due to activation of complement by the immune complex mechanisms; that of polymyositis and inclusion body myositis is destruction of muscle by T_{CTL} cells. In dermatomyositis, the inflammatory lesions are predominantly perivascular and are predominantly B cells and $CD4^+$ T cells. Deposits of the membrane attack complex of complement in the capillaries are the earliest and most specific lesion and precede mononuclear cell infiltration, and destruction of muscle occurs by microinfarction. In contrast, the cellular infiltrate of polymyositis and inclusion body myositis is primarily in the connective tissue fascicles surrounding individual muscle fibers, not perivascular, and the predominant cell infiltrate is $CD8^+$. Destruction of individual muscle fibers is by the action of T_{CTL} cells. There is increased expression of class I MHC, which is recognized by T_{CTL} cells, as well as increased expression of costimulatory molecules CTLA4 and CD28 on muscle cells, further supporting the pathogenic role of cytotoxic lymphocytes. There is also a difference in cytokines: IL-1β is active in inclusion body myositis and TGF-β is active in dermatomyositis. Inclusion body myositis also features granular inclusions containing whorls of membranes, which are dissolved by the usual process of paraffin embedding. An experimental disease, experimental allergic myositis with features similar to polymyositis, may be produced in animals by immunization with xenogeneic muscle tissue in complete Freund's adjuvant.

Autoantibodies

A number of antinuclear and anticytoplasmic autoantibodies have been found in myositis patients. However, there is no consistent pattern that permits them to be used for diagnosis, and their role in pathogenesis is doubtful. One antibody, JO-1, directed against histidyl-tRNA synthetase, is found in 50% of patients with lung involvement (Table 10.8).

Therapy

The disease frequently has remissions and exacerbations, but the natural course is progressive. Corticosteroid therapy provides effective relief, and death from progressive muscular weakness producing respiratory failure occurs rarely. Long-term prednisone therapy (5 to 20 mg daily) may be required to control the disease. Nonsteroidal immunosuppressive drugs (cyclophosphamide, cyclosporine) have been reported to induce remissions in some steroid-resistant cases, but the response is generally disappointing. More recently, intravenous immunoglobulin has been shown to be effective in patients who have steroid lesions, and it may allow lowering of steroid doses.

Progressive Systemic Sclerosis (PSS, or Scleroderma)

Diagnosis

PSS is a disease of unknown etiology that is characterized by fibrotic thickening (sclerosis) of connective tissue in association with mild to moderate mononuclear cell infiltration. Scleroderma refers to scarring of the skin, the only lesion in some cases; but systemic involvement of synovia, gastrointestinal tract, kidneys, heart, and lungs, as well as muscles and viscera, may occur and lead to a number of symptoms (Table 10.13). PSS may be roughly classified into three groups: (i) diffuse systemic, (ii) localized cutaneous (CREST), and (iii) overlap, in which symptoms of other connective tissue diseases occur along with PSS. One of the major complications of PSS is the loss of mobility of the gastrointestinal tract, most often the esophagus, leading to an inability to take food properly. Vascular complications are also frequent, with a high incidence of Raynaud's phenomenon, rapid vasconstriction of the arteries of the fingers followed by painful vasodilation. In severe cases, this may result in infarcts of parts of the fingers. The etiology of PSS is unknown. No clear-cut environmental factor

Table 10.13 Symptoms and lesions of PSS

Classic PSS
Pulmonary: dyspnea, cough, failure
Gastrointestinal: dysphagia, dysmobility, constipation, malabsorption
Renal: proteinuria, azotemia, hypertension, failure
Musculoskeletal: polyarthralgia, contractures, myositis
Cardiovascular: cardiac arrhythmias, failure
CREST complex
Calcinosis in subcutaneous connective tissue
Raynaud's phenomenon (temporary vasospasm of fingers)
Esophageal dysmobility (dysphagia)
Sclerodactyly (thickening of the skin of the fingers)
Telangiectasia (hyperplasia of small blood vessels in skin and mucous membranes)

has been identified. The claimed association of PSS with silicone implants in American women has not been epidemiologically verified.

The five major findings that make up the CREST complex designate a more benign form of the disease that is usually limited to cutaneous manifestations. Females are affected approximately twice as frequently as males. Skin thickening is usually first noted on the fingers, then on the upper extremities and upper torso. The skin loses its flexibility and becomes taut and shiny. The dermis of the skin or the muscular wall of the gastrointestinal tract is replaced with compact bundles of collagen. Inability to move fingers and difficulty in swallowing may be prominent symptoms. Arthralgia is usually present. Joint lesions show focal collections of chronic inflammatory cells; the appearance may essentially be identical to that of early rheumatoid arthritis. The kidneys have concentric intimal thickening of small renal arteries and sometimes fibrinoid necrosis of the arterial wall. The concentric subendothelial intimal proliferation (proliferative endarteritis) is similar to that seen in PAN but has a characteristic looser "myxoid" appearance.

Pathogenesis

The course of the disease may be rapidly progressive or slowly evolving over a number of years. Progression of the disease occurs in three phases: edematous, indurative, and atrophic. Eventually, the skin has a hidebound appearance with a loss of wrinkles and folds. The major feature is the overproduction of connective tissue. Histologically, the skin has a markedly thinned epidermal layer, a loss of rete pegs, and an extensive increase in dermal collagen. The mechanism for this is not known, but there is some evidence that lymphocytes or mast cells from scleroderma patients may produce soluble factors that enhance synthesis of collagen by fibroblasts. Prime candidates are IL-1, which stimulates fibroblast proliferation, and TGF-β, which stimulates fibroblasts to synthesize collagen, but conclusive evidence of an increase in these factors has not been reported. The similarity of the lesions of PSS to chronic graft-versus-host disease after allogeneic bone marrow transplantation in humans and laboratory animals has led to the proposal that a similar mechanism involving an autoimmune self-versus-self reaction may cause PSS. The finding of persistent fetal cells in the circulation of parous females has led to the suggestion that persistent fetal cells may be causing PSS (microchimerism). Although classically the lack of cellular infiltrate has been stressed, earlier lesions have been noted to contain mononuclear infiltrate, including lymphocytes, plasma cells, macrophages, and fibroblastic cells in the dermis and subcutaneous tissues of patients with either localized or systemic disease. Recently, increased expression of β_1- and β_2-integrins on lymphocytes and ELAM-1 and ICAM-1 on endothelial cells has been found in the skin. This may explain increased inflammatory cell accumulation in scleroderma, but the factors that lead to the increased expression have not been defined. On the basis of the finding of increased IL-6 production by fibroblasts from affected skin sites, it has been postulated that increased cytokine production by scleroderma fibroblasts may initiate inflammation.

Autoantibodies

A variety of serologic abnormalities occur, including the presence of LE factors, antinuclear antibodies (especially Scl-70, centromere, Pm-Scl, and nucleolar), RFs, and other autoantibodies. Scl-70 is DNA topoisomerase I, which is localized in the nucleus and is catalytically active in transcription. Antibodies to Scl-70 are highly specific for scleroderma and may inhibit the enzymatic activity of topoisomerase I. A conclusive association with a particular HLA type has not been found, and familial PSS is rare. In a mouse model of SS (tsk1 mouse), there is duplication in the fibrillin-1 gene and production of autoantibodies to fibrillin-1. Some patients with SS also have high levels of anti-fibrillin-1 antibodies. There is evidence that PSS patients have chromosomal instability, as evidenced by chromosomal breaks, but a correlation of chromosomal instability with fibrillin-1 antibodies in humans has not yet been shown.

Treatment

Treatment for PSS is largely symptomatic. Local application of retinoids may alleviate some of the skin stiffening. Trials with systemic administration of drugs have largely been inconclusive. Octreotide, a prokinetic agent that stimulates muscle motility, may elevate gastrointestinal immobility. Experimental trials of iloprost, a prostaglandin G_2 analog that modulates vascular tone and increases circulation, have shown some promising results in loosening skin lesions, and the effect may be increased in combination with cyclosporin A. Trials of "photopheresis" are now under way for treatment of scleroderma as well as some other autoimmune diseases and for treatment of graft rejection. In this approach, whole blood is removed from patients who have previously ingested the photosensitizing agent 8-methoxypsoralen (8-MOP), followed by leukapheresis and exposure of the 8-MOP-containing white blood cells extracorporeally to ultraviolet light (UVA) and return of the cells to the patient. In preclinical experimental graft-versus-host scleroderma models in mice, anti-TGF-β prevents skin and lung fibrosis. In addition, bleomycin injected into the skin of mice produces fibrotic lesions similar to scleroderma, and these can be inhibited by administration of superoxide dismutase.

Shulman's Syndrome

Shulman's syndrome (diffuse fasciitis with eosinophilia) is a very rare disease consisting of diffuse fasciitis of rapid onset, hypergammaglobulinemia, and eosinophilia associated with sclerodermalike lesions with firm taut skin and contractures. There is often a dramatic response to prednisone therapy. There is an absence of Raynaud's phenomenon or visceral involvement, but immune-mediated aplastic anemia and/or thrombocytopenia may occur. Immunoglobulin and C3 are localized in the affected fascia.

Mixed Connective Tissue Disease and Overlap Syndromes

In 1972, G. C. Sharp described a syndrome characterized by features of various rheumatic diseases that has been designated mixed connective tissue disease. This disease is defined by a very high speckled ANA titer and antibodies to U1 snRNP, increased frequency of HLA-DR4, and, in the one-third of patients with progressive disease, death due to pulmonary hypertension. Although these patients may exhibit a variety of symptoms in common with other connective tissue diseases, the disease should not be considered the same as what is referred to as "overlap syndromes." Overlap syndrome patients have a variety of clinical features of connective tissue diseases, which overlap with those of SLE. Thus, patients with SLE may develop features of dermatomyositis, RA, and scleroderma, including arthritis and arthralgia, Raynaud's phenomenon, myositis, serositis, splenomegaly, anemia, leukopenia, hyperglobulinemia, and glomerulonephritis. As mentioned above, some SS patients develop SLE, and some SLE patients develop SS. In addition, patients with SLE may manifest multiple sclerosis, autoimmune thyroiditis, autoimmune hemolytic anemia, and diabetes mellitus. However, well-defined mixed connective tissue disease characteristics rarely evolve into SLE or SS. Low-dose steroids or immunosuppressive drugs (cyclophosphamide or cyclosporine) may arrest developing lesions.

Thrombotic Microangiopathies

Thrombotic microangiopathies, while not included in the connective tissue disease group, have vascular lesions that must be differentiated from connective tissue lesions. The thrombotic microangiopathies include hemolytic-uremic syndrome (HUS), thrombotic thrombocytopenic purpura (TTP), and peripartum HUS. The disorders are mainly secondary to thrombocytopenia (decreased number of blood platelets) and include hemolytic anemia, hemorrhagic skin lesions (purpura), and central nervous system signs and symptoms secondary to thrombosis. TTP usually occurs in adults and has a high mortality rate if not treated, whereas HUS occurs in young children and postpartum, is usually self-limiting, and features renal failure, which is rare in TTP. Autopsy of TTP patients reveals widespread thrombotic occlusion of arterioles and capillaries by hyaline masses that are usually located beneath the endothelium. The central nervous system symptoms are presumably due to microvascular occlusions. The anemia is microangiopathic (secondary to mechanical destruction of erythrocytes by physical trauma of contact with the altered vascular walls). The etiology of the vascular lesions is unknown, but they may be caused by a form of toxic complex or autoantibody deposits leading to focal fibrinoid necroses and hyaline scarring or by activation of the clotting mechanism by toxic complexes. Some cases are associated with antiphospholipid antibody. Plasmapheresis (plasma exchange) may be effective treatment.

Summary

Connective tissue (collagen-vascular) diseases are believed to be caused by autoantibodies and mediated primarily by immune complex mechanisms, but chronic progressive forms of these diseases are driven by cell-mediated immunity. The connective tissue diseases are PAN, RA, SLE, SS, dermatomyositis, and PSS (scleroderma). The shared lesions include fibrinoid necrosis, glomerulonephritis, and vasculitis. Other immune effector mechanisms (neutralization, cytotoxic, DTH, and granulomatous reactions) play a pathogenic role in some lesions seen in these diseases, but most of the major acute manifestations are due to immune complex reactions, and chronic stages are caused by cell-mediated immunity. The etiology of these diseases is not known. Most hypotheses include the possibility of a genetically determined immune reaction to some infectious agent, but none has been clearly identified. There is clear evidence of inherited tendencies and HLA association in the case of RA and SLE. The symptoms may be quite variable, with many very mild limited cases but also, unfortunately, many severe life-threatening ones. Fulminant manifestations may be controlled by anti-inflammatory drugs or steroids, but chronic progression is usual in severe cases.

Other Immune Complex Diseases

In addition to the renal glomerulus, other organs of the body also contain capillary basement membrane exposed to circulating blood: the lung (see Goodpasture's disease above), synovial capillaries, the choroid plexus of the brain, and the uveal tract of the eye. These organs are susceptible to anti-basement membrane antibody attack and deposition of immune complexes.

Cellular Interstitial Pneumonia

Immune complex deposition and subsequent inflammation may also cause an interstitial inflammation in the lung. These lesions have been identified morphologically as an infiltration of the lung with different cellular elements. Cellular interstitial pneumonia is often found associated with various collagen diseases. Immunoglobulin and complement have been identified in the lungs of patients with active interstitial disease in a manner similar to that of an experimental systemic immune complex-induced pneumonitis in rabbits. In addition, circulating immune complexes have been found in the serum of patients with interstitial pneumonias. A chronic form of interstitial pneumonia (diffuse fibrosis) is not associated with circulating immune complexes. This may be a later stage of a cellular interstitial pneumonia, when complexes are no longer present, or there may be a different pathogenesis. Patients with active stages of the disease (when immune complexes are present) are responsive to steroid therapy. The spectrum of interstitial pneumonias resembles the stages of glomerulonephritis described above. It is also possible that immune complex formation is secondary to, and not the cause of, cellular interstitial inflammation.

Arthritis

Subsynovial capillaries are also a site for immune complex deposition. Transient arthritis is seen in many infectious diseases (reactive arthritis) and is also often associated with collagen diseases. A classic example is the arthritis seen during acute attacks of rheumatic fever. It is likely that such transient arthritis episodes are due to immune complex-initiated inflammation.

Choroid Plexus Deposition

The choroid plexus is a frequent site of immune complex deposition in laboratory animals injected with immune complexes and with infections associated with circulating immune complexes. In humans, depositions of immune complexes in the choroid plexus are found in some diseases, such as SLE. In the choroid plexus, the endothelial cells are fenestrated so that, in contrast to other parts of the cerebral vasculature, there is not a tight blood-brain barrier. Immune complexes pass through the endothelial cells to lie between the endothelial and epithelial cells. The epithelial cells overlying the basement membrane are tightly joined and prevent increased filtration after complex deposition, such as is seen in renal glomeruli. The role of these immune complexes in producing the neurological symptoms of SLE remains undefined.

Uveitis

Some forms of uveitis may be caused by deposition of immune complexes in the ocular basement membrane. In rabbits, circulating immune complexes may deposit in ocular tissue and be responsible for inflammation of the uveal tract (iris, ciliary body, and choroid). However, in a rat model, two different mechanisms, one involving endotoxin activation of macrophages and a second implicating a delayed-type hypersensitivity reaction to ocular melanin, have been observed. In humans, uveitis is associated with circulating immune complexes, and immune complexes and Th1-type cytokines (IL-2, IFN-γ) have been detected in the aqueous humor of the anterior chamber of the eye. Thus, the uveal tract may also be a preferential site for immune complex deposition and subsequent inflammation, but other forms of uveitis may be caused by cellular autoimmunity to uveal antigens.

Evaluation of Circulating Immune Complexes

There are a number of laboratory assays for immune complexes, but the assays currently used have limited value for diagnosing or aiding therapeutic decisions and are not done routinely in clinical immunology laboratories.

Summary

Immune complex reactions are caused by immunoglobulin antibody reacting with tissue antigens, by formation of antibody-antigen complexes that deposit in vessel walls or basement membrane of capillaries, or by antibodies that react with basement membrane antigens. Tissue destruction is mediated by lysosomal enzymes released from PMNs attracted and activated by complement components (C3a and C5a). Acute lesions consist of tissue digestion by enzymes, whereas chronic lesions may be caused by deposition of large amounts of immune complexes or scarring. Typical diseases caused by this mechanism include serum sickness, glomerulonephritis, vasculitis, collagen diseases, and many types of skin eruptions. The antigens involved may be host tissue antigens (autoimmune reaction) or foreign (bacterial or viral) antigens.

Bibliography

Immune Complex Injury

Cochrane, C. G., and D. Koffler. 1973. Immune complex disease in experimental animals and in man. *Adv. Immunol.* **16:**185–264.

Heller, T., J. E. Gessner, R. E. Schmidt, A. Klos, W. Bautsch, and J. Kohl. 1999. Cutting edge: Fc receptor type I for IgG on macrophages and complement mediate the inflammatory response in immune complex peritonitis. *J. Immunol.* **162:** 5657–5661.

Oldham, K. T., K. S. Guice, P. A. Ward, and K. J. Johnson. 1988. The role of oxygen radicals in immune complex injury. *Free Radical Biol. Med.* **4:**387–397.

Arthus Reaction

Arthus, M. 1903. Injections répétées de sérum de cheval chez le lapin. *C. R. Soc. Biol.* (Paris) **55:**817.

Steil, A. A., C. F. Teixeira, and S. Jancar. 1999. Platelet-activating factor and eicosanoids are mediators of local and systemic changes induced by immune-complexes in mice. *Prostaglandins Other Lipid Mediat.* **57:**35–48.

Serum Sickness

Bielory, L., P. Gascon, T. J. Lawley, N. S. Young, and M. Frank. 1988. Human serum sickness: a prospective analysis of 35 patients treated with equine anti-thymocyte globulin for bone marrow failure. *Medicine* **67:**40–57.

Dixon, F. J., J. J. Vasquez, W. O. Weigle, and C. G. Cochrane. 1958. Pathogenesis of serum sickness. *Arch. Pathol.* **65:**18–28.

Gaig, P., P. Garcia-Ortega, E. Enrique, A. Benet, B. Bartolome, and R. Palacios. 1999. Serum sickness-like syndrome due to mosquito bite. *J. Investig. Allergol. Clin. Immunol.* **9:**190–192.

von Pirquet, C. F., and B. Schick. 1951. *Serum Sickness* (B. Schick, trans.). The Williams & Wilkins Co., Baltimore, Md. [Reprint of 1905 article.]

Vozianova, Z. I., and K. I. Chepilko. 1999. Serum sickness in diphtheria. *Lik. Sprava.* **3:**126–128.

Winter, G., and W. J. Harris. 1993. Humanized antibodies. *Trends Pharmacol. Sci.* **14:**139–143.

Glomerulonephritis

Andres, G., J. R. Brentjens, P. R. B. Caldwell, G. Camussi, and S. Matsuo. 1986. Biology of disease. Formation of immune deposits and disease. *Lab. Investig.* **55:**510–520.

Bruijn, J. A., P. J. Hoedemaeker, and G. J. Fleuren. 1989. Pathogenesis of anti-basement membrane glomerulonephritis and immune-complex glomerulonephritis: dichotomy dissolved. *Lab. Investig.* **61:**480–488.

Feintzeig, I. D., J. E. Dittmer, A. V. Cybulsky, and D. J. Salant. 1986. Antibody, antigen and glomerular capillary wall charge interactions: influence of antigen location on in situ immune complex formation. *Kidney Int.* **29:**649–657.

Foster, M. H., and V. R. Kelly. 1999. Lupus nephritis: update on pathogenesis and disease mechanisms. *Semin. Nephrol.* **19:**173–181.

Hudson, B. G., J. Wieslander, B. J. Wisdom, and M. E. Noelken. 1989. Goodpasture syndrome: molecular architecture and function of basement membrane antigen. *Lab. Investig.* **61:**256–269.

Julian, B. A., M. Tomana, J. Novak, and J. Mestecky. 1999. Progress in the pathogenesis of IgA nephropathy. *Adv. Nephrol. Necker Hosp.* **29:**53–72.

Kitching, A. R., S. R. Holdsworth, and P. G. Tipping. 1999. INF-gamma mediates crescent formation and cell-mediated immune injury in murine glomerulonephritis. *J. Am. Soc. Nephrol.* **10:**752–759.

Krane, N. K., and P. Gaglio. 1999. Viral hepatitis as a cause of renal disease. *South. Med. J.* **92:**354–360.

Muda, A. O., S. Feriozzi, S. Rahimi, E. Ancarani, and T. Faraggiana. 1999. Spatial arrangement of subepithelial deposits in lupus and nonlupus membranous nephropathy. *Am. J. Kidney Dis.* **34:**85–91.

Rychlik, I., K. Andrassy, R. Waldherr, I. Zuna, V. Tesar, E. Jancova, A. Stejskalova, and E. Ritz. 1999. Clinical features and natural history of IgA nephropathy. *Ann. Med. Interne* (Paris) **150:**117–126.

Ryffel, B., H. Eugster, C. Haas, and M. Le Hir. 1998. Failure to induce anti-glomerular basement membrane glomerulonephritis in TNF α/β deficient mice. *Int. J. Exp. Pathol.* **79:**453–460.

Schneider, A., U. Panzer, G. Zahner, U. Wenzel, G. Wolf, et al. 1999. Monocyte chemoattractant protein-1 mediates collagen deposition in experimental glomerulonephritis by transforming growth factor-beta. *Kidney Int.* **56:**135–144.

Vasculitis

Behçet, H. 1937. Über rez'diverende Aphtose durch ein Virus verursachte Geschwure am Mund, am Auge und an den Genitalen. *Dermatol. Wochenschr.* **105:**1152.

Clark, J. A. 1995. Unraveling the mystery: clues to systemic vasculitic disorders. *AACN Clin. Issues* **6:**645–656.

Csernok, E., A. Muller, and W. L. Gross. 1999. Immunopathology of ANCA-associated vasculitis. *Intern. Med.* **38:**759–765.

Curtis, N., and M. Levin. 1998. Kawasaki disease thirty years on. *Curr. Opin. Pediatr.* **10:**24–33.

Ghate, J. F., and J. L. Jorizzo. 1999. Behçet's disease and complex aphthosis. *J. Am. Acad. Dermatol.* **40:**1–18.

Hunder, C. G., J. T. Lie, J. J. Goronzy, and C. M. Weyand. 1993. Pathogenesis of giant cell arteritis. *Arth. Rheum.* **36:**757–761.

Laupland, K. B., and H. Dele Davies. 1999. Epidemiology, etiology, and management of Kawasaki disease: state of the art. *Pediatr. Cardiol.* **20:**177–183.

LeRoy, E. C. (ed.). 1992. *Systemic Vasculitis: the Biologic Basis.* Marcel Dekker, Inc., New York, N.Y.

Mochizuki, M. 1997. Immunotherapy for Behçet's disease. *Int. Rev. Immunol.* **14:**49–66.

Piette, J. C. C. Fieschi, and Z. Amoura. 1999. Classification of vasculitis. *N. Engl. J. Med.* **341:**1174–1175.

Rheumatic Fever

Brandt, E. R., and M. F. Good. 1999. Vaccine strategies to prevent rheumatic fever. *Immunol. Res.* **19:**89–103.

Froude, J., A. Gibofsky, D. R. Buskirk, A. Khanna, and J. B. Zabriskie. 1989. Cross-reactivity between streptococcus and human tissue: a model of molecular mimicry and autoimmunity. *Curr. Top. Microbiol. Immunol.* **145:**5–26.

Groves, A. M. 1999. Rheumatic fever and rheumatic heart disease: an overview. *Trop. Doct.* **29:**129–132.

McCarty, M., and W. Lewis. 1985. Waunamaker in the campaign against rheumatic fever. *Zentbl. Bakteriol. Hyg. A* **260:**151–164.

Stollerman, G. H. 1991. Rheumatogenic streptococci and autoimmunity. *Clin. Immunol. Immunopathol.* **61:**131–142.

Connective Tissue Diseases

Benedek, T. G. 1987. A century of American rheumatology. *Ann. Intern. Med.* **106:**304–312.

Farid, N. R. 1990. *The Immunogenetics of Autoimmune Diseases.* CRC Press, Boca Raton, Fla.

Klemperer, P. 1961. The concept of collagen diseases in medicine. *Am. Rev. Respir. Dis.* **83:**331–339.

Polyarteritis Nodosa

Guillevin, L. 1999. Treatment of classic polyarteritis nodosa in 1999. *Nephrol. Dial. Transplant.* **14:**2077–2079.

Kussmaul, A., and R. Maier. 1866. Ueber eine bisher nicht beschriebene eigenthumliche Arterienerkrankung (Periarteritis Nodosa), die mit Morbus Brightii and rapid fortschreitender allgemeiner Muskellahmung einhergeht. *Dtsch. Arch. Klin. Med.* **1:**484.

McCombs, R. P. 1965. Systemic "allergic" vasculitis: clinical and pathological relationships. *JAMA* **194:**1059–1064.

Phanuphak, P., and P. F. Kohler. 1980. Onset of polyarteritis nodosa during allergic hypersensitization treatment. *Am. J. Med.* **68:**479–485.

Soufir, N., V. Descamps, B. Crickx, V. Thibault, A. Cosnes, P. A. Becherel, et al. 1999. Hepatitis C virus infection in cutaneous polyarteritis nodosa: a retrospective study of 16 cases. *Arch. Dermatol.* **135:**1001–1002.

Trepo, C. G., J. Thivolet, and A. M. Prince. 1972. Australia antigen and polyarteritis nodosa. *Am. J. Dis. Child.* **123:**390–392.

Rheumatoid Arthritis

Arnett, F. C. 1986. Immunogenetics and arthritis, p. 405. *In* D. J. McCarty (ed.), *Arthritis and Allied Conditions.* Lea & Febiger, Philadelphia, Pa.

Felson, D. T., J. J. Anderson, M. Boers, C. Bombardier, M. Chernoff, et al. 1993. The American College of Rheumatology preliminary core set of disease activity measures for rheumatoid arthritis clinical trials. *Arth. Rheum.* **36:**729–740.

Lipsky, P. E., L. S. Davis, J. J. Cush, and N. Oppenheimer-Marks. 1989. The role of cytokines in the pathogenesis of rheumatoid arthritis. *Springer Semin. Immunopathol.* **11:**123–162.

Lockwood, C. M., J. D. Elliott, L. Brettman, G. Hale, P. Rebello, et al. 1999. Anti-adhesion molecular therapy as an interventional strategy for autoimmune inflammation. *Clin. Immunol.* **93:**93–106.

Mellbye, O. J., O. Forre, T. E. Mollnes, and L. Kvarnes. 1991. Immunopathology of subcutaneous rheumatoid nodules. *Ann. Rheum. Dis.* **50:**909–912.

Moore, T. L., and R. W. Dorner. 1993. Rheumatoid factors. *Clin. Biochem.* **26:**75–84.

Pincus, T., J. R. O'Dell, and J. M. Kremer. 1999. Combination therapy with multiple disease-modifying antirheumatic drugs in rheumatoid arthritis: a preventive strategy. *Ann. Intern. Med.* **131:**768–774.

Shimoyama, Y., J. Nagafuchi, N. Suzuki, T. Ochi, and T. Sakane. 1999. Synovial infiltrating T cells induce excessive synovial cell function through CD28/B7 pathway in patients with rheumatoid arthritis. *J. Rheumatol.* **26:**2094–2101.

Vaughn, J. H. 1993. Pathogenic concepts and origins of rheumatoid factor in rheumatoid arthritis. *Arth. Rheum.* **36:**1–6.

Zvailfer, N. J. 1974. Rheumatoid synovitis. An extravascular immune complex disease. *Arth. Rheum.* **17:**297–305.

Spondyloarthritis

Gonzalez, S., J. Martinez-Borra, and C. Lopez-Larrea. 1999. Immunogenetics, HLA-B27 and spondyloarthropathies. *Curr. Opin. Rheumatol.* **11:**257–264.

Marker-Hermann, E., and T. Hohler. 1999. Pathogenesis of human leukocyte B27-positive arthritis. Information from clinical materials. *Rheum. Dis. Clin. N. Am.* **24:**865–881.

Ringose, J. H. 1999. HLA-B27 associated spondyloarthropathy, an autoimmune disease based on crossreactivity between bacteria and HLA-B27? *Ann. Rheum. Dis.* **58:**598–610.

Scofield, R. H., W. L. Warren, G. Koelsch, and J. B. Harley. 1973. A hypothesis for the HLA-B27 immune dysregulation in spondyloarthropathy: contributions from enteric organisms, B27 structure, peptides bound by B27, and convergent evolution. *Proc. Natl. Acad. Sci. USA* **90:**9330–9334.

Taurog, J. D., S. D. Maika, N. Satumtira, M. L. Dorris, I. L. McLean, H. Yanagisawa, et al. 1999. Inflammatory disease in HLA-B27 transgenic rats. *Immunol. Rev.* **169:**209–223.

Systemic Lupus Erythematosus

Arnett, F. C. 1985. HLA and genetic predisposition to lupus erythematosus and other dermatologic disorders. *J. Am. Acad. Dermatol.* **13:**472–481.

Blatt, N. B., and G. D. Glick. 1999. Anti-DNA autoantibodies and systemic lupus erythematosus. *Pharmacol. Ther.* **83:**125–139.

Brooks, E. B., and M. H. Liang. 1999. Evaluation of recent clinical trials in lupus. *Curr. Opin. Rheumatol.* **11:**341–347.

Foster, M. H., and V. R. Kelley. 1999. Lupus nephritis: update on pathogenesis and disease mechanisms. *Semin. Nephrol.* **19:**173–181.

Hargraves, M. M., H. Richmond, and R. Morton. 1948. Presentation of 2 bone marrow elements: the "tart" cell and the "LE" cell. *Mayo Clin. Proc.* **23:**25–31.

Rubin, R. L. 1999. Etiology and mechanisms of drug-induced lupus. *Curr. Opin. Rheumatol.* **11:**357–363.

Southeimer, R. D. 1996. Photoimmunology of lupus erythematosus and dermatomyositis: a speculative review. *Photochem. Photobiol.* **63:**583–594.

Steinberg, A. D. 1992. Concepts of pathogenesis of systemic lupus erythematosus. *Clin. Immunol. Immunopathol.* **63:**19–22.

Sullivan, K. E. 1998. Complement deficiency and autoimmunity. *Curr. Opin. Pediatr.* **10:**600–606.

Tan, E. M., A. S. Cohen, J. F. Fries, A. T. Masi, D. J. McShane, et al. 1982. The 1982 revised criteria for the classification of systemic lupus erythematosus. *Arth. Rheum.* **25:**1271–1277.

Sjögren's Syndrome

Bell, M., A. Askari, A. Bookman, S. Frydrych, J. Lamont, J. McComb, C. Muscoplat, and A. Slomovic. 1999. Sjögren's syndrome: a critical review of clinical management. *J. Rheumatol.* **26:**2051–2061.

Fox, R. I., J. Tronwell, and P. Michelson. 1999. Current issues in the diagnosis and treatment of Sjögren's syndrome. *Curr. Opin. Rheumatol.* **11:**364–371.

Hadden, W. B. 1888. On "dry mouth," or suppression of the salivary buccal secretions. *Trans. Clin. Soc. Hand* **21:**176.

Humphreys-Beher, M. G., and A. B. Peck. 1999. New concepts for the development of autoimmune endocrinopathy derived from studies with the NOD mouse model. *Arch. Oral Biol.* **44**(Suppl. 1)**:**S21–S25.

Mikulicz, J. 1937. Concerning a peculiar symmetrical disease of the lacrimal and salivary glands, p. 137–186. *In Medical Classics,* vol. 2. The Williams & Wilkins Co., Baltimore, Md. [Reprint of 1892 article.]

Sjögren, H. 1933. Zur Kenntnis der keratoconjunctivitis sicca (keratitis filiformus bei Hypofunktion der Tränendrüsen). *Acta Ophthalmol.* (Copenhagen) **11:**1.

Voulgarelis, M., U. G. Dafni, D. A. Isenberg, and H. M. Moutsopoulos. 1999. Malignant lymphoma in primary Sjögren's syndrome: a multicenter, retrospective, clinical study by the European Concentrated Action on Sjögren's syndrome. *Arth. Rheum.* **42:**1765–1772.

Xanthou, G., N. I. Tapinos, M. Polihronis, I. P. Nezis, L. H. Margaritis, and H. M. Moutsopoulos. 1999. CD4 cytotoxic and dendritic cells in the immunopathologic lesion of Sjögren's syndrome. *Clin. Exp. Immunol.* **118:**154–163.

Dermatomyositis

Dalakas, M. C. 1998. Molecular immunology and genetics of inflammatory muscle diseases. *Arch. Neurol.* **55:**1509–1512.

Dalakas, M. C. 1999. Intravenous immunoglobulin in the treatment of autoimmune neuromuscular diseases: present status and practical therapeutic guidelines. *Muscle Nerve* **22:**1479–1497.

Vogel, H. 1998. Inclusion body myositis—a review. *Adv. Anat. Pathol.* **5:**164–169.

Wagner, E. 1886. Ein Fall von akuter Polymyositis. *Dtsch. Arch. Klin. Med.* **11:**241.

West, J. E., and A. M. Reed. 1999. Analysis of HLA-DM polymorphism in juvenile dermatomyositis (JDM) patients. *Hum. Immunol.* **60:**255–258.

Progressive Systemic Sclerosis (Scleroderma)

Brautbar, N., A. Vojdani, and A. W. Campbell. 1992. Silicone implants and systemic immunological disease: review of the literature and preliminary results. *Toxicol. Ind. Health* **8:**231–237.

Claman, H. N., B. D. Jafee, J. C. Huff, and R. A. F. Clark. 1985. Chronic graft vs. host disease as a model for scleroderma. *Cell. Immunol.* **94:**73–84.

Kaal, S. E., F. H. Ven Den Hoogen, E. M. de Jong, and H. E. Vietor. 1999. Systemic sclerosis: new insights in autoimmunity. *Proc. Soc. Exp. Biol. Med.* **222:**1–8.

Kerin, K., and J. H. Yost. 1998. Advances in the diagnosis and management of scleroderma-related vascular complications. *Comp. Ther.* **24:**574–581.

LeRoy, E. C., C. Black, R. Fleischmajer, S. Jablonska, et al. 1988. Scleroderma (systemic sclerosis): classification, subsets and pathogenesis. *J. Rheumatol.* **15:** 202–205.

Lock, G., A. Holstege, B. Lang, and J. Scholmerich. 1977. Gastrointestinal manifestations of progressive systemic sclerosis. *Am. J. Gastroenterol.* **92:**763–771.

Nelson, J. L. 1998. Microchimerism and the pathogenesis of systemic sclerosis. *Curr. Opin. Rheumatol.* **10:**564–571.

Mixed Connective Tissue Disease

Alarcon-Segovia, D. 1981. Mixed connective tissue disease—a decade of growing pains. *J. Rheumatol.* **8:**535–540.

Brandt, M. A., R. W. Hoffman, S. L. Deutscher, G. S. Wang, J. C. Johnson, and G. C. Sharp. 1999. Long-term outcome in mixed connective tissue disease: longitudinal clinical and serologic findings. *Arth. Rheum.* **42:**899–909.

Kasukawa, R. 1999. Mixed connective tissue disease. *Intern. Med.* **38:**386–393.

Thrombotic Thrombocytopenia Purpura

Brain, M. C., and P. B. Neame. 1983. Thrombotic thrombocytopenic purpura and the hemolytic uremic syndrome. *Semin. Thromb. Hemost.* **8:**186–197.

Moake, J. L. 1999. Thrombotic thrombocytopenic purpura today. *Hosp. Pract.* **34:**53–59.

Other Immune Complex Diseases

Brentjens, J. R., D. W. O'Connel, I. B. Pawlowski, K. C. Hsu, and C. A. Andres. 1974. Experimental immune complex disease of the lung: the pathogenesis of a laboratory model resembling certain interstitial lung diseases. *J. Exp. Med.* **140:**105–125.

Maumenee, A. E., and A. M. Silverstein (ed.). 1964. *Immunopathology of Uveitis.* The Williams & Wilkins, Co., Baltimore, Md.

Murray, P. I., C. D. Clay, C. Mappin, and M. Salmon. 1999. Molecular analysis of resolving immune responses in uveitis. *Clin. Exp. Immunol.* **117:**455–461.

Smith, J. R., P. H. Hart, and K. A. Williams. 1998. Basic pathogenic mechanisms operating in experimental models of acute anterior uveitis. *Immunol. Cell. Biol.* **76:**497–512.

Atopic and Anaphylactic Reactions (Allergy)

11

Introduction

Definitions

The term *anaphylaxis* was coined by Portier and Richet in 1902 to indicate adverse reactions in dogs to a toxin derived from the sea anemone. They expected that repeated injections of the toxin would lead to a neutralization of the toxic effect by antibody but instead found lethal responses to doses of the toxin that were previously innocuous. Although the word anaphylaxis literally means "without protection," the term as used by Portier and Richet implied a reaction that is the opposite of prophylaxis, a destructive rather than a protective reaction, as a result of previous exposure to an agent. Coca applied the term *atopy* in the 1920s for a variety of reactions in humans, at the time not yet described in other species. The origin of this term is from the Greek word *atopia,* meaning strangeness. These reactions are now included in the term "allergy." The word *allergy* was introduced by von Pirquet in 1906 to designate "altered reactivity" as a result of previous exposure. The term allergy is now mostly used for atopic or anaphylactic reactions but is also used as a general term for reactions of discomfort of unknown origin. Although the association of seasonal allergic rhinitis *(catarrhus aestivus)* with grass pollen in England and with ragweed in the United States *(autumnal catarrh)* was reported in 1872, the name now applied to this group of diseases was not forthcoming until much later.

The effects produced by atopic or anaphylactic reactions are the result of a two-phase system initiated by mediators that are released by the reaction of antigen with effector cells passively sensitized by immunoglobulin E (IgE) antibody (Fig. 11.1). Antigens that elicit these responses are also called *allergens.* The mast cell (tissue) or basophil (peripheral blood) is the major effector cell for acute reactions, whereas T cells and eosinophils play important roles in persistent asthma. Mast cells are stimulated to develop from bone marrow precursors by stem cell factor and interleukin-4 (IL-4). Cells in the mast cell (basophil) lineage migrate to sites in the tissues where smooth muscles (e.g., blood vessels, bronchi) are located. It is at these sites where release of mast cell mediators produce effects on smooth muscle.

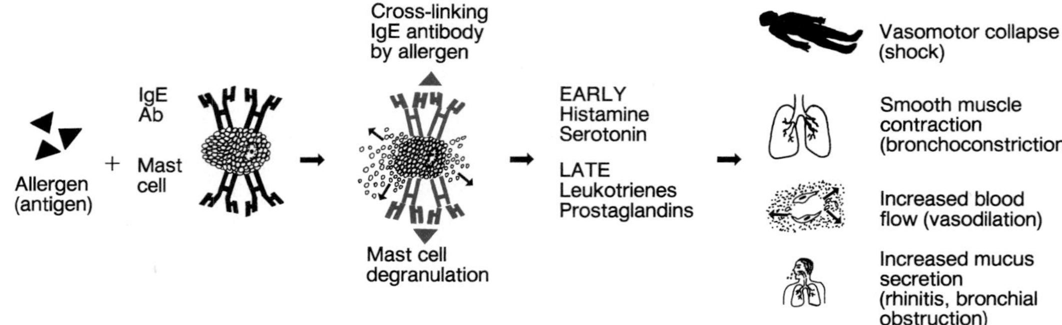

Figure 11.1 Atopic or anaphylactic reactions. Reaction of antigen (allergen) with reaginic antibody (IgE) fixed to effector (mast) cells causes release of pharmacologically active agents stored in cytoplasmic granules (degranulation of mast cells). These released mediators, primarily histamine and serotonin, cause contraction of endothelial cells and bronchial smooth cells and produce edema and bronchoconstriction. Cell membrane-associated arachidonic acids also released from mast cells are converted to other inflammatory mediators—leukotrienes and prostaglandins—which are responsible for later stages of the reactions. The acute effects are termed anaphylactic; the more chronic effects, atopic.

Histamine Receptors

Following reaction with allergens, mast cells release a number of biologically active substances, including histamine, heparin, and serotonin (early-phase reaction), as well as arachidonic acid, which is converted by other cells into prostaglandins and leukotrienes responsible for the later-phase inflammation reactions. The acute phase is characterized by immediate smooth muscle constriction or dilation. On one hand, the smooth muscle of arterioles is stimulated to dilate by reaction of histamine with H_2 receptors (blocked by cimetidine), causing increased blood flow (erythema). On the other hand, the smooth muscle of pulmonary bronchi, gastrointestinal tract (asthma), and the genitourinary system (cramps and diarrhea), as well as endothelial cells (edema), are stimulated to contract by action of histamine on H_1 receptors (blocked by anti-histamines) (Table 11.1). The clinical effect of treatment with antihistamines for treatment of bronchoconstriction is through H_1 receptor antagonism, as well as by blocking histamine release from mast cells. The effects of the immediate anaphylactic mediators include contraction of bronchi, increased vascular permeability, early increase in vascular resistance followed by collapse (shock), and increased gastric, nasal, and lacrimal secretion. The type of lesion observed depends upon the dose of antigen, the route of contact with antigen, the

Table 11.1 Allergic symptoms and receptors: five organ systems

Histamine receptor	Reactive tissue	Constriction	Dilation	Symptom
H_2	Vascular		X	Shock
H_1	Pulmonary	X		Asthma
	Gastrointestinal	X		Vomiting and diarrhea
	Genitourinary	X		Involuntary urination
	Endothelium	X		Edema

frequency of contract with antigen, the tendency for a given organ system to react (shock organ), and the degree of sensitivity of the involved individual. This final factor may be genetically controlled or may be altered by environmental conditions (temperature), unrelated inflammation (presence of a viral upper respiratory infection), or the emotional state of the individual. Some of the reactions seen clinically are urticaria (wheal and flare, hives), hay fever, asthma, eczema, angioedema, and anaphylaxis.

Comparison of Anaphylactic and Atopic Reactions

Acute reactions (wheal and flare, systemic shock) are generally referred to as anaphylactic; chronic recurring reactions (hay fever) are called atopic. However, this distinction is not always made, and there is considerable overlap in the use of the terms atopic and anaphylactic. An atopic individual is one who is prone to develop this type of allergic reaction. Although in the Western world, these reactions are largely pathologic, in the tropics the capacity to produce an IgE response may be protective against worm (helminthic) infections (see below).The early-phase reaction consists of edema (extravasation of the fluid component of blood into the tissues) and bronchoconstriction, and it occurs within minutes of exposure to antigen. The late phase occurs 6 to 12 h after antigen exposure, and is characterized by a more prolonged reaction involving infiltration by neutrophilic, eosinophilic, and basophilic polymorphonuclear cells, as well as lymphocytes, and macrophages. This late phase causes an indurated, erythematous, painful reaction in the skin or, in the lung, a more prolonged deterioration in airflow as compared with the rapidly appearing wheal-and-flare skin reaction or asthma characterized by rapidly reversible bronchoconstriction in the immediate or early phase. The inflammatory properties of prostaglandins and leukotrienes are discussed in more detail in chapter 3. These mediators cause infiltration of polymorphonuclear leukocytes (PMNs) and other hallmarks of acute inflammation. In turn, PMN granules contain defensins, which induce mast cell degranulation, providing a pathway of communication between PMNs and basophils. Prostaglandin E is a potent dilator of bronchial smooth muscle, and prostaglandin F is a potent constrictor. Leukotriene E_4 (slow-reacting substance of anaphylaxis) causes later vasoreactions, whereas leukotriene B_4 is chemotactic for acute inflammatory cells. Another pathway is IL-5-mediated eosinophil infiltration. A better understanding of the production, release, and effects of these mediators may lead to improved therapeutic approaches.

Chronic reactions such as hay fever and persistent asthma are accompanied by a lowering of the threshold to atopic stimuli. This hyperreactivity is associated with chronic tissue infiltration with mast cells, macrophages, T cells, B cells, and eosinophils. The increased numbers of inflammatory cells, as well as smooth muscle hyperplasia, sets up conditions whereby lower levels of allergen exposure may trigger fits of sneezing or asthmatic attacks. One school of thought implies that Th2 cell stimulation of eosinophil differentiation by IL-3, IL-5, and granulocyte-macrophage colony-stimulating factor leads to production and release of leukotrienes (C_4 and D_4) and platelet-activating factors that contribute to the chronic inflammation in atopic conditions. However, the relative importance of this mechanism to those of the other possible mechanisms remains to be clarified. The role of non-IgE-mediated reactions in asthma is presented in more detail below.

Allergens

Allergic Sensitization

The antigens that induce and elicit allergic reactions, allergens, have no unique features to distinguish them as a subset of antigenic molecules. Induction of IgE antibody appears to be favored by things such as route, dose, or presence of a modifying agent. Thus, inhalation or ingestion of an antigen predisposes to IgE formation, as does low dose or the presence of adjuvants such as alumina gel or *Bordetella pertussis*. The injected allergenic components of bee venom or mosquito bites also reach the immune system in very small doses, as do ingested allergenic compounds in foods. Inhaled allergens include pollen, fungi, dander and dust, which are usually inhaled at very low doses. Larger pollen particulate allergens (20-μm diameter) tend to deposit in the upper airway and produce allergic rhinitis (hay fever), whereas smaller particles are inhaled into the bronchi, where they may cause asthma.

Induction of IgE antibodies depends on the maturation of IgE-producing B cells after exposure to antigen. In humans, allergic sensitization to allergens, such as ragweed antigen, is associated with genetic factors (HLA). In addition, infections in early childhood may protect against development of allergies later in life. Immunologic factors that appear to determine if IgG or IgE B cells will be formed during induction of antibody formation are the relative balance of interleukins. This lymphokine balance is, in turn, related to the activation of different T-helper-cell populations. In the mouse, there are two subpopulations of T-helper cells: Th1 and Th2. Th1 cells secrete IL-2, gamma interferon (IFN-γ), and lymphotoxin but not IL-4; Th2 cells secrete IL-4, IL-5, and IL-6 but not IFN-γ. Th1 cell products drive B cells toward production of complement-fixing IgG antibodies responsible for immune complex reactions; Th2 cell products drive B cells to IgE and IgA production and stimulate differentiation of mast cells. Thus, IgE antibody production is determined by genetically controlled factors as well as dose, route, frequency of exposure, and presence of infections that act to direct antigen presentation to Th2 cells.

Chemistry of Allergens

Analysis of the pollen allergens in ragweed, as an example of a pollen allergen, indicates at least six different allergenic polypeptides with molecular weights from 5,000 to 38,000 (Table 11.2). There is little or no cross-reactivity among the pollens of different plants, but there may be extensive cross-reactivity within related species, such as with allergies to grass. Sequential (primary sequence) determinants appear to be relatively unimportant for

Table 11.2 Some properties of highly purified short ragweed *(Ambrosia artemisifolia)* antigens

Systematic name	Original name	M_r	No. of amino acids	% Allergen in dry pollen
Amb aI	AgE	37,800	337	0.48
Amb aII	AgK	38,200	331	0.12
Amb aIII	Ra31	12,300	101	0.08
Amb aIV	RaIV(BPA-R)	22,800	189	0.1
Amb aV	RaV	4,990	45	0.3
Amb aVI	Ra6	11,500	108	0.12

most allergens. Conformational structures are recognized by IgE antibody, so denaturation of allergens results in loss of antibody binding. Cooking may greatly alter the allergenic potential of dietary allergens. Anaphylactic reactions to drugs are increasingly common and are discussed below. *Allergoids* are allergens that have been chemically modified so that the allergenic reactivity has been greatly reduced, but the capacity to induce IgG antibody has been retained. Such modification has been attempted by formaldehyde, glutaraldehyde, and polyethylene glycol treatment. Allergoids have been shown to induce IgG antibodies in rodents, with little IgE antibody formation, but clinical trials in humans have not been successful.

Natural Distribution of Allergens

Atopic reactions may occur to very unusual antigens. Systemic anaphylactic reactions have been unleashed by ingestion of beans, rice, shrimp, fish, milk, beer, cereal mixes, potatoes, Brazil nuts, tangerines, etc. Allergy to birch tree pollen may be manifested by reactions to cross-reacting allergens in fruits and vegetables, such as cherries, apples, pears, celery, and carrots. Peanut allergy has become a major problem because of the inclusion of peanut products in many different food items. Genetic engineering that introduces defense proteins into plants may result in allergic reactions not previously seen, in particular because of cross-reactions between plant defensins and latex; a more general allergy to various fruits (bananas, avocados, chestnuts, etc.) is found in those with latex allergy. Men have complained about being allergic to their wives, but usually they are reacting to some component of makeup, hair spray, or other cosmetic agent. Rarely, women have developed systemic anaphylactic symptoms shortly after intercourse, due to an IgE-mediated reaction to a seminal plasma protein. About 10% of individuals who work with laboratory animals develop anaphylactic reactions to the dander or urinary and serum proteins from these animals that is severe enough to prevent them from further work with the animals. The incidence of such sensitivity increases with the amount of contact with the animals. During the days of cavalry, many officers and troops had to be discharged or moved to different tasks because of an allergic reaction to horse dander. As many as 20% of the cavaliers were involved. Documentation of allergic reactions of horses to humans has not been found. Several laundry detergents contain allergenic enzymes derived from *Bacillus subtilis,* which may cause severe reactions to laundry detergent in occasional unsuspecting users. With the widespread use of gloves for protection of health workers against AIDS, an increase in allergic reactions to latex has been seen.

Reaginic Antibody

IgE contributes less than 0.001% of the total circulating immunoglobulins but has a major biologic effect as reaginic antibody. Reaginic antibody has a special ability to bind to skin or other tissues. The term *atopic reagin* was adopted to refer to the particular tissue-fixing antibody found in the serum of patients with hay fever and asthma. The original use of the word reagin was to designate the reacting serum component responsible for the Wassermann reaction, the serologic test for syphilis. The Wassermann reagin is a peculiar serum reactant found in individuals infected with syphilis. The Wassermann reagin is demonstrable by its ability to combine with an antigen extracted from ungulate heart muscle (cardiolipin) and has no relation to anaphylactic or atopic reactions. It has been reported that atopic reaginic antibody may be found in all the major immunoglobulin groups (IgA, IgG, IgM). However, in essentially all cases, reagin is found only in IgE. In humans, it may be assumed that atopic or anaphylactic reactions are due to IgE antibody, but it is possible that some release of mast cell mediators may be mediated by complement fixing antibodies.

IgE Antibody

IgE antibody is termed "skin fixing" because it binds to mast cells in skin and sensitizes these cells to react to allergen. IgE anaphylactic antibodies have structures on the Fc piece of the molecule that fit receptors of the mast cell. There are two Fcϵ receptors, FcϵRI and FcϵRII. FcϵRI is the highest-affinity Fc receptor known, is found only on mast cells and basophils, and is responsible for transmission of the mast cell degranulation signal upon reaction of Fc-bound IgE antibody with allergen. FcϵRI is a tetramer and a member of the immunoglobulin supergene family. FcϵRII is a low-affinity receptor also found on macrophages, lymphocytes, eosinophils, and platelets. It is not well defined chemically and is believed to be involved in control of IgE synthesis and in antibody-dependent cell-mediated parasite killing. The average number of FcϵRIs on a mast cell is estimated to be 10,000 to 40,000. The number of FcϵRI cell-bound IgE antibody molecules determines the sensitivity of mast cells to an allergen. IL-4 and IgE act synergistically to increase expression of FcεRI on mast cells to increase mediator release. However, the amount of mediators released from a given cell also depends on enzyme systems that regulate the biochemical mechanisms of mediator release. Antigen cross-linking of two adjacent IgE molecules on the cell surface initiates events leading to mediator release. Mediator release may also be initiated by reaction of cross-linking anti-IgE antibodies with IgE on the cell surface. This induces activation of mitogen-activated protein kinase and Janus-3 kinase, as well as phosphokinase C pathways of activation (see chapter 3).

Passive Anaphylaxis

The reaginic activity of an immunoglobulin is determined by its ability to fix to skin of the same species. If serum from a sensitive individual is passively transferred to the skin of a normal recipient, the classic wheal-and-flare reaction can be elicited at this site upon application of the antigen (Prausnitz-Kustner test). In 1921, Carl Prausnitz (a professor) and Heinz Kustner (a medical student) reported the passive transfer of anaphylactic reactions both systemically and cutaneously by injection of serum from a patient sensitive to fish into a normal individual (Kustner). Because the antibody fixes to the skin, the transfer site may be tested up to 45 days later and still elicit a positive reaction. In contrast, with local passive transfer of nonreaginic antibody (passive Arthus reaction), the skin site must be tested within a few hours to obtain a positive reaction before the non-skin-fixing IgG antibody diffuses away (Table 11.3).

The passive transfer of atopic or anaphylactic reactions may be accomplished by a variety of methods, all of which depend upon the ability of reagins or IgE antibodies to fix to tissue mast cells. Most of these methods are now only used in laboratory animals.

1. For the local passive cutaneous anaphylaxis transfer (Prausnitz-Kustner) test, antibody-containing serum is injected into the skin, and after an appropriate period of time (usually several days) the same skin site is challenged with antigen.

Table 11.3 Passive transfer of antibody-mediated skin reactions

Method	No. of days after antibody transfer	Time after antigen challenge to reaction	Reaction	Histology
Passive cutaneous anaphylaxis (Prausnitz-Kustner)	Up to 90	15 min	Wheal and flare	Edema and congestion, spongiosis[a]
Passive cutaneous Arthus reaction	1–2	5–6 h	Induration and erythema	Vasculitis

[a]Spongiosis: intercellular epidermal edema.

2. For systemic passive cutaneous anaphylaxis, either the antibody is injected intravenously and the antigen intradermally, or the antibody is injected intradermally and the antigen intravenously.
3. Transfer of a systemic reaction (passive systemic anaphylaxis) is best elicited by injection of the antibody intravenously, followed by injection of the antigen intravenously 24 h later.
4. Reverse passive cutaneous anaphylaxis may be elicited if the antigen fixes to skin; in this instance, the antibody does not require tissue-fixing capacities. For reverse reactions, the antigen is injected into the skin, and after a suitable period the antibody is injected intravenously or at the same site. Reverse tests are useful for determining the skin-fixing properties of the immunoglobulins of one species for the skin of another species.

In most species studied, the antibody that fixes to the skin of the same species (e.g., human reagin fixing to human skin) belongs to a special class of immunoglobulin with properties similar to those of human IgE. If a given antibody in a species fixes to the skin of individuals of the same species, it is termed *homocytophilic*. In some instances, the immunoglobulins that fit tissue receptors of another species belong to a class other than IgE. For instance, human IgG antibodies may fix to guinea pig skin, but IgA, IgM, or IgE does not fix to guinea pig skin. Immunoglobulins that fix to the skin of a species different from their source are termed *heterocytophilic*.

IgE (reaginic) antibody has other properties different from usual antibody: it does not fix complement in the usual manner, and its skin-fixing capacity is heat labile (56°C for 30 min). IgE antibody can precipitate with antigen if sufficient amounts of antibody can be obtained. However, the amount of IgE antibody present in the serum of a sensitive individual is usually much too small to be detected by precipitation but can be detected by more sensitive techniques involving the anaphylactic response.

Clinical Antibody Tests (In Vivo)

Because of the unusual properties noted above, there is no simple test for reagin, even at the elevated levels found in atopic individuals. The most commonly used clinical test is the skin test. Suspected allergens are injected into the skin of an individual to test for cutaneous anaphylaxis. In this way, allergenic antigens may be identified. Skin testing must be done under careful supervision because systemic anaphylactic shock may be induced. Although the incidence of severe reaction is very low (approximately 1 fatality per 2 million doses per year in the United States), antianaphylactic drugs (e.g., epinephrine) must be kept on hand for rapid use, if necessary. The local transfer of skin-fixing antibody may be used to demonstrate reaginic activity in serum (passive) cutaneous anaphylaxis. This is the basis of the Prausnitz-Kustner test (see chapter 4). This test is no longer used because of the possibility of transmitting hepatitis or human immunodeficiency virus infection.

Another in vivo test that is extremely sensitive is bronchoprovocation. Inhalation of small amounts of the allergen will elicit acute bronchospasm (asthma). This test is rarely done except in well-controlled settings because of the obvious danger of inducing fatal anaphylaxis.

Laboratory Tests (In Vitro)

In vitro laboratory tests for specific reaginic antibody include the Schultz-Dale test, histamine release by mast cells (degranulation), and the radioallergosorbent test (RAST). The radioimmunoabsorbent test (RIST) is used to measure total serum IgE.

The Schultz-Dale Test

The Schultz-Dale test utilizes organs containing smooth muscle (guinea pig intestine or rat uterus) in an organ bath. When the organ is taken from a sensitized animal or incubated with serum from a sensitized individual, contraction will occur when the specific antigen is added. The extent of this contraction may be measured with a kymograph. Contraction may also be induced by the addition of mediators (histamine, leukotrienes).

Histamine Release

Histamine release from mast cells in vitro may be induced by contact of sensitized mast cells with antigen. The amount of histamine release may be determined spectrophotometrically or by morphologic observation of mast cell degranulation. Nonsensitized mast cells may be passively sensitized by incubation with reagin-containing serum. The passive leukocyte-sensitizing (PLS) activity of a given serum is determined by incubating a reaginic serum with blood leukocytes from nonallergic donors for about 2 h. The cells are then washed and treated with antigen for 1 h. The amount of histamine present in the supernatant is then determined photometrically. The extent of histamine release is used as an index of the serum reagin content. The PLS activity of ragweed-sensitive individuals is highest in the early fall (during the pollen season) and lowest in summer just before the pollen season.

The RAST

The RAST depends upon the binding of IgE antibody to specific antigen and the subsequent binding of radiolabeled anti-IgE to the IgE antibody-antigen complex. Fluorescent and enzyme-labeled antibodies are also used. The suspected antigen is first covalently bound to insoluble particles, or, in the case of more commonly used clinical tests, to paper discs. The insoluble antigen is then added to samples of serum. Those sera containing antibodies to the antigen will have antibody immunoglobulin that binds to the insoluble antigen. Antibody of classes other than IgE may also bind so that excess insoluble antigen is used. Antigen fixed to paper or particles is incubated with test sera, washed, and incubated with a labeled antibody to IgE. The labeled anti-IgE will bind to the IgE antibody, which is bound to the insoluble antigen. By determining the amount of labeled anti-IgE bound, an estimate of the IgE antibody to the specific antigen may be made. At present, the indiscriminate use of the RAST to diagnose allergy has resulted in many false-positive results that do not correlate with in vivo testing. Reliable allergists conduct careful history taking and skin testing before attempting immunotherapy.

The RIST

For total IgE, the RIST is most commonly used. Sera is added to anti-IgE-coated beads so that the IgE is bound to the beads. After washing, labeled anti-IgE is added. The amount of labeled anti-IgE bound is directly proportional to the amount of IgE in the unknown serum sample.

Mediator Release from Mast Cells

Two types of mechanisms may operate for release of mediators from mast cells or basophils: nonlytic, in which mast cell lysosomal membranes fuse with each other and with the cell surface membrane, resulting in release of lysosomal contents (degranulation), and lytic, in which antibody-antigen complexes on the surface of mast cells bind complement components and lyse the mast cell. Nonlytic release is the usual mechanism active in anaphylactic reactions involving reaginic antibody. The mast cell is not destroyed, and granules re-form. Lytic release provides a mechanism whereby cytolytic allergic reactions mediated by IgG or IgM may produce anaphylactic symptoms. The mechanism by which reaction of antigen with reaginic antibody on mast cells or basophils causes the release of mediators is described in chapter 3.

Anaphylaxis

Anaphylaxis is edema and congestion due to vasodilation and increased vascular permeability that may occur locally (cutaneous anaphylaxis) or a systemic shock reaction (systemic anaphylactic shock) due to massive vasodilation and loss of blood pressure.

Cutaneous Anaphylaxis

Cutaneous anaphylaxis (urticaria, wheal and flare, or hives) is elicited in a sensitive individual by skin test (scratch or intradermal injection of antigen). Grossly visible manifestations are erythema; a pale, soft, raised wheal; pseudopods; and a spreading flare, reaching a maximum in 15 to 20 min and fading in a few hours. Early, there is edema, with essentially no cellular infiltration until 12 to 18 h. The mechanism is the same as that in systemic anaphylaxis, but the reaction is localized because of antibody fixation in the skin and release of histamine or histaminelike substances into the skin with local changes in vascular permeability. Cutaneous anaphylaxis should be differentiated from the Arthus reaction in both time of appearance and morphology of the reaction (Table 11.3).

Systemic Anaphylaxis

Systemic anaphylaxis or anaphylactic shock is a generalized reaction elicited in a sensitized animal by the intravenous injection of antigen or in a human by natural exposure or iatrogenic injection of an allergen. It was discovered in 1902 following the injection of an extract of sea anemone into a dog. The injection was tolerated the first time but caused sudden death when injected into the same dog several weeks later. The use of horse serum as diphtheria antitoxin produced anaphylactic shock in humans and resulted in a renewed interest in anaphylaxis. This interest has been renewed again by the number of such reactions to antilymphocyte globulin used to suppress transplantation rejection, to penicillin, and to other drugs, including chymopapain used to digest the nucleus pulposus of herniated intervertebral disks. In highly sensitive individuals, a severe systemic reaction to small doses of the allergen placed on the skin (scratch or patch test) may occur. For this reason, the clinical allergist must be prepared to administer epinephrine (β-adrenergic stimulation) to any patient during skin testing. This counteracts the systemic effects of the anaphylactic reaction. The nature of the systemic reaction is species dependent. In all species, bronchial and gastrointestinal smooth muscle contraction is prominent, as well as increased permeability of small vessels, leukopenia, fall in temperature, hypotension, slowing of the heart rate, and decreased serum complement levels. However, different species have somewhat different fatal systemic anaphylactic reactions.

Guinea Pigs

Death occurs in 2 to 5 min, with prostration, convulsions, respiratory embarrassment, involuntary urination, defecation, itching, sneezing, and coughing. At autopsy, the lungs are inflated because of bronchiolar constriction with air trapping.

Rabbits

Death occurs in minutes; the course is similar in other respects to that in the guinea pig, except for the absence of respiratory difficulty. Autopsy shows right heart failure attributed to obstruction of the pulmonary circulatory.

Dogs

Death occurs after 1 to 2 h. There is a profound prostration with vomiting and bloody diarrhea, as well as liver engorgement from hepatic vein obstruction.

Rats

Death occurs in 30 min to 5 h. There is congestion of the small intestine and midzonal and periportal necrosis of the liver.

Humans

Humans exhibit a combination of the above reactions; death is not common but may occur upon exposure to high levels of the allergen. For instance, the description of systemic anaphylaxis by Prausnitz and Kustner after skin injection of fish muscle extract into a patient with fish allergy in 1921 is as follows.

> After half an hour: itching of the scalp, neck, lower abdomen, dry sensation in the throat; soon afterwards swelling and congestion of the conjunctivae, severe congestion and secretion of the respiratory mucous membranes, intense fits of sneezing, irritating cough, hoarseness merging into aphonia, and marked inspiratory dyspnoea. The skin of the entire body, especially the face, becomes highly hyperemic, and all over the skin of the body there appear numerous very itching wheals, 1 to 2 cm large, which show a marked tendency to confluence. Increased perspiration has not been noted. After about 2 hours heavy salivation starts and is followed by vomiting, after which the symptoms very gradually fade away. Temperature, cardiac and renal function have always been normal. After 10 or 12 hours all the symptoms have disappeared; only a feeling of debility persists for a day or so. After each attack there is a period of oliguria and constipation; this may be due to dehydration and vomiting.

Circulatory shock with dizziness and faintness may be the only manifestation, but collapse, unconsciousness, and death can occur within 16 to 120 min. There is obstruction and edema of the upper respiratory tract, laryngeal edema, and increased eosinophils in sinusoids of spleen and liver.

Acute systemic anaphylaxis in humans is often iatrogenic, i.e., produced by injection of drugs (penicillin) or biologics (gamma globulin), but can occur naturally after insect (bee, wasp) stings.

Idiopathic Anaphylaxis

Idiopathic anaphylaxis refers to acute systemic anaphylaxis not caused by any identifiable external antigen. Treatment requires prednisone, β-agonists, and H_1 blockers, but is not always successful. The mechanism is not clear, but it is important that this form of anaphylaxis be recognized clinically so that treatment may be effected.

Atopic Allergy

Atopic allergy is a term applied to a group of chronic human allergies to natural antigens, including asthma, hay fever, allergic rhinitis, urticaria (hives), eczema, serous otitis media, conjunctivitis, and chronic food allergy. The mechanisms are essentially the same as those involved in systemic and cutaneous anaphylaxis. Anaphylaxis is included by many under the general term of atopy.

The general clinical features of atopic allergy are itching and whealing, sneezing, and respiratory embarrassment. The pathologic features include edema, smooth muscle contraction, and leukopenia. The pharmacologic characteristics are repeated episodes of histamine release and partial protection by antihistamines as well as involvement of leukotrienes and prostaglandins. The type of reaction seen clinically depends upon four factors, described below.

Route of Access of Antigen

If contact occurs via the skin, hives (wheal and flare) predominate; if contact is via respiratory mucous membranes, asthma and rhinitis occur; if contact occurs via the eyes, conjunctivitis will predominate, or if through the ears, serous otitis; if contact occurs via the gastrointestinal tract, food allergy, with cramps, nausea, vomiting and diarrhea, results.

Dose of Antigen

The rarity of death from most atopic allergies, in contrast to anaphylaxis, is most likely because of the dose and route of access of the antigen. In systemic anaphylaxis, inadvertently large doses of antigen are usually given intravenously; in atopic allergy, the doses are low and contact is across mucous membranes. Such a conclusion is justified by the observation that anaphylactically sensitized guinea pigs exposed to small amounts of antigen by inhalation develop typical asthmatic symptoms. However, in highly sensitive individuals, minute doses of allergen may elicit fatal reactions, and in sensitized individuals injected with relatively large doses of allergen in the form of drugs, severe, sometimes fatal, anaphylactic reactions may occur.

"The Shock Organ"

Individual differences in reactivity depend upon individual idiosyncrasy, pharmacologic abnormality of the target tissue (increased numbers of mast cells or increased H receptors on target organs), or increased susceptibility of a given organ because of nonspecific irritation or inflammation. Many affected individuals commonly have an atopic reaction involving one organ system (asthma) without involvement of other organs.

Familial Susceptibility (Genetics)

One of the most fascinating questions about atopic diseases is why some individuals make an IgE response to the same antigen to which other individuals make an IgG response or no response. While some of the differences may be explained by dose, route, and number of exposures, there has long been evidence that heredity plays a major role. In 1872, Wyman reported that allergies were higher in family members than in nonallergic families, but that the expression of the allergy could differ, e.g., asthma or allergic rhinitis. Later, it was concluded that children inherit an "allergic predisposition" about equally from both parents and that the prevalence of an allergic family history is about three times greater in allergic patients than history of a nonallergic family.

Exposure is also critical. If a genetically allergy-predisposed individual is not exposed to a given allergen, or a cross-reacting allergen, then the allergy will never become manifested. For instance, in primitive villages of Papua New Guinea, a marked increase in mite allergy (asthma) correlated with the introduction of blankets, which become infested with mites. Before this, mite allergy was not seen in this population.

The genetic regulation of atopic responses may involve at least three major mechanisms: (i) specific IgE antibody HLA-related immune response control, (ii) non-HLA-linked overall IgE synthesis regulation, and (iii) genetic control of factors that regulate end-organ (bronchial) responsiveness. It is well known that control of specific immune responses is HLA-linked. For example, individuals of HLA type DW2 tend to form IgE antibodies to ragweed pollen extract. However, a clear relationship between the propensity to form allergic responses and HLA phenotype has not been confirmed.

Overall IgE levels also appear to be genetically controlled, but this control is not linked to HLA. The serum IgE concentrations of pairs of monozygotic twins are significantly more similar to each other than are the levels of otherwise comparable pairs of dizygotic twins. In addition, the concept of genetic control of basal IgE levels in humans is supported by statistical analysis of serum IgE levels in normal adults. It is possible, although not yet established, that genetic control of the immune responses by immune response genes may extend to the IgE immunoglobulin class; certain individuals inherit genes that select an IgE antibody response to a given antigen rather than a response with another immunoglobulin class. Elevated serum IgE levels during the first year of life frequently occur in infants who develop atopic disease later, suggesting the early expression of a genetically controlled propensity of atopic individuals to produce IgE immunoglobulin.

The compounding variables of genetic control of mast cell numbers, mast cell distribution in tissues, and mediator release illustrate the multifactorial nature of the genetics of allergic reactions. In addition, it appears that late T-cell-dependent asthmatic reactions may be HLA-linked but separate from early IgE-mediated reactions.

Asthma

The word *asthma* is derived from a Greek word meaning panting, a general term for difficulty in breathing. The problem was believed by Galen to be caused by secretions dripping from the brain into the lung: "phlegm doth fall upon the lung." This, as well as other errors of Galen's concepts, was not disproved until the 17th century. Clinically, asthma must be differentiated from chronic bronchitis and emphysema. Asthma presents clinically as reversible acute respiratory distress from airway obstruction. Osler described presentation "with a distressing sense of want of breath and a feeling of great oppression of the chest. Soon the respiratory efforts become violent, and all of the accessory muscles are brought into play. In a few minutes the patient is in a paroxysm of the most intense dyspnea." After a gradual decline, the incidence of mortality due to asthma has been increasing since the mid-1980s. The reason for this increase is not clear. Some factors considered are air pollution or indoor living related to urban environment, overuse of β_2-agonists (see below), and changed therapy. Airway obstruction is a complex event due to constriction of the smooth muscles of the small bronchi (bronchospasm), inflammation, and mucus secretion. Chronic inflammation not only contributes to airflow obstruction, but also to bronchial hyperresponsiveness to allergens.

Predisposing Factors

A number of factors predispose to development of allergic asthma, the most important being repeated exposure to the allergen. Other correlations with an allergic proclivity are listed in Table 11.4. There are at least two forms of asthma: one clearly mediated by the anaphylactic mechanism and one that is not mediated by known immune reactions. The immune (allergic) mediated form is caused by the activation of effector cells (mast cells) sensitized by IgE antibody. Allergic asthma is termed extrinsic because of the clear identification of an exogenous eliciting antigen in most cases. The mechanism of activation of the nonallergic form of asthma is not well understood but is probably due to an imbalance of the physiologic control of smooth muscle tone (see below). Immune mechanisms are not believed to be involved, and a specific eliciting antigen cannot be identified. Drugs that block β-adrenergic effects used for treatment of angina pectoris, cardiac arrhythmias, hypertension, glaucoma, migraine headache, and other diseases are contraindicated in patients with bronchial asthma.

Table 11.4 Factors believed to predispose to development of allergic disease[a]

1. Heredity: positive family history (HLA-DW2)
2. Prenatal effects (high cord blood IgE levels, prenatal exposure to allergens)
3. High postnatal IgE serum level
4. Birth during pollen season
5. Birth in urban environment
6. Stressful perinatal period
7. Early diet, early exposure to eggs, wheat, and bovine products (cow's milk versus breast feeding)
8. Low serum IgA levels at 3 months of age
9. Low levels of T lymphocytes at 3 months of age
10. Early surgery or hospitalization
11. Exposure to animals, molds, tobacco smoke, and pollen
12. Primarily indoor living
13. Frequent infections

[a]Items 4, 5, 6, and 10 are questionable. Table modified from D. E. Johnston, *Ann. Allergy* **49**:257, 1982.

Intrinsic Asthma

Intrinsic asthma presents as chronic recurrent asthma attacks without a clearly identifiable exposure to an antigen. This may be because the antigen is just not detectable or because there is no antigen (nonimmune asthma). One possible explanation is that intrinsic asthma is caused by sensitivity to a chronic infecting organism, but proof of this hypothesis is lacking. Allergic asthma is usually seasonal, although it is year-round in parts of the world where pollen allergens are present for most of the year (e.g., Bermuda grass pollen in southern California) or if nonpollen allergens such as animal dander are responsible. Occasional outbreaks of asthma may be associated with the sudden release of an allergen. Since 1981, 26 outbreaks of asthma have occurred in Barcelona, Spain, affecting 687 persons. The outbreaks have been traced to inhalation of soybean dust released during the unloading of soybeans at the city harbor. In contrast, intrinsic asthma occurs throughout the year without seasonal exception. A condition of intrinsic asthma may evolve from a background of seasonal asthma or from a nonatopic background of chronic bronchitis. In addition, a wide variety of agents have been identified as causing work-related asthma in selected populations (Table 11.5). For example, isocyanates, such as toluene diisocyanate used as an industrial solvent, may be the principal cause of occupational asthma in the Western world. IgE antibody has been detected in some affected workers. An increasing problem for medical workers is allergic reactions to latex resulting from increased use of latex gloves for protection against human immunodeficiency virus transmission.

Nonimmune Asthma

Constriction of bronchial smooth muscle may be triggered by a variety of nonimmune mechanisms, including chemical irritation, change in temperature, physical activity, and emotional stress, as well as by a variety of respiratory infections. In cases of nonimmune asthma, no exogenous eliciting antigen can be identified, and no IgE antibodies can be demonstrated. Mast cells have receptors for adenosine, and it is possible that adenosine released from metabolically active cells causes mast cell degranulation as well as direct bronchoconstriction. Chronic hyperreactivity may also result from a modification of the reactivity of the bronchial epithelium secondary to air pollutants, viral infections, or chronic exposure to allergens. The level of nitric oxide in the exhaled air may be used as a measure of the degree of chronic inflammation in the lung.

One form of nonimmune asthma is caused by exposure to aspirin and other nonsteroidal anti-inflammatory agents through blocking of the cyclooxygenase pathway for metabolism of arachidonic acid and increased production of leukotrienes, which cause chronic airway inflammation and bronchial constriction. As stated above, it is believed that chronic inflammation with infiltration of the bronchial mucosa with inflammatory cells and hyperplasia of bronchial smooth muscle leads to a lowering of the threshold for a bronchospastic response to a variety of stimuli.

Pathologic Changes

A number of pathologic changes have been found in the lungs of patients with either type of asthma. In the acute attack, which may be fatal because of acute asphyxiation, there is marked constriction of the bronchi and occlusion of the bronchi with a particularly thick mucus secretion (mucus

Table 11.5 Agents causing asthma in selected occupations[a]

Occupation or occupational field	Agent
Laboratory animal workers, veterinarians	Dander and urine proteins
Food processing	Shellfish, egg proteins, pancreatic enzymes, papain, amylase
Dairy farmers	Storage mites
Poultry farmers	Poultry mites, droppings, and feathers
Granary workers	Storage mites, aspergillus, indoor ragweed, and grass pollen
Research workers	Locusts
Fish food manufacturing	Midges
Detergent manufacturing	*B. subtilis* enzymes
Silk workers	Silkworm moths and larvae
Exposure to plant proteins	
Bakers	Flour amylase
Food processing	Coffee bean dust, meat tenderizer (papain), tea
Farmers	Soybean dust
Shipping workers	Grain dust (molds, insects, grain)
Laxative manufacturing	Ispaghula, psyllium
Sawmill workers, carpenters	Wood dust (western red cedar, oak, mahogany, zebrawood, redwood, Lebanon cedar, African maple, eastern white cedar)
Electric soldering	Colophony (pine resin)
Cotton textile workers	Cotton dust
Nurses	Psyllium, latex
Exposure to inorganic chemicals	
Refinery workers	Platinum salts, vanadium
Plating	Nickel salts
Diamond polishing	Cobalt salts
Manufacturing	Aluminum fluoride
Beauty shop	Persulfate
Welding	Stainless steel fumes, chromium salts
Exposure to organic chemicals	
Manufacturing	Antibiotics, piperazine, methyl dopa, salbutamol, cimetidine
Hospital workers	Disinfectants (sulfathiazole, chlormine, formaldehyde, glutaraldehyde)
Anesthesiology	Enflurane
Poultry workers	Aprolium
Fur dyeing	Paraphenylene diamine
Rubber processing	Formaldehyde, ethylene diamine, phthalic anhydride
Plastics industry	Toluene diisocyanate, hexamethyl diisocyanate, dephenylmethyl isocyanate, phthalic anhydride, triethylene tetramines, trimellitic anhydride, hexamethyl tetramine
Automobile painting	Dimethyl ethanolamine diisocyanate
Foundry workers	Reaction product of furan binder

[a]From *International Consensus Report on Diagnosis and Management of Asthma* (National Heart, Lung, and Blood Institute, Bethesda, Md. [National Institutes of Health publication no. 92-3091], 1992).

plugs). In chronic asthma, the pulmonary changes are (i) marked thickening of the basement membrane of the bronchial mucosa, (ii) hypertrophy of the bronchial smooth muscle, (iii) hypertrophy of the bronchial mucous glands, (iv) eosinophils, chronic inflammatory cells in the bronchial wall with a substantial increase over normal in the number of mast cells, and (v) the presence of mucus in the bronchi containing large numbers of eosinophilic leukocytes. In addition, T cells are prominent in the lung of chronic asthmatics. The thickened basement membrane may contain deposits of IgG or IgM, but IgE has not been detected often. Eosinophil degranulation may contribute to epithelial desquamation. Repairing epithelium has the potential to contribute to disease chronicity through production of inflammatory mediators and adhesion molecules. Other stigmata of chronic inflammation and airway obstruction not specific for asthma, including focal fibrosis and scarring, emphysema, and atelectasis, may be found in the periphery of the lung. In experimental models, repeated inhalation of antigens by sensitized animals leads to pathologic changes similar to asthma and bronchial hyperresponsiveness to acetylcholine. Since repeated asthma attacks are also associated with increased susceptibility to pulmonary infections, some of the pathologic changes may be due to repeated bronchopneumonia. Mild asthmatics have histologic changes similar to those with severe asthma but to a lesser degree. It is now possible to follow patients with mild asthma using endobronchial biopsies and monitor the degree of inflammation. Severe asthma correlates with an increase in the number of activated IL-5-positive lymphocytes, not the number of eosinophils or mast cells. If inflammation persists, treatment with anti-inflammatory drugs may be warranted even though there are no immediate symptoms.

Therapy

The increasing incidence of asthma has stimulated the formation of an international asthma management committee, which has recommended a six-part program treatment:

1. Educate the patient to develop a partnership in asthma management.
2. Assess and monitor asthma severity with objective measures of lung function.
3. Avoid or control asthma triggers.
4. Establish medication plans for chronic management.
5. Establish plans for managing exacerbations.
6. Provide regular follow-up care.

This therapy program emphasizes three critical aspects of asthma: first, determining the extent of the disease and the motivation of the patient to control the manifestations; second, attempting to limit predisposing inflammation; and third, identifying the specific allergen.

Specific therapy for asthma depends on whether or not a specific eliciting antigen can be identified. If it can, the best treatment is avoidance of the antigen. Immunotherapy by injection of the antigen in a manner that will change the reactivity of the patient may also be successful. Drugs that produce bronchodilation or that alter the state of activation of effector mast cells may be effective in both extrinsic and intrinsic allergy, and prompt administration by aerosol or injection may be required to prevent death in an acute attack. Inhibition of production of leukotrienes by 5-lipoxygenase inhibitors, such as A64077, may decrease airway hyperresponsiveness that predisposes to asthma attacks. Psychotherapy may be effective in some cases, because the extent of a given attack may be increased by anxiety; the frequency of asthma is higher for individuals in emotional distress. Breathing exercises may reduce symptoms, especially in growing children. Intermittent short-term steroid therapy (up to 7 days) will produce dramatic relief of severe asthmatic symptoms (see below). On the other hand, long-term steroid administration may lead to secondary adrenal insufficiency, which at times of stress may be fatal in patients with otherwise severe but controlled asthma. In addition, all antiasthmatic medications have the potential to produce life-threatening reactions. For instance, aerosol bronchodilators (primarily β_2-adrenergic agonists) and theophylline together may produce significant cardiovascular effects. A more comprehensive discussion of the prevention and treatment of allergic reactions is presented below.

The following is recommended by the *International Consensus Report on Diagnosis and Management of Asthma* (National Institutes of Health publication no. 92-3091, 1992):

1. Mild asthma: Inhalant β_2-agonist as needed, oral cromolyn
2. Moderate asthma: Add anti-inflammatory agents (e.g., nedocromil), inhalant low-dose steroid as required, theophylline if needed
3. Severe asthma: High-dose steroids

Atopic Reactions

Hay Fever (Seasonal Allergic Rhinitis)

Seasonal upper respiratory reactions to pollen are commonly referred to as hay fever. Nonseasonal "perennial" allergic rhinitis is caused by animal danders, house dust, house dust mites, and molds that cause a reaction in the nasal passages and eyes of affected individuals. In temperate climates, seasonal allergic rhinitis is caused by nonflowering, wind-pollinated plants. Larger pollen particles (>10 μm) are efficiently filtered out by the nasal mucosa and cause rhinitis, whereas smaller particles, less than 1 to 2 μm, pass into the tracheobronchial tree and cause asthma. Hay fever symptoms include sneezing, nasal congestion, watery discharge from the eye, conjunctival itching, and cough with mild bronchoconstriction. Similar symptoms may be exhibited by *vasomotor rhinitis,* caused by parasympathetic hyperactivity, a foreign body, and infection—in particular, the common cold. The diagnosis is usually made by history of nasal itching, sneezing, nasal discharge, and difficulty breathing, particularly during the pollen season. A calendar of some common airborne allergens is shown in Table 11.6.

Examination of an allergic rhinitis patient, particularly a child, may reveal a transverse wrinkle across the middle of the nose caused by the *allergic salute.* The allergic salute is delivered by placing the palm of the hand against the tip of the nose and pushing up. This is done to relieve the obstruction to the nasal air passages caused by swollen nasal mucosae.

Table 11.6 Calendar of some common airborne allergens in a temperate climate (England)[a]

Allergen	February	March	April	May	June	July	August	September
Alder and hazel	---	---	---					
Oak, ash, poplar		---	---	---				
Plane, birch			---	---	---			
Mixed grasses				---	---	---	---	
Nettle					---	---	---	---
Plantain, mugwort						---	---	---
Cladosporium				---	---	---	---	---
Alternaria						---	---	---
Ragweed							---	---

[a]The timing of allergen exposure varies with climate. Table modified from P. H. Howarth, *Respir. Med.* **83**:179, 1989.

Pathologic changes are not extensive. Usually, there is edema of the submucosal tissue with an infiltration of eosinophils that is reversible. The degree of reaction and severity of symptoms are directly related to the amount of exposure to the allergen responsible. The lesion is caused by release of mediators from mast cells in the nasal mucosa—histamine, serotonin, eosinophil and neutrophil chemotactic factors, and mast cell proteases—as well as newly formed, membrane-derived lipid mediators such as prostaglandin D_2 and other arachidonic acid metabolites (Table 11.7). These mediators produce vasodilation, mucosal edema, mucus secretion, stimulation of itch receptors, and reduction in the threshold for sneezing. The most effective approach to prevent allergic rhinitis is avoidance of the allergen, if possible. Repeated episodes of rhinitis lead to increased numbers of mast cells in the nasal mucosa and establishment of a state of nasal hyperresponsiveness to provoking stimuli. Treatment consists of antihistamines, H_1 receptor blockers (e.g., astemizole), adrenergic drugs that produce vasoconstriction (xylometazoline or oxymetazoline), disodium cromoglycate (reduces mast cell mediator release), and topical glucocorticoids administered by aerosol (beclomethasone, flunisolide, etc.). Steroids may take several days or a week to produce effects but are usually more effective than disodium cromoglycate or antihistamines. Specific immunotherapy (see below) may be effective if the allergen has been identified and is available but is usually reserved for those patients whose symptoms are poorly controlled by optimal medical management. Psychological factors may determine the degree of discomfort considerably. Hay fever may progress to asthma, but usually the severity of symptoms gradually diminishes with aging.

Nasal Polyps

Nasal polyps are tumorlike masses that form in the nasal air passages, causing chronic airway obstruction and rendering nasal breathing difficult or impossible. These masses can be removed surgically but usually recur promptly. The relationship between nasal polyps and allergic rhinitis is uncertain; they are frequently found in patients with perennial rhinitis. There is some evidence that chronic rhinitis and sinusitis, as well as polyps, may be caused by bacterial allergy. Nasal polyps characteristically show marked edema, swelling of hydrophilic ground substance, and scattered eosinophilic infiltration. Eosinophilic PMNs are associated with se-

Table 11.7 Mediators and symptoms of allergic rhinitis[a]

Symptom	Pathology	Proposed mediators[b]
Pruritus	Sensory nerve stimulation	Histamine (H_1), prostaglandins
Obstruction	Mucosal edema due to vascular permeability and vasodilation	Histamine (H_1), kinins, LTC_4, LTD_4, LTE_4, TNF-α, neuropeptides (calcitonin gene-related peptide; substance P)
Sneezing	Sensory nerve stimulation	Histamine (H_1), LTC_4, LTD_4, LTE_4
Rhinorrhea	Mucus secretion	Histamine (muscarinic reflex), LTC_4, LTD_4, LTE_4, substance P, vasoactive intestinal polypeptide
Hyperactivity and prolonged congestion	Late-phase reaction	Cytokines (IL-1, IL-5, IL-6, IL-8, and TNF-α), eicosanoids

[a]Modified from M. V. White, and M. A. Kaliner, *J. Allerg. Clin. Immunol.* **90:**699–704, 1992.
[b]Abbreviations: LTC, leukotriene C; LTD, leukotriene D; LTE, leukotriene E; IL, interleukin; TNF, tumor necrosis factor.

vere persistent allergic rhinitis, and it has been suggested that persistent contact with small amounts of antigen leads to the characteristic picture. The prolonged nature of the swelling may be explained by continued production of hydrophilic ground substance by tissue fibroblasts.

Food Allergy

Ingestion of allergens may lead to remarkable gastrointestinal reactions known collectively as food allergy. The relationship of the gastrointestinal reaction to atopic sensitivity is not clear. Many individuals with positive skin reactions to an allergen do react to ingestion of the allergen, whereas individuals with repeated episodes of vomiting or diarrhea that occur on eating a given food may not produce a skin reaction to the food. Food allergens are most likely to be those that survive the process of digestion (Table 11.8) or to drugs added to foods as preservatives. Allergy to cow's milk is the most frequently suspected gastrointestinal reaction to food in infants. Milk contains over 16 proteins that might be allergenic, and skin reactions to a number of these proteins occur in some sensitive children. It is thought that intact milk proteins are more likely to be absorbed through the child's intestine than the adult's. In addition, unsuspected bovine food additives, such as penicillin, may be present in milk and elicit allergic reactions. Food allergy may lead to hypoproteinemia from the loss of protein in the gastrointestinal tract and persistent diarrhea. Other manifestations of food allergy are extensive skin eruptions (urticaria or eczema) or systemic shock. Avoidance of the allergen is the primary therapy, and artificial diets are sometimes required to prevent food allergy reactions. Individuals with known severe food allergy should carry epinephrine and be instructed on how to use it if an anaphylactic attack is imminent. It has been recognized for many years that breast feeding results in a dramatic reduction in the incidence of food allergy in children, in particular, of allergic eczema.

Insect Allergy

Atopic or anaphylactic reactions to insects may be divided into three groups: inhalant or contact reactions to insect body parts or products, skin reactions (wheal and flare) to biting insects, and systemic shock reactions to stinging insects. Asthmatic or hay fever-like reactions may occur after airborne exposure of a sensitive individual to large numbers of insects or their body parts. This happens outdoors with insects that periodically appear in large numbers, such as locusts or grasshoppers, and indoors, more chronically, with beetles, flies, and spiders. IgE antibody in individuals with insect allergy reacts most frequently with gastrointestinal epithelium.

Table 11.8 Some purified water-soluble food antigens[a]

Allergen	Source	Mol wt	Composition	Characteristics
Antigen M	Codfish	12,328	113 amino acids to 1 glucose	A parvalbulin, chelates calcium, acid and protease resistant
Antigen II	Shrimp	38,000	96% protein	Heat stable
Peanut I	Peanut		91% protein	Acid and protease resistant
Trypsin inhibitor	Soybean	20,500	Polypeptide	Acid and protease resistant

[a]Modified from D. D. Metcalfe, M. Sampter, and J. J. Condemi, p. 1165, *in* M. Sampter et al., ed., *Immunological Diseases,* Little, Brown & Co., Boston, Mass., 1988.

Bites

Biting insects may produce delayed-type hypersensitivity or acute wheal-and-flare skin reactions. A delayed reaction to insect bite may convert to an anaphylactic one with aging of the individual. The common reaction to a mosquito or flea bite is a localized cutaneous anaphylactic reaction. Although allergy may play a role, it is thought that local release of histamine triggered by the bite is the cause of such reactions. Delayed-type hypersensitivity reactions to mosquito bites may also occur. Serious effects of a reaction to biting insects occur in parts of the world where large numbers of mosquitoes appear in waves; multiple mosquito bites to a sensitive individual may produce systemic effects.

Stings

Fatalities occur more frequently from stinging insects, such as bees and wasps. More people die each year as a result of being stung by an insect than from being bitten by a snake—about 40 documented deaths in the United States per year. This is expected to increase with the influx of Africanized honeybees. Deaths from stinging insects are caused by systemic anaphylaxis and usually occur within 1 h of being stung. Therefore, immediate therapy is required. This may be provided by injection of epinephrine (see below). Immunotherapy may prevent subsequent severe reactions. People who raise bees may permit a bee to sting them and limit the amount of venom injected; by increasing the amount on subsequent stings, the degree of reaction to a larger dose becomes less. The amount of protein material injected in a sting is actually very small—about 50 μg for a honeybee and 2 to 20 μg for a wasp.

The venom of honeybees and wasps contains a number of biologically active agents, such as histamine, serotonin, and other biologic amines that directly produce vascular reactions, as well as phospholipase, hyaluronidase, and acid phosphatase. The peptides include melittin, which has a unique amipathic structure that incorporates into biomembranes; apamin, which blocks Ca^{2+}-dependent ion channels; and mast cell degranulating peptide, which causes release of histamine. The main ingredient of fire ant venom is phospholipase. Thus, the venom itself produces a marked acute and delayed inflammatory reaction that may be magnified by an allergic reaction to the venom. Most of the insect venom allergens are proteins of 20 to 50 kDa and cross-react with similar proteins of other species (Table 11.9). It is possible that some susceptible people are sensitized to cross-reacting antigens and then react to minute doses of these antigens in insect venom.

Table 11.9 Some arthropod allergens and common proteins of known sequence similarity or antigen cross-reactivity[a]

Venom allergen	Other protein(s)
Honeybee phospholipase A_2	Bovine, porcine, and human pancreatic phospholipase A_2
Honeybee venom melittin	Calmodulin-binding protein, phospholipase A_2-stimulating protein
Hornet venom antigen 5	Tobacco and tomato leaf pathogenesis-related protein
Major mite antigen	Human cathepsin B and other cysteine proteases
Midge antigen	Human hemoglobin alpha chain

[a]Modified from T. P. King, *Monogr. Allergy* **28:**84, 1990.

Protective Role of Anaphylactic Reactions to Insects

It is not clear what survival advantage these acute allergic reactions to insect bites and stings provide. It has been postulated that the reaction induces immediate avoidance behavior and may limit the exposure of a bitten individual to a dose of a toxic venom that could be even more damaging. On the other hand, a systemic anaphylactic reaction to an insect sting may be interpreted as an immune mechanism that should be protective but is instead deleterious and potentially fatal.

Atopic Eczema-Atopic Dermatitis

In 1892, Brocq and Besnier described a familial, pruritic skin disease beginning in infancy and often occurring in association with hay fever and asthma. The term *atopic dermatitis* was coined by Wise and Sulzberger in 1933. Eczema refers to the weeping phase of early lesions, and dermatitis refers to the more chronic dry, hyperkeratotic lesions. Atopic dermatitis is a chronic skin eruption of varied etiology that usually occurs in young individuals who develop atopic reactions (asthma or hay fever) at a later age. In children, the typical lesions are located in the antecubital and popliteal areas with variable involvement of the neck, wrist, and ankles. The pathologic changes in the skin are consistent with those of a severe contact dermatitis. Erythema, papules, and vesicles are accompanied by intense pruritus. There is perivascular accumulation of mononuclear cells followed by infiltration into the epidermis with epidermal spongiosis. As the affected child becomes older, thickening of the skin of the affected areas occurs (lichenification). Atopic dermatitis features thickened patches with frequent, acute itching episodes. Identification of an antigen that elicits the eczema is very difficult, but in some cases there is evidence that the antigens are those that also elicit other allergic reactions (pollen, house dust, animal dander). Atopic eczema is morphologically more like a reaction of cellular or delayed-type hypersensitivity but is discussed here because of its association with atopic conditions.

The pathogenic mechanism of atopic dermatitis remains unclear. Patients with atopic dermatitis will produce wheal-and-flare reactions when challenged with allergen and this reactivity is IgE-mediated. On the other hand, cutaneous antigen exposure does not elicit the skin lesion characteristic of atopic dermatitis. Atopic dermatitis patients frequently have increased delayed-type hypersensitivity skin reactivity and decreased in vitro blast transformation responses to various test antigens; thus, it has been suggested that atopic dermatitis is caused by immune deviation from delayed-type hypersensitivity to IgE production. The role of certain food allergies in accentuation of severe eczema has been found in double-blinded food challenges.

An allergic etiology of all eczema must be questioned, because typical eczema may occur in children with severe combined immune deficiency. Therefore, although proven eczema of atopic allergic origin exists, eczema-like (eczematoid) skin lesions may be produced in other ways. Abnormalities in the activation, production, or inactivation of arachidonic acid metabolites have been considered as possibilities.

Aspirin Intolerance

Aspirin, one of the world's most widely used drugs, was once generally thought to be almost completely devoid of undesirable effects when used within a therapeutic dose range. However, aspirin is now known to be responsible for a variety of atopic and anaphylactic reactions, including asthma, rhinitis, nasal polyps, and even anaphylactic shock. Aspirin intolerance may develop in children or appear in adults with no previous history of atopy. In adults, the symptoms of aspirin intolerance appear suddenly with a watery rhinorrhea followed by development of nasal polyps, chronic asthma, and in some cases even shock reactions to ingestion of aspirin. The chronic asthma related to aspirin intolerance responds well to drug therapy, but, of course, avoidance of aspirin is the obvious treatment. This is easier said than done, because aspirin is included in many drug mixtures, where it is unsuspected, and other cross-reacting haptens may elicit reactions in aspirin-sensitive individuals. Yellow food color number 5 contains such a related hapten. Desensitization to aspirin intolerance can be obtained by giving small doses of aspirin until symptoms disappear and then increasing dosage. This happens in all aspirin-sensitive individuals but is reversible and must be maintained by daily aspirin treatment.

Aspirin and widely different nonsteroidal anti-inflammatory drugs act through a common pharmacologic mechanism, i.e., inhibition of cyclooxygenase, and the dose of drug required to elicit sensitivity is directly related to its ability to cause this inhibition. The present hypotheses regarding the mechanism of aspirin sensitivity are based on this action. One idea is that these drugs produce a relative deficiency in cyclooxygenase products, so that prostaglandin E_2 (a bronchodilator) is produced relatively less than prostaglandin $F_{2\alpha}$ (a bronchoconstrictor). Although such an imbalance in effect has not been demonstrated with aspirin treatment, this idea is supported by the observation that inhibition of thromboxane synthase, which does not decrease prostaglandin E_2 synthesis, does not induce asthma in aspirin-sensitive individuals. Another idea is that inhibition of the cyclooxygenase pathway diverts arachidonic acid metabolism to the 5-lipoxygenase pathway and production of bronchoconstrictive leukotrienes. This mechanism does not explain why aspirin sensitivity is limited to a subpopulation of asthmatic patients. Although an accepted mechanism has not yet been found, it appears likely that some individuals have an increased sensitivity to inhibition of cyclooxygenase, perhaps because of inflammation of the bronchi such as that caused by a virus infection, that predisposes them to aspirin sensitivity. Further understanding of the interaction of cyclooxygenase inhibition and inflammatory cells, such as platelets, mast cells, and eosinophils, may provide a better explanation of the mechanism of aspirin intolerance than is now available.

Urticaria and Angioedema

Urticaria is a condition of red or pale, itchy edematous swellings of the skin (hives), usually short-lived; angioedema is a more extensive swelling of the subcutaneous tissues and mucous membranes. Urticaria and angioedema may coexist and are believed to have similar mechanisms. The types of urticaria and angioedema may be arbitrarily classified into physical (see anaphylactoid reactions below), immunological, hereditary, and idiopathic. Urticaria (hives) is usually due to release of mediators from mast cells as a result of allergen reacting with IgE-bound antibody, by bites of insects, by physical trauma (dermatographia), by exercise, heat, cold, sunlight, etc. Angioedema is a diffuse pale swelling of the skin or mucous membrane that may be associated with other forms of allergic reactions. Some of the more common physically induced urticarial and angioedema reactions are listed in Table 11.10. In some cases, these reactions are caused by physical stimulation inducing antigens that react with IgE; in others, there is an increased number or sensitivity of mast cells or increased parasympathetic stimulation; in others, the etiology is not immunological or is unknown. Recent evidence indicates that up to 50% of patients with chronic urticaria may have autoantibodies to the high-affinity IgE receptor on mast cells.

Anaphylactoid Reactions

Any event causing histamine release may cause atopic symptoms that can be confused with a true allergic reaction. Anaphylactoid shock is produced in normal (nonimmune) animals by injection of a variety of agents capable of releasing histamine or activating arachidonic acid metabolism without the mediation of an antigen-antibody reaction. The resulting clinical, physiologic, and pathologic picture is virtually indistinguishable from true anaphylaxis but is not produced by immune reaction. Physical agents (heat or cold), trauma (dermatographia), emotional disturbances, or exercise may evoke pharmacologic mechanisms that mimic allergic reactions. However, there is increasingly convincing evidence that most of these reactions are IgE-mediated.

Dermatographia literally means "writing on the skin." Stroking the skin results in whealing at the contact points of the stroke. Pressure urticaria is closely related. Swelling may occur at the wrists or ankles if tight clothing is worn, or over the buttocks if the individual sits for long periods of time. Dermatographia and pressure urticaria may be caused by the release of anaphylactic mediators from mast cells by a degree of physical trauma that does not induce a reaction in normal individuals. In at least 50% of cases, passive-transfer studies have demonstrated an IgE-dependent mechanism. However, such a reaction may confuse the results of skin testing, because a wheal may result from insertion of a needle alone.

Table 11.10 Major urticarial and angioedematous reactions induced by physical stimuli

Physical agent	Immunological findings	Pathophysiology
Cold		
Idiopathic	IgE-dependent passive transfer, cold-induced skin antigen?, IgG, IgM, auto-anti-IgE	Histamine, prostaglandin G_2, cytophilic factors, edema, urticaria
Cryoprotein	Cold-dependent autoantibodies	Anaphylatoxin, vasculitis, edema
Others	None consistent	Histamine, edema
Exercise		
Urticaria	Increased acetylcholine receptors (cholinergic)	Parasympathetic activation of cholinergic nerves, histamine, etc.
Anaphylaxis	?Food allergy	Increased lung mast cells, histamine
Heat	?Heat-induced autoantigen	Histamine, urticaria, cytophilic
Pressure		
Dermatographia	50% IgE-dependent	Histamine, increased mast cells
Delayed	None	Histamine, kinins, vasculitis
Solar	IgE-transferable, non-IgE complement activation	Sun-activated antigen?, histamine, porphyrin photosensitization

In some patients, a reaction to a physical agent may actually have an immune basis. A physical agent may cause release or production of altered tissue antigens to which a patient is sensitive. The reaction of idiopathic cold urticaria may be transferred with IgE from many patients, and it is possible that this reaction is caused by reaction of an IgE autoantibody to a cold-dependent skin antigen. Reactions to light (photoallergy) may be caused by agents activated by sunlight that are applied to the skin to form haptens. Such reactions are usually contact dermatitis reactions (see chapter 12). Cholinergic urticaria is believed to be produced by an abnormal response to acetylcholine released from efferent nerves after emotional stress, physical activity, or trauma. Cholinesterase levels of the skin may be reduced in cholinergic urticaria, leading to prolonged survival of acetylcholine that may act to release histamine from tissue mast cells. These anaphylactoid reactions may be mediated by nonimmunologic mediator release, an imbalance of the sympathetic nervous system or hyperreactivity of end-organ smooth muscles.

Hereditary Angioedema

Hereditary angioedema is a specific form of angioedema, first reported in 1882, that involves a defect in the ability to inactivate the first component of complement. Massive swellings may involve the eyelids, lips, tongue, and areas of the trunk. Involvement of the gastrointestinal tract may produce symptoms of acute abdominal distress, but the symptoms almost always disappear in a few days without surgical intervention. Sonography reveals marked mucosal thickening and edema of the bowel and may be useful in preventing unnecessary surgery. The most significant life-threatening complication is severe pharyngeal involvement, which may lead to asphyxia. The pathologic alteration is firm, nonpitting edema of the dermis and subcutaneous tissue, which can be differentiated from a wheal-and flare reaction by the absence of erythema. In addition, antihistamines have no effect upon hereditary angioedema, and the lesions cause a burning or stinging sensation rather than itching.

Angioedema is inherited as an autosomal dominant trait. Biochemically, there is a deficiency of C1 esterase inhibitor (C1-INH), or C1-INH esterase inhibitor is present in an inactive form. C1 esterase is the active form of the first component of complement. If normal serum is incubated at 37°C, there is a gradual "spontaneous" loss of complement activity. In patients with angioedema, this spontaneous decrease may not occur because of a lack of C1-INH. During attacks, the C4 and C2 levels in the serum are decreased, indicating that activation of the complement system is important in this phenomenon. The injection of C1 esterase into the skin of normal individuals produces a wheal-and-flare reaction, but the injection of C1 esterase into the skin of patients with angioedema produces a firm, nonpitting induration with no flare (localized angioedema). Production of the lesions of angioedema must involve factors other than lack of C1-INH. C1-INH is a γ_2 neuroaminoglycoprotein that is a serine esterase inhibitor. It is effective not only on activated C1 but also on plasmin, activated Hageman factor (XIIa), and kallikrein. Thus, interactions of different inflammatory systems due to C1-INH deficiency may be responsible for the clinical picture observed.

It has been claimed that attacks of hereditary angioedema may be terminated by the injection of fresh-frozen plasma from normal individuals, presumably because of the presence of C1-INH in such preparations. However, this observation has not been generally reproducible. Episodes of local angioedema may follow surgical procedures such as dental extractions. It thus becomes important to prevent such attacks. Short-term administration of tranexamic acid does prevent these attacks. It is believed that tranexamic acid may inhibit plasmin-dependent conversion of the product of C1, C4, and C2 interaction to a pathologically active peptide. Androgenic steroids raise the serum level of C1-INH and are used extensively in postpubertal pediatric patients with angioedema. This reversal of C1 esterase serum deficiency by drug therapy suggests a regulatory gene defect.

Acquired Angioedema

Acquired angioedema with C1-INH deficiency is caused by development of antibodies to C1-INH. This is very rare and may be associated with lymphoproliferative diseases.

Angiotensin-Converting Enzyme (ACE) Inhibitor-Associated Angioedema

About 20% of patients with angioedema of the face without urticaria develop angiodema due to treatment with ACE-mediated metabolism of bradykinin. ACE inhibitor is kininase II, which inactivates bradykinin, and high levels of bradykinin have been reported during active attacks. C1-INHs are usually normal in ACE-dependent angioedema, and administration of ACE inhibitor to C1-INH-deficient patients may exacerbate angioedema. ACE inhibitors appear to facilitate angioedema in predisposed subjects, rather than causing it.

Immunotherapeutic Modification of Atopic Allergy

Atopic or anaphylactic conditions may be treated by injecting small amounts of the offending allergen and increasing the amount of antigen over a protracted period of time. "Desensitization" therapy for hay fever was introduced in England in 1911 by L. Noon. He was following the lead of Louis Pasteur, who had success in "vaccination" against infectious disease. Many farmers in England at that time developed severe reactions to hay during the harvest season and were unable to continue farming. Noon prepared aqueous extracts of hay, "immunized" the affected farmers, and obtained significant beneficial effects. The major factors contributing to successful immunotherapy are the proper antigen and adequate doses of the antigen, as well as the high motivation and enthusiasm for the therapy by the patient. Immunotherapy for ragweed, for example, is now largely successful because there is a known available major antigen (antigen E), an immune response to the antigen can be measured, and the skin tests are reproducible. In the case of asthma, these criteria are difficult to meet, and the efficacy of immunotherapy for asthma is questionable. During the application of inoculation therapy in office practice, frequently not enough of the allergen is given to be effective, but the placebo effect (estimated to be up to 30%) deludes the physician and patient that the low doses of allergen are effective. Controlled clinical trials demonstrate up to 70% effective use with high-dose immunotherapy for required allergy, but only 10 to 20% with low doses (the placebo effect). Effective immunotherapy has been accomplished by using various preparations of plant antigens, insect venoms, cat dander, and, more recently, fire ant toxin, but the proper antigens for immunotherapy of insect or animal dander reactions remain controversial. Purified allergen preparations must be used; "whole-body" insect extracts are not effective. In a long-term study, pharmacotherapy was found to be more effective during the first 2 years, but after 5 years, those who had received immunotherapy had better treatment results.

The mechanism of the beneficial effect of immunotherapy of allergies is not always clear. Possible mechanisms include hyposensitization (blocking), desensitization, tolerance, and suppression (Fig. 11.2).

Hyposensitization

The production of blocking antibody is referred to as hyposensitization. By careful immunization with the offending allergen, it may be possible to induce the formation of nonreaginic, precipitating IgG antibody. Since the precipitation antibody reacts with the same antigen as the reaginic antibody, the precipitating antibody will compete with the reaginic antibody in the reaction with antigen and help prevent atopic symptoms. The formation of precipitating antigen-antibody complexes may also produce tissue changes, but many more molecules of precipitating antibody reacting with antibody are needed to produce a reaction of clinical significance than molecules of reaginic antibody. Such blocking antibody may be demonstrated in vitro by its ability to inhibit the release of anaphylactic mediators from sensitized mast cells upon exposure to antigen, and passive transfer of IgG antibody under controlled conditions reduces anaphy-

Figure 11.2 Immunotherapy of atopic allergies. Immunotherapy of atopic reactions by injection of the specific allergen is known to be effective, particularly for alleviation of the symptoms of hay fever. The mechanism of reduction of allergic symptoms is unclear. At least four possibilities are **(1)** hyposensitization, production of IgG blocking antibody; **(2)** desensitization, consumption of IgE antibody by repeated small doses of allergen; **(3)** tolerance, a loss or significant decrease in IgE antibody production to the allergen; and **(4)** production of suppressor T cells specific for IgE B cells. Another possible mechanism not yet identified as being due to specific immunotherapy is the production of nonspecific IgE that might block the effector cell receptors for IgE allergen-specific antibody.

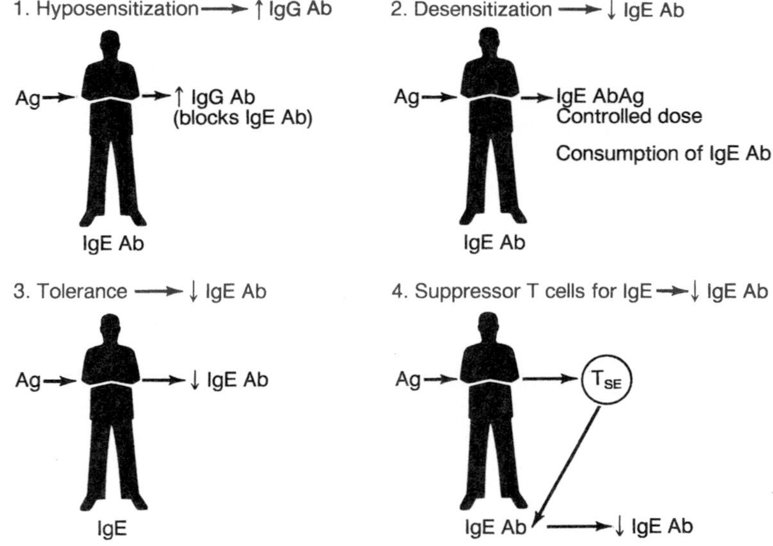

lactic responses to bee venom. However, in some individuals who have had a beneficial response to injection therapy, no blocking antibody is demonstrable. Another possibility is that IgA antibodies in nasal or bronchial secretions may block IgE-mediated reaction, but the small changes in mucosal IgA levels measured do not account for the marked beneficial effect seen. Thus, the decrease in sensitization of many individuals must be due to some other mechanism.

Hyposensitization effect may be explained by changing the balance of Th1 and Th2 responses (see above). Since Th1 responses result in production of complement-fixing IgG antibodies, whereas Th2 responses produce IgE antibodies (as well as IgA and non-complement fixing IgG), hyposensitization may be explained by shifting the balance of cytokines from a Th2 to a Th1 pattern.

Desensitization

Desensitization may be produced by providing enough antigen in small doses to combine with the IgE antibody so that IgE antibody is not available for reactive tissue mast cells. Upon subsequent exposure to allergen, mediator release does not occur. Desensitization may occur with injection therapy for hay fever. Frequently, a series of injections of allergen bind the available antibody as it is produced without producing significant symptoms. With cessation of injections, continued IgE antibody production is able to overcome the antigen and become available for tissue sensitization.

Tolerance

Tolerance may be defined as the specific deletion of responding T or B cells for a given antigen. Specific deletion of responding cells has been difficult to demonstrate. However, it is possible that specific immunotherapy might produce a temporary loss of responsiveness by specific deletion. Experimental studies suggest that such lack of responsiveness is due to the action of T suppressor cells.

Suppression

Suppressor T cells specific for IgE production have been found by several investigators using mouse model systems. In an animal model, $CD3^+$ $T_{\gamma\delta}$ cells have been shown to downregulate IgE responses to inert protein antigen delivered via epithelial surfaces. Suppressor T cells for IgE may be preferentially induced by controlled immunization. Factors selecting for IgE suppressor activity over IgE production include high doses (1 mg versus 1 ng) of allergen, use of particulate antigens such as alum precipitates, conjugation of antigens with polyethylene glycol, intramuscular or intraperitoneal injection of antigens rather than aerosol exposure via mucous membranes, and the use of large carrier antigens such as bacterial or parasitic extracts. Suppressor activity may be demonstrated by passive transfer of T cells from suppressed donors to primed B cells in culture or to syngeneic recipient animals. Suppressor cells may actually turn off ongoing IgE antibody responses. There is evidence that there are separate populations of T-helper cells for different Ig classes of B cells. IgE-specific T-suppressor cells may act on T-helper cells for IgE, IgE B cells, or T-B cell interactions, perhaps by production of a specific suppressor factor. IgE-specific B cells may be more susceptible to T-cell suppression than are IgG-specific B cells. IgE-specific T-suppressor cells appear to control the degree of responsiveness of high and low IgE responder strains of mice, thus providing an explanation for the observation of the role of heredity in determining the class of immunoglobulin response to a given antigen. It is not clear that the same phenomenon is being studied in these experimental systems, because some investigators find that the T-suppressor cells for IgE are antigen-specific, whereas others do not. T cells of humans have type 1 and type 2 histamine receptors. T cells bearing histamine type 2 receptors are activated by reaction with histamine to express suppressor function. This subclass of T cells appears to be lower in allergic individuals than normal, and allergic individuals are less able to generate histamine induced suppressor activity. The role of this activity in controlling allergy is not known.

Increased Serum IgE

The presence of high concentrations of an IgE that does not bind a particular antigen (nonantibody IgE) could saturate mast cell binding sites and prevent the functional sensitization of mast cells by IgE with specific antibody activity. This would be an IgE "blocking" effect, that is, nonantibody IgE blocking IgE antibody. Support for this concept comes from observations that laboratory animals with helminth infections that have high serum IgE concentrations have a decreased incidence of "allergic" reactions. On the other hand, in Venezuela in areas where intestinal helminthiasis is endemic, there is a decreased incidence of allergies in rural populations as compared with urban populations, even though both have elevated serum IgE concentrations as compared with other populations. A final possibility that must be considered is a decrease in the threshold for activation of mast cells or decreased numbers of mast cells in effector organs, such as the bronchial and nasal submucosa, but the evidence for such changes is not consistent. Hyperimmunoglobulin-IgE is a clinical syndrome consisting of an immune deficiency manifested as dermatitis, very high serum levels of IgE, and recurrent staphylococcal infections of the skin and lung, associated with a defect in neutrophil chemotaxis. The role of IgE in this syndrome is not clear, but it is possible that IgE or IgE-immune complexes may affect neutrophil function adversely.

Anti-IgE

In clinical trials, regular injections of humanized monoclonal antibodies to IgE will reduce allergic symptoms. These anti-IgE antibodies are produced by combining the Fab of a mouse monoclonal antibody to human IgE with the Fc portions of human IgG1. These anti-IgE antibodies bind to the Fc regions of IgE and form immune complexes at ratios of two or three molecules of anti-IgE to two or three molecules of IgE. To be effective, these antibodies must (i) have a high affinity for IgE, (ii) not bind to IgE already on the FcεRI receptor on mast cells, and (iii) bind to membrane IgE on B cells. Administration of anti-IgE with these properties will neutralize circulating IgE, will not activate mast cells already sensitized with IgE, and will inhibit production of IgE by B-cells. In addition, the effective anti-IgEs form small soluble immune complexes that do not fix complement and thus do not produce immune complex lesions. On the other hand, the small complexes are not rapidly cleared from the circulation and can still bind to allergens, so they may effectively compete with unbound IgE, which has a much shorter half-life.

Pharmacologic Control of Atopic Reactions

The severity of reaction by an anaphylactically sensitized individual upon exposure to the specific allergen depends not only upon the amount of allergen and reaginic antibody but also upon the reactivity of mast cells, the excitability of the end organ (smooth muscle), and the effect of the autonomic nervous system (Fig. 11.3). Imbalance of these homeostatic control mechanisms explains how exposure to nonimmunologic stimuli, such as heat, cold, physical exercise, or light, may, in some individuals, serve to excite physiologic reactions that mimic allergic reactions (anaphylactoid reactions).

Figure 11.3 Pharmacologic control of atopic-anaphylactic reactions. Effects of atopic or anaphylactic reactions are mediated by biologically active mediators released by mast cells that affect end-organ smooth muscle. The amount of mediators released and reactivity of end organ to mediators are controlled by cellular messenger systems. Mast cell sensitivity depends on the amount of reaginic antibody sensitizing the cell and on relative intracellular levels of cyclic AMP (cAMP) and cyclic GMP (cGMP). cAMP and cGMP levels are controlled by adrenergic receptors. Stimulation of α-receptors causes a decrease of cAMP, an increase of cGMP, and increased reactivity; stimulation of β-receptors activates adenyl cyclase and produces increased cAMP, decreased cGMP, and decreased reactivity. A similar mechanism is operative for end-organ smooth muscle. The degree of mast cell and end-organ excitability may be modified by pharmacologic agents that operate through adrenergic or autonomic systems. cAMP is broken down to 5′-AMP by phosphodiesterase, so inhibition of phosphodiesterase activity by methylxanthines increases cAMP and decreases sensitivity of mast cell and end organs. Epinephrine stimulates both α- and β-receptors but generally has the pronounced ability to reverse acute allergic reactions at the usual therapeutic dose. Disodium cromoglycate and diethylcarbamazine inhibit histamine release from mast cells. Excitation of end organs is controlled by a balance of the autonomic nervous system. Parasympathetic effects are similar to anaphylactic effects (bronchial constriction, endothelial contraction, increased peristalsis, dilatation of the bladder sphincter, and so on), whereas sympathetic effects are the opposite. Certain situations may result in temporary imbalance of these systems and increase severity of reaction, as in patients with chronic asthma.

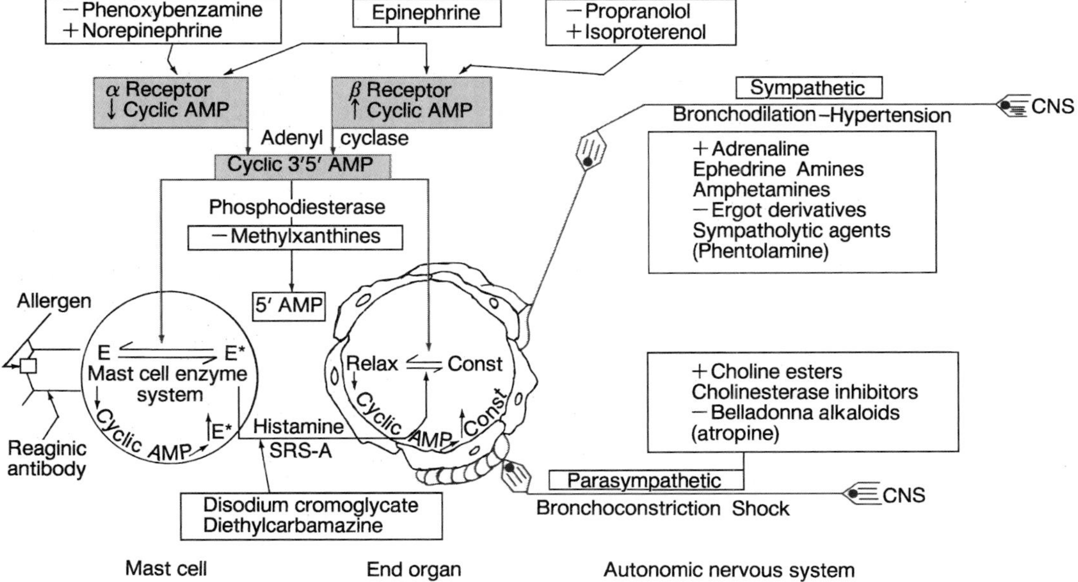

In fact, it has been estimated that over 80% of asthma in adults is caused not by extrinsic antigen exposure but by physiologic imbalance of the responsive smooth muscle end organs. The role of cyclic nucleotides as "second messengers" in controlling cellular responses has led to a theoretic appreciation of the mechanisms controlling anaphylactic reactions (β-adrenergic blockage theory of asthma).

Mast Cells

Control or sensitivity of mast cells to allergen (the amount of mediators released by sensitized mast cells following contact with allergen) is accomplished by balanced adrenergic receptors (α- and β-receptors) that control the cellular level of enzyme systems, such as methyltransferase phosphorylating enzymes and phospholipases, the activation of which leads to mediator release. Contact of the sensitized mast cell with antigen causes activation of the enzyme system and release of mediators. The amount of enzyme available is determined by the cellular level of cyclic AMP (cAMP), which in turn is controlled by the stimulation of the α- and β-receptors. Stimulation of β-receptors activates adenyl cyclase and causes increased cAMP and decreased reactivity, whereas activation of the β-receptors results in decreased cAMP and increased reactivity. cAMP is normally broken down to 5′-AMP by phosphodiesterase, so inhibition of phosphodiesterase leads to increased cAMP and decreased reactivity. The extent of reaction of mast cells to antigen may be controlled by stimulating or blocking the controlling receptors. Norepinephrine stimulates α-receptors, which results in a decrease in cellular cAMP (increased enzymes and increased sensitivity to allergen), whereas isoproterenol stimulates β-receptors (decreased sensitivity to allergen). Phenoxybenzamine blocks both α- and β-receptors but has a more profound effect on β-receptors, and selective stimulation may be achieved by the use of epinephrine combined with one of the blocking drugs. Methylxanthines (theophylline) inhibit phosphodiesterase and thus prevent cAMP breakdown (decreased sensitivity to antigen). Two drugs block the release of mediators after contact of sensitized mast cells with allergen. The way that these drugs, diethylcarbamazine and disodium chromoglycate, inhibit histamine release is not known. Specific desensitization of sensitized cells occurs as patients treated with sodium cromolyn and challenged with antigen remain refractory to subsequent challenge with the same antigen but not a different antigen when retested after 5 h.

End-Organ Sensitivity

The unleashing of severe atopic reactions is not only controlled at the mast cell level but also depends upon the balance between homeostatic α- and β-end-organ (smooth muscle) adrenergic receptors. The cAMP levels of the end-organ cells may be controlled in a similar manner as described above for mast cells. Thus, stimulation of α-receptors leads to a decrease in cAMP and increased anaphylactic effects; stimulation of β-receptors leads to increased cAMP and decreased end-organ effects. The β-adrenergic theory states that atopic individuals do not have the normal adrenergic end-organ homeostatic mechanism. Activation of α-receptors in normal nonatopic individuals does not produce significant anaphylactic symptoms, because such activation is counterbalanced by activation of the β-adrenergic system. Thus, according to this theory, bronchial asthma is not primarily an immunologic disease but is due to an abnormality in the β-adrenergic end-organ system. The marked beneficial effect of epinephrine on anaphylactic symptoms is due to its apparent stimulation of end-organ β-receptors and not because of its effect on mast cells.

The Autonomic Nervous System

The excitability of the end-organ smooth muscle (bronchial muscles, arterioles, gastrointestinal muscles) is also controlled by the autonomic nervous system and is maintained by a balance of sympathetic (adrenergic) and parasympathetic (cholinergic) effects. In general, parasympathetic effects are similar to anaphylactic effects (bronchial constriction, increased gastrointestinal peristalsis, dilatation of the bladder sphincter, dilatation of arteries, and pupil constriction), whereas sympathetic effects are the opposite (bronchial and pupil dilatation and arterial and sphincter constriction). In a normal individual, the effects of the two components of the autonomic system are usually in balance, with a tendency to sympathetic dominance. It is known that certain situations may result in a temporary imbalance of these systems. Thus, stimulation of the parasympathetic system by injection of Mecholyl or acetylcholine in a normal individual results in a temporary drop in blood pressure. Immediately after this effect, the individual may be hyperresponsive to sympathetic stimulation, so-called sympathetic tuning. A permanent imbalance may be produced in laboratory animals by producing lesions in the pituitary. Ablation of areas of the anterior pituitary that reduces parasympathetic discharge protects against the lethal effects of anaphylaxis. Anaphylactically sensitized individuals may have a permanent imbalance of autonomic control that predisposes them to increased reactivity to mediator release. The shock organ effect (i.e., selective reactivity of certain organs) may be explained by a local imbalance of autonomic effects. Anaphylactoid reactions may be overreactions of this balancing system induced by physiologic change. Because the autonomic nervous system is indirectly connected through neuronal synapses to higher areas of the brain, it is possible for emotional conditioning to affect the autonomic balance. Thus, emotional states may lead to parasympathetic tuning with resultant atopic or anaphylactic symptoms (cholinergic urticaria).

An imbalance of any or all of three levels (mast cells, end organ, or autonomic nervous system) may explain the increased sensitivity of atopic individuals to anaphylactic mediators. Atopic individuals injected with small doses of histamine have a much greater reaction than nonatopic individuals. It has been shown that the lymphocytes of atopic individuals have a decreased ability to respond to certain stimuli by increased cAMP levels. Thus, atopic individuals may be unable to balance the effects of α-stimulation or allergen contact.

Autoantibodies to β-Adrenergic Receptors

Some individuals with high risk for development of asthma have autoantibodies for β_2-adrenergic receptors. Since such antibodies might block β_2-adrenergic receptors, it is possible that this blockade could increase mast cell sensitivity to IgE-mediated degranulation (β_2-adrenergic receptor stimulation decreases mast cell sensitivity). Auto-anti-β_2-adrenergic receptors might also affect end-organ responsiveness. At the time of this writing, only clinical correlations have been made; i.e., such antibodies are found in 10% of severe asthmatics but not in sera of nonasthmatic individuals. Questions regarding the role that these antibodies play in the pathogenesis of asthma, how they arise (for instance, are they stimulated by therapy with synthetic β-adrenergic ligand?), and whether or not they have any prognostic value remain to be answered.

Figure 11.4 Levels of possible therapeutic or preventive intervention in allergy. **(1)** Avoidance of contact with the allergen is the most effective means of preventing atopic allergic reactions, thus removing antigen activation of IgE receptors. Avoidance is not always feasible and other methods must be used. **(2)** The amount of IgE antibody may be reduced by hyposensitization, desensitization, or tolerance as the result of injection therapy (see above) or by treatment with humanized anti-IgE antibody. **(3)** The sensitivity of the mast cell upon reaction of IgE receptors with allergen may be controlled by the amount of cAMP available. This level may be affected by drugs as indicated in Fig. 11.3. If mast cell cAMP can be increased by the methods indicated above, the extent of mast cell mediator release upon reaction of sensitized cells with allergen may be decreased and atopic symptoms controlled. **(4)** Two drugs, diethylcarbamazine and disodium chromoglycate (cromines), significantly decrease the release of mediators from mast cells upon contact with allergen. **(5)** The effect of mast cell mediators may be partially controlled by drugs that interfere with histamine activity (antihistamines). The fact that antihistamines are only partially effective in decreasing atopic symptoms indicates that other mediators play an important role. **(6)** The rapidly increasing understanding of the role of arachidonic acid metabolites in allergic reactions could well lead to more effective therapy. In particular, nonsteroidal anti-inflammatory agents or agents that could control the balance of effects of prostaglandin E (bronchodilation) and prostaglandin F (bronchoconstriction) could have great potential beneficial effects. Steroids are used only as a last resort. **(7)** The sensitivity of the end organ (smooth muscle) to atopic mediators also depends upon β-adrenergic control of cellular cAMP levels. If end-organ cAMP can be increased, then atopic symptoms should be decreased. **(8)** Sympathetic stimulation or parasympathetic blockade may also have a significant beneficial effect upon atopic reactions through the effect of the autonomic nervous system upon organ excitability (Fig. 11.3). **(9)** It is well known that severity of atopic reactions (particularly asthma) depends upon the emotional state of the individual. Anxious or insecure patients have more severe symptoms than more secure or stable patients. Thus, the emotional state of the reactive individual should be evaluated and treated with psychotherapy, if necessary. Other experimental agents that block cytokines, chemokines, cell adhesion, signal transduction, or nuclear transcription may affect different stages of IgE production or IgE-mediated reactions.

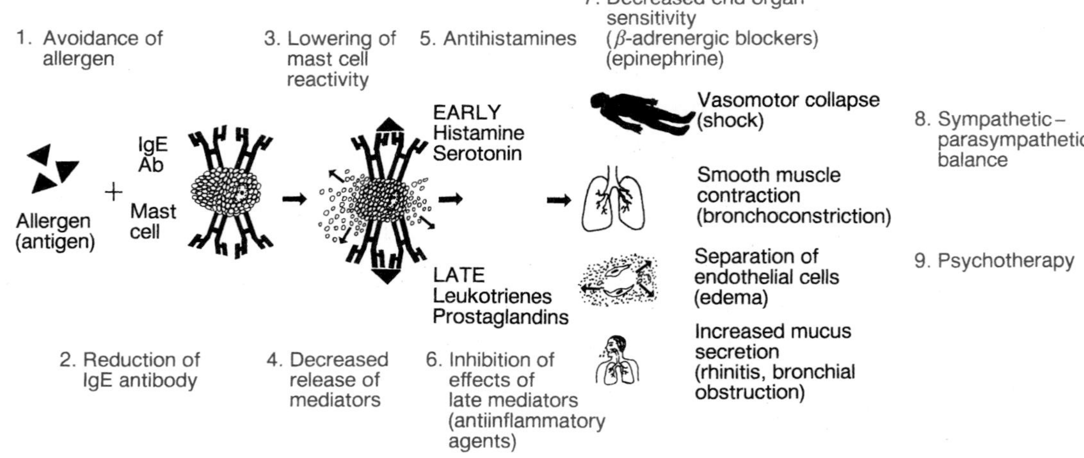

Table 11.11 Pharmacologic agents used in treatment of mast cell-mediated allergic reactions

Class	Example(s)	Mechanism(s) of action	Result
Antihistamines	Diphenhydramine (H_1), cimetidine (H_2)	Block action of histamine on H_1 or H_2 receptors in surrounding tissue	Block mediator effects on target organs
β-Adrenergic drugs	Isoproterenol	Increase cAMP through activation of adenylate cyclase	Decrease mediator release; counteract mediator effects on target organs
Corticosteroids	Prednisone	Inhibit phospholipases, increase β-receptor number	Inhibit mediator synthesis, mediator secretion, chemotaxis, and cell adherence
Methylxanthines	Theophylline	Increase cAMP by inhibition of phosphodiesterase	Decrease mediator release; counteract mediator effects on target organs
Nonsteroidal anti-inflammatory agents	Aspirin, indomethacin	Inhibit cyclooxygenase pathway	Inhibit prostaglandin production
Cromolynlike drugs	Sodium cromolyn, doxantrazole	Inhibit phosphodiesterase; decrease Ca^{2+} flux across mast cell membrane	Inhibit mediator release

Treatment of Allergies

Therapeutic procedures to prevent or decrease atopic reactions may be applied at the various levels of the reaction: contact with antigen, IgE receptor, sensitivity of the mast cell to stimulation, degranulation of mast cell, mast cell mediator activity, sensitivity of end-organ cell, autonomic nervous system balance, and emotional state of the reactive individual (Fig. 11.4).

Drugs that counteract the effects of mast cell mediators upon target cells or decrease the release of mediators from mast cells are under active development and clinical investigation by pharmaceutical companies (Table 11.11). There is every reason to believe that new pharmacologic approaches will be able to decrease or inhibit allergic reactions with few or no side effects. The effectiveness of currently available therapeutic drugs for atopic diseases is listed in Table 11.12. There is clearly a need for new treatments to deal with asthma that is not controlled by inhaled steroids and for a generally effective approach for treatment of all atopic diseases.

Protective Role of IgE

The protective role of atopic or anaphylactic reactions has been the subject of considerable speculation. The most popular hypothesis is that anaphylactic reactions open small blood vessels via endothelial cell contraction and thus permit the exudation of other immunoglobulin classes of antibodies or inflammatory cells into the tissue containing the offending

Table 11.12 Current therapies for atopic diseases[a]

Therapy	Asthma	Allergic rhinitis	Eczema	Atopic conjunctivitis	Anaphylaxis
Topical steroids	+++	+++	++	+++	−
Bronchodilators	+++	−	−	−	+++ (Epinephrine)
Theophylline	++	−	−	−	−
Cromones	+	+	−	++	−
Antihistamines	−	++	+	−	+
Antileukotrienes	+	−	−	−	−

[a]From J. Barnes, *Nature* **402**(Suppl.):B31–B38, 1999. −, not effective; + to +++, increasing degrees of effectiveness.

antigen, the "gatekeeper effect." In immunized animals containing IgG anti-diphtheria toxin antibodies, the simultaneous injection of ragweed antigen and diphtheria toxin into the skin results in an increase in toxin neutralization if the skin site is prepared by previous sensitization with reaginic antibody for the ragweed antigen. It is concluded that the increased toxin-neutralizing capacity of the local skin sites in passively immunized animals is due to increased transudation of serum IgG antibody into the skin test sites ("gatekeeper effect").

Bacterial Infections

Antibody-mediated protection against bacterial infections involves cooperative effects of different mechanisms. IgE-mediated increased vascular permeability allows rapid delivery of other antibodies into infected tissues. Activation of mast cells by IgE-mediated reactions serves to increase vascular permeability (endothelial cell contraction), permitting egress of blood-borne antibody or inflammatory cells into the site of infection.

Intestinal Parasites

The protective action of an individual with a parasitic gastrointestinal worm infestation is to expel the worms from the gastrointestinal tract. Our understanding of how this is accomplished is based largely on studies in rodents and is still incomplete. In the human disease trichinosis, cysts of *Trichinella* are digested in the gastrointestinal tract, liberating larvae that mature into adult worms. Female adult worms release larvae that penetrate the intestinal wall and lodge in muscle tissue, where they encyst. The invasion of the muscle is associated with an intense inflammatory reaction, causing fever and muscle pain and swelling, but some larvae survive this attack and encyst. These cysts are protected niches where the encysted larvae may remain viable for many years. When uncooked meat containing these cysts is eaten, the infection is repeated.

It is believed that intestinal larvae or worms are eliminated as their microenvironment deteriorates as a consequence of immune-mediated inflammation. Mast cell mediators are involved in elimination of larval forms by producing effects such as local acidosis, hypermotility, and epithelial cell changes as well as increased blood flow, edema, and attraction of other inflammatory cells, particularly eosinophils. Eosinophils contain major basic protein, which is not only toxic for worms but also attracts more mast cells. In addition, eosinophils may release leukotrienes, platelet-activating factor, and oxygen radicals that kill adult worms. Dead organisms in tissue are usually surrounded by large numbers of eosinophils. Production of IL-13 by Th2 cells may stimulate increased mucin production by hyperplastic goblet cells and produce dislodgement of established worms or prevent attachment of larvae. Antibody and complement in mucus may increase this effect. However, the understanding of how these mechanisms are induced and how they effect protection remains incomplete.

The ability of previously infected individuals to resist reinfection indicates that effective immunity to reinfection can be induced and that immunization with worm products might prevent primary infection through rapid expulsion of larvae. However, immunization with dead organisms or extracts has failed to induce immunity. Thus, biological interactions between the living parasite and the host appear to be required to induce effective immunity, perhaps by expression of antigens specific for developmental stages in vivo. Effective vaccines for veterinary use have been produced by using irradiated larvae, and studies are under way in an attempt to produce vaccines for human nematodes. IgE-mediated nitric oxide release that involves CD23 on macrophages may also play a role in the protective reaction in cutaneous leishmaniasis.

Avoidance of Allergy

Acute anaphylactic reactions may force the sensitized individual to avoid further exposure to the offending allergen. By avoiding exposure to the antigens, more prolonged extensive immune-mediated damage may be prevented. Avoidance may prevent formation of immune complex disease or delayed-type hypersensitivity to the same antigen, since anaphylactic reactions may be elicited by extremely small doses of an antigen.

Allergic Bronchopulmonary Aspergillosis

Anaphylactic reactions to fungal or bacterial antigens are not uncommon and may be responsible for pathologic effects rather than protection (the double-edged sword). For example, several laundry detergents contain enzymes from *B. subtilis* that may elicit acute allergic reactions. A more serious problem is allergic reaction to fungi in the tracheobronchial flora (e.g., *Aspergillus fumigatus*). "Aspergillus" comes from the Latin word *aspere,* to scatter. An aspergill is a brush to sprinkle (scatter) holy water during the asperges, a short service in the Roman Catholic Church before a High Mass. The name is applied to the *Aspergillus* fungus because of the resemblance of the conidiospores to the aspergill. The term aspergillus is also applied to a medieval weapon consisting of a spiked ball on the end of a chain.

The syndrome of allergic bronchopulmonary aspergillosis includes wheezing, fever, occasional expectoration of golden brown plugs that contain mycelia, systemic eosinophilia, elevated serum IgE concentrations, and the presence of antibodies to *Aspergillus* spp. in the serum. Invasive *Aspergillus* infection may be diagnosed by detection of circulating fungal DNA in serum by enzyme immunoassay after expansion by polymerase chain reaction. *A. fumigatus* is one of the most common airborne saprophytic fungi and is constantly inhaled during normal life. In normal individuals, the fungus is cleared by immune mechanisms. Invasive infection may occur in immune-deficient individuals, and allergic bronchopulmonary aspergillosis may occur in patients with asthma or cystic fibrosis. The syndrome is caused by prolonged anaphylactic reactions to aspergillus antigens (Fig. 11.5). Allergic aspergillosis most likely begins with the inhalation and trapping of aspergillial conidia in the viscous secretions present in the bronchi of an asthmatic. The spores germinate and form mycelia; antigens released from mycelia react with IgE on mast cells in the bronchial walls, resulting in greatly increased mucus secretion and bronchospasm. Allergic bronchopulmonary aspergillosis differs from most other forms of asthma in that the supply of inciting antigen is continuously replenished by replication within the bronchi and bronchioles. The anaphylactic reaction to *Aspergillus* in bronchi may lead to formation of mucus plugs containing fungi, produce protracted constriction of bronchial smooth muscle, and cause death by asphyxiation.

Almost all affected patients will react with a wheal-and-flare skin response to dermal injection of aspergillus antigens (IgE). Many patients also have precipitating IgG antibodies and may have pulmonary vasculitis, presumably due to immune complexes. Nonallergic patients may develop

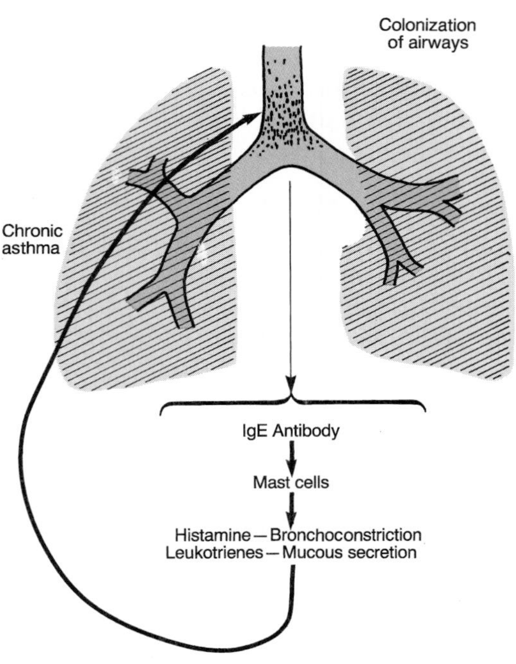

Figure 11.5 Allergic bronchopulmonary aspergillosis. Anaphylactic reaction to *Aspergillus* infection in the bronchi causes secondary pathologic effects leading to repeated asthmatic attacks and plugging of airways with thick mucus plugs.

Aspergillus infections, which usually present as single lesions (fungus ball) in areas of previously damaged lung tissue. Invasive *Aspergillus* in which mycelia actually extend into tissue is different from allergic bronchopulmonary aspergillosis and is seen in patients with immune deficiency diseases.

Summary

Anaphylactic (acute) or atopic (chronic) reactions are caused by activation of mast cells via reaction of reaginic antibody fixed to the mast cell surface. Reaginic antibody belongs to a unique class of immunoglobulin, IgE, which has the capacity to bind to receptors on mast cells ("fix.") Mast cells are stimulated by reaction with allergen to release pharmacologically agents stored in cytoplasmic granules (degranulation) such as histamine and serotonin, which produce acute reactions. In addition, arachidonic acid from membrane phospholipids is converted to leukotrienes and prostaglandins, which produce or cause later inflammatory lesions. These released mediators act on smooth muscle cells and endothelial cells, causing constriction. This in turn produces clinical symptoms because of bronchoconstriction (asthma), loss of intravascular fluid (edema, cutaneous anaphylaxis, shock), or chronic accumulation of mucus (hay fever, nasal polyps). The degree of reactivity of the system is controlled by a balance between adrenergic and cholinergic receptors, and the extent of these reactions may be controlled by drugs that affect this physiologic balance. Many allergic symptoms are believed to be the result of an imbalance of this controlling system rather than an exposure to allergen. The extent of production of reaginic (IgE) antibody may be influenced by specific immunization (immunotherapy). The mechanism of action of immunotherapy remains poorly defined. Experimental models indicate that $T_{\gamma\delta}$-suppressor cells specific for IgE production may be active.

Anaphylactic reactions may serve a protective role in providing rapid egress of other antibodies or cells into sites of antigen deposition by inducing endothelial cell separation. However, allergic reactions cause problems for a large number of people and constitute the basis for the practice of a major clinical specialty: that of the allergist.

Bibliography

Introduction

Befus, A. D., C. Mowat, M. Gilchrist, J. Hu, S. Solomon, and A. Bateman. 1999. Neutrophil defensins induce histamine secretion from mast cells: mechanisms of action. *J. Immunol.* **163:**947–953.

Blackley, C. H. 1873. *Experiments and Researches on the Causes of Nature of Catarrhus Aestivus.* Balliere, London, England.

Coca, A. F., and E. F. Grove. 1925. Studies on hypersensitiveness. XIII. A study of the atopic reagins. *J. Immunol.* **10:**445–464.

Cuss, F. M. 1999. Beyond the histamine receptor: effect of antihistamines on mast cells. *Clin. Exp. Allergy* **29**(Suppl. 3)**:**54–59.

Friedman, M. M., and M. A. Kaliner. 1987. Human mast cells and asthma. *Am. Rev. Respir. Dis.* **135:**1157–1164.

Hamelmann, E., K. Tadeda, A. Oshiba, and E. W. Gelfand. 1999. Role of IgE in the development of allergic airway inflammation and airway hyperresponsiveness—a murine model. *Allergy* **54:**297–305.

Hiraoka, S., Y. Furumoto, H. Koseki, Y. Takagaki, M. Taniguchi, K. Okumura, and C. Ra. 1999. Fc receptor beta subunit is required for full activation of mast cells through Fc receptor engagement. *Int. Immunol.* **11:**199–207.

Howarth, P. H. 1999. Assessment of antihistamine efficacy and potency. *Clin. Exp. Allergy* **29**(Suppl. 3)**:**87–97.

Ishizaka, T., K. Ishizaka, S. G. O. Johansson, and H. Bennich. 1969. Histamine release from human leukocytes by anti-E antibodies. *J. Immunol.* **102:**884.

Lynch, N. R., I. A. Hagel, M. E. Palenque, M. C. DiPrisco, J. E. Escudero, et al. 1998. Relationship between helminthic infection and IgE response in atopic and nonatopic children in a tropical environment. *J. Allergy Clin. Immunol.* **101:**217–221.

O'Sullivan, S. 1999. On the role of PDG2 metabolites as markers of mast cell activation in asthma. *Acta Physiol. Scand. Suppl.* **644:**1–74.

Wyman, M. 1872. *Autumnal Catarrah; Hay Fever.* Hurd and Houghton, Cambridge, Mass.

Allergens

Baldo, B. A. (ed.). 1988. Molecular approaches to the study of allergens. *Monogr. Allergy* **28.**

Figueredo, E., S. Quirce, A. del Amo, J. Cuesta, I. Arrieta, C. Lahoz, and J. Sastre. 1999. Beer-induced anaphylaxis: identification of allergens. *Allergy* **54:**630–634.

Marsh, D. G., L. Goodfriend, T. P. King, H. Lowenstein, and T. A. E. Platts-Mills. 1988. Allergen nomenclature. *Clin. Allergy* **18:**201–207.

Moneret-Vautrin, D. A. 1999. Cow's milk allergy. *Allerg. Immunol.* (Paris) **31:** 201–210.

Park, J. W., S. H. Ko, C. W. Kim, S. W. Bae, and C. S. Hong. 1999. Seminal plasma anaphylaxis: successful pregnancy after intravaginal desensitization and immunodetection of allergens. *Allergy* **54:**990–993.

Svanes, C., D. Jarvis, S. Chinn, and P. Burney. 1999. Childhood environment and adult atopy: results from the European community respiratory health survey. *J. Allergy Clin. Immunol.* **103:**415–420.

Warner, J. O. 1999. "Peanut allergy" a major public health issue. *Pediatr. Allergy Immunol.* **10:**14–20.

Reaginic Antibody

Anonymous. 1999. Current issues relating to in vitro testing for allergen-specific IgE: a workshop report. *Ann. Allergy Asthma Immunol.* **82:**407–412. (Editorial.)

Baumruker, T., R. Csonga, D. Jaksche, V. Novotny, and E. E. Prieschl. 1999. TNF-alpha and IL-5 gene induction in IgE plus antigen-stimulated mast cells require common and distinct signaling pathways. *Int. Arch. Allergy Immunol.* **118:**108–111.

Corry, D. B., and F. Kheradmand. 1999. Induction and regulation of the IgE response. *Nature* **402**(Suppl.)**:**B18–B23.

Holgate, S. T. 1999. The epidemic of allergy and asthma. *Nature* **402**(Suppl.)**:**B2–B4.

Holt, P. G., C. Macaubas, S. L. Prescott, and P. D. Sly. 1999. Microbial stimulation as an aetiologic factor in atopic disease. *Allergy* **54**(Suppl. 49)**:**12–16.

Ishizaka, K., T. Ishizaka, and M. H. Hornbrook. 1966. Physico-chemical properties of human reaginic antibody. IV. Presence of a unique immunoglobulin as a carrier of reaginic activity. *J. Immunol.* **97:**75–85.

Malavija, R., and F. M. Uckun. 1999. Genetic and biochemical evidence for a critical role of Janus kinase (JAK)-3 in mast cell-mediated type I hypersensitivity reactions. *Biochem. Biophys. Res. Commun.* **257:**807–813.

Marone, G., G. Spadaro, C. Palumbo, and G. Condorelli. 1999. The anti-IgE/anti-FcεRIα autoantibody network in allergic and autoimmune diseases. *Clin. Exp. Allergy* **29:**17–27.

Metzger, H. 1992. The receptor with high affinity for IgE. *Immunol. Rev.* **125:**37.

Prausnitz, C., and H. Kustner. 1921. Studies on sensitivity. *Zentbl. Bakteriol. Orig.* **86:**160. (English translation in P. G. H. Gell and R. R. A. Coombs, p. 808, *Clinical Aspects of Immunology,* Davis, Philadelphia, Pa., 1963.)

Reid, M. J., R. F. Lockey, P. C. Turkeltaub, and T. A. E. Platts-Mills. 1993. Survey of fatalities from skin testing and immunotherapy, 1985–1989. *J. Allergy Clin. Immunol.* **92:**6–15.

Turner, H., and J.-P. Kinet. 1999. Signalling through the high-affinity IgE receptor FcεRI. *Nature* **402**(Suppl.)**:**B24–B30.

Valyasevi, M. A., D. E. Maddox, and J. T. Li. 1999. Systemic reactions to allergy skin tests. *Ann. Allergy Asthma Immunol.* **83:**132–136.

Genetics

Coleman, R., R. E. Trembath, and J. I. Harper. 1997. Genetic studies of atopy and atopic dermatitis. *Br. J. Dermatol.* **136:**1–5.

Haselden, G. M., K. A. Barry, and M. Larche. 1999. Immunoglobulin E-independent major histocompatibility complex-restricted T cell peptide epitope-induced late asthmatic reactions. *J. Exp. Med.* **189:**1885–1894.

Orgel, H. A., and R. N. Hamburger. 1975. Development of IgE and allergy in infancy. *J. Allergy Clin. Immunol.* **56:**296–307.

Stephan, V., J. Kuehr, A. Seibt, H. Saueressig, S. Zingsem, et al. 1999. Genetic linkage of HLA-class II locus to mite-specific IgE immune responses. *Clin. Exp. Allergy* **29:**1049–1054.

Anaphylaxis

Burks, A. V., H. A. Sampson, and R. H. Buckley. 1986. Anaphylactic reactions after gamma globulin administration in patients with hypogammaglobulinemia. Detection of IgE antibodies to IgA. *N. Engl. J. Med.* **314:**560.

Patterson, R., and K. E. Harris. 1999. Idiopathic anaphylaxis. *Allergy Asthma Proc.* **20:**311–315.

Portier, R. H., and C. Richet. 1902. De l'action anaphylactique de certains venims. *C. R. Soc. Biol.* **54:**170.

Quinke, H. 1882. On acute localized edema of the skin. *Monatsh. Prakt. Dermatol.* **1:**129.

Reunala, T., A. I. Koskimies, F. Bjorksten, J. Janne, and A. Lassus. 1977. Immunoglobulin E-mediated severe allergy to human seminal plasma. *Fertil. Steril.* **28:**832–835.

Shadick, N. A., M. H. Liang, A. J. Partridge, C. Bingham, E. Wright, A. H. Fossel, and A. L. Sheffer. 1999. The natural history of exercise-induced anaphylaxis: survey results from a 10–year follow-up study. *J. Allergy Clin. Immunol.* **104:** 123–127.

Snell, D. 1961. How it feels to die. *Life,* May 26.

Atopic Allergy

Bahna, S. L. 1992. Factors determining development of allergy in infants. *Allergy Proc.* **13:**21–25.

Botham, P. A., G. E. Davies, and E. L. Teasdale. 1987. Allergy to laboratory animals: a prospective study of its incidence and of the influence of atopy on its development. *Br. J. Ind. Med.* **44:**627.

Cookson, W. 1999. The alliance of genes and environment in asthma and allergy. *Nature* **402**(Suppl.)**:**B5–B9.

Hunskaar, S., and R. T. Fosse. 1990. Allergy to laboratory mice and rats: a review of the pathophysiology, epidemiology and clinical aspects. *Lab. Anim. Sci.* **24:**358–374.

Juliusson, S., U. Pipkorn, G. Karlsson, and L. Enerback. 1992. Mast cells and eosinophils in the allergic mucosal response to allergen challenge: changes in distribution and signs of activation in relation to symptoms. *J. Allergy Clin. Immunol.* **80:**898–909.

Lamblin, C., P. Gosset, F. Sallez, L. M. Vandezande, T. Perez, et al. 1999. Eosinophilic airway inflammation in nasal polyposis. *J. Allergy Clin. Immunol.* **104:**85–92.

Levy, D. A., D. Charpin, D. Pecquet, F. Leynadier, and D. Vervloet. 1992. Allergy to latex. *Allergy* **47:**579–587.

Ludman, B. G. 1999. Human seminal plasma protein allergy: a diagnosis rarely considered. *J. Obstet. Gynecol. Neonatal Nurs.* **28:**359–363.

Simons, F. E. 1999. Allergic rhinobronchitis: the asthma-allergic rhinitis link. *J. Allergy Clin. Immunol.* **104:**534–540.

Asthma

Aalbers, R., M. Smith, and W. Timens. 1993. Immunohistology in bronchial asthma. *Respir. Med.* **87**(Suppl. B)**:**13–21.

Ashutosh, K. 2000. Nitric oxide and asthma: a review. *Curr. Opin. Pulm. Med.* **6:**21–25.

Barnes, P. J. 1999. Therapeutic strategies for allergic diseases. *Nature* **402** (Suppl.)**:**B31–B38.

Beasley, R., C. Burgess, J. Crane, N. Pearce, and W. Roche. 1993. Pathology of asthma and its clinical implications. *J. Allergy Clin. Immunol.* **92:**148–154.

Bjornsdottir, U. S., and D. M. Cypcar. 1999. Asthma: an inflammatory mediator soup. *Allergy* **54**(Suppl. 49)**:**55–61.

Cui, Z. H., B. E. Skoogh, T. Pullerits, and J. Lotvall. 1999. Bronchial hyperresponsiveness and airway wall remodelling induced by exposure to allergen for 9 weeks. *Allergy* **54:**1074–1082.

Custovic, A., A. Simpson, and A. Woodcock. 1998. Importance of indoor allergens in the induction of allergy and elicitation of allergic disease. *Allergy* **53**(Suppl. 48)**:**115–120.

Fish, J. E., and S. P. Peters. 1999. Airway remodeling and persistent airway obstruction in asthma. *J. Allergy Clin. Immunol.* **104:**509–516.

Forsyth, P., and M. Ennis. 1999. Adenosine, mast cells and asthma. *Inflamm. Res.* **48:**301–307.

Osler, W. 1892. *The Principles and Practice of Medicine,* p. 499. Appleton & Low, New York, N.Y.

Rothenberg, M. E., N. Zimmerman, A. Mishra, E. Brandt, L. A. Birkenberger, S. P. Hogan, and P. S. Foster. 1999. Chemokines and chemokine receptors: their role in allergic airway disease. *J. Clin. Immunol.* **19:**250–265.

Wardlaw, A. J. 1993. *Asthma.* Bios Sci Publishers, Oxford, England.

Hay Fever and Nasal Polyps

LaForce, C. 1999. Use of nasal steroids in managing allergic rhinitis. *J. Allergy Clin. Immunol.* **103:**S388–S394.

Lieberman, P. 1999. Management of allergic rhinitis with a combination antihistamine/anti-inflammatory agent. *J. Allergy Clin. Immunol.* **103:**S400–S404.

Mygind, N., and R. M. Nacierio. 1993. *Allergic and Non-allergic Rhinitis: Clinical Aspects.* The W. B. Saunders Co., Orlando, Fla.

Raphael, G. D., J. N. Baraniuk, and M. A. Kaliner. 1991. How and why the nose runs. *J. Allergy Clin. Immunol.* **87:**457–467.

Winkerwerder, W. L., and L. N. Gay. 1937. Perennial allergic rhinitis: an analysis of 198 cases. *Bull. Johns Hopkins Hosp.* **2:**90–100.

Food Allergy

Aas, K. 1988. The biochemistry of food allergens: what is essential for future research?, p. 1. *In* E. Schmidt (ed.), *Food Allergy,* Nestle's nutrition workshop series, vol. 17. Vevry/Raven Press, Ltd., New York, N.Y.

Burks, W., G. A. Bannon, S. Sicherer, and H. A. Sampson. 1999. Peanut-induced anaphylactic reactions. *Int. Arch. Allergy Immunol.* **119:**165–172.

Oehling, A., M. Fernandez, H. Cordoba, and M. L. Sanz. 1997. Skin manifestations and immunological parameters in childhood food allergy. *J. Investig. Allergol. Clin. Immunol.* **7:**155–159.

Rance, F., G. Kanny, G. Dutau, and D. A. Moneret-Vautrin. 1999. Food hypersensitivity in children: clinical aspects and distribution of allergens. *Pediatr. Allergy Immunol.* **10:**33–38.

Rowe, A. H., and A. Rowe, Jr. 1972. *Food Allergy.* Charles C Thomas, Springfield, Ill.

Savilahti, E. 1981. Cow's milk allergy. *Allergy* **36:**73–88.

Insect Allergy

Barr, S. E. 1971. Allergy to hymenopteria stings—review of the world literature: 1953–1970. *Ann. Allergy* **29:**49–66.

Frazier, C. A. 1969. *Insect Allergy.* Green, St. Louis, Mo.

King, T. P. 1990. Insect venom allergy. *Monogr. Allergy* **28:**84–100.

Reisman, R. E. 1992. Stinging insect allergy. *Med. Clin. N. Am.* **76:**883–894.

Vetter, R. S., P. K. Visscher, and S. Camazine. 1999. Mass envenomations by honey bees and wasps. *West. J. Med.* **170:**223–227.

Zwick, H., W. Popp, K. Sertl, H. Rauscher, and T. Wanke. 1991. Allergic structures in cockroach hypersensitivity. *J. Allergy Clin. Immunol.* **87:**626–630.

Atopic Dermatitis

Brocq, L., and L. Jacquet. 1891. Notes pour servie a l'histoire des neurodermites; du lichen circumscriptus des anciens auteurs, ou lichen simplex chronique du M. le Dr. E. Vidal. *Ann. Derm. Syphilgr.* **2:**97.

Hanifin, J. M. 1984. Atopic dermatitis. *J. Allergy Clin. Immunol.* **73:**211–226.

Klein, P. A., and R. A. Clark. 1999. An evidence-based review of the efficacy of antihistamines in relieving pruritus in atopic dermatitis. *Arch. Dermatol.* **135:**1522–1525.

McNally, N. J., D. R. Phillips, and H. C. Williams. 1998. The problem of atopic eczema: aetiologic clues from the environment and lifestyles. *Soc. Sci. Med.* **46:**729–741.

Rajka, G. 1975. *Atopic Dermatitis.* The W. B. Saunders Co., London, England.

Aspirin Intolerance

Abrishami, M. A., and J. Thomas. 1977. Aspirin intolerance—a review. *Ann. Allergy* **39:**28–37.

Davies, R. J., J. Wang, M. M. Abdelaziz, M. A. Calderon, O. Khair, J. L. Devalia, and C. Rusznak. 1997. New insights into the understanding of asthma. *Chest* **111**(Suppl. 2)**:**2S-10S.

Farr, R. S. 1970. Presidential message. *J. Allergy* **45:**321–328.

Urticaria and Angioedema

Agostoni, A., M. Cicardi, M. Cugno, L. C. Zingale, D. Gioffre, and J. Nussberger. 1999. Angioedema due to angiotensin-converting enzyme inhibitors. *Immunopharmacology* **44:**21–25.

Cohen, G., and A. Peterson. 1972. Treatment of hereditary angioedema with frozen plasma. *Ann. Allergy* **30:**690–692.

D'Incan, M., A. Tridon, D. Ponard, C. Dumestre-Perard, M. Ferrier-Le Bouedec, et al. 1999. Acquired angioedema with C1 inhibitor deficiency: is the distinction between type I and type II still relevant? *Dermatology* **199:**227–230.

Ebken, R. K., F. A. Bauschard, and M. I. Levin. 1968. Dermatographism: its definition, demonstration, and prevalence. *J. Allergy* **41:**338–343.

Friedmann, P. S. 1999. Assessment of urticaria and angio-edema. *Clin. Exp. Allergy* **29**(Suppl. 3)**:**109–115.

Kaplan, A. P. 1988. Urticaria and angioedema, p. 667. *In* J. L. Gallin, I. M. Goldstein, and R. Snyderman (ed.), *Inflammation: Basic Principles and Clinical Conditions.* Raven Press, Ltd., New York, N.Y.

Kumar, S. A., and B. L. Martin. 1999. Urticaria and angioedema: diagnostic and treatment considerations. *J. Am. Osteopath. Assoc.* **99**(Suppl. 3)**:**S1–S4.

Leenutaphong, V., E. Holze, and G. Plewig. 1989. Pathogenesis and classification of solar urticaria: a new concept. *J. Am. Acad. Dermatol.* **21:**237–240.

Sofia, S., A. Casali, and L. Bolondi. 1999. Sonographic findings in abdominal hereditary angioedema. *J. Clin. Ultrasound* **27:**537–540.

Immunotherapy

Ebner, C. 1999. Immunological mechanisms operative in allergen-specific immunotherapy. *Int. Arch. Allergy Immunol.* **119:**1–5.

Hurst, D. S., B. R. Gordon, J. A. Fornadley, and D. H. Hunsaker. 1999. Safety of home-based and office allergy immunotherapy: a multicenter prospective study. *Otolaryngol. Head Neck Surg.* **121:**553–561.

Ishizaka, K. 1984. Regulation of IgE synthesis. *Annu. Rev. Immunol.* **2:**159–182.

Karl, S., and J. Ring. 1999. Pro and contra of specific hyposensitization. *Eur. J. Dermatol.* **9:**325–331.

Malling, H. J. 1999. Allergen-specific immunotherapy. Present state and directions for the future. *Allergy* **54**(Suppl. 50)**:**30–33.

Noon, L. 1911. Prophylactic inoculation against hay fever. *Lancet* **i:**1572.

Ohashi, Y., Y. Nakai, A. Tanaka, Y. Kakinoki, Y. Washio, et al. 1998. A comparative study of the clinical efficacy of immunotherapy and conventional pharmacological treatment for patients with perennial allergic rhinitis. *Acta Otolaryngol. Suppl.* **538:**102–112.

Ohman, J. L. 1989. Allergen immunotherapy in asthma: evidence for efficacy. *J. Allergy Clin. Immunol.* **84:**133–140.

Stewart, G. E., and R. F. Lockey. 1992. Systemic reactions from allergen immunotherapy. *J. Allergy Clin. Immunol.* **90:**567.

van Neerven, R. J. 1999. The role of allergen-specific T cells in the allergic immune response: relevance to allergy vaccination. *Allergy* **54:**552–561.

Pharmacology of Atopic Reactions

Church, M. K., M. A. Lowman, P. H. Pees, and R. C. Benyon. 1989. Mast cells, neuropeptides and inflammation. *Agents Action* **27:**8–16.

Haahtela, T. 1999. Advances in pharmacotherapy of asthma. *Curr. Prob. Dermatol.* **28:**135–152.

Morley, J. (ed.). 1984. *Beta-Adrenergic Receptors in Asthma,* Academic Press, New York, N.Y.

Sibley, D. R., and R. J. Lefkowitz. 1985. Molecular mechanisms of receptor desensitization using the β-adrenergic receptor coupled adenylate cyclase system as a model. *Nature* **317:**124–129.

Szentivanyi, A. 1968. The beta adrenergic theory of the atopic abnormality in bronchial asthma. *J. Allergy* **42:**203–232.

Willis, T. 1684. *Pharmaceutic Rationalis on the Operations of Mechanics in Humane Bodies,* p. 78–85, sect. 1, pt. 2. Dring, London, England.

Treatment of Atopic Allergy

Buckle, D. R., and H. Smith (ed.). 1984. *Development of Anti-Asthma Drugs.* Butterworths, London, England.

Chang, T. W. 2000. The pharmacological basis of anti-IgE therapy. *Nat. Biotechnol.* **18:**157–162.

Dahl, R., and T. Haahtela. 1992. Prophylactic pharmacologic treatment of asthma. *Allergy* **47:**588–593.

Kay, A. B., K. F. Austen, and L. M. Lightenstein (ed.). 1984. *Asthma: Physiology, Immunopharmacology and Treatment.* Academic Press, New York, N.Y.

Platts-Mills, T. A. E., and M. D. Chapman. 1987. Dust mites: immunology, allergic disease and environmental control. *J. Allergy Clin. Immunol.* **80:**755–775.

Protective Role of Atopic Reactions

Cockrill, B. A., and C. A. Hales. 1999. Allergic bronchopulmonary aspergillosis. *Annu. Rev. Med.* **50:**303–316.

Else, K. J., and F. D. Finkelman. 1998. Intestinal nematode parasites, cytokines and effector mechanisms. *Int. J. Parasitol.* **28:**1145–1158.

Rothwell, T. L. W. 1989. Immune expulsion of parasitic nematodes from the alimentary tract. *Int. J. Parasitol.* **19:**139–168.

Infectious Disease

Latge, J. P. 1999. *Aspergillus fumigatus* and aspergillosis *Clin. Microbiol. Rev.* **12:**310–350.

Moqbel, R., and D. I. Pritchard. 1990. Parasites and allergy: evidence for a "cause and effect" relationship. *Clin. Exp. Allergy* **20:**611–618.

Mossalayi, M. D., M. Arock, D. Mazier, P. Vincendeay, and I. Vouldoukis. 1999. The human immune response during cutaneous leishmaniasis: NO problem. *Parasitol. Today* **15:**342–345.

Pritchare, D. I., C. Hewitt, and R. Moqbel. 1997. The relationship between immunological responsiveness controlled by T-helper 2 lymphocytes and infections with parasitic helminths. *Parasitology* **115**(Suppl.)**:**S33–S44.

Stebbings, J. H., Jr. 1974. Immediate hypersensitivity: a defense against arthropods. *Perspect. Biol. Med.* **17:**233–239

T-Cell-Mediated Cytotoxicity

12

Cell-Mediated Immunity

The term "cell-mediated immunity" (CMI) was first used to refer to the effects of specifically sensitized lymphocytes after reaction with antigen or target cells in vitro. Specifically sensitized lymphocytes are generated in response to antigenic stimulation and bear receptors for the specific antigen. It was not until the mid-1960s that most immunologists began to consider CMI a biologically important immune effector mechanism. Before that, essentially all that was known was the peculiar delayed-type hypersensitivity skin reaction that was elicited in certain infectious diseases, in particular tuberculosis, to extracts of organisms (delayed-type hypersensitivity skin test). It is now known that CMI, in the form of T-cell killing and/or delayed-type hypersensitivity, is the major defense mechanism against many infectious diseases, as well as the effector mechanism in homograft rejections and many autoimmune diseases. It differs from the immune reactions mentioned previously in this book in that no humoral antibody is involved, and reactivity cannot be transferred by serum, only by cells; the time course of the development of the lesion is usually much more prolonged than in antibody-mediated reactions; and the gross appearance and microscopic appearance are different. Cell-mediated reactions feature infiltrations of tissues by mononuclear cells (lymphocytes and macrophages). The importance of CMI in infectious diseases has been brought to the forefront by the variety and number of opportunistic infections with viruses, protozoa, fungi, and mycobacteria in AIDS patients who have defective T-cell-mediated immunity.

T_{CTL}, T_{DTH}, and Natural Killer Cells

In the 1960s, the term cell-mediated immunity was extended to two types of T-cell-mediated effects in vitro: T-cell killing and T-cell-mediated delayed-type hypersensitivity. Cytotoxic T cells (T_{CTL} cells) lyse or "kill" target cells expressing specific antigens in vitro; T cells that mediate delayed-type hypersensitivity (T_{DTH} cells) release "lymphokines" with biologic activity after reaction with specific antigens in vitro. T-cell killing is initiated by a $CD8^+$ subpopulation of specifically sensitized T_{CTL} cells that react with cell surface antigens associated with class I major histocompatibility complex (MHC) markers and destroy the target cells. Delayed-type hypersensitivity is a local inflammatory reaction caused by the release of lymphokines from $CD4^+$

T_{DTH} cells that are induced through antigen processing in the context of class II MHC markers. T_{DTH} cells may be activated by reaction with soluble protein antigens, such as purified protein derivative of *Mycobacterium tuberculosis*. T_{CTL} cells may be induced by class I MHC antigen processing in any nucleated cell (endogenous processing), whereas T_{DTH}-cell induction requires exogenous processing by class II MHC-positive antigen-presenting cells (macrophages, B cells). MHC restriction is mediated by the receptors of T cells, which contain recognition sites for both antigens and MHC molecules. Natural killer (NK) cells are related to T_{CTL} cells but do not require antigenic stimulation for generation. They are present naturally.

T-Cell Killing

Upon reaction with antigens in association with class I MHC on tissue cells, T_{CTL} cells are activated to kill the target cell. $CD8^+$ T_{CTL} cells kill target cells through two distinct but not mutually exclusive mechanisms, (i) granule exocytosis (perforin and granzymes) and (ii) the Fas-ligand cell death system (Fig. 12.1).

Granule Exocytosis

T_{CTL} cells contain multicomponent cytoplasmic granules containing cytolytic molecules such as perforin, proteoglycans, and serine proteases (granzymes), which, in the presence of calcium, mediate lysis of target cells. These enzymes are also active in NK-cell-mediated killing. Thus, the mechanisms of cell lysis by T_{CTL} and NK cells appear to be very similar. However, it was found that some T_{CTL}-cell line hybridomas lacking detectable perforin, granzymes, and lytic granules are still able to lyse target cells in vitro, suggesting an additional mechanism of T_{CTL}-cell-mediated cytotoxicity. This mechanism was identified as the Fas system.

Fas

The Fas gene codes for a cell surface receptor in the tumor necrosis factor receptor family (Fas receptor). When this receptor reacts with the Fas ligand (FasL), a "ready-to-go" cell death system is activated. Reaction of T_{CTL} cells through the T-cell receptor leads to activation of the Fas ligand gene and expression of FasL on the surface of the T cell. Many potential target cells, including liver, heart, keratinocytes, as well as tumor cells, express Fas and thus can react with FasL on T_{CTL} cells and activate the Fas death gene system. The effectiveness of T_{CTL}-cell killing is related to the expression of cell adhesion molecules, such as H-CAM (CD44) and $\alpha_4\beta_1$-integrin (VLA-4), which determine the ability of the T_{CTL} cell to bind to target cells. Both $CD8^+$ and $CD4^+$ (Th1) cells may express the FasL, but $CD4^+$ cells do not express the granule system. The subset of $T_{\gamma\delta}$ $CD4^-CD8^-$ cells, which makes up 1 to 2% of circulating T cells, also expresses FasL and may serve as an "early-warning" rapid-response T_{CTL}-cell system. These cells may act to hold infections in check during the first few days after exposure. These cells are constitutively activated and can kill target cells in vitro without being activated by interleukin-2 (IL-2).

NK Cell Killing

NK cells may also take part in what may be considered a mirror image of T_{CTL} cell-mediated cytolytic mechanisms. T_{CTL} cells recognize foreign peptides complexed to class I MHC and are activated to kill the cells; NK cells recognize class I MHC molecules complexed with self-protective peptides and do not kill the cells. Potential target cells are protected against NK lysis by binding protective peptides, such as heat shock protein, elongation factor 2, histone H3, and ribosomal proteins. These proteins occupy

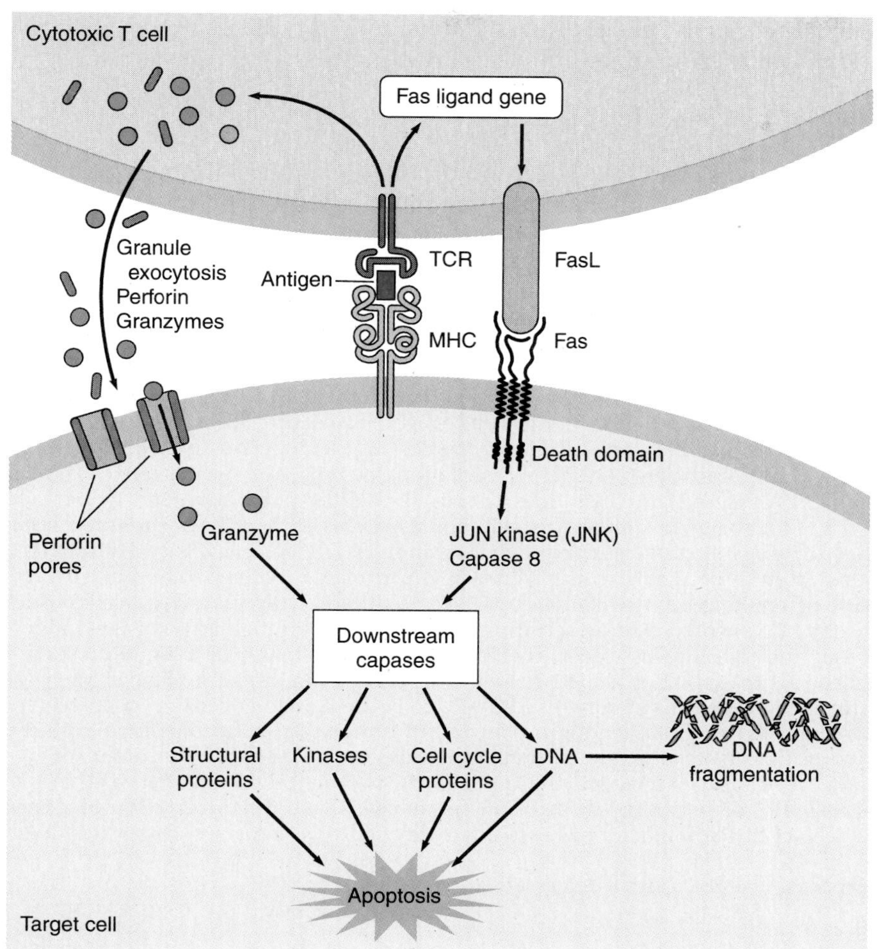

Figure 12.1 Two pathways of T_{CTL} cell killing of target cells. T_{CTL} cell killing is mediated through endogenous proteases (capases) in the target cell. Upon binding of the T_{CTL}-cell receptor (TCR) to antigen of the class I MHC of the target cells, T_{CTL} cells activate two killing systems: Fas ligand and granule exocytosis (perforin and granzymes). Fas ligand on the T cells contains an intracellular "death domain" that binds to at least five intracellular signaling molecules. This activates JUN kinases (JNK) and capase 8. These in turn activate a series of downstream capases. Perforin reacts with the target cell membrane to produce "holes" in the membrane, permitting granzymes to enter the target cell. Upon entering the cytoplasm, granzymes also activate downstream capases. The active capases act on a variety of substrates, including but not limited to structural proteins (laminin, G-actin, etc.), kinases, cell cycle-controlling proteins (Rb and mdm-2), and DNA. This latter action results in the fragmentation of DNA characteristic of apoptosis.

a pocket in the MHC groove. Cells with abnormal MHC class I expression or insufficient protective peptide binding, such as tumor cells or cells infected with virus, are subject to lysis by NK cells. The conserved protective peptides appear to be similar to peptides encoded by infectious agents (e.g., viruses), but the peptides produced by infectious agents have critical amino acid substitutions that do not confer protection. Upon infection, peptides from the infectious agent compete with self peptides for presentation by MHC molecules. Complexes of these peptides with MHC prevent self-recognition by the NK receptor, rendering an infected cell susceptible to NK lysis. Although there is considerable interest in the adaptation of NK cells for tumor immunotherapy, it is not clear what role NK cells play during naturally occurring immune responses in vitro.

Induction of T-Cell Immunity

As presented in part I, the selection of which immune effector systems will predominate after induction of immunity depends upon the type of antigen processing, the nature of the antigen-processing cell, and the characteristics of the T-helper cells that are activated. A simplified presentation of this concept is presented in Fig. 12.2. After exogenous antigen processing

Figure 12.2 Summary of factors determining selection of immune effector systems. Selection of which immune effector mechanisms will predominate after an immune response depends on the location of the antigen-presenting cell (follicular or parafollicular), the type of antigen processing (endogenous or exogenous), the class of MHC-associated antigen presentation, the presence of accessory cells (mast cells, NK cells, etc.), the cytokines produced, and the population of T-helper cells activated. Exogenous antigen presentation by professional antigen-presenting cells (dendritic or follicular cells) leads to activation of Th1 or Th2 cells and stimulation of antibody production. In this figure, it is postulated that separation of Th1 activation from helping B cells make antibody to differentiation into T_{DTH} cells, which mediate delayed-type hypersensitivity, is dependent on the nature of the antigen-presenting cells. Procession of antigen by dendritic or follicular antigen-presenting cells leads to activation of Th1 helper cells; processing by parafollicular interdigitating reticulum cells stimulates Th1 cells to become effector cells for delayed-type hypersensitivity. Endogenous processing of antigen by nonprofessional antigen-presenting cells results in presentation by class I MHC to $CD8^+$ precursors of T_{CTL} cells. T_{CTL} cells recognize antigens on surfaces of other cells and produce molecules (granzymes or perforins) that kill the target cells. T_{DTH} cells release lymphokines, which act through macrophages to effect delayed-type hypersensitivity reactions.

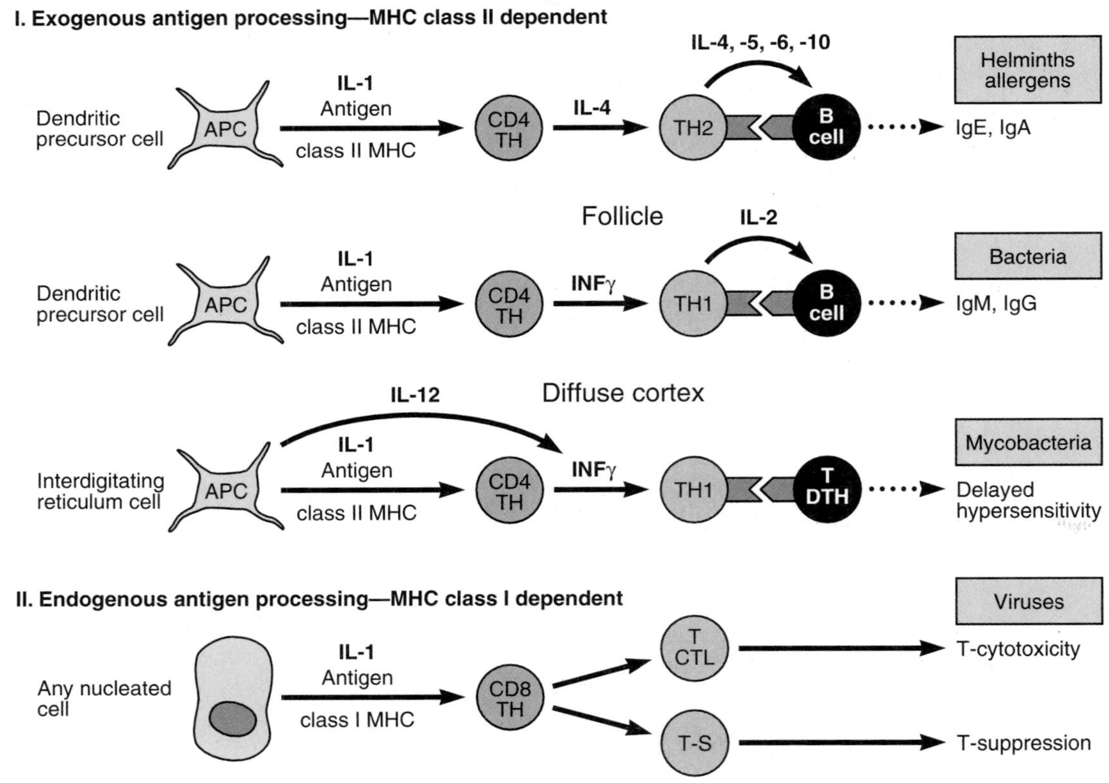

by follicular dendritic cells, if Th1 cells predominate, there will be preferential production of immunoglobulin M (IgM) and IgG antibody by B cells; if Th2 cells predominate, IgE and IgA antibodies will be formed. Although the Th1/Th2 paradigm states that Th1 cells are active in induction of T_{DTH} cells, it seems unlikely that dendritic cells process antigen for T_{DTH} cells since the site of delayed-type hypersensitivity induction is in the lymph node paracortex and not in the follicles. Therefore, induction of T_{DTH} cells is more likely to be determined by exogenous antigen processing by interdigitating reticulum cells in the paracortex. T_{CTL} cells are produced after endogenous antigen processing by any nucleated cell in association with class I MHC surface molecules. Although discounted by many immunologists, so-called T-suppressor cells may also be activated by endogenous antigen processing, resulting in a temporary state of nonreactivity (a form of tolerance). What determines which process of immune induction will predominate is not well understood. Some of the factors are genetically determined; others are related to the form (i.e., nature of the infectious agent), route, and dose of the antigen.

T_{CTL}-Cell Reactions In Vitro

The first appreciation of T-cytotoxic activity came from the recognition that T_{CTL} cells could "kill" specific target cells in vitro. The interaction of sensitized lymphocytes and target cells can be studied morphologically by observing the effect of sensitized lymphocytes on target cells growing in monolayers. Plaques or holes occur in the monolayer when sensitized lymphocytes are added. Sensitized lymphocytes surround the target cells and eventually cause their detachment from the monolayer. Figure 12.3 depicts the destruction of monolayer target cells. As long as the target cells

Figure 12.3 Reaction of sensitized lymphocytes with target cells in vitro. T lymphocytes from a sensitized donor infiltrate and surround monolayer target cells, seemingly without effect on viability or morphologic appearance of target cells. As a result of this infiltration, monolayer cells become separated from each other and from the culture surface. Monolayer cells that retain contact with the monolayer remain viable, but when separated from other monolayer cells, morphologic changes consistent with cell death occur. These alterations do not occur in tissue culture cells that become separated from the monolayer in the presence of normal lymphocytes. Fluids and washings taken from monolayers treated with sensitized lymphocytes cannot be used to initiate new cultures, whereas fluids or washings of cultures treated with normal lymphocytes can. (Modified from P. Biberfield, G. Holm, and P. Perlmann, *Exp. Cell Res.* **52:**672, 1968. Copyright Academic Press.)

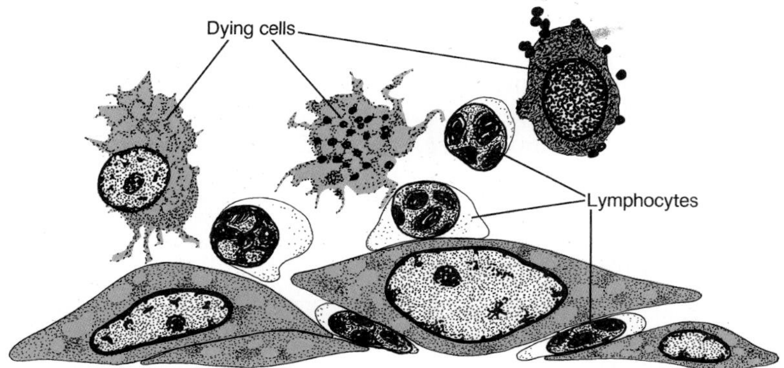

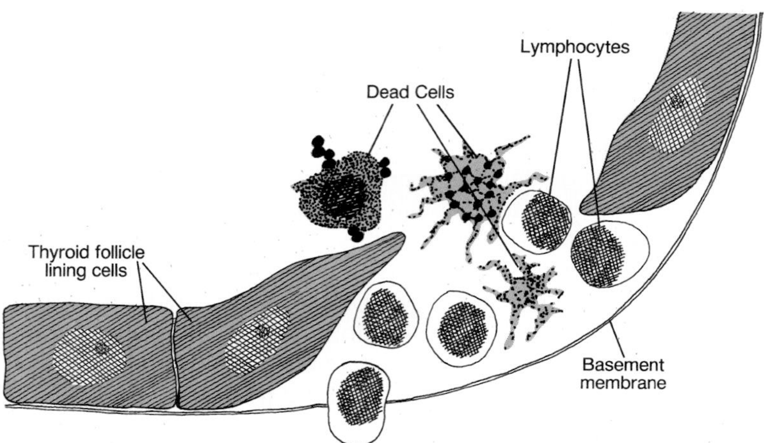

Figure 12.4 Reaction of sensitized lymphocytes with target cells in vivo (morphologic changes in experimental renal graft rejection or allergic thyroiditis). Changes similar to those observed in reactions of sensitized lymphocytes with tissue culture monolayers occur during renal homograft rejection or with thyroid follicle-lining cells in allergic thyroiditis. Mononuclear cells appear first in perivenular areas and then invade stroma of organ. Invasion of tubules or follicles follows. Lymphocytes appear to pass through basement membrane, separating renal tubule or thyroid follicle-lining cells from basement membrane and from other follicular cells. Death of lining cells occurs when these cells are isolated from basement membrane and from other tubule or follicular cells. (Modified from M. H. Flax, *Lab. Investig.* **12:**199, 1963.)

remain attached to the monolayer, they appear to be viable; however, upon separation from the monolayer, the target cell undergoes morphologic alterations indicative of cell death. These alterations include vacuolization and disintegration of the cytoplasm and condensation of nucleus and cytoplasm. Although close contact between the sensitized lymphocytes and target cells occurs, the exact mechanism of target cell death remains unclear.

An identical type of interaction between lymphocytes and target cells may occur in vitro in tissue reactions mediated by lymphocytes. Figure 12.4 shows the pathologic changes occurring during the cell-mediated rejection of a renal allograft or development of experimental allergic thyroiditis. As in the target cell monolayer system, lymphocytes pass across the basement membrane of the renal tubule or the thyroid follicle. The T_{CTL} cells pass between the renal tubule cells or the thyroid follicular cells, causing them to separate from each other and from the basement membrane, eventually destroying the renal tubule or thyroid follicle cells. The basement membrane appears intact during the development of the lesion. Infiltration of mononuclear cells, with separation, isolation, and destruction of target cells, is seen in contact dermatitis and viral exanthems, as well as in many autoimmune diseases and during tissue graft rejections.

T_{CTL}-Cell Reactions In Vivo

Contact Dermatitis

Contact dermatitis (contact eczema; also formerly called dermatitis venenata) is exemplified by the common "allergic" reaction to *poison ivy*. It also occurs as a response to a wide variety of simple chemicals in such things as ointments, clothing, cosmetics, dyes, rubber products, antiseptics, and adhesive tape, as well as metals, such as nickel in sewing thimbles. The antigens are usually highly reactive chemical compounds capable of combining with proteins; they are also lipid-soluble and can penetrate the epidermis. The antigen often is an incomplete antigen (hapten) that combines with some constituent of the epidermis to form a complete antigen. Sensitization occurs by exposure of the skin once or repeatedly to sufficiently high concentrations of antigen to induce an immune response. Langerhans cells within the epidermis are believed to play an important role in antigen processing and delivery of the antigen to the draining lymph node, where sensitization takes place. In addition, epidermal keratinocytes express class I MHC antigens and may be able to present antigen directly to class I MHC-restricted T_{CTL}-cell precursors.

Every person is susceptible if exposed to the antigen in sufficient amounts. For instance, poison ivy is not found in Great Britain. When native Britons are first exposed to poison ivy, they do not show the typical contact allergic reaction, because they have not been sensitized. However, after a sensitizing exposure, poison ivy will elicit contact dermatitis. A greater amount of antigen is needed for sensitization than for elicitation of skin reaction in an already sensitive individual. When U.S. soldiers moved into Japan after World War II, the military medical dispensaries noticed the widespread occurrence of a skin rash with the appearance of contact dermatitis. It was the distribution of the rash that was most unusual: it occurred on the elbows and buttocks. After diligent sleuthing, it was discovered that the bars and toilet seats of certain Japanese public establishments were coated with a lacquer made from the sap of a tree that contained small amounts of a substance closely related to the poison ivy antigen. The amounts of this related antigen were not great enough to sensitize the native Japanese but were sufficient to elicit the characteristic dermatitis in the American soldiers, who were sensitive because of previous exposure to poison ivy. Also related are the oleoresins of the cashew nut shell, the rind of the mango, the ginkgo tree fruit pulp, and Indian-marking nut resin. All of these plants belong to the family Avacardiaceae and produce oleoresins called urushiols that cross-react in skin tests of sensitive patients.

The characteristic skin reaction is elicited in sensitized individuals by exposing the skin to the antigen (natural exposure or patch tests). The reaction is a sharply delineated, superficial skin inflammation, beginning as early as 24 h after exposure and reaching a maximum at 48 to 96 h (Fig. 12.5). It is characterized by redness, induration, and vesiculation. The reaction may take longer to reach a maximum than the tuberculin skin test (see below), because of the longer time required for the antigen to penetrate the epidermis, and may persist for longer times because of the time required to remove the antigen from the epidermis. Histologically, the dermis shows perivenous accumulation of lymphocytes and monocytes and some edema. The epidermis is invaded by these cells and shows intraepidermal edema (spongiosis), which progresses to vesiculation and death of epidermal cells. A histopathologically similar reaction may be observed in irritant contact dermatitis, in which there is chemical injury of epidermal cells not caused by an immune mechanism. In lesions, there is upregulation of the cell adhesion molecule ICAM-1 on keratinocytes that are associated with lymphocyte function-associated antigen 1 (LFA-1)-positive lymphocytes. Thus, these cell adhesion molecules may play an important role in the T_{CTL} cell-keratinocyte interaction.

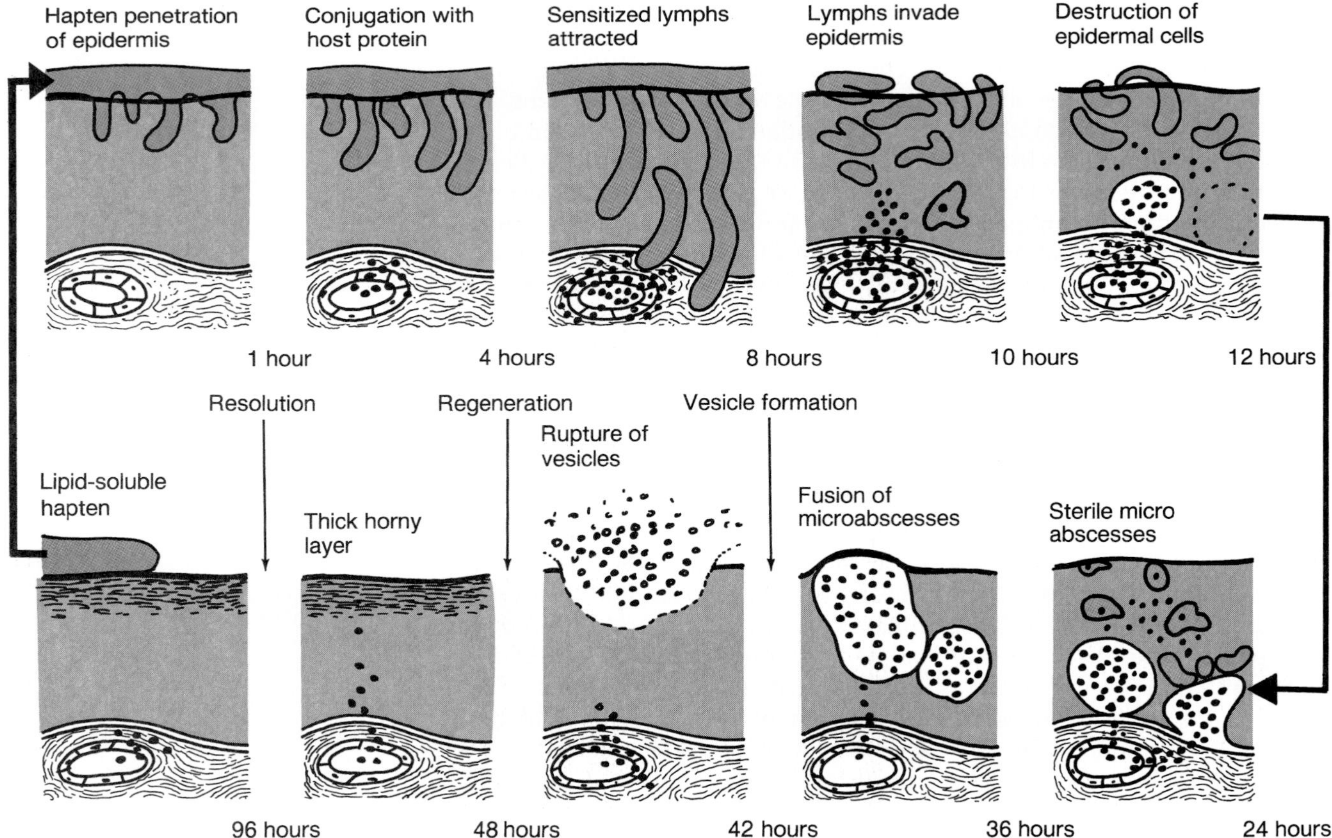

Figure 12.5 Evolution of contact dermatitis reaction. A contact-sensitizing hapten such as dinitrophenol or poison ivy oleoresin needs to be in either a lipid-solvent or lipid-soluble form to penetrate the epidermis. In so doing, the contact-sensitizing hapten joins to host proteins to become a complete antigen. In a sensitive individual, penetration of the epidermis brings the antigen into contact with specifically sensitized T_{CTL} cells that react with the antigen and initiate a cell-mediated reaction that destroys the epithelial cells.

It was once assumed that the lesion was the result of sensitization of the epidermal cells themselves. However, no reaction occurs when the local vascular supply is interrupted, and careful histologic study shows that infiltration of the epidermis with lymphocytes precedes the epidermal cell damage. Since antibody is not involved, it is clear that hematogenous cells are the carriers of sensitivity, and epidermal death is comparable to the destruction of parenchyma (i.e., of the cells bearing the antigen) in homograft rejection and cell-mediated autoimmune lesions. Sensitivity can be passively transferred with lymphocytes but not with antiserum. In addition, contact reactivity is suppressed by depleting the circulating lymphocytes in laboratory animals by radiation or by specific antiserum to lymphocytes.

The characteristics of the eliciting antigen determine the nature of the reaction. In poison ivy reactions, for example, because the lipid-soluble antigen is mainly present in the epidermis, it takes about 2 days for the reacting mononuclear cells (mainly lymphocytes) to invade from the dermis and react with the antigen. As a result of this invasion and reaction, epidermal cells are destroyed, and small foci (sterile microabscesses) are formed, eventually leading to vesicle formation that can be seen on the skin as small, fluid-filled blebs. Since all of the hapten may not be degraded in the vesicles, rupture of the vesicles by scratching may spread the antigen to uninvolved areas of the skin and provoke new reactions. Proliferation of the basal epidermal cells results in eventual sloughing of the affected epidermal cells. This process may take up to a week to 10 days, depending on the amount of antigen present and the degree of sensitization of the individual. Poison ivy or poison oak oleoresin may remain stable in the dry state for long periods of time, so indirect exposure may occur from touching clothes, tools, or animals that are contaminated with dried plant resins.

Tissue Graft Rejection

The replacement of the lost function of a diseased organ by transplantation of a healthy organ from one individual to another has been considered as a possibility for many years, but in practice, it has become clinically useful only during the last 30 years (Table 12.1). Now transplantation can be used to supply a missing gene as well as to replace a diseased organ. Transplantation of a number of solid organs, including kidney, liver, heart, and lung; sheets of skin; and cell suspensions, such as bone marrow, pancreatic islet cells, and fetal brain cells has met with different levels of clinical success. The practical obstacles to transplantation are the availability of donor organs and the cost. A national system of organ procurement has been established but still falls short of meeting the needs of identified recipients. The expense of organ transplantation adds greatly to the national health costs. In 1992, the costs of an individual organ transplant at a Houston hospital with a major transplant service were $55,000 for a kidney transplant, $163,000 for a heart transplant plus $30,000 for the first year follow-up, and $234,000 for a liver transplant (*The Houston Post*, December 30, 1992). The number of solid organ transplantations has increased over threefold during the last 10 years. This increase is driven both by the improved clinical success and by the willingness of third-party payers to reimburse hospitals and physicians for these services. As a result, more transplant centers are created each year. The main biological obstacles to successful transplantation are control of immune rejection of the transplanted organ or cells and prevention of infections. This requires extensive follow-up of transplant patients, involving hundreds of hours of professional care and hundreds of laboratory tests.

Table 12.1 A brief history of clinical transplantation

1942	Skin grafts in war casualties
1954	First kidney transplant in identical twins
1962	First successful kidney transplant in unrelated individuals
1965–1975	Discovery of HLA system and development of tissue typing
1975	25,000 kidney transplants worldwide
1978	Introduction of cyclosporine
1981	4,885 kidney, 62 heart, and 26 liver transplants
1987	8,967 kidney, 1,512 heart, and 1,182 liver transplants

Classic tissue graft rejection is usually caused by CMI to alloantigens. Graft rejection is principally determined by differences in the histocompatibility antigens between the donor and the recipient, mainly antigens of the MHC (see chapter 5). Control of the rejection reaction is accomplished by matching donor and recipient as well as by immunosuppressive treatment of the recipient. Both direct killing of target cells by $CD8^+$ class I MHC-restricted T_{CTL} cells and release of lymphokines from $CD4^+$ class II MHC-restricted T_{DTH} cells that attract and activate macrophages are involved in immune destruction of a tissue graft. In addition, humoral antibody can activate complement-mediated inflammation and destruction of a graft. Antibody-mediated graft rejection usually becomes important when cellular immunity is controlled by immunosuppressive therapy. In the absence of immunosuppressive therapy, rejection of tissue grafts is associated with mononuclear cell infiltrate. For skin, kidney and liver grafts, for example, the major target antigens are on differentiated epithelial cells: the squamous epithelium of the skin, the tubule-lining cells of the kidney, and the bile duct cells of the liver. Early histologic signs of rejection feature the infiltration of lymphocytes across the basement membrane into and between the epithelial cells with killing of individual keratinocytes, tubule cells, or bile duct cells. The major cellular infiltrate in the epithelial cells is made up of $CD8^+$ cells; $CD4^+$ cells are seen in the interstitial connective tissues. Cell-mediated rejection of the kidney, for example, is characterized by tubulitis: the infiltration of lymphocytes, usually $CD8^+$ cells, into the renal tubules. Interstitial infiltrates of mononuclear cells are not specific for graft rejection. Thus, the major mechanism of rejection of solid organs in untreated recipients is due to the cytotoxicity of T_{CTL} cells for epithelial cells.

Humoral antibody may contribute to rejection of a tissue allograft. Perhaps the first evidence that circulating antibody did play a role in graft rejection was provided by Chandler Stetson, who demonstrated an acute necrotic rejection of skin allograft when specific antiserum to the graft was injected directly into the site of the skin graft. The failure of any circulation to be established resulted in complete ischemic necrosis—the *white graft rejection*. The interplay of antibody-mediated and cellular reactions in graft rejection is illustrated by the stages of rejection observed in human renal allografts (see below).

Immunopathology of Graft Rejection

Skin Grafts. The pathology of rejection reactions is perhaps best illustrated by the behavior of two skin grafts from the same donor to the same recipient, with the second graft placed about 1 month after the first graft (Fig. 12.6).

First-set rejection. During the second or third day following the first grafting procedure (first-set rejection), revascularization begins and is complete by the sixth or seventh day. A similar response is observed for autografts, synografts, allografts, or xenografts, in that each type of graft becomes vascularized. However, at about 1 week, the first signs of rejection appear in the deep layers of the allograft or xenograft. A perivascular (perivenular) accumulation of mononuclear cells occurs similar to that seen in the early stages of a tuberculin skin reaction. The infiltration steadily intensifies, and edema is grossly visible. Migration of lymphocytes into the epithelial layer of the skin is associated with separation and

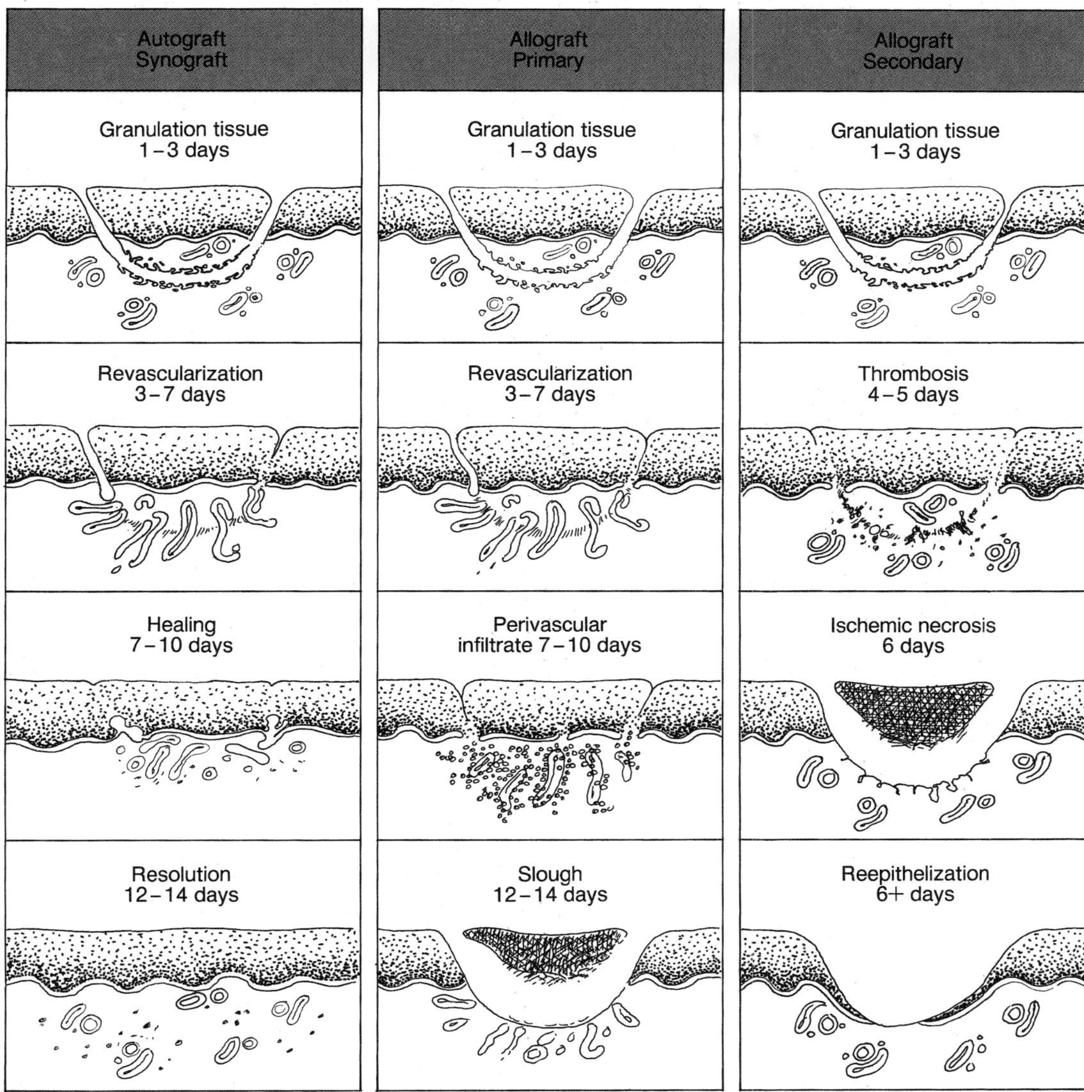

Figure 12.6 Stages of skin graft rejection. The type of rejection of an allogeneic skin graft depends upon immune reactivity. An autograft or synograft will "take," that is, survive and heal into the grafted site. An allograft to an unsensitized individual will be rejected after a stage of vascularization by a mononuclear cell infiltrate. An allograft to a sensitized recipient will not become vascularized and will be rejected by ischemic necrosis within a few days after transplantation. (See text for details.)

death of epithelial cells. T_{CTL} cells are the major effector cells for epithelial cell destruction, whereas lymphokines released by T_{DTH} cells may contribute to the vascular inflammation and thrombosis. Monoclonal antibodies to LFA-1 block interaction between T_{CTL} cells and target cells in vitro, and in vitro administration prolongs skin graft survival. At about 10 days, thrombosis of the involved vessels occurs, with necrosis and sloughing of the graft. This entire process usually requires 11 to 14 days. The synograft or autograft does not undergo this process but remains viable with little or no inflammatory reaction.

Second-set rejection. When a second graft is transplanted from the same genetically unrelated donor who provided the rejected first graft, a more rapid and more vigorous rejection occurs (second-set rejection). For the first 3 days after transplant, the second-set graft looks essentially the same as the first graft. However, vascularization is abruptly halted at 4 to 5 days, with a sudden onset of ischemic necrosis. Because the graft never becomes vascularized, and the blood supply is cut off by the second-set rejection, there is little chance for cellular infiltration to occur. The primary target for the second-set rejection appears to be the capillaries taking part in revascularization. Essentially the same events follow grafting of other solid organs, such as kidney or heart.

Renal Grafts. The effect of specific antibody and of sensitized cells in allograft rejection is illustrated by different stages of rejection of kidney grafts recognized in humans. The possible fates of renal allografts are depicted in Fig. 12.7 and Table 12.2.

First-set rejection (acute rejection). The morphology of renal graft rejection across major histocompatibility barriers in untreated recipients is entirely consistent with classic cellular mechanisms. The main feature is the accumulation of a mononuclear cell infiltrate. Within a few hours, small lymphocytes collect around small venules; later, many more mononuclear cells appear in the stroma. After a few days, these mononuclear cells are much more varied in structure, with many small and large lymphocytes, immature blast cells, and more typical mature plasma cells. Both T_{CTL} and T_{DTH} cells are active, but many non-T cells are also present. Irreversible graft injury is associated with activation of infiltrating cells and secretion of IL-2. HLA class I-reactive $CD8^+$ T_{CTL} cells react against vascular endothelium as well as tubular epithelial class I MHC antigens. Invasion of the renal tubular cells occurs, with isolation, separation, and death of these cells occurring in a way very similar, if not identical, to that described for

Table 12.2 Stages of renal allograft rejection[a]

Type of rejection	Principal target(s)	Primary mechanism(s)	Secondary mechanism(s)
Hyperacute rejection	Vascular endothelium	Antibodies to alloantigens (especially HLA and ABO) from previous sensitization, also T cell?	Complement, neutrophils, and coagulation system, leading to acute vascular insufficiency
Acute rejection			
Cellular allograft rejection	Vascular endothelium Tubular epithelium Other cells	HLA class I reactive T8 cells HLA class II reactive T4 cells May act via lymphokines or direct cytotoxicity	Monocytes/macrophages, basophils, other granulocytes, clotting system (chiefly nonthrombotic); small vessel injury; ischemic and direct cytotoxic injury
Fibrinoid allograft arteritis	Arterial endothelium	Humoral antibody cytotoxic to cells in vessel wall	Complement, clotting system, neutrophils
Chronic rejection			
Chronic allograft arteritis	Arterial endothelium and media	Probably combination of T cell- and antibody-mediated injury damage	Scarring, organization of mural thrombi, intimal proliferation superimposed hypertension
Chronic allograft interstitial nephritis	As for cellular allograft rejection	Repeated episodes of cellular allograft rejection or with a much slower pace	As for cellular allograft rejection plus ischemia from chronic allograft arteritis

[a]From P. S. Russell, *in* M. Sampter, ed., *Immunological Diseases,* 4th ed., Little, Brown & Co., Boston, Mass., 1988.

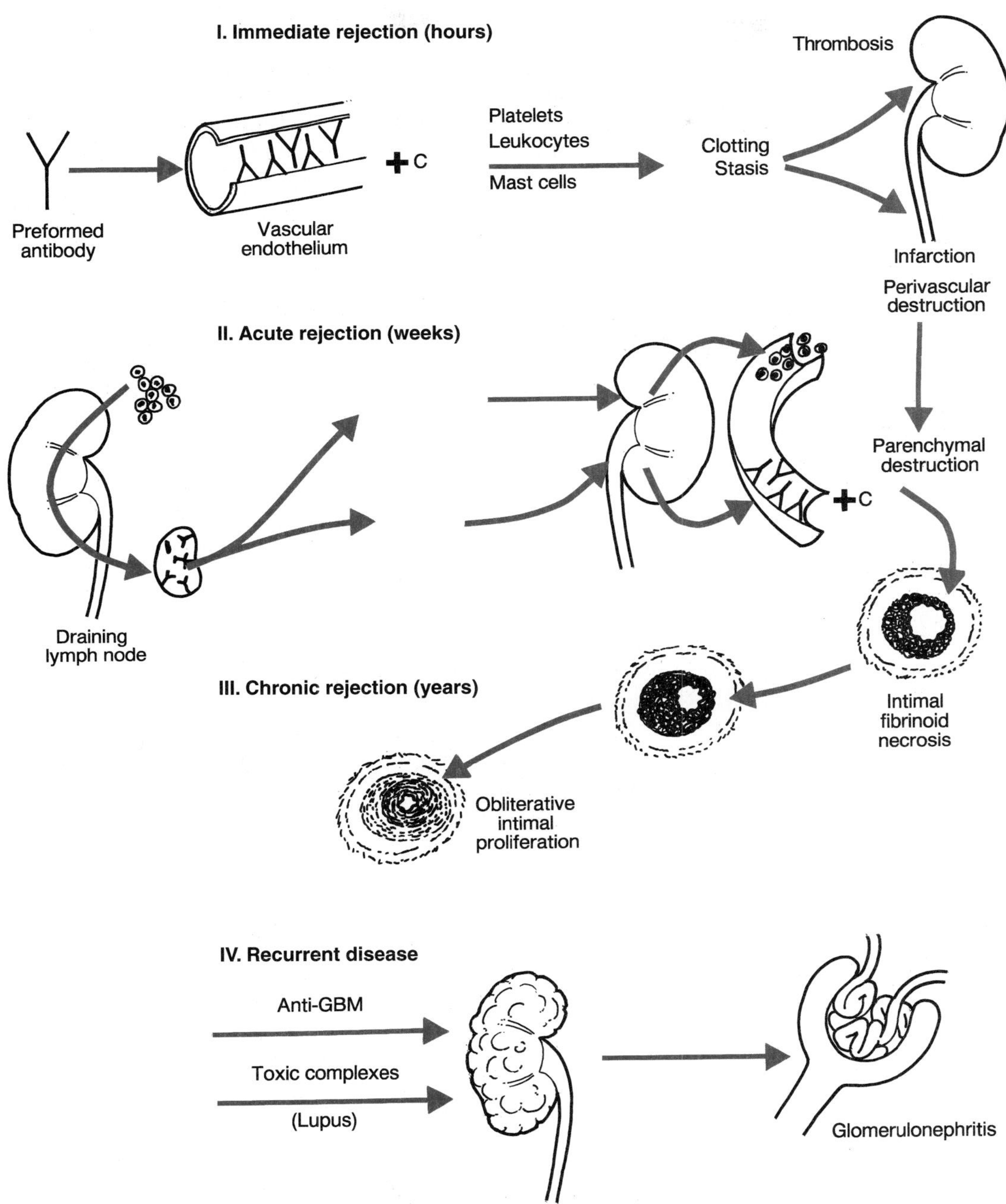

Figure 12.7 Some fates of human renal allografts. Renal allografts are subject to immune rejection as well as to recurrence of the original disease. Long-term uncomplicated survival essentially only occurs with completely matched donor and recipient, such as with identical twins. Immune rejection may be caused by either antibody or cell-mediated reactions. Immediate rejection is caused by reaction of preformed antibody with vascular endothelium and activation of the clotting system. Acute rejection is caused mainly by mononuclear cell infiltration (T_{CTL}-cell-mediated tubulitis). Chronic rejection occurs as a result of continuing low-grade endarteritis because of long-term deposition of antibody or immune complexes. Recurrence of the original disease may occur if the predisposing cause is not controlled. Anti-GBM, anti-glomerular basement membrane.

the effects of T_{CTL} cells on tissue culture monolayers and thyroid follicular cells. The interstitial tissue of the rejecting kidney accumulates large quantities of fluid (edema). Finally, the afferent arterioles and small arteries become swollen and occluded by fibrin and white cell thrombi. Occasionally, these vessels show fibrinoid necrosis and contain immunoglobulins and complement consistent with deposition of antibody-antigen complexes. Therefore, the first-set renal allograft rejection by an untreated recipient appears to occur primarily via cellular mechanisms, although there is evidence that humoral antibody may contribute. For practical purposes, infiltration of the renal tubules by lymphocytes (tubulitis) is the most important criterion used for diagnosis of acute rejection.

Second-set renal graft rejection (hyperacute rejection). A second renal allotransplant from the same donor who provided the first graft is rejected much more rapidly (within 1 to 3 days). There is little mononuclear cell infiltrate, presumably because adequate circulation necessary for the accumulation of blood mononuclear cells is never established. Morphologically, the main features are destruction of peritubular capillaries and fibrinoid necrosis of the walls of the small arteries and arterioles. The glomeruli may contain intercapillary deposition of fibrin clots similar to those observed in the systemic Shwartzman reaction. By 24 h, there is widespread tubular necrosis, and the kidney never assumes functional activity. Perfusion of a renal homotransplant with plasma from an animal hyperimmunized against the donor of the kidney produces a similar reaction. Therefore, the hyperacute second-set rejection of renal allograft appears to be mediated by preformed circulating antibodies. This type of rejection has been observed in humans when grafting was attempted across ABO blood group types. A renal allograft from a B or A to an O recipient may lead to complete failure of circulation in the graft. There is distention and thrombosis of afferent arterioles and glomerular capillaries with sludged red cells, presumably owing to the action of cytotoxic anti-blood group antibodies upon blood group antigens located in the vasculature of the grafted kidney.

Late rejection. Immunosuppressive therapy is very effective in controlling allograft rejection, and the use of immunosuppressive agents has resulted in a prolonged survival of human renal allografts. Some patients with renal allografts survive for many years before rejection results in loss of function of the transplant. Morphologically, the major finding in such late-rejected kidneys is a marked intimal proliferation and scarring of the walls of medium-sized arteries. The appearance is much like that of healed or late-stage polyarteritis nodosa. This late proliferative obliterative endarteritis is the result of a chronic antibody-mediated toxic complex reaction causing scarring of the intimal of the arteries.

Recurrent disease. An important factor in the survival of a renal transplant is the original disease that caused renal failure. The most frequent diseases for which renal transplantation is done include diabetic renal disease, pyelonephritis, and glomerulonephritis. Of these, patients with diabetes (usually males) generally have less success after transplantation than do patients without diabetes. Patients with pyelonephritis will have recurrence of pyelonephritis if the factors predisposing to pyelonephritis are still present. Those recipients whose renal failure resulted from glomerulonephritis may develop glomerulonephritis in the transplanted kidney, but in practice this rarely occurs, indicating that the original situation producing glomerulonephritis is no longer present. In diabetes and other diseases associated with chronic deposition of immune complexes, recurrent glomerulonephritis will occur if production of the complexes is not controlled. For instance, recurrence of immune complex nephritis is to be expected in patients with lupus nephritis if the immune complexes are still present.

Other Organs. During the last 20 years, transplantation of hearts, livers, and other organs has emerged as an acceptable therapy for end-stage organ failure. Each of these organs has its own characteristic features of rejection, but essentially the same reactions that occur in renal transplants are seen. In the heart, classic rejection is associated with a diffuse infiltration of the myocardium with mononuclear cells. In the liver, the main cellular attack is on the biliary ductular system. In each organ system, improved survival is related to recipient selection, donor-recipient matching, and patient management; in particular, more carefully controlled immunosuppressive posttransplant therapy reduces the death rate due to infection. Infectious complications accounted for more than 50% of patient deaths during the early era of organ transplantation. This percentage has been greatly reduced with carefully titrated immunosuppression using steroids, antimetabolic drugs, cyclosporine, and FK 506.

The most important factors now limiting liver and heart transplantation are the cost and the availability of donor organs. The number of well-trained transplant surgeons now exceeds the availability of donor organs. Extensive networks have been organized to identify potential donors, obtain donor organs, and deliver them to undersupplied transplant centers. However, it is doubtful that any public health service system can support organ transplantation on a large scale.

The possibility of brain transplantation has titillated the imagination of science fiction writers for many years, and mammalian neural transplantation in laboratory animals has recently been demonstrated to be feasible. The brain is an immunologically privileged site, so the usual graft rejection mechanisms may not be active in neural transplantation. In experimental models, it has been possible to transplant neuronal cells to re-enervate damaged zones of the host brain. In these studies, small grafts of fetal brain cells can be placed in zones of damage induced in the brain. Small groups of only a few thousand cells are able to restore some neuroendocrine deficits, cognitive disorders, and motor dysfunctions in young adult rodents, and neuroendocrine cells can integrate into brains of aged rodents and improve behavioral performance.

Human applications of neural transplantation are directed toward correction of neurotransmitter defects in Parkinson's disease or Alzheimer's disease. In Parkinson's disease, patients lose dopamine-producing cells in a part of the brain called the substantia nigra. Theoretically, these cells could be replaced with fetal brain cells, and preliminary results demonstrate some benefit in patients given fetal ventral mesencephalic implants. Although in one study, only 5 to 10% of the cells injected into four patients with Parkinson's disease survived, three of four patients had improved mobility. Although many questions remain unanswered, the results of more recent studies have resulted in cautious optimism that this approach will eventually work, and clinical trials are now under way.

Other possible uses are to restore some function in patients with Alzheimer's disease and to replace defects in damaged spinal cord by transplantation of fetal spinal cord cells that stimulate growth of host axons and reconstitution of synaptic complexes within the transplant. Lifting of the ban on the use of fetal tissue for research in the United States should result in an acceleration of the clinical development of these approaches. In animals, transplantation of the photoreceptor layer of the retina has been successful in restoring retinal degeneration.

Diagnosis of Graft Rejection

One of the critical factors in long-term survival of a graft is the ability of the physician to predict when a rejection episode may occur. Increased immunosuppressive therapy can usually reduce the effects of such an episode, but the effectiveness of this therapy is directly related to how long the rejection reaction has been going on. It is important to be able to monitor transplant patients for possible rejection reactions. The most important methods for diagnosing transplant rejections are listed in Table 12.3.

Factors Affecting Graft Survival

The survival rates for patients with organ transplants have steadily increased over the last 15 to 20 years (Table 12.4). The survival of a functioning solid organ graft is dependent upon multiple factors, including the original disease and condition of the recipient, tissue matching, organ source, time between organ removal from the donor and placement in the recipient, effectiveness of organ preservation techniques, choice of immunosuppressive treatment, and surgical skill. However, from a pragmatic standpoint, the most important factors for successful grafting are careful pretransplant work-up and conditioning, and thorough and painstaking posttransplant follow-up of the patient by his or her physicians, including psychiatric counseling. Recently, local (regional) immunotherapy has been directed to eliminating infiltrating lymphocytes that may mediate graft rejection by maintaining a high drug level within the grafted organ. Regional immunosuppression is accomplished by infusion of drugs, such as cyclosporine, into blood vessels that supply the organ (renal artery, portal vein) or as aerosols into the lung. Because of the

Table 12.3 Methods used to evaluate transplant function or rejection[a]

Transplant	Clinical tests of organ function	Radiological method(s)	Gross physiological assessment	Biopsy
Kidney	Creatinine, BUN, urine, Na^+ concn (+++)	Scan, ultrasound, angiogram (++)	Urine output, blood pressure (+++)	+++
Heart	Enzyme determinations (++)	±	Blood pressure, heart sounds (++)	++++
Liver	Enzymes, bilirubin (+++)	Scans, cholangiogram (++)	Bile production, jaundice (++)	++
Heart-lung	Enzymes (++)	Chest films (+)	As for heart transplant (++)	++++
Pancreas	Glucose levels, levels in urine of C-peptide fragment of insulin (++)	Scans (+)	±	±
Lung	±	++	++	±

[a]Interpretation: applicability and success of each approach ± (lowest) to ++++ (highest). BUN, blood urea nitrogen. From P. S. Russell, *in* M. Sampter et al., ed., *Immunological Diseases,* 4th ed., Little, Brown, & Co., Boston, Mass., 1988.

Table 12.4 Survival rates for transplanted solid organs

Transplanted organ	% Survival after transplantation	
	1 yr	5 yr
Kidney (HLA-matched)	95	85
Kidney (HLA-mismatched)	80	75
Heart	80	72
Liver	75	39
Lung, heart/lung	79	55
Pancreas	70	

nature of the data, the fact that transplantations are done at many different centers, and the presence of multiple uncontrolled variables, many of the results reported on human organ transplantation are difficult to evaluate. The increasing success of solid organ transplantation is a tribute to the immense research effort that has gone into advancing transplant technology. For the major organs—the kidneys, liver, heart, and lungs—the technical limitations of transplantation are well on the way to resolution. However, wider application of this technology is limited by social and economic considerations and above all by the availability of donor organs.

Pregnancy: a Tolerated Graft

The Fetus as a Graft

Since the fetus acquires half of its genetic endowment from the father, it is a *semiallogeneic* tissue graft from the immunologic view of the mother. The potential reaction of the maternal immune response in pregnancy to fetal antigens has been the subject of extensive investigation and speculation. Except for matings within inbred strains of animals, a fetus in utero is a graft of tissue containing transplantation antigens to which the mother can react. Paternal histocompatibility antigens are present on spermatozoa and are represented in fetal tissue. Despite this potential for immune rejection as an allograft, the fetus is not usually affected. The fetus survives much longer in the uterus than other foreign tissue grafts, and gestation is terminated by nonimmune events. In fact, there is statistical evidence from human studies that HLA differences between parents may increase fetal survival. In addition, histocompatible gestations have smaller birth weights and placental sizes than histoincompatible gestations. Thus, HLA differences may actually contribute to fetal growth and survival; HLA sharing may adversely affect pregnancy outcome. Cytokines, such as IL-1, tumor necrosis factor alpha, gamma interferon, and colony-stimulating factors, may actually aid blastocyst attachment and placentation. However, increased spontaneous abortion rates may be associated with specific MHC haplotypes or antigens. There is evidence for a spontaneous abortion susceptibility region (SAR) in, or linked to, the HLA region on chromosome 6. The relationship of this SAR to immune interactions between mother and fetus is not clear.

Whereas in general it has been impossible to induce a graft-versus-host reaction by immunization of the mother to fetal antigens, such runting can be observed under special circumstances. Female rats of one strain who rejected skin grafts from another produced runted offspring (offspring with graft-versus-host disease) if mating to fathers of the other strain took place at the time of rejection of the graft. If rejection of the graft took place 2 weeks before mating, runting was not observed. Runting is believed to be due to the presence of large numbers of lymphoid cells sensitized to fetal antigens at a time when no humoral antibody is present and the fetus is particularly susceptible to a graft-versus-host reaction; rejection of a graft 2 weeks before mating does not interfere with pregnancy. Thus, fetal rejection may occur if the mother has large numbers of specifically reactive T cells to fetal antigens at critical times during gestation.

Mechanisms of Tolerance of Fetal Grafts

The means by which the fetus avoids immune rejection is not fully understood. Some of the mechanisms proposed are listed in Table 12.5. Although considerable controversy remains, the most likely explanation for the survival of the semiallogeneic fetal graft is the *placenta*. The placenta serves as a selective barrier between the mother and the fetus. During implantation, fetal tissue, the trophoblast, actually invades the endometrial wall of the uterus and comes into direct contact with the maternal circulation. Trophoblastic tissue does not appear to be immunogenic and is not rejected if transplanted into sites outside the uterus. In fact, the developing fetus may

Table 12.5 Possible mechanisms of tolerance of the fetus as a homograft

Mechanism	Comment
Paternal antigens are not present on embryonal or fetal tissues	Paternal antigens are present on embryonal and fetal cells at all stages of development in sufficient amounts to be killed by sensitized lymphocytes in vitro.
Half of fetal MHC antigens are common with those of the mother	This is true, but a mother will reject skin grafts of fetal skin, and surrogate mothers will support ova from unrelated parents when transplanted in utero.
The mother does not become immunized to fetal tissues	This is unlikely, because mothers will develop antibodies to fetal antigens; one of the common sources of HLA typing sera is multiparous women. There is hypertrophy of the draining lymph nodes during pregnancy. Pregnancy is not affected if the mother is preimmunized to fetal or paternal antigens before pregnancy.
The uterus is an immunologically privileged site	Skin grafts from F_1 or paternal strains will be rejected if placed in the uterus of a histoincompatible female, even if the recipient is hormonally prepared and the uterus has undergone a decidual reaction (i.e., the uterus is hormonally prepared for acceptance of a fertilized ovum). In addition, delayed-type hypersensitivity reactions can be elicited in the uterus by injection of antigen into the uterus.
Humoral (blocking) antibody prevents cell-mediated immunity to fetal antigens	In humans, the incidence of spontaneous abortions is higher in couples that share MHC markers than in those who don't, and antibodies to paternal class II MHC are absent in sera of spontaneous aborters.
Soluble factors may interfere with immune effector mechanisms	Factors include alpha-fetoprotein, pregnancy-associated proteins, alpha regulatory globulin, etc. However, pregnant animals are not immunosuppressed. In fact, in mice, pregnancy actually increases immune responses to injected antigens. Factors might block effector mechanisms at the fetal-maternal interface.
An immune response by the fetus eliminates the small number of maternal lymphocytes that cross the placenta	Fetal liver-derived lymphoid progenitors are largely $T_{\gamma\delta}$ cells that can give rise to $CD8^+$ cells, which are cytotoxic for maternal class I MHC antigens on T-cell lines. Maternal cells that cross the placenta may produce a graft-versus-host reaction in fetuses that are not yet sufficiently immunologically competent to reject the maternal cells. In humans, most instances of neonatal graft-versus-host disease are associated with an immune deficiency of the fetus.
The placenta serves as a barrier to immunization and maternal immune effector cells	The fetus is contained in a fluid-filled cyst of fetal origin, the amniotic sac, which separates the mother from the fetus except at the point of attachment of the placenta. This appears to be the most likely mechanism (see text).

actually be maintained in the abdominal cavity outside the uterus until nonimmune complications develop (ectopic pregnancy). Trophoblastic cells do not contain H, A, or B blood group antigens; the endothelium of the vessels of the placenta and umbilical cord have only the basic H structure. In contrast, the endothelial cells of the fetus have a high amount of these antigens. The lack of ABH antigens in trophoblast prevents attack by maternal AB isoantibodies. The trophoblastic cells contain a large amount of glycocalyx, a cell coating of carbohydrate that masks transplantation antigens and repels lymphocytes. However, small numbers of maternal lymphocytes do cross the placenta, but evidently not in sufficient numbers to cause rejection of the fetus. That the placenta may contain lymphocytes that might attack the fetus is supported by the finding that placental size and lymphocyte content is increased in proportion to the degree of immunity of the mother to the fetus. One possible protective mechanism for the placenta is the high expression of FasL on trophoblast cells within the maternal decidua that may protect these cells against activated maternal T_{CTL} cells, which react with target cells through FasL. It is also possible that the placental tissue may contain histocompatibility antigens distributed in such a way that specifically sensitized lymphocytes react with placental tissue with minimal effect on placental function but are prevented from passing into the fetal circulation. There appear to be regulatory mechanisms that suppress the synthesis of both class I and class II MHC antigens in the placenta. Maternal lymphocytes that do cross the placenta may not be reactive to fetal tissue antigens. Passively transferred antibody to fetal tissues is rapidly absorbed from the maternal circulation, most likely by the placenta. Thus, the placenta may act not only to provide a simple barrier but also to remove and inactivate immune reactants.

Other mechanisms that have not been ruled out as playing a role, but are less likely, include immunological immaturity of the conceptus, selective and local immunosuppression, some qualitative difference in the immune response of the mother during pregnancy that promotes rather than hinders fetal survival, and reactivity of fetal immune cells to maternal cells that cross the placenta. There does not appear to be an immunological explanation for the natural termination of pregnancy after 9 months. This is most likely an endocrinologically determined event.

Transplantation Summary

Transplantation of tissues from one genetically different individual to another (allograft) is subject to cell-mediated and antibody-directed graft rejection. The major mechanism is T-cell cytotoxicity against major histocompatibility antigens, and in some instances humoral antibody may actually protect a graft from cellular rejection (graft facilitation). Transplantation rejection can be controlled by chemical immunosuppression or by matching the major histocompatibility antigens of the donor tissue to those of the recipient. Suppression of CMI allows long-term survival of solid tissue grafts, but chronic rejection may be caused by antibody-mediated scarring of blood vessels. In the last few years, the introduction of new immunosuppressive agents (e.g., cyclosporine and FK 506) has led to a much better prognosis for kidney, heart, liver, and other organ grafts. The major limitation to the clinical application of solid organ transplantation is the availability of donor organs. During pregnancy, immune rejection of the fetus is mainly prevented by the barrier of the placenta, but a number of other mechanisms may play a role.

Viral Exanthems

Cell-mediated reactions to viral infections illustrate the "double-edged sword" of protective and destructive effects of immunity. CMI to viral antigens may be either protective by limiting viral infections or destructive by destroying functioning host cells that are expressing viral antigens. On the one hand, CMI is responsible for destruction of virus-infected cells and recovery from infections such as measles, mumps, and chickenpox. On the other hand, CMI to viral antigens on vital host cells may lead to loss of tissue function, or viral infections may lead to reaction of CMI to self tissue antigens (autoimmunity).

An exanthem is a disease or fever associated with eruptive skin lesions. von Pirquet in 1907 observed that the local lesion following smallpox vaccination (vaccinia virus) consisted of a two-stage reaction. Early (first 8 days), there is a papular vesicular lesion because of the growth of the inoculated virus; later (8 to 14 days), an indurated erythematous (take) reaction follows. The take reaction corresponds to the development of CMI and is interpreted as evidence that protective immunity has been established. Similar lesions appear at the same time on different parts of the body, even though the different areas are inoculated with the virus at different times. Animal experiments have shown that protection against the virus is associated with T_{CTL} cells and that the infective virus disappears from the local lesion when systemic CMI is maximal. The same concept was considered valid by von Pirquet for other viral exanthems (measles and varicella) in which multiple, disseminated lesions occur as a result of T_{CTL}-cell reaction to viruses located at the sites of lesions. Some of the lesions of the viral exanthems may be modified by humoral antibody reacting with viral antigens to produce an Arthus-like reaction in the skin or T_{DTH}-cell reaction producing delayed-type hypersensitivity reactions; however, T_{CTL}-cell-mediated killing of virus-infected cells is the major mechanism. Lesions are caused by destruction of infected epithelial cells.

Smallpox

The history of immunization against smallpox is presented in chapter 5. Immunity to the smallpox virus is mediated by T_{CTL} cells. Vaccination against smallpox is accomplished by inoculation into the skin of a related virus (vaccinia virus) that usually produces only a local lesion. The local lesion, called a take, is produced by T-cell cytotoxicity to vaccinia virus antigens that are shared with the virulent smallpox virus. The take reaction consists of a focal necrotic reaction produced by infiltrating T_{CTL} cells killing virus-infected epithelial cells (Fig. 12.8). Some data suggest that the introduction of smallpox vaccination into Europe contributed greatly to an unprecedented growth of the population.

Viral Hepatitis

Viral hepatitis (inflammation of the liver) is caused by both destruction of liver cells by virus and reaction of T_{CTL} cells with viral antigens on infected hepatocytes. Hepatitis is caused by at least five viruses: hepatitis A virus (infectious hepatitis), hepatitis B virus (serum hepatitis), and hepatitis C, D, and E viruses (Table 12.6). The first association of a specific virus with hepatitis was made possible by the study of Australia antigen, now known as hepatitis B surface antigen (HBsAg). HBsAg is the coat or surface antigen of hepatitis B virus. Another antigen, the core antigen,

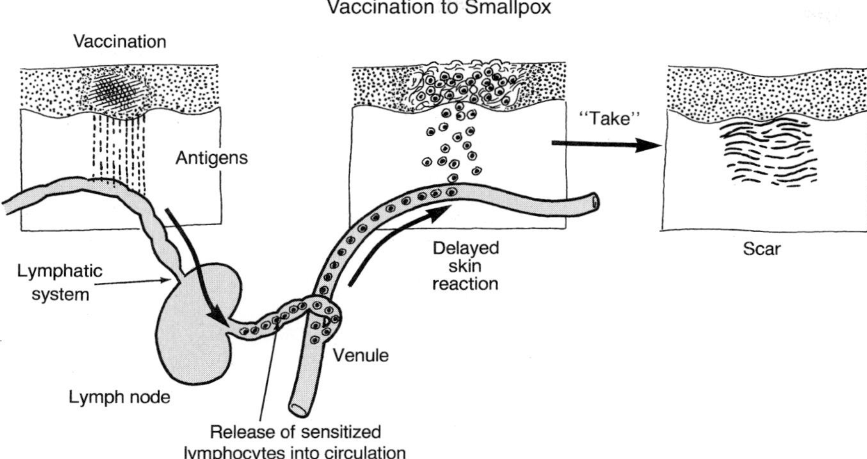

Figure 12.8 Vaccination against smallpox. Introduction of vaccinia virus into the skin results in proliferation of organisms in epithelial cells followed by development of T_{CTL} cells and destruction of infected cells. Viral antigens are carried by lymphatics to draining lymph nodes, where primary T-cell response results in production of sensitized cells. The sensitized cells return to attack virus-infected epithelial cells, producing a take, i.e., a necrotic delayed skin reaction. The take reaction indicates establishment of protective immunity to reinfection.

HBcAg, contains double-stranded circular DNA with DNA polymerase activity and is antigenically distinct from HBsAg. The core virus infects and replicates within the hepatocyte nucleus. It then migrates to the cytoplasm, where it is ensheathed in a coat made by the liver cell under the direction of the viral genome.

The time of appearance of hepatitis B virus antigens and the immune response is exemplified in Fig. 12.9. The viral surface antigen, HBsAg, is detected in the serum of hepatitis patients or antigen carriers by reaction with anti-HBsAg. The association with hepatitis was first made when a

Table 12.6 Hepatitis viruses[a]

Name	Mode of transmission	Yr of discovery	Disease	Genome	Family
A	Enteric	1979	Serum hepatitis, self-resolving	ss linear RNA	*Picornaviridae*
B	Parenteral	1968	Infectious hepatitis, most serious worldwide infectious agent	ds circular DNA	*Hepadnaviridae*
C	Parenteral	1988	NANB hepatitis, transfusion associated	ss linear RNA	Flaviviruslike?
D	Parenteral	1977	Increases severity of hepatitis B	ss circular RNA	Defective virus
E	Enteric	1990	NANB hepatitis	ss linear RNA	*Caliciviridae*?
G	Parenteral	1995	Non-A–E hepatitis?	ss linear RNA	Flaviviruslike?

[a]ss, single-stranded; ds, double-stranded; NANB, non-A, non-B. Table modified from N. L. Dock, *Clin. Microbiol. Newsl.* **13**:17,1991.

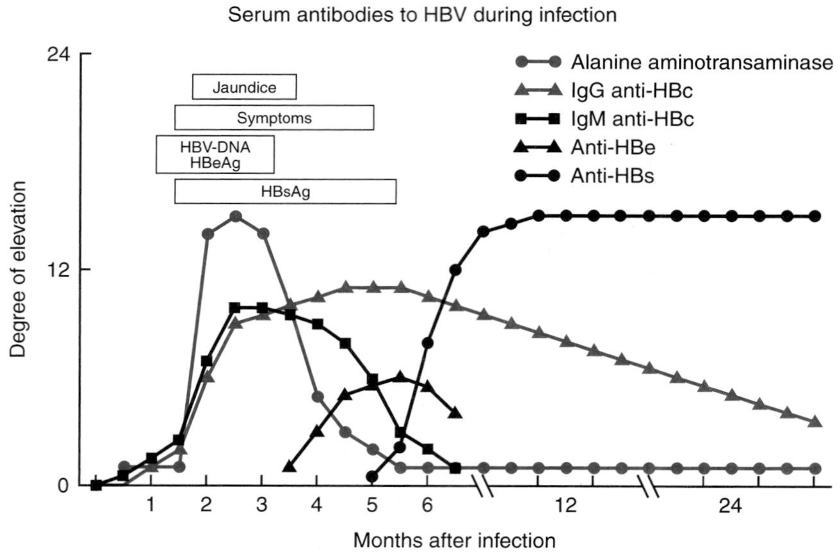

Figure 12.9 Antigen, antibody, and immune response during the course of hepatitis B virus infection. Within 2 months after infection, systemic symptoms and jaundice are associated with the presence of hepatitis B virus DNA and hepatitis B virus antigens in the blood and elevations of alanine aminotransaminase, which is an indicator of liver cell injury. Antibodies to HBc (core) antigens appear at about the same time. Anti-HBsAg may not become elevated until 6 months after the initial infection. Failure to produce anti-HBsAg is associated with a prolonged carrier state and continued production of infectious virus.

patient previously found to be lacking the HBsAg antigen was found to possess the antigen at the time of development of hepatitis. A systematic survey then demonstrated a high incidence of HBsAg antigen among patients with acute viral hepatitis and disappearance of the antigen upon their clinical recovery. Viral antigen may be identified within the liver cells of infected individuals using immunofluorescence, and viral particles may be obtained from the blood of some patients during active stages of the disease. The blood-borne particles consist mainly of viral coat particles, whereas whole viral particles (coat and nucleoprotein core) are rarely found. The detection of HBsAg antigen is now used to confirm the clinical diagnosis of hepatitis. A third antigen, the e antigen, which is distinct from HBsAg and HBcAg, may be present in long-term carriers. The presence of the e antigen is associated with chronic active hepatitis, cirrhosis, and with an infectious carrier state.

T_{CTL} CMI to viral antigens expressed on the surface of infected liver cells in association with class I MHC molecules occurs 5 months to a year after infection and is a major mechanism of liver cell destruction leading to elimination of virus-infected cells. Cytokines released by T cells may downregulate virus replication, resulting in control of the infection without hepatocyte destruction. In the infected cells, the capsular antigen is found in the cytoplasm and the core antigen in the nucleus. The acute lesion is formed by destruction of hepatocytes (liver cell necrosis), most likely directly produced by virus infection; later lesions are associated with a marked infiltration of mononuclear cells. Chronic hepatitis may evolve from acute hepatitis or may arise without an obvious acute phase and is most likely due to immune lymphocytes (T_{CTL} cells) attacking virus-infected liver cells.

Antibodies to core antigens (anti-HBc) appear earlier in the disease than anti-surface (anti-HBsAg) antibodies. Humoral antibody and HBsAg-antibody complexes are present in the sera of patients during or recovering from the disease. Whereas humoral antibody may act to neutralize the virus, the presence of HBsAg-antibody complexes may lead to systemic toxic complex disease; polyarteritis has been found in patients with HBsAg-antibody complexes in their sera (see chapter 10). The passive transfer of antibody to HBsAg has been used not only for prevention of disease in exposed individuals but also for therapy for patients with active viral hepatitis. A pregnant patient with fulminant HBsAg-positive hepatitis was treated successfully with plasmapheresis and anti-HBsAg plasma.

In summary, the acute destructive lesions of viral hepatitis are most likely due to direct destruction of liver cells by the virus, whereas chronic destruction is caused by a cellular reaction to the virus, killing virus-infected cells. Protection may be effected by humoral antibody, which probably acts to prevent spread of the infection from cell to cell. However, circulating HBsAg-antibody complexes may cause systemic immune complex disease. Type 1 cytokines released by $CD4^+$ and $CD8^+$ T cells may downregulate virus replication, resulting in control of the infection without killing the infected hepatocytes.

Warts

Cutaneous warts in humans are caused by a human papillomavirus that, like animal papillomaviruses, most commonly causes lesions in young individuals. Spontaneous regression frequently occurs and is associated with the appearance of IgG serum antibodies but is mediated by T_{CTL} cells. Patients with recurring warts are characterized by a weak or nonexistent specific immune response. Thus, a wart is a virus infestation that is effectively controlled by an immune response and only occurs persistently in individuals with an inadequate immune response to the virus.

The situation with *genital warts* is essentially similar, but some of these patients may develop progressive proliferative lesions and genital cancer. The replication cycle of genital papillomaviruses is tightly linked to keratinocyte differentiation. The virus infects the basal cells, but virus replication and assembly are restricted to the superficial epithelial cells. Thus, viral replication occurs in cells that are destined to die. However, in many cases of genital warts, virus-infected cells are eventually eliminated, and the lesions regress. Treatment of genital warts with topical imiquimod cream produces a marked upregulation of genes for type I cytokines as well as a marked decrease in viral load. Approximately 50% of women with cervical papillomavirus infections develop invasive cervical cancer, and 50% have spontaneous regression.

Autoimmune Disease

Autoimmune diseases are caused by a damaging effect of an *endogenous immune response to an endogenous antigen* (self antigen). Normally, the immune system of our bodies is able to distinguish our own tissue antigens (self) from foreign tissue antigens (nonself). The essential mechanism of autoimmunity is the failure of the immune system to recognize our own tissues as self and to react to self as a foreign antigen. When the hypothetical results of an autoimmune attack to self were first considered by Paul

Ehrlich at the turn of the century, he considered the outcome so disastrous that he introduced the term *horror autotoxicus* for such a possibility. Sir MacFarlane Burnet, in work for which he shared the Nobel Prize with Sir Peter Medawar in 1960, called the immune cells responsible for autoimmunity *forbidden clones*. He postulated that these forbidden clones of reactive immune cells should normally be eliminated during development (neonatal tolerance). However, we now recognize that autoimmune responses are not unusual, and in many individuals autoantibodies may be found without manifestations of an autoimmune disease. Some autoantibodies may be a normal part of the regulation of the immune system or take part in the turnover and catabolism of effete molecules. On the other hand, a large number of diseases caused by autoimmunity are now recognized. Myasthenia gravis, acquired hemolytic anemia, idiopathic thrombocytopenic purpura, experimental allergic glomerulonephritis, and lupus erythematosus are examples of autoimmune diseases caused by humoral autoantibodies discussed in previous chapters. Juvenile diabetes mellitus and rheumatoid arthritis are diseases in which both humoral antibodies and CMI play a role. Many other autoimmune diseases are the result of CMI, initiated by specifically reactive $CD4^+$ T_{DTH} cells and/or $CD8^+$ T_{CTL} cells. Demyelinating diseases (e.g., multiple sclerosis) are caused by T_{DTH}-cell activation of macrophages that phagocytose and destroy myelin (see chapter 13). Thyroiditis is an example of an autoimmune disease caused by T_{CTL} cells; destruction of thyroid epithelial cells is due to invasion and interaction with T_{CTL} cells, which kill the thyroid follicle cells.

Thyroiditis

Thyroiditis is one of the most extensively studied experimental autoimmune diseases and is mainly mediated by T_{CTL} cells. It occurs 6 to 14 days after immunization of a laboratory animal with thyroid extract or thyroglobulin in complete Freund's adjuvant. The evolution of the disease is shown in Fig. 12.10. The lesion begins as a perivenous infiltration of lymphocytes, and destruction of the thyroid follicular epithelium is accomplished by the invasion of specifically sensitized cells similar to the lesion of contact dermatitis. Thus, the major effector mechanism for the disease appears to be T_{CTL} cell-mediated lysis of thyroid follicular cells. $CD4^+$ cells are more active in passive transfer of the experimental disease, but $CD8^+$ cells are found in situ in the lesions and are able to kill follicular cells in vitro. In active lesions, secretion of IFN-γ induces expression of ICAM-1 and class I MHC on thyroid cells. This may contribute to binding of T_{CTL} cells between ICAM-1 and $\alpha_1\beta_2$-integrin (LFA-1) and maintenance of the inflammatory response to autoantigens on thyroid cells by T_{DTH} cells. Of interest is the finding that about 20% of cancer patients treated with IL-2 or IFN-α develop hypothyroid symptoms and evidence of autoimmune thyroiditis.

The experimental disease almost always resolves, although some instances of chronic lesions have been reported. The severity and course of the disease are not related to antibody titer but do correlate with delayed-type hypersensitivity skin tests. Experimental thyroiditis may be transferred both with cells and with antiserum in rabbits. Antibody may play a role in initiation of lesions by increasing the permeability of venules to lymphocytes, permitting the passage of sensitized cells that make contact with the target cells. In humans, a disease of unknown etiology, *Hashimoto's thyroiditis,* is characterized by intense lymphocytic infiltration and formation of lymphocytic follicles with prominent germinal centers.

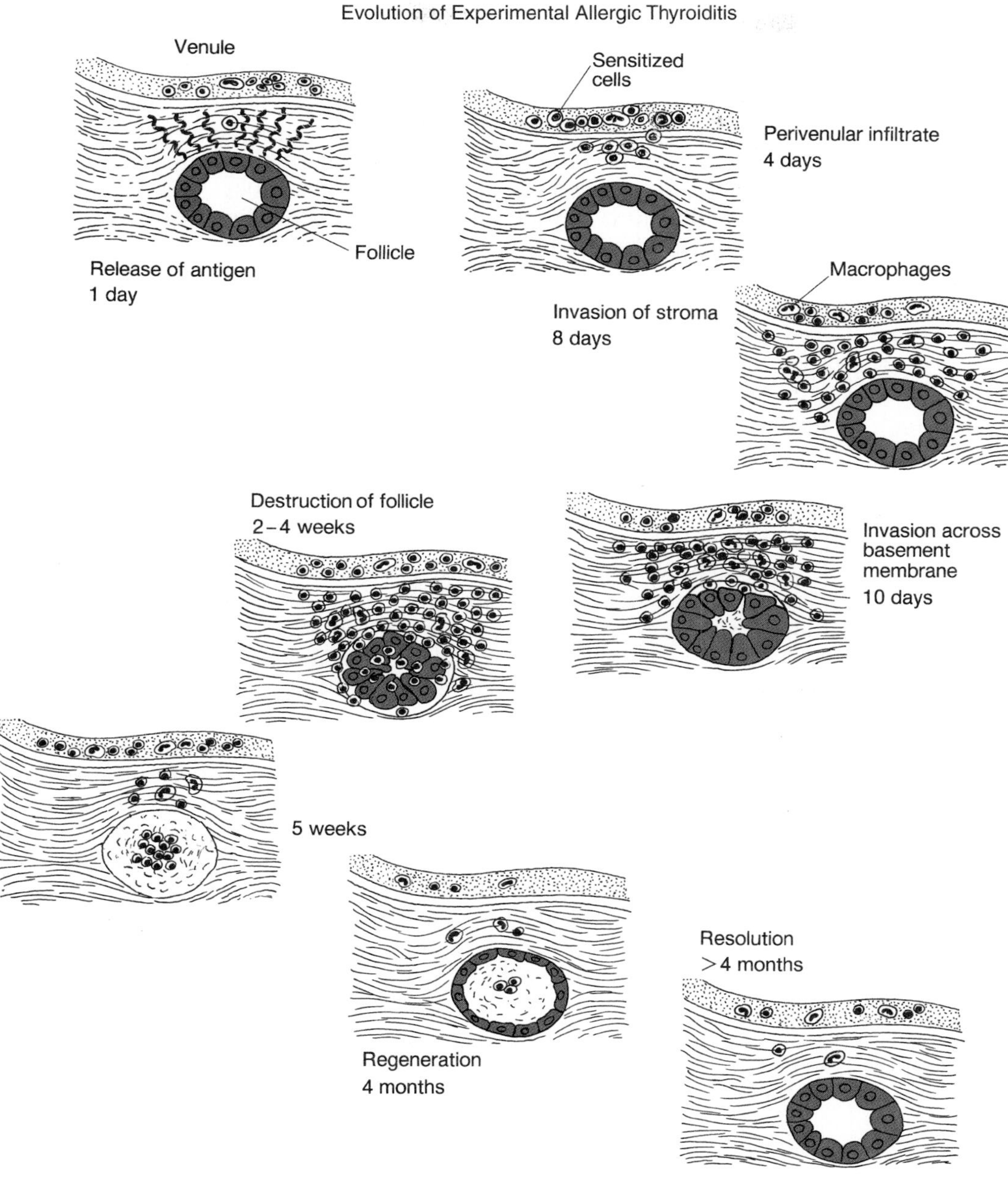

Figure 12.10 Evolution of experimental allergic thyroiditis. The lesions begin as perivascular infiltrates that extend through the interfollicular stroma to invade the follicular lining cells. Destruction of the lining cells occurs wherever mononuclear cells invade. Before destruction, the lining cells may enlarge and become more densely stained in histologic sections (Hurthle or Askanazy cells). After the follicular lining cells are destroyed, the follicles may be filled with mononuclear cells (Askanazy body). In experimental allergic thyroiditis, the lesions always resolve, presumably because of regeneration of the follicular lining cells similar to that of epithelial cells after contact dermatitis.

There are certain histologic similarities between Hashimoto's thyroiditis and experimental allergic thyroiditis, and there is a high incidence of antibodies in thyroglobulin and other thyroid antigens in patients with this disease.

Comparison of Experimental and Human Autoimmune Diseases

Autoimmune lesions are produced in laboratory animals by immunizing an individual with constituents of its own tissues. Humoral antibody-induced disease is produced when the autoantibodies react with self antigens, neutralizing the function of the antigen (myasthenia gravis), causing lysis of cells (autoimmune hemolytic anemia), or producing immune complex-mediated inflammation (lupus erythematosus). Cell-mediated autoimmune disease is caused by reaction of specifically self-reactive T_{CTL} or T_{DTH} cells with tissue antigen. When the hypersensitive state appears, inflammatory reactions occur where antigen is situated. Cell-mediated lesions have been produced by immunization with tissues such as lens, uvea, central nervous system myelin, peripheral nervous system myelin, thyroid, adrenal, testis, and salivary gland tissues. Antibody has been produced, but no lesions have been observed, with breast and pancreas tissues. Cell-mediated lesions are irregularly distributed in regions of high antigen concentration (the white matter of the central nervous system in experimental allergic encephalomyelitis). Local inflammatory reactions occur around small veins and consist of lymphocytes, histiocytes, and other mononuclear cells. Necrosis, hemorrhage, and polymorphonuclear leukocyte infiltration occur only in very severe reactions and only in some species. Parenchymal destruction is coexistent with inflammation (i.e., demyelination, destruction of uvea pigment). Byron Waksman has stressed that within the involved tissue, the lesion distribution is determined by blood-tissue barriers. There is a high correlation between the sites at which lesions appear and the passage of injection of large colloids, such as trypan blue from the blood into the tissues. Thus, in the testes, the most severe (though, not the only) involvement is in the epididymis and the rete testes, both areas provided with numerous veins that permit passage of trypan blue.

Experimental cell-mediated autoimmune diseases are of great interest because they provide useful models for the human diseases of unknown etiology listed in Table 12.7. The human diseases in general are chronic relapsing processes, since the antigen is consistently present in the tissues, and the hypersensitive state may persist or be boosted from time to time by further immunization. The acute monocyclic disease may result from

Table 12.7 Relation of cell-mediated experimental autoimmune diseases to human diseases[a]

Experimental disease	Tissue involved[b]	Histologically similar human disease	
		Acute monocyclic	Chronic relapsing
Allergic encephalomyelitis	Myelin (CNS)	Postinfectious encephalomyelitis	Multiple sclerosis
Allergic neuritis	Myelin (PNS)	Guillain-Barré polyneuritis	
Phacoanaphylactic endophthalmitis	Lens		Phacoanaphylactic endophthalmitis
Allergic uveitis	Uvea	Postinfectious iridocyclitis	Sympathetic ophthalmia
Allergic orchitis	Germinal epithelium	Mumps orchitis	Nonendocrine chronic infertility
Allergic thyroiditis	Thyroglobulin	Mumps thyroiditis	Subacute and chronic thyroiditis
Allergic sialoadenitis	Glandular epithelium	Mumps parotitis	Sjögren's syndrome
Allergic adrenalitis	Cortical cells		Cytotoxic contraction of adrenal gland
Allergic gastritis	Gastric mucosa		Atrophic gastritis
Experimental allergic nephritis[c]	Glomerular membrane	Acute glomerulonephritis	Chronic glomerulonephritis

[a]Modified from B. H. Waksman, *Int. Arch. Allergy Appl. Immunol.* **14**(Suppl.), 1959.
[b]CNS, central nervous system; PNS, peripheral nervous system.
[c]Experimental allergic nephritis is caused by antibody to glomerular basement membrane.

allergic reactions to viruses or to combinations of bacterial products and tissues. The morphologic similarity of the acute infection-related human lesions to the experimental autoimmune lesions is evidence that the same hypersensitivity response is involved in the production of lesions in both instances, even though the antigens may be different. Most of these diseases are mediated by T_{CTL} cells but may also involve other effector mechanisms. Glomerular autoimmune disease (glomerulonephritis, chapter 10) is mainly caused by antibodies, whereas experimental allergic encephalomyelitis is caused by delayed-type hypersensitivity (see chapter 13).

Summary

Cell-mediated immune reactions are initiated by the reaction of specifically sensitized lymphocytes with antigen in tissues. Two major T-lymphocyte populations are involved: T_{CTL}-cell killing of antigen-bearing target cells and T_{DTH} cells. When activated by antigen, T_{DTH} cells release lymphocytic mediators that produce tissue inflammation mainly by attracting and activating macrophages. Most of the tissue damage seen in vivo is mediated by macrophages. Examples of T_{CTL}-cell-mediated reactions presented in this chapter include contact dermatitis, viral exanthems (smallpox), tissue graft rejections, and autoimmune diseases, such as thyroiditis.

Bibliography

T_{CTL} and NK Cells

Berke, G. 1997. Killing mechanisms of cytotoxic lymphocytes. *Curr. Opin. Hematol.* **4:**32–40.

Biberfield, P., G. Holm, and P. Perlmann. 1968. Morphologic observations on lymphocyte peripolesis and cytotoxic action in vitro. *Exp. Cell Res.* **52:**672–677.

Flax, M. H. 1971. Experimental allergic thyroiditis in the guinea pig. II. Morphologic studies on the development of the disease. *Lab. Investig.* **12:**199–207.

Kos, F. J. 1998. Regulation of adaptive immunity by natural killer cells. *Immunol. Res.* **17:**303–312.

Richards, S. J., and C. S. Scott. 1992. Human NK cells in health and disease: clinical, functional, phenotypic and DNA genotypic characteristics. *Leuk. Lymphoma* **7:**377–399.

Versteeg, R. 1992. NK cells and T cells: mirror images? *Immunol. Today* **13:**244.

Contact Dermatitis

Basketter, D. A. 1998. Chemistry of contact allergens and irritants. *Am. J. Contact Dermat.* **9:**119–124.

Coutant, K. D., P. Ulrich, H. Thomas, A. Cordier, and A. Brugerolle de Fraissinette. 1999. Early changes in murine epidermal cell phenotype by contact sensitizers. *Toxicol. Sci.* **48:**74–81.

Epstein, W. L. 1994. Occupational poison ivy and oak dermatitis. *Dermatol. Clin.* **12:**511–516.

Fisher, A. A. 1992. Allergic contact reactions in health personnel. *J. Allergy Clin. Immunol.* **90:**729–738.

Held, E., J. D. Johansen, T. Agner, and T. Menne. 1999. Contact allergy to cosmetics: testing with patients' own products. *Contact Dermat.* **40:**310–315.

Kalish, R. S., and K. L. Johnson. 1990. Enrichment and function of urushiol (poison ivy)-specific T lymphocytes in lesions of allergic contact dermatitis to urushiol. *J. Immunol.* **145:**3706–3713.

Krasteva, M., J. Kehren, M. Sayag, M. T. Duclezeau, M. Dupuis, J. Kanitakis, and J. F. Nicolas. 1999. Contact dermatitis. II. Clinical aspects and diagnosis. *Eur. J. Dermatol.* **9:**144–159.

Martin, B. G. 1999. Contact dermatitis: evaluation and treatment. *J. Am. Osteopath. Assoc.* **99**(Suppl. 3)**:**S11–S14.

Vestergaard, L., O. J. Clemmensen, F. B. Sorensen, and K. E. Andersen. 1999. Histological distinction between early allergic and irritant patch test reactions: follicular spongiosis may be characteristic of early allergic contact dermatitis. *Contact Dermat.* **41:**207–210.

Skin Grafts

Mason, D. 1998. The roles of T cell subpopulations in allograft rejection. *Transplant. Proc.* **20:**239–242.

Mayer, T. G., A. K. Bhan, and H. J. Winn. 1988. Immunohistochemical analysis of skin graft rejection in mice: kinetics of lymphocyte infiltration in grafts of limited immunogenetic disparity. *Transplantation* **46:**890–899.

Nakamura, H., and R. E. Grees. 1990. Graft rejection by cytotoxic T cells. *Transplantation* **49:**453–458.

Renal Grafts

Barry, J. M. 1992. Immunosuppressive drugs in renal transplantation: a review of the regimens. *Drugs* **44:**554–566.

Guttmann, R. D. 1992. Long-term problems of renal transplantation. *Transplant. Proc.* **24:**1741–1743.

Kirk, A. D., M. A. Ibrahim, R. R. Bollinger, D. V. Dawson, and O. J. Finn. 1992. Renal allograft-infiltrating lymphocytes. *Transplantation* **53:**329–338.

Kuypers, D. R., J. R. Chapman, P. J. O'Connell, R. D. Allen, and B. J. Nankivell. 1999. Predictors of renal transplant histology at three months. *Transplantation* **67:**1222–1230.

Porter, K. A., J. B. Dossetor, T. L. Marchioro, W. S. Peart, J. M. Rendall, T. E. Starzl, and P. I. Terasaki. 1967. Human renal transplants. *Lab. Investig.* **16:**153–181.

Tanabe, K., K. Takahashi, K. Sonda, T. Tokumoto, N. Ishikawa, et al. 1998. Long-term results of ABO-incompatible living kidney transplantation: a single-center experience. *Transplantation* **65:**224–228.

Other Organs

Carrel, A., and C. Guthrie. 1905. The transplantation of veins and organs. *Am. Med.* **10:**1101.

Hering, B. J., C. C. Browatzki, A. Schultz, R. G. Bretzel, and K. F. Federlin. 1993. Clinical islet transplantation—registry report, accomplishments in the past and future research needs. *Cell Transplant.* **2:**269–282.

Kahan, B. D. 1996. Concepts and challenges in solid organ transplantation, p. 1593–1607. *In* R. R. Rich (ed.), *Clinical Immunology: Principles and Practice.* The C. V. Mosby Co., St. Louis, Mo.

Ricordi, C. 1992. *Pancreatic Islet Cell Transplantation.* CRC Press, Boca Raton, Fla.

Neural Transplantation

Bjornson, C. R. R., R. L. Rietze, B. A. Reynolds, M. C. Magli, and A. L. Vescovi. 1999. Turning brain into blood: a hematopoietic fate adopted by adult neural stem cells in vivo. *Science* **283:**534–537.

Freed, W. J. 1993. Neural transplantation: a special issue. *Exp. Neurol.* **122:**1–4.

McDonald, J. W., X.-Z. Liu, Y. Qu, S. Liu, S. K. Mickey, D. Turetsky, D. I. Gottlieb, and D. W. Choi. 1999. Transplanted embryonic stem cells survive, differentiate and promote recovery in injured rat spinal cord. *Nat. Med.* **5:**1410–1412.

Pregnancy

Chaouat, G. 1992. *Immunology of Pregnancy.* CRC Press, Boca Raton, Fla.

Hill, J. A. 1992. Cytokines considered critical in pregnancy. *Am. J. Reprod. Immunol.* **28:**123–126.

Loke, Y. W., and A. King. 1996. Evolution of the fetal-maternal immunological relationship. *Am. J. Reprod. Immunol.* **35:**256–257.

Ober, C. 1992. The maternal-fetal relationship in human pregnancy: an immunologenic perspective. *Exp. Clin. Immunogenet.* **9:**1–14.

Rinkevich, B. 1998. Immunology of human implantation: from the invertebrates' point of view. *Hum. Reprod.* **13:**455–459.

Szulman, A. E. 1972. The A, B and H blood group antigens in the human placenta. *N. Engl. J. Med.* **286:**1028–1031.

Wegmann, T. G., and G. A. Carlson. 1977. Allogenic pregnancy as immunoabsorbent. *J. Immunol.* **119:**1659–1663.

Smallpox

Bonanni, P. 1999. Demographic impact of vaccination: a review. *Vaccine* **17**(Suppl. 3)**:**S120–S125.

von Pirquet, C. F. 1907. *Klinische Studien über Vakzination und vakzinale Allergie.* Deuticke, Leipzig, Germany.

Viral Hepatitis

Desmet, V. J. 1991. Immunopathology of chronic viral hepatitis. *Hepatogastroenterology* **38:**14–21.

Dmochowski, L. 1976. Viral type A and type B hepatitis: morphology, biology, immunology and epidemiology. *Am. J. Clin. Pathol.* **65:**741–786.

Guidotti, L. G., R. Rochford, J. Chung, M. Shapiro, R. Purcell, and F. V. Chisari. 1999. Viral clearance without destruction of infected cells during acute HBV infection. *Science* **284:**825–829.

Hodgson, P. D., M. D. Grant, and T. I. Michalak. 1999. Perforin and Fas/Fas ligand-mediated cytotoxicity in acute and chronic woodchuck viral hepatitis. *Clin. Exp. Immunol.* **118:**63–70.

Koziel, M. J. 1999. Cytokines in viral hepatitis. *Semin. Liver Dis.* **19:**157–169.

Muller, C. 1999. The hepatitis alphabet—hepatitis A–G and RRV. *Wien. Klin. Wochenschr.* **111:**461–468.

Robaczewska, M., L. Cova, A. J. Podhajska, and B. Falkiewicz. 1999. Hepatitis G virus: molecular organization, methods of detection, prevalence, and disease association. *Int. J. Infect. Dis.* **3:**220–233.

Storch, W. 1988. Immunopathology and humoral autoimmunity in chronic active hepatitis. *Scand. J. Gastroenterol.* **23:**513–516.

Warts

Harwood, C. A., P. J. Spink, T. Surentheran, I. M. Leigh, E. M. de Villers, J. M. McGregor, C. M. Proby, and J. Breuer. 1999. Degenerate and nested PCR: a highly sensitive and specific method for detection of human papillomavirus infection in cutaneous warts. *J. Clin. Microbiol.* **37:**3545–3555.

Sonnex, C. 1998. Human papillomavirus infection with particular reference to genital disease. *J. Clin. Pathol.* **51:**643–648.

Stanley, M. 1998. The immunology of genital human papilloma virus infection. *Eur. J. Dermatol.* **8**(Suppl. 7)**:**8–12.

Viac, J., J. Thivolet, and Y. Chardonnet. 1977. Specific immunity in patients suffering from recurring warts before and after repetitive intradermal tests with human papilloma virus. *Br. J. Dermatol.* **97:**365–370.

Thyroiditis

Askanasy, M. 1898. Pathologische-anatomische Beitrage zur Kenntnies des Morbus basedouri, insbesondere über die dabie auftretende Muskelerkrankung. *Dtsch. Arch. Klin. Med.* **61:**118–186.

Bernet, V., and K. Burman. 1996. Autoimmune thyroid disease, p. 1482–1502. *In* R. R. Rich (ed.), *Clinical Immunology: Principles and Practice.* The C. V. Mosby Co., St. Louis, Mo.

Borgerson, K. L., J. D. Bretz, and J. R. Baker, Jr. 1999. The role of Fas-mediated apoptosis in thyroid autoimmune disease. *Autoimmunity* **30:**251–264.

Flax, M. H. 1963. Experimental allergic thyroiditis in the guinea pig. II. Morphologic studies on the development of the disease. *Lab. Investig.* **12:**119.

Hashimoto, H. 1912. Zur Kenntnis der lymphomatosen Veränderung der Schilddrüse (Struma lymphomatosa). *Arch. Klin. Chir.* **97:**219.

Huang, W., and G. D. Kukes. 1999. Hashimoto's thyroiditis: an organ-specific autoimmune disease—pathogenesis and recent developments. *Lab. Investig.* **79:**1175–1180.

Marino, M., F. Latrofa, G. Barbesino, and L. Chiovato. 1999. Pathogenetic and clinical aspects of autoimmune thyroiditis. *Exp. Clin. Endocrinol. Diabetes* **107**(Suppl. 3)**:**S79–S83.

Witebsky, E., N. R. Rose, K. Terplan, et al. 1957. Chronic thyroiditis and autoimmunization. *JAMA* **64:**1439–1447.

General Autoimmunity

Alferink, J., S. Aigner, R. Reibke, G. J. Hammerling, and B. Arnold. 1999. Peripheral T-cell tolerance: the contribution of permissive T-cell migration into parenchymal tissues of the neonate. *Immunol. Rev.* **169:**155–261.

Burnet, F. M. 1991. The Nobel Lectures in Immunology: 1960, immunologic recognition of self. *Scand. J. Immunol.* **33:**3–13.

Coutinho, A., and M. Kazatchkine (ed.). 1993. *Autoimmunity: Physiology and Disease.* Wiley-Liss, New York, N.Y.

Ehrlich, P. 1900. On autoimmunity with special reference to cell life. *Proc. R. Sci. Biol. (Lond.)* **66B:**424.

Shoenfeld, Y., and D. Isenberg. 1990. *The Mosaic of Autoimmunity.* Elsevier Science Publishing, Inc., New York, N.Y.

Staerz, U. D., and Y. Qi. 1999. Treatment of an autoimmune disease with "classical" T cell veto: a proposal. *J. Clin. Immunol.* **19:**195–202.

Waksman, B. H. 1962. Autoimmunization and the lesions of autoimmunity. *Medicine* **41:**93–141.

Delayed-Type Hypersensitivity

13

T_{DTH}-Cell Reactions: Delayed-Type Hypersensitivity

Delayed-type hypersensitivity (DTH) reactions are variations on a theme of chronic inflammation; they are in vivo reactions, which, because of the time course and complexity of the different cell types involved, cannot be duplicated in vitro (see chapter 3). The reactions are initiated by specific $CD4^+$ T cells that are attracted to gradients of antigen released from tissues. Specifically sensitized T cells that mediate DTH (T_{DTH} cells) are also activated to proliferate upon contact with antigen (blast transformation), resulting in an increased number of specifically sensitized cells. This response has been used as an in vitro test for the presence of T cells specifically responsive to antigen. DTH reactions begin with endothelial adhesion of lymphocytes, followed by perivascular accumulation of lymphocytes and monocytes at the tissue site where the antigen is located. On reaction with antigen, specific T_{DTH} cells upregulate receptors for ligands on endothelial cells and then interact with endothelial cells through reaction of lymphocyte receptors (L-selectin [LAM-1], $\alpha_4\beta_1$-integrin [VLA-4], $\alpha_L\beta_2$-integrin [LFA-1], and H-CAM [CD44]) with ligands (E-selectin, VCAM-1, ICAM-1, and carbohydrates) on endothelial cells (see Fig. 3.16). T_{DTH} lymphocytes then pass through the endothelial cells of venules and react with soluble antigens in the adjacent tissue. This reaction leads to lymphocyte activation and release of lymphokines, such as tumor necrosis factor (TNF), interleukin-2 (IL-2), gamma interferon (IFN-γ), and other inflammatory initiating factors (see Table 3.20). The main function of these factors is to attract and activate macrophages (Fig. 13.1). One in vitro test for this effect is the inhibition of the migration of macrophages cultured in agar when supernatants of cultures of activated T_{DTH} cells are added. This is caused by a factor, produced by activated T_{DTH} cells, known as migration inhibitory factor. Evidence obtained by using labeled, specifically sensitized cells transferred to normal donors indicates that only a few of the infiltrating cells are specifically sensitized. The reaction of these few sensitized cells with the antigen in the tissue causes large numbers of unlabeled cells to infiltrate the area. Dendritic cells in the blood may be particularly recruited into the skin through selectin interactions. If the antigen is expressed or secreted by infecting organisms, the "activated" macrophages phagocytose and digest the organisms. Activated macrophages also phagocytose and digest cells and tissue debris and produce TNF-α, IL-1,

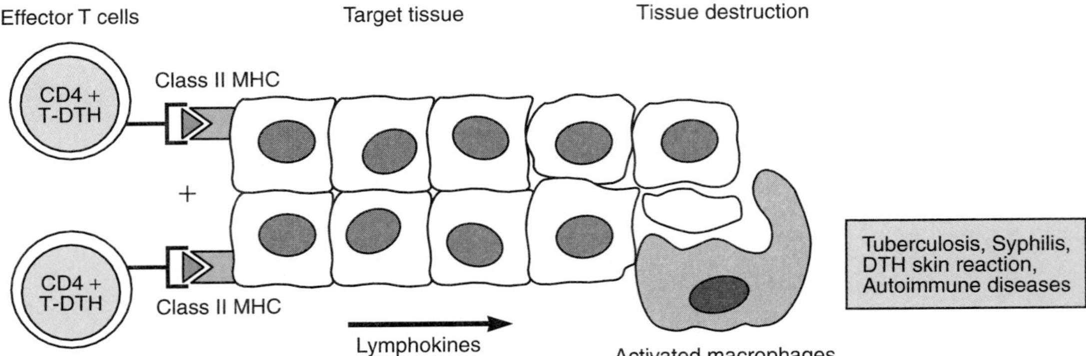

Figure 13.1 DTH reactions. Specifically sensitized T_{DTH} cells are activated by reaction with antigen on cells or soluble antigen to release interleukins (TNF, IL-2, and IFN-γ), which attract and activate macrophages. Activated macrophages produce TNF-α, IL-1, IL-6, and prostaglandin E_2, which contribute to the late phase of the DTH reactions as well as phagocytose and digest cells and tissue debris. The activation of the macrophages is effective in clearing macrophages of intracellular infections, such as tuberculosis, leprosy, leishmaniasis, and viruses, as well as for phagocytosis and destruction of extracellular infections, such as in syphilis and candidiasis.

IL-6, and prostaglandin E_2, which contribute to the late phase of the DTH reaction and may lead to tissue destruction.

DTH reactions are particularly effective against intracellular parasites that can replicate within macrophages, such as mycobacteria and listeria, as well as against other organisms for which the major clearing mechanism is activation of macrophages, such as *Candida albicans, Treponema pallidum* (which causes syphilis), and many viruses. The products of activated T_{DTH} cells enable infected macrophages to destroy the organisms they harbor or activate macrophages to phagocytose and digest extracellular parasites. Of particular importance is the ability of activated T_{DTH} cells to produce IFN-γ. Mice with inactive IFN-γ genes are particularly susceptible to parasites, such as *Mycobacterium bovis* and *Listeria monocytogenes,* which are parasites of macrophages.

The term "delayed" is applied because of the time course of the inflammatory skin reaction that follows intradermal injection of antigen into an individual who has been sensitized (see below). The reaction takes several days to peak, in contrast to cutaneous anaphylactic reactions, which reach their peak in a few minutes, and the Arthus reaction, which occurs in hours. The term "tuberculin-type hypersensitivity" is used because for many years the study of this type of immune response was essentially the study of the delayed hypersensitivity immune response to tuberculin proteins extracted from cultures of *Mycobacterium tuberculosis* and infection with tubercle bacilli.

T_{DTH}-Cell Activation and Superantigens

A group of toxins produced by various strains of *Staphylococcus aureus* and related toxins (Table 13.1) produces food poisoning, and one of these toxins is responsible for tampon-related toxic shock. These toxins are also called *superantigens* because they directly activate major histocompatibility complex (MHC) class II-restricted T_{DTH} cells. These molecules are not

Table 13.1 Diseases caused by superantigens[a]

Superantigen/toxin	Source	Disease
Staphylococcal enterotoxins	*S. aureus*	Food poisoning, shock
Toxic shock syndrome toxin I	*S. aureus*	Toxic shock syndrome
Exfoliating toxins A and B	*S. aureus*	Scalded skin syndrome
Pyrogenic exotoxins A, B, and C	*Streptococcus pyogenes*	Rheumatic fever, scarlet fever
Mycoplasma arthritidis supernatant	*M. arthritidis*	Arthritis, shock

[a]Modified from P. Marrack and J. Kappler, *Science* **248:**705, 1990.

processed to smaller peptides but bind to class II MHC molecules as whole molecules. The toxins/superantigens are intermediate-sized proteins that bind to the V_β region of the T-cell receptor in association with the class II DR protein, outside the peptide binding cleft (Fig. 13.2), and directly activate T cells. The most likely pathogenesis of symptoms is that the toxins produce massive T-cell stimulation and consequent release of T-cell-derived lymphokines such as IL-2 and TNF. Large amounts of these lymphokines released in the body cause the food poisoning/toxic shock reaction. It is also possible that toxins could stimulate macrophages through class II MHC binding, but experimental studies in mice that lack T cells but have normal macrophage activity indicate that activation of macrophages is not sufficient to produce disease. However, studies on human cells in vitro show not only that both monocytes and T cells are required but also that the monocytes and T cells must be in contact with each other. In addition, superantigen immune stimulation may increase expression of monocyte chemoattractant protein 1 and RANTES in epithelial cells, which could then serve as chemokine attractants for T cells. IL-1

Figure 13.2 Hypothetical reaction of staphylococcal enterotoxin with the class II MHC T-cell receptor. The toxins (superantigens) react with the class II MHC β chain, away from the antigen-binding groove and the V_β chain of the T-cell receptor, and act as a clamp, bringing into close apposition the surfaces of the T-cell receptor and the MHC. This mimics the effect of the contact that occurs during T-cell recognition of antigen through conventional binding in the antigen groove of the MHC. J, D, V, chains of the cell receptor; α and β, chains of the MHC; Ag, the antigen-binding groove of class II MHC.

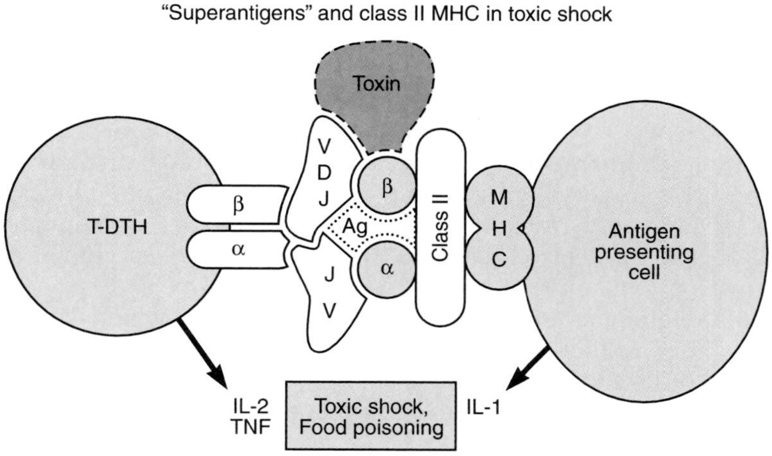

(produced by macrophages) is elevated after toxin stimulation of human cells but may not be sufficient to produce shock by itself.

Delayed-Type Hypersensitivity Skin Reaction

The classic example of a DTH skin test is the delayed-type tuberculin skin reaction (Fig. 13.3). It is elicited in sensitive individuals by intradermal injection of tuberculoprotein antigens. A delayed skin reaction to tubercle bacilli was noted in 1890 by Robert Koch, who injected live tubercle bacilli into guinea pigs previously infected with tuberculosis. Redness and swelling were noted 24 h after injection. The lesion progressed to local tissue necrosis. This reaction was not observed in previously uninfected animals but could be demonstrated in infected animals with the use of killed bacilli or extracts of the bacilli. The extract originally used was called old tuberculin (OT), a crude extract of cultures of tubercle bacilli. This was replaced by a more purified protein derivative (PPD) of cultures. Because the reaction occurred in hypersensitive animals, not in nonsensitized animals, and appeared much later after testing than the Arthus reaction, it was called delayed hypersensitivity.

After injection of antigen into the skin of a sensitized individual, there is little or no reaction for 4 to 6 h. The grossly visible induration and swelling usually reach a maximum at 24 to 48 h. Histologically, there is accumulation of mononuclear cells around small veins. Later, mononuclear cells may be seen throughout the area of the reaction, with extensive infiltration in the dermis. Polymorphonuclear cells constitute fewer than one-third of the cells at any time, and usually few are present at 24 h or later unless the reaction is severe enough to cause necrosis. There may also be infiltration and degranulation of basophils, perhaps contributing to the increased vascular permeability and edema observed. The $CD4^+$ and $CD8^+$ subsets of T cells in the perivascular areas are in the same ratio as in the peripheral blood, but the cells in the diffuse infiltrate in the dermis are predominantly $CD4^+$ T cells. The perivascular infiltrate may include nonspecifically attracted cells, whereas the diffuse infiltrate includes more specifically sensitized T_{DTH} cells. There are similarities in both mechanism and morphology between the late stages of allergen-induced anaphylactic reactions and classic DTH skin reactions.

The role of lymphocyte mediators in DTH reactions may be explained as follows. Upon contact with antigen, lymphocytes release migratory-inhibitory, skin-reactive, macrophage-specific chemotactic and macrophage activation factors, each of which serves to attract and hold macrophages in the reaction site. The number of specifically sensitized cells may be increased by lymphocyte-stimulating factors, which induce proliferation of lymphocytes. Cytotoxic factors may cause the death of tissue cells in the reactive area; proliferative-inhibitory factor may inhibit nonlymphoid cell growth, and lymphocyte-permeability factor may increase the magnitude of the inflammatory reaction by causing more cells to accumulate. An early 2-h phase of delayed reactions in the mouse has been shown to require a vasoactive amine-dependent T-cell activity. This early effect leads to the vasodilation necessary for the later phase of the reaction. It has been suggested that antigen-dependent T-cell factors are released by early-acting T_{DTH} cells and sensitize mast cells to release serotonin after antigen challenge. However, other studies do not support a role for the mast cell in DTH.

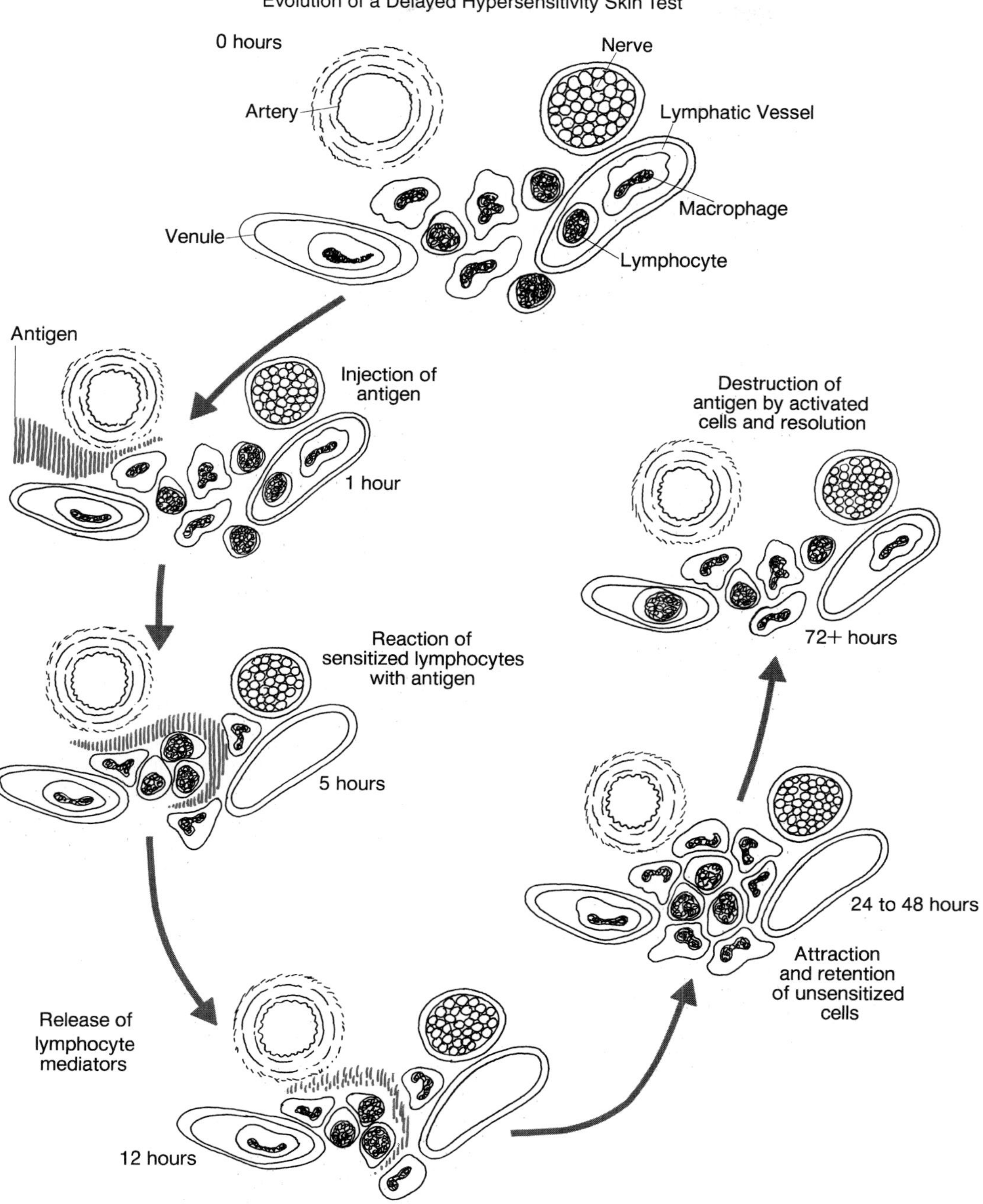

Figure 13.3 Evolution of the delayed skin reaction. In normal skin, lymphocytes pass from venules through the dermis to lymphatics, which return these cells to the circulation. Development of a delayed skin reaction involves recognition of antigen by sensitized lymphocytes (T cells), immobilization of lymphocytes at the site, production and release of lymphocyte mediators, and accumulation of macrophages with eventual destruction of antigen and resolution of the reaction. This results in an accumulation of cells seen at 24 to 48 h after antigen injection. Macrophages degrade the antigen. When the antigen is destroyed, the reactive cells are either destroyed or returned via the lymphatics to the bloodstream or draining lymph nodes. In this way, specifically sensitized lymphocytes may be distributed throughout the lymphoid system after local stimulation with antigen.

The evolution of the delayed skin reaction is presented in Fig. 13.3. This description incorporates the function of the lymphocyte mediators and macrophages. A simpler explanation is that the lymphocyte initiates the reaction, and the macrophage cleans it up.

Cutaneous Basophil Hypersensitivity

The term cutaneous basophil hypersensitivity (CBH) is used to denote a group of lymphocyte-mediated basophilic reactions that differ histologically from classic DTH reactions. Basophils may be found in a variety of cellular-mediated reactions, including skin graft rejection, tumor rejection, reactions to viral infections, and contact allergy. CBH reactions require specifically sensitized lymphocytes. In contact dermatitis, infiltration of lymphocytes precedes basophils by at least 12 h, probably releasing a lymphokine responsible for attracting basophils. The function of the basophilic infiltrate is not known, but it might serve as a phagocytic cell that supplements the macrophage.

The term *Jones-Mote reaction* originally referred to the reappearance of a delayed type of sensitivity to serum proteins after the development and regression of an Arthus reaction, noted in humans by Jones and Mote in 1934. This term was extended to cover the transient form of delayed skin reaction to protein antigens occurring before antibody production in laboratory animals, a finding also previously observed in humans. With a better appreciation of the basophilic nature of these reactions, the term cutaneous basophil hypersensitivity has been applied. Immunologically, the significance of CBH-type reactions remains unclear. Since the presence of basophils in varying numbers has been described in human tuberculin as well as in Jones-Mote reactions, it may be that basophils are not really a distinguishing feature but are a variable constituent of delayed hypersensitivity reactions or other delayed immune reactions, such as late stages of cutaneous anaphylactic reactions. Some experimental evidence suggests that tissue mast cells must be present in the dermis for antigens to elicit a DTH reaction. The mast cells may function to permit vasodilation and increased vascular permeability. However, typical DTH cutaneous reactions have been elicited in strains of mice lacking tissue mast cells.

Transfer Factor

In the 1950s, Jerry Lawrence reported that DTH reactions could be transferred from one individual to another with lysates from a population of highly sensitized lymphocytes, termed *transfer factor.* Previous passive transfer studies had required viable cells. Transfer factor is dialyzable, has a molecular weight of 10,000, is antigen-specific, but is not genetically restricted. Transfer factor-containing dialysates have been used to restore cell-mediated immunity in patients with a deficiency in cell-mediated immunity and have been used to help control infections in patients with chronic mucocutaneous candidiasis. It may even be possible to administer transfer factor orally, although this has not been tested in clinical trials. The chemical nature of transfer factor has not been determined. It appears that transfer factor acts on cells that have receptors for a related specific antigen and may interact with the variable regions of the T-cell receptor to change their avidity and affinity for the antigen.

Delayed-Type Hypersensitivity and Infection

For many years, the study of immunity was directed to the role of humoral antibody-mediated effects. During the 1960s, the importance of cell-mediated immunity in defense against viral, fungal, protozoal, and parasitic diseases became increasingly recognized. The opportunistic infections seen in AIDS (see chapter 19) have driven home the significance of cellular immunity, especially DTH. The major immune deficit in AIDS is a lack of function of $CD4^+$ T cells. Humoral antibody can prevent infections from first exposures, but once a virus infection has become established intracellularly, it must be combated by immunity mediated by either T_{CTL} cells or T_{DTH} cells. The effects of cell-mediated immunity in the pathogenesis of syphilis and viral infections (encephalomyelitis) will now be covered as an example of the "double-edged sword" of immunity, i.e., the sword that protects against infection with one edge but causes tissue destruction and disease with the other. The role of T_{DTH} cells is also critical for the pathogenesis of tuberculosis and is covered in chapter 14.

Syphilis

The tissue-clearing mechanism resulting in the healing of primary (chancre) and secondary syphilis lesions is T_{DTH}-cell-mediated delayed hypersensitivity. The host-parasite relationship in syphilis has been the subject of study for 500 years, ever since syphilis was introduced into Europe by sailors returning with Christopher Columbus. By 1498, syphilis was ravaging Europe, killing up to 30% of infected individuals in the acute (primary) stage. The association of syphilis with sexual activity become readily apparent and is believed by some to have been the major factor in the change of sexual mores that occurred in the 16th and 17th centuries, giving rise to Puritanism. The social effects of syphilis in the late 15th century resemble the effects of AIDS in the late 20th century.

Natural History

The natural history of the disease syphilis has changed, presumably as the less-resistant population was killed off. Today, we recognize primary, secondary, latent, and tertiary disease, each of which is determined largely by the immune response of the host. The evolution of the primary lesion, the chancre, the first clinical manifestation of primary syphilis, closely follows the pattern of a delayed hypersensitivity reaction in the skin. It lasts from 1 to 5 weeks, is initiated by sensitized T cells reacting with antigen, and is resolved by phagocytosis and digestion of organisms by macrophages (Fig. 13.4). Protection against reinfection may be partially mediated by antibody neutralization of organisms, but macrophages activated by a delayed hypersensitivity reaction appear to be the most effective way of killing the organism. Immunity to infection (chancre immunity) is established only by active infection for at least 3 months. The relative contribution of different immune mechanisms to "chancre immunity" is not clear at this time.

The skin and mucous membrane lesions of secondary syphilis, which appear 2 weeks to 6 months after primary infection, also appear to be a delayed hypersensitivity reaction at sites of dissemination and replication of *T. pallidum.* The cellular reaction is similar to that of primary lesions, although plasma cells are more prominent. Although vasculitis has been described in secondary lesions, it is an exception to the rule. Thus, there is lit-

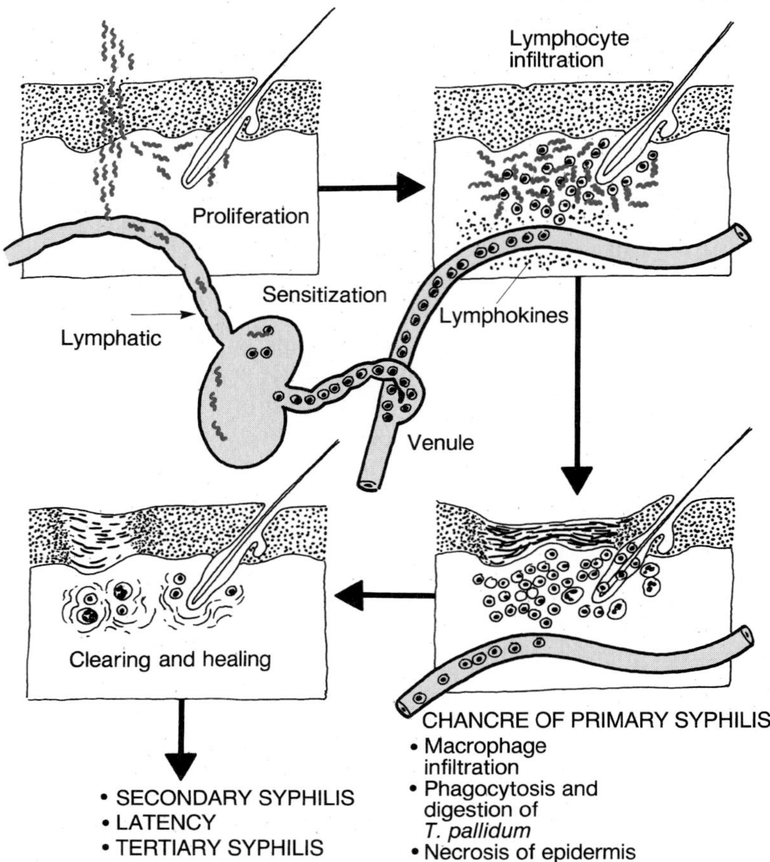

Figure 13.4 Progression of the primary chancre of syphilis. Infection with *T. pallidum* occurs by inoculation through abraded skin or mucous membrane. After inoculation, there is systemic dissemination of the organisms as well as local proliferation at the site of infection. Hyperplasia of draining lymph nodes (lymphadenopathy) signifies an active immune response. Both sensitized cells and humoral antibody are produced. The primary lesion, which is a firm, elevated skin lesion with central necrosis, is a manifestation of a delayed hypersensitivity reaction. T cells infiltrate first, followed by macrophages, which phagocytose and destroy the infecting organisms. Viable organisms remain in "protective niches" in the body, giving rise to secondary, latent, and tertiary disease.

tle evidence for immune complex-mediated vasculitis in syphilitic lesions. The lesions heal spontaneously, and the patient enters a period of latency.

In latent syphilis, there is no clinical evidence of infection. However, some *T. pallidum* organisms survive the immune attack of the host and remain viable. There does not appear to be any abnormality of the immune system; indeed, persons with latent syphilis are resistant to reinfection; that is, they are immune yet are infected (concomitant immunity).

The destructive lesions characteristic of tertiary syphilis are granulomatous reactions (gummas), which occur in areas where spirochetes apparently persist during latency, e.g., the brain, skin, bones, or viscera. Because no differences in immune potential distinguish patients who develop tertiary disease from those who do not, it is not known why some patients move from latency to tertiary disease. Development of tertiary lesions could result either from an increased state of hypersensitivity, causing more intense inflammation, or from a decreased state of reactivity that permits organisms to proliferate and initiate a destructive reaction.

At present, no vaccine for syphilis is available. The major problem is that more than 100 antigens have been identified in *T. pallidum,* but those that might be effective in induction of protective immunity have not been identified.

T_{DTH}-Cell-Mediated Autoimmune Disease

Experimental Allergic Encephalomyelitis

Experimental allergic encephalomyelitis (EAE) is produced by the injection of central nervous system tissue incorporated into complete Freund's adjuvant, an immunization procedure that produces a high level of DTH. In rats, hind leg paralysis occurs after 2 to 3 weeks and is associated with a disseminated focal perivascular accumulation of inflammatory cells in the white matter of the brain involving small veins or venules. The inflammatory cells, which accumulate within the vessel wall and in the perivascular space, are usually mononuclear, but polymorphonuclear leukocytes may be prominent in very acute reactions. Demyelination occurs in intimate association with the focal vasculitis and most likely is a result of the action of macrophages activated by specifically sensitized T_{DTH} cells; toxic complex activation of polymorphonuclear neutrophils may be responsible for acute lesions. The antigen, encephalitogenic protein, has been studied extensively, and the amino acid sequence has been determined. The major encephalitogenic determinant is a nonapeptide with the amino acid sequence Phe-Ser-Trp-Gly-Ala-Glu-Gly-Gln-Lys, the important amino acids being Trp and Gln. The astrocytes in the central nervous system and Schwann cells in peripheral nerves are able to present antigen to T cells, and the endogenous myelin basic protein may be presented to autoreactive T cells that constantly move through the nervous system. Study of T-cell clones that are active in passive transfer of EAE indicates that the T-cell receptors employed for EAE are highly restricted, using only two V_{α}, one J_{α}, two V_{β}, and two J_{β} gene segments and a highly conserved, third hypervariable region, V_{β} gene segment. Reactivity of the encephalitogenic peptide with reactive T-cell clones can be blocked by anti-$V_{\beta 8}$ monoclonal antibody, suggesting that such an antibody may be used to treat demyelinating lesions. In the experimental model, immunization with the putative myelin basic protein peptide binding region of the T-cell receptor appears to result in the production of a cytotoxic T cell that reacts with the T-cell receptor of the encephalitogenic T cell and prevents reaction of the encephalitogenic T cell with the myelin basic protein in vivo, blocking development of EAE.

Although the reaction of specifically sensitized cells with myelin antigen and subsequent attraction of macrophages are believed to be the major pathological event (T cells are required for transfer of the disease, and monoclonal antibodies to activated T cells block development of the disease in laboratory animals), humoral antibody and T_{CTL} cells may also play important effector roles. Because of the blood-brain barrier, the venules of the brain do not permit lymphocytes to pass through, as they do in other organs. Humoral antibody may react with myelin antigens released from the brain normally or as the result of a viral infection. The antibody-antigen reaction may activate anaphylactic or complement mediators, causing contraction and separation of endothelial cells, thus permitting extravasation of lymphocytes into brain tissue (Fig. 13.5). In

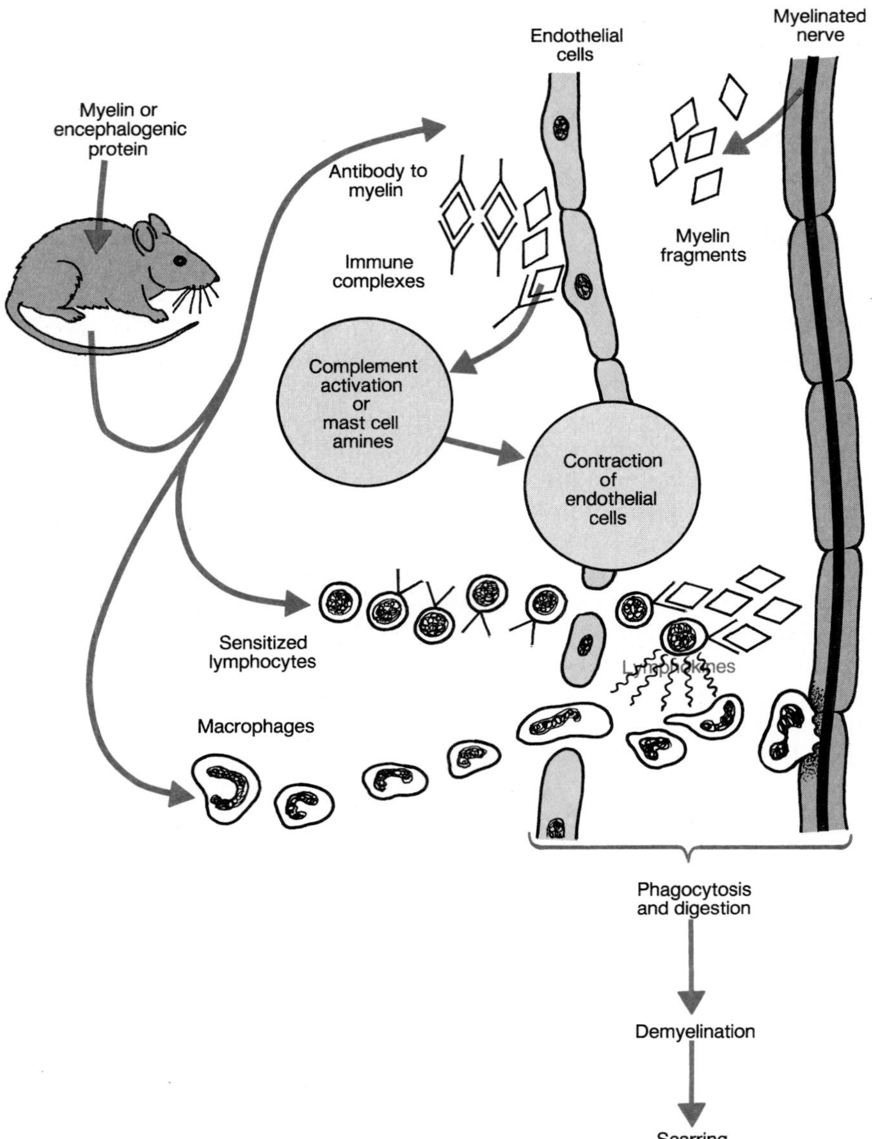

Figure 13.5 Pathogenic events in experimental allergic encephalomyelitis. Immunization of experimental animals with myelin or encephalitogenic protein results in production of humoral antibody and specifically sensitized cells, which together lead to demyelination by macrophages. Antibody reacting with myelin released into circulation through endothelial venules in white matter (i.e., myelinated area of brain and spinal cord) activates either anaphylatoxin (complement) or mast cell (immunoglobulin E) degranulation. Contraction of endothelial cells opens up gaps in small venule walls. Sensitized small T_{DTH} lymphocytes move into white matter, react with myelin antigen, and release lymphocyte mediators. Macrophages, attracted and activated by these mediators, phagocytose and digest antibody-coated myelin or myelin affected by reaction with sensitized lymphocytes. If zones of demyelination are large, fibrosis will occur, and permanent loss of function will result.

addition, demyelination may occur secondary to upregulation of expression of class I MHC antigens on oligodendrocytes without involvement of antibody or T cells. Transgenic mice expressing increased class I MHC antigens on oligodendrocytes have extensive demyelination in the brain and spinal cord without T-cell infiltrate.

The prominent tissue lesion is perivascular infiltration of the white matter of the brain and spinal cord with lymphocytes. Antigen-reactive T_{DTH} cells may first recognize myelin antigens on vascular cells at the blood brain interface and release cytokines that activate the central nervous system endothelium to express cell adhesion and chemoattractant molecules. However, activated T cells appear to be able to cross the blood-brain barrier, whereas cells not in the blast phase do not. The phenotype of the cells in experimental lesions is mainly $\alpha\beta$ T-cell receptor-positive, $CD4^+$ T cells. T-cell infiltration is followed by migration of macrophages into tissue containing myelinated nerve fibers and stripping of myelinated fibers by macrophages, culminating in phagocytosis and digestion of the myelin. Toxic products of activated T_{DTH} cells appear to have a role, because treatment of recipient mice with antibodies to lymphotoxin (TNF-β) and TNF-α prevents cell-mediated passive transfer of the disease. IL-6 may also be involved, because EAE is inhibited in IL-6-knockout mice.

Human Encephalomyelitis and Multiple Sclerosis

The human disease takes three forms: acute hemorrhagic encephalomyelitis, acute disseminated encephalomyelitis, and multiple sclerosis.

Acute Hemorrhagic Encephalomyelitis

Acute hemorrhagic encephalomyelitis is a rare disease that shows necrosis and fibrin deposits within the walls of venules, hemorrhages through the venule walls with intense polymorphonuclear infiltration, and demyelination in areas of the infiltration. This disease is similar to the acute forms of EAE.

Acute Disseminated Encephalomyelitis

Acute disseminated encephalomyelitis has two variants. The form that was associated with rabies vaccination occurred 4 to 15 days after injection of killed rabies virus and was histologically identical to EAE. The lesion was caused by an allergic reaction to the brain tissue used to culture the virus from which the vaccine was prepared. This type of vaccine has been replaced by one prepared from human tissue, and no proven case of post-rabies inoculation encephalomyelitis has been reported since introduction of the new vaccine. The second type of acute disseminated encephalomyelitis occurs after smallpox vaccination or infection with rubella, varicella, or variola (see above). The clinical course of some cases suggests that acute hemorrhagic encephalomyelitis may progress to acute disseminated encephalomyelitis and then to multiple sclerosis.

Multiple Sclerosis

Multiple sclerosis may be considered the end stage or chronic form of the encephalitides. There is a pathogenic similarity between multiple sclerosis and chronic EAE. However, animals that survive the acute stages of the experimental disease do not go on to develop the chronic scarring lesions typical of multiple sclerosis. SCID mice receiving mononuclear cells from the cerebrospinal fluid of patients with multiple sclerosis developed demyelinated lesions. In addition, upregulation of vascular adhesion molecules for lymphocytes (ICAM-1 and H-CAM) occurs on postcapillary venules in periplaque white matter, and studies in an experimental model indicate that reactions between CD40 and CD154 (CD40L) may direct T-cell migration and activation by microglial cells. It is possible that the chronic lesions of multiple sclerosis are caused by stimulation of glial cell or fibroblast proliferation after abnormal production or response to growth factors. (A "glial cell stimulating factor" produced by lymphocytes has been described.) The lesions are multiple, sharply defined gray plaques, measure up to several centimeters in diameter, and are composed of microglial cells, lymphocytes, and plasma cells usually located around small veins. At later stages, scarring may obscure the small veins, and plaques may be found with no vascular component. One of the diagnostic features of multiple sclerosis is the presence of oligoclonal immunoglobulins in the cerebrospinal fluid. However, EAE may be consistently transferred with cells but not with antiserum. Viral infections may produce an immunizing event leading to cellular sensitivity to myelin antigens.

Therapy is directed to limiting the progression of the disease. Treatment with corticosteroids and other anti-inflammatory agents has not proved effective. Clinical trials are now under way using two drugs, IFN-β and copolymer I (a synthetic polypeptide resembling myelin basic protein). Interferon may reduce the relapse rate, but the results are not yet conclusive. In animal experiments, synthetic peptides reduced the lesions of EAE. Although early results suggested that copolymer I treatment significantly reduced progression, similar effects were seen with placebo treatment. In patients with multiple sclerosis, a positive attitude may be as effective as these specific treatments.

Experimental Allergic Neuritis

Experimental allergic neuritis is induced by the injection of peripheral nervous tissue in complete Freund's adjuvant. The lesions are limited to the peripheral nervous tissue; none are found in the central nervous system. The experimental disease is similar to a demyelinating syndrome, *Guillain-Barré syndrome,* that follows infection with certain microorganisms. It is postulated that there is immunological cross-reactivity between neural and viral antigens, resulting in breaking of tolerance to self neural antigens following a viral infection. Guillain-Barré syndrome is an acute or subacute monophasic progressive ascending muscle weakness, usually self limiting and reversible but sometimes culminating in quadriplegia. Myelin destruction is confined to loci of nerve roots that are infiltrated by mononuclear inflammatory cells (demyelinating inflammatory polyradiculoneuropathy). More than 75% of affected patients have a well-documented antecedent infection, usually viral, but sometimes from mycoplasmas, salmonellae, or other bacteria. Guillain-Barré syndrome can also occur after smallpox or rabies vaccination. A role for autoantibody in the pathogenesis is suggested by clinical improvement following plasmapheresis of treatment with anti-idiotypic antibodies to presumptive anti-peripheral nerve antigens.

Experimental Allergic Sympathetic Neuritis

Experimental allergic sympathetic neuritis may be induced by immunization with antigens obtained from sympathetic ganglia. The inflammatory lesions are limited to the sympathetic nervous system.

Viral Encephalitis

T_{CTL}-cell killing of virus-infected cells appears to be the most efficient way of eliminating virus-infected cells. However, if virus-infected cells, such as neurons, perform a vital irreplaceable function, their loss results in manifestations of the disease (encephalitis). This loss may be caused directly by the virus itself or may be secondary to the destruction of the infected cells by T_{CTL} or T_{DTH} cells. In many cases of chronic encephalitis, the lesions are caused by autoimmune T_{DTH}-cell-mediated reactions to myelin, as described above.

Animal Models of Viral Encephalitis

Animal models of virus-induced inflammation of the central nervous system (encephalomyelitis) illustrate important differences in pathogenesis involving immune mechanisms (Table 13.2).

Lymphocytic Choriomeningitis

The role of T_{CTL} cells in producing the lesions of some infectious diseases is exemplified by a viral disease of mice and humans, lymphocytic choriomeningitis (LCM). Certain features of the experimental disease suggest that the brain lesions are due not just to the presence of the virus itself but also to a T_{CTL}-cell reaction to the viral antigens located on cells in the brain. Systemic infection may produce immunity that prevents infection of the brain. Intracranial injection of the virus results in much more severe disease than does intracutaneous injection. If a sublethal intracutaneous injection is followed by a lethal intracranial injection, the eventual outcome depends upon the interval between the cutaneous and cranial injections. If the cranial injection follows the cutaneous injection by fewer than 4 days, the outcome is invariably fatal, and the course of the disease is more rapid than when the virus is given only intracranially. If 7 days intervene between the cranial and cutaneous injections, the animals survive. The interpretation is that the sublethal cutaneous injection produces an immune response to the virus. If immunity is developed (7-day interval) when the cranial injection is administered, specific immunity prevents dissemination and growth of virus. However, if the virus is already distributed before the immune reaction develops, the reaction of the specifically sensitized T_{CTL} cells with the localized virus produces the lesions. In the 4-day interval, the cutaneous injection initiates the development of immunity so that it is partially developed but not active (in the induction period) when the cranial injection is given. Since T cytotoxicity is already

Table 13.2 Pathogenesis of some virus-related encephalitides of animals

Disease	Species	Suspected mechanism(s)
Lymphocytic choriomeningitis	Mouse	T_{CTL}-cell reaction to virus antigens on neurons
Mouse hepatitis virus encephalitis	Mouse	Viral destruction of myelin
Canine distemper	Dog	Postinfectious T_{DTH}-cell autoimmunity to myelin or slowly progressing virus destruction
Theiler's virus myelitis	Mouse	Postinfectious autoimmunity to myelin
Marek's disease	Chicken	Postinfectious autoimmunity to myelin
Visna	Sheep	Primary infection of monocytes, T_{DTH}-cell destruction of myelin

partially developed, the onset of symptoms caused by reaction of T_{CTL} cells with viral antigens on infected cells occurs earlier than when the induction of generalized immunity and the cranial injection of the virus occur at the same time. Further evidence that T_{CTL} cells are the mechanism responsible for the actual production of lesions is that procedures that suppress it (administration of immunosuppressive drugs, irradiation, thymectomy at birth, or antilymphocyte serum) markedly suppress the development of the symptoms of LCM. Some of the mice so treated may remain completely asymptomatic, even though viable virus can be isolated from brain tissue. However, these mice may develop immune complex-mediated disease because of the production of humoral antibody to LCM virus and the formation of circulating antibody-antigen complexes.

The role of histocompatibility (MHC) restriction in killing of virus-infected target cells was worked out by Rolf Zinkernagel and Peter Doherty using the LCM model. Specifically sensitized T_{CTL} cells will not lyse LCM virus-infected target cells unless the T_{CTL} cells also recognize class I MHC antigens on the target cells. Adoptive immunization (passive transfer) of T_{CTL} cells sensitized to LCM virus or to immunosuppressed LCM virus-infected mice causes a fatal reaction within 2 to 4 days. The fatal disease occurs only when the T_{CTL} cells can recognize both viral antigens and MHC antigens on the target cells. Thus, cell injury in LCM is mediated by class I MHC-restricted T_{CTL} cells.

Mouse Hepatitis Virus Encephalitis

Virus-induced demyelination that does not depend upon an immune response is exemplified by mouse hepatitis virus. Mouse hepatitis virus infects oligodendrocytes and produces plaques of demyelination. Viral antigens are detectable in glial cells, which are intimately associated with myelin. Demyelination is believed to be caused by virus infection. In contrast to LCM, immunosuppressive treatment increases the rate of mortality in infected mice. Demyelination occurs randomly with no relation to blood vessels, in contrast to what is observed in EAE. Lymphocyte infiltration is scanty and rarely detected before demyelination. Thus, this infection illustrates that some virus infections may cause demyelination directly without the action of immune cells.

Canine Distemper

The relationship of an inadequate or inappropriate immune response to a virus-induced disease is seen in a naturally occurring infectious disease of dogs, canine distemper. The canine distemper paramyxovirus is closely related to human measles virus and produces a disease in dogs similar to human measles and the related neurologic diseases acute encephalitis, postinfectious encephalitis, and subacute sclerosing panencephalitis (SSPE) (see below). Canine distemper produces an acute systemic disease from which most animals recover. Following this disease, however, a certain proportion of the affected animals go on to develop a demyelinating postinfectious encephalomyelitis, the pathology of which is similar to that of EAE. The chronic phase of distemper is called "old dog encephalitis" and bears similarities to human SSPE. The distemper virus enters the brain during the acute systemic viremia, and viral inclusions can be found in glial cells. The postinfectious disease develops suddenly after a latent period of several weeks, even though it can be assumed that the virus particles are in the brain throughout the latent period. Although the role of immunopathologic mechanisms in the disease remains unclear, antibodies to viral antigens and to myelin appear in high titers in the sera of affected dogs. Since the virus does not appear to cause tissue destruction, it is likely that the demyelination is due to sensitized lymphocytes reacting to either viral antigens present in myelinated tissue or to myelin antigens rendered immunogenic from the viral infection. Humoral antibody may play a role in initiating vascular reactions or may actually be protective (e.g., blocking antibody).

Theiler's Myelitis

Theiler's myelitis is an inflammatory demyelination of the spinal cord of mice occurring 1 to 3 months after infection with Theiler's mouse encephalitis virus. After initial involvement of the gray matter, patchy demyelination occurs. The pathologic picture is similar to that of EAE (see above) and is used as a model of multiple sclerosis. In this model, deletion of $CD4^+$ T cells but not of $CD8^+$ T cells greatly increases the degree of demyelination, suggesting a T_{CTL}-cell demyelination mechanism that may be controlled by $CD4^+$ cells. Immunosuppression increases the virus particles, but they are not present in the areas of demyelination. This demyelination is believed to be caused by postinfectious autosensitization to myelin.

Marek's Disease

Marek's disease is a herpesvirus-induced lymphoproliferative disease of chickens that also induces paralysis associated with perivascular infiltration of mononuclear cells and demyelination. It is postulated that there is an autosensitization to myelin, and a number of observations indicate that the demyelination is T cell dependent. The mechanism of autosensitization in this disease is not known, but the lesions are similar to those of EAE in animals and Guillain-Barré syndrome.

Visna

Visna is a primary infection of macrophages and lymphocytes of sheep with a lentivirus with properties similar to those of human immunodeficiency virus (HIV). In contrast to HIV, however, there is little evidence of immune suppression. Usually, the infected sheep mount a strong immunoprotective response. However, in some cases there is a progressive meningitis and periventricular inflammation associated with perivascular mononuclear cell infiltration and demyelination. $CD4^+$ cells predominate immediately perivascularly, but $CD8^+$ cells are seen infiltrating the parenchyma, suggesting that T_{CTL} cells are the main effector cells.

Viral Encephalitides of Humans

The viral encephalitides of humans occur in a variety of forms, depending upon the nature of the infecting agent and the type and intensity of the immune response. The disorders are classified as acute, postinfectious, latent, chronic, and slow (Table 13.3).

In the acute encephalitides (poliomyelitis, rabies, and herpes simplex), the virus destroys nerve cells directly in a predictable fashion. The immune response is protective in the sense that it blocks the destructive aspects of the disease by elimination of the virus.

Postinfectious encephalomyelitis follows a mild virus infection and is caused by an autoimmune reaction of sensitized cells with myelin,

Table 13.3 Viral encephalitides of humans

Type	Example(s)	Mechanism(s)
Acute	Polio, rabies, herpes, equine encephalitis	Virus destruction of cells, immune response protective
Postinfectious	Postvaccinial, postvirus infection	Lymphocyte-mediated destruction (autoimmune?; mumps, measles, multiple sclerosis?)
Latent	Progressive multifocal leukoencephalopathy	Inadequate protective immunity because of secondary immune deficiency (leukemia or lymphoma), T_{CTL} cell-mediated attack on virus-infected cells.
Chronic or slow	SSPE, kuru, Creutzfeldt-Jakob disease, amyotrophic lateral sclerosis?	Persistent infection because of lack of protective response, alteration of specialized function of infected cells

presumably because of the presence of altered host antigen or virus antigen-host myelin combinations. The virus alone does not produce significant destruction. Such reactions may follow infections such as mumps, measles, or distemper or rabies or vaccinia virus vaccination.

Latent viral infections are caused by a change in the relation of the host's immune response to a virus infection that has not produced clinical manifestations, so that clinical symptoms become manifest. This may occur because of an increase or a decrease in the host's immune state. Progressive multifocal leukoencephalopathy occurs in patients whose immune state is lowered (leukemia or lymphoma). Destruction of brain cells occurs in the absence of significant inflammation. Cytomegalic inclusion disease, a systemic virus infection, also occurs in patients with depressed ability to mount an immune response, (e.g., patients with AIDS or kidney transplant recipients undergoing immunosuppression with drugs). On the other hand, symptoms related to lymphocytic choriomeningitis may be produced in laboratory animals with latent infections by increasing their immune response to lymphocytic choriomeningitis virus. The lesions contain numerous mononuclear inflammatory cells. Because of an immune response to the virus, not only virus infected cells but also uninfected cells in the areas of inflammation may be destroyed (innocent bystander reaction). Human T-cell leukemia virus type 1 (HTLV-1) encephalitis is also believed to be caused by immune destruction of infected cells. HTLV-1-associated demyelination mimics the progressive form of multiple sclerosis. The blood and spinal fluid contain antibodies to HTLV-1 and high precursor frequencies of $CD8^+$, MHC class I-restricted T_{CTL} cells specific for HTLV-1 proteins that correlate with the degree of disease. The major pathologic findings are chronic meningitis and perivascular mononuclear cell infiltrates. The most likely pathogenesis is destruction of HTLV-1-infected cells by specific T_{CTL} cells. HIV encephalopathy often has histopathologic features typical of viral inflammation, including perivascular round cell infiltrate and glial nodules containing virus but may also be associated with neuronal loss or no change (see chapter 19).

Chronic encephalomyelitis features an irregular protracted course with variation in immune reactivity and brain cell destruction by virus. The condition of subacute sclerosing panencephalitis is believed to be a later manifestation in adults following measles infection in childhood. Affected patients have brain cell inclusions and high antibody titers to measles virus. Some change in the relation between protective immunity and virus infection is believed to occur, but it is not clear whether the allergic reaction or the virus itself is the cause of the destruction. Multiple sclerosis is a chronic remitting disease with the occurrence of repeated attacks, whereas subacute SSPE is an unremitting progressive disease caused by the dissemination of a defective yet replicating virus. SSPE is probably caused by an inadequate protective immune response to the virus, whereas multiple sclerosis may be caused by a delayed hypersensitivity response to myelin.

Slow virus infections, such as kuru and Creutzfeldt-Jakob disease, have a regular protracted fatal course following a long latent period. These diseases are characterized by abnormal membrane accumulations. The responsible agents have not been characterized but appear to consist of "prion proteins" with characteristics of membrane proteins with no RNA or DNA component. No inflammatory response or immune reactivity of the host can be demonstrated; the course of the disease is determined by characteristics of the agent. Kuru occurs in certain native tribes of New Guinea. Its incidence has decreased sharply since the discontinuation of ritual cannibalism, which involved removal of the brain and widespread contamination of those preparing the brain for consumption with tissue containing millions of infective doses of kuru. Kuru is caused by the progressive proliferation and dissemination of an agent that provokes no immune response and is normally not infective but becomes so if large amounts of the agent are introduced through the skin, such as occurs during preparation of brains for ritual eating.

Amyotrophic lateral sclerosis is a disease of unknown origin associated with destruction or injury of anterior cells in the spinal cord and pyramidal cells in the cerebral cortex. Persistent infection with a virus, such as LCM virus, can alter luxury functions of certain cells without affecting vital functions. Viral infections of neural cells may not actually destroy the cells but can alter their neurotransmitter function. Thus, although the function of these cells is lost, the infected cells are not destroyed by either virus or immune response to the virus. Patients with amyotrophic lateral sclerosis often have circulating immune complexes. Identification of the antigen in these complexes may give an important clue to the etiologic agent.

T_{CTL} and T_{DTH} Cells, Tuberculosis, and Leprosy

Because granulomas are a major feature of tuberculosis and leprosy, the role of T_{DTH} cell-mediated immunity in the pathogenesis and protection to tuberculosis is covered in chapter 14. However, since T-cell-mediated immunity is paramount in these diseases, they are mentioned briefly here. Although the reaction to tuberculosis or leprosy has been considered to be a classic example of a DTH reaction whereby T_{DTH} cells react with tubercular or lepromatous antigens and release lymphokines (IFN-γ, IL-2, etc.) that activate macrophages to kill bacilli that have been ingested by macrophages, T_{CTL}-cell-mediated cytotoxicity may also be called into play. T_{CTL} cells may lyse incompetent macrophages that contain bacilli that they are unable to digest. The microorganisms are thus released into a toxic extracellular environment or are made available for phagocytosis by fully competent macrophages. In this way, intracellular organisms that may persist in a protected niche are booted out and destroyed. Failure of this mechanism to operate may result in long-standing "latent" infections that may become reactivated by changing immune status with age or immunosuppressive therapy.

Summary

DTH reactions are unleashed when antigens react with $CD4^+$ T_{DTH}-sensitized cells. The tissue lesions are caused by macrophages that are attracted and activated through the release of lymphokines such as IFN-γ, MIF, and IL-2. Activated macrophages phagocytose and destroy foreign organisms in protective responses but may also destroy host tissue cells in immunopathologic reactions. DTH reactions discussed as examples of this reactivity are delayed-type skin test reactions (tuberculin), immune response to syphilis infection, and autoimmune and virus-related encephalomyelitis. T_{CTL}- and T_{DTH}-cell activity is called into play in the intracellular infections with mycobacteria.

Bibliography

General

Ahmed, A. R., and D. A. Blox. 1983. Delayed-type hypersensitivity skin testing. A review. *Arch. Dermatol.* **119:**934–945.

Cohen, S. 1986. Symposium on cell mediated immunity in human disease. *Hum. Pathol.* **17:**111–178.

Dvorak, H. F., M. C. Mihm, Jr., A. M. Dvorak, R. A. Johnson, E. J. Manseau, et al. 1974. Morphology of delayed type hypersensitivity reactions in man. I. Quantitative description of the inflammatory response. *Lab. Investig.* **31:**111–130.

Ferreri, N. R., I. Millet, V. Paliwal, W. Herzog, D. Solomon, R. Ramabhadran, and P. W. Askenase. 1991. Induction of macrophage TNFα, IL-1, IL-6 and PGE_2 production by DTH-initiating factors. *Cell. Immunol.* **137:**389–405.

Gell, P. G. H., and B. Benacerraf. 1961. Delayed hypersensitivity to simple protein antigens. *Adv. Immunol.* **1:**319–343.

Seabrook, T., B. Au, J. Dickstein, X. Zhang, B. Ristevski, and J. B. Hay. 1999. The traffic of resting lymphocytes through delayed hypersensitivity and chronic inflammatory lesions: a dynamic equilibrium. *Semin. Immunol.* **11:**115–123.

Simon, F. A., and F. F. Rackeman. 1934. The development of hypersensitiveness in man. I. Following intradermal injection of the antigen. *J. Allergy* **5:**439–450.

Turk, J. L. 1967. *Delayed Hypersensitivity.* John Wiley & Sons, Inc., New York, N.Y.

Waksman, B. H. 1960. Delayed hypersensitivity: a growing class of immunological phenomena. *J. Allergy* **31:**468–475.

Superantigens

Cantor, H., A. L. Crump, V. K. Raman, H. Liu, J. S. Markowitz, M. J. Grusby, and L. H. Glimcher. 1993. Immunoregulatory effects of superantigens: interactions of staphylococcal enterotoxins with host MHC and non-MHC products. *Immunol. Rev.* **131:**27–42.

Gerwien, J., M. Neilsen, T. Labuda, M. H. Nissen, A. Svejgaard, C. Beisler, C. Ropke, and N. Odum. 1999. Cutting edge: TCR stimulation by antibody and bacterial superantigen induces Stat3 activation in human T cells. *J. Immunol.* **163:**1742–1745.

Herman, A., J. W. Kappler, P. Marrack, and A. M. Pullen. 1991. Superantigens: mechanism of T-cell stimulation and role in immune responses. *Annu. Rev. Immunol.* **9:**745–772.

Krakauer, T. 1999. Immune response to staphylococcal superantigens. *Immunol. Res.* **20:**163–173.

Lavoie, P. M., J. Thibodeau, F. Erard, and R. P. Sekaly. 1999. Understanding the mechanism of action of bacterial superantigens from a decade of research. *Immunol. Rev.* **168:**257–269.

Li, H., A. Llera, E. L. Malchiodi, and R. A. Mariuzza. 1999. The structural basis of T cell activation by superantigens. *Annu. Rev. Immunol.* **17:**435–466.

DTH Skin Reaction

Koch, R. 1890. Weitere Mittheilungen über ein Helmittel gegen Tuberculose. *Dtsch. Med. Wochenschr.* **16:**1029.

Pais, T. F., R. A. Silva, B. Smedegaard, R. Appelberg, and P. Andersen. 1998. Analysis of T cells recruited during delayed-type hypersensitivity to purified protein derivative (PPD) versus challenge with tuberculosis infection. *Immunology* **95:**69–75.

Seiter, S., P. Engel, N. Fohr, and M. Zoller. 1999. Mitigation of delayed-type hypersensitivity reactions by a CD44 variant isoform v3–specific antibody: blockade of leukocyte egress. *J. Investig. Dermatol.* **113:**11–21.

Tsicopoulos, A., O. Fahy, and A. B. Tonnel. 1999. Delayed-type hypersensitivity reactions to nominal protein antigens and to environmental allergens: similarities and differences. *Eur. J. Dermatol.* **9:**261–268.

Youmans, G. P. 1975. Relation between delayed hypersensitivity and immunity in tuberculosis. *Am. Rev. Respir. Dis.* **111:**109–118.

Cutaneous Basophil Hypersensitivity

Askenase, P. W., and J. E. Atwood. 1976. Basophils in tuberculin and "Jones-Mote" delayed reactions of humans. *J. Clin. Investig.* **58:**1145–1154.

Irani, A. M., C. Huang, H. Z. Xia, C. Kepley, A. Nafie, E. D. Fouda, S. Craing, B. Zweiman, and L. B. Schwartz. 1998. Immunohistochemical detection of human basophils in late-phase skin reactions. *J. Allergy Clin. Immunol.* **101:**354–362.

Jones, T. D., and J. R. Mote. 1934. The phases of foreign sensitization in human beings. *N. Engl. J. Med.* **210:**120–123.

Mote, J. R., and T. D. Jones. 1936. The development of foreign protein sensitization in human beings. *J. Immunol.* **30:**149–167.

Richerson, H. B., H. F. Dvorak, and S. Leskowitz. 1969. Cutaneous basophil hypersensitivity: a new interpretation of the Jones-Mote reaction. *J. Immunol.* **103:**1431–1434.

Transfer Factor

Dwyer, J. M. 1996. Transfer factor in the age of molecular biology: a review. *Biotherapy* **9:**7–11.

Kirkpatrick, C. H. 1996. Activities and characteristics of transfer factors. *Biotherapy* **9:**13–16.

Lawrence, H. S. 1955. The transfer in humans of delayed skin sensitivity to streptococcal M protein and to tuberculin with disrupted leucocytes. *J. Clin. Investig.* **34:**219–230.

Syphilis

Chesney, A. M. 1926. Immunity in syphilis. *Medicine* **5:**463–547.

Dennie, C. C. 1962. *A History of Syphilis.* C C Thomas, Springfield, Ill.

Jones, J. A. 1981. *Bad Blood.* Macmillan Publishing Co., New York, N.Y.

Sell, S., and S. J. Norris. 1983. The biology, pathology, and immunology of syphilis. *Int. Rev. Exp. Pathol.* **24:**203–276.

Turner, T. B., and D. H. Hollander. 1957. *Biology of the Treponematoses.* World Health Organization, Geneva, Switzerland.

Experimental Allergic Encephalomyelitis, Multiple Sclerosis, and Neuritis

Allen, I., and B. Brankin. 1993. Pathogenesis of multiple sclerosis—the immune diathesis and the role of viruses. *J. Neuropathol. Exp. Neurol.* **52:**95–105.

Dalakas, M. C. 1996. Autoimmune peripheral neuropathies, p. 1377–1394. *In* R. Rich (ed.), *Clinical Immunology,* The C. V. Mosby Co., St. Louis, Mo.

Deber, C. M., and S. J. Reynolds. 1991. Central nervous system myelin: structure, function and pathology. *Clin. Biochem.* **24:**113–134.

Gran, B., B. Hemmer, and R. Martin. 1999. Molecular mimicry and multiple sclerosis—a possible role for degenerate T cell recognition in the induction of autoimmune responses. *J. Neural Trans. Suppl.* **55:**19–31.

Hickey, W. F. 1991. Migration of hematogenous cells through the blood-brain barrier and the initiation of CNS inflammation. *Brain Pathol.* **1:**97–105.

Lampert, P. W. 1969. Mechanism of demyelination in experimental allergic neuritis: electron microscopic studies. *Lab. Investig.* **20:**127–138.

Martin, R., H. F. McFarland, and D. E. McFarlin. 1992. Immunological aspects of demyelinating diseases. *Annu. Rev. Immunol.* **10:**153–187.

Noronha, A., and B. Arnason. 1996. Demyelinating diseases, p. 1364–1376. *In* R. Rich (ed.), *Clinical Immunology,* The C. V. Mosby Co., St. Louis, Mo.

Ropper, A. H. 1992. The Guillain-Barré syndrome. *N. Engl. J. Med.* **326:**1130–1136.

Waksman, B. H. 1959. Experimental allergic encephalomyelitis and the "autoallergic" diseases. *Int. Arch. Allergy Appl. Immunol. (Suppl.)* **14.**

Viral Encephalitides of Animals

Doherty, P. C., and R. M. Zinkernagel. 1975. Capacity of sensitized thymus-derived lymphocytes to induce fatal lymphocyte choriomeningitis is restricted by the H_2 gene complex. *J. Immunol.* **114:**30–33.

Georgsson, G., S. Torsteinsdottir, G. Petursson, P. Palsson, and O. S. Andresson. 1993. Role of immune response in visna, a lentiviral central nervous system disease of sheep, p. 183–195. *In* P. Racs, N. L. Letvin, and J. C. Gluckman (ed.), *Animal Models of HIV and Other Retroviral Infections.* S. Karger, Basel, Switzerland.

Hotchin, J. E. 1962. The biology of lymphocytic choriomeningitis infection: virus-induced immune disease. *Cold Spring Harbor Symp. Quant. Biol.* **14:**479–486.

Inoue, A., C. S. Koh, M. Yamazaki, M. Ichiwara, M. Isobe, Y. Ishihara, H. Yagita, and B. S. Kim. 1997. Anti-adhesion molecule therapy in Theiler's murine encephalomyelitis virus-induced demyelinating disease. *Int. Immunol.* **9:**1837–1847.

Lampert, P. W., R. Garrett, and H. Powell. 1977. Demyelination in allergic and Marek's disease virus induced neuritis, comparative electron microscopic studies. *Acta Neuropathol.* (Berlin) **40:**103–114.

Murray, P. D., K. D. Pavelko, J. Leibowitz, X. Lin, and M. Rodriquez. 1998. CD4(+) and CD8(+) T cells make discrete contributions to demyelination and neurologic disease in a viral model of multiple sclerosis. *J. Virol.* **72:**7320–7329.

Weiner, L. P. 1978. Viral models of demyelination. *Neurology* **28:**111–114.

Viral Encephalitides of Humans

Burgoon, M. P., G. P. Owens, T. Smith-Jensen, D. Walker, and D. H. Gilden. 1999. Cloning the antibody response in humans with inflammatory central nervous system disease: analysis of the expressed IgG repertoire in subacute sclerosing panencephalitis brain reveals disease-relevant antibodies that recognize specific measles virus antigens. *J. Immunol.* **163:**3496–3502.

Diener, T. O. 1987. PrP and the nature of the scrapie agent. *Cell* **49:**719–721.

Gajdusek, D. C. 1977. Unconventional viruses and the origin and disappearance of kuru. *Science* **197:**943–960.

Garen, P. D., T. F. Tsai, and J. M. Powers. 1999. Human eastern equine encephalitis: immunohistochemistry and ultrastructure. *Mod. Pathol.* **12:**646–652.

Lampert, P. W. 1978. Autoimmune and virus-induced demyelinating diseases. *Am. J. Pathol.* **91:**176–183.

Schneider-Schaulies, S., and V. ter Meulen. 1999. Pathogenic aspects of measles virus infections. *Arch. Virol. Suppl.* **15:**139–158.

Whitley, R. J., and D. W. Kimberlin. 1999. Viral encephalitis. *Pediatr. Rev.* **20:**192–198.

Granulomatous Reactions

14

The Nature of Granulomas

Granulomas (Fig. 14.1) are identified by focal collections of inflammatory and connective tissue cells in tissue, including macrophages, histiocytes, fibroblasts, epithelioid cells, and giant cells, as well as lymphocytes and plasma cells, surrounded by varying amounts of fibrous tissue. Granulomas progress from highly cellular reactions, which are eventually replaced by fibrous scars (Fig. 14.2). Although it is not always possible using morphological criteria alone, these reactions should be differentiated from nonspecific chronic inflammatory reactions in which lymphocytes, plasma cells, and eosinophils accumulate.

Granulomatous reactions are cellular responses to irritating, persistent, and poorly soluble substances. These reactions are characteristically initiated by sensitized lymphocytes reacting with antigen but may also occur to poorly catabolizable antigen-antibody complexes that persist locally. However, not all granulomas have their origin in an immune response. Common granulomatous reaction may surround insoluble suture material, urate deposits in gouty lesions, or other poorly degradable foreign bodies. Antibody-antigen complexes may provide a stimulus for granuloma formation if the complex is insoluble and relatively indigestible. Antigen complexed to insoluble particles, such as latex beads, will produce granulomas when injected into immunized animals. Granulomatous hypersensitivity reactions may evolve over weeks or even months owing to the persistent nature of the stimulus.

Epithelioid cells in granulomas have an appearance similar to that of epithelial cells, such as keratinocytes. The origin of this most characteristic cell of granulomatous hypersensitivity reaction is from a phagocyte that has ingested foreign material but cannot digest or exocytose the material. This cytoplasmic foreign material takes on the appearance of cytokeratin, thus giving the cell an epithelial appearance. Multinuclear giant cells form from fusion of macrophages or epithelioid cells. *T-cell factors* that modulate granuloma formation have been identified. (i) Interleukin-4 (IL-4) causes aggregation and fusion of macrophages. (ii) Gamma interferon (IFN-γ) causes inhibition of macrophage migration and fusion of monocytes. (iii) Tumor necrosis factor beta (TNF-β) plays a role in local organization of granulomas. In addition, macrophage-derived factors, including IL-1 and TNF-α, stimulate fibrosis and scarring

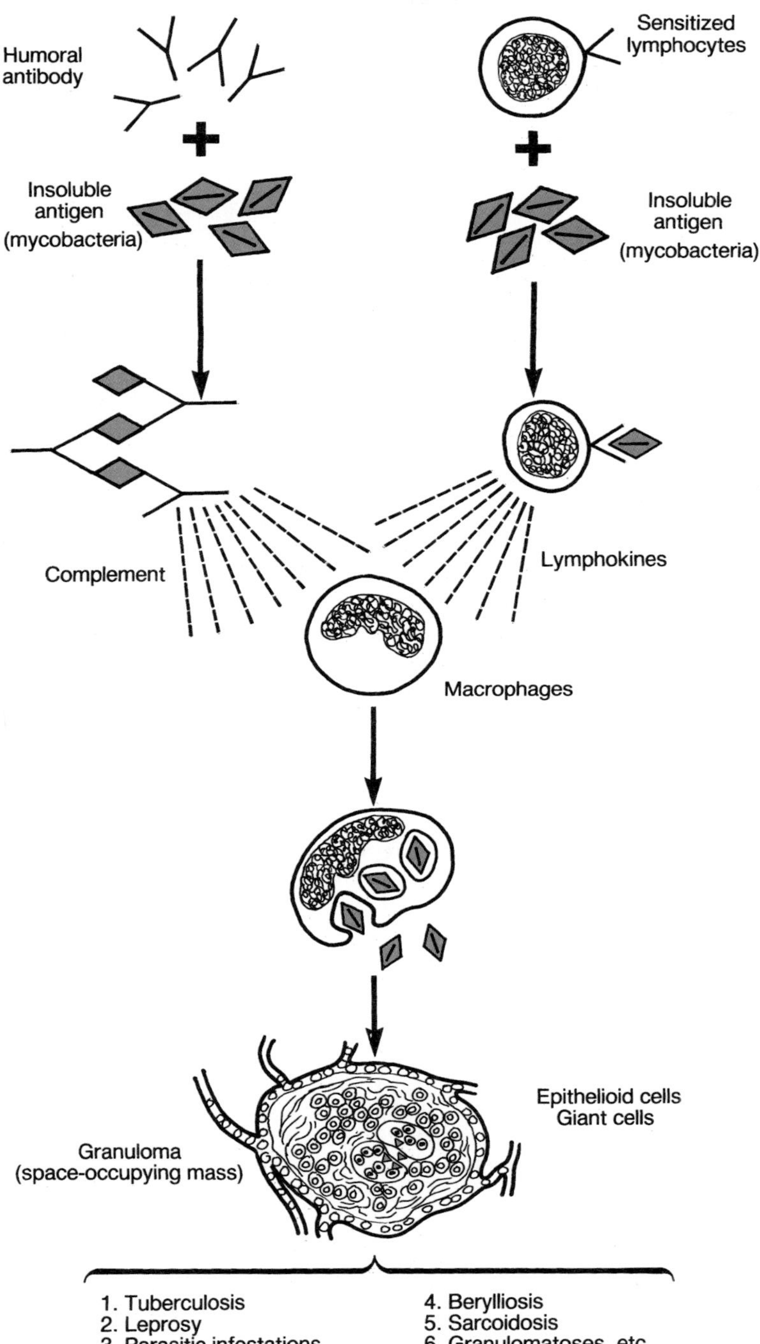

Figure 14.1 Granulomatous hypersensitivity reactions. Granulomatous reactions can be identified morphologically by the appearance of reticuloendothelial cells, including histiocytes, epithelioid cells, giant cells, and lymphocytes, arranged in a characteristic round or oval laminated structure called a granuloma. Hypersensitivity granulomas form as a variation of DTH or antibody reactions. Sensitized lymphocytes react with antigens, releasing lymphokines that attract and activate macrophages. The activated macrophages are unable to "clear" the poorly degradable antigens, accumulate in the tissues, form epithelioid and giant cells, and organize into granulomas. Granulomas may also form in response to poorly degradable antibody-antigen complexes in tissue, where complement-mediated inflammation results in accumulation of macrophages unable to degrade the antigen.

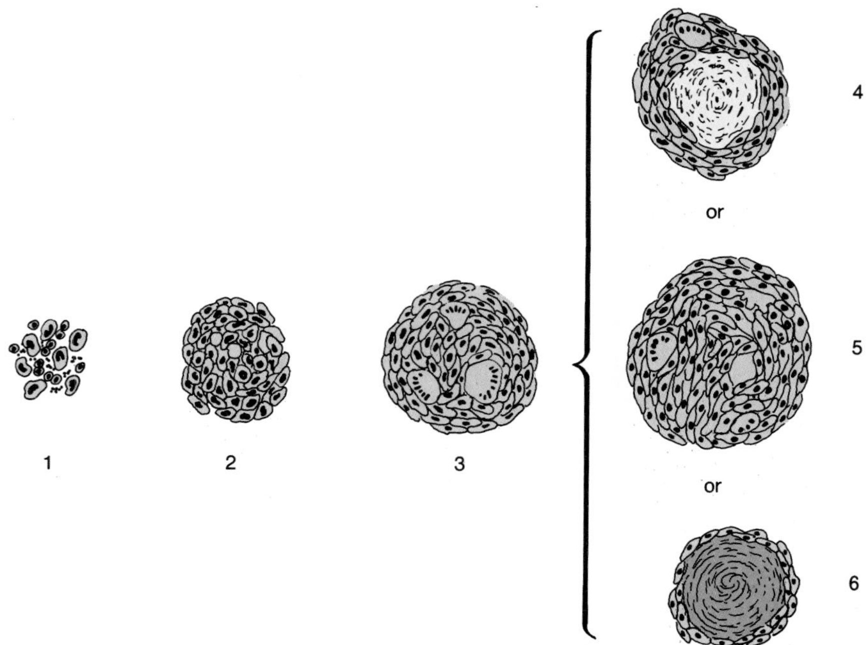

Figure 14.2 Progression of granulomas. **(1)** Granulomas begin as small collections of lymphocytes and macrophages that form around poorly degradable antigens. **(2)** Macrophages change to epithelioid cells and become organized into a cluster of cells. **(3)** Further progression results in ball-like clusters of cells and fusion of macrophages into giant cells. Further progression may include the following: **(4)** development of necrosis in the center as characteristic of chronic tuberculosis, **(5)** continued enlargement and replacement of normal tissue (progressive disease), or **(6)** fibrosis with scar formation, characteristic of "healed" sarcoidosis.

Figure 14.3 Spectrum of association of granulomatous reactions and vasculitis. The lesions of Loeffler's syndrome and eosinophilic granuloma are essentially granulomas; those of the vasculitis found with polyarteritis nodosa and collagen diseases are almost pure arteritis. On the other hand, a number of diseases, such as some connective tissue diseases (see chapter 10) and Wegener's granulomatosis, demonstrate a mixture of granulomatous reactions and vasculitis. In these lesions, which are difficult to classify, it is possible that the granulomatous reactions are secondary to tissue damage initiated by another mechanism.

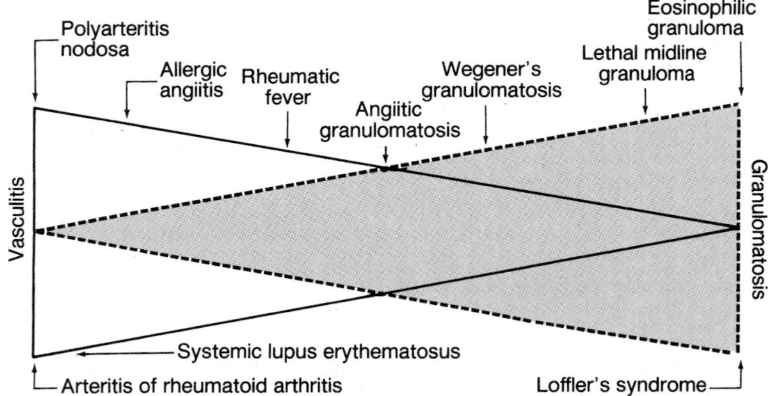

in granulomas. (For more details on the roles of various factors in chronic inflammation, see chapter 3.)

Many diseases demonstrate both granulomatous reactions and *vasculitis,* varying from essentially pure granulomatous lesions to pure vasculitis (Fig. 14.3). "Allergic granulomatosis," or Churg-Strauss syndrome, includes necrotizing vasculitis, extravascular granulomas, and tissue infiltration with eosinophils, which occur in a setting of bronchial asthma. A common feature of granulomas, such as Wegener's granulomatosis and Churg-Strauss syndrome, is the presence of anti-neutrophil cytoplasmic antibodies (ANCA), which reflect disease activity.

Granulomatous Diseases

Granulomatous diseases include infectious diseases, such as tuberculosis, leprosy, and parasitic infestations; responses to known antigens, such as zirconium granuloma, berylliosis, and extrinsic alveolitis; and other diseases of unknown etiology in which epithelioid granulomas are the primary lesion. Epithelioid granulomas occur in other diseases such as tertiary syphilis, fungus infections, and some foreign body reactions (e.g., around urate deposits in gout). Granulomas are also a prominent feature of early asbestosis and silicosis.

Infectious Diseases

Tuberculosis

Tuberculosis, "the white plague," has had a long and devastating relationship with humankind. Lesions of tuberculosis have been found in Egyptian mummies, and the disease was described clinically in pre-Christian times. Until the discovery of antituberculosis drugs in the 1950s, tuberculosis was a major public health problem. In the early 1800s, mortality may have been as high as 1 in 100 adults per year in large American and European cities. The story line in many novels revolved around the tragic fate of the hero or heroine with fatal tuberculosis. The infectious nature of tuberculosis was discovered in 1882 by Robert Koch, who cultured the organism and satisfied his famous set of postulates (Table 14.1) to prove that the isolated organism caused the clinical manifestations of tuberculosis. The organism, now known as *Mycobacterium tuberculosis,* was first called Koch's bacillus. Eight years later, Koch announced that he had discovered a cure for tuberculosis. Koch claimed that injection of "tuberculin" could rapidly reverse advanced symptoms of tuberculosis. Within a few months, his spectacular claims were debunked, and his reputation was seriously damaged. Fortunately, we remember Koch's solid contributions and not his unproven claims. Even though there was a gradual decline in the disease related to improved living standards, pasteurization of milk, vaccination of children with the bacterial strain BCG (see below), improved diagnostic and public health procedures, and isolation of infected individuals in sanatoria, most large cites in the first half of the 20th century still had entire hospitals dedicated to the care of tuberculosis patients.

The dramatic effect of the antituberculosis drugs isoniazid (in the early 1950s) and rifampin (in the 1960s) led to optimism that tuberculosis would finally be brought under control. However, to check the growth of the bacillus in infected individuals, it was necessary to continue treatment for at least 9 months. The biggest problem in attempts to eradicate tuberculosis

Table 14.1 Koch's postulates: a statement of the experimental evidence required to establish the etiologic relationships of a given microorganism to a given disease

1. The microorganism must be observed in every case of the disease.
2. It must be isolated and grown in pure culture.
3. The pure culture must, when inoculated into a susceptible animal, reproduce the disease.
4. The microorganism must be observed in, and recovered from, the experimentally diseased animal.

was that many patients discontinued treatment when they began to feel better, allowing drug-resistant strains to develop. In the early 1990s, the incidence of tuberculosis increased dramatically; the increase coincided with the increased susceptibility of the elderly, alcoholics, drug users, AIDS patients, and immigrants from third world countries. At the time of this writing, the disease is again declining, largely owing to public health measures. However, the drugs once believed to be the means to eradicate tuberculosis are now relatively ineffective because of the emergence of drug-resistant strains. Patients who have been previously treated and then relapse are particularly likely to be harboring drug-resistant organisms.

Natural history of tuberculosis. Tuberculosis is the classic example of mixed protective and pathogenic effects of immune and nonimmune inflammatory reactions to a single agent. Primary infection begins by inhalation of a droplet containing a viable bacillus and implantation in the lung, usually in a lower lobe. This leads to a local infection (primary focus) of acute inflammation that spreads by drainage to the hilar lymph nodes and eventually to the blood (bacteremia).

For pulmonary tuberculosis, four stages of infection can be identified at the cellular level. In stage 1, the bacillus is ingested by alveolar macrophages. The bacillus is usually destroyed by the macrophage; if not, it grows in the macrophage and eventually destroys it. At this stage, $T_{\gamma\delta}$ cells may act on infected macrophages to kill them. It is estimated that only 3 to 5% of humans who contact the bacillus will progress to later stages of infection. A positive delayed-type hypersensitivity (DTH) skin reaction indicates that an individual has been exposed and reacted to a tuberculosis infection. Conversion from negative to positive is used to make a preliminary diagnosis of tuberculosis infection, which should be followed up for radiologic evidence of lesions. However skin tests are not useful in patients with immune defects, such as AIDS, when DTH is suppressed.

In stage 2, the bacilli grow logarithmically within immature macrophages that arrive from the bloodstream. *Miliary tuberculosis* results from acute infection or reinfection, and blood-borne dissemination results in multiple small granulomas in many organs. However, these granulomas are poorly formed, being mostly made up of macrophages with a few lymphocytes and epithelioid cells, and may contain large numbers of viable organisms. In miliary tuberculosis, cell-mediated immunity to tuberculin antigens is often lacking, and the immune response is unable to check the spread of the infection. Cell-mediated immunity recovers in patients with miliary tuberculosis who are successfully treated with antibiotics.

In stage 3, the number of bacilli becomes stationary as their growth is inhibited by the immune response (bacteriostasis). In this stage, newly arriving immature macrophages may continue to support growth of the bacilli, whereas activated macrophages inhibit multiplication and destroy the organisms. Arrest at this stage depends upon the ability of macrophages to be activated. If the infection is checked, the primary infection site and the hilar lesions heal by granuloma formation, leading to formation of a *Ghon complex*. The Ghon complex consists of a healed granuloma or scar on the pleural surface of the middle lobes of the lung and granulomas in the draining hilar lymph nodes. The Ghon complex suggests that the patient resisted a previous tuberculosis infection by a granulomatous reaction.

In stage 4, bacilli multiply extracellularly in the center of granulomas protected from the host's immune defenses. The center of tubercular granulomas frequently becomes necrotic, resulting in a gross appearance similar to that of cheese. This is referred to as *caseous necrosis*. Caseous necrosis may also occur in other granulomatous diseases but is most often seen in tuberculosis. Viable organisms may multiply to enormous numbers within the "protected niche" provided by the liquefied center of a caseous granuloma. Rupture of the infected granuloma allows these viable organisms to enter the bronchial tree. The course of the infection then depends on whether the quantity of bacilli exceeds the capacity of the host's immune system to limit reinfection. Alterations in the host's immune response with aging or malnutrition may cause breakdown of the granuloma and allow auto-reinfection with persisting viable organisms *(reactivation tuberculosis).* This also provides a source for spreading the infection to others, because large numbers of viable tubercle bacilli are released through coughing and provide an aerosol of potentially infective organisms for others.

Infection with tubercle bacilli may result in different types of immune responses, including nonspecific $T_{\gamma\delta}$ cytotoxic cells active during the first few days after infection, circulating antibody, T-cytotoxic (T_{CTL}) cells directed against infected monocytes, T-delayed-type hypersensitivity (T_{DTH}) cell-mediated classic DTH, increased macrophage activity (immune phagocytosis), and granulomatous inflammation. Cell-mediated immunity is accepted by most as the main line of specific defense. There is little evidence that immunoglobulin antibody plays an important role. In the majority of cases, cell-mediated immunity to *M. tuberculosis* can be demonstrated by positive DTH skin tests to tuberculoproteins within 2 to 4 weeks after infection.

The granulomatous "lesions" of tuberculosis are the result of the host-parasite immune interaction. Clearly, a granulomatous reaction represents a not always successful defensive reaction on the part of an infected individual. T_{DTH} cells secrete lymphokines that enable activated macrophages to limit dissemination of the organism. T_{CTL} cells are activated and actually kill infected macrophages. This reaction may certainly contribute to the necrosis seen, but the protective effect of macrophage destruction in tuberculosis is not clear. It is postulated that T_{CTL}-mediated destruction of infected macrophages allows activated macrophages to phagocytose and digest the organisms, thus clearing the intracellular infection. This process would require T_{DTH} cells reacting with antigens on the bacilli and releasing factors that attract and activate macrophages (Fig. 14.4). If the infiltrating macrophages are not activated, lysis of infected macrophages may be a weakness in the battle against tuberculosis, contributing to spread of the

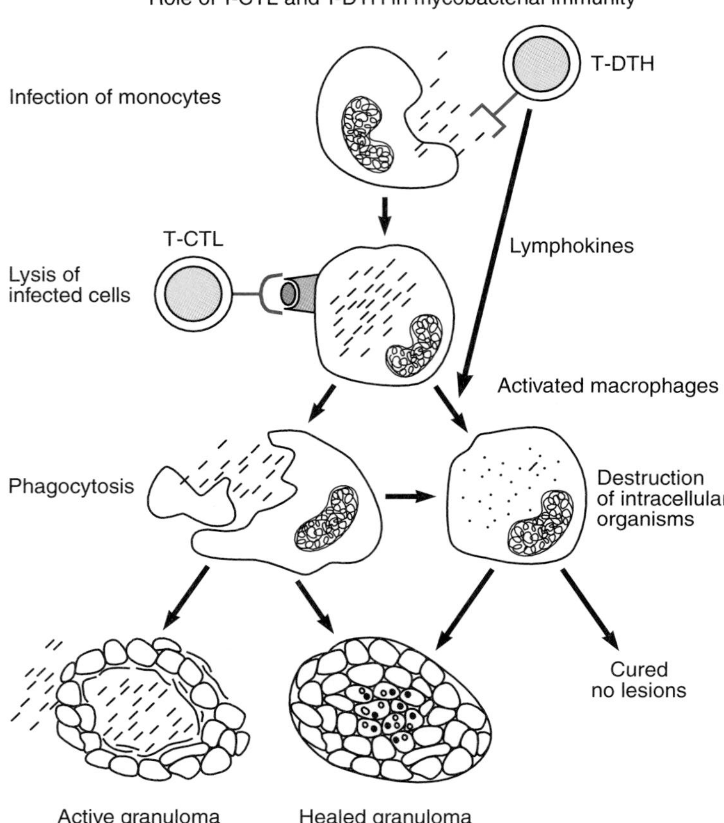

Figure 14.4 Postulated role of cell-mediated immunity to tuberculosis.

infection to other macrophages. If extensive, proliferation of macrophages and accumulation of granulomas as the result of ongoing chronic infection lead to eventual loss of organ function as the normal tissue is replaced by granulomas.

Both T_{CTL} and T_{DTH} cells are believed to play important roles in immunity to tuberculosis. Infection is initiated by uptake of bacilli into macrophages. Key to the progression of the infection is the ability of the bacilli to replicate within the macrophages. In over 90% of infected individuals, bacilli are unable to replicate in infected macrophages. This effect may be due to rapid reaction of $T_{\gamma\delta}$ cells with infected macrophages. If infection persists, specific cell-mediated immunity is induced with production of specifically sensitized T_{DTH} and T_{CTL} cells. Specific T_{DTH} cells react with mycobacterial antigens and release mediators, such as IL-2, TNF, and IFN-γ, that activate macrophages to digest the intracellular bacilli. T_{CTL} cells react with infected macrophages and lyse them. The released bacilli may then either be phagocytosed and destroyed by activated macrophages or reinfect immature macrophages. Four possible outcomes are cure with no residual lesions (most common), cure with residual lesions (Ghon complex), arrest with healed granulomas, or progression with active granulomas.

Many believe the answer to controlling tuberculosis lies in finding ways to improve the effectiveness of the immune defenses to the infection.

Individuals with depressed cell-mediated immunity are particularly susceptible. Previously, tuberculosis was noted in high incidence in the elderly and patients on immunosuppressive therapy; now AIDS patients are highly susceptible to progressive tuberculosis. New approaches to both therapy and prevention are urgently needed. One approach is to apply advances in molecular biology and tissue culture to identify and clone the genes responsible for the production of the protective epitopes of *M. tuberculosis* and to introduce these into specifically designed vectors to produce vaccines that might provide protective immunity. Regardless of the availability of new medical approaches, reinstitution of stringent isolation procedures, careful supervision of antibiotic treatment, and public health-directed education may be the most effective measures.

Because of the worldwide impact of tuberculosis, many countries have introduced mandatory immunization with BCG. Today, BCG holds the interesting position of being one of the most widely used, most poorly understood, and most controversial vaccines. BCG stands for bacillus Calmette-Guérin, a strain of *Mycobacterium bovis,* attenuated between 1906 and 1919 by Léon Calmette and Camille Guérin. The use of BCG had a shaky start. Calmette was an abrasive French nationalist who disliked Germans and was uneasy with the English. In addition, he greatly exaggerated his early results. Guérin, who lived much longer than Calmette, appears to have been much less abrasive but an ineffectual promoter of the vaccine. After years of animal experiments, human trials were carried out in 1921, and by 1924 the French government had adopted the vaccine for mass use. In the 1950s, BCG vaccination against tuberculosis came into widespread use throughout the world, except for the United States and The Netherlands, through the sponsorship of the World Health Organization. In 1939, it was shown that BCG inoculation also induced a positive Mitsuda reaction (skin reaction to leprosy antigens). The efficacy of BCG immunization has been found to vary in different studies from 0 to 80% for tuberculosis and from 20 to 80% for leprosy. Explanations for this variation in efficacy include the following: (i) infection with other atypical mycobacteria that impart some protection against tuberculosis in control groups, (ii) differences in immunogenicity among BCG preparations, (iii) differences in the natural history of the disease in different populations, (iv) methodological differences in the trials, and (v) nutritional or other environmental effects, such as incidence of infections with other agents. These problems led 14 of the 32 countries using the vaccine to discontinue BCG immunization programs. In England and Wales, BCG inoculation is not required but is offered to high-risk neonates in most districts.

The protective epitopes of BCG are poorly understood, but older studies suggested that the most important immunogens are polysaccharides. Thus, recombinant techniques will most likely not work, but the immunizing polysaccharide epitope can be synthesized and conjugate methodology used to produce an effective acellular vaccine. Using reactive cloned T-cell lines, which do not necessarily identify a protective immunogen, it appears that the most likely candidate is a 65-kDa antigen, but other evidence implicates larger proteoglycans. Immunization with BCG stimulates type 1 T cells with production of $CD4^+$ T_{DTH} cells, as well as complement-fixing antibodies. One clinical effect is conversion to a positive tuberculin skin test, so a positive skin test in a person who has been immunized with BCG cannot be used as an indication of exposure to tuberculosis.

Leprosy

Leprosy is another mycobacterial infection clearly known since biblical times. The clinical features of leprosy depend upon the immune reaction of the infected individual; a form of *immune deviation,* in which some individuals predominantly express cell-mediated immunity and others predominantly express humoral immunity. The immune characteristics of various clinical classifications of leprosy are presented in Table 14.2.

At one pole of the leprosy spectrum, patients have little manifestation of the disease other than one or more well-defined erythematous or hypopigmented anesthetic plaques or macules on the skin. This is the high-resistance or *tuberculoid* form. Histologic examination reveals sarcoidlike dermal granulomatous lesions with prominent Langhans giant cells, epithelioid cells, and many lymphocytes. Few, if any, *Mycobacterium leprae* organisms can be found in the tissues. However, in early cases of neuritic leprosy, the visually normal skin or nasal mucosa may show nonspecific inflammation or granulomas with small numbers of organisms. Because of a tendency to involve peripheral nerves with loss of sensory function, this is also known as the anesthetic form. The neural fibrosis appears to be related to production of fibroblastic stimulatory factors by activated macrophages. Affected individuals develop secondary traumatic injury owing to loss of pain sensation. There is hyperplasia of the paracortical areas of the lymph nodes, a prominent delayed skin reaction to injection of lepromin, and little or no humoral antibody to mycobacterial antigens.

At the other pole of the clinical spectrum is *lepromatous leprosy*. This form is the low-resistance type. It is known as the nodular form because of a prominence of skin and lymph node involvement and gross nodule for-

Table 14.2 Immunologic characteristics of leprosy[a]

Characteristic	Form of leprosy[b]		
	Tuberculoid	**Borderline**	**Lepromatous**
Mycobacterium leprae in tissues	− or ±	+ or ++	++++
Granuloma formation	++++	+++	−
Lymphocytic infiltration	+++	−	−
Lymph node morphology			
Paracortical lymphocytes	++++	++	−
Paracortical histiocytes	−	++	++++
Germinal center formation	+	++	++++
Plasma cells	±	+	+++
Lepromin test	+++	−	−
DTH, % reactivity to:			
Dinitrochlorobenzene	90	75	50
Hemocyanin	100	100	100
Antimycobacterial antibodies (% of patients with precipitins in serum)	11–28	82	95
Autoantibodies in serum (%)	3–11		30–50
Immune complex disease (erythema nodosum leprosum)	−	±	+++

[a] Modified from J. L. Turk and A. D. M. Bryceson, *Adv. Immunol.* **13:**209–266, 1971.
[b] − to ++++ indicates the extent of the observation noted.

mation. There is massive infiltration of tissues with large macrophages filled with numerous mycobacteria. There is extensive skin involvement that can produce marked disfigurement (leonine faces). The cellular infiltrate in the dermis is separated from the basal layer of the skin by a band of foamy macrophages (Virchow cells) filled with acid-fast organisms (Grenz zone). The lymph nodes of lepromatous patients have hyperplastic germinal centers, yet the cell-mediated immune defense against these organisms is diminished. The paracortical areas have a paucity of lymphocytes and are often filled with large macrophages containing organisms. There are few, if any, lymphocytes in the tissue lesions, the lepromin skin test is negative, and antibodies to mycobacterial antigens are common (Table 14.2). In addition, patients with lepromatous leprosy develop a number of autoantibodies, most likely because of polyclonal B-cell responses in this form of the disease. Antibodies to cross-reacting antigens between human skin and *M. leprae* have been identified and may play a role in the chronic destruction of the skin seen in this disease. In addition, the production of antinuclear factor and rheumatoid factor (anti-immunoglobulin) may cause rheumatic manifestations.

The spectrum of leprosy includes many patients who have characteristics that are essentially mixtures of the tuberculoid and lepromatous forms. Between the two polar forms of the disease are intermediate forms progressing from the paucibacillary (tuberculoid) form to the multibacillary (lepromatous) form: TT (full tuberculoid) → BT (borderline tuberculoid) → BB (borderline) → BL (borderline lepromatous) → LL (full lepromatous). The manifestations of *M. leprae* infection are therefore quite variable and range from severe tissue destruction to only locally depigmented areas of the skin. This latter form is frequently found in the natives of Baja California. Europeans tend to be resistant, and South Americans develop little immune response but frequently manifest only depigmented skin, whereas Southeast Asians usually develop lepromatous leprosy.

The protective function of granulomatous reactivity is exemplified by the spectrum of reactions to *M. leprae* in leprosy. Resistance is associated with granuloma formation and a high degree of DTH, whereas low resistance is associated with lack of granuloma development and prominence of antibody formation. The position that a given patient occupies on the clinical spectrum frequently changes. A shift from a lepromatous form to a tuberculoid form is associated with a definite clinical improvement.

When the bacterial load diminishes, tissues that contain residual organisms undergo hypersensitivity reactions. There is swelling and erythema of skin lesions associated with fever. The skin lesions show infiltration with lymphocytes. The foamy macrophages lose their content of organisms and become more epithelioid. Although patients with polar tuberculoid or polar lepromatous leprosy usually remain in their part of the spectrum, frequent shifts in the borderline groups occur. Effective chemotherapy frequently precipitates a reversal reaction. Chemotherapy of leprosy with 4,4-diaminodiphenylsulfone may produce a reduction in the antigenic load and permit poorly reactive patients to express a granulomatous reaction. More recently, a vaccine for leprosy based on immunization with an autoclaved cultured strain of *Mycobacterium* (*Mycobacterium* w) was shown to cause conversion of lepromin from negative to positive in phase III trials as an adjunct to chemotherapy.

To produce an effective granulomatous reaction, both macrophages and T cells are required. Cytologic analysis indicates segregation of T_{DTH}

cells within the aggregate of macrophages and T_{CTL} cells in the mantle of tuberculoid granulomas, whereas T_{DTH} and T_{CTL} cells are admixed among the undifferentiated macrophages of lepromatous lesions. The formation of a tuberculoid granuloma appears to require activated T_{DTH} cells, which produce soluble factors that activate macrophages to kill the intracellular organisms and stimulate giant cell formation. Granulomas from tuberculoid leprosy contain large numbers of cells containing IL-1β, TNF-α, and TNF-γ. Without this lymphokine-mediated activation of macrophage killing, the infected macrophages serve as the permissive cell for proliferation of the organisms. In lepromatous leprosy, T_{CTL} cells may not be able to act against *M. leprae* cells, which are protected by their intracellular location, and the few T_{DTH} cells present are unable to produce sufficient interleukins to activate the infected macrophages to kill the bacilli they harbor.

The development of a granuloma is mediated through the action of T-helper and T-suppressor cells on T_{DTH}-cell activity. T cells from patients with lepromatous leprosy fail to respond to *M. leprae* antigens in vitro and not only fail to produce IL-2 but also do not express IL-2 receptors. There is compelling evidence, both in experimental and human leprosy, that activation of a T-cell suppressor mechanism explains the *immune deviation* responsible for the lack of cell-mediated immunity in lepromatous leprosy. In lepromatous lesions, the CD4/CD8 ratios are markedly reduced when compared with lesions of tuberculoid leprosy. Addition of blood lymphocytes from patients with lepromatous leprosy to cultures of lymphocytes from patients with tuberculoid leprosy greatly reduces the mitogen response to *M. leprae* antigens. Secretion of a "suppressor factor" that inhibits development of granulomas has been reported. In borderline lepromatous leprosy, removal of $CD8^+$ cells can partially restore the mitogen response; however, in polar lepromatous leprosy, the lymphocytes fail to respond even when $CD8^+$ (suppressor) cells are removed. Thus, T-suppressor cells cannot account for the entire lack of cell-mediated immunity in lepromatous leprosy; a deletion of leprosy-specific $CD4^+$ T_{DTH} cells also occurs.

The macrophages of lepromatous leprosy patients have a decreased capacity for destroying various target cells as well as other microorganisms (decreased cell-mediated immunity) and decreased IL-1 production. Treatment of mice with agents that increase the phagocytic and metabolic activity (digestive capacity) of macrophages will prevent the development of experimental infection. Leprosy infection is always limited in normal mice but assumes a more virulent course in thymectomized or anti-lymphocyte serum-treated mice who have depressed cell-mediated immunity. Patients with lepromatous leprosy have a decreased capacity to respond to a variety of cell-mediated reactions, including mitogen activation of lymphocytes, sensitization to contact sensitivity agents, and decreased production of lymphokines.

The *lepromin test* is a skin reaction to extracts of *M. leprae*. It consists of a two-stage reaction. The first is a typical DTH reaction that occurs 24 to 48 h after injection of the antigen (the Fernandez reaction); the second (Mitsuda reaction) appears between 2 and 4 weeks after testing and is an indurated skin nodule caused by the formation of a granuloma. This nodule is over 4 mm in diameter and usually ulcerates. The 24- to 48-h Fernandez reaction is positive in a large number of persons who have no history of ever contacting leprosy. This is probably because of exposure to cross-reacting antigens of other bacteria. Therefore, the lepromin reaction cannot be used to indicate active or acute infection with *M. leprae*. The clinical importance of the lepromin test in determining the reactivity of infected patients is as a prognostic test. A positive Mitsuda granulomatous reaction is associated with high resistance to the infection and a good prognosis.

Better laboratory tests are being developed to aid in the diagnosis of leprosy. Attempts to use so-called *M. leprae*-soluble antigens as skin test antigens have had limited success—about 50% of cases of tuberculoid leprosy are negative using these antigens. Serological tests include a fluorescence test (FLA-ABS), an enzyme-linked immunosorbent assay (ELISA), and an ELISA inhibition test. The ELISA-based tests measure antibody to a *M. leprae*-specific terminal disaccharide (PGL-1) or to specific epitopes on different protein antigens. These are consistently positive in lepromatous leprosy (multibacillary form) but negative in tuberculoid leprosy (paucibacillary form).

Erythema nodosum leprosum is an immune complex-mediated vascular skin reaction (Arthus reaction) found in patients with lepromatous leprosy and antibody to mycobacterial antigens. Crops of red nodules appear in the skin, last for 24 to 48 h, and may be associated with systemic manifestations, such as arthritis, inflammation of the eye or testes, pain along nerves, fever, and proteinuria. The lesions in the skin show a fibrinoid vasculitis with polymorphonuclear infiltrate. The frequent occurrence of these reactions during chemotherapy suggests that they are related to the release of mycobacterial antigens and deposition of immune complexes in affected tissues. Similar lesions may also be seen in patients with progressive tuberculosis, erythema nodosum tuberculosum. One final feature of lepromatous leprosy is the high incidence of autoantibodies. These include antinuclear factor, rheumatoid factor, antithyroglobulin antibodies, and false-positive serologic tests for syphilis. Most of these autoantibodies do not seem to produce lesions or symptoms in affected patients. The high incidence of autoantibodies in leprosy may be due to an adjuvant effect of the organisms, continued tissue destruction releasing potential autoantigens, or altered activity of suppressor cells.

Parasitic Infections

Granulomatous reactions occur in response to many parasitic infections, particularly those of fungi and certain helminths, and may be responsible for the pathogenesis of the chronic forms of the diseases. It is not possible to include the many different infections here. Histoplasmosis, schistosomiasis, and filariasis will be mentioned briefly.

Histoplasmosis. Histoplasmosis is a common respiratory infection caused by the yeast *Histoplasma capsulatum.* The course and lesions are very similar to those of tuberculosis, and it is a major differential diagnosis alternative for tuberculosis. Histoplasmosis may be diagnosed by the presence of pulmonary lesions and antibody to *H. capsulatum* antigens. Following inhalation of the conidia of the yeast into the lung, the micro- and macroconidia germinate into yeastlike forms that cause a nonimmune specific inflammatory reaction, including polymorphonuclear leukocytes, natural killer cells, and macrophages. This usually inhibits the progression of the infection. The development of an immune response with antibody and T-cell activation further limits the infection. Protection against primary infection in experimental models is associated with IFN-γ production, whereas inhibition of progressive disease requires TNF-α. In immunocompromised individuals, especially those with chronic obstructive pulmonary disease, there may be compromise of the local inflammatory reaction, particularly if there is a large inoculum. This leads to local growth of the fungus, which cannot be cleared, and then to the formation of an encircling granuloma. This granuloma may resolve in about 10% of patients or may progress to increasing granuloma formation. Treatment with amphotericin B is usually effective in arresting the progress of the disease.

Schistosomiasis. In infestations with *Schistosoma mansoni,* the eggs are released into the portal bloodstream and lodge in the portal veins of the liver. Here, the eggs evoke a severe granulomatous inflammatory reaction that may gradually increase and lead to extensive fibrosis of the portal areas (pipe stem fibrosis). If the liver involvement is severe, collateral circulation of the portal system develops as the branches of the portal vein in the liver become obstructed. The eggs may then pass from the portal system through collateral channels to the pulmonary arteries, resulting in multiple, small granulomatous lesions resembling miliary tuberculosis (pseudotubercles). The eggs of other schistosomes (*S. hematobium* and *S. japonicum*) are deposited in large numbers in the subepithelial connective tissue of the urinary bladder. A severe granulomatous reaction may occur, resulting in obstruction of urinary flow.

The granulomas associated with schistosomiasis appear to depend on the balance of Th1- and Th2-type immune reactions. Thus, granulomas in schistosomiasis result from type 2 reactions against the poorly degradable antigens in the face of a lack of macrophage stimulation by Th1-type cytokines. A key inflammatory cell is the eosinophil. The extent of granulomatous inflammation may actually decrease in chronic infection, at least in laboratory animals. This amelioration of the disease state is termed modulation and may occur because of an active suppressor mechanism mediated by both cellular and humoral systems or a change from a type 2 to type 1 immune response and decreased production of IL-4, IL-10, and IL-13. This may allow activation of macrophages and clearing of infected tissues.

Filariasis. Host reactions to filarial infections determine the type and progression of lesions. Filariae are roundworms with complex life cycles that live in the subcutaneous or lymphoreticular tissues and have been called connective tissue parasites. They are highly specialized parasites that are narrowly restricted as to their sites of infection and reproduction. As higher-order parasites, they have traded in fast reproductive rates and genetic modulation, which are characteristic of viruses and trypanosomes, for greater individual longevity and reproductive complexity. Filariform larvae are transmitted to humans by a biting insect that serves as the intermediate host. The larvae penetrate the skin and may pass into the lymphatic system. All of the eight filariids known to infect humans may evoke allergic reactions (Table 14.3); however, only three cause serious disease: *Wuchereria bancrofti*, *Brugia malayi*, and *Onchocerca volvulus*.

The manifestations of filariasis clearly reflect the state of immune responsiveness of the host (Table 14.4). Chronic, asymptomatic filaremia is associated with specific hyporesponsiveness to filarial antigens. It is a host-parasite relationship that permits prolonged production of microfilar-

Table 14.3 Human filarial infections

Species	Site of infection	Immune effector mechanism	Geographical distribution
Wuchereria bancrofti	Lymphatic	Multiple	Tropics
Brugia malayi	Lymphatic	Multiple	Southeast Africa
Brugia timori	Lymphatic	Multiple	Indonesia
Onchocerca volvulus	Subcutaneous	Cellular	Africa, South America, Central America
Loa loa	Subcutaneous	Anaphylactic	Africa
Dipetalonema perstans	Subcutaneous	Anaphylactic	Africa, South America
Mansonella sp.	Subcutaneous	Not known	South America
Dracunculus medinensis[a]	Connective tissue	Anaphylactic	Tropics

[a]This organism is often grouped with the filariae but is actually in a different, though related family.

iae, which are cleared from the circulation by the lungs, liver, and spleen without evoking symptoms. The lack of an immune response in asymptomatic microfilaremia may be due to specific tolerance, major histocompatibility complex-linked unresponsiveness, or suppressive mechanisms. Evidence has been presented that favors the presence of a suppressive mechanism, but specific tolerance based on anergy is considered possible in some cases.

Endemic normals are individuals who have no signs of infection but who have immunoglobulin G (IgG) antibody and T-cell blastogenic responses to filarial antigens. The existence of such individuals argues that immunization resulting in a high T-cell sensitivity could provide effective protection against infection. In occult filariasis, there are neither symptoms nor microfilariae in the blood. Such individuals may be very difficult to differentiate from endemic normals, but some individuals have minimal evidence of infection, such as subconjunctival adult worms in *Loa loa* infection and symptomatic episodes of lymph node enlargement and respiratory complaints in *W. bancrofti* and *B. malayi* infections. IgG antibodies may be responsible for the rapid, apparently complete clearance of organisms from the blood and the resulting asymptomatic latency. The comparison of endemic normals and occult filariasis with other forms of the disease indicate that both antibody and cellular immunity are important for complete control of the infection.

However, immune responses that apparently cure the infection may actually lead to disease. Thus, filarial fevers are an indication that an immune response has been activated, most likely involving immune complexes. The manifestations of tropical eosinophilia, attacks of bronchial asthma with in-

Table 14.4 Classification and immunopathologic mechanisms in filariasis

Disease state	Age at infection	Immune mechanism
Asymptomatic microfilaremia	Infants	Tolerance
Endemic normal	Infants	IgG antibody and T cells
Occult filariasis	Infants	IgG antibody
Tropical eosinophilia	Adult, acute	Anaphylactic
Lymphadenitis	Adult, chronic	Delayed hypersensitivity
Lymphatic obstruction	Adult, chronic	Granulomatous

terstitial inflammation of the lungs, are consistent with an IgE response and the formation of immune complexes. A cellular (granulomatous) response is implicated in the pathogenesis of lymphadenitis and lymphatic obstruction leading to massive edema (elephantiasis).

The development of more benign host-parasite relationships is related to the age when exposure to the parasite occurs. When previously unexposed adults are infected, there is a tendency to develop acute inflammation with pain, urticaria, angioedema, and marked lymphangitis, which disappear without sequelae if exposure is terminated. However, if exposure continues, the disease progresses rapidly from temporary to permanent lymphatic obstruction. Thus, continued exposure to the organism in sensitized individuals is required for the development of lymphatic obstruction by granulomas formed around killed microfilariae. In contrast, residents of regions of endemicity who contact filariae early in life may develop less frequent and less severe manifestations of the disease. In some unknown way, the immune response of such persons is either specifically suppressed or restricted to IgG antibody production, resulting in an asymptomatic carrier state or occult filariasis. Adults from outside the area of endemicity tend to produce IgE antibody or cellular hypersensitivity when infected. This intriguing host-parasite relationship clearly deserves further study.

Granulomatous Responses to Known Antigens

Zirconium Granulomas

Some 6 months after the marketing of stick deodorants containing zirconium salts, individuals were observed with axillary granulomas. The injection of zirconium into the skin of such patients resulted in the delayed appearance of a typical epithelioid granuloma. Some type of hypersensitivity was suspected, because relatively few individuals who used such deodorants actually developed lesions. When the use of zirconium was discontinued, lesions no longer occurred.

Berylliosis

Two forms of lung disease are associated with inhalation of beryllium: an acute chemical inflammation caused by heavy exposure and a chronic progressive pulmonary disease following low exposure that features multiple small, noncaseating granulomas, first reported in 1946. The conclusion that a type of hypersensitivity is involved in the latter is based on the observations that only a small number of the exposed individuals actually develop the disease and that there may be a delay of months or years from the time of exposure to the development of berylliosis. Beryllium was once used for the manufacture of fluorescent light bulbs, and many exposed individuals remained symptomless. Beryllium is no longer used for this purpose, and the incidence of the disease has been greatly reduced. Berylliosis has been reported more recently following low exposure in precious-metal refining, and beryllium is still used in the aircraft industry. Cases have been reported following exposure to levels previously believed to be safe. The chronicity of the disease may also be due to the fact that beryllium tends to remain in the tissue indefinitely. It has been reported that patients with berylliosis give positive patch test reactions with the antigen, but the validity of this observation has been questioned. Further studies have shown that beryllium is an active inducer of contact (delayed-type) sensitivity, and a beryllium patch test measures DTH. A more relevant test is the production of a granuloma upon intradermal application of beryllium in patients with berylliosis. Application of beryllium in a patch test most likely does not stimulate a granulomatous reaction, which requires deposition of the eliciting antigen in tissues. $CD4^+$ T cells accumulate in the lungs, and the lymphocytes of patients with berylliosis will transform in vitro upon exposure to beryllium sulfate, further suggesting that cellular sensitization to beryllium occurs. Zirconium as well as beryllium may bind serum proteins and function as a hapten in the production of contact sensitivity. However, the relation of this mechanism to the development of granulomas remains obscure. Berylliosis may be considered an example of hypersensitivity pneumonitis.

Hypersensitivity Pneumonitis (Extrinsic Allergic Alveolitis)
Allergic reactions to organic dusts, bacteria, or mold products in the lung are believed to cause a certain type of interstitial pneumonitis, designated extrinsic allergic alveolitis by J. Pepys (Table 14.5). Frequently, the diagnosis is made after acute respiratory distress develops 4 to 12 h after exposure to an eliciting "antigen." With repeated exposure, progressive pulmonary fibrosis (farmer's lung) occurs, with the main tissue lesion being granulomatous; however, the frequent coexistence of other types of reactions, such as anaphylactic, toxic complex, or delayed, may produce a complex clinical and pathologic picture in a given patient. Viral infections may augment the progression of the disease. The pathologic reaction is mixed, but inflammation of the alveolar walls is the primary feature, usually consisting

Table 14.5 Source and type of antigen-producing extrinsic allergic alveolitis[a]

Disease	Source of antigen	Antigen against which precipitating antibody is present
Farmer's lung	Moldy hay	*Micropolyspora faeni, Thermoactinomyces vulgaris*
Bagassosis	Moldy bagasse[b]	*T. vulgaris*
Mushroom worker's lung	Mushroom compost	*M. faeni, T. vulgaris*
Fog fever in cattle	Moldy hay	*M. faeni*
Suberosis	Moldy oak bark, cork dust	Moldy cork dust
New Guinea lung	Moldy thatch dust	Thatch
Maple bark pneumonitis	Moldy maple-bark	*Cryptostroma (Coniosporium)*
Malt worker's lung	Moldy barley, malt dust	*Aspergillus clavatus, Aspergillus fumigatus*
Bird fancier's lung	Pigeon, budgerigar, parrot, or chicken droppings	Serum protein, droppings
Pituitary snuff-taker's lung	Heterologous pituitary powder	Serum protein, pituitary antigens
Wheat weevil disease	Infested wheat flour	*Sitophilus granarius*
Sequoiosis	Moldy sawdust	Graphium *Aureobasidium pullulans* (pullularia)
Mollusk shell pneumonitis	Mollusk shell dust	Pearl oyster shells
Cheese washer's lung	Moldy cheese	*Penicillium* spp.

[a]Modified from J. Pepys, *Monogr. Allergy*, **4**:1–147, 1969.
[b]Residue of sugarcane after extraction of syrup.

of epithelioid cell granulomas. Plasma and lymphoid cell infiltration (a high ratio of $CD8^+$ to $CD4^+$ T cells) may also be prominent, and granulomas are not always present. In fact, a variety of lymphoid cell infiltrates and inflammatory reactions may be found in the lung, suggesting that a mixture of different types of immune or allergic reactions may be manifested at any given time. In many cases, precipitating antibodies may be demonstrated to test antigens. However, vasculitis is not a prominent feature, although there are notable exceptions. Patients with these chronic pulmonary diseases often have acute attacks of asthma on exposure to the antigen; these may be caused by the existence of anaphylactic antibodies. Experimental hypersensitivity pneumonitis models in animals also support a combined role of immune complexes and cell-mediated immunity in the pathogenesis of this disease, but $CD4^+$ Th1 cells appear to be most important.

Diseases of Unknown Etiology

Sarcoidosis

Boeck's sarcoidosis is a systemic, noncaseating, granulomatous process of unknown etiology prominently involving the lymph nodes, lungs, eyes, and skin, with lesions that may be indistinguishable from those of tuberculosis, fungus infections, or other granulomatous hypersensitivity reactions. The term "sarcoid" was coined by Caesar Boeck in 1899 for the skin lesions; later systemic involvement was recognized by Schaumann in 1917. The clinical presentation of sarcoidosis may masquerade as acute rheumatoid arthritis, tuberculosis, erythema nodosum, or Crohn's disease but usually appears as pulmonary masses and bilateral hilar adenopathy on a chest X ray of a young adult black male with dyspnea. Berylliosis and sarcoidosis may be almost identical in their clinical presentation. Because of the frequent involvement of the eye, conjunctival biopsy is a cost-effective diagnostic procedure. About 80% of patients with sarcoidosis will resolve spontaneously; 20% will progress without treatment and 5% will die from complications of the disease. Rarely, sarcoidosis will present in an explosive picture by the appearance of erythema nodosum, polyarthritis, iritis, and fever (Lofgren's syndrome), but the onset is usually insidious, with lesions often being found in asymptomatic individuals. Progressive loss of pulmonary function is the major cause of disability and death; sudden death from sarcoid lesions in the conducting system of the heart is a rare but recognized possibility. Corticosteroids are the drugs of choice but should not be used unless disease progression is noted. The serum levels of angiotensin-converting enzyme are elevated in patients with sarcoidosis, and the serum level of this enzyme may be used to monitor disease activity. Sarcoidosis is noted for its geographic prevalence in the southeastern United States and its relative rarity in the western United States. The highest incidence is in Sweden, where 64 persons per 100,000 have radiologic evidence of the disease. In the 1960s, this geographic distribution was used to argue effectively that sarcoidosis was caused by an "allergy" to pine pollen, which contains acid-fast waxy material similar to *M. tuberculosis.* However, a number of studies showed that a variety of infectious agents and fatty acids could produce granulomas in laboratory animals identical to those of sarcoidosis. The nonspecificity of granuloma production led to dismissal of the pine pollen hypothesis.

A cutaneous granulomatous reaction may be elicited 3 to 4 weeks after the subcutaneous injection of crude extracts of spleen or lymph nodes from patients with sarcoidosis. This test was first reported in 1935 by Williams and Nickerson but has become known as the *Kveim-Sitzbach reaction*. The specificity of this reaction and its use as a diagnostic test are controversial. The diagnostic accuracy of the Kveim test depends on the preparation of "antigen" used; new extracts must be tested on known positive and negative controls before being used to test patients suspected of having sarcoidosis.

An infectious agent is suspected, but as yet no specific agent has been identified. The characteristic noncaseating granuloma is not pathognomonic; identical histopathologic lesions may be seen with mycobacterial and fungal infections, brucellosis, mineral dust exposure, hypersensitivity pneumonitis, and Wegener's granulomatosis. The granuloma has a central zone with tightly packed cells, including epithelioid cells, macrophages, and giant cells, surrounded by a peripheral zone with more loosely arranged mononuclear cells. The giant cells may contain concentrically laminated basophilic structures (Schaumann bodies), and smaller spindle-shaped inclusions with radiating spines (asteroid bodies) may be found at the outer edge of the central zone of the granuloma. The granulomas ultimately resolve, leaving no morphologic lesion, or undergoes fibrosis and contraction. The lesions are believed to be caused by T-cell activation leading to accumulation, fusion, and epithelioid changes in macrophages, but the "antigen" responsible for the T-cell activation has not been identified. The epithelioid cells in the granulomas and the alveolar macrophages may act as antigen-presenting accessory cells. Patients with sarcoidosis generally exhibit a depression of delayed-type hypersensitivity and increased levels of circulating antibody. The relationship of these findings to the disease process remains unclear, but an imbalance in the immune system, with a relatively incompetent T-cell system, is suspected. This could be because of a redistribution of T cells in the inflammatory process or to an inherent loss of T-cell activity. The reason for the polyclonal activation of B cells is not known, but it may be secondary to production of interleukins by activation of T-helper cells during granuloma formation or to a form of immune deviation. Th1 cells and the cytokines IFN-γ and IL-12 predominate early in the disease, but Th2, transforming growth factor β (inhibitor of IL-12 and IFN-γ production), and suppressor T cells ($CD8^+$) predominate during regression of the granulomas. Shifting of Th1 and Th2 predominance may allow remodeling of the granulomatous lesions. Recently, $T_{\gamma\delta}$ cells have been reported to be elevated in the blood and lungs of patients with sarcoidosis. Could it be that hyperactivity of this nonspecific "early warning system" is part of the pathogenesis of sarcoidosis?

Wegener's Granulomatosis

Wegener's granulomatosis is a triad of granulomatous arteritis, glomerulonephritis, and sinusitis. The presentation of the disease is variable: glomerulonephritis may or may not be present, and the granulomas may be disseminated but are usually prominent in the lungs, nasal and oral cavities, and spleen. The granulomatous lesions are destructive and contain fibroblastic proliferation, necrosis, and prominent Langhans giant cells. This disease may be related to polyarteritis nodosa, and some authors have called it polyarteritis of the lungs or a type of hypersensitivity angiitis. However, the lesions of Wegener's granulomatosis are distinctive enough to warrant a separate diagnosis. An unusual finding is granulomatous glomerulonephritis, believed to be caused by a reaction to fibrin mixed with immune complexes in gaps in Bowman's capsule, leading to the destruction of Bowman's capsule and surrounding granulomatous inflammation. The natural history of the disease is invariable rapid progression with destruction of the upper respiratory system. Treatment with low-dose cyclophosphamide combined with alternate-day corticosteroids has led to a high rate of temporary remissions, but relentless progression occurs in some patients. In some cases, exacerbation of the disease is closely associated with infection, and treatment of the infection with antibiotics may be associated with remission of the granulomatous lesions. The relation of Wegener's granulomatosis to other necrotizing granulomatous processes, such as midline lethal granuloma of the face, is not clear. No infectious agent has been consistently isolated from patients with any of these diseases.

Recently, antibodies to neutrophils, called ANCA, have been found in patients with Wegener's granulomatosis. Two types of ANCA are recognized: cytoplasmic ANCA (cANCA) and perinuclear ANCA (pANCA). cANCA reacts with proteinase-3 and gives a diffuse staining of the cytoplasm of neutrophils; pANCA reacts with myeloperoxidase and gives a perinuclear pattern. cANCA has a sensitivity of 78 to 96% for Wegener's granulomatosis but is not diagnostic, because positive cANCA is also found in related diseases such as polyarteritis nodosa, rapidly progressive glomerulonephritis, and Churg-Strauss syndrome. Rising cANCA titers are highly suggestive of relapse. pANCA is found in patients with disease limited to the kidneys, especially idiopathic concentric glomerulonephritis, whereas cANCA predominates in patients with respiratory disease. Although a pathogenic role for ANCA has not been established, it is possible that infections (such as pneumonitis) cause degranulation of neutrophils and release of lysosomal enzymes that elicit an autoimmune response. Excessive stimulation of neutrophils by ANCA and the proteolytic effects of released lysosomal enzymes may then cause endothelial damage and tissue necrosis.

Granulomatous Hepatitis

Circumscribed granulomas consisting of epithelioid cells surrounded by plasma cells and lymphocytes may be seen in the liver and are associated with a variety of diseases, including hepatitis C infection, coccidiomycosis, histoplasmosis, tuberculosis, cirrhosis, lymphomas, Wegener's granulomatosis, immune deficiency diseases, and malignant tumors, as well as with BCG immunization and drug reactions. However, in a substantial number of patients, there is no specific disease association (*idiopathic granulomatous hepatitis*). It is likely that the reaction is an allergic reaction to a drug or a response to an unidentified infectious agent.

Regional Enteritis

Regional enteritis (Crohn's disease) and ulcerative colitis are chronic destructive inflammatory diseases of unknown etiology involving the bowel, so-called inflammatory bowel disease (IBD). Ulcerative colitis primarily involves the colon; Crohn's disease may involve the colon, the small intestine, or both. The clinical characteristics of both are abdominal pain and diarrhea. The primary feature of regional enteritis is lymphedema, thickening and scarring of the intestinal wall that may occur at any level of the gastrointestinal tract but usually involves the terminal ileum. Histologically, the inflammatory changes vary from those consistent with a DTH reaction (dense infiltration of mononuclear lymphoid follicles, often containing germinal centers) to those of granulomatous hypersensitivity (typical epithelioid granulomas with prominent giant cells, essentially identical to the pulmonary lesions of sarcoidosis). The lesions appear to begin as accumulations of lymphocytes and plasma cells around intestinal crypts. Later, macrophages are seen associated with destruction of the crypt *(crypt abscess)* followed by formation of epithelial cells and then granulomas (Fig. 14.5). The T-cell ratios in mature lesions are 2:1 $CD4^+/CD8^+$, about the same as in control tissues, but active lesions show a predominance of Th1-type cytokines, in particular, IL-12. The mononuclear inflammation of regional enteritis may be the result of the development of DTH, and granulomatous inflammation may result from failure of lymphatics to drain foreign material from the intestinal wall and chronic reactivity to these potential antigens.

In ulcerative colitis, there are superficial mucosal ulcers, vascular and lymphatic congestion, edema, hemorrhage, and a mixed infiltration of polymorphonuclear leukocytes, activated T and B lymphocytes, plasma cells, and eosinophils characteristic of these lesions. The lesions of IBD have been described as similar to those of graft-versus-host lesions in the colon of laboratory animals. Associated with IBD are hypergammaglobulinemia, a prevalence of atopic sensitivities, a prominent occurrence of other autoimmune diseases, antibodies to colonic tissue, and increased levels of some cytokines. However, the antibody is not cytotoxic in vitro, and "anticolon" antibodies are not infrequently found in individuals without IBD. In addition, the cytotoxic capacity of intestinal lymphocytes is less than that of peripheral blood lymphocytes, and there is no evidence that intestinal lymphocytes from IBD patients have increased

Figure 14.5 Sequence of tissue changes in evolution of granulomas in regional enteritis. Lesions begin with pericryptal mononuclear cell infiltration. This is followed by destruction of the epithelial cells (crypt abscess). Macrophage reaction converts the lesion to a granuloma. (Modified from P. Schmitz-Moorman and H. Becker, p. 76, *in* A. S. Pera, et al., ed., *Recent Advances in Crohn's Disease,* Martinus Nijhoff Publishers, The Hague, The Netherlands, 1981.)

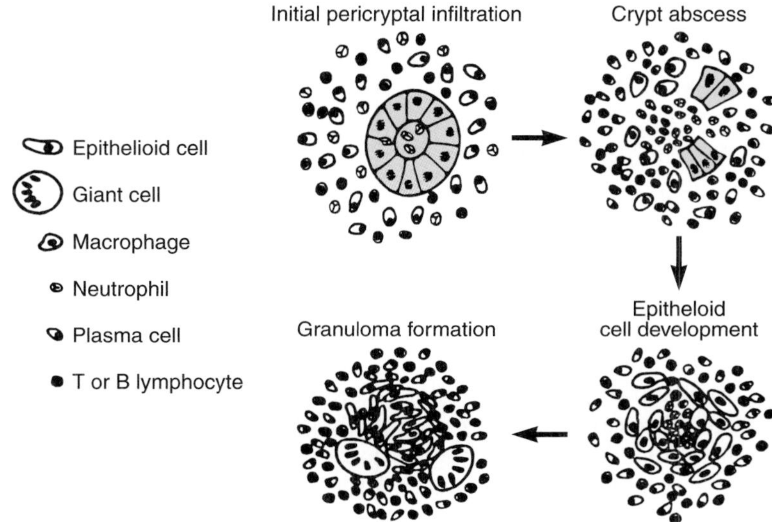

killing for intestinal epithelial cells. Specific colon antigens to which an autoimmune response might be directed have not been identified, and etiologic agents for these diseases have not been convincingly demonstrated. Although there are higher rates for IBD in family members than in the general population, there is no clear correlation with HLA antigens, except for the high association of HLA-B27 in patients with IBD and ankylosing spondylitis. *Auer's colitis* is a hemorrhagic necrotic lesion of the colon, with a cellular infiltrate at the base of the crypts and perivascular polymorphonuclear leukocyte accumulation produced experimentally by the injection of antigen (egg albumen) into the colonic cavity of sensitized rabbits (Arthus reaction).

Autoimmune Gastritis

Autoimmune inflammation of the stomach is an infrequent lesion in humans, but when it occurs, it is often associated with other autoimmune diseases. This disease was first recognized by the identification of autoantibodies to intrinsic factor and gastric parietal cells in patients with pernicious anemia (see chapter 8). There is a high association of gastritis with the parietal cell antibody. Autoimmune gastritis may be induced in laboratory animals by immunization with crude gastric mucosal antigens. Gastric parietal cell and chief cell destruction is associated with marked mucosal lymphocytic infiltration, and cell transfer studies indicate that T cells are the primary mediators of the lesions. Infection with *Helicobacter pylori* is the major cause of chronic gastritis in humans, but this infection is not highly associated with autoimmune gastritis.

Intestinal Villous Atrophy

An extremely rare intractable diarrhea and membranous glomerulonephritis in children appears to be caused by an autoantibody to small intestinal mucosa and renal epithelial cells. There is a common 55-kDa antigen in small bowel and kidney with which the antibody reacts.

Immune Deficiency Diseases

Granulomatous Disease of Children

Granulomatous disease of children consists of chronic pulmonary disease, recurrent suppurative lymphadenitis, and chronic dermatitis with scattered granulomas in many organs. This disease is due to a defect in NADPH that prevents the phagocytic cell from producing free radicals necessary to kill bacteria following phagocytosis (see chapter 18).This results in formation of nonallergic granulomas, which consist of collections of large macrophages in affected tissues.

Protective Functions of Granulomatous Reactions

The formation of a granuloma is a way that the body deals with substances that it finds difficult to eliminate by the usual process of phagocytosis and digestion by macrophages. The fixed macrophages within tissues and the monocytes that infiltrate sites of inflammation are primarily scavenger cells that are able to break down most infectious agents, as well as foreign bodies and residua of inflammation, by an array of toxic effector molecules and hydrolytic enzymes (see chapter 3). It is ironic that a number of infectious agents, including protozoa, bacteria, fungi, mycobacteria, and viruses, preferentially infect and replicate within these same cells. Complex signals generated through the products of activated T cells as well as other cytokines induce a state of activation in the infected cell that kills the intracellular parasites. In addition, T_{CTL} cells that react with antigens of the infecting organisms expressed on macrophages may attack and kill infected cells, with subsequent destruction of the extracellular organisms by phagocytosis and digestion by other activated macrophages. The major killing mechanism of activated macrophages may be through generation of nitrogen oxides derived from L-arginine. How cytokines activate the pathway of L-arginine conversion to L-citrulline with formation of nitrogen oxides remains unclear.

Granulomas form because of the sometimes massive load of organisms or poorly digestible breakdown products of the organisms. When the system is functioning, activation of macrophages by cytokines prevents proliferation of the infecting organisms, and the infection may be cleared early on with little residual evidence in the tissues that infection ever occurred. Positive DTH skin tests provide evidence of previous infection in some individuals with no evidence of disease. However, if the infecting organisms are allowed to multiply, the macrophage system may be faced with an incredible cleanup job, and continued survival and multiplication of some organisms may continue even when there is massive destruction of most of the infecting agents. This results in a sometimes lifelong, life-and-death struggle between the host and the infection. Prolonged chemotherapy may hold replication of the organisms in check and allow the immune response to get the upper hand. However, if therapy is stopped too soon, or the immune system is weakened by age, immunosuppressive drugs, or other infections, recurrence of active infection is the expected course.

Summary

Granulomatous reactions are characterized by the accumulation of oval collections of modified mononuclear cells in tissue. The typical tissue lesion contains large mononuclear cells that look like epithelial cells (epithelioid cells), multinucleated giant cells, lymphocytes, and plasma cells. Granulomatous reactions may be a variant of DTH reactions to insoluble antigens but also frequently occur in association with vasculitis or in response to nonantigenic foreign bodies. It is likely that poorly degradable antigens or insoluble antibody-antigen complexes produce granulomas, whereas soluble complexes cause vasculitis or glomerulonephritis. The mechanism of granulomatous reactivity is not clear, but the inability of macrophages to digest antigens is believed to be a major pathogenic feature. Granulomatous reactions may be initiated by antibody-mediated inflammatory reactions as well as cell-mediated immune reactions or nonimmune inflammation (foreign bodies). Granulomatous tissue reactions serve to isolate infectious agents such as tubercle bacilli, leprosy bacilli, or parasites. Deleterious effects of these reactions occur because of the displacement of normal tissue by granulomas and healing by fibrosis, leading to a loss of normal function.

Bibliography

General

Bean, A. G., D. R. Roach, H. Briscoe, M. P. France, H. Korner, J. D. Sedgwick, and W. J. Britton. 1999. Structural deficiencies in granuloma formation in TNF gene-targeted mice underlie the heightened susceptibility to aerosol *Mycobacterium* *tuberculosis* infection, which is not compensated for by lymphotoxin. *J. Immunol.* **162:**3504–3511.

Boros, D. L. 1981. *Basic and Clinical Aspects of Granulomatous Disease.* Elsevier/North-Holland Publishing Co., New York, N.Y.

Csernok, E., A. Muller, and W. L. Gross. 1999. Immunopathology of ANCA-associated vasculitis. *Intern. Med.* **38:**759–765.

Eustace, J. A., T. Nadasdy, and M. Choi. 1999. Disease of the month. The Churg Strauss syndrome. *J. Am. Soc. Nephrol.* **10:**2048–2055.

Langhans, T. 1868. Über Riesenzellen mit Mandestandigen Kernen in Tuberkeln und die fibrose Form des Tuberkels. *Virchows Arch. Pathol. Anat. Physiol. Kim. Med.* **42:**382.

Muller, J. 1838. *Ueber den Feineren Bau formen der Krankhaften Geschwulste.* Berlin, Germany.

Orme, I. M., and A. M. Cooper. 1999. Cyto/chemokine cascades in immunity to tuberculosis. *Immunol. Today* **20:**307–312.

Savige, J., D. Gillis, E. Benson, D. Davies, V. Esnault, R. J. Falk, E. C. Hagen, D. Jayne, J. C. Jennette, B. Paspaliaris, W. Pollock, C. Pusey, C. O. Savage, R. Silvestrini, F. van der Woude, J. Wieslander, and A. Wiik. 1999. International Consensus Statement on Testing and Reporting of Antineutrophil Cytoplasmic Antibodies (ANCA). *Am. J. Clin. Pathol.* **111:**507–513.

Turk, J. L. 1980. The role of delayed hypersensitivity in granuloma formation: *Res. Monogr. Immunol.* **1:**275–298.

Infectious Diseases

Tuberculosis

Burke, D. S. 1993. Of postulates and peccadilloes: Robert Koch and vaccine (tuberculin) therapy for tuberculosis. *Vaccine* **11:**795–804.

Casarini, M., F. Ameglio, L. Alemanno, P. Zangrilli, P. Mattia, G. Paone, A. Bisetti, and S. Giosue. 1999. Cytokine levels correlate with a radiologic score in active pulmonary tuberculosis. *Am. J. Respir. Crit. Care Med.* **159:**143–148.

Collins, F. M. 1991. Antituberculous immunity: new solution to an old problem. *Rev. Infect. Dis.* **13:**940–950.

Hoft, D. F., E. B. Kemp, M. Marinaro, O. Cruz, H. Kiyono, J. R. McGhee, J. T. Belisle, T. W. Milligan, J. P. Miller, and R. B. Belshe. 1999. A double-blind, placebo-controlled study of Mycobacterium-specific human immune responses induced by intradermal bacille Calmette-Guérin vaccination. *J. Lab. Clin. Med.* **134:**244–252.

Orme, I. M., E. S. Miller, A. D. Roberts, S. K. Furney, J. P. Griffin, K. M. Dobos, D. Chi, B. Rivoire, and P. J. Brennan. 1992. T lymphocytes mediating protection and cellular cytolysis during the course of *Mycobacterium tuberculosis* infection. *J. Immunol.* **148:**189–196.

Power, C. A., G. Wei, and P. A. Bretcher. 1998. Mycobacterial dose defines the Th1/Th2 nature of the immune response independently of whether immunization is administered by the intravenous, subcutaneous, or intradermal route. *Infect. Immun.* **66:**5743–5750.

Rich, A. R. 1951. *The Pathogenesis of Tuberculosis.* C C Thomas, Springfield, Ill.

Weissler, J. C. 1993. Tuberculosis—immunopathogenesis and therapy. *Am. J. Med. Sci.* **305:**52–65.

Leprosy

Arnoldi, J., J. Gerdes, and H. D. Flad. 1990. Immunohistologic assessment of cytokine production of infiltrating cells in various forms of leprosy. *Am. J. Pathol.* **137:**749–753.

Fine, P. E. M. 1989. Immunological tools in leprosy control. *Int. J. Leprosy* **57:**671.

Garcia-de la Torre, I. 1993. Autoimmune phenomena in leprosy, particularly antinuclear antibodies and rheumatoid factor. *J. Rheumatol.* **20:**900–903.

Mahaisavariya, P., K. Kulthanan, S. Khemngern, and S. Pindaew. 1999. Lesional T-cell subset in leprosy reaction. *Int. J. Dermatol.* **38:**345–347.

Sharma, P., H. K. Kar, R. S. Misra, A. Mukherjee, H. Kaur, R. Mukherjee, and R. Rani. 1999. Induction of lepromin positivity following immuno-chemotherapy with Mycobacterium w vaccine and multidrug therapy and its impact on bacteriological clearance in multibacillary leprosy: report on a hospital-based clinical trial with the candidate antileprosy vaccine. *Int. J. Lepr. Mycobact. Dis.* **67:**259–269.

Sieling, P. A., D. Jullien, M. Dahlem, T. F. Tedder, T. H. Rea, R. L. Modlin, and S. A. Porcelli. 1999. CD1 expression by dendritic cells in human leprosy lesions: correlation with effective host immunity. *J. Immunol.* **162:**1851–1858.

Skinsnes, O. K. 1973. Immunopathology of leprosy: the century in review—pathology, pathogenesis and the development of classification. *Int. J. Leprosy* **41:**329–360.

Suneetha, S., S. Arunthathi, A. Job, A. Date, N. Kurian, and C. J. Shacko. 1998. Histologic studies in primary neuritic leprosy: changes in the nasal mucosa. *Lepr. Rev.* **69:**358–366.

Turk, J. L., and A. D. M. Bryceson. 1971. Immunological phenomena in leprosy and related disease. *Adv. Immunol.* **13:**209–266.

Histoplasmosis

Deepe, G. S., Jr., and R. A. Seder. 1998. Molecular and cellular determinants of immunity to *Histoplasma capsulatum*. *Res. Immunol.* **149:**397–406.

Newman, S. L. 1999. Macrophages in host defense against *Histoplasma capsulatum*. *Trends Microbiol.* **7:**67–71.

Vanek, J., and J. Schwartz. 1971. The gamut of histoplasmosis. *Am. J. Med.* **50:**89.

Schistosomiasis

Chiaramonte, M. G., D. D. Donaldson, A. W. Cheever, and T. A. Wynn. 1999. An IL-13 inhibitor blocks the development of hepatic fibrosis during a T-helper type 2–dominated inflammatory response. *J. Clin. Investig.* **104:**777–785.

Mola, P. W., I. O. Farah, T. M. Kariuki, M. Nyindo, R. E. Blanton, and C. L. King. 1999. Cytokine control of the granulomatous response in *Schistosoma mansoni*-infected baboons: role of exposure and treatment. *Infect. Immun.* **67:**6565–6571.

Rumbley, C. A., H. Sugaya, S. A. Zekavat, M. El Refaei, P. J. Perrin, and S. M. Phillips. 1999. Activated eosinophils are the major source of Th2–associated cytokines in the schistosome granuloma. *J. Immunol.* **162:**1003–1009.

Warren, K. S. 1977. Modulation of immunopathology and disease in schistosomiasis. *Am. J. Trop. Med. Hyg.* **26:**113–119.

Yang, J. Q., K. Tsaka, C. K. Chuang, H. Yoshikawa, and Y. Nakajima. 1999. Dynamic analysis of T-lymphocyte function in relation to hepatopathologic changes and effect of interleukin-12 treatment in mice infected with *Schistosoma japonicum*. *J. Parasitol.* **85:**257–262.

Filariasis

King, C. L., V. Kumaraswami, R. W. Poindexter, S. Kumari, K. Kayaraman, D. W. Alling, E. A. Ottesen, and T. B. Nutman. 1992. Immunologic tolerance in lymphatic filariasis. Diminished parasite-specific T and B lymphocyte precursor frequency in the microfilaremic state. *J. Clin. Investig.* **89:**1403–1410.

Maizels, R. M., and R. A. Lawrence. 1991. Immunological tolerance: the key feature in human filariasis? *Parasitol. Today* **7:**271–274.

Nutman, T. B. 1989. Protective immunity in lymphatic filariasis. *Exp. Parasitol.* **68:**248–252.

Philipp, M., T. B. Davis, N. Storey, and C. K. Carlow. 1988. Immunity in filariasis: prospectives for vaccine development. *Annu. Rev. Microbiol.* **42:**685–716.

Von Lichtenberg, F. 1987. Inflammatory responses to filarial connective tissue parasites *Parasitology* **94:**S101–S122.

Zirconium Disease

Montemarano, A. D., P. Sau, F. B. Johnson, and W. D. James. 1997. Cutaneous granulomas caused by an aluminum-zirconium complex: an ingredient of antiperspirants. *J. Am. Acad. Dermatol.* **37:**496–498.

Werfel, U., J. Schneider, K. Rodelsperger, J. Kotter, W. Popp, H. J. Woitowitz, and G. Zieger. 1998. Sarcoid granulomatosis after zirconium exposure with multiple organ involvement. *Eur. Respir. J.* **12:**750.

Beryllium Disease

Cullen, M. R., J. R. Kominsky, M. D. Rossman, M. G. Cherniack, J. A. Rankin, J. R. Balmes, J. A. Kern, R. P. Daniele, L. Palmer, G. P. Naegel, et al. 1987. Chronic beryllium disease in a precious metal refinery. Clinical, epidemiologic and immunologic evidence for continuing risk from exposure to low level beryllium fume. *Am. Rev. Respir. Dis.* **135:**201–208.

Deodhar, S. D., B. Barna, and H. S. Van Ordstrand. 1973. A study of the immunologic aspects of chronic berylliosis. *Chest* **63:**309–313.

Fontenot, A. P., B. L. Kotzin, C. E. Comment, and L. S. Newman. 1998. Expansions of T-cell subsets expressing particular T-cell receptor variable regions in chronic beryllium disease. *Am. J. Respir. Cell. Mol. Biol.* **18:**581–589.

Rossman, M. D. 1996. Chronic beryllium disease: diagnosis and management. *Environ. Health Perspect.* **104S:**945–947.

Hypersensitivity Pneumonitis

Ando, M., M. Suga, and H. Kohrogi. 1999. A new look at hypersensitivity pneumonitis. *Curr. Opin. Pulm. Med.* **5:**299–304.

Gudmundsson, G., M. M. Monick, and G. W. Humminghake. 1999. Viral infection modulates expression of hypersensitivity pneumonitis. *J. Immunol.* **162:**7397–7401.

Pepys, J. 1969. Hypersensitivity diseases of the lungs due to fungi and organic dusts. *Monogr. Allergy* **4:**1–147.

Sarcoidosis

Agostini, C., and G. Semenzato. 1998. Cytokines in sarcoidosis. *Semin. Respir. Infect.* **13:**184–196.

Boeck, C. 1899. Multiple benign sarkoid of the skin. *J. Cutan. Genit. Urin. Dis.* **17:**543.

Iwai, K., T. Tachibana, T. Takemura, Y. Matsui, M. Kitaichi, and Y. Kawabata. 1993. Pathological studies on sarcoidosis autopsy. I. Epidemiological features of 320 cases in Japan. *Acta Pathol. Jpn.* **43:**372–376.

James, D. G., and W. J. Williams. 1985. *Sarcoidosis and Other Granulomatous Disorders.* The W. B. Saunders Co., Philadelphia, Pa.

Kveim, A. 1941. En ny og spesifik Kulan-reackjon ved Boeck's sarcoid. *Nord. Med.* **9:**169.

Leavitt, J. A., and R. J. Campbell. 1998. Cost-effectiveness in the diagnosis of sarcoidosis: the conjunctival biopsy. *Eye* **12:**959–962.

Moller, D. R. 1999. Cells and cytokines involved in the pathogenesis of sarcoidosis. *Sarcoidosis Vasc. Diffuse Lung Dis.* **16:**24–31.

Siltzbach, L. E. 1967. The international Kveim test study, 1960–1966, p. 201–213. *In* T. Turial and J. Chabot (ed.), *Proceedings of the Fourth International Conference on Sarcoidosis.* Masson et Cie, Paris, France.

Allergic Granulomatosis/Wegener's Granulomatosis

Alarcon-Segovia, D., and A. L. Brown. 1964. Classification and etiologic aspects of necrotizing angiitis. An analytic approach to a confused subject with a critical review of the evidence for hypersensitivity in polyarteritis nodosa. *Mayo Clin. Proc.* **39:**205–222.

Gross, W. L., W. H. Schmit, and E. Csernok. 1993. ANCA and associated diseases; immunologic and pathogenetic aspects. *Clin. Exp. Immunol.* **91:**1–12.

Hoffman, G. S., G. S. Kerr, R. Y. Leavitt, C. W. Hallahan, R. S. Lebovics, W. D. Travis, M. Rottem, and A. S. Fauci. 1992. Wegener granulomatosis: an analysis of 158 patients. *Ann. Intern. Med.* **116:**488–498.

Leavitt, R. Y., A. S. Fauci, D. A. Bloch, B. A. Michel, G. G. Hunder, W. P. Arend, L. H. Calabrese, J. F. Fries, J. T. Lie, R. W. Lightfoot, Jr., et al. 1990. The American College of Rheumatology 1990 criteria for the classification of Wegener's granulomatosis. *Arth. Rheum.* **33:**1101.

Granulomatous Hepatitis

Ozakkaloglu, B., O. Tunger, S. Surucuoglu, M. Lekili, and A. R. Kandiloglu. 1999. Granulomatous hepatitis following intravesical bacille Calmette-Guérin therapy. *Int. Urol. Nephrol.* **31:**49–53.

Sabharwal, B. D., N. Malotra, R. Garg, and V. Malhotra. 1995. Granulomatous hepatitis: a retrospective study. *Indian J. Pathol. Microbiol.* **38:**413–416.

Regional Enteritis (Crohn's Disease)

Berrebi, D., M. Besnard, G. Fromont-Hankard, R. Paris, J.-F. Mougenot, P. de Lagausie, D. Emilie, J.-P. Cezard, J. Navarro, and M. Peuchmaur. 1999. Interleukin-12 expression is focally enhanced in the gastric mucosa of pediatric patients with Crohn's disease. *Am. J. Pathol.* **152:**667–672.

Brynskov, J., O. H. Nielsen, I. Ahnfelt-Ronne, and K. Bendtzen. 1992. Cytokines in inflammatory bowel disease. *Scand. J. Gastroenterol.* **27:**897–906.

Crohn, B. B., L. Ginzburg, and G. D. Openheimer. 1932. Regional ileitis: a pathologic and clinical entity. *JAMA* **99:**1323–1329.

Kakazu, T., J. Hara, T. Matsumoto, S. Nakamura, N. Oshitani, T. Arakawa, A. Kitano, K. Nakatani, F. Kinjo, and T. Kuroki. 1999. Type 1 T-helper cell predominance in granulomas of Crohn's disease. *Am. J. Gastroenterol.* **94:**2149–2155.

Granulomatous Disease of Children

Landing, B. H., and H. S. Shirkey. 1957. A syndrome of recurrent infection and infiltration of viscera by pigmented lipid histiocytes. *Pediatrics* **20:**431–438.

Segal, B. H., T. L. Leto, J. I. Callin, M. I. Malech, and S. M. Holland. 2000. Genetic, biochemical, and clinical features of chronic granulomatous disease. *Medicine* **79:**170–200.

Interplay of Inflammatory and Immunopathologic Mechanisms, Immune Defense, and Evasion of Immune Defense Mechanisms during Infection

15

In any inflammatory reaction, both immune and "nonimmune" mechanisms may be activated. In the preceding chapters, the distinguishing characteristics of individual immune-mediated pathogenic mechanisms were emphasized. In many immune defense or disease processes, more than one immune and nonimmune mechanism may be playing a part sequentially, at the same time, or both. Thus, not only are the clinical manifestations and pathologic lesions associated with a given immune-mediated disease determined by more than one mechanism, but also different mechanisms share common components of the inflammatory process, such as cytokine release or upregulation of adhesion molecules.

Nonimmune Inflammation

Inflammation may be activated by nonimmune factors such as tissue necrosis (infarct), release of bacterial products, or trauma. Such stimuli may activate complement, kinin, coagulation, or mast cell inflammatory mediators, as well as cause upregulation of vascular adhesion molecules, leukocyte selectins and integrins, and/or cytokines that are also activated by immune effector mechanisms (see chapter 3). The tissue manifestations may include acute or chronic inflammatory changes that in some cases are indistinguishable from the lesions caused by immune mechanisms. Chronic noninflammation in the skin may be manifested by a perivascular mononuclear infiltrate that looks like a delayed-type hypersensitivity (DTH) reaction; "nonimmune" granulomatous reactions to foreign bodies may be very similar, if not identical, to granulomatous "hypersensitivity" reactions activated by immune mechanisms.

Immune Inflammation

Histologic similarities between lesions of immune- and nonimmune-mediated inflammation are not surprising, since the same basic inflammatory mechanisms are utilized, and immunization often results in production of different classes of antibody as well as cellular immunity to the same antigens. $CD4^+$ T-helper cells not only produce factors that help B cells make antibody but also are precursors for T-delayed-type hypersensitivity (T_{DTH}) cells. In addition, different immune mechanisms share some of the same inflammatory mediators, or one immune mechanism may activate another through cross-activation of effectors. In serum sickness, more than 50 serum protein antigens are potentially available to react with different antibodies or T cells. Thus, anaphylactic and cell-mediated lesions as well as immune complex lesions may coexist in the acute phase of serum sickness as reactions to different horse serum protein antigens.

In addition, the reaction of an antibody with an antigen in vivo may result in activation of more than one immune mechanism. For example, immune complex-like inflammatory reactions may activate or be activated by each of the other immune mechanisms (Fig. 15.1). Antibody reacting with a biologically active antigen may not only cause neutralization but also lead to the formation of soluble immune complexes and immune complex lesions. In fact, neutralization reactions may be considered a specialized form of immune complex reaction wherein the biologic activity of the antigen adds an additional dimension to the effects of an antibody-antigen reaction. Binding of antibody-antigen complexes to red cells may result in their destruction by activation of complement (the innocent bystander reaction), and soluble complexes released by lysed cells may contribute to an immune complex effect. The activation of complement or release of enzymes from polymorphonuclear neutrophils as a result of an immune complex reaction may cause mast cell lysis and activation of anaphylactic mechanisms. The reaction of immune complexes with platelets may induce serotonin release, which causes increased vascular permeability and upregulation of cell adhesion molecules, polymorphonuclear infiltrate, with subsequent tissue damage, followed by lymphocyte and macrophage invasion and further inflammation or healing. Anaphylactic mediators released from mast cells may cause separation of endothelial

Figure 15.1 Possible interactions of immune complex and other immunopathologic mechanisms. See text for description.

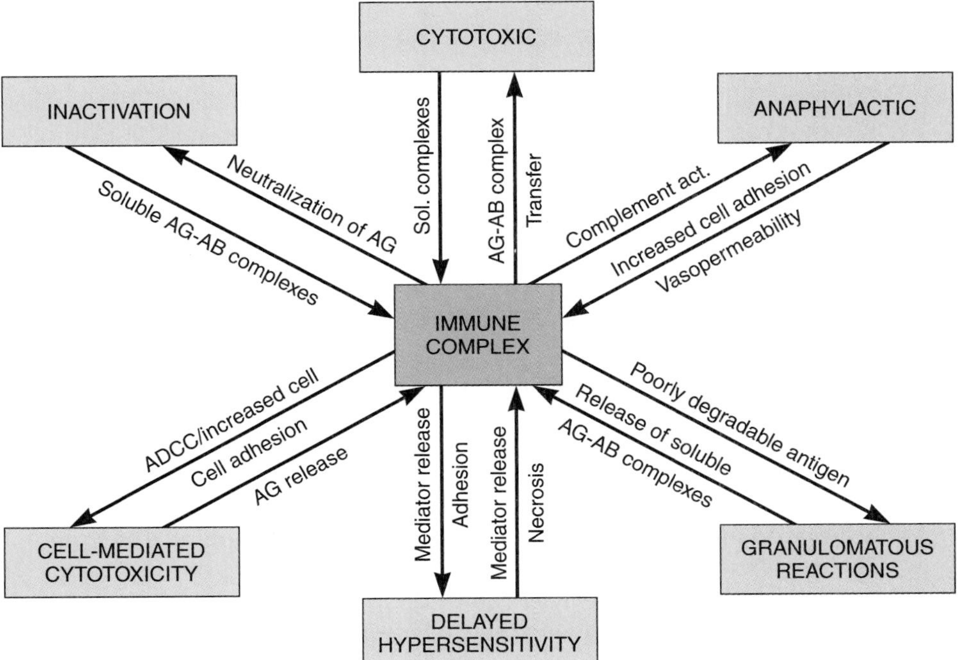

cells, exposing the basement membrane and thus forming foci where immune complexes can lodge and initiate basement membrane damage by an Arthus mechanism, or allow sensitized cells, which initiate DTH, to pass through the vessels into tissue spaces. Both immunoglobulin antibody and sensitized cells may play a role in the lesions seen in autoimmune diseases such as thyroiditis, encephalomyelitis, or orchitis. Upregulation of adhesion molecules on endothelial cells in the brain as a result of formation of myelin-antimyelin complexes leads to lymphocyte margination and emigration of mononuclear cells into the brain.

The roles of immune complex reactivity, cell-mediated immunity, macrophage activation, and the chronic proliferative response in the pathogenesis of a progressive lesion are illustrated by rheumatoid arthritis. Chronic immune complex-mediated injury leads to mononuclear cell proliferation and activation of pannus formation by macrophage products. Immune complex vasculitis may lead to upregulation of cell adhesion molecules and lymphocyte infiltration characteristic of cell-mediated reactions. Tissue damage or cell destruction caused by T-cell cytotoxicity or DTH may activate cytokines that attract and activate polymorphonuclear cells. The formation of poorly degradable antibody-antigen complexes may initiate granuloma formation, whereas tissue-antibody or breakdown products produced by granulomatous reactions may lead to toxic complex glomerulonephritis. Granulomatous lesions frequently occur in association with immune complex vasculitis and/or anaphylactic type reactions.

Other immune effector mechanisms may also interact. Complement-induced mast cell lysis (cytotoxic reaction) may cause anaphylactic symptoms as a result of release of mediators, and pharmacologic mediators and vascular reactions may contribute to cytotoxic effects. Cytotoxic antibody may contribute to cell-mediated tissue destruction (e.g., aspermatogenesis); antibody-dependent cell-mediated cytotoxic cells or cytotoxic factors released by activated lymphocytes may produce lysis of cells. Chronic asthmatic lesions are characterized by infiltration with activated T cells that lower the threshold for reactivity by increased cytokine release. Interleukin-1 (IL-1) released from activated macrophages during a DTH reaction upgrades expression of adhesion molecules and major histocompatibility complex (MHC) class II antigens on endothelial cells, leading to granulocyte and lymphocyte margination, respectively. Lymphocyte mediators may contribute to the evolution of a granulomatous reaction by attracting and activating macrophages; release of lymphocyte-stimulating factors from granulomatous inflammatory sites may contribute to the cellular component of such reactions. Finally, granulomatous lung diseases (such as farmer's lung) frequently have asthmatic (anaphylactic) components.

Granulomatous inflammation may increase the number of mast cells present, and tissue destruction by anaphylactic mechanisms may contribute to granuloma formation. Mixtures of vasculitis, glomerulonephritis, cellular lesions, and granulomas, such as those seen in Wegener's granulomatosis and some infectious diseases, are among the most complex diseases to analyze from the immunopathologic standpoint. The granulomas associated with schistosomiasis appear to depend on the balance of Th1- and Th2-type immune reactions. Thus, progressive granulomas result from Th2-type reactions (anaphylactic) against the poorly degradable antigens in the face of a lack of macrophage stimulation by Th1-type cytokines. Th1-type immune responses, complement-fixing antibody, and T_{DTH} cells appear to activate macrophages and lead to eventual clearing of the infection.

Interaction of Immune and Nonimmune Inflammation

Other systems, such as the blood-clotting and kinin systems, may be activated during the evolution of an inflammatory reaction that also involves allergic reactions. For example, the role that Hageman factor (factor XII of the blood sequence) plays in involvement of other systems is illustrated in chapter 3. Conversion of plasminogen to plasmin produces activation of complement that may induce lytic or inflammatory reactions. Kinins increase vascular permeability and may expose basement membranes for toxic complex deposition. Reaction of α_2-macroglobulin with prekallikrein forms a temperature-sensitive complex that produces increased capillary permeability and chronic inflammation in the skin. Complement may be activated by nonimmunologic mechanisms (see "Alternate Pathway," chapter 3).

Interaction of these "nonimmune" inflammatory mechanisms with allergic (immune) mechanisms may make it difficult to evaluate the role of different immune mechanisms responsible for an inflammatory process taking place in a given patient. However, it is critical for diagnosis and therapeutic decisions to identify the type of inflammatory or immunopathologic reactions responsible for disease in a given patient. In most cases, nonimmune inflammatory reactions or the clotting system are activated secondary to tissue damage caused by immunopathologic mechanisms, and successful treatment may be directed to both the primary immunopathologic process and the secondary inflammatory process.

Immune-Specific Protection against Infection

The specific immune effector mechanisms responsible for protection against infectious agents are the same as those that cause immune-mediated disease. Although it has become popular to define the immunity to infectious diseases on the basis of the type of T-helper subsets (e.g., Th1 for DTH and Th2 for IgE-mediated reactions), it must be kept in mind that T-helper subsets are used for hypothetical explanations for induction of various types of immunoglobulin antibody responses based on observations of the types of lymphokines produced by various T-cell lines in vitro. They do not act, as often postulated, at the level of effector mechanisms. The type of protective mechanism differs with different infectious agents (Table 15.1). With some notable exceptions, the mechanisms mediated by humoral antibody (immunoglobulin) are effective against infectious agents that exist extracellularly, such as bacteria, whereas cell-mediated reactions (T_{CTL}, T_{DTH}, and granulomatous reactions) are effective against intracellular parasites, such as viruses and mycobacteria. T_{CTL} cells react with antigens on virus-infected cells and kill the cells infected with virus as well as the virus. T_{DTH} cells activate macrophages to kill organisms that they have internalized and are most effective against parasite diseases, such as tuberculosis, leprosy, candidiasis, and leishmaniasis, in which the organisms infect macrophages.

Table 15.1 Major immune defense mechanisms for infectious diseases

Type of infection	Major immune defense mechanism(s)
Bacterial	Antibody
Viral	Antibody and T_{CTL} cell
Mycobacterial	DTH, T_{CTL} cell, and granulomatous
Protozoal	DTH and antibody
Helminth	Anaphylactic and granulomatous
Fungal	DTH and granulomatous

Bacterial Infections

Specific immunity to the destructive effects of bacteria or bacterial products is usually mediated by humoral antibody. The mechanisms of antibody-mediated and cell-mediated protection against bacterial infections are illustrated in Fig. 15.2. Some bacteria produce disease not by direct effects of the organism but by the release of products called toxins, which may have severe destructive effects distant from the site of infection. Destructive bacterial toxins are rendered harmless by reaction with antibody (neutralization reaction). For instance, anti-toxin antibodies inactivate toxins of diphtheria or tetanus (see below). In addition, IgA antibodies in the gastrointestinal tract may be able to block the production of watery diarrhea by *Vibrio cholerae* infection of the intestinal tract by preventing the toxin from binding to gastrointestinal lining cells (neutralization). Destruction of infecting organisms in connective tissues is accomplished by the activation of complement following the reaction of antibody with the organism. This leads to increased susceptibility of the organism to phagocytosis (toxic complex reaction) or destruction by insertion of the terminal components of complement into the bacterial cell membrane and lysis (cytotoxic reaction). Activation of mast cells by IgE-mediated reactions serves to increase vascular permeability (endothelial cell contraction), permitting egress of blood-borne antibody or inflammatory cells into the site of infection. Specific T_{CTL} and T_{DTH} cells may also gain access to the site of infection through the contracted endothelial cells. T_{DTH} cells may also be activated by bacterial antigens and release lymphokines, which attract and activate macrophages. The activated macrophages clear the site of inflammation by phagocytosis and digestion of dead bacteria, neutrophils, and necrotic tissue, and prepare the site for healing through the release of monokines that stimulate fibroblastic proliferation and wound healing.

As an example of the role of different immune mechanisms in protection against a bacterial infection, let us assume that an anaerobic, gram-negative bacillus of the genus *Bacteroides,* which is a normal inhabitant of the intestine, gains access to the peritoneal cavity. The organism starts to multiply, and the body recognizes that something is wrong. The initial host response consists of polymorphonuclear cells (PMN), which are attracted to the site by the release of chemoattractants from the damaged tissue along with C5a, since desialylated *Bacteroides* lipopolysaccharide endotoxin (LPS) can fix complement by the alternate pathway. Another powerful PMN attractant is formylated peptides, which are the leader sequences of bacterial protein synthesis. As the PMN and resident macrophages attack the bacterial cells, antigens are released and delivered by lymphatics to lymph nodes. In the lymph nodes, macrophages present

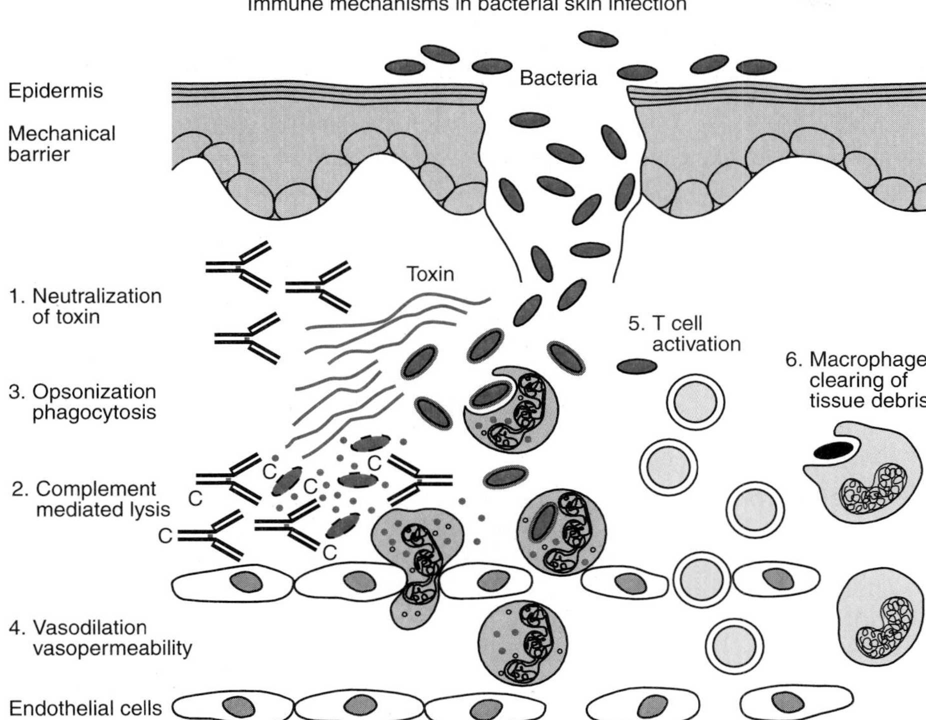

Figure 15.2 Antibody-mediated and cell-mediated mechanisms of protection against bacterial infections. Bacterial infections may be resisted by each of the antibody-mediated immune mechanisms, including **(1)** neutralization of bacterial toxins, **(2)** cytotoxic lysis by antibody and complement, **(3)** acute polymorphonuclear infiltration (Arthus reaction) and opsonization of bacteria leading to increased phagocytosis, and **(4)** acute anaphylactic vascular events permitting exudation of inflammatory cells and fluids. During the chronic stage of the infection, cell-mediated immunity is activated: **(5)** T_{CTL} cells that react with antigens on the surface of virus-infected cells and cause their destruction. **(6)** T_{DTH} cells that react with bacterial antigens may infiltrate the site of infection, become activated, and release lymphokines that attract and activate macrophages. The activated macrophages phagocytose and degrade necrotic bacteria and tissue, preparing the lesion for healing. Granulomas form when organisms cannot be destroyed by macrophages, walling off the infection from the rest of the host.

the processed antigens to T and B cells, stimulating them to become specific effector cells (T cells) or to produce specific antibody (B cells). The specific antibody reacts with antigens on the surface of the *Bacteroides* organisms and fixes complement, which may kill the cell, allow for more efficient phagocytosis, or produce inflammatory fragments (C3a and C5a), which increase circulation to the site and attract more inflammatory cells. Specific T_{CTL} or T_{DTH} cells gain access to the site owing to the increased vascular permeability and also react with specific antigens. Activated T_{DTH} cells release lymphokines, which further contribute by attracting and activating macrophages. The macrophages then phagocytose and clear the site of the dead organisms as well as the products of inflammation and release monokines to activate the healing process.

Immune complex-mediated reactions are responsible for the boils or abscesses of cutaneous infection with *Staphylococcus aureus*. The organisms initially invade the hair follicles of the skin, causing folliculitis. This is painless and may be as far as the infection goes. However, the infection may penetrate into the subcutaneous connective tissue. The infected zone becomes filled with fibrin, PMNs, and lymphocytes. The inflammatory reaction is driven by IgG or IgM serum antibodies, which diffuse into the tissues and react with the staphylococcal antigens, fixing complement and attracting more inflammatory cells. *S. aureus* produces serine proteases that cleave human immunoglobulins, thus contributing to the virulence of the infection. The infected zone becomes ringed with leukocytes and collagen, limiting the spread of infection. Necrosis of the involved tissue occurs when the PMNs release the contents of their lysosomes into the infected area. The lesions heal after they open to the surface and lose the necrotic core of tissue. The resulting defect is filled with connective tissue, leaving a scar that is usually inapparent.

Viral Infections

Immune resistance to viral infections is mainly mediated by cell-mediated immunity, but humoral antibody also plays a role by preventing virus from attaching to cell receptors (Fig. 15.3). Viruses live within the host's cells and can spread from cell to cell. To be effective in attacking intracellular organisms, an immune mechanism must have the capacity to react with cells in solid tissue. This is a property of cell-mediated reactions, in particular those mediated by T_{CTL} cells, but not of antibody-mediated reactions. Many cells infected with a virus will, at some stage of the infection, express viral antigens on the cell surface. It is at this stage that specifically sensitized T_{CTL} cells can recognize cell surface-expressed viral antigens in association with class I MHC molecules and destroy the virus-infected cells. Transgenic mice lacking class I MHC-restricted T cells have decreased resistance to viral infections. Adverse effects of this reaction occur if the cell expressing the viral antigens is important functionally, as is the case for certain viral infections of the central nervous system (see below). If the virus infects macrophages, lymphokines from reactive T_{DTH} cells can activate the macrophages to kill the intracellular viruses. Transgenic knockout mice that lack gamma interferon (IFN-γ) receptors are susceptible to virus infections. Humoral antibody can prevent the entry of virus particles into cells by interfering with the ability of the virus to attach to a host cell, and secretory IgA can prevent the establishment of viral infections of mucous membranes. However, once the virus is within cells, it is not susceptible to the effects of antibody. Patients with deficiencies in antibody production alone usually do not have serious viral infections but develop life-threatening bacterial infections. Patients with defects in cell-mediated immunity develop serious virus infections (see chapter 18).

Mycobacterial Infections

Mycobacterial infections, such as tuberculosis and leprosy, are resisted by cellular mechanisms, including T_{CTL} cells, T_{DTH} cells, and granulomatous hypersensitivity. T_{CTL} cells destroy highly infected macrophages that are unable to cleanse themselves of intracellular infections, resulting in uptake of organisms by other macrophages. T_{DTH} cells release lymphokines that activate macrophages to destroy intracellular organisms, including those released from macrophages destroyed through the action of T_{CTL} cells. IFN-γ appears to be critical for production of macrophage killing, because IFN-γ-deficient mice (IFN-γ knockout mice) are susceptible to sublethal in-

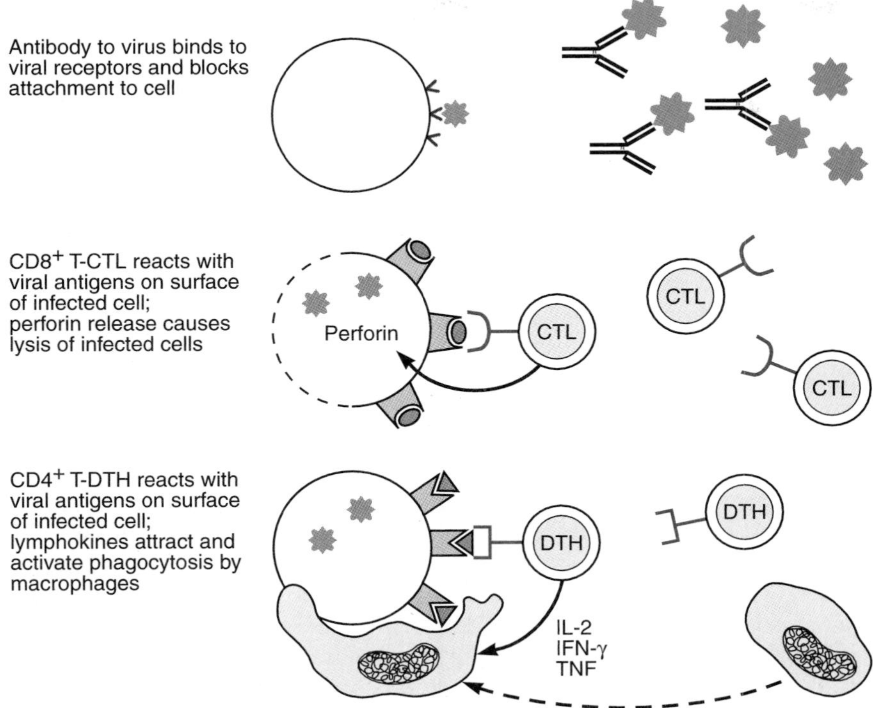
Antibody to virus binds to viral receptors and blocks attachment to cell
CD8+ T-CTL reacts with viral antigens on surface of infected cell; perforin release causes lysis of infected cells
Perforin
CTL
CTL
CTL
CD4+ T-DTH reacts with viral antigens on surface of infected cell; lymphokines attract and activate phagocytosis by macrophages
DTH
DTH
IL-2
IFN-γ
TNF

Figure 15.3 Cellular and antibody-mediated mechanisms of protection against viral infections. Circulating immunoglobulin antibody (usually IgG) or secretory antibody (usually IgA) reacts with surface antigens on the virus and prevents the virus from attaching to cells (neutralizing antibody), thereby inhibiting spread of the infection. Sensitized T_{CTL} cells may destroy virus-infected cells that express viral antigens associated with class I MHC molecules on the surface. T_{DTH} cells reacting with viral antigens release lymphokines that activate macrophages to eliminate intracellular viral infections of macrophages.

fections with *Mycobacterium bovis.* Granulomatous reactions isolate infected sites in tissues and prevent dissemination. At one time, it was thought that the tissue lesions of tuberculosis required the effect of DTH. The term "hypersensitivity" was coined because animals with cellular immune reactivity to tubercle bacilli developed greater tissue lesions after reinoculation of bacilli than did animals injected for the first time. The granulomatous lesions seen in tuberculosis do depend upon immune mechanisms for their formation. However, these lesions are not really the cause of the disease but an unfortunate effect of the protective mechanisms; the granulomatous inflammatory reaction to the infective mycobacteria results in destruction of normal tissue. In the lung, for instance, extensive damage done by the formation of large granulomas in response to a tuberculosis infection can result in respiratory failure. The granulomatous immune response produces the lesion, but the mycobacterium causes the disease. For more details, see chapters 13 and 14.

Protozoal Infections

The mechanism of protection against protozoal infections, like viral infections, depends upon the location of the agent in the host. Protozoa are unicellular organisms that may be located intracellularly, extracellularly in the blood, both intracellularly and in the blood, or primarily in the gastrointestinal tract. Intracellular protozoans, such as *Leishmania,* are eliminated by delayed and granulomatous reactions similar to the response evoked by leprosy. In certain types of leishmaniasis, the organism is limited to focal inflamed areas of the skin. This response has histologic characteristics of a DTH reaction. If this DTH is lost, dissemination of the organisms may occur. Trypanosomiasis is an example of a blood-borne extracellular parasite that may also be found intracellularly; the major defense appears to be via humoral antibody, because rising titers of antibody are associated with containment of symptoms. However, as discussed below, the organisms of African trypanosomiasis are able to change surface antigens in a cyclic fashion, resulting in growth of new clones in successive waves of parasitemia. Malaria protozoa multiply intracellularly but disseminate through release into the bloodstream. Malarial immunity is mediated both by IgG antibody, which can effectively attack the blood-borne organism, and by T_{CTL} and T_{DTH} cells, which are effective against the intracellular stage in liver cells. Therefore, humoral immunity is effective only during a short period of the malarial protozoal life cycle. Even highly immune infected persons may be unable to clear the parasites completely because of the inability of antibody to affect the intracellular stages. The number of organisms present in the body may be controlled by antibody, and the host lives in balance with the infection. Preventive immunity to malaria may be mediated by antibodies to the sporozoite stage introduced by the mosquito vector or by preventing initial infection of hepatocytes (see below for details). *Entamoeba histolytica* is an intestinal protozoan that infects humans. Although antibodies are produced, the protective effect of these antibodies remains to be demonstrated; immunity may be mediated by cell-mediated immunity or IgA antibody.

Helminth (Worm) Infections

The response to worm infections also depends upon the location of the infestation. Worms are located in the intestinal tract and/or tissues. Tapeworms, which exist in the intestinal lumen, isolated from the tissues of the infected host, promote no protective immunologic response. On the other hand, worms with larval forms that invade tissue do stimulate an immune response. The tissue reaction to *Ascaris* and *Trichinella* consists of an intense infiltrate of PMNs, with a predominance of eosinophils. Eosinophil granules contain basic proteins that are toxic to worms. Eosinophils are directed to attack worms by antibody-dependent cellular cytotoxicity. Anaphylactic antibodies (IgE) are also frequently associated with helminth infections, and intradermal injection of worm extracts elicits a wheal-and-flare reaction. Children infested with *A. lumbricoides* have attacks of urticaria, asthma, and other anaphylactic or atopic types of reactions presumably associated with dissemination of *Ascaris* antigens. An eosinophilic pulmonary infiltrate (pneumonia) may be found associated with migration of helminth larvae through the lung. In experimental models, expulsion of parasitic worms from the gastrointestinal tract occurs following the induction of peristalsis and diarrhea from intestinal IgE-mediated anaphylactic reactions to worms (see below). In tissues, the egg forms of schistosomes elicit a granulomatous response in which both DTH (IL-2 and TNF-γ) and anaphylactic (IL-4, IL-5, and eosinophils) responses play a prominent role.

Fungal Infections

Cellular immunity, primarily T_{DTH}-mediated activation of macrophages, appears to be the most important immunologic factor in resistance to fungal infections, although humoral antibody certainly may play a role. The importance of cellular reactions is indicated by the intense mononuclear infiltrate and granulomatous reactions that occur in tissues infected with fungi and by the fact that fungal infections are frequently associated with depressed immune reactivity of the delayed type (opportunistic infections). Chronic mucocutaneous candidiasis refers to persistent or recurrent infection by *C. albicans* of mucous membranes, nails, and skin. Patients with this disease generally have a form of immune deviation, i.e., a depression of cellular immune reactions, with high levels of humoral antibody (see below), similar to lepromatous leprosy. Fungi appear to be resistant to the effects of antibody, so cell-mediated immunity is needed for effective resistance.

Insect Stings

Immune reactions to insect bites or stings are generally believed to be responsible for most of the irritating skin reactions that follow the bite or sting. Individuals vary markedly in their immune reactions to insect stings. Clearly, the reaction of a given person to an insect sting depends upon the dominant type of immune response. Most people react to insect stings or bites, including mosquito bites, by acute cutaneous anaphylactic reactions. Systemic shock and death from wasp or bee stings, while infrequent, may develop in hyperreactive individuals. Two possible protective functions of anaphylactic reactions to insect stings are possible: (i) immediate avoidance behavior by the recipient serves to reduce antigen contact, and (ii) anaphylactic reactions may help prevent toxic complex reactions or DTH reactions. Since potentially fatal anaphylactic reactions require much less antigen contact than other allergic reactions, the latter mechanism seems unlikely. In fact, hyposensitization via the production of blocking IgG antibodies is attempted clinically to reduce the possibility of anaphylactic reactions to insect bites (see chapter 11). An anaphylactic reaction to insect stings may be protective in producing avoidance behavior. However, in all likelihood, anaphylactic reactions to insect bites are not protective reactions but examples of potentially protective immune reactions being applied inappropriately.

Summary of the Role of Immune Mechanisms in Protection against Infections

From the preceding discussion, it can be appreciated that each of the seven types of allergic reactions responsible for immune disease also has important functions in resistance to infection.

1. Neutralization or inactivation of biologically active toxins by antibodies is highly desirable. This is precisely what is accomplished by immunization with diphtheria toxoid.
2. Cytotoxic or cytolytic reactions directed against the infecting organisms cause their death, resulting in cure of the infection.
3. The inflammatory effect of antigen-antibody complexes in the Arthus mechanism results in chemotaxis and stickiness of leukocytes, platelets, and endothelium and increases permeability. These effects promote defense by localization and diapedesis of

leukocytes. At the dose level of a usual infection, this effect is not harmful to the host. Precipitating antibody and complement, as means of enhancing phagocytosis (opsonization), are responsible for protection against many bacterial infections.

4. The effect of histamine release (the anaphylactic mechanism) at the usual dose level results in slight vasodilation and increased capillary permeability, both effects interpreted in classic pathology as aiding defense. Eosinophilic infiltrates may be toxic to worm infestations in tissues. Smooth muscle contraction and diarrhea induced by the anaphylactic mechanism may cause expulsion of intestinal parasites.
5. T-cytotoxic reactions are protective when directed against virus-infected cells, but the loss of these cells may be the critical factor in a disease. In addition, T_{CTL} cells directed against host cells is a major mechanism for autoimmune lesions.
6. DTH at the dose level that occurs in infection results in local mobilization and activation of phagocytes and effective destruction of infecting agents. DTH is particularly effective against infectious agents that proliferate inside macrophages; such organisms thrive in the absence of DTH but are eliminated by DTH-activated macrophages.
7. Granulomatous hypersensitivity may serve to isolate or localize insoluble toxic materials or organisms.

Interaction of Immune Mechanisms in Some Infectious Diseases

A major thesis of this book is that the same nonimmune-specific and immune-specific effector mechanisms that cause disease also protect us from disease. Thus, the interactions of various immune effector mechanisms are also seen in infectious diseases in roles of protection and pathogenesis. For example, the effects of different types of immune effector mechanisms in different forms of filariasis are described in chapter 14. Many other infectious diseases have similar, if not so complicated, mixtures of immunoprotective and immunopathologic mechanisms. A few examples are presented here.

Lyme Disease

Lyme disease is manifested by various stages of inflammation for which the immune response to the infecting organism, *Borrelia burgdorferi,* is responsible for the lesions. The lesions resemble those of other immunopathological diseases, e.g., demyelination, similar to postvaccinial encephalomyelitis; inflammation of the heart and heart block, similar to rheumatic fever; arthritis, similar to rheumatoid arthritis; and vasculitis, consistent with immune complex disease. Circulating immune complexes containing *B. burgdorferi* antigens are present in most patients with active lesions. The name Lyme disease comes from the recognition of a geographic clustering of children with what was thought to be a peculiar form of juvenile arthritis in Lyme, Connecticut, in 1977. *B. burgdorferi* is a spirochete related to *Treponema pallidum,* the causative agent of syphilis. It is transmitted to humans through the bite of certain species of ticks. Following infection, there may be an inapparent infection or development of a complex series of lesions, first involving the skin and then extending to a systemic disease (Table 15.2). Recently, various strains of *B. burgdorferi* have been identified, and different strains may be associated with different clinical manifestations.

Table 15.2 Clinical manifestations of Lyme disease[a]

	Clinical manifestation(s)		
System	**Localized (stage 1)**	**Disseminated (stage 2)**	**Persistent (stage 3)**
Skin	Erythema migrans	Annular lesions, malar rash, diffuse erythema, or urticaria	Acrodermatitis chronica atropicans, localized sclerodermalike lesions
Musculoskeletal		Migratory joint and bone pain, transient arthritis, myositis	Prolonged arthritis
Neurologic		Meningitis, cranial neuritis, Bell's palsy, myelitis, chorea	Chronic encephalomyelitis, spastic paraparesis, ataxia, dementia, etc.
Lymph	Lymphadenopathy	Lymphadenopathy, splenomegaly	Lymphoma
Heart		Nodal block, pancarditis	
Eyes		Conjunctivitis, iritis, choroiditis, retinal detachment, ophthalmitis	Keratitis
Liver		Mild or recurrent hepatitis	
Respiratory		Sore throat, nonproductive cough, adult respiratory distress syndrome	
Kidney		Mild hematuria or proteinuria	
Genitourinary		Orchitis	
Constitutional	Minor	Severe malaise and fatigue	Fatigue

[a]Modified from A. C. Steere, *N. Engl. J. Med.* **321**:586–596, 1989.

The disease begins with the appearance of a pathognomonic skin lesion, *erythema chronicum migrans,* first described in 1909 by Arvid Afzelius in Sweden; it was not until 1982 that the spirochete *B. burgdorferi* was isolated from these skin lesions. Erythema migrans begins as a red macule or papule that expands to form a large ring of erythema with a bright red outer border and partial central clearing. This is sometimes accompanied by fever, minor constitutional symptoms, and regional swelling in the lymph nodes (lymphadenopathy). Without this characteristic lesion, the diagnosis may be very difficult to make.

The next stage of the disease, *early infection,* evolves after spread of the spirochete through the blood to other organs. The major characteristics of the second stage are skin rashes, migratory joint pains, meningitis, lymphadenopathy, and severe malaise and fatigue. By this time, serum immunoglobulin M (IgM) antibody has usually appeared, and its detection may be used to aid in the diagnosis. In addition, lymphocytes respond to *B. burgdorferi* antigens by blastogenesis, and IL-1 and tumor necrosis factor (TNF) levels increase.

Late infection (stage 3), usually seen during the second or third year after infection, features prolonged episodes of arthritis, similar to rheumatoid arthritis. Synovial lesions show hypertrophy with increases in mononuclear cells and plasma cells. In a few cases, Lyme disease spirochetes have been isolated from synovial fluid, and the IL-1 level is elevated. At this stage, a few spirochetes may be found around lesions of obliterative endarteritis (chronic immune complex vasculitis). Thus, although the exact pathogenesis of Lyme disease is not clear, there appear to be many similarities to other immune-mediated diseases involving both antibody- and cell-mediated mechanisms. Cross-reactivity (molecular mimicry) between *B. burgdorferi* antigens and host tissues may be responsible for many of the lesions (central nervous system, heart, joint) that are similar to those of other presumed autoimmune diseases.

The diverse manifestations can make the diagnosis of Lyme disease very difficult. In the United States, Lyme disease is seen in the summer with the appearance of erythema marginatum, accompanied by flulike or meningitislike symptoms. Weeks or months later, neurologic or heart problems, migratory arthritis, or musculoskeletal pain may occur, and more than a year after onset, some patients have chronic joint, skin, or neurologic abnormalities. However, the course of the disease may vary greatly in different patients. In particular, the late neurologic symptoms are not completely codified but should be different from those of multiple sclerosis, amyotrophic lateral sclerosis, or Alzheimer's disease. The more vague constitutional symptoms may be confused with those of chronic fatigue syndrome, but careful analysis can lead to the correct differential diagnosis in most cases. After the first several weeks, almost all patients develop specific antibody. However, serologic testing is complicated by the fact that the tests for antibody are not yet fully standardized and differ from laboratory to laboratory. Thus, serologic testing, such as enzyme-linked immunosorbent assays for specific antibody, is the most practical laboratory aid in diagnosis, but results must be interpreted with caution. Diagnosis is important, because *B. burgdorferi* is highly sensitive to tetracyclines, and oral treatment is effective in stage 1 or 2; its effectiveness in stage 3 has not been determined.

The life cycle of *B. burgdorferi* depends on ticks, which in turn depend on certain types of mice. In the United States, the primary host for the ticks is the white-footed mouse. This mouse is tolerant of the infection and supports large numbers of *B. burgdorferi* without apparent untoward effects. The ticks can also feed on a number of other wild animals and birds without causing disease. However, humans and domestic animals, such as dogs and cattle, are not natural hosts and develop disease. Lyme disease is worldwide but in particularly high incidence in New England and Europe. The marked increase seen during the last 15 years in New England is explained by the conversion of farmland to woodland, with measures to protect deer, which also protect white-footed mice, and the expansion of suburban populations into these woodland areas.

Vaccines against *B. burgdorferi* using recombinant outer surface proteins as antigens have been tested and found to be highly immunogenic and well tolerated. Most of the cases of Lyme disease in the United States appear to be caused by one strain of *Borrelia,* whereas in Europe, several subspecies are pathogenic, and a more complicated vaccine will be required for complete coverage. The monovalent vaccine (rOspA) is now recommended for those with a high risk of exposure in the United States.

Strongyloides Hyperinfection

An example of the role of DTH (granulomatous reactivity) and anaphylactic mechanisms in controlling intestinal nematode infection is the occurrence of "hyperinfection" by *Strongyloides stercoralis* in immune-suppressed individuals. Infestations with *S. stercoralis* were first noted in French soldiers returning from Vietnam in 1876. It is estimated that 100 million to 200 million people in the tropics and subtropics have *S. stercoralis* infections. *S. stercoralis* is also found in the southeastern United States. In one study, 4% of patients in a New Orleans hospital were found to contain eggs or larvae in their stools.

Unique among the intestinal nematodes of humans is the ability of invasive larvae of *S. stercoralis* to mature within the gastrointestinal tract (Fig. 15.4). This allows autoinfection. Infected individuals with normal im-

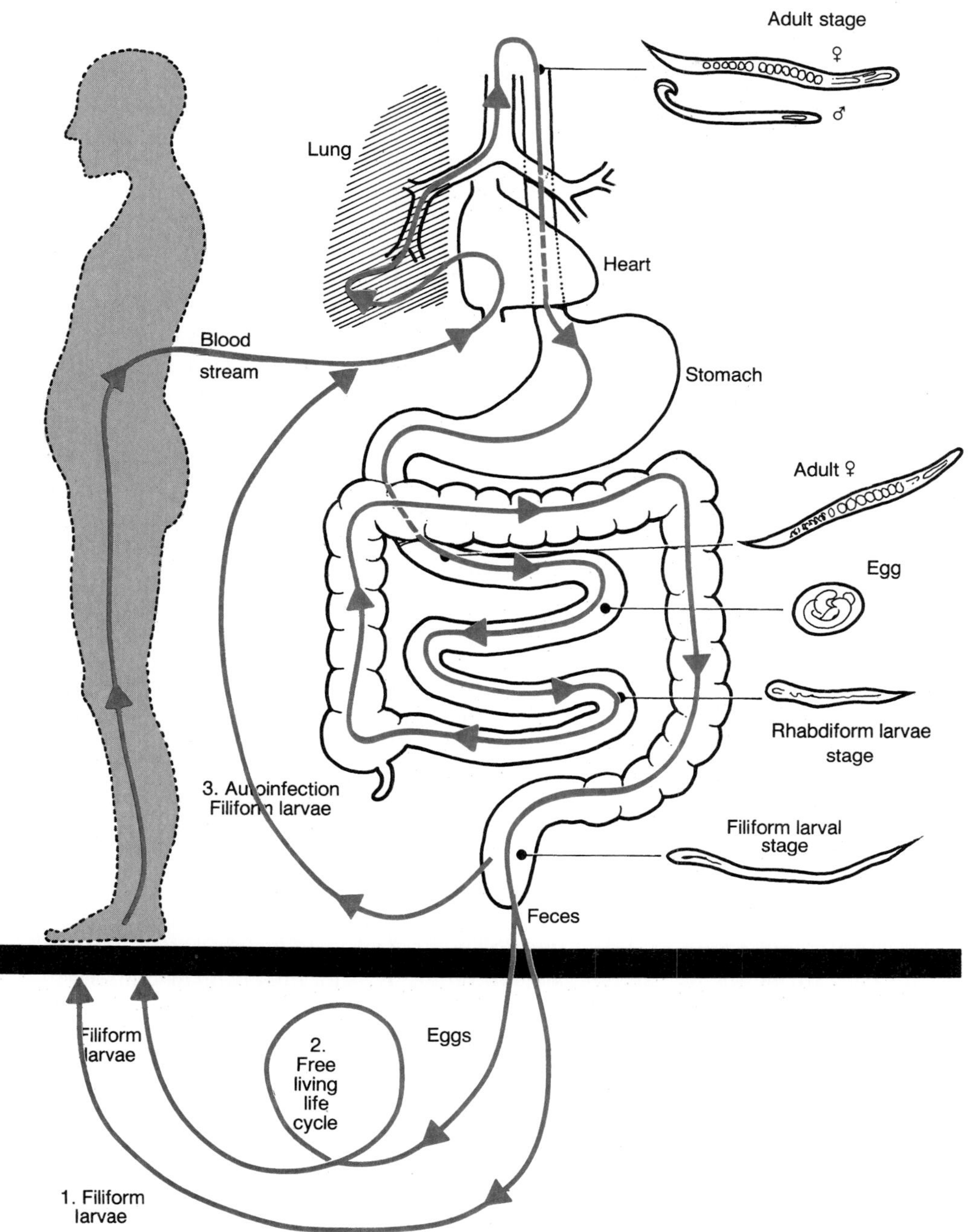

Figure 15.4 The life cycle of *S. stercoralis* provides three routes of human infection: **(1)** infection by invasive filiform larvae excreted into the soil, **(2)** maturation of invasive filiform larvae from free-living organisms in the soil, and **(3)** autoinfection from filiform larvae that mature in the gastrointestinal tract of the host. Filiform larvae invade skin, enter the venous circulation, and pass to the alveolar capillaries. In the lung, the adolescent worms mature to adult male and female worms. The adult worms pass to the gastrointestinal tract, presumably by being coughed up and swallowed. The females lodge in the mucosa of the gastrointestinal tract, set up housekeeping, and lay many eggs; the male is no longer needed and most likely is passed out in the feces. In the gastrointestinal tract, eggs may mature to rhabdiform larvae and to filiform larvae. All of these forms may be passed into the soil. In addition, filiform larvae may invade the intestinal mucosa, particularly at the anal canal, permitting autoinfection.

mune function remain essentially asymptomatic; the immune system provides a barrier to autoinfection. However, in immunosuppressed individuals, hyperinfection occurs.

Hyperinfected individuals are most likely asymptomatic bearers of *S. stercoralis* until a natural disease (e.g., Hodgkin's disease, lymphoma, debilitation, leprosy) or immunosuppressive therapy, such as steroids or cytotoxic drugs for graft recipients, results in depressed immunity. It is believed that anaphylactic and DTH mechanisms are primarily responsible for maintenance of the asymptomatic state. Evidence for this is the association of poor prognosis with a lack of eosinophilia and the finding of hyperinfection in patients with lepromatous leprosy who have a selective deficiency in DTH. In hyperinfected patients, there is a failure to develop granulomas in infected organs; such granulomas are characteristic of lesions in infected individuals with normal immune function.

The apparent pathogenesis of hyperinfection is loss of intestinal barriers to invasion of filiform larvae secondary to immunodeficiency and decreased intestinal motility, allowing more time for filiform larvae to develop from eggs and rhabdiform larvae. Patients with strongyloides hyperinfection develop inflammatory changes in the intestine associated with diarrhea and ileus. Massive infiltration leads to severe inflammation in the lung, and larvae may be seen in the liver, lung, brain, and meninges. Also associated is sepsis by enteric organisms leading to fatal meningitis. Invasion of the strongyloides larvae opens the way for organisms in the gut to enter the body of an already immunosuppressed individual. A definitive diagnosis is made by identification of the organisms in biopsies of the gastrointestinal tract.

Evasion of Immune Defense Mechanisms

The many different immune effector mechanisms most likely evolved as a means for defending us against many different infectious agents. In return, infectious organisms have evolved many "ingenious" ways to avoid immune defense mechanisms (Table 15.3). Organisms may locate in niches not accessible to immune effector mechanisms or may mask themselves by acquiring host molecules. They may change their surface antigens, hide within cells, produce factors that inhibit the immune response, fool the immune system into responding with an ineffective effector mechanism, or actually use part of the immune response to increase infectivity or growth of the infectious agent. The ultimate end point of coevolution of the human host and its infectious organisms results in an eventual mutual coexistence. No better evidence of this is the loss of this coexistence when the immune mechanisms do not function properly. Then organisms that do not normally cause disease become virulent. These are known as opportunistic infections. One of the many lessons of the AIDS epidemic is that new infectious organisms will become dominant when introduced into a previously unexposed population. Previous examples of this are the devastating effects of tuberculosis and smallpox introduced to previously unexposed American Indians and of syphilis introduced into Europe in the 1490s. The genetic diversity of immune responsiveness in populations is responsible for both the inability of some individuals to develop an immune response to a new infectious agent and the ability of other individuals to make a protective response and survive. If genetic diversity in immune responsiveness is not

Table 15.3 Some mechanisms of evasion of immune defenses by infectious agents

Mechanism	Example(s)
Localization in protective niches	Latent syphilis, herpes simplex virus, tapeworm *(Echinococcus)*
Extracorporeal location	*Clostridium tetani, Ascaris lumbricoides*
Intracellular location	Histoplasmosis, viruses (human immunodeficiency virus [HIV]), *Chlamydia, Listeria monocytogenes*
Resistance to phagocytosis	*Streptococcus pneumoniae*
FasL expression (blocks T_{CTL}-cell killing)	Tuberculosis, Epstein-Barr virus, tumors
Killing of activated $CD4^+$ T cells	HIV
Blocking production of memory T cells	Malaria
Killing of activated $CD8^+$ T cells	Herpes simplex virus
Ineffective activated $CD8^+$ T cells	Lymphocytic choriomeningitis virus
Suppression of $CD8^+$ T-cell production	Hepatitis C virus
Downregulation of CD1	Tuberculosis
Complement misdirection	Schistosomiasis, vaccinia virus, herpesviruses, trypanosomiasis
Loss of cell surface antigens	Schistosomiasis
Antigenic modulation	Malaria, trypanosomiasis, *Helicobacter pylori*
Stearic hindrance of receptor sites (the canyon hypothesis)	Influenza virus, rhinoviruses, HIV?
Fc receptor induction (bipolar bridging)	Herpes simplex virus, cytomegalovirus, *Staphylococcus,* syphilis
Antibody-mediated infection	Malaria
Immunosuppression	Malaria, measles, HIV, tuberculosis (anergy)
MHC-restricted recognition of antigens	*Ascaris lumbricoides,* malaria
Downregulation of class I MHC	Adenovirus
Blocking of death ligands (inhibit apoptosis)	Adenovirus
Degradation of class II MHC	Cytomegalovirus
Dendritic cell maturation inhibition	Vaccinia virus
Inappropriate immune response (immune deviation)	Lepromatous leprosy, chronic mucocutaneous candidiasis
Competing soluble cytokine receptors	Poxviruses (IL-1R, TNF receptor)
Suppressive lymphokines	Epstein-Barr virus (IL-10)
Multiple mechanisms	Leishmaniasis

present, a new infectious agent could annihilate a genetically unresponsive population. In a fully evolved, mature relationship host and infectious agent coexist without detrimental affects. Thus the ultimate evolution of the host parasite relationship is not "cure" of an infection by complete elimination of the parasite, but is mutual coexistence without deleterious effects of the parasite on the host. In fact, in many human infections, the infectious agent is never fully destroyed and the disease enters a latent state, that can be reactivated under different conditions, such as decreased immunity with aging or the effect of superinfection with another agent.

Most infectious agents use more than one mechanism for evading immunity. To illustrate some examples of how the host's immunity is avoided during an infection the following will be briefly presented: echinococcosis, human immunodeficiency virus (HIV), *Chlamydia, Streptococcus,* tuberculosis, schistosomiasis, vaccinia virus, trypanosomiasis, measles, influenza virus, herpesvirus, malaria, *Ascaris,* adenovirus, cytomegalovirus, leprosy and syphilis, poxviruses, Epstein-Barr virus, and leishmaniasis.

Echinococcosis: Protected Niche

Echinococcosis is initiated by ingestion of eggs of the dog tapeworm *Echinococcus granulosus*. The eggs hatch in the human intestine and release embryos (oncospheres) that penetrate the gut wall, enter the bloodstream, and disseminate to deep organs, such as liver, kidney, and lung, where the larvae mature and produce cysts called hydatid cysts. Cystic hydatid disease of humans consists of multiple unilocular fluid-filled cysts containing viable larvae. The mature larvae (metacestode) may survive for many years in the cyst, even though the infected individual is resistant to reinfection (concomitant immunity). The larvae are protected from immune attack by an acellular laminated external layer or cuticle as well as by a thick capsule of connective tissue that walls off the site of infection, similar to what occurs in the granulomas of chronic tuberculosis. Thus, the organisms survive in a protected niche, while the infected individual has a high titer of circulating antibody and is protected from newly acquired infection.

HIV: Intracellular Location and Immunosuppression

The pathogenesis of AIDS and HIV infection is covered in detail in chapter 19. HIV is carried inside monocytes and lymphocytes in the form of integrated DNA, where it is hidden from immune attack for long periods of time during latent infection. In addition, lentiviruses downregulate cell surface expression of CD4 and class I MHC. These events preserve infectivity and prevent immune recognition by T_{CTL} cells. Transmission of infection from one individual to another is mediated by passage of living infected cells during intimate body contact through open lesions in the skin or mucous membranes. Even if circulating antibody to HIV antigens is present in the recipient of the infected cells, no HIV antigens are on the infected cells to which the antibody could react. The immune response does appear to be able to hold in check manifestations of the infection, but since one of the most important cells of the immune system, the $CD4^+$ T cell, is also the prime target for HIV infection, eventually the cytolytic HIV destroys enough of the $CD4^+$ T cells to produce a severe immunodeficiency. This allows not only expansion of the HIV infection but also opportunistic infections by other organisms.

Chlamydia trachomatis: Endosomes

Chlamydia trachomatis is a prokaryotic obligate intracellular parasite (bacterium) that causes keratoconjunctivitis and pelvic inflammatory disease. The organisms are taken into epithelial cells by receptor-mediated endocytosis and multiply within the host cell in membrane-delimited endosomes. Within the host cell, the organisms are protected from host immune defenses. Large numbers of infective particles are released when the host cell dies.

Streptococcus pneumoniae: Resistance to Phagocytosis

S. pneumoniae has a thick capsule of polysaccharide that enables the bacteria to resist phagocytosis by either resident pulmonary macrophages or recruited neutrophils. Inhaled organisms are cleared by the microvilli of the respiratory epithelium. The incidence of infection is greatly increased in individuals who have defective clearing mechanisms (e.g., smokers, persons with chronic bronchitis, and persons with asthma). In such individuals, organisms are able to colonize the nasopharynx and spread to the pulmonary alveoli. Reaction of antibodies to antigens of the cell wall activates complement, but because of the capsule, neither the Fc of IgG nor the C3b on the cell surface is able to interact with receptors of phagocytic cells. In the absence of antibody to the capsular polysaccharide, phagocytosis and killing do not occur. Activation of the inflammatory peptides of complement, particularly C5a, causes an intense polymorphonuclear reaction, and along with other mediators, such as IL-1, endogenous pyrogens and pneumolysin (a toxin produced by pneumococci), causes a self-perpetuating inflammatory reaction that is largely responsible for symptoms and signs of the disease. In contrast to antibodies to the cell wall, antibodies to the capsular polysaccharides are extremely effective in opsonizing the organisms. Immunization with capsular polysaccharides stimulates antibodies that cause agglutination and a marked swelling of the capsule (the quellung reaction) and protect against challenge in laboratory animals. Pneumococcal vaccination is recommended for individuals at risk for infection and is likely to offer a substantial degree of protection.

Mycobacterium tuberculosis: FasL Expression

In tuberculosis granulomas, some macrophages may contain large numbers of mycobacteria but appear to be protected from T-cell killing. These infected macrophages have a markedly increased expression of Fas ligand (FasL). A major component of T_{CTL}-cell killing is reaction of FasL on T_{CTL} cells with Fas on target cells. Expression of FasL on the infected macrophages protects these cells from T-killer cells. Infected cells may also downregulate CD1, thus inhibiting antigen recognition.

Schistosomiasis: Protective Niche, Masking of Surface Antigens, Complement Misdirection, and Th1-versus-Th2 Response

The life cycle of the schistosomes that infect humans provides stages that express little if any antigens recognizable by infected individuals and stages that are highly immunogenic. Infection begins when motile aquatic cercariae released from the snail intermediate invade the skin of a human host. These larvae penetrate blood vessels, pass through the lung, and circulate selectively to the venous sinusoids of the gastrointestinal wall (*Schistosoma japonicum* and *Schistosoma mansoni*) or bladder wall (*Schistosoma haematobium*), where maturation to adult worms occurs in the venous sinuses. The adults may live for over a decade in this location. The female releases eggs, which pass through the gastrointestinal wall or bladder, where they are excreted into fresh water to infect the intermediate snail host.

The adult worms survive in the circulation of the host in the face of high titers of circulating antibodies to schistosomal antigens. This paradox has been attributed to several possible mechanisms, including very low surface antigen expression on the adult organism so that IgG antibody is unable to from aggregates to fix complement; absorption of host molecules, such as blood group glycolipids, MHC glycoproteins, fibronectin, and immunoglobulin bound through the Fc regions, that disguise schistosomal antigens; shedding or endocytosis of surface antigens without destruction of the organisms; or membrane pumps that compensate for the ion imbalance that might be produced by immune attack. A more recent explanation is that schistosomula acquire resistance to alternate pathway-mediated complement killing by shedding glycoproteins that activate complement. This protects the organisms not only directly but also indirectly. The released glycoproteins bind to the C3 receptors on effector cells, such as eosinophils or neutrophils, damage the effector cells, and further protect the organisms. Regardless of the mechanisms, the adult organisms develop a tegument resistant to immune attack, which is not the case for the egg or larval forms.

Individuals who are infected are resistant to reinfection even though they carry live adults in their veins (concomitant immunity). There is a strong cellular immune response to antigens on the eggs that is shared with the invading larvae. The outcome of this immunity depends on the balance of Th1 versus Th2 response. The Th1 response appears to protect against infection and, although contributing to granuloma formation, will eventually destroy the organisms. On the other hand, the Th2 response also induces extensive granulomatous inflammation in the liver or bladder wall to eggs that are deposited there, but the cytokines released from reacting Th1 cells, such as IL-10, IL-4, and transforming growth factor beta, may actually inhibit destruction of parasites by blocking nitric oxide metabolism of macrophages. The presence of concomitant immunity indicates that appropriate immunization of uninfected individuals with egg antigens should produce immunity to primary infection.

Vaccinia Virus: Control of Complement Activation

Vaccinia virus secretes a complement control protein (VCP) that has homology to eukaryotic regulators of complement. VCP is also identified as CD55. VCP (CD55) can inhibit both classical and alternate pathways of complement activation. VCP binds to both C4b and C3b and accelerates the decay of complement convertases. Although the lesion of vaccinia is clearly cell-mediated, complement-mediated neutralization decreases the pathogenic effects of the virus, presumably by limiting the spread of infection. In rabbits, lesions caused by wild-type and mutant viruses lacking the gene for VCP are similar for the first 5 days, but after that, the lesions of the mutant virus decrease in size, whereas those of the wild type do not. Antibody to virus appears at about day 5. Thus, wild-type virus is able to avoid antibody-mediated attack, whereas virus lacking VCP is not. In addition, vaccinia virus appears to prevent maturation of infected dendritic cells, thus inhibiting T-cell activation.

Trypanosomiasis: Antigenic Modulation

Trypanosomes avoid immune attack by changing the antigens that they express (antigenic variation). This mechanism is also used by other organisms, but trypanosomes have the most sophisticated system of antigenic variation known. A relatively large portion of the trypanosome genome (approximately 2%) is devoted to antigenic variation. *Trypanosoma brucei* has been estimated to have 1,000 different antigen genes. The maximum number of antigen types actually identified in one clone of a trypanosome is 101. Thus, when an infected individual produces an antibody to one antigen, the organism shifts to expression of a new antigen and avoids immune attack.

The genetic mechanisms for antigen switching include the following.

1. Gene conversion, by which the activated gene is replaced by a copy of another gene, so that the original gene activation site acts on a different gene
2. Differential activation, in which an activation factor binds to a different controlling region, activating another gene
3. Partial gene conversion, in which part of an inactive gene replaces part of an active gene
4. Reciprocal recombination, by which an inactive gene gains access to an active controlling site by unequal crossing over
5. Point mutation

Many of the variable surface glycoprotein antigen genes are found in repeat sequences at chromosomes' ends (telomeres). Telomeres with extensive regions of repeated sequences are recombination hot spots. In addition, a telomeric transcription site allows activation of a series of alternative telomeres on different chromosomes.

In the blood, antigen types succeed each other in different parasitemia waves (Fig. 15.5). Analysis of clones reveals the presence of different DNA rearrangements within a clone, suggesting a high rate of recombination or polyclonal activation. The timing of antigenic variation is important for long-term survival of the organism, since otherwise it would be possible to exhaust the antigenic repertoire and eliminate the infection. The succession of antigen types appears to be conserved in a given strain, but the mechanism controlling the sequence of antigen expression is not known.

Measles: Immunosuppression

Measles was the first virus infection shown to cause a generalized immune deficiency; HIV (see chapter 19) produces even more profound effects. Measles was first described in Baghdad by Rhazes in the 6th century. It is

Figure 15.5 Antigenic variation during trypanosomiasis infection. Successive waves of different clones expressing different surface glycoproteins (VSG, variable surface glycoproteins) of the parasite are characteristic of trypanosomiasis. After infection, one clone of parasites, most of which carry a particular VSG, proliferates in the bloodstream. Antibody is produced to this VSG and kills most of the parasites. A few individuals survive by expressing a new VSG. This clone then expands until antibody to the new VSG is produced and kills most of the second wave. This process is repeated over and over again as new clones are produced. (From J. E. Donelson and M. J. Turner, *Sci. Am.* **252:**44, 1985.)

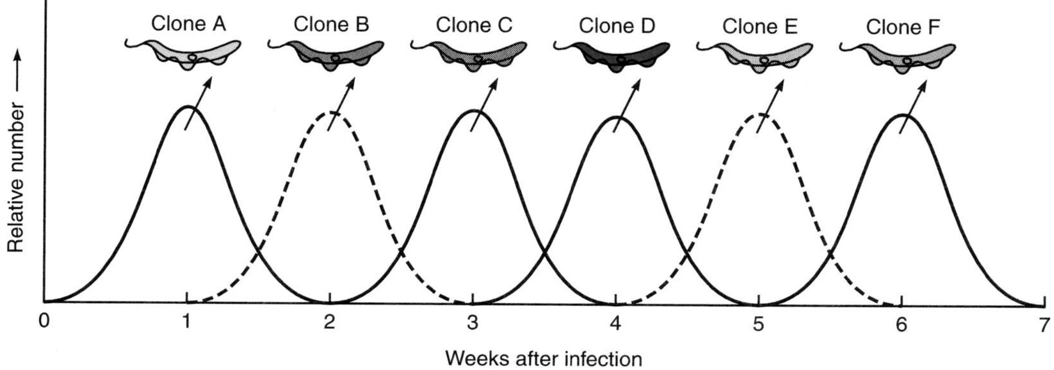

believed to have evolved in Africa from an animal virus. It was spread into Europe in the 8th century by the Saracen invasion, where it produced vast numbers of fatalities from opportunistic infections, as well as by activation of latent tuberculosis or superinfection with tuberculosis. In 1908, von Pirquet first noted a loss of cutaneous tuberculin reactions in children who had the measles rash. Like many other infectious agents, measles produces high death rates in virgin populations but is much less virulent in exposed populations.

Measles infection is associated with depressed cellular immunity. This is not specific for measles, as there is depression of skin test reactivity to other test antigens and depressed lymphoproliferative responses to antigens and mitogens in individuals with more severe manifestations, such as measles pneumonia. In vitro, the virus will infect T cells of both CD4 and CD8 subsets as well as B cells and macrophages. However, the exact nature of the immunosuppression in vivo is not well understood. There appears to be decreased production of IL-1 and IL-2 by macrophages or lymphocytes, elevation of IgE, and evidence for spontaneous suppressor cell activity. Thus, even with major advances in analyzing immune functions, the pathogenesis of measles immunodeficiency remains unclear.

Influenza Virus: Stearic Hindrance

Influenza virus has conserved structures required for infectivity as well as rapidly modulating structures that are recognized by antibodies produced by the infected host. To survive in the face of development of immunity in a population, the virus is able to undergo modification of those structures that are recognized by antibody without changing the structure required to bind to the specific cell receptor. Influenza virus, as well as most other animal viruses, initiates infection by specific binding of a receptor to a site on the host cell. For influenza virus, the binding site is sialyl-lactose. The virus binding site is located in a depression in the hemagglutinin spike on the surface of the virus that is too narrow for antibody binding to occur. Thus, neutralizing antibodies react with determinants on the surface of the spike and not with the specific cell-binding domain. Human flu epidemics occur because of the appearance of new strains of influenza virus that have different surface epitopes, whereas the cell-binding structure remains unmodified (Fig. 15.6). This is known as the canyon hypothesis.

Herpes Simplex Virus: Intracellular Location, Bipolar Bridging, and Complement Inhibition

Herpes simplex virus (HSV) is endemic in all human populations. It generally remains dormant but may be frequently activated. Although the precise role of cellular and humoral immunity in protection and pathogenesis of HSV infection has not been clearly established, it is protected against immune effector mechanisms by its intracellular location and its ability to infect and eliminate activated T cells. In addition, HSV induces Fc receptors (FcR) on infected cells. The receptors provide protection against lysis by IgG antibody and complement. Binding of the Fab domains of IgG antibodies to virus antigens expressed on the surface of infected cells has the potential to fix complement through binding of C1 to aggregated Fcs of the bound antibodies. However, infection of human cells with HSV is associated with the appearance of a novel FcR so that the Fc portion of IgG antibodies that react with the infected cells is bound to this receptor and is

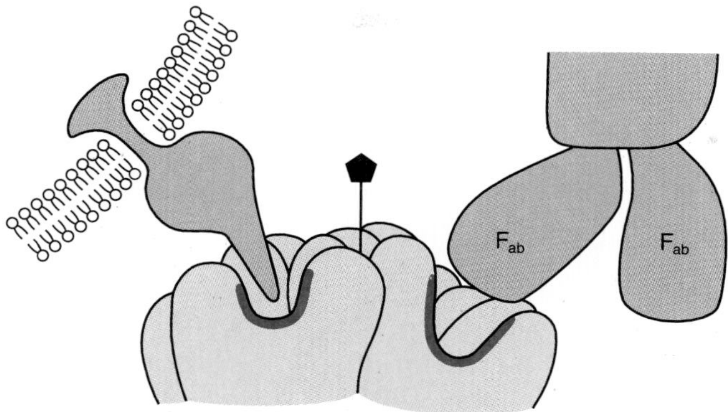

Figure 15.6 The canyon hypothesis. This hypothesis states that the virus-binding site for a cell surface receptor for the virus is located in a depression of the viral spikes on the surface of the virus particles and that this location, while able to receive the cell surface receptor (R), sterically prevents larger antibody paratopes (P) from reacting. This allows for conservation of the virus binding site while at the same time permitting evolution of new serotypes by mutating epitopes about the rim of the canyon. (Modified from M. Luo, G. Vriend, G. Kamer, I. Minor, E. Arnold, M. G. Rossmann, U. Boege, D. G. Scraba, G. M. Duke, and A. C. Palmenberg, *Science* **235:**182–191, 1987.)

not available to react with C1. This is termed bipolar bridging (Fig. 15.7). FcR expression is also associated with other infectious agents, including cytomegalovirus, *S. aureus*, *Trypanosoma*, *Leishmania*, and *S. mansoni*. Staphylococcal protein A binds the $C\gamma2$ and $C\gamma3$ domains of IgG and impairs antibody-dependent complement-mediated killing. Induction of FcR by cytomegalovirus renders cells susceptible to infection by HIV bound to antibody. HSV also produces a glycoprotein C (gC) that binds complement and inhibits complement-mediated virus neutralization and lysis of infected cells.

Malaria: FasL Expression, Antibody-Mediated Infection, and Peptide Inhibition of Antigen Presentation

Malaria parasites infect liver cells and red blood cells. Clearing of infected liver cells is thought to be mediated mainly by T_{CTL}-cell lysis. This may be inhibited by increased expression of FasL, which blocks binding of the FasL on T_{CTL} cells to the liver cells (see below). In addition, antibody to merozoites in the blood may actually increase infectivity for red cells. In an experimental model, malaria merozoites treated with bivalent antibodies IgG or $F(ab')_2$ to surface protein MSA2 increased the proportions of red cells infected. This effect was not seen using univalent (Fab) fragments. It is thought that merozoites cross-linked by bivalent antibody are more effectively attached to and subsequently invade the same cell. In addition, malaria infections may result in production of modified peptides that antagonize with immunogenic peptides to prevent induction of T-cell immunity.

Ascaris lumbricoides: Extracorporeal Location and MHC-Restricted Recognition

In addition to the location of the adult worms within the gastrointestinal tract lumen, where they essentially do not come into contact with the host's immune system, there is MHC-related restriction of recognition of the antigens of the tissue-invading larval stages of *Ascaris*. In mice, the

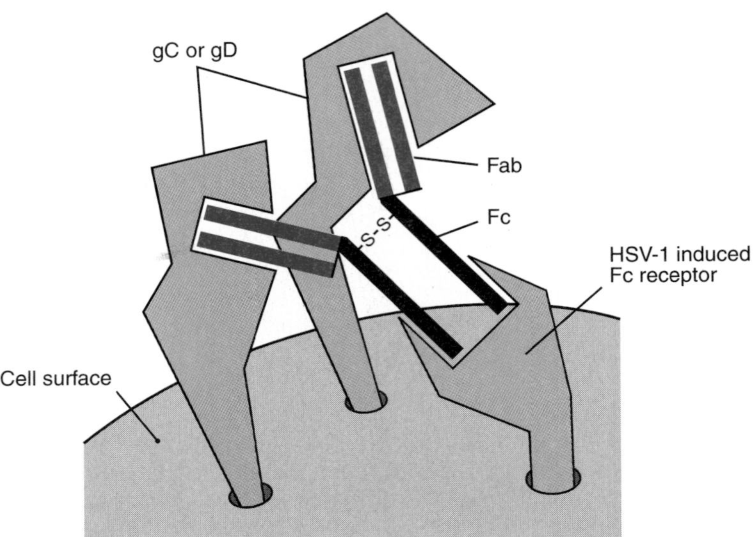

Figure 15.7 Bipolar bridging prevents complement activation. HSV infection induces Fc receptors on the surface of infected cells that tie up the Fc domain of antibody that binds to either of the dominant antigens of HSV-1, gC or gD, through the antigen-binding site (paratope) on the Fab domain. This prevents aggregation of the Fc regions of antibodies on the surface of the cell and prevents binding of C1 of complement. (Modified from I. Frank and H. M. Friedman, *J. Virol.* **63:**4479, 1989.)

ability to recognize and produce antibody to the external excretory/secretory material of the larvae is under the control of H2 loci, not only in regard to the epitopes recognized but also in the class of antibody produced. For instance, mouse strains differ markedly in the level of IgE production, eosinophilia, and the capacity of the immune response to inhibit migration of the larvae to the lungs, a necessary stage of the life cycle of *Ascaris*. MHC-controlled heterogeneity in the immune response explains, at least in part, the variation in disease patterns produced by infection of humans by a number of infectious agents.

Adenovirus: Downregulation of Class I MHC and Inhibition of Apoptosis

Adenovirus product E19 causes intracellular retention of the class I MHC heavy chain by direct binding to the protein and to the transporter associated with antigen processing (TAP), which is involved in class I peptide loading, thus protecting infected cells from T_{CTL}-cell killing. Adenoviruses also encode proteins that block responses to interferons, inhibit apoptosis, and inhibit killing by death ligands TNF, FasL, and TRIAL. Viral products appear to control apoptosis—preventing apoptosis during active replication of the virus but triggering apoptosis in order to release infective viral particles after replication is complete.

Cytomegalovirus: Class I and II MHC Degradation and Molecular Decoys

Human cytomegalovirus (HCMV) establishes lifelong latent infections and, after periodic reactivation from latency, may become activated, especially in immunosuppressed individuals. HCMV downregulates cell surface class I MHC, presumably protecting cells from T_{CTL}-cell killing. However, downregulation of class I MHC may render infected cells more susceptible to natural killer cell recognition. Natural killer cells recognize aberrant expression of class I MHC molecules. HCMV appears to produce viral proteins that serve as molecular decoys, which mimic the ability of normal class I MHC to inhibit natural killer reaction but avoid T_{CTL}-cell recognition. HCMV also produces a protein, US2, that degrades two essential proteins in the MHC class II antigen presentation pathway: HLA-DR-α and DM-α. This may affect recognition of infected macrophages by $CD4^+$ T_{DTH} cells and prevent macrophage activation.

Leprosy and Syphilis: Immune Deviation

Immune deviation or split tolerance is defined as the dominance of one immune response mechanism over another for a specific antigen and has been implicated in the tendency for certain individuals to develop IgE (allergy) antibodies rather than IgG antibodies. In addition, for reasons that are unclear but may be genetically determined, some individuals tend to make strong cellular immune responses but weak antibody response to certain antigens, whereas other individuals will have the opposite response. The course of leprosy depends upon the immune reaction of the patient (see chapter 14). Leprosy may be classified into three overlapping groups: tuberculoid, borderline, and lepromatous. In tuberculoid leprosy, there are prominent, well-formed granulomatous lesions, many lymphocytes, and few if any organisms. DTH skin tests are intact, and there is predominant hyperplasia of the diffuse cortex (T-cell zone) of the lymph nodes. The level of antibodies is low. In lepromatous leprosy, granulomas are not formed, there are few or no lymphocytes, and lesions consist of large macrophages filled with viable organisms. DTH skin tests are depressed, and there is marked follicular hyperplasia in the lymph nodes with little or no diffuse cortex. The levels of antibodies are high, and vascular lesions due to immune complexes (erythema nodosum leprosum) are seen. Borderline leprosy has intermediate findings. The prognosis in tuberculoid leprosy is good, and the response to chemotherapy is excellent. In borderline leprosy, a good response to therapy is associated with a conversion to the tuberculoid form. The prognosis in lepromatous leprosy and the response to chemotherapy are poor. The example of the forms of leprosy illustrates the role of cellular immunity (DTH) in controlling the infection and the lack of protective response provided by humoral antibodies. This concept is also considered valid for immunity to *Candida albicans*. Depressed cellular immunity is associated with chronic mucocutaneous candidiasis, a condition in which the infected individual is unable to clear candida infections. It is now proposed that the same holds for the clinical stages of syphilis.

A diagram illustrating the relationship of the degree of cellular and humoral immune response to the stages of syphilis and leprosy is shown in Fig. 15.8. In this model, the primary chancre of syphilis is considered to be a DTH reaction that essentially clears the site of infectious organisms. If the cellular immune mechanism is dominant, the infection will be cured. If the cellular immune mechanism is not able to clear the infection, replication of the organisms in multiple sites will stimulate secondary reactions, which again are manifestations of DTH. Because of the large number of organisms now present, it may take weeks to clear the lesions, and many organisms will remain in protected niches. However, if cellular

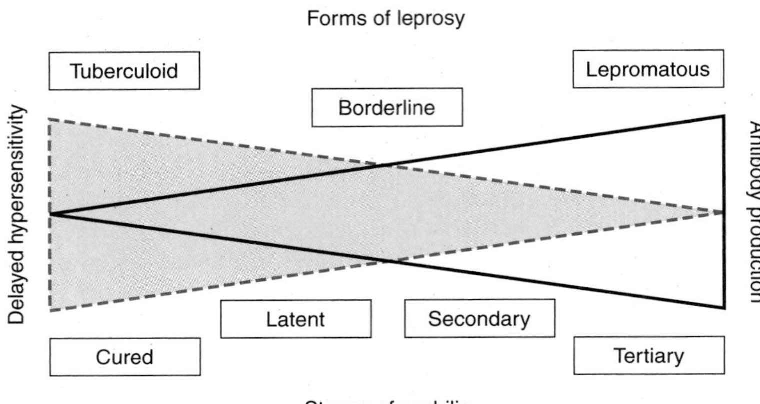

Figure 15.8 A comparison of the association of DTH and antibody production in the clinical forms of leprosy and in the clinical stages of syphilis. The overlapping triangles indicate the relative strength of DTH and antibody production. The cross-hatched triangle indicates DTH; the open triangle, antibody production. High levels of DTH are associated with cure; weak DTH is associated with progressive disease; balanced DTH and antibody production are associated with borderline leprosy and latent syphilis. Progression of syphilis to the tertiary stage is most likely more related to depressed T-cell immunity, with or without high levels of antibody. The nature of the antigen-presenting cell may determine if Th1 cells are activated to help in antibody production or in development of DTH. Antibody production is stimulated by antigens processed by dendritic follicular cells; DTH is stimulated by antigens processed by interdigitating reticulum cells.

immunity remains strong, no further lesion development will occur, and latent infection will be maintained. If the cellular immune response declines, organisms will increase, and lesions of tertiary syphilis will appear, even in the face of high antibody titers in the serum or in the cerebral spinal fluid. In the experimental model in the rabbit, cellular immunity is able to clear dermal or testicular infection, and lesions of secondary and tertiary syphilis do not occur. Penicillin treatment of secondary or tertiary syphilis is able to reduce the number of organisms so that the low level of cellular immunity present is able to reestablish control of the infection. However, if suppression of the cellular immune response is induced by immunosuppression or AIDS, latency may be terminated more rapidly and produce a systemic infection requiring high doses of penicillin.

Poxviruses: Effector Modulation and Soluble Receptors

Poxviruses, such as cowpox virus and vaccinia virus, produce soluble receptors for IL-1, and Shope fibroma/myxoma virus, which produces tumorlike lesions in rabbits, produces soluble forms of receptors for TNF and gamma interferon. These receptors intercept their respective cytokines and prevent reaction with the cell surface receptor, thus preventing the decoyed mediator from binding to its cellular receptor and destroying virus-infected cells.

Epstein-Barr Virus: IL-10

Epstein-Barr virus (EBV) produces a homolog of IL-10, which normally downregulates the antiviral T-cell response and also stimulates B cells that EBV infects. In this way, IL-10 production by EBV-infected B cells not only "auto-upregulates" virus production but also blocks the T_{CTL}-cell response to infected B cells. In addition, EBV-infected cells increase expression of FasL and thus avoid T_{CTL}-cell killing.

Leishmaniasis: Complement-Mediated Endocytosis, Inhibition of Macrophage Killing, Modulation of T-Cell Immunity, and Immune Deviation

Perhaps no organism better exemplifies the multiple ways that parasites can evade or even use the host immune system to its advantage than *Leishmania donovani*. Other species of *Leishmania,* such as *L. major, L. aethiopica,* and *L. mexicana,* do not have these evasive mechanisms and usually cause only local cutaneous lesions that are controlled by DTH reactions, with destruction by phagocytosis and digestion by macrophages. However, infection with *L. donovani* leads to a systemic, eventually lethal disease, kala-azar, because of its ability to evade macrophage-mediated killing. The three major evasion mechanisms used by *L. donovani* are (i) use of complement receptors on macrophages for endocytosis, (ii) inhibition of intracellular killing by macrophages, and (iii) modulation of T-cell immunity (immune deviation) (Fig. 15.9). The major pathologic feature of kala-azar is intracellular accumulation of organisms in macrophages, which leads to massive hepatosplenomegaly and stimulation of monocyte hyperplasia in the bone marrow.

In pathogenic leishmaniae, the surface lipophosphoglycan (LPG) can serve as an acceptor for the third component of complement. After binding to the acceptor, C3 is converted to C3b, and the "opsonized" parasites bind to the CR1 or CR3 of the host's macrophages, which then endocytose the parasite. The effect of this is not only to protect the organism from lysis by antibody and complement activated in the classical pathway but also to facilitate the entry of the parasite into their permissive host cells.

In progressive leishmaniasis, the infecting organisms are able to survive within macrophages by the ability of the parasite to avoid the oxidative and enzymatic destructive mechanisms of the macrophage. Binding to CR1/CR3 inhibits the oxidative burst usually associated with phagocytosis. Once inside the cell, the acid phosphatase on the surface of the parasite downregulates oxygen-dependent killing, and other enzymes, as well as the surface LPG, are able to scavenge toxic oxygen metabolites. In addition, LPG and other surface molecules inhibit digestive enzymes of phagolysosomes, and the pathogenic organisms are able to maintain a neutral intercellular milieu despite the acidic environment inside the phagolysosome. Through these mechanisms, the parasite is able to convert the macrophage into a permissive cell for its survival and propagation.

Finally, in progressive disease, leishmaniae are able to modulate the T-cell immune response so that T_{DTH} cells are not induced to activate the macrophages (immune deviation), similar to what occurs in lepromatous leprosy. The parasite may downregulate a Th1-specific costimulatory molecule (M150) on the surface of infected macrophages. Antigen presentation by macrophages infected by leishmaniae is directed to activation of Th2 cells in preference to Th1 cells. Epidermal Langerhans cells internalize *L. major* and deliver processed antigens to the T-cell zones of draining lymph nodes. In mice, proliferation of organisms in dendritic macrophages in the lymph nodes correlates with the induction of Th2 cells, whereas resistance correlates with the induction of Th1 cells. The release of IL-3, IL-4, and GM-CSF by Th2 cells stimulates bone marrow hyperplasia and the release

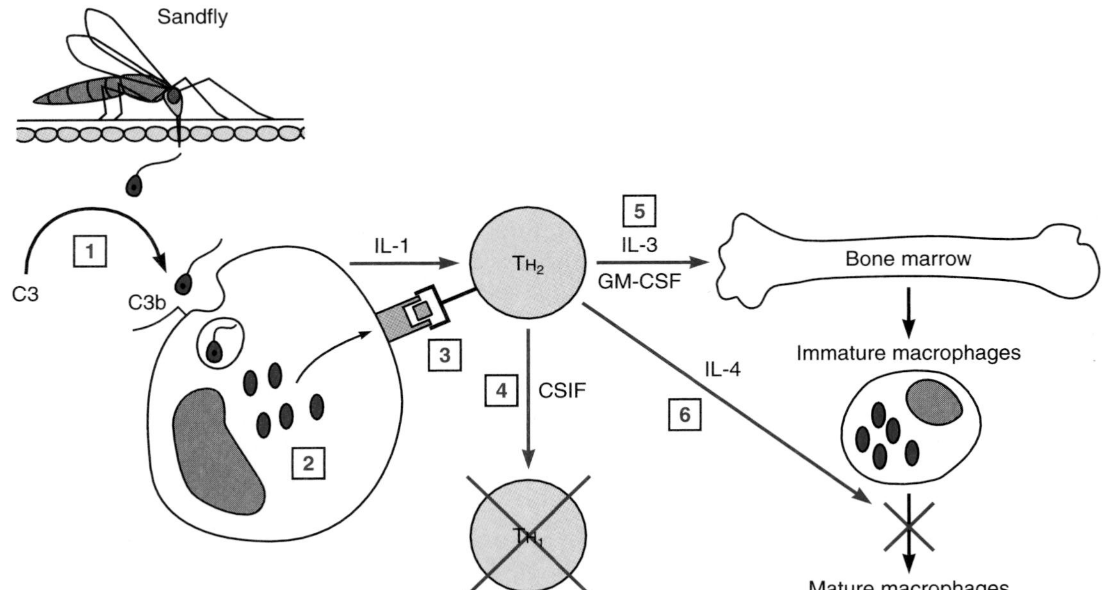

Figure 15.9 Immune evasion during *L. donovani* infection. **(1)** Motile promastigotes injected by the bite of the infected sandfly are able to activate C3 to C3b, bind to macrophages through C3b and CR1/CR3, and are endocytosed without a fatal oxygen burst. **(2)** Inside the cell, the promastigotes transform into amastigotes that are resistant to the oxygen-dependent and enzymatic killing process of the phagocyte. **(3)** Infected macrophages in T-cell zones of lymph nodes present antigens preferentially to Th2 helper cells, which release colony-stimulating inhibitory factor (CSIF), IL-3, granulocyte-macrophage colony-stimulating factor (GM-CSF), and IL-4. **(4)** CSIF inhibits activation of Th1 helper cells and prevents development of T_{DTH} cells and DTH. **(5)** IL-3 and GM-CSF stimulate the bone marrow to produce immature monocytes, which are permissive for parasite replication. **(6)** IL-4 inhibits maturation of monocytes to a state of being able to resist parasite infestation.

of immature macrophages from the bone marrow that are unable to destroy endocytosed organisms, providing more permissive cells for infection. In addition, factors from Th2 cells (colony-stimulating inhibitory factor) further inhibit Th1 cells. The inhibition of IL-2 and gamma interferon release from Th1 cells prevents not only induction of T_{DTH} cells, but also macrophage activation, resulting in immunosuppression as well as inhibition of the killing potential of macrophages.

In conclusion, the host-parasite relationship between infectious agents and their supportive hosts has evolved to allow ways for the infecting parasite to avoid immune attack of the host. There are three general ways that this is accomplished: (i) anatomic (protective niches, intracellular location of the infection, and extracorporeal location), (ii) antigenic change or masking of the infectious agent (antigenic modulation, absorption of host molecules, formation of external cuticles or coats with low antigenicity, and location of important surface structures in "canyons" inaccessible to antibodies), and (iii) variations of the host's immune response (immune suppression, immune deviation, MHC-controlled epitope recognition, and production of competitive inhibitors of cytokines). Each of these approaches is used effectively with many variations to suit the characteristics and life cycles of the infecting organisms.

Summary

Immune and nonimmune inflammatory mechanisms may interact to produce either tissue lesions (immunopathology) or protection against infections (the double-edged sword of immunity). Each immune effector mechanism has a relatively well defined way to effect tissue lesions or defensive functions. In defense, antibody-mediated effector mechanisms generally operate against bacteria or bacterial products; cellular effector mechanisms protect against viral, mycobacterial, or fungal diseases. A list of postulated specific effector mechanisms for selected infectious diseases is given in Table 15.4. In many infectious diseases, more than one mechanism may be active, particularly if the organism exists in different stages. The activation

Table 15.4 Postulated specific immune defense mechanisms in some infectious diseases

Disease	Agent	Site of infection	Defense mechanism
Viral (RNA)			
Influenza	Paramyxovirus	Lung	Antibody blocks cell attachment
Mumps	Paramyxovirus	Parotid gland	T_{CTL} cells kill infected cells
Measles (rubeola)	Paramyxovirus	Skin systemic	T_{CTL} cells kill infected cells
Rabies	Rhabdovirus	Brain cells	T_{CTL} cells kill infected cells
Polio	Picornavirus	Systemic, neurons	Antibody blocks cell attachment
Yellow fever	Flavivirus	Viscera	Antibody blocks cell attachment
Viral (DNA)			
Herpes	Herpesvirus	Skin, mucous membranes	T_{CTL} cells kill infected cells
Smallpox	Poxvirus	Skin	T_{CTL} cells kill infected cells
Hepatitis B	Hepatitis B virus	Liver	Antibody blocks cell attachment
Rickettsial			
Rocky Mountain spotted fever	*Rickettsia rickettsii*	Vascular endothelium	T_{CTL} cells kill infected cells
Typhus	*Rickettsia prowazekii*	Vascular endothelium	T_{CTL} cells kill infected cells
Bacterial			
Botulism	*Clostridium botulinum*	Exotoxin	Neutralization by antibody
Tetanus	*Clostridium tetani*	Exotoxin	Neutralization by antibody
Diphtheria	*Corynebacterium diphtheriae*	Exotoxin	Neutralization by antibody
Pertussis (whooping cough)	*Bordetella pertussis*	Endo- and exotoxin	Neutralization, opsonization
Cholera	*Vibrio cholerae*	Enterotoxin	IgA neutralization of toxin
Staphylococcal	*Staphylococcus aureus*	Connective tissue, pyogenic abscess	Antibody neutralization of toxin, opsonization
Streptococcal	*Streptococcus,* beta-hemolytic	Connective tissue, cellulitis	Antibody neutralization of toxin, opsonization
Pneumonia	*Streptococcus pneumoniae*	Lungs	Antibody opsonization, cytotoxicity
Meningitis	*Neisseria meningitidis*	Meninges, IgA protease	Antibody opsonization, protease neutralization
Gonorrhea	*Neisseria gonorrhoeae*	Mucous surface	Antibody, opsonization, protease neutralization
Influenza	*Haemophilus influenzae*	Lung, endotoxin	Antibody, opsonization, neutralization
Infantile diarrhea	*Escherichia coli*	GI tract, endotoxin	Antibody blocks cell attachment, neutralization, opsonization
Typhoid fever	*Salmonella typhi*	GI tract, systemic endotoxin	Antibody neutralization, DTH, macrophage activation

(continued)

Table 15.4 Postulated specific immune defense mechanisms in some infectious diseases *(continued)*

Disease	Agent	Site of infection	Defense mechanism
Mycobacterial			
Tuberculosis	*Mycobacterium tuberculosis*	Lung	Granulomatous, DTH
Leprosy	*Mycobacterium leprae*	Dermis	Granulomatous, DTH
Spirochetal			
Syphilis	*Treponema pallidum*	Connective tissue	DTH, antibody opsonization?
Lyme disease	*Borrelia burgdorferi*	Skin, systemic	Antibody, immune complex, DTH
Fungal			
Actinomycosis	*Actinomyces* spp.	Connective tissue	Immune complex opsonization, granulomatous
Aspergillosis	*Aspergillus* spp.	Lung	Immune complex, granulomatous
Candidiasis	*Candida albicans*	Skin, mucous membranes	DTH, granuloma
Coccidioidomycosis	*Coccidioides immitis*	Lung	DTH, granulomatous
Cryptococcosis	*Cryptococcus neoformans*	Lung	Granulomatous
Histoplasmosis	*Histoplasma capsulatum*	Inside macrophages	DTH, macrophage activation
Protozoal			
Amebiasis	*Entamoeba histolytica*	GI mucosa	Immune complex, inflammation
Malaria	*Plasmodium* spp.	Inside cells, free in blood	Cytotoxic, immune complex opsonization, T_{CTL} cells kill infected cells
Leishmaniasis	*Leishmania* spp.	Inside macrophages	DTH, activated macrophages
Toxoplasmosis	*Toxoplasma gondii*	Intracellular	Immune complex opsonization
Chagas' disease	*Trypanosoma cruzi*	Free in blood, intracellular	Cytotoxic, immune complex opsonization
Sleeping sickness	*Trypanosoma rhodesiense, Trypanosoma gambiense*	Free in blood	Cytotoxic, immune complex opsonization
Giardiasis	*Giardia lamblia*	GI tract	IgA antibody
Helminthic			
Schistosomiasis	*Schistosoma* spp.	Veins	Eosinophil ADCC[a]
Fascioliasis	*Fasciola*	Biliary ducts	Eosinophil ADCC, granulomatous
Trichinosis	*Trichinella spiralis*	Muscle	Eosinophil ADCC, DTH
Strongyloidiasis	*Strongyloides stercoralis*	GI tract	Eosinophil ADCC, DTH
Filiariasis	*Wuchereria bancrofti*	Lymphatics	Eosinophil ADCC, granulomatous
	Onchocerca volvulus	Dermis	Immune complex, granulomatous
Taeniasis	*Taenia*	GI tract	Eosinophil ADCC, GI motility

[a]ADCC, antibody-dependent cell-mediated cytotoxicity.

of more than one effector mechanism may lead to marked complication of tissue reactions, which can be understood if the role of each mechanism is considered separately and then the effect of combinations of mechanisms is analyzed.

Examples of the destructive capacity of immune responses to some selected infectious agents have also been presented. Tissue lesions caused by immune reactions to infectious agents usually occur when an inappropriate mechanism is activated. Thus, in leprosy antibody causes problems due to immune complex formation but has no protective effect against the intracellular bacilli; granulomatous reactivity is protective but may cause tissue damage if activated after large numbers of organisms have already been disseminated. The relative contribution of different immune mechanisms to the pathogenesis of other infectious diseases reflects even more variations in the interplay between immune effector mechanisms in protection and pathogenesis. The ability of many organisms to cause disease depends upon their ability to evade the immune defenses. For as many different immune defense mechanisms that can be recognized, infectious agents have been able to evolve ways to avoid the defenses and even ways to use the immune system to their advantage.

Bibliography

General

Bayon, Y., A. Alonso, M. Hernandez, M. L. Nieto, and M. Sanchez Crespo. 1998. Mechanisms of cell signaling in immune mediated inflammation. *Cytokines Cell Mol. Ther.* **4:**275–286.

Cochrane, C. G. 1968. Immunologic tissue injury mediated by neutrophilic leukocytes. *Adv. Immunol.* **9:**97–162.

Marx, J. L. 1982. The leukotrienes in allergy and inflammation. *Science* **215:**1380–1388.

Movat, H. Z. 1979. The kinin system and its relation to other systems. *Curr. Top. Pathol.* **68:**111–134.

Owen, C. H., and E. J. W. Bowie. 1976. *The Intravascular Coagulation-Fibrinolysis Syndromes in Obstetrics and Gynecology.* Upjohn, Kalamazoo, Mich.

Pober, J. S. 1999. Immunobiology of human vascular endothelium. *Immunol. Res.* **19:**225–232.

Ryan, G. B., and G. Majno. 1977. Acute inflammation. A review. *Am. J. Pathol.* **86:**183–276.

Lyme Disease

Brown, S. L., S. L. Hansen, and J. J. Langone. 1999. Role of serology in the diagnosis of Lyme disease. *JAMA* **282:**62–66.

Burgdorfer, W. 1986. Discovery of Lyme disease spirochete: a historical review. *Zentbl. Bakteriol. Hyg. A* **263:**7–10.

Centers for Disease Control and Prevention. 1999. Recommendations for the use of Lyme disease vaccine. Recommendations of the Advisory Committee on Immunization Practices. *Morb. Mortal. Wkly. Rep.* **48:**1–17, 21–25.

Duray, P. H. 1987. The surgical pathology of human Lyme disease. *Am. J. Surg. Pathol.* **11**(Suppl. 1)**:**47–60.

Hayner, M. S., M. M. Grunske, and L. E. Boh. 1999. Lyme disease prevention and vaccine prophylaxis. *Ann. Pharmacother.* **33:**723–729.

Schutzer, S. E., P. K. Coyle, P. Reid, and B. Holland. 1999. *Borrelia burgdorferi*-specific immune complexes in acute Lyme disease. *JAMA* **282:**1942–1946.

Steere, A. C. 1989. Lyme disease. *N. Engl. J. Med.* **321:**586–596.

Strongyloides

Al Samman, M., S. Haque, and J. D. Long. 1999. Strongyloidiasis colitis: a case report and review of the literature. *J. Clin. Gastroenterol.* **28:**77–80.

Gill, C. V., and D. R. Bell. 1979. Strongyloides stercoralis infection in Far East prisoners of war. *Br. Med. J.* **2:**572–574.

Purtillo, D. T., W. M. Meyers, and D. H. Conner. 1974. Fatal strongyloidiosis in immunosuppressed patients. *Am. J. Med.* **56:**488–493.

Van der Feltz, M., P. H. Slee, P. A. van Hees, and M. Tersmette. 1999. Strongyloides stercoralis infection: how to diagnose best? *Neth. J. Med.* **55:**128–131.

Immune Evasion

Bloom, B. R. 1979. Games parasites play: how parasites evade immune surveillance. *Nature* **279:**21–26.

Bogdan, C., M. Rollinghoff, and W. Solbach. 1990. Evasion strategies of *Leishmania* parasites. *Parasitol. Today* **6:**183–187.

Brodsky, F. M., L. Lem, A. Slache, and E. M. Bennett. 1999. Human pathogen subversion of antigen presentation. *Immunol. Rev.* **168:**199–215.

Cameron, C. E., C. Castro, S. A. Lukehart, and W. C. Van Voorhis. 1998. Function and protective capacity of *Treponema pallidum* subsp. *pallidum* glycerophosphodiester phosphodiesterase. *Infect. Immun.* **66:**5763–5770.

Craig, P. S. 1988. Immunology of human hydatid disease, p. 95–100. *In ISI Atlas of Science: Immunology*. Institute for Scientific Information, Philadelphia, Pa.

Das, G., H. Vohra, B. Saha, J. N. Agrewala, and G. C. Mishra. 1998. Leishmania donovani infection of a susceptible host results in apoptosis of Th1-like cells: rescue of anti-leishmanial CMI by providing Th1-specific bystander costimulation. *Microbiol. Immunol.* **42:**795–801.

Domian, R. T. 1997. Parasite immune evasion and exploitation: reflections and projections. *Parasitology* **115**(Suppl.)**:**S169–S175.

Donelson, J. E., K. L. Hill, and N. M. Il-Sayed. 1998. Multiple mechanisms of immune evasion by African trypanosomes. *Mol. Biochem. Parasitol.* **91:**51–66.

Engelmayer, J., M. Larsson, M. Subklewe, A. Chahroudi, W. I. Cox, R. M. Steinman, and N. Bhardwaj. 1999. Vaccinia virus inhibits the maturation of human dendritic cells: a novel mechanism of immune evasion. *J. Immunol.* **163:**6762–6768.

Farrell, H. E., and N. J. Davis-Poynter. 1998. From sabotage to camouflage: viral evasion of cytotoxic T lymphocyte and natural killer cell-mediated immunity. *Semin. Cell. Dev. Biol.* **9:**369–378.

Frank, I., and H. M. Friedman. 1989. A novel function of the herpes simplex virus type 1 Fc receptor: participation in bipolar bridging of antiviral immunoglobulin G. *J. Virol.* **63:**4479–4488.

Fruh, K., A. Gruhler, R. M. Krishna, and G. J. Schoenhals. 1999. A comparison of viral immune escape strategies targeting the MHC class I assembly pathway. *Immunol. Rev.* **168:**157–166.

Good, M. F., and D. L. Doolan. 1999. Immune effector mechanisms in malaria. *Curr. Opin. Immunol.* **11:**412–419.

Handman, E. 1999. Cell biology of Leishmania. *Adv. Parasitol.* **44:**1–39.

Isaacs, S. N., G. J. Kotwal, and B. Moss. 1992. Vaccinia virus complement-control protein prevents antibody-dependent complement-enhanced neutralization of infectivity and contributes to virulence. *Proc. Natl. Acad. Sci. USA* **89:**628.

Johnson, D. C., and A. B. Hill. 1999. Herpesvirus evasion of the immune system. *Curr. Top. Microbiol. Immunol.* **232:**149–177.

Jones, N. L., and P. M. Sherman. 1999. On/off antigenic variation in *Helicobacter pylori*: a clue to understanding immune evasion in the host. *J. Pediatr. Gastroenterol. Nutr.* **28:**233–234.

Large, M. K., D. J. Kittlesen, and Y. S. Hahn. 1999. Suppression of host immune response by the core protein of hepatitis C virus: possible implications for hepatitis C virus persistence. *J. Immunol.* **162:**931–938.

Lubinski, J. M., L. Wang, A. M. Soulika, R. Burger, R. A. Wetsel, H. Colten, et al. 1999. Herpes simplex virus type 1 glycoprotein gC mediates immune evasion in vivo. *J. Virol.* **72:**8257–8263.

Mahr, J. A., and L. R. Gooding. 1999. Immune evasion by adenoviruses. *Immunol. Rev.* **168:**121–130.

McKerrow, J. H. 1997. Cytokine induction and exploitation in schistosome infections. *Parasitology* **115**(Suppl.)**:**S107–S112.

Medici, M. A. 1972. The immunoprotective niche—a new pathogenic mechanism for syphilis, the systemic mycoses and other infectious diseases. *J. Theor. Biol.* **36:**617–625.

Mustafa, T., S. Phyu, R. Nilsen, G. Bjune, and R. Jonsson. 1999. Increased expression of Fas ligand on *Mycobacterium tuberculosis* infected macrophages: a potential novel mechanism of immune evasion by *Mycobacterium tuberculosis? Inflammation* **23:**507–521.

Ohshima, K., J. Suzumiya, M. Sugihara, S. Hagafuchi, S. Ohga, and M. Kikuchi. 1999. CD95 (Fas) ligand expression of Epstein-Barr virus (EBV) infected lymphocytes: a possible mechanism of immune evasion in chronic active EBV infection. *Pathol. Int.* **49:**9–13.

Piguet, V., O. Schwartz, S. Le Gall, and D. Trono. 1999. The down regulation of CD4 and MHC-I by primate lentiviruses: a paradigm for the modulation of cell surface receptors. *Immunol. Rev.* **168:**51–63.

Plebanski, M., E. A. Lee, and A. V. Hill. 1997. Immune evasion in malaria: altered peptide ligands of the circumsporozoite protein. *Parasitology* **115**(Suppl.)**:**S55–S66.

Raftery, M. H., C. K. Behrens, A. Muller, P. H. Krammer, H. Walczak, and G. Schonrich. 1999. Herpes simplex virus type I infection of activated cytotoxic T cells: induction of fratricide as a mechanism of viral immune evasion. *J. Exp. Med.* **190:**1103–1114.

Ramasamy, R., S. Yasawardena, R. Kanagaratnam, E. Buratti, F. E. Baralle, and M. S. Ramasamy. 1999. Antibodies to a merozoite surface protein promote multiple invasion of red blood cells by malaria parasites. *Parasite Immunol.* **21:**397–407.

Rossman, M. G. 1989. The canyon hypothesis. *Viral Immunol.* **2:**143–161.

Roulston, A., R. C. Marcellus, and P. E. Branton. 1999. Viruses and apoptosis. *Annu. Rev. Microbiol.* **53:**577–628.

Stenger, S., N. R. Niazi, and R. L. Modlin. 1998. Downregulation of CD1 antigen on presenting cells by infection with *Mycobacterium tuberculosis. J. Immunol.* **161:**3582–3588.

Sweet, C. 1999. The pathogenicity of cytomegalovirus. *FEMS Microbiol. Rev.* **23:**457–482.

Tomazin, R., J. Roname, N. R. Degde, D. M. Lewinsohn, Y. Altschuler, et al. 1999. Cytomegalovirus US2 destroys two components of the MHC class II pathway, preventing recognition by CD4+ T cells. *Nat. Med.* **5:**1039–1043.

Wold, W. S., K. Doronin, K. Toth, M. Kuppuswamy, D. L. Lichtenstein, and A. E. Tollefson. 1999. Immune responses to adenoviruses: viral evasion mechanisms and their implication for the clinic. *Curr. Opin. Immunol.* **11:**380–386.

Wurzner, R. 1999. Evasion of pathogens by avoiding recognition or eradication by complement, in part via molecular mimicry. *Mol. Immunol.* **36:**249–260.

Zajac, A. J., J. N. Blattman, K. Murali-Krishna, D. J. Sourdive, M. Suresh, J. D. Altman, and R. Ahmed. 1998. Viral immune evasion due to persistence of activated T cells without effector function. *J. Exp. Med.* **188:**2205–2213.

Immune-Mediated Skin Diseases

16

The Skin Immune System

This chapter on immune mechanisms in skin diseases is included to illustrate, in an organ system, the effects of various immune effector mechanisms. In other chapters, different skin reactions are used to demonstrate typical examples of these mechanisms (Table 16.1). The skin provides an ideal window on how different immune mechanisms produce different immunopathologic lesions.

The skin is a major lymphoid organ as well as a mechanical barrier to foreign invasion; it is a complex lymphoepithelial organ that takes an active part in both nonspecific (innate) and specific (acquired) immune reactivity. This complex is called the skin immune system, or skin-associated lymphoid tissues. The skin immune system components include antigen-processing Langerhans cells (class II major histocompatibility complex [MHC]), subcutaneous dendritic cells (class II MHC), and keratinocytes (class I and class II MHC); antigen-reactive T and B cells; and granulocytes, mast cells, endothelial cells, and fibroblasts. Langerhans cells are unique antigen-presenting cells. Langerhans cells are the precursors of dendritic cells in the lymph nodes. So-called "veiled cells" in the afferent lymphatics are believed to be derived from Langerhans cells and to migrate to the lymph node. In this way, Langerhans cells process antigen and play a key role in induction and maintenance of immunity through activation of T and B cells. Keratinocytes have emerged as major producers of cytokines (Table 16.2). Keratinocytes may provide continuing physiological signals for response to external stimuli with the production of inflammatory cytokines, adhesion molecules, and chemotactic factors for inflammatory cells.

The Perivascular Unit

Located in the skin close to the endothelial cells are mast cells, macrophages, T cells, and dermal dendritic cells, which form a perivascular unit that can rapidly expand into a collection of inflammatory cells (perivascular cuff) in response to a variety of inflammatory stimuli. The vascular endothelial cells produce cytokines and adhesion molecules that are critical for inflammatory reactions. Many of the T cells in the skin express phenotypes of activated or memory T cells; thus, the skin contains T cells that appear to be highly trained and ready for action (frontline

Table 16.1 Comparison of immune-mediated skin reactions[a]

Immune mechanism	Time of reaction	Lesion or reaction observed
Neutralization	Variable	Inactivation of toxin (Schick test)
Cutaneous anaphylaxis	5–10 min	Wheal and flare (edema and vasodilation)
Arthritis (immune complex)	5–6 h	Acute arteritis, fibrinoid necrosis
Contact dermatitis (T_{CTL} cells)	24–48 h	Vesiculation and blebbing, apoptosis, lymphocytes in epidermis
Delayed-type hypersensitivity (T_{DTH} cells)	24–48 h	Lymphocytes in dermis, venules
Granuloma	Weeks	Granulomas in dermis

[a]A skin test reaction for an antibody-mediated cytotoxic reaction has not yet been reported.

troops). The presence of E-selectin (ELAM-1) on the dermal endothelial cells may act as an adhesion molecule for skin homing of memory T cells. A feature of many infectious and immune diseases is perivascular cuffing of inflammatory cells in the skin.

Functions of the Skin Immune System

The effector function of the skin immune system is realized by a combination of signals from keratinocytes that prepare the dermal perivascular units for specific and nonspecific responses to injury. Langerhans cells and dermal dendritic cells are well situated to contact and process antigens that enter through the skin. The perivascular unit provides chemoattractive and adhesion molecules that signal inflammatory cells to enter the skin. Dermal T cells are situated to provide a rapid response to recall antigens and initiate cell-mediated immunity. Dermal macrophages are activated to phagocytose and clear away products of inflammation as well as provide proliferation signals to dermal fibroblasts and endothelial cells for repair. It is not surprising that the skin is the site of immune reactions representing all of the major immunopathologic mechanisms.

The skin is the largest organ of the body and the most common site for manifestations of immune reactions. Immune skin lesions may be classified by the different immunopathologic mechanisms, such as the cytotoxic destruction of epidermal cell contacts in pemphigus, immune complex-mediated vasculitis, the acute wheal-and-flare or hive reaction of cutaneous anaphylaxis, or delayed skin reactions and intraepithelial T-cytotoxic (T_{CTL})

Table 16.2 Cytokines produced by human keratinocytes in vitro[a]

Family	Cytokines[b]
Interleukins	IL-1α, IL-Iβ, IL-6, IL-8
Colony-stimulating factors	IL-3, GM-CSF, G-CSF, M-CSF
Interferons	IFN-α, IFN-β
Tumor necrosis factor	TGF-α, TGF-β
Transforming growth factors	TGF-α, TGF-β
Growth factors	PDGF, FGF

[a]Modified from J. D. Bos and M. L. Kapsenberg, *Immunol. Today* **14:**75, 1993.
[b]Abbreviations: CSF, colony-stimulating factor; FGF, fibroblast growth factor; G, granulocyte; IFN, interferon; IL, interleukin; M, macrophage; PDGF, platelet-derived growth factor; TGF, transforming growth factor.

Table 16.3 Immune mechanisms in some skin diseases[a]

Reaction and disease	Lesion	Association	Mechanism
Inactivation			
Pemphigus	Intraepithelial bullae	Autoallergic diseases	Autoantibody to desmosome protein
Pemphigoid	Subepidermal bullae	Neoplasm, autoallergy	Autoantibody to basement membrane
Epidermolysis bullosa	Subepidermal bullae	Autoimmunity	Autoantibody to basement membrane
Cytotoxic			
Dermatitis herpetiformis	Subepidermal bullae	Gluten enteropathy	IgA, alternate pathway activation?
Herpes gestationis	Subepidermal bullae	Pregnancy	Properdin, C3 in basement membrane
Cutaneous lupus	Basement membrane degeneration	Systemic and discoid lupus	Ig and C3 in basement membrane
Dermatomyositis	Microvascular injury	Myositis, lupus	C5b-C9 in vessels
Vitiligo	Depigmentation	Autoallergic diseases	Antibody to melanocytes
Alopecia areata	Focal hair loss	Endocrinopathy	Antibody to hair bulb capillaries
Immune complex			
Erythema nodosum	Subcutaneous vasculitis	Infection, systemic lupus erythematosus	Immune complex
Erythema marginatum	Subcutaneous vasculitis	Rheumatic fever	Immune complex
Cutaneous vasculitis	Subcutaneous vasculitis	Infections	Immune complex
Temporal arteritis	Temporal vasculitis	Actinic damage	Immune complex?
Anaphylactic reactions			
Mastocytosis	Whealing and anaphylaxis	Neoplasia	Increase in tissue mast cells
Cutaneous anaphylaxis	Wheal-and-flare	Allergic reaction	IgE-mediated mast cell degranulation
Giant urticaria	Large whealing	Allergy	Mast cell degranulation, IgE?
Angioedema	Nonpitting edema	Injury	Decrease in C1 esterase inhibitor
Hypocomplementemic urticarial vasculitis	Urticaria, vasculitis	Injury	C1q activation
Atopic dermatitis	Pruritic skin rash	Allergy	IgE, activation of macrophages
T_{CTL} cells			
Contact dermatitis	Spongiosis, vesiculation	Poison ivy, oak	T_{CTL}-cell reaction to hapten
Graft-versus-host	Intraepithelial necrosis	Bone marrow transplant	T_{CTL}-cell reaction to epithelial antigens
Viral exanthems	Intraepithelial necrosis	Virus infection	T_{CTL}-cell reaction to viral antigens
Erythema multiforme	Intraepithelial necrosis	Drugs, infection (herpes simplex virus)	T_{CTL} cells, antigens on endothelial cells
T_{DTH} cells			
DTH skin tests	Lymphocytic vasculitis	Skin test antigens	T_{DTH}-cell reaction to antigen, lymphokines
Syphilis	Perivascular and diffuse	*Treponema pallidum* infection	T_{DTH}-cell reaction to *T. pallidum* antigens
Psoriasis	Corneum parakeratosis	Rheumatoid arthritis	Th1, IFN-γ, TNF-α, keratinocyte lymphokines
Toxic epidermal necrosis	Epidermal necrosis	Drugs	Macrophage activation, TNF-α
Granulomatous reactions			
Leprosy	Subcutaneous granulomas	*Mycobacterium leprae* infection	T_{DTH} cells, granuloma formation
Gumma	Granulomas, various	*T. pallidum* infection	T_{DTH} cells, granuloma formation
Zirconium granuloma	Axillary granulomas	Stick deodorants	Granulomas
Sarcoidosis	Internal granulomas	Sarcoid	Granulomas, unknown

[a]Modified from S. Sell, p. 87–100, *in* R. E. Jordon, ed., *Immunologic Diseases of the Skin,* Appleton & Lange, Norwalk, Conn., 1991.

effects of cell-mediated immunity. A classification of skin diseases according to immune effector mechanisms is given in Table 16.3.

Antibody-Mediated Skin Diseases

The role of antibodies in human skin diseases has been unraveled largely by immunohistological localization of immunoglobulin and complement in different locations in the skin (Fig. 16.1). These findings, along with the participation of various inflammatory cell types, have implicated antibody-mediated mechanisms.

Inactivation or Activation

The reaction of antibodies with cell surface components of epithelial cells may result in phosphorylation of these proteins and loss of intercellular adhesiveness. Thus, activation of phosphorylation leads to loss of function. The basal layer of the epidermis, the basement membrane, and the subdermal connective tissue are connected by a complex of proteins (Fig. 16.2). Abnormalities or alterations of these connecting proteins produce spaces or bullae either in the epidermal layer or at the basement membrane. These diseases are caused by antibodies that react with the proteins that connect the basal cells to the basement membrane, maintain the integrity of the basement membrane, or connect the basement membrane to the dermis or by inherited deletions or abnormalities in these proteins (Table 16.4).

Pemphigus and Pemphigoid

Pemphigus and *pemphigoid* are skin lesions caused by denudation of the epidermis. In pemphigus, the epidermal cells separate above the basal layer, resulting in either formation of large fluid-filled spaces (pemphigus vulgaris) or stripping of the upper (horny and granular) layer of epidermis (pemphigus foliaceus). In pemphigoid, separation occurs between the basal layer of

Figure 16.1 Diagrammatic representation of lesion location and deposits of immunoglobulin and complement cell infiltrates in some skin diseases.

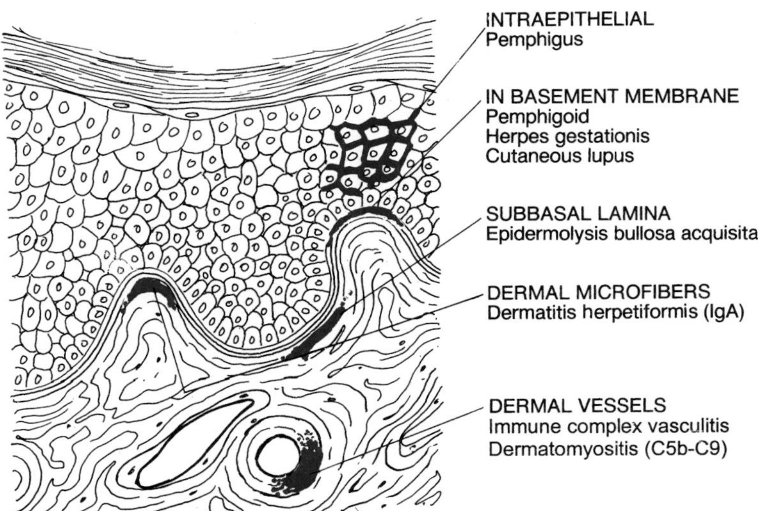

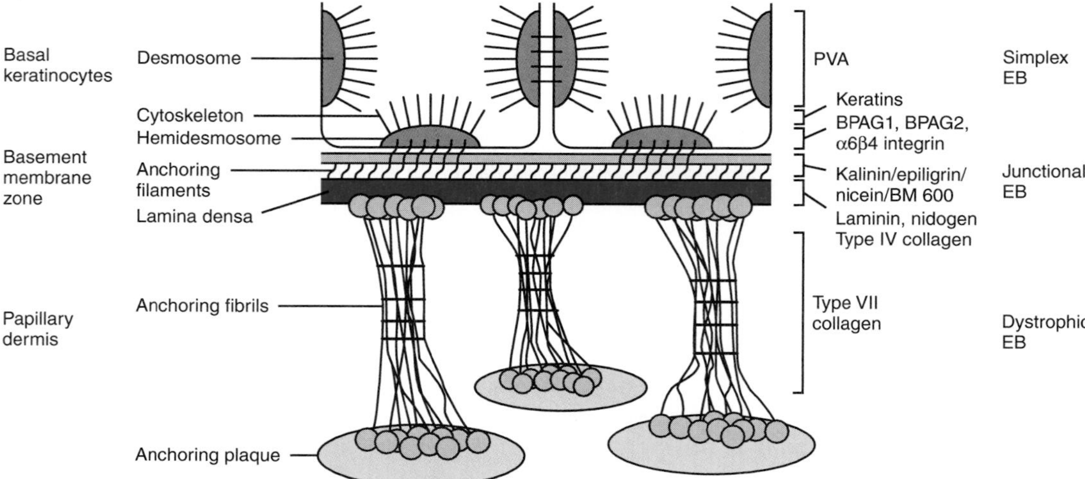

Figure 16.2 Schematic drawing of the connecting structures of the skin. Depicted are basal cells overlying the papillary dermis with the basement membrane separating them. Morphologic structures are shown on the left: the proteins making up these structures are shown on the right. (Modified from J. Uitto and A. M. Christiano, *J. Clin. Investig.* **90:**687, 1992.)

the epidermis and the dermis, leading to the formation of subepidermal bullae. Antibodies to desmosomes, adhesion molecules in the stratified epithelium, are found in the sera of patients with pemphigus; in contrast, antibodies to subepidermal basement membrane components are found in patients with pemphigoid. Thus, pemphigus antibodies attack the epithelial cells in the stratified layers, leading to their separation from each other, cell death, and bullae formation, whereas pemphigoid antibodies attack the basement membrane separating the epidermis from the dermis and producing subepidermal bullae. In bullous pemphigoid, there is also infiltration of neutrophils and eosinophil, indicating that complement-mediated inflammation is also involved in these lesions.

Table 16.4 Level of lesions and connecting proteins in blistering skin diseases

Disease	Tissue level	Protein(s)
Antibody-mediated acquired diseases		
Pemphigus vulgaris	Intraepidermal, suprabasilar	Desmoglein 3
Pemphigus foliaceus	Intraepidermal, superficial	Desmoglein 1
Bullous pemphigoid	Lamina lucida	BP Ag1 (type XVII collagen) and/or BP Ag2
Herpes gestationis	Lamina lucida	BP Ag2 ($\alpha_6\beta_4$-integrin)
Epidermolysis bullosa (EB) acquisita	Sublamina densa	Type VII collagen
Heritable diseases		
EB simplex	Basal keratinocytes	Keratins 5 and 14
EB junctional	Lamina lucida	Anchoring filaments
EB dystrophic	Sublamina densa	Type VII collagen
Epidermolytic hyperkeratosis	Intraepidermal, suprabasilar	Keratins 1 and 10

Evidence that antiepithelial autoantibodies cause the lesions includes the following facts: the patient's own immunoglobulin binds to his or her skin cells; both immunoglobulin G (IgG) and complement are demonstrable in the lesions; and the site of the lesion, either intraepithelial or subepithelial, is directly related to the site of immunoglobulin binding in pemphigus and pemphigoid. Lesions similar to those of the human may be induced by injection of pemphigus antibodies into monkey mucosa, and anti-epidermal cell surface antibody from pemphigus patients detaches viable epidermal cells from tissue culture dishes.

The antigens involved are listed in Table 16.4. The reaction of antibodies with these antigens may change their biologic behavior. For example, the pathogenic autoantibody of pemphigus vulgaris reacts with desmoglein 3 (Dsg 3), a specific desmosomal constituent. Reaction with the pemphigus vulgaris antibody induces phosphorylation of Dsg 3 and causes dissociation of Dsg 3 from plakoglobin, another desmosomal component, resulting in loss of intercellular binding of desmosomes. Autoantibodies to desmoglein 1 play a similar role in pemphigus foliaceous. Either of these antibodies may be found in patients with a variant of pemphigus called herpetiform pemphigus. There is evidence that an increase in desmoglein autoreactive T-helper cells may upregulate the production of autoantibodies in these diseases. Several clinical courses are recognized, from rapidly fatal to relatively benign. Activation of complement-mediated cell destruction or immune complex-mediated inflammation may add to the pathogenesis of these diseases. Corticosteroid and immunosuppressive therapy has been highly efficacious in severe cases. Successful therapy not only reverses the skin lesions but also causes a reduction in the titer of autoantibodies. Pemphigoid lesions are frequently associated with other autoimmune diseases and antitissue antibodies.

Epidermolysis Bullosa Acquisita

Epidermolysis bullosa acquisita is a rare skin disease characterized by blisters and extreme fragility of the skin due to subepidermal bullae similar in appearance to bullous pemphigoid. There are two major forms: hereditary and acquired. In the hereditary forms, separation may occur between the basal cells and the basement membrane (simplex form), within the basement membrane (junctional form), or below the basement membrane (dystrophic form). The hereditary forms of epidermolysis bullosa appear to be caused by genetic abnormalities in the proteins that join the basal keratinocytes to the basement membrane and the basement membrane to the dermis. For the acquired form, as in bullous pemphigoid, linear depositions of immunoglobulin and complement are seen along the dermal epidermal junction. However, by immune-electron microscopy, these depositions are localized below the subbasal lamina-anchoring fibril zone of the basement membrane, whereas in bullous pemphigoid the deposits are localized within the lamina lucida. The autoantibody in this disease is directed to type VII procollagen (anchoring fibrils).

Cytotoxic or Cytolytic Reactions

Cytotoxic effects of antibodies to epithelial cell or basement membrane antigens could also produce separation and destruction of the cells or destruction of the basement membrane. The diseases listed in this section have complex features and most likely are due to an interplay of additional pathogenic mechanisms. They have in common the finding of deposition of complement components in their lesions.

Dermatitis Herpetiformis and Gluten-Sensitive Enteropathy (Sprue, or Celiac Disease)

Dermatitis herpetiformis is a blistering skin lesion with papillary edema, microabscesses containing polymorphonuclear cells in dermal papillae, and subepidermal blisters. There may be intense burning and itching. Immunoglobulin A and complement are prominent in microfibers in the dermal papillae, and some patients have a bandlike granular deposition of IgA and complement in the dermal papillae along the epidermal basement membrane. IgA activates complement by the alternate pathway, and C3 is regularly found in areas of IgA deposition. Patients with celiac disease have a high incidence of IgA antibody to endomyosin. There are also IgA antibodies to gliadin and reticulin but at a lower incidence. Endomyosin is the intermyofibril substance of smooth muscle. Patients with dermatitis herpetiformis usually have sprue, a *gluten-sensitive enteropathy* (an inability to absorb nutrients from the gastrointestinal tract), and increased amounts of gastrointestinal IgA. Gluten is a gelatinous protein found in wheat and other grains. Elimination of gluten from the diet frequently results in reversal of the gastrointestinal lesions as well as the skin lesions. The IgA antibodies to gliadin and reticulin completely disappear on withdrawal of gluten from the diet, whereas antiendomyosin persists. These antibodies are all directed against the connective tissue of the surface of smooth muscle cells. It is postulated that gluten protein activates production of IgA antibodies in the gut-associated lymphoid tissues. With villous atrophy of the gut because of gluten-sensitive enteropathy, more gluten is absorbed, and more IgA antibodies are produced and released into the circulation. IgA antibodies may then circulate and deposit preferentially in the dermal microfibers in the skin because of its mucosal origin or genetically determined characteristics.

Herpes Gestationis

Herpes gestationis is a rare, blistering skin disease associated with pregnancy and the postpartum period. The skin lesions are large subepidermal bullae. C3 and properdin have been identified in the epidermal basement membrane, indicating that the alternate pathway of complement is activated. However, IgG may be identified by more sensitive techniques, and a more recent interpretation is that IgG antibody is involved but may not be identified by the usual immunofluorescent techniques. The antigen-binding specificity of the IgG deposited remains unknown.

Lupus Erythematosus

The skin lesions associated with *lupus erythematosus* are quite variable and most likely are due to different pathogenic mechanisms. The term lupus refers to the wolflike appearance of individuals with the full-blown facial rash; lupus erythematosus means "red-faced wolf." In chronic discoid lupus, there is extensive accumulation of keratin in hair follicles (keratotic plugging). The epidermis is atrophic and there is a patchy mononuclear cell infiltrate near the hair follicles. In systemic lupus erythematosus (SLE), the epidermis is atrophic with dissolution of the basal layer (liquefaction degeneration). There is less inflammatory filtrate, usually limited to a perivascular cuffing, and less keratotic plugging than that seen in discoid lupus. There may be small vacuoles within, above, and below the basement membrane, and marked thickening of the basement membrane occurs in chronic lesions. Immunoglobulin and complement are found in the walls of blood vessels and at the dermal-epidermal junction. The characteristic lesion is described as a band of immunoglobulin at the dermal-epidermal junction and may be seen before development of positive antibody-based laboratory tests. Granular depositions of immunoglobulin and/or complement may help predict those patients with glomerulonephritis, even when clinically the skin is not involved. It is likely that in lupus, deposition of antinuclear antibody-antigen complexes occurs in epidermal basement membrane as well as in renal glomerular basement membrane, but autoantibodies to basement membrane of the skin are also present. Thus, complement-mediated destruction of the basement membrane may be only one part of a complex process.

Dermatomyositis

The skin lesions of *dermatomyositis* (DM) are similar to those of SLE. However, microvascular injury appears to be the pathogenic basis of both the muscle inflammation (myositis) and skin lesions of DM. The membrane attack complex C5b-C9 of complement is found in the dermal vessels in DM associated with endothelial injury, vascular ectasia, and vascular fibrin deposition. This may distinguish DM from SLE. Along with the relative lack of polymorphonuclear infiltrate and fibrinoid necrosis characteristic of immune complex lesions, the deposit of the membrane attack complex suggests direct cytotoxic action of complement on dermal vessels as the pathogenesis.

Vitiligo

Vitiligo is sharply delineated patches of depigmentation of the skin that occur in various sizes and shapes. Histologically, all that can be identified is an absence of melanin pigment and a decrease in or complete loss of melanocytes. The occurrence of vitiligo is associated with autoimmune diseases and a variety of autoantibodies. Autoantibodies to melanin are seen in some patients with vitiligo, and cytotoxic T cells and complement deposits have been found. Therefore, an autoimmune etiology of vitiligo is postulated. However, loss of melanocytes could be due to a metabolic defect in melanocytes, deficiency in an unidentified melanocyte growth factor, oxidative stress, or lack of a melanocyte receptor.

Alopecia

Alopecia is a loss of hair in either circumscribed areas (alopecia areata) or the entire body (alopecia totalis). There is a loosely arranged nonspecific inflammatory infiltrate around the lower third of the hair follicle. Later, the hair follicle becomes atrophic, and the inflammatory infiltrate disappears. An association between alopecia and endocrine disease has been noted. An antibody that reacts with the capillary endothelium of the hair bulb has been reported to be eluted from lymphocytes in these patients, suggesting an antibody-dependent cell-mediated mechanism.

Immune Complex Reactions

Immune complex reactions are responsible for a variety of vascular reactions in the skin. Most lesions are secondary to deposition of immune complexes in dermal vessels.

Erythema Nodosum

The lesions of *erythema nodosum* are painful red nodules that appear bilaterally on the shins. The lesions occur predominantly in women in the fall and winter months. Their appearance is usually associated with an infection, a reaction to a drug, or a granulomatous disease such as sarcoidosis. In particular, erythema nodosum is associated with SLE and leprosy (erythema nodosum leprosum). The major pathologic finding is a subcutaneous vasculitis featuring a polymorphonuclear infiltrate of small veins or arterioles. Erythema nodosum is generally believed to be caused by a toxic complex allergic reaction. The skin reactions usually fade and do not require treatment.

Erythema Marginatum

Erythema marginatum is an uncommon feature of rheumatic fever. Classic erythema marginatum is described as a bright pink, ringlike lesion that spreads irregularly through a pale skin. It is flat and is not pruritic or painful. The center fades as the peripheral pink edge spreads. The lesions change appearance quite rapidly (in hours or even minutes) and may fade and reappear within a few minutes. Erythema marginatum is associated with cardiac involvement and may go on intermittently for months, even when all other signs of rheumatic fever are gone. The pathology is not well documented, although a nonspecific perivascular mononuclear infiltrate is sometimes seen. The lesions may be mediated by the vasomotor activity of anaphylatoxin as well as by inflammatory cells. Erythema chronicum migrans, which resembles erythema marginatum, follows a tick bite that introduces the *Borrelia* organism responsible for Lyme disease.

Cutaneous Vasculitis in Infectious Diseases

A variety of skin lesions may be associated with infections such as viral hepatitis, infective endocarditis, infectious mononucleosis, and a number of bacterial infections, in particular, streptococcal and pseudomonal. In some cases, immunoglobulin and complement have been identified in cutaneous vessels, and circulating immune complexes are present. Often, these patients have glomerular or pulmonary lesions as well.

Anaphylactic Reactions

Wheal-and-flare reactions and urticarial skin eruptions are common occurrences, not only on contact with allergens but also during the course of infectious diseases or drug treatment. In cases of naturally occurring diseases, it is now generally accepted that the occurrence of cutaneous anaphylactic reactions is the result of a preferential activation of Th2 helper cells over Th1 helper cells, stimulating, in particular, the production of IgE antibodies.

Mastocytosis

Mastocytosis is a mixed group of diseases in which there is a marked increase in the number of mast cells in tissues. Mastocytosis may occur as a localized lesion in the skin or as a systemic disease (Table 16.5).

The initial report of the typical lesions of mastocytosis, in 1889, described the production of a wheal by stroking the skin over a localized skin lesion. Lesions may be solitary or disseminated, indolent or progressive, benign or malignant, depending on the location and progression of

Table 16.5 Classification of mastocytosis[a]

I. Indolent mastocytosis
A. Skin only
Urticaria pigmentosa
Diffuse cutaneous mastocytosis
B. Systemic
II. Mastocytosis associated with hematologic diseases
III. Mast cell leukemia
IV. Lymphadenopathic mastocytosis with eosinophilia

[a]Modified from D. D. Metcalfe, *J. Investig. Dermatol.* **96**:2S, 1991.

the disease, but all have tissue infiltration with mast cells as a result of disorders of mast cell and basophil proliferation. The preponderance of symptoms are due to the release of mast cell mediators and include flushing episodes, whealing, and anaphylaxis.

Cutaneous Anaphylaxis

Cutaneous anaphylaxis (urticaria, wheal-and-flare, or hive) is an IgE antibody–allergen-activated mast cell-mediated skin reaction consisting of erythema, itching, a pale, soft, raised wheal, pseudopods, and a spreading flare, reaching a maximum in 15 to 20 min and fading in a few hours. The reaction is a vascular response to release of histamine or histaminelike substances into the skin with local changes in vascular permeability. A typical example of cutaneous anaphylaxis is a mosquito bite caused by histamine release from mast cells as a toxic reaction to mosquito saliva (see chapter 11).

Giant Urticaria

Giant urticaria is manifested by the widespread development of firm, raised wheal-like lesions over large areas of the skin. They are superficial, erythematous, and intensely pruritic, with raised serpiginous edges and blanched centers. Individual lesions last about 48 h, but new eruptions may appear for an indefinite period. Although allergic mechanisms may be operative, identification of an eliciting allergen is not possible in most instances, and nonimmunologic stimuli such as heat, cold, or sunlight frequently initiate urticarial lesions. However, in some instances the lesions of cold urticaria can be transferred with serum factors—either IgM, suggesting the involvement of a cryoimmunoglobulin, or IgE, indicating that an IgE-mediated reaction can cause giant urticaria.

Angioedema

Angioedema is a hereditary deficiency of C1 esterase inhibitor that allows extensive edema and swelling upon activation of C1. The lesion may involve the eyelids, lips, tongue, and areas of the trunk. Involvement of the gastrointestinal tract may produce symptoms of acute abdominal distress, but the symptoms almost always disappear in a few days without surgical intervention. The most significant life-threatening complication is severe pharyngeal involvement, which may lead to asphyxia. The pathologic alteration is firm, nonpitting edema of the dermis and subcutaneous tissue, which can be differentiated from a wheal-and-flare reaction by the absence of erythema.

Hypocomplementemic Vasculitic Urticarial Syndrome

A 7S protein that precipitates C1q (C1q-activating factor) is believed to activate complement and produce urticaria, leukoclastic vasculitis, arthritis, and neurologic abnormalities.

Atopic Dermatitis

The diagnosis of atopic dermatitis is based on three findings: (i) a focal or generalized maculopapular pruritic skin rash on the flexural area of the extremities and the face and neck, (ii) a chronic or chronic relapsing course, and (iii) a family history of asthma or eczema. Patients with atopic dermatitis have the following immune dysfunctions: elevated serum IgE, positive wheal-and-flare skin tests to many antigens, reduced responsiveness to contact allergens, and lack of delayed-type hypersensitivity (DTH) reactivity to intradermally administered microbial antigens. These are all consistent with increased Th2 activity. The skin lesions are infiltrated by activated $CD4^+$ interleukin-4 (IL-4)-producing T cells and IgE-bearing dendritic reticular cells and macrophages and T cells. These Th2-type helper cells express cutaneous lymphocyte antigen and may represent a specific subset of "skin-homing lymphocytes" that react with E-selectin on endothelial cells in the dermis. One of the effects of IL-4 and IL-13 produced by these cells is to upregulate the FcϵII receptor on mononuclear cells; another is to increase the number of eosinophil in the lesions. Although the pathogenesis of these lesions remains unclear, it is thought that they may be caused by effector mononuclear cells bearing FcϵII receptors. Binding of IgE antibodies through these receptors could lead to activation by a variety of antigens, such as aeroantigens, food allergens, bacterial and fungal allergens, and autoantigens. Although lesion severity correlates with the number of eosinophils, the role of eosinophils is not clear.

Cell-Mediated Reactions

Skin reactions mediated by sensitized cells can be divided into those primarily due to T_{CTL} cells and those mediated by T-delayed-type hypersensitivity (T_{DTH}) cells. Contact dermatitis and viral exanthems are presented as reactions mainly mediated by T-killer/T-cytotoxic cells that cross into the epidermis and cause the death of epithelial cells. The tuberculin skin test and the primary chancre are presented as reactions initiated by T_{DTH} cells, which release lymphokines that attract and activate macrophages. Although T_{CTL} and T_{DTH} cells represent the different effector arms of cell-mediated immunity, both effector arms may be active in different degrees in other reactions.

T-Cytotoxic Reactions

Contact Dermatitis

Contact dermatitis, or contact allergy, is exemplified by the common allergic reaction to poison ivy. The characteristic skin reaction is elicited in sensitized individuals by exposing the skin to the oleoresins of poison ivy or poison oak. The reaction is a sharply delineated, superficial skin inflammation, beginning as early as 24 h after exposure and reaching a maximum at 48 to 96 h. It is characterized by redness, induration, and vesiculation caused by the invasion of T_{CTL} cells into the epidermis, where they react with antigen on epidermal cells and kill them. In active lesions, keratinocytes have marked increased expression of intercellular adhesion molecule 1 and lymphocyte function-associated antigen 1-positive lymphocytes in the epidermis. The finding of dead keratinocytes associated with one or more satellite lymphocytes, so-called satellite cell necrosis, is a common feature of skin lesions believed to be mediated by T_{CTL} cells.

GVH Reaction

Graft-versus-host (GVH) reaction is a life-threatening complication of bone marrow transplantation when progeny of transplanted cells react with tissue antigens in the gastrointestinal tract, biliary tract of the liver, and skin. GVH reactions in the skin are particularly noticeable and occur to some extent in up to 70% of recipients of bone marrow transplantation. The acute phase of the skin reaction shows diffuse lymphocytic infiltrates in the upper dermis with destruction of keratinocytes (satellite necrosis). Similar findings are seen in drug reactions and viral exanthems, from which GVH reactions are very difficult to distinguish histologically. Both $CD4^+$ (T_{DTH}) and $CD8^+$ (T_{CTL}) lymphocytes may be found in the epidermis. At this time, there is some disagreement about the relative roles of these T-cell effector populations, with both T_{CTL}-cell- and T_{DTH}-cell-mediated damage possible. In support of T_{CTL} cells are the presence of activated T_{CTL} cells associated with apoptotic keratinocytes and the ability to transfer the lesions in experimental models in mice with $CD8^+$ cells. In support of T_{DTH} cells are the findings of high numbers of $CD4^+$ lymphocytes and activated dendritic cells in the lesions.

Viral Exanthems

The early (first 8 days) papular vesicular lesion of cutaneous viral infections (i.e., measles) is most likely caused by the growth of the virus, and the later (8 to 14 days) inflammatory reaction (rash) is caused by T_{CTL}-cell invasion and destruction of virus-infected epidermal cells. Similar lesions appear at the same time on different parts of the body, even though the different areas are inoculated with the virus at different times. For more details, see chapter 12.

Erythema Multiforme

Erythema multiforme lesions may vary from a mild skin eruption consisting of erythematous or edematous flat plaques to widespread eruptions with bullous formation and extensive sloughing of the surface of the skin. The skin lesions consist of large circular macules or papules with a central blue depression and an elevated red periphery. The variety of types of lesions is reflected in the term "erythema multiforme." Vesicles and bullae may occur, and new crops of lesions may appear in the center of the fading plaques, resulting in a targetlike appearance. These eruptions usually resolve in a few weeks, but a mortality rate of up to 20% occurs with the more severe form of the disease. Histologically, solitary and clustered necrotic keratinocytes in conjunction with lymphocytes are characteristic of erythema multiforme lesions. The occurrence of the disease is associated with infections and the use of certain drugs. Recently, a T_{CTL}-cell reaction to herpes simplex virus infection was implicated in many cases of recurrent erythema multiforme as herpes simplex virus DNA was identified in lesions by polymerase chain reaction. Evidence of an allergic reaction includes (i) a latency period of 10 to 12 days between initial exposure to a drug and development of the disease, (ii) the appearance of lesions in a few hours on second exposure to the drug, (iii) recurrence of the disease after subsequent exposure to the offending drug, (iv) changes in the small blood vessels consistent with the allergic vasculitis, and (v) skin tests with a suspected antigen that elicit the cutaneous lesion. No circulating autoantibodies to epidermal or dermal antigens have been demonstrated, and immunoglobulin and complement are not present in the lesions. Thus, erythema multiforme is believed to be a T_{CTL}-cell-mediated destruction of virus-infected or drug-haptenized cells in the skin.

Delayed-Type Hypersensitivity Reactions

Tuberculin Test

The classic delayed-type tuberculin skin reaction is elicited in sensitive individuals by intradermal injection of tuberculoprotein antigens (purified protein derivative [PPD] and old tuberculin [OT]). Redness and swelling occur 24 h after injection. Because the reaction requires previous sensitization and occurs much later after testing than cutaneous anaphylaxis or the Arthus reaction, it is called a delayed-type hypersensitivity reaction. Specifically sensitized T_{DTH} cells react with the antigen in the tissue and release lymphokines that attract and activate macrophages, and the activated macrophages phagocytose and digest the antigen (see chapter 13).

Syphilis

The primary lesion of *syphilis,* the chancre, is the result of a DTH reaction to organisms in the skin. It lasts from 1 to 5 weeks, is initiated by sensitized T_{DTH} cells reacting with antigen, and is resolved by phagocytosis and digestion of organisms by macrophages. Infection with *Treponema pallidum* occurs by inoculation through abraded skin.

The skin and mucous membrane lesions of secondary syphilis, which appear 2 weeks to 6 months after primary infection, appear to be a mixture of DTH and antibody-mediated immune complex reactions at sites of dissemination and replication of *T. pallidum*. The cellular reaction is similar to that of primary lesions, although plasma cells and vasculitis may be more prominent. Many systemic effects of secondary syphilis may be the result of immune complexes or cytokine release.

Psoriasis

Psoriasis is a chronic, brownish, scaly, sharply demarcated skin lesion associated with arthritis. Psoriasis is characterized by an abnormality in keratinization with elongation of dermal papillae, epidermal proliferation, parakeratosis (imperfect keratinization), and intraepithelial collections of polymorphonuclear leukocytes. The pathogenesis is believed to be caused by an exaggerated cytokine response to injury (Table 16.6). High numbers of $CD4^+$ T cells producing gamma interferon are present in the early lesions. The T_{DTH}-cell lymphokines activate macrophages and dermal dendritic cells, and the resulting cytokines lead to hyperplasia of the basal layer of the skin. Inhibition of T-cell activation leads to resolution of the lesions. There is immunoglobulin deposition in the epidermal layer that has a characteristic intracellular and diffuse staining pattern in the stratum

Table 16.6 Postulated pathogenic steps in psoriasis

1. Th1 lymphokines are released from activated $CD4^+$ TH1 T_{DTH} cells
2. IFN-γ activates keratinocytes to release monocyte chemotactic and activating factors
3. Activated monocytes accumulate and release TNF-α
4. TNF-α increases ICAM[a] expression on keratinocytes; T cells bind to ICAM and produce TGF-α
5. TGF-α and IL-8 stimulate keratinocyte proliferation and angiogenesis typical of psoriasis

[a]ICAM, intercellular adhesion molecule.

corneum. A pathogenic role of stratum corneum antibody in psoriasis is implied but not established.

TEN

A mechanism similar to that of psoriasis, but in a more acute form with bullous necrosis, may be responsible for the full-thickness skin loss seen in *toxic epidermal necrosis* (TEN). TEN is an infrequent complication of drug treatment (in particular, treatment with sulfonamides, anticonvulsants, or nonsteroidal anti-inflammatory drugs) or of severe GVH reactions. Histologically, the skin of TEN shows sparse inflammatory cell infiltrate. The cell-poor infiltrate of TEN contains macrophages and dendritic cells with a strong immunoreactivity for tumor necrosis factor alpha (TNF-α). Mortality is relatively high compared with that of other bullous skin diseases owing to renal or pulmonary complications. The pathologic mechanism is not well characterized but activation of macrophages and overproduction of TNF-α appears likely.

Granulomatous Lesions

Granulomatous lesions in the skin result from the accumulation of macrophages and reactive fibrosis to poorly degradable phagocytosed debris. The reactions may be initiated by antibody to T cells reacting with antigen or to foreign bodies that are not immunogenic. The characteristic lesion is a space-occupying mass of epithelioid macrophages with various amounts of lymphocytic infiltration and fibrosis.

Gumma

The destructive lesions characteristic of tertiary syphilis are granulomatous reactions (gummas), which occur in areas where spirochetes apparently persist during latency, e.g., brain, skin, bone, or viscera.

Zirconium Granulomas

Stick deodorants containing zirconium salts may induce axillary granulomas in apparently sensitized individuals. When the use of zirconium was discontinued, lesions no longer occurred.

Leprosy

The clinical features of *leprosy* are presented in detail in chapter 14. At one pole of the clinical spectrum are prominent granulomatous lesions with epithelioid cells and many lymphocytes and few, if any, *Mycobacterium leprae* organisms in the tissues (tuberculoid leprosy). At the other pole is massive infiltration of tissues with large foamy macrophages filled with numerous mycobacteria with few lymphocytes and limited fibrosis (lepromatous leprosy).

Sarcoidosis

Boeck's sarcoidosis is a systemic granulomatous process prominently involving the lymph nodes, lungs, eyes, and skin, with lesions that may be indistinguishable from those of tuberculosis, fungus infections, or other granulomatous hypersensitivity reactions. A cutaneous granulomatous reaction may be elicited 3 to 4 weeks after the subcutaneous injection of crude extracts of sarcoid lymph nodes in patients with sarcoidosis (Kveim reaction). The specificity of this reaction and its use as a diagnostic test are questionable.

Disorders of Coagulation

A common manifestation of lesions of small vessels in the skin is purpura. Purpura refers to purple lesions caused by extravasation of blood. Purpura is caused by inflammatory lesions of blood vessels, such as "palpable purpura" found in association with immune complex vasculitis in the skin (see chapter 10) or by thrombosis of dermal vessels. *Purpura fulminans* is a sudden onset of massive bleeding into the skin, followed by necrosis, and is often fatal. The bleeding is secondary to necrosis of endothelial cells. The lesion is initiated by the development of microvascular thrombosis, such as that associated with disseminated intravascular coagulation, in particular, with endotoxin. Cytokines such as IL-1 and TNF are released by inflammatory cells exposed to endotoxin, and attraction of granulocytes followed by release of lysosomal enzymes further contributes to the necrotic reaction. This may be considered an extensive cutaneous Shwartzman reaction.

Summary

Immune-mediated cutaneous lesions are examples of diseases caused by different immunopathologic mechanisms. Cytotoxic reactions produce blistering diseases; immune complex reactions, vascular lesions; anaphylactic reactions, whealing lesions; cell-mediated reactions, chronic infiltrative diseases; and granulomatous reactions, destructive mass lesions of the skin. In addition, many other disease processes, such as disorders of coagulation, are manifested in the skin. Thus, the skin is a "window" through which immunopathologic processes may be viewed.

Bibliography

General

Jordon, R. E. 1991. *Immunologic Diseases of the Skin.* Appleton & Lange, Norwalk, Conn.

Stone, J. 1985. *Dermatologic Immunology and Allergy.* The C. V. Mosby Co., St. Louis, Mo.

The Skin Immune System

Bos, J. D. 1997. *Skin Immune System,* 2nd ed. CRC Press, Boca Raton, Fla.

Steinman, R. M. 1991. The dendritic cell system and its role in immunogenicity. *Annu. Rev. Immunol.* **9:**271–296.

Neutralization or Inactivation

Aoyama, Y., M. K. Owada, and Y. Kitajima. 1999. A pathogenic autoantibody, pemphigus vulgaris-IgG, induces phosphorylation of desmoglein 3, and its dissociation from plakoglobin in cultured keratinocytes. *Eur. J. Immunol.* **29:**2233–2240.

Beutner, E. H., R. E. Jordon, and T. P. Shorzelski. 1968. The immunopathology of pemphigus and bullous pemphigoid. *J. Investig. Dermatol.* **51:**63–80.

Ishii, K., M. Amagai, A. Komai, T. Ebihara, T. P. Chorzelski, S. Jablonska, K. Ohya, T. Nishikawa, and T. Hashimoto. 1999. Desmoglein 1 and desmoglein 3 are the target autoantigens in herpetiform pemphigus. *Arch. Dermatol.* **135:**943–947.

Karpati, S., M. Amagai, R. Prussick, K. Cehrs, and A. R. Stanley. 1993. Pemphigus vulgaris antigen, a desmoglein type of cadherin, is localized within keratinocyte desmosomes. *J. Cell Biol.* **122:**409–415.

Kowalczyk, A. P., E. A. Bornslaeger, S. M. Norvell, H. L. Palka, and K. J. Green. 1999. Desmosomes: intercellular adhesive junctions specialized for attachment of intermediate filaments. *Int. Rev. Cytol.* **185:**237–302.

Riechers, R., J. Grotzinger, and M. Hertl. 1999. HLA class II restriction of autoreactive T cell responses in pemphigus vulgaris: review of the literature and potential applications for the development of specific immunotherapy. *Autoimmunity* **30:**183–196.

Stanley, J. R. 1989. Pemphigus and pemphigoid as paradigms of organ-specific, autoantibody-mediated diseases. *J. Clin. Investig.* **83:**1443–1448.

Cytotoxic or Cytolytic Reactions

Crowson, A. N., and C. M. Magro. 1996. The role of microvascular injury in the pathogenesis of cutaneous lesions of dermatomyositis. *Hum. Pathol.* **27:**15–19.

Hall, R. P. 1992. Dermatitis herpetiformis. *J. Investig. Dermatol.* **99:**873–881.

Magro, C. M., and A. N. Crowson. 1997. The immunofluorescent profile of dermatomyositis: a comparative study with lupus erythematosus. *J. Cutan. Pathol.* **24:**543–552.

Mascaro, J. M., Jr. G. Hausmann, C. Herrero, J. M. Grau, M. C. Cid, J. Palou, and J. M. Mascaro. 1995. Membrane attack complex deposits in cutaneous lesions of dermatomyositis. *Arch. Dermatol.* **131:**1386–1392.

Ortonne, J.-P., and S. K. Bose. 1993. Vitiligo: where do we stand? *Pigment Cell Res.* **6:**61–72.

Scott, J. E., and A. R. Ahmed. 1998. The blistering diseases. *Med. Clin. N. Am.* **82:**1239–1283.

Volta, U., N. Molinare, M. Fusconi, F. Cassani, and F. B. Bianchi. 1991. IgA antiendomysial antibody test: a step forward in celiac disease screening. *Dig. Dis. Sci.* **36:**752–756.

Immune Complex Reactions

Lotta, T. M., C. Comacchi, and I. Ghersetich. 1999. Cutaneous necrotizing vasculitis. Relation to system disease. *Adv. Exp. Med. Biol.* **455:**115–125.

Patterson, R., and A. Tripathi. 1999. Stevens-Johnson syndrome: getting ready for the year 2000 and beyond. *Ann. Allergy Asthma Immunol.* **83:**339–340.

Tan, E. M., and H. G. Kunkel. 1966. An immunofluorescent study of the skin lesions in systemic lupus erythematosus. *Arth. Rheum.* **9:**37–46.

Thomas, B. A. 1950. The so-called Stevens-Johnson Syndrome. *Br. J. Med.* **1:**1393.

Anaphylactic Reactions

Church, M. K., and G. F. Clough. 1999. Human skin mast cells: in vitro and in vivo studies. *Ann. Allergy Asthma Immunol.* **83:**471–475.

Cicardi, M., L. Bergamaschini, M. Cugno, A. Beretta, L. C. Zingale, M. Colombo, and A. Agostini. 1998. Pathogenetic and clinical aspects of C1 inhibitor deficiency. *Immunobiology* **199:**366–376.

Greaves, M. 2000. Chronic urticaria. *J. Allergy Clin. Immunol.* **105:**664–672.

Grewe, M., C. A. Bruijnzeel-Koomen, E. Schopf, T. Thepen, A. G. Langeveld-Wildschut, T. Ruziecka, and J. Krutmann. 1998. A role for Th1 and Th2 cells in the immunopathogenesis of atopic dermatitis. *Immunol. Today* **19:**359–361.

Karnam, U., and A. Rogers. 1999. Systemic mastocytosis. *Dig. Dis.* **17:**299–307.

Maurer, D., E. Fiebiger, B. Reinger, B. Wolff-Winiski, M. H. Jouvin, O. Kilgus, J. P. Kinet, and G. Stingl. 1994. Expression of functional high affinity immunoglobulin E receptors (FcεRI) on monocytes of atopic individuals. *J. Exp. Med.* **179:**745–750.

Cell-Mediated Reactions

T_{CTL} Cells

Bedi, T. R., and H. Pinkus. 1976. Histopathologic spectrum of erythema multiforme. *Br. J. Dermatol.* **95:**243–250.

Budinger, L., and M. Hertil. 2000. Immunologic mechanisms in hypersensitivity reactions to metal ions. *Allergy* **55:**108–115.

Chosidow, O. 1994. Drug rashes: what are the targets of cell-mediated cytotoxicity? *Arch. Dermatol.* **130:**627–629.

Darragh, T. M., B. M. Egbert, T. G. Berger, and T. S. B. Yen. 1991. Identification of herpes simplex virus DNA in lesions of erythema multiforme by the polymerase chain reaction. *J. Am. Acad. Dermatol.* **24:**23–26.

Kohler, S., M. R. Hendrickson, N. J. Chao, and B. R. Smoller. 1997. Value of skin biopsies in assessing prognosis and progression of acute graft-versus-host disease. *Am. J. Surg. Pathol.* **21:**988–996.

McCracken, S. 1999. Latex glove hypersensitivity and irritation: a literature review. *Probe* **33:**13–15.

Miyauchi, H., H. Hosokawa, T. Akaeda, H. Iba, and Y. Asada. 1991. T-cell subsets in drug-induced toxic epidermal necrolysis: possible pathogenic mechanism induced by CD8-positive T cells. *Arch. Dermatol.* **127:**851–855.

Nikaein, A., T. Poole, R. Fishbeck, G. Ordonez, L. Dombrausky, M. J. Stone, R. H. Collins, Jr., and J. W. Fay. 1994. Characterization of skin-infiltrating cells during acute graft-versus-host disease following bone marrow transplantation using unrelated marrow donors. *Hum. Immunol.* **40:**68–76.

Paquet, P., A. Nikkels, J. E. Arrese, A. Vanderkelen, and G. E. Pierard. 1991. Macrophages and tumor necrosis factor in toxic epidermal necrolysis. *Arch. Dermatol.* **127:**851–855.

Willis, C. M., C. J. M. Stephens, and J. D. Wilkinson. 1991. Selective expression of immune-associated surface antigens by keratinocytes in irritant contact dermatitis. *J. Investig. Dermatol.* **96:**505–511.

Yoo, Y. H., B. S. Park, D. Whitaker-Menezes, R. Korngold, and G. F. Murphy. 1998. Dermal dendrocytes participate in the cellular pathology of experimental acute graft-versus-host disease. *J. Cutan. Pathol.* **25:**426–434.

T_{DTH} Cells

Arnason, B. G., and B. H. Waksman. 1964. Tuberculin sensitivity: immunologic considerations. *Adv. Tuberc. Res.* **13:**1.

Chase, M. C. 1976. Developments in delayed type hypersensitivity 1950–1975. *J. Investig. Dermatol.* **67:**136–148.

Paquet, P., and G. E. Peirard. 1997. Erythema multiforme and toxic epidermal necrolysis: a comparative study. *Am. J. Dermatopathol.* **19:**127–132.

Stone, N., S. Sheerin, and S. Burge. 1999. Toxic epidermal necrolysis and graft vs. host disease: a clinical spectrum but a diagnostic dilemma. *Clin. Exp. Dermatol.* **24:**260–262.

Turk, J. L. 1975. *Delayed Hypersensitivity,* 2nd ed. Elsevier/North-Holland Publishing Co., Amsterdam, The Netherlands.

Granulomas

Epstein, W. L. 1983. Granulomatous inflammation in the skin, p. 21–59. *In* H. L. Ioachim (ed.), *Pathology of Granulomas.* Raven Press, New York, N.Y.

Stiltzbach, L. E. (ed.). 1976. *Seventh International Conference on Sarcoidosis and Other Granulomatous Disorders.* New York Academy of Sciences, New York, N.Y.

Turk, J. L., and A. D. M. Bryceson. 1971. Immunological phenomena in leprosy and related diseases. *Adv. Immunol.* **13:**209–266.

Disorders of Coagulation

Adcock, D. M., J. Brozna, and R. A. Marlar. 1990. Proposed classification and pathologic mechanisms of purpura fulminans and skin necrosis. *Semin. Thromb. Hemostasis* **16:**333–340.

Henoch, E. 1887. Über purpura fulminans. *Berl. Klin. Wochenschr.* **24:**8.

Immunoproliferative Diseases

17

The term "immunoproliferative diseases" refers to abnormalities that result in an increase in the number of lymphocytes, macrophages, or polymorphonuclear cells in the body. Enlargement of lymphoid organs and marked increases in the white cells in the blood result from an imbalance in the rate of proliferation relative to the rate of destruction of the cells in the hematopoietic/lymphoid lineage. Immunoproliferative diseases include both inflammatory (self-limited, reversible) and malignant (progressive) increases in numbers of cells.

Leukemias and Lymphomas

The term "malignant lymphoma" was first proposed by Billroth in 1871, to differentiate malignant tumors from inflammatory reactions or benign hyperplasia. The suffix "-oma" means mass (or lump); thus, "lymphoma" means an increase in the mass of a lymphoid organ. According to the standard nomenclature for cancer, malignant tumors of lymphoid cells should be called "lymphosarcomas" to indicate their malignant nature, and benign lymphoid tumors should be called lymphomas. However, in practice, the term lymphoma is used for malignant tumors.

Leukemia means "white blood." In patients with cancers of the circulating white blood cells, the large numbers of malignant leukemic white blood cells give the normally red blood a whitish color. Thus, "lymphoma" is used for malignant proliferation of white cells in lymphoid organs; "leukemia" is used for malignant increases in white cells in the blood.

Lymphomas and leukemias are progressively growing tumors that mimic the appearance normal lymphoid cells. Until recently, the classification and understanding of these diseases were based mainly on morphological observations and clinical correlations. The identification of cell surface markers for various lymphocyte populations has led to a much better understanding of lymphocyte differentiation and to the reclassification of immunoproliferative diseases on the basis of T-cell, B-cell, or macrophage (histiocyte) lineage. Older classifications are confusing because the terminology presumed a cell type of origin on the basis of morphology, which may not have been valid. For instance, the terms "reticulum cell sarcoma" and "histiocytic lymphoma," implying a macrophage origin, were used for tumors that are now known to express B-cell markers. These tumors are now classified as poorly differentiated forms of diffuse B-cell lymphoma.

Maturation of Blood-Forming Cells and Leukemia

A diagram of the normal maturation of blood cells with the stages of development at which maturation arrest becomes manifest for various leukemias and lymphomas is presented in Fig. 17.1. Pluripotent stem cells are present in the bone marrow and give rise to other cell types by differentiation. Before maturation, these cells do not express T- or B-cell markers but differentiate into cells that migrate to other lymphoid organs. Mature cells in each series normally die at the same rate as new cell types in each series are produced, resulting in a constant number of each cell type. In lymphomas and leukemias, differentiation of a given cell lineage is arrested, so increasing numbers of relatively homogeneous, less mature cells appear. As a result of the differentiation block, cells in a given lineage that normally would differentiate into cells that would die to make way for newly formed cells (i.e., terminally differentiate) do not die and continue to accumulate in tissues. This results in the "forcing out" of normal cells, leading to loss of function of blood cells and disease manifestations such as anemia (loss of red blood cells), bleeding (loss of platelets), susceptibility to infection (loss of lymphocytes and granulocytes), and wasting. Arrest at an early stage of differentiation produces acute "blastic" tumors; arrest at a mature stage of differentiation results in chronic "well-differentiated" tumors.

Lymphoid Tissue Structure and Lymphoproliferative Disease

To understand the morphology, growth patterns, manifestations, and tissue alterations characteristic of human lymphoproliferative diseases, the localization of normal lymphoid cells in lymphoid organs and phenotypic markers reflecting differentiation of lymphocytes must be considered.

Tissue Localization of Lymphoid Cells

Most human lymphocytic tumors (lymphomas) are of B-cell lineage. Tumors of lymphoid cells usually are first located in lymphoid organs in areas where cells of the same lineage are normally found (Fig. 17.2)—T cells in the thymus-dependent or diffuse lymphoid zones, B cells in follicular zones. Macrophages are found in follicular zones as well as being prominent in medullary zones. Some lymphoid cells normally circulate and are found in peripheral blood. The major difference between lymphomas and leukemias is the lack of cell surface homing markers on leukemic cells that react with endothelial cells; these cells do not "home" to lymphoid organs, as do cells of lymphomas. Thus, B-cell tumors in the blood are leukemias, and B-cell tumors in tissues are lymphomas.

Nonmalignant Lymphoproliferation

Physiologic stress may result in reversible increased production of a given cell type (hyperplasia). When production exceeds terminal differentiation, the number of cells will increase. At high altitudes, the production of erythrocytes will increase, resulting in higher numbers of erythrocytes;

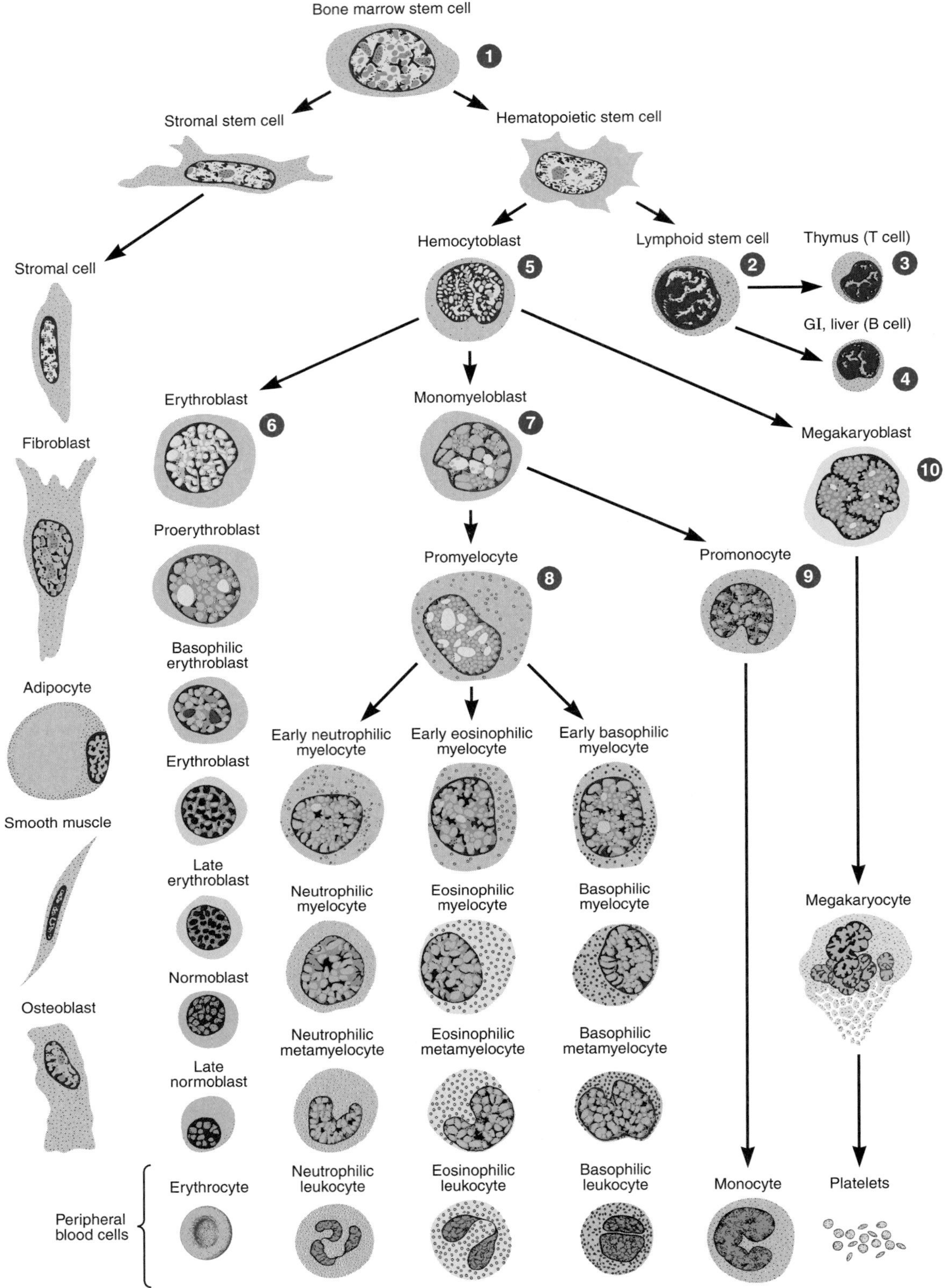

Figure 17.1 Maturation of blood cells during hematopoiesis and postulated sites of maturation arrest in lymphomas and leukemias. **(1)** Acute undifferentiated leukemia. **(2)** Acute lymphocyte leukemia. **(3)** T-cell leukemia (acute lymphocytic leukemia) (in blood), T-cell lymphoma (in tissues). **(4)** B-cell leukemia (acute lymphocytic leukemia, chronic lymphocytic leukemia) (in blood), B-cell lymphoma (in tissues), multiple myeloma (in plasma cells), Hodgkin's disease (lymphocyte predominant). **(5)** Polycythemia rubra vera. **(6)** Acute erythroid leukemia. **(7)** Acute myeloblastic leukemia. **(8)** Chronic granulocytic leukemia. **(9)** Monocytic leukemia (in blood), true histiocytic lymphoma (in tissue), Hodgkin's disease (other types). **(10)** Acute megakaryocyte leukemia.

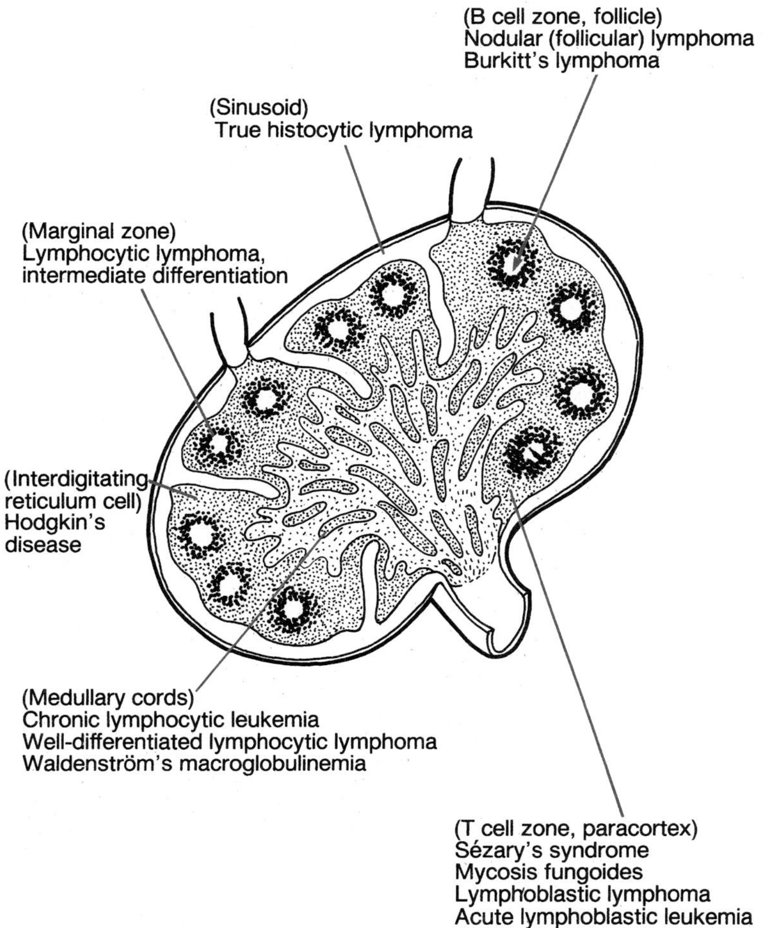

Figure 17.2 Structure of lymph node and origin of lymphomas. Drawing of lymph node illustrating anatomic localization of B cells (follicles), T cells (diffuse, paracortex, and deep cortex) and macrophages (medullary cords). B-cell tumors arise in the cortex and are often follicular in structure but sometimes diffuse. T-cell lymphomas arise in the paracortex and deep cortex and are always diffuse. Tumors of macrophages arise in the medulla and are diffuse. In general, the structure of the tumor reflects the normal morphology of the cell type from which it arises. (Modified from R. S. Mann, E. S. Jaffe, and C. W. Berard, *Am. J. Pathol.* **94:**105–192, 1979.)

during a chronic infection, production of granulocytes will increase. With removal of the stimulus for hyperplasia, production will return to normal, and the number of cells dying will exceed production until normal cell numbers are again attained.

Benign (nonmalignant) hyperplasia of lymphoid tissue usually occurs in response to inflammatory stimuli or infections (Table 17.1). Both benign and malignant lymphoproliferative diseases may present with enlarged lymph nodes or spleen associated with fever, so it is often not a simple matter to differentiate benign from malignant lymphadenopathy or splenomegaly (enlarged lymph nodes or spleen). If an obvious source of infection is present, such as inflamed tonsils associated with cervical lymphadenopathy, and if this responds to appropriate therapy by antibiotics,

Table 17.1 Nonmalignant lymphoid hyperplasias (lymphadenopathies)

Lymphoproliferative condition	Features	Example(s)
Suppurative lymphadenitis	Draining a zone of acute infection. Polymorphonuclear leukocytes early, macrophages later. Basic lymph node structure intact.	Tonsillitis
Postvaccinial and viral lymphadenitis	Mixed cellular response; mainly paracortical (T-cells); also blast cells, giant cells	Vaccination
AIDS-related lymphadenopathy	Early polyclonal follicular (B-cell) and diffuse (T-cell) hyperplasia; later mixture of follicular hyperplasia and diffuse hypoplasia; terminally, marked lymphocyte depletion; sometimes Epstein-Barr virus-associated B-cell lymphoma	HIV
Drug-induced lymphadenopathy	Loss of normal architecture with a pleomorphic cell infiltrate: blasts, eosinophils, neutrophils, and plasma cells; history of drug exposure; also skin rash and fever	Diphenylhydantoin, mephenytoin
Sinus histiocytosis with massive lymphadenopathy	Massive cervical lymphadenopathy, fever, and leukocytosis; subcapsular and medullary sinusoids filled with proliferating histiocytes that phagocytose normal lymphocytes	Rosai-Dorfman disease
Lymphodermatitis (dermatopathic lymphadenitis)	Mixed inflammation: granulomas, histiocytosis, follicular hyperplasia, polymorphonuclear exudation	Tuberculosis, sarcoidosis, cat scratch disease, contrast media reaction
Giant lymph node hyperplasia	Hyaline vascular (i) and plasma cell (ii) varieties: (i) hyalinized blood vessels in small follicules; (ii) sheets of plasma cells in the interfollicular tissue	Castleman's disease
Infectious mononucleosis	Immature mononuclear cells in the peripheral blood; polyclonal Epstein-Barr virus-driven B-cell and reactive T-cell proliferation; fatigue, general malaise, and loss of appetite	Epstein-Barr virus infection

malignancy may be considered unlikely. However, it is advisable to obtain a lymph node biopsy to rule out malignancy. If an invasive procedure is to be performed, every effort should be made to obtain a satisfactory diagnostic tissue specimen. It is important to obtain the largest nodes accessible to the surgeon, not just some nodal tissues, because frequently not all nodes in a group will be involved. Histologically, inflammatory hyperplasias are not monoclonal or limited to one cell type, as are most lymphomas. The cells involved will be a mixture of T, polyclonal B, null, as well as polymorphonuclear cells and macrophages. Malignant tumors demonstrate a relative uniformity of cell type and replacement of normal structures; whereas hyperplasias contain a mixture of cell types and an exaggeration of normal structure.

Malignant Lymphomas

Human lymphomas are cancers of lymphoid cells: T cells, B cells, or macrophages. The major clinical classification consists of two types, non-Hodgkin's and Hodgkin's lymphoma, because the response to therapy and clinical course of Hodgkin's diseases and other lymphomas are critically different. The cellular origin of Hodgkin's disease has been the subject of controversy, but recent evidence suggests that one form of these tumors arises from B cells, whereas others arise from a particular macrophage subpopulation, the interdigitating reticulum cells (see below). Non-Hodgkin's lymphomas usually are derived from lymphocytes. Also of critical importance is the characterization of the growth potential and clinical course as acute or chronic.

Non-Hodgkin's Lymphomas

Three major characteristics determine the ability to predict the growth behavior of a malignant lymphoma, non-Hodgkin's type: the pattern of tissue replacement, the morphology of the cells, and the extent of organ involvement. A general principle of neoplastic disease is that cancer tissue is a caricature of the normal tissue from which it arises. Lymphomas are tumors of lymphoid organs, and the morphologic structure reflects the lymphoid cell organ. The most useful working morphologic classification of non-Hodgkin's lymphomas reflects this relationship.

Classification

Nodular or diffuse. The major morphologic differentiation of non-Hodgkin's lymphomas is nodular (follicular) or diffuse. Nodular lymphomas reflect the morphology of lymphoid follicles and are composed of B cells. Diffuse lymphomas reflect the structure of the diffuse cortex of lymph nodes and appear as sheets of cells without follicular structure and may be of B-cell, T-cell, or true histiocytic (macrophage) origin. Nodular tumors have a much better prognosis than diffuse tumors.

Cell size. The second major morphologic feature is the size of the nuclei of the cells that make up the tumor. The size of the nucleus is a reflection of the number of cells in the growth cycle. Resting cells have small nuclei, whereas the nuclei of cells in the cell cycle enlarge as RNA and DNA are synthesized. Therefore, the size of the cells in a given lymphoma is an indication of the growth fraction, i.e., the proportion of actively proliferating cells. Tumors made up of small cells have a better prognosis than tumors made up of large (undifferentiated) cells. Tumors made up of a mixture of large, intermediate, and small cells have an intermediate prognosis.

Organ involvement. The third major prognostic factor is the extent of organ involvement by the tumor. This is known as clinical staging and is described in more detail below. In general, the more tissue that is involved with lymphoma cells when the diagnosis is made, the poorer the prognosis.

The Rappaport System

The morphologic features are incorporated into the classic classification of non-Hodgkin's lymphomas proposed by Henry Rappaport in 1956 (Table 17.2). In this classification, "histiocytic" refers to a large lymphocytic type of tumor, now known usually to be composed of B cells and not histiocytes. Rappaport used the term "histiocytic lymphoma" because the large cells looked like tissue histiocytes. Over the last 30 years, this classification has provided a valuable method of evaluating non-Hodgkin's lymphomas. Although there have been a number of attempts to improve upon this classification, the general rule is that patients with tumors of small cells do better than patients with tumors of large cells, and patients with nodular tumors do better than those with diffuse tumors. In 1982, a reclassification called the Working Formulation was devised by an international group of authorities. Since then, a number of different classifications have been proposed, none of which has received universal acceptance. In

Table 17.2 Morphologic classification of non-Hodgkin's lymphomas[a]

Topography or tissue pattern
Nodular
Diffuse
Cell type
Lymphocytic, well differentiated (small)
Lymphocytic, poorly differentiated (intermediate)
Histiocytic[b] (reticulum cell sarcoma) (large)
Mixed histiocytic and lymphocytic (mixed)
Undifferentiated (blast) (very large)

[a]Modified from H. Rappaport et al., *Cancer* **9**:792, 1956.
[b]Histiocytic refers to large cells and does not necessarily imply macrophage origin.

this chapter, a simplified classification of B-cell, T-cell, and macrophage tumors is used. This classification is relatively easy to understand but most likely unsatisfactory to many practicing pathologists because it is not sufficiently complicated.

B-Cell Tumors

B-cell tumors make up 90% of chronic lymphocytic leukemias, several kinds of nodular or diffuse lymphomas, and tumors of plasma cells (e.g., multiple myeloma), as well as Hodgkin's disease (see below). The cells of these tumors reflect their B-cell origin by expressing either cell surface immunoglobulin (sIg), cytoplasmic monoclonal immunoglobulin, rearranged Ig genes, or cell surface markers of B-cell lineage. The major characteristics of some B-cell tumors are listed in Table 17.3. All these tumors arise from

Table 17.3 Characterization of B-cell tumors[a]

Tumor	Phenotypic markers	Characteristics
Bone marrow origin		
Chronic lymphocytic leukemia (CLL)	Mature B-cell, sIg^+, $CD5^+$	Mature B cells, small lymphocytes, blood involved, indolent course
CLL (prolymphocytoid)	Like CLL, but with immature cells	>10% large (immature B) cells, accelerating course
Acute lymphocytic leukemia	Immature B, sIg^{+++}, $CD5^{+/-}$	Large cells, spleen prominently involved, rapid progression, responds to chemotherapy
Multiple myeloma	Cytoplasmic Ig, monoclonal Ig, rearranged Ig gene	Plasma cell tumors, arise in bone marrow; usually high levels of monoclonal Ig in serum and less often monoclonal Ig light chain in urine
Lymph node origin		
Follicular lymphoma	sIg^{+++}, Bcl-2 rearranged, $CD5^-$	Atypical lymphocytes, germinal center type; prominent node and spleen involvement, variable course, usually follicular but may progress to diffuse tissue pattern
Mantle zone lymphoma	$sIgM^{+++}$, Bcl-1 rearranged, $CD5^+$	Usually cleaved lymphocytes, lymph node and spleen involvement, variable course
Hairy cell leukemia	sIg^{+++}, $CD5^-$, $IL\text{-}2R^+$	Splenomegaly; serum contains IL-2R
Burkitt's lymphoma	sIg^{++}, $CD5^-$, c-myc translocation	Small noncleaved cells, jaw mass, Epstein-Barr virus

[a]Modified from G. P. Schecter, p. 1734, *in* R. H. Rich, ed., *Clinical Immunology, Principles and Practice,* The C. V. Mosby Co., St. Louis, Mo., 1996.

cells at different stages of B-cell development and thus reflect the tissue distribution and surface characteristics of normal B cells at similar stages. The incidence of B-cell tumors is much higher in elderly individuals (50 to 70 years of age) than in people younger than 50 years of age. Monoclonal immunoglobulins are sometimes found in persons with other diseases, such as nonlymphoid tumors, and in elderly persons. The significance of these elevations remains uncertain. The presence of a monoclonal immunoglobulin (gammopathy) in an otherwise normal person suggests that covert myeloma is present and will become manifest if the person lives long enough (see below). Most B-cell tumors arise in the bone marrow (leukemias) or in the germinal centers of lymph nodes (lymphomas). Tumors of plasma cells (multiple myeloma) arise in the bone marrow but usually do not give rise to circulating cells.

B-cell leukemias. In general, B-cell leukemias occur in two major forms, acute lymphoblastic leukemia (ALL) and chronic lymphocytic leukemia (CLL), with intermediate forms.

Acute B-cell leukemias are the most common leukemias of childhood but also occur in adults. In these diseases, the point of arrested maturation is essentially at lymphoid stem cell level in the bone marrow, and the leukemias may have either B- or T-cell phenotypes. Thus, B-cell lymphoblastic leukemias will express CD19, terminal deoxytransferase (TdT), CD79a, and sometimes sIg and CD10, whereas the much rarer T-cell lymphoblastic leukemias will be sIg^-, $CD7^+$, $CD3^+$, and TdT^+. Because the arrested stage of maturation is at the blast cell stage, most of the cells in these leukemias are in cycle, i.e., there is a very high growth fraction. Because of this, the natural history is a very rapid course. On the other hand, since chemotherapeutic drugs act on cells in cycle, the clinical response to chemotherapy usually is initially good. In general, there are two types of acute B-cell leukemia. Infants under 1 year of age with acute B-cell leukemia usually have a rearrangement of the myeloid/lymphoid, or mixed-lineage, leukemia gene (MLL) transcription factor at 11q23. They respond poorly to chemotherapy and are generally scheduled for bone marrow transplantation after the first remission. After 1 year of age, children with ALL generally respond better to chemotherapy and may have long first remissions without bone marrow transplantation.

Chronic lymphocytic leukemia is a protracted disease consisting of a marked increase in small lymphocytes in the bone marrow and blood. Lymph node and spleen involvement may occur late in the disease, with diffuse infiltration of small lymphocytes. The tumor cells express monoclonal sIg or rearranged Ig gene in 90% of cases but also express a T-cell marker, CD5. These cells are referred to as $CD5^+$ B cells. The disease most likely starts in the bone marrow. Later in the course of disease, large numbers of mature lymphocytes extend from the bone marrow to the blood and visceral organs, giving the appearance of diffuse lymphocytic lymphoma. The course of the disease is relatively long, and patients with this disease often die of infection or from some unrelated disease.

Normally, $CD5^+$ B lymphocytes appear early in development and represent a high proportion of fetal and neonatal B cells. They are not found in the normal adult bone marrow but represent about 20% of circulating lymphocytes in adults. Nonmalignant $CD5^+$ B cells belong to a special category of cells that spontaneously secrete IgM autoantibodies. $CD5^+$ B cells are believed to play a role in the first line of defense against infection, as well as in many autoimmune diseases. Leukemic $CD5^+$ B cells also express the α chain of the C3bi receptor, and many of these CLLs possess "cross-reactive" idiotypes, i.e., immunoglobulin epitopes shared by different tumors. In contrast, the idiotypes of human myelomas are not shared, i.e., are unique for each tumor. Thus, 20 to 30% of CLLs from different patients may express the same idiotype. This raises the possibility of anti-idiotypic directed passive immunotherapy in which one monoclonal antibody reagent could be used for many different tumors.

Hairy cell leukemia (leukemic reticuloendotheliosis) is a disease characterized by the appearance of an unusual mononuclear cell in the peripheral blood, associated with splenomegaly and a decrease in other cellular elements of the blood. The disease progresses slowly, and severe infections appear to be related to the decreased number of normally functioning monocytes in the blood. The hairy cell is the size of normal, nonlymphocytic mononuclear cells, has a markedly convoluted cytoplasm (hairy by scanning electron microscopy), has monoclonal cytoplasmic and surface Ig, and is capable of phagocytosis. Thus, it is a B cell with some features of macrophages and most likely represents an immature B-cell type. T-cell variants of hairy cell leukemia have also been reported, but rearrangements of Ig genes have been found in all cases of hairy cell leukemia so far studied in this manner. Hairy cell leukemia is particularly susceptible to treatment with alpha interferon.

B-cell lymphomas. Two major forms of B-cell lymphoma are recognized topographically: follicular and diffuse. Either follicular or diffuse B-cell lymphomas may contain small and large lymphocytes in different proportions and are usually found in lymph nodes, spleen, or gastrointestinal tract. The growth pattern of follicular lymphomas mimics the nodular arrangement of cells in lymphoid follicles—hence the designation of follicular or nodular.

Follicular center cells. In 1971, Lukes and Collins refined the cellular classification of non-Hodgkin's lymphomas. They recognized that the cells of most non-Hodgkin's lymphomas resembled cells seen in germinal centers and postulated that these cells represented different stages of the cell cycle of B cells, regardless of whether the lymphoma was nodular or diffuse. This concept is presented in Fig. 17.3. Lukes and Collins also postulated that the shape of the nuclei of the cells of a lymphoma (cleaved or not cleaved) reflected the stage of maturation of the cells in the tumor and that there is evolution of B-cell lymphomas (small cleaved → large cleaved → small noncleaved → large noncleaved) associated with progression to more malignant behavior. Unfortunately, the fine morphologic characteristics used in this classification are subject to subtle changes in tissue fixation and processing and are not easily defined, even by experienced pathologists; the reproducibility of this classification at different centers has not been uniform. In the 1970s, a number of classification systems of non-Hodgkin's lymphomas were proposed, generating considerable debate and confusion. These classifications, while still useful, have largely been superseded by the use of other cellular markers, but morphologic classification of small, large, intermediate, and mixed-cell type is still critical in determining the prognosis of lymphoma. Small cell types progress very slowly. Large cell types progress more rapidly and may respond initially to chemotherapy. Unfortunately, they frequently develop resistance to chemotherapy and are often fatal.

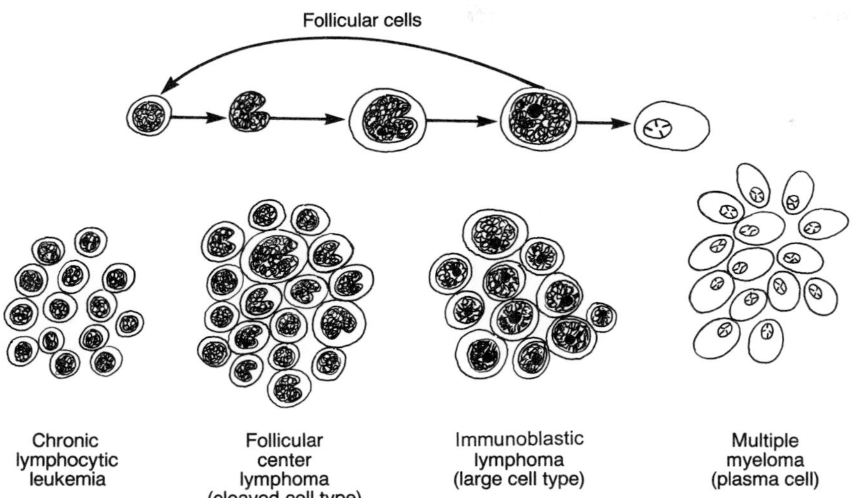

Figure 17.3 Histologic features of B-cell lymphomas as related to morphology of germinal center B cells. During the cell cycle, B cells change from small round cells to large "blast cells" and divide to form small cells. Differentiation results in production of plasma cells. The nucleus of the early activated B cell is cleaved, whereas the nuclei of the small resting cell and the cells in later stages of B-cell differentiation are not cleaved. Chronic lymphocyte leukemia represents a maturation arrest at the small noncleaved stage; multiple myeloma at the plasma cell stage; follicular lymphomas at the activated B-cell stage (cleaved), and large-cell lymphomas at the immunoblastic B-cell stage (large noncleaved cells). (Modified from R. J. Lukes and R. D. Collins, *Cancer Treatment Rep.* **61:**971–979, 1977, and C. R. Taylor, *Arch. Pathol. Lab. Med.* **102:**549–554, 1978.)

Tissue pattern. In contrast to normal lymph follicles, which are found in the cortex of a lymph node, neoplastic follicles are found throughout the node, with obliteration of the normal node architecture (Fig. 17.4). Diffuse B-cell lymphocytic lymphoma consists of small- to medium-sized lymphocytes, which do not form follicles and diffusely infiltrate and replace lymph node and spleen structures. The variations in follicular and diffuse patterns of B-cell lymphomas and the progression from follicular to diffuse are illustrated in Fig. 17.5. Analysis of the immunoglobulin genes of diffuse and follicular areas in a given lymphoma indicates that diffuse B-cell tumors represent tumor progression by a single clone of malignant cells. Diffuse large-cell lymphomas are made up of large cells, sometimes resembling reticulum cells or macrophages, which replace lymphoid organs as sheets of malignant cells. This tumor has a much worse prognosis than the diffuse lymphocytic lymphoma, which consists of small cells. Fine tuning of the cellular morphology of diffuse B-cell tumors permits more accurate prognosis. For example, intermediate lymphocytic lymphoma has cytologic features and a prognosis that lie between those of small lymphocytic lymphoma and diffuse, small, cleaved-cell lymphoma.

Phenotypic markers. The stage of maturation arrest in the B-cell lineage may be deduced from the phenotypic expression of immunoglobulins produced by B-cell tumors and rearrangements of immunoglobulin genes or by expression of developmentally related cell surface markers. The major distinguishing feature of B-cell tumors (Table 17.3) is monoclonality, i.e., the presence or production of only one class of immunoglobulin and/or one light-chain type by all the cells of the tumor. In contrast, the B cells or

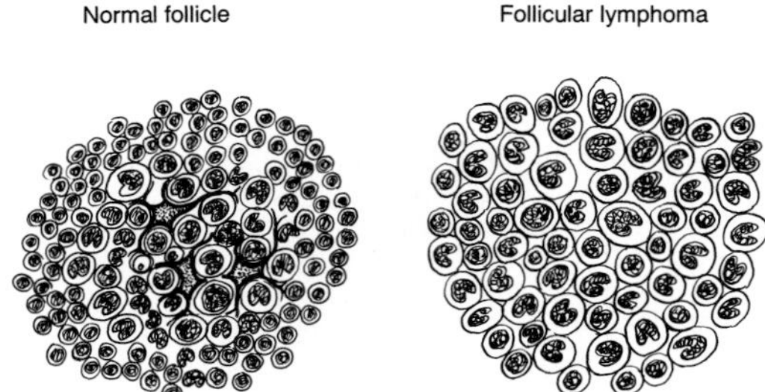

Figure 17.4 Patterns of normal polyclonal and neoplastic B-cell follicles. Normal secondary or germinal centers contain a mixture of different cell types, including not only polyclonal B cells but also macrophages and T cells, and are surrounded by a rim of polyclonal cells. On the other hand, malignant B-cell tumors may form follicles or replace the node structure diffusely with a homogeneous cell type. Malignant follicles are made up of cells of a single clonal line, do not contain T cells or macrophages, and are not surrounded by a rim of polyclonal cells. Malignant follicles efface the other components of the lymph node (paracortex, medulla) and extend diffusely into adjacent tissue, with loss of the structure of capsule and subcapsular sinus, whereas in nonmalignant hyperplasia, these areas, although relatively less conspicuous, are preserved.

plasma cells that make up normal or benign lymphoproliferation are mixtures of cells with different Ig classes and light chains. A simple test for monoclonality is immune labeling of tissue for kappa and lambda light chains of immunoglobulin. If all of the cells contain one light-chain type, then the criterion for monoclonality is met. If some cells express the kappa chain and others express the lambda chain (usually a 60:40 ratio), then polyclonality is established.

Ig gene rearrangements. Rearrangement of immunoglobulin genes may be used to differentiate B-cell tumors from nonneoplastic proliferation, T-cell tumors, or nonlymphoid tumors that morphologically resemble B-cell tumors. As described in chapter 4, the first step in B-cell differentiation that can be detected is rearrangement of the immunoglobulin genes. B-cell lymphoma rearrangements can be differentiated from normal polyclonal rearrangements by the presence of a single band on polyacrylamide gel fractionation of DNA digested with appropriate restriction enzymes. Selected enzymes cut the DNA at specific points in the sequence of bases. Polyclonal B-cell DNA contains multiple gene arrangements that produce a diffuse, nondistinct pattern when labeled with a specific cDNA probe for the Ig gene probe. In contrast, the DNA from a clonal proliferation will be cleaved at the same site, giving rise to discrete bands. In this manner, clonal B cells that make up only 2 to 5% of a heterogeneous tissue sample may be detected, and diagnosis of lymphoma within a mixture of polyclonal cells can be made accurately. In addition, undifferentiated carcinomas or atypical hyperplasia of lymphocytes can be differentiated from B-cell lymphomas. An unexpected finding is that some B-cell leukemias have rearranged T-cell receptor genes. However, the nature of the T-cell receptor gene in B-cell tumors does not correlate with response to therapy.

B-cell differentiation markers. B-cell surface markers identified by monoclonal antibodies to lymphocyte differentiation markers may also be used to evaluate the stage of differentiation of B-cell lymphomas and leukemias

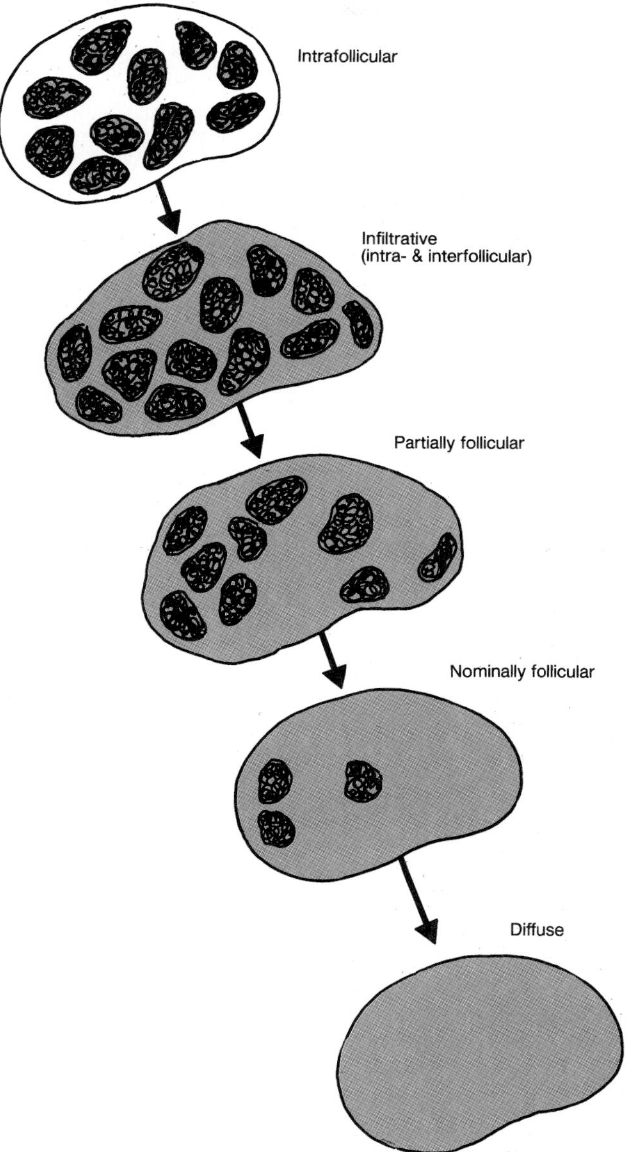

Figure 17.5 Evolution of B-cell lymphomas. Increased malignancy or the progression toward more aggressive tumor is associated with a change from more follicular to more diffuse, as well as with cell size and morphology. Small, cleaved follicular tumors have the best prognosis. Large, noncleaved diffuse tumors have the worst prognosis. Approximately 30% of patients followed carefully demonstrate progression from less malignant to more malignant forms.

(Fig. 17.6). By international agreement, the differentiation markers on lymphoid cells are termed "cluster designations" or "clusters of differentiation" (CD). A CD number refers to a group of epitopes identified by a set of monoclonal antibodies that are present on a subset of lymphocytes. These epitopes are markers of normal differentiation or activation states but also appear on leukemia and lymphoma cells (see chapter 4).

So far, classification of B-cell lymphomas by phenotypic markers has not contributed greatly to determination of prognosis or choice of therapy,

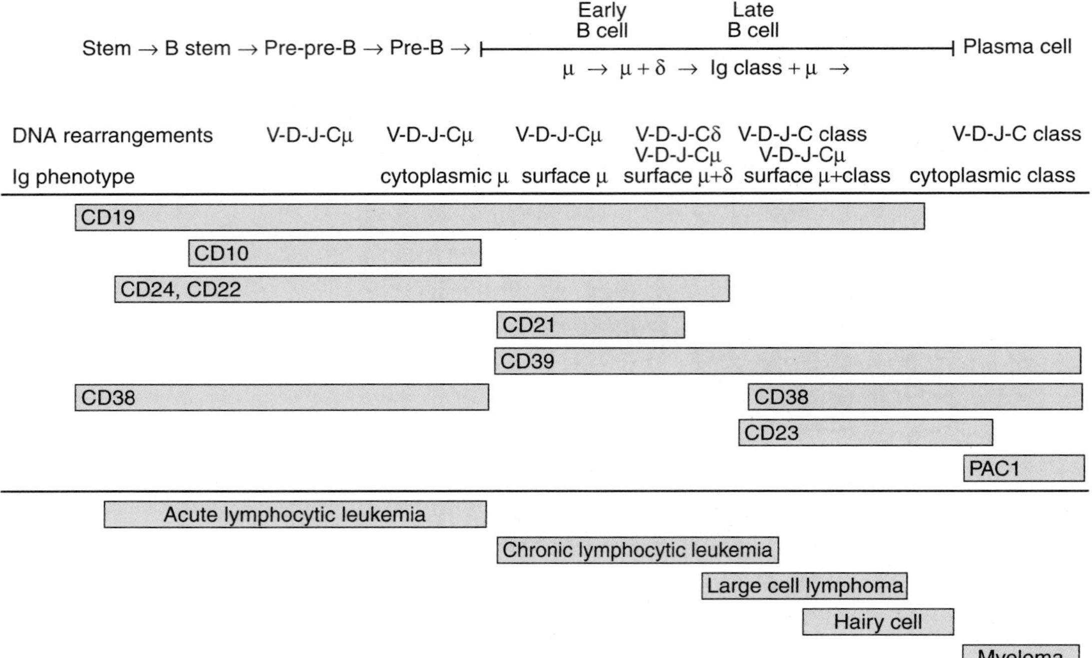

Figure 17.6 Expression of CD markers during B-cell development and on B-cell tumors. (i) Stem cell: CDs 19 and 38; sometimes CDs 22 and 24; no Ig gene rearrangements; no Ig expression. (ii) Pre-pre-B cell: gain of CD 10; VDJCμ rearrangement; no Ig expression. (iii) Pre-B cell: same CDs as above; VDJCμ rearrangement; cytoplasmic μ chain. (iv) Early B cell: loss of CD 10 and 38, gain of CD 21 and 39; μ or μ and δ surface positive. (v) Late B cell: loss of CD 21, gain of CDs 23 and 38; VDJC class gene rearrangements; μ, γ, ϵ, or δ surface positive. (vi) Plasma cell: loss of CDs 19, 22, 23, and 24; gain of PCA1 (plasma cell antigen 1); cytoplasmic Ig of a single class. The expression of these markers on various B-cell tumors is indicated at the bottom of the figure.

except that, in general, B-cell tumors respond better to treatment than do T-cell tumors, and expression of markers of mature B cells is associated with better prognosis and expression of markers of immature B cells with poor prognosis. For instance, expression of CD23, a marker of late B-cell differentiation, and the lack of early B-cell differentiation markers, such as CD38, indicate longer disease-free survival than the reverse. The expression of CD markers on B cells frequently disobeys the differentiation patterns. Thus, CD21 and CD23, markers of different stages of normal differentiation, are often found on the same tumor cells. Unfortunately, analysis of CD expression does not provide better prognostic information than does conventional histology or clinical features. An exception to this is the proliferation antigen called Ki-67. Monoclonal antibody to Ki-67 reacts with a nuclear antigen expressed during the cell cycle but not on resting cells. In a recent comparison to histologic grading, the percentages of Ki-67-positive cells correlated to grade, as shown in Table 17.4.

Gene expression profiling. The levels of hundreds to thousands of mRNAs in tissues may be estimated using cDNA microarray analysis. When this method was used to compare gene expression in diffuse large B-cell lymphomas, two distinct patterns of expression were found. Ap-

Table 17.4 Correlation between histiocytic grade and Ki-67 positivity

Grade	% Ki-67 positive	Examples
Low	14	Small cell, follicular
Intermediate	43	Mixed, follicular
High	58	Large cell, diffuse

proximately 40% of patients with a relative good prognosis have a pattern similar to that of germinal center B cells, whereas 60% with a poor prognosis have a gene expression pattern similar to that seen in proliferating B cells in vitro (activated B cells). Thus, this approach is able to differentiate between different types of large B-cell lymphomas.

Multiple myeloma. The final step in differentiation of B cells is the plasma cells that synthesize and secrete immunoglobulin. Tumors of plasma cells almost always arise in the bone marrow as leukemias do, but, except in rare cases, the tumor cells do not appear in the blood in large numbers, i.e., do not produce leukemia. The tumor is termed multiple myeloma because of many sites (multiple) of masses (-oma) of the tumor cells found in the bone marrow (myel-). The cells of multiple myeloma are plasma cells that usually contain or secrete a single type of immunoglobulin molecule (monoclonal). These may belong to any of the major immunoglobulin classes and may, but usually do not, demonstrate antigen-binding capacity. A variant form of myeloma that produces IgM and that has slightly different morphological and clinical features is termed Waldenstrom's macroglobulinemia.

Monoclonal immunoglobulin refers to a uniform, homogeneous, molecular species of immunoglobulin, in contrast to the heterogeneous array of immunoglobulins present in sera of normal persons. This homogeneous immunoglobulin is often referred to as myeloma paraprotein. Electrophoretic or immunoelectrophoretic analysis of sera from myeloma patients reveals a characteristic peak of protein in about 80% of cases (myeloma spike). The myeloma proteins are usually complete immunoglobulin molecules. In some cases, one part of the molecule (e.g., light chain or heavy chain) may be produced in excess or may be the only myeloma paraprotein found. The light-chain paraprotein is usually rapidly cleared from the circulation by filtration through the kidney and appears in the urine as Bence Jones protein. Bence Jones protein (light chains) classically precipitates in acidified urine when heated to 50 to 60°C and redissolves at 100°C. Free, excess heavy chains may also be the only secreted myeloma paraprotein identified in the serum of affected patients (H-chain disease). In about 1% of cases, no myeloma paraprotein can be detected, even though myeloma plasma cells are present in the bone marrow and contain monoclonal immunoglobulin. Kappa light chains are present in myeloma proteins at a slightly higher frequency than lambda light chains (55 versus 45%), and patients with kappa-type myeloma proteins tend to have longer survival. The degree of elevation of a paraprotein in a given patient may be used to monitor therapeutic effects (e.g., chemotherapy). Symptoms related to the excess immunoglobulin may appear, e.g., hyperviscosity of the blood because of the high intrinsic viscosity of the myeloma protein, insolubility in the cold (cryoglobulinemia) or formation of immunoglobulin complexes by paraprotein interactions. These symptoms lead to circulatory disturbances and microvascular occlusions. IgM production is associated with a cell type that is generally less differentiated than the plasma cell. This disease is called Waldenstrom's macroglobulinemia. The cell type is more like that seen in CLL.

Monoclonal gammopathies (MGs) are various conditions in which an increase in a monoclonal immunoglobulin is found. In 1985, a classification of four types of MG was made: (i) B-cell malignancies, (ii) B-cell benign neoplasia, (iii) MG in immunodeficiencies with a T/B-cell imbalance, and (iv) MG due to infection or antigenic stimulation. By following patients in these categories and relating the course of the related disease to animal models, it has been tentatively concluded that MG may arise as a result of four interacting mechanisms: genetic instability of B cells leading to selected oncogene activation, chronic antigen stimulation with resulting cytokine stimulation of B cells, restricted clonality of the B cells in certain individuals producing oligoclonal dominance of stimulated B-cell populations, and defective T-cell control. The development of the malignant B cells appears to be related to gene instability in certain individuals.

Ig idiotypes and therapy. The myeloma idiotype not only serves as a marker for all cells in the myeloma but also may be used as a target for specific immunotherapy. In experimental models, immunization of mice with a myeloma idiotype can produce resistance to transplanted myeloma cells bearing the idiotype. There appears to be more than one mechanism for control of myeloma cell growth. The resistance may be mediated by antibodies to the idiotype (antibody-directed complement-dependent killing, opsonization, or antibody-dependent cell-mediated immunity) or by T cells (specific T-suppressor cells for the idiotype or T-killer cells directed to the idiotype). In human clinical trials, mouse monoclonal anti-idiotypic infusion has had limited success. Most recipients demonstrated no effect, whereas approximately 20% had a definite antibody-related remission. Clinical trials using drug-conjugated anti-idiotypic antibodies are now under way. Biological problems in anti-idiotypic therapy include the ability of some tumors to switch idiotype expression and escape idiotype-directed control mechanisms, the ability of tumor cells to modulate cell surface expression of antigenic molecules, and, if mouse monoclonal anti-human idiotypic antibodies are used, a host response resulting in neutralizing human anti-mouse immunoglobulin.

Burkitt's lymphoma. *Burkitt's lymphoma* features cytoplasmic and surface Ig, receptors for C3, and surface viral antigens of Epstein-Barr (EB) virus. Burkitt's lymphoma was first identified in African children residing in high-rainfall areas of Africa, where mosquitoes are abundant. Cases of Burkitt's lymphoma have now been identified throughout the world, and the relationship to the self-limiting disease infectious mononucleosis, which is common in Western nations, has attracted considerable attention. In African patients, the jaw is involved, with a diffuse, rapidly growing lymphoid tumor composed of blast cells. In Americans, abdominal, pelvic, and bone marrow involvement is more common. Chemotherapy with cyclophosphamide can produce sustained remissions in 80% of patients with African Burkitt's lymphoma. These tumors are also very responsive to radiotherapy and may undergo spontaneous remission. This supports the concept of a viral etiology, because virus-induced tumors of animals are often self-limiting or responsive to therapy in adults but grow progressively in newborns.

The presence of EB virus antigens on the cell surface provides a relatively strong potential tumor antigen to which the human host may respond. Both cell-mediated and humoral antibody responses may occur to EB virus antigens in patients with Burkitt's lymphoma. Some antigens are found on Burkitt's lymphoma cells that are not viral antigens but are new antigenic specificities unique to early EB virus-transformed cells. Since antibodies to these antigens are found before antibodies to viral antigens, they have been termed early EB virus antigens. Antibody responses are complicated—high titers of antibody to "early antigen" expressed on Burkitt's lymphoma cells are associated with relapses, whereas responses to viral capsid antigens may be protective. Antibodies to capsid antigens are found in tumor-free relatives of patients with Burkitt's lymphoma. A reduction of antibody to early antigens is associated with the development of delayed-type hypersensitivity to early antigens. The relationship of antibody against capsid antigens or appearance of delayed-type hypersensitivity in the course of the disease remains uncertain, but it is believed to be protective. Production of the EBNA 1 product of the EB virus by the tumor cells may contribute to the development of the lymphoma, because transgenic mice expressing this product develop lymphomas. There is increasing evidence that EB virus may also be involved in malignant transformation in Hodgkin's disease (see below) and that Burkitt's lymphoma may be more closely related to Hodgkin's disease than to other B-cell lymphomas.

Transplantation-associated lymphoproliferation. Patients who are heavily immunosuppressed, in particular, recipients of cardiac or hepatic grafts, are at risk for developing an unusual lymphoproliferation lesion. The cells resemble those of large-cell lymphoma, often occur outside of lymphoid organs (muscle and fat), and may progress rapidly. Although the disease progresses with the features of a true malignancy, marker studies demonstrate a polyclonal B-cell proliferation that frequently contains EB virus. Studies on the immunoglobulin gene arrangements in these lesions often indicate a spectrum of proliferation ranging from polymorphic polyclonal proliferation with the features of a virus infection to monomorphic and monoclonal proliferation with all the features of a non-Hodgkin's lymphoma.

T-Cell Tumors

T-cell tumors include thymoma, lymphoblastic lymphoma, acute lymphoblastic leukemia (20 to 30%), mycosis fungoides (Sézary syndrome), and rare diffuse non-Hodgkin's lymphomas and leukemias (Table 17.5). Most T-cell tumors seem to arise in the bone marrow, with only rare diffuse T-cell lymphomas arising in the lymph nodes or spleen.

T-cell markers. Monoclonal antibodies to T-cell populations are now being applied to define T-cell tumors (Fig. 17.7). These monoclonal antibodies identify T-cell differentiation markers. Previously, phenotypic markers, such as E-rosette formation (the sheep erythrocyte receptor is now defined as CD2), lack of sIg, presence of TdT, lack of surface HLA-D antigens, and reactivity with heteroantisera to T cells, were used. Of these, E rosettes (in the form of CD2) and TdT remain the most useful markers. In addition,

Table 17.5 Characterization of T-cell tumors[a]

Tumor	Phenotypic markers[b]	Characteristics
Bone marrow origin		
T-cell ALL	Heterogeneous; most $CD1^+$, $CD4^-$, $CD8^-$, TdT^+, acid phosphatase$^+$, $CD2^-$(ER, sheep erythrocyte receptor)	Bone marrow origin; rapid course; poor response to chemotherapy compared with that of B-cell tumors
T-cell CLL	Mature T-cell ($CD4^+$, $CD5^-$, sIg^-, TdT^-, $CD1^-$, $CD3^+$), rare $CD8^+$, $CD2^+$	Very rare; most CLLs are $CD5^+$ B cells; worse prognosis than B-cell CLL
IgG FcR^+ (T_G) lymphoproliferative disease	Large granular lymphocytes; mature T-cell phenotype; natural killer activity; $CD2^+$	Anemia, hypogammaglobulinemia, recurrent infections; benign course; natural killer-large granular lymphoma is aggressive
Mycosis fungoides/Sézary syndrome	Mature Th ($CD9^-$, $CD4^+$, $CD8^-$, $CD1^-$, $CD2^+$)	Skin (mycosis fungoides); blood (Sézary syndrome); associated with dermatitis; survival varies with stage from 1 to 12 years
T-cell type of hairy cell leukemia	Mature T-cell phenotype	Usually B-cell tumor; splenomegaly
Adult T-cell leukemia/ lymphoma	Mature Th ($CD9^-$, $CD4^+$, $CD8^-$, $CD1^-$, $CD2^+$), also HLA-$B5^+$ (shared with HTLV-1)	Skin, hypercalcemia, often aggressive HTLV-1 associated; Japan, Caribbean
Thymoma	Immature: $CD1^+$, $CD4^-$, $CD8^-$, $CD2^-$	Anterior mediastinum: usually epithelial with nonmalignant T cells; true thymic lymphoma very rare
Lymph node		
T-lymphoblastic lymphoma	Heterogeneous; most express immature thymocyte phenotype; TdT^+, sIg^-, $CD2^+$	Rare, usually in children; begins in thymus, extends to other organs and blood
T-cell non-Hodgkin's lymphoma	Mature T-cell phenotype	Rare, diffuse lymphoma, usually B-cell tumors

[a]Modified from E. A. Harden, T. J. Polker, and B. F. Haynes, *in* S. Sell and R. Reisfeld, ed., *Monoclonal Antibodies in Cancer,* Humana Press, Totowa, N.J., 1985.
[b]Many variations in phenotyic expression are seen.

T-cell malignancies may be phenotyped by monoclonal antibodies (Table 17.5). Many of these antibodies, such as CD1, CD5, CD10, transferrin receptor, HLA-A, B, and C, and HLA-DR, are not particularly useful for delineation of T-cell lineage since they also appear on non-T-cell tissue. Others, such as CD2, CD3, CD4, CD7, and CD8, are essentially T-cell-specific. These markers define T-cell lineage and stages of maturation arrest (Fig. 17.7). However, the clinical relevance of the phenotypic identification of T-cell tumors is not yet clear. On the other hand, some adults with acute myelogenous leukemia (AML) have blasts that express T-cell marker CD2 or B-cell marker CD19; these patients have a more favorable prognosis than patients with AML that do not express these markers. The major feature of malignancies is the monoclonal nature of the malignant cells (all the cells in a tumor have the same markers) as compared with normal, nonmalignant, polyclonal T-cell populations. Phenotypic characterization may be carried out on cell suspensions, such as those from leukemic blood or effusions, as well as on frozen tissue sections. The future application of such analysis depends upon clinical correlations yet to be made.

Macrophage Tumors

"Malignant histiocytosis" and "histiocytosis X" are terms used for tumors of macrophages. Malignant histiocytosis is a family of diseases including Letterer-Siwe disease, Hand-Schüller-Christian disease, and eosinophilic granuloma of bone (Table 17.6). These tumors consist of space-occupying lesions filled by mature histiocytes with abundant cytoplasm. Hand-

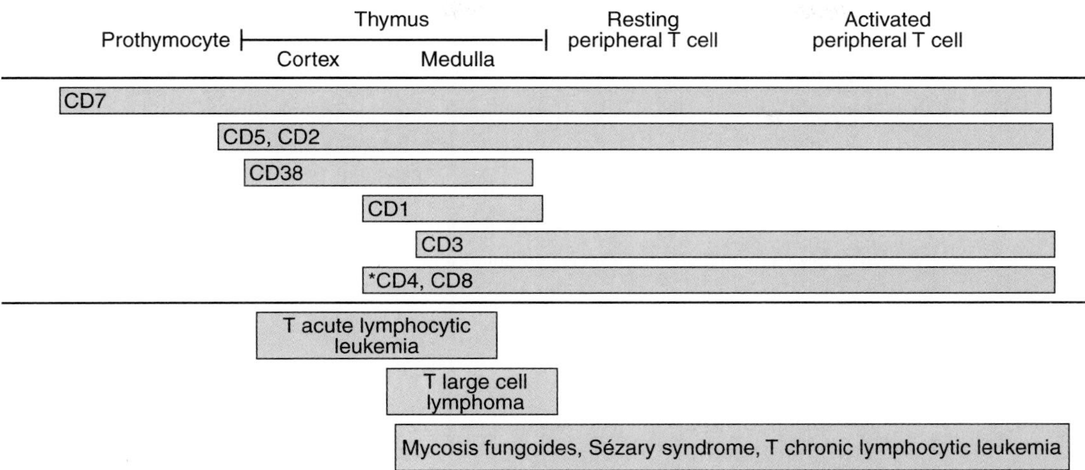

Figure 17.7 T-cell differentiation markers and T-cell lymphomas. The boxes in the top half of the figure indicate the appearance of T-CLL markers detected by monoclonal antibodies at the stages of normal T-cell development. The boxes in the bottom half of the figure indicate the expression of these markers on T-cell tumors.

Schüller-Christian disease and eosinophilic granuloma occur in bone, with the former also occurring predominantly in spleen and lymph node. Letterer-Siwe disease involves the skin, lymph nodes, and spleen. The cells in these diseases contain a distinctive rod-shaped inclusion also found in intraepithelial monocytes (Langerhans cells). Note that in the Rappaport classification, the term histiocytic lymphoma has been used for a B-cell tumor, not a true histiocytic (macrophage) tumor. True histiocytic lymphomas are believed to arise from fixed histiocytes.

Hodgkin's Lymphoma

Hodgkin's disease is a malignant tumor of lymphoid organs composed of mixed lymphoid cell types. Hodgkin's disease has been known in some form or another for over 150 years; however, the original description by Hodgkin in 1832 of seven patients with "tumors of the absorbent glands" included lesions now believed to be tuberculosis. Although significant advances have been made in the diagnosis and treatment of Hodgkin's disease, the etiology remains unknown. Major theories of the nature of Hodgkin's disease include that it is a form of lymphoma, an inflammatory response, or a viral infection.

Table 17.6 Classification of macrophage-histiocyte-derived tumors

Histiocyte type	Normal tissue distribution	Putative malignant tumor
Free histiocytes	Circulating monocytes	Monocytic leukemia
Fixed histiocytes	Reticuloendothelial cells	True histiocytic lymphoma
Dendritic histiocytes	Follicular, lymph node cortex	Hand-Schüller-Christian disease
Langerhans cells	Intraepithelial	Letterer-Siwe disease
Macrophage stem cells	Bone marrow	Eosinophilic granuloma

Table 17.7 Histopathologic classification of Hodgkin's disease[a]

Type of tumor	Features	Relative prognosis
Lymphocyte predominance	Mainly small lymphocytes, few R-S cells	Most favorable
Modular sclerosis	Lymphoid nodules separated by fibrous bands	Favorable
Mixed cellularity	Numerous R-S cells in pleomorphic stroma	Guarded
Lymphocyte depletion	Diffuse irregular fibrosis; anaplastic R-S cells	Least favorable

[a]From R. J. Lukes and J. J. Butler, *Cancer Res.* **26:**1063–1083, 1966.

Histopathologic Classification

The major feature of Hodgkin's disease is the pleomorphism (different cell types) of the tumor lesions, in contrast to the more homogeneous cell types of the non-Hodgkin's lymphomas. Tentative agreement on the classification of Hodgkin's disease was reached at a conference in Rye, New York, in 1966. This classification scheme is important, because the histologic forms of each type correlate with the clinical course (Table 17.7). The characteristic large, binuclear cell of Hodgkin's disease was described independently in the United States by Dorothy Reed, a pathology resident at Johns Hopkins University, and a famous German pathologist, C. Sternberg. In the United States, these cells are referred to as Reed-Sternberg (R-S) cells; in Europe, they are called Sternberg-Reed cells (Fig. 17.8).

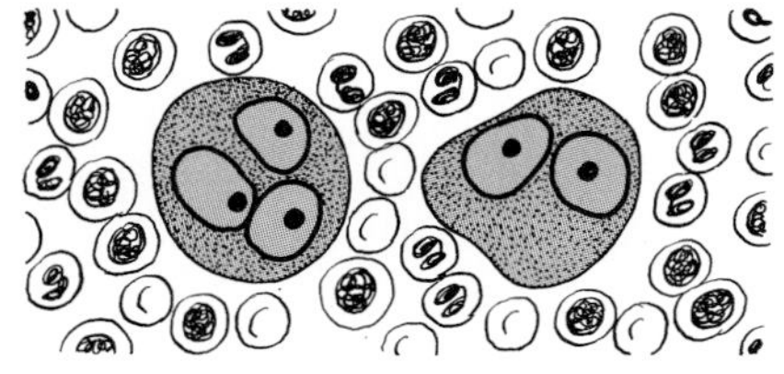

Figure 17.8 Reed-Sternberg cells are large multinucleated "giant" cells considered essential for the diagnosis of Hodgkin's disease.

The histopathologic classification is based on the relative proportion of lymphocytes, fibrosis, and R-S cells in relation to other cells (neutrophils, eosinophils, plasma cells) in the pleomorphic tumor. R-S cells are of particular diagnostic significance for Hodgkin's disease (Fig. 17.9).

Cellular origin. The cellular origin of the R-S cells has been a continuing story. In the past, the origin has been attributed to T cells, B cells, and dendritic cells, in particular, interdigitating reticulum cells. At present, the evidence indicates that Hodgkin's disease is of B-cell origin. First, cy-

Figure 17.9 Drawing of cell types in Hodgkin's disease. Depicted is a drawing modified from a textbook by William Osler published in 1914, illustrating the different cell types seen in mixed-cellularity Hodgkin's disease. The diagnosis depends on the identification of Reed-Sternberg cells in a lesion containing a mixture of other cell types. Lymphocytes and eosinophils are often prominent.

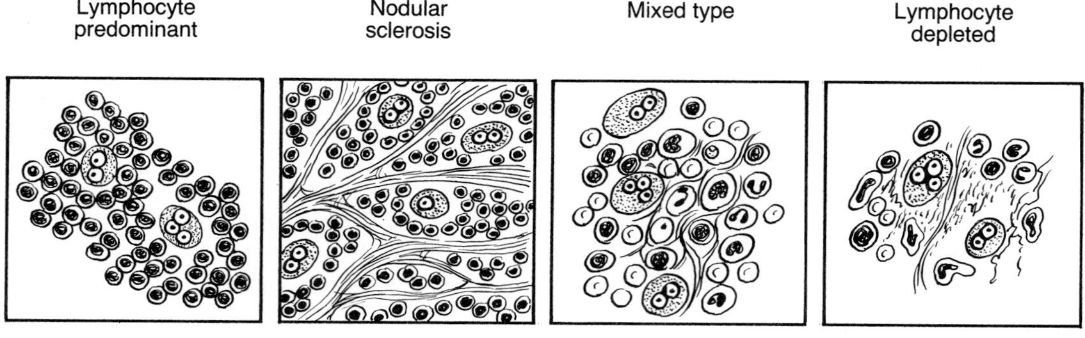

togenetic analysis of R-S cells demonstrates that the R-S cells in a given patient arise from a single clone. Second, genetic analysis of the DNA of individual R-S cells obtained from tissue sections by microdissection reveals rearrangement of the VDJ immunoglobulin genes. The nature of these rearrangements indicates that R-S cells are derived from germinal center B cells that have undergone "crippling" rearrangements in the framework regions of potentially functional V region genes. Normally, B cells in the germinal center undergo somatic mutation. B cells that express high-affinity antigen receptors are selected for proliferation and differentiation, whereas those that undergo crippling rearrangements are eliminated by apoptosis. According to a theory developed by Klaus Rajewsky, in Hodgkin's disease these crippled B cells are rescued by latent EB virus infection. If this theory holds up, it will turn out that classic Hodgkin's disease is a B-cell tumor caused by EB virus infection and, as stated above, closely related to Burkitt's lymphoma. An exception to this is lymphocyte-predominant Hodgkin's disease. The R-S cells in these cases have productive Ig gene rearrangements, express cell sIg, and do not have evidence of EB virus infection. Also unexplained is the ectopic expression of cell markers by classic R-S cells. Classic R-S cells express markers of interdigitating reticulum cells, including morphologic similarities, similar levels of HLA-DR antigen, esterase, and acid phosphatase, reactivity with monoclonal antibody LeuM1 (CD15), which identifies an epitope on interdigitating reticulum cells, and CD30 (Ki-1), which does not react with T cells or B cells.

The "nonneoplastic" components of Hodgkin's disease, the accompanying lymphocytes, plasma cells, eosinophils, and other cells, also proliferate and contribute to the cellular composition of the lesions but are not truly malignant cells. The proliferation of these cells may be stimulated by monokines produced by the Hodgkin's (R-S) cells. It has been reported that R-S cells in Hodgkin's disease secrete interleukin-1 (IL-1), IL-5, IL-6, IL-9, tumor necrosis factor alpha, macrophage colony-stimulating factor, transforming growth factor beta, and, less frequently, IL-4 and granulocyte colony-stimulating factor, but it is not clear that the cells used in these studies are truly R-S cells. With some exceptions, most non-Hodgkin's disease lymphoma cells do not secrete cytokines. Exceptions are the so-called T-cell-rich B-cell lymphomas, in which the tumor B cells secrete IL-4, which is responsible for the T-cell infiltrate, and angioimmunoblastic lymphadenopathy-type T-cell lymphomas, in which the tumor T cells secrete IL-6, which is responsible for the plasma cell reaction. The large number of cytokines secreted by Hodgkin's tumor cells may be responsible for the varied types of nontumor cells included within the mass of the Hodgkin's lymphomas. Why B-cell tumors are secreting such a variety of growth factors is not known.

Staging. The clinical course of Hodgkin's disease is dependent on the extent of the disease when first diagnosed. The exact relationship between the extent of disease (stage) and prognosis is not clear, but prognosis generally becomes worse as the extent of the disease increases (Fig. 17.10).

Treatment. The treatment of Hodgkin's disease with high-dose radiation to the total lymphoid tissue involved with tumor has led to substantial increases in survival times and essential cure of some patients. Clearly, early-stage Hodgkin's disease can be treated with limited field radiation,

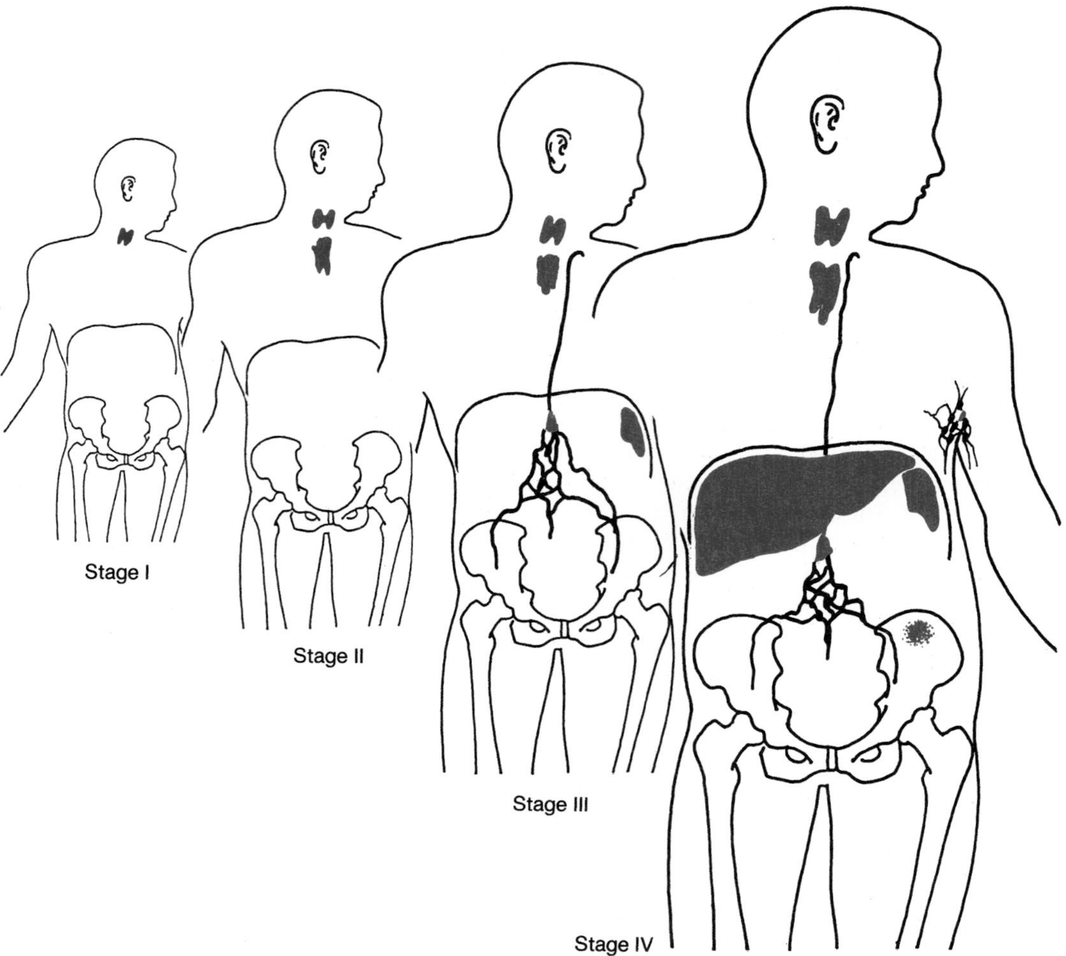

Figure 17.10 Clinical staging of Hodgkin's disease. Staging correlates well with prognosis and helps in deciding the selection of therapy. The same clinical staging is also applicable to the non-Hodgkin's lymphomas. Stage I: involvement of a single lymph node region. Stage II: involvement of two or more lymph node regions on the same side of the diaphragm. Stage III: involvement of lymphatic structures on both sides of the diaphragm. Stage IV: diffuse or disseminated involvement.

whereas late-stage disease requires more extensive radiation. In addition, combined drug chemotherapy has yielded up to 80% complete remission, even in patients with far advanced disease, and has induced remission in patients who relapse after radiotherapy. Patients with Hodgkin's disease frequently demonstrate immunodeficiencies, particularly of the cellular immune system, and may develop infectious complications.

Angioimmunoblastic Lymphadenopathy

Angioimmunoblastic lymphadenopathy is associated with clinical findings similar to those seen in Hodgkin's disease (fever, sweats, weight loss, skin rash, and so on). There may also be hypergammaglobulinemia (polyclonal). Histologically, there is a marked increase in small blood vessels (particularly endothelial hyperplasia) in the involved nodes, with numerous blasts and plasma cells, epithelial cells, and large numbers of dying and degenerating cells. The lesion resembles a florid proliferation of the B-cell system, although T cells may also be involved. Most patients demonstrate a rapid downhill course, with death occurring after 1 to 2 years. It is not yet clear if this condition is truly a malignant tumor. Some investigators consider it to be a nonneoplastic progressive immune reaction, but the progressive clinical course is consistent with malignancy. A variant is angioimmunoblastic lymphadenopathy with dysproteinemia. These patients usually have partial or complete displacement of lymph nodes with diffuse lymphoplasmacytic proliferation and evidence of autoimmune or immune complex disease. As stated above, the plasma cell proliferation and differentiation in these tumors may be due to lymphokines secreted by the tumor cells.

Etiology of Lymphomas

Gene Rearrangements

Cells from lymphomas and leukemias demonstrate a variety of nonrandom chromosome translocations that may bring "promoter" areas of one gene into juxtaposition with proto-oncogene DNA sequences (Table 17.8). The activation of these proto-oncogenes plays a key role in producing neoplastic activation of the cells. For example, in Burkitt's lymphoma, the *myc* oncogene in chromosome 8 is transposed to Ig heavy-chain locus on chromosome 14, resulting in activation of the oncogene (Fig. 17.11). Another critical example is the arrangement in AML that leads to constitutive activation of IL-3. As shown in Fig. 2.8, IL-3 is involved in activation of proliferation at many stages of myelocytic development, from the hematopoietic stem cell through the erythrocytic, megakaryocytic, and myelocytic lineages. It is not surprising that this rearrangement leads to accumulation of cells in these lineages, because there is a continual signal for proliferation and no competing signal for cell death. A different mechanism is the activation of expression of *bcl-2* in B-cell lymphomas, which blocks cell death (apoptosis). Overexpression of *bcl-2* results in prolonged survival of the affected cells, because the lymphoma cells that are produced do not die.

An exception, so far, to the gene rearrangement etiology of leukemias is the absence of gene rearrangements in CLL. Other possible etiologies for these tumors include loss of immunoregulation or viral infection.

Loss of Immunoregulation

Patients who are administered drugs that depress immune responses, such as recipients of allografted organs, display an extremely high incidence of

Table 17.8 Some gene rearrangements in human malignant lymphomas and leukemias

Tumor type	Chromosomal rearrangement
Chronic myelogenous leukemia	t9;22 *bcr/abl* (Philadelphia chromosome); chromosomal region/*abl* (mutated tyrosine kinase)
Acute myelogenous leukemia	IL-3 rearrangement (activated tyrosine kinase)
Acute lymphoblastic leukemia	t12;22, t9;12 (fusion transcription factors)
Burkitt's (B-cell) lymphoma	t8;14 IgG/*myc* (nuclear transcription factor)
B-cell lymphoma	t14;22 IgG/*bcl-2* (inhibits apoptosis)
Chronic lymphocytic leukemia	None

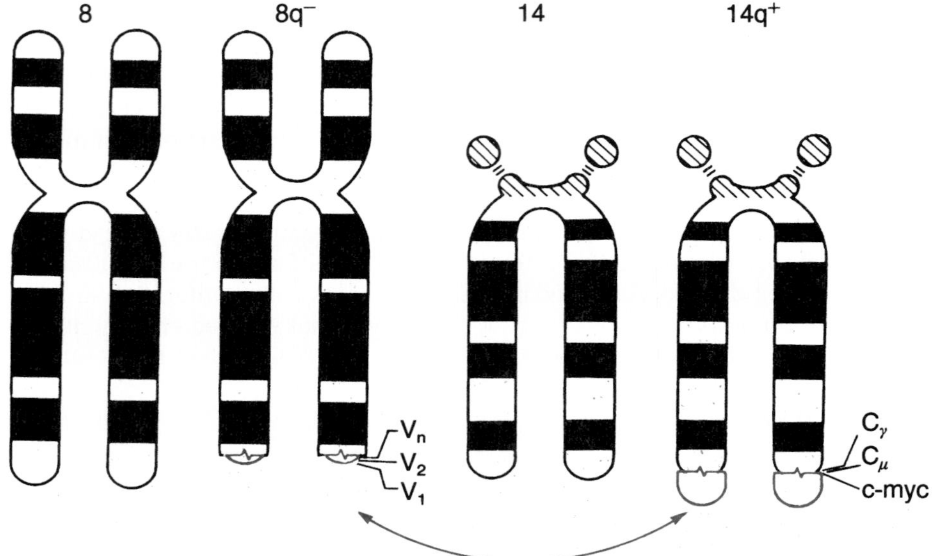

Figure 17.11 Diagram of the t(8;14) translocation in Burkitt's lymphoma cells. The c-*myc* gene on chromosome 8 translocates next to the C and Cγ genes on chromosome 14. (From J. Erikson, A. ar-Rushdi, H. L. Drwinga, P. C. Nowell, and C. M. Croce, *Proc. Natl. Acad. Sci. USA* **80:**820–824, 1983.)

lymphoid malignancies but a normal incidence of other nonlymphoid tumors. Thus, patients receiving immunosuppressive therapy may lose the ability to regulate proliferation of clones of cells that would normally be suppressed by immune regulatory mechanism cells. Further support for this concept is the observation that the incidence of many of the lymphoid tumors increases with age. Aging is also associated with involution of the thymus, autoantibody production, and other evidence of loss of immunoregulation. In addition, the incidence of lymphoid tumors, particularly those of B-cell origin, is increased in patients with naturally occurring immune deficiency diseases such as ataxia telangiectasia. It is postulated that immune deficiencies are associated not only with losses of responding cells (T-helper and B cells) but also with losses of controlling cell populations (suppressor or regulatory cells). This imbalance permits inadequately controlled proliferation of the remaining lymphoid cells.

Viral Infection

Although many tumors of animals are known to be caused by viral infection, a viral etiology for most human cancers has been difficult to demonstrate. As described above, infection with EB virus is implicated in Burkitt's lymphoma, posttransplant lymphoma, and, now, Hodgkin's disease. In addition, human T-cell leukemia virus type 1 (HTLV-1) clearly causes leukemias in southern Japan, the Caribbean, and other areas of the world that were frequented by sailing ships involved in the slave trade. The role of viruses in other human lymphomas remains conjectural. In contrast, many of the lymphoid tumors of animals are virus-induced. These are usually fast-growing tumors that are more frequent in young animals than in older ones. Virus-induced tumors of animals are similar to the acute lymphoid tumors of children, whereas the lymphoid tumors of adults are generally more chronic and may reflect loss of immune control.

Infections Associated with Lymphoproliferative Diseases

Patients with lymphoproliferative disease are subject to an increased incidence of clinically significant infections. This may be caused by the nature of the disease or, secondarily, by the type of treatment usually employed, chemotherapy or irradiation. Abnormalities of immune function are frequently found in patients with lymphoproliferative diseases. These include increased production of abnormal immunoglobulins, found with immunoglobulin-secreting tumors, and a variety of autoantibodies as well as depressed immune reactivity. Some reasons for increased susceptibility to infections in these diseases are as follows: (i) replacement of normally functioning immune cells with tumor cells that function poorly, (ii) production of secreted products that inhibit inflammatory or immune reactions; (iii) appearance of cells (suppressor cells) that suppress normal immune function; and (iv) loss of normal homeostatic mechanisms (loss of suppressor cells), permitting overproduction of some immune products and underproduction of others.

Summary

Both benign and malignant proliferation of lymphoid cells may lead to enlargement of lymph nodes and spleen, increases in lymphoid cells in the peripheral blood, and systemic symptoms (fever, sweats, and weight loss). Benign lymphoproliferative lesions are usually made up of a heterogeneous population of lymphoid cells that may cause enlargement of lymphoid organs, but the basic structures of the organs (cortex, follicles, medulla) are usually, but not always, maintained. Malignant lymphoid tumors result from an arrest in maturation of a single cell lineage and usually consist of a homogeneous cell type that replaces or destroys the normal architecture of the organ. Malignant tumors of white cells in the blood are known as leukemias; those in organs, lymphomas. Strict morphological criteria are not adequate for acceptable diagnosis of lymphoproliferative disease; immune characteristics and phenotypic markers of the cell type determined by flow cytometry provide critical additional information in regard to diagnosis, prognosis, and selection of chemotherapeutic agents. In many instances, the growth pattern of the tumor reflects the cell type of origin (B cells produce follicular tumors; T cells, diffuse tumors), but considerable deviation from predicted growth patterns occurs in individual patients.

B-cell tumors may be considered to occur at various stages of B-cell development, from small lymphocytes to large "blast" cells to well-differentiated plasma cells, with multiple myeloma representing the most differentiated stage. Although the most impressive cellular component of multiple myeloma is the differentiated plasma cell, clearly, tumor cells in different stages of the cell cycle and at different levels of differentiation must be present in the malignant population, including dividing, less-differentiated plasma cells. The cells in myelomas, like B-cell tumors, have sIg. Since the immunoglobulin produced by these cells is monoclonal, each sIg-bearing cell will contain immunoglobulin with antigens specific for that molecule (idiotype). $CD5^+$ B cells that give rise to CLL most likely represent a separate lineage of B cells.

Tumors of T cells and macrophages are much less frequent than tumors of B cells, and the resulting malignant cells reflect the morphology and marker phenotype of the cell lineage from which they arise. Many lymphoid malignancies result from gene rearrangements that lead to constitutive activation of proliferation or loss of normal cell maturation processes. Novel methods of interfering with these processes are now being studied to develop therapeutic strategies to block these processes.

Bibliography

Lymphoid Tissue Structure and Lymphomas

Lukes, R. J., and R. D. Collins. 1973. New observations in follicular lymphoma. *Gann Monogr. Cancer Res.* **15:**209.

Mann, R. B., E. S. Jaffe, and C. W. Berard. 1979. Malignant lymphomas—a conceptual understanding of morphologic diversity. *Am. J. Pathol.* **94:**105.

Warnke, R. A., et al. 1995. *Tumors of the Lymph Nodes and Spleen.* AFIP Press, Washington, D.C.

Classification of Lymphomas

Baird, S. 1993. The usefulness of cell surface markers in predicting the prognosis of non-Hodgkin's lymphomas. *Crit. Rev. Clin. Lab. Sci.* **30:**1–28.

Frizzera, G., G. D. Wu, and G. Inghirami. 1999. The usefulness of immunophenotypic and genotypic studies in the diagnosis and classification of hematopoietic and lymphoid neoplasms. An update. *Am. J. Clin. Pathol.* **111:**S13–S39.

Harris, N. L., E. S. Jaffe, H. Stein, P. M. Banks, J. K. Chan, M. L. Cleary, G. Delsol, C. De Wolf-Peeters, B. Falini, and K. C. Gatter. 1994. A revised European-American classification of lymphoid neoplasms. A proposal from the International Lymphoma Study Group. *Blood* **84:**1361–1392.

Hauke, R. J., and J. O. Armitage. 2000. A new approach to non-Hodgkin's lymphoma. *Intern. Med.* **39:**197–208.

Isaacson, P. G. 2000. The current status of lymphoma classification. *Br. J. Haematol.* **109:**258–266.

Jaffe, E. S., N. L. Harris, J. Diebold, and H. K. Muller-Hermerlink. 1999. World Health Organization classification of neoplastic diseases of the hematopoietic and lymphoid tissues: a progress report. *Am. J. Clin. Pathol.* **111:**S8–S12.

Nonmalignant Lymphoproliferation

Frizzera, G. 1985. Castleman's disease: more questions than answers. *Hum. Pathol.* **16:**202–205.

Neiman, R. S., P. Dervan, C. Haudenschild, and R. Jaffe. 1978. Angioimmunoblastic lymphadenopathy. *Cancer* **41:**507–518.

Phatak, P. D., J. S. Janas, R. L. Sham, B. Yirinec, and V. J. Marder. 1997. Disorders that resemble lymphomas. *Am. J. Hematol.* **56:**63–68.

AIDS-Related Lymphadenopathy

Ciacci, J. D., C. Tellez, J. VonRoenn, and R. M. Levy. 1999. Lymphomas of the central nervous system in AIDS. *Semin. Neurol.* **12:**213–221.

Ioachim, H. L. 1989. *Pathology of AIDS.* J. B. Lippincott Co., Philadelphia, Pa.

Levine, A. M. 1992. Acquired immunodeficiency syndrome-related lymphoma. *Blood* **80:**8–20.

Spina, M., E. Vaccher, A. Carbone, and U. Tirelli. 1999. Neoplastic complications of HIV infection. *Ann. Oncol.* **10:**1271–1286.

Infectious Mononucleosis

Kawa, K. 2000. Epstein-Barr virus-associated diseases in humans. *Int. J. Hematol.* **71:**108–117.

Purtilo, D. T., R. S. Strobach, M. Okano, and J. E. Davis. 1992. Epstein-Barr virus-associated lymphoproliferative disorders. *Lab. Investig.* **67:**5–23.

B-Cell Tumors

Alizadeh, A. A., M. B. Eisen, R. E. Davis, C. Ma, I. S. Lossos, A. Rosenwald, J. C. Boldrick, H. Sabet, T. Tran, X. Yu, J. I. Powell, L. Yang, G. E. Marti, T. Moore, J. Hudson, Jr., L. Lu, D. B. Lewis, R. Tibshirani, G. Sherlock, W. C. Chan, T. C. Greiner, D. D. Weisenburger, J. O. Armitage, R. Warnke, L. M. Staudt, et al. 2000. Distinct types of diffuse large B-cell lymphoma identified by gene expression profiling. *Nature* **403:**503–511.

Bouroncle, B. A. 1994. Thirty-five years in the progress of hairy cell leukemia. *Leukemia Lymphoma* **14:1–12.**

Cheson, B. D. 1992. *Chronic Lymphocytic Leukemia.* Marcel Dekker, Inc., New York, N.Y.

Norton, A. J., J. Matthews, V. Pappa, J. Shamash, S. Love, A. Z. Rohatiner, and T. A. Lister. 1995. Mantle cell lymphoma: natural history defined in a serially biopsied population over a 20 year period. *Ann. Oncol.* **6:**249–256.

Rozman, C., and E. Montserrat. 1995. Chronic lymphocytic leukemia. *N. Engl. J. Med.* **333:**1052–1057.

Stevenson, G. T., and M. S. Cragg. 1999. Molecular markers of B-cell lymphoma. *Semin. Cancer Biol.* **9:**139–147.

Zelenetz, A. D., T. T. Chen, and R. Levy. 1991. Histologic transformation of follicular lymphoma to diffuse lymphoma represents tumor progression by a single malignant B cell. *J. Exp. Med.* **173:**197–207.

Multiple Myeloma

Durie, B. G. M., and S. E. Salmon. 1975. Cellular kinetics, staging and immunoglobulin synthesis in multiple myeloma. *Annu. Rev. Med.* **26:**283–288.

Oken, M. M. 1997. Multiple myeloma: prognosis and standard treatment. *Cancer Investig.* **15:**57–64.

Oken, M. M. 1998. Management of myeloma: current and future approaches. *Cancer Control* **5:**218–225.

Waldenstrom, J. 1964. The occurrence of benign, essential monoclonal (M type), non-macromolecular hyperglobulinemia and its differential diagnosis. *Acta Med. Scand.* **176:**345.

Burkitt's Lymphoma

Baumforth, K. R., L. S. Young, K. J. Flavell, C. Constandinou, and P. G. Murray. 1999. The Epstein-Barr virus and its association with human cancers. *Mol. Pathol.* **52:**307–322.

Burkitt, D. P., and D. H. Wright. 1970. *Burkitt's Lymphoma.* E and S Livingston, Edinburgh, United Kingdom.

Van Hasselt, E. J., and R. Broadhead. 1995. Burkitt's lymphoma: a case study of 160 patients treated in Queen Elizabeth Central Hospital from 1988 to 1992. *Paediatr. Haematol. Oncol.* **12:**283.

Transplant-Associated Lymphoma

Knowles, D. M. 1999. Immunodeficiency-associated lymphoproliferative disorders. *Mod. Pathol.* **12:**200–217.

Penn, I. 1981. Malignant lymphomas in transplant recipients. *Transplant. Proc.* **13:**736–739.

Swerdlow, A. H. 1992. Post-transplant lymphoproliferative disorders: a morphologic, phenotypic and genotypic spectrum of the disease. *Histopathology* **20:**373–385.

T-Cell Tumors

Jaffe, E. S. 1996. Classification of natural killer (NK) and NK-like T cell malignancies. *Blood* **87:**1207–1210.

Loughran, T. P. 1993. Clonal diseases of large granular lymphocytes. *Blood* **82:**1–14.

Pandolfi, F., R. Zambello, A. Cafaro, and G. Semenzato. 1992. Biologic and clinical heterogeneity of lymphoproliferative diseases of peripheral mature T lymphocytes. *Lab. Investig.* **67:**274–302.

Reis, M. D., H. Griesser, and T. W. Mak. 1989. T cell receptor and immunoglobulin gene rearrangement in lymphoproliferative disorders. *Adv. Cancer Res.* **52:**45–80.

Weinberg, J. M., C. Jaworsky, B. M. Benoit, B. Telegan, A. H. Rook, and S. R. Lessin. 1995. The clonal nature of circulating Sézary cells. *Blood* **86:**4257–4262. (Erratum, **87:**4923, 1996.)

Macrophage Tumors

Cline, M. J. 1994. Histiocytes and histiocytosis. *Blood* **84:**2840–2853.

Hodgkin's Disease

Hodgkin, T. 1832. On some morbid appearance of the absorbent glands and spleen. *Med. Chir. Dig.* **17:**68.

Hsu, S.-M., J. W. Waldron, P.-L. Hsu, and A. J. Hough. 1993. Cytokines in malignant lymphomas: review and prospective evaluation. *Hum. Pathol.* **24:**1040–1057.

Kaplan, H. S. 1981. Hodgkin's disease: biology, treatment, prognosis. *Blood* **57:**813–822.

Kuppers, R., and K. Rajewsky. 1998. The origin of Hodgkin and Reed/Sternberg cells in Hodgkin's disease. *Annu. Rev. Immunol.* **16:**471–494.

Pan, L. X., T. C. Diss, H. Z. Peng, A. J. Norton, and P. G. Isaacson. 1996. Nodular lymphocyte predominance in Hodgkin's disease: a monoclonal or polyclonal B cell disorder? *Blood* **87:**2428–2434.

Rather, L. J. 1972. Who discovered the pathognomonic giant cell of Hodgkin's disease. *Bull. N. Y. Acad. Med.* **48:**943–950.

Treatment

Bierman, P. J. 2000. Allogeneic bone marrow transplantation for lymphoma. *Blood Rev.* **14:**1–13.

Kernan, N. A., G. Bartsch, R. C. Ash, P. G. Beatty, R. Champlin, A. Filipovich, J. Gajewski, J. A. Hansen, J. Henslee-Downey, J. McCullough, et al. 1993. Analysis of 462 transplantations from unrelated donors facilitated by the national marrow donor program. *N. Engl. J. Med.* **328:**593–602.

Mertelsmann, R., and F. Herrmann. 1990. *Hematopoietic Growth Factors in Clinical Applications.* Marcel Dekker, Inc., New York, N.Y.

Petz, C. D., and K. G. Blume (ed.). 1983. *Clinical Bone Marrow Transplantation.* Churchill Livingstone, Ltd., New York, N.Y.

Thomas, E. D. 1999. Bone marrow transplantation: a review. *Semin. Hematol.* **36:**95–103.

Chromosomal Translocations

Heim, S., and F. Mitelman. 1995. *Cancer Cytogenetics,* Alan R. Liss, New York, N.Y.

Rowley, J. D. 1999. The role of chromosomal translocations in leukemogenesis. *Semin. Hematol.* **36:**59–72.

Rowley, J. D. 2000. Molecular genetics in acute leukemia. *Leukemia* **14:**513–517.

Immunoregulation

Kinlen, L. 1992. Immunosuppressive therapy and acquired immunological disorders. *Cancer Res.* **52**(Suppl.):5474S-5476S.

Kolb, H. J., G. Socie, T. Duell, M. T. Van Lint, A. Tichelli, et al. 1999. Malignant neoplasms in long-term survivors of bone marrow transplantation. *Ann. Intern. Med.* **131**:738–744.

Virus Infection

Blattner, W. A. 1999. Human retroviruses: their role in cancer. *Proc. Assoc. Am. Physicians* **111**:563–572.

Li, J., H. Shen, K. L. Himmel, A. J. Dupuy, D. A. Largaespada, et al. 1999. Leukaemia disease genes: large-scale cloning and pathway predictions. *Nat. Genet.* **23**:348–353.

Immunodeficiency Diseases

18

Immune Deficiencies and Infections

The occurrence of repeated or unusual infections in an individual may reflect a deficiency in defense mechanisms against infection (Table 18.1). Such deficiencies must be especially considered if the infecting organism is one that is not usually responsible for human diseases (opportunistic infection). The type of infection observed is determined by the kind of immune abnormality present. In general, antibody deficiencies are associated with bacterial infections, and cell-mediated immunity deficiencies are associated with viral, fungal, protozoal, and mycobacterial infections. Immune deficiency diseases are classified as primary or secondary. Primary immune deficiencies result from genetic or developmental abnormalities in the acquisition of immune maturity. Secondary deficiencies are caused by diseases that interfere with the expression of a mature immune system.

Both immune and nonimmune specific levels of defensive reactions must be considered in evaluating resistance to infection. Since the major role of inflammation is defense against infection and repair of injury, any alteration in the inflammatory response or defect in the natural barriers to infectious organisms may lead to an increase in infections. For instance, infections are a major complication of burn patients who have lost their external barrier to infection. The depression of pulmonary clearing mechanisms due to the loss of the ciliary activity of bronchial lining cells that is associated with exposure to cigarette smoke is another example. In addition, there is a genetic disorder resulting in a microtubule defect that affects the mobility of cilia, the *immotile cilia syndrome*. Affected male patients also have immobile sperm and chronic respiratory infections, frequent *Haemophilus influenzae* infection, and abundant mucous secretions. Because of the complexity of immune deficiencies and the diverse clinical presentation of deficiency states, a careful systematic diagnostic work-up must be carried out in order to select appropriate therapy.

There are more than 70 different kinds of primary immunodeficiencies involving B cells (antibodies), T cells (cell-mediated immunity), phagocytic cells, and complement proteins. In general, 1 in 10,000 individuals has some primary immunodeficiency. Although the incidence of a selective immunoglobulin A (IgA) deficiency is the most common (1 in 500), it

Table 18.1 Characteristics of infections associated with immunodeficiency diseases

Increased frequency
Increased severity
Prolonged duration
Unexpected complications and unusual manifestations
Significant infection with agents with low infectivity and/or pathogenicity

is not usually associated with any clinical manifestations. In the United States, approximately 370 infants are born annually with a clinically significant primary immunodeficiency, distributed as follows:

Antibody (B-cell) immunodeficiencies	50%
Cellular (T-cell) immunodeficiencies	40%
Combined with antibody deficiency	30%
T-cell only	10%
Phagocytic deficiencies	6%
Complement deficiencies	4%

Immune Response of Immature Animals

Fetal and neonatal animals may be induced to form antibody or develop high levels of immunoglobulin if given strong antigenic stimuli, but they often have a delayed or blunted response to T-dependent antigens. Neonatal animals normally are protected by maternal antibody received by placental transfer or by absorption of colostral antibodies shortly after birth (Fig. 18.1). The newborn animal begins to produce its own antibodies owing to natural stimulation within the first 3 months after birth. The development of "normal" lymphoid tissue and "normal" immunoglobulin levels depends upon contact with antigen; germfree animals that have a markedly reduced antigenic load maintain only very low levels of serum immunoglobulin and have undeveloped, immature lymphoid tissue. However, germfree animals have genetically normal immune systems and can respond to appropriate antigenic stimuli. In contrast, children with severe congenital immune deficiencies, who have been maintained in germfree isolators with the hope of acquiring immune maturity later in life, have died from infection or complications of bone marrow transplantation when removed from the germfree environment.

Hypogammaglobulinemia of Infancy

A temporary functional delay in the production of immunoglobulin by a newborn may cause a transient hypogammaglobulinemia of infancy. Hypogammaglobulinemia occurs when the normal catabolism of placentally transferred maternal IgG commencing after birth is associated with an abnormal delay in the onset of the immunoglobulin synthetic capacity by the infant. This temporary immunoglobulin deficiency usually terminates between 9 and 18 months of age. Since it is only temporary, hypogammaglobulinemia of infancy is not considered a primary immune deficiency disease. If it continues, a true permanent immune deficiency disease must be considered.

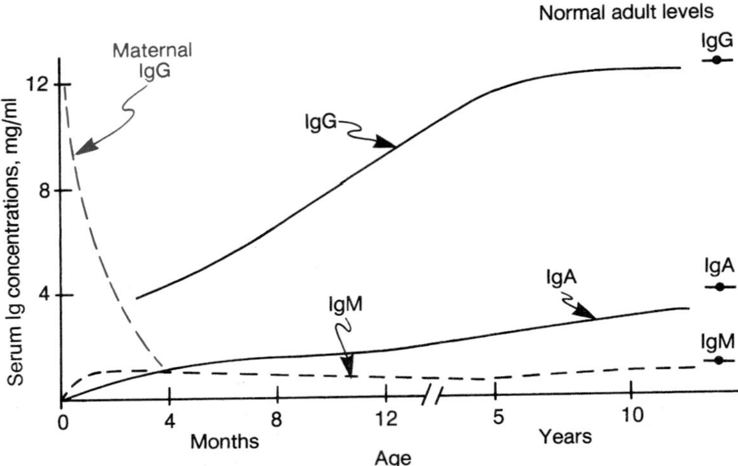

Figure 18.1 Serum immunoglobulin levels during normal life. The newborn human has high levels of serum IgG because of maternal transfer of IgG across the placenta. Colostrum provides additional immunoglobulin, particularly gastrointestinal IgA. During infancy, serum IgM becomes elevated within 1 month, serum IgG becomes elevated between 4 and 8 months, and serum IgA rises gradually over the first 10 years of life because of synthesis by the child. Neonates also have decreased cellular immune responses even though the $CD4^+$ T-cell count may be >1,500/mm^3, most likely owing to immature immune regulation.

Neonatal Wasting Syndrome (TORCH)

"Wasting" of newborn infants is seen following infection in utero with a number of organisms that are able to cross the placenta from the mother to the fetus (i.e., rubella virus) or with infection at birth because of organisms in the birth canal (herpes simplex virus). A newborn infant with low birth weight, microencephaly, eye abnormalities, and liver and other visceral abnormalities may reflect the effects of congenital infection with a number of otherwise unrelated agents given the term TORCH. TORCH refers to *Toxoplasma*, rubella virus, cytomegalovirus, and herpes simplex virus, in recognition of the infectious organisms most frequently recognized as the causative agents. Other infectious agents, such as *Treponema pallidum* (congenital syphilis) or *Listeria monocytogenes*, may produce similar findings, so that the "O" in TORCH may be considered to stand for "other" infectious agents. In addition, congenital infection with human immunodeficiency virus (HIV) can cause congenital acquired immune deficiency syndrome (AIDS), so the "H" may also stand for HIV, as well as herpes. The chronic infectious state is the result of immaturity of the infant's immune system at the time of infection. Such infections are not able to be controlled by the infant's immune system or by passively transferred immunity from the mother, resulting in chronic wasting disease. In addition to immune deficiencies, congenitally infected infants frequently also have other developmental abnormalities, such as blindness, mental retardation, and heart defects.

Primary Immunodeficiencies

Primary immunodeficiencies are due to inherited genetic abnormalities that result in failure of maturation or function of cells or components of the immune system. These may occur in both T cells and B cells (combined immune deficiencies), T cells alone, B cells alone, phagocytic cells, as well as in inflammatory mediators or in complement components (Table 18.2). In addition to recurrent infections, the clinical manifestations of primary immunodeficiencies may include autoimmune diseases, cancer, and allergic reactions. The clinical expression may range from relatively mild to life-threatening. Some, such as severe combined immunodeficiency (SCID), are manifested early in life, whereas others, such as common variable immunodeficiency, Ig subclass deficiencies, and complement component deficiencies most often do not occur until later in life.

Mouse Models of Primary Immunodeficiencies

Understanding of heritable human immunodeficiency diseases has been aided by a number of genetic defects in the mouse that produce effects similar to those of human immunodeficiencies (Table 18.3).

Severe Combined Immunodeficiencies

SCID has an incidence of 1 in 100,000 births and may have several etiologies, including a failure in recombinase activating genes, mutation in the gene for the γ chain of the interleukin-2 (IL-2) receptor, and inborn errors of metabolism in which purine synthesizing enzymes are inactive or defective (Table 18.2). Patients with these diseases develop severe recurrent infections with multiple agents at an early age and generally do not survive early childhood unless treated with a bone marrow transplant (see below). Symptoms may appear within the first few days of life, but in most cases infectious complications do not appear until 4 to 6 months of age. Early clinical developments are persistent oral candidiasis (thrush), chronic diarrhea, pneumonia otitis media, and recurrent sepsis, associated with failure to thrive (wasting). Patients with SCID are susceptible to a wide variety of infections and developed progressive vaccinia when smallpox immunizations were done, or BCGosis if immunized with *Mycobacterium bovis* BCG. All major immunoglobulin groups (IgG, IgA, and IgM) are severely depressed (total, <0.25 mg/ml) and there is a striking deficiency of lymphocytes in the blood (<1,000/ml). At autopsy, only a few plasma cells and lymphocytes are found, and the thymus is atrophic and lacks Hassall's corpuscles. A deficiency in the reactivity of lymphocytes from patients with SCID can be demonstrated by the lack of in vitro stimulation by mitogens. The presence of epithelial remnants in the thymus in most types of SCID associated with an absence of lymphocytes suggests a defect in the production of prothymocytes as well as of B stem cells, i.e., a defect at the level of the lymphoid stem cell that gives rise to both T- and B-cell lineages.

Maternal transfer of some cellular immune function, as well as immunoglobulin, occurs and may partially protect the infant or contribute to wasting. Children with SCID frequently develop a skin rash, consistent with that of a graft-versus-host reaction, believed to be caused by maternal lymphoid cells. Maternal lymphocytes may cross the placenta during gestation. Normally, such placentally transferred cells are rejected by the immune system of the fetus. However, if the fetus is unable to react to them, the foreign cells may proliferate in the immune-deficient child and produce a graft-versus-host reaction. Such cells may also provide some cellular immunity and protect the child from fulminant viral infections during the first 4 to 6 months of life.

Table 18.2 Human primary immunodeficiencies[a]

Type Name	Inheritance	Molecular defect	Phenotype: Ig[b]	T cells	B cells	NK	Other	Treatment	Autoimmunity	Malignancy
Severe combined immunodeficiencies										
Reticular dysgenesis	AR	?	–	–	–	–	–	BMT	?	?
Alymphocytosis	AR	RAG-1, RAG-2	–	–	–	+	+	BMT	+	–
Hyper-B syndrome	X-linked	γ chain, IL-2R	–	–	+	–	+	BMT	+	–
	AR	*Jak3*	–	–	+	–	+	BMT	?	?
Adenosine deaminase deficiency	AR	ADA	–	–	–	–	+	BMT, gene transfer	+	–
Purine nucleoside phosphorylase deficiency	AR	PNP	–	–	+	–	+	BMT	+	–
Omenn syndrome	AR	5′ nucleotidase	–	↑	–	–	↑Eos	BMT	+	–
T-cell activation deficiencies										
MHC deficiencies										
MHC class II	AR	CIITA/RFX5	+/–	+	+	+	+	BMT	+	+
MHC class I	AR	TAP2	+/–	+	+	+	+	BMT	?	?
CD3 deficiency	AR	γ, ϵ CD3	+/–	↓CD3	+	+	+	BMT?	+	+
Zap-70 deficiency	AR	Zap-70	+/–	↓CD8	+	+	+	BMT	+	+
Calcium influx deficiency	AR	?	+/–	+	+	+	+	?	?	?
IL-2 deficiency	AR	IL-2 synthesis	+/–	+	+	+	+	BMT	+	+
Down's syndrome	Sporadic	Trisomy 21	+	–	+	–	–	?	+	+
Defects in DNA repair (T-cell defects)										
Ataxia telangectasia	AR	*ATM* gene	+/–	+	+	+	+	IVIg	+	++
Bloom's syndrome	AR	*BLM*	+/–	+	+	+	+	IVIg	–	++
Nijmegen syndrome	AR	?	+/–	+	+	+	+	IVIg	–	++
Xeroderma pigmentosum	AR	?	+	+	+	+	+	IVIg	–	++
Others										
Wiskott-Aldrich syndrome	X-linked, AR	WASP	+/–	+/–	+	+	↓Plat	BMT/splenectomy	+	+
DiGeorge's syndrome	Sporadic	del22q11	+/–	+/–	+	+	+	BMT/thymus	–	–
Hyper-IgM syndrome	X-linked, AR	CD40L	–↑IgM	+	+	+	+	IV-Ig/BMT	+	+

B-cell defects										
Bruton's agammaglobulinemia	X-linked	BTK	–	+	–	+	+	IVIg	–	–
Common variable immunodeficiency	Sporadic	?	–	+	+/–	+	+	IVIg, IL-2	+	+
IgA deficiency	Sporadic, AR, AD	?	+↓IgA	+	+	+	+	Abx	+	–
IgG	AR	?	+↓IgG	+	+	+	+	IVIg	+	+
Antipolysaccharide deficiency	Sporadic	?	+	+	+	+	+	IVIg	–	–
Hyper-IgE syndrome	AR	?	+↑IgE	+	+	+	↑Eos	Abx	–	–
Lymphoproliferative syndrome										
X-linked	X-linked	SAP	+	+	+	+	+	BMT	–	+
Autoimmune										
Ia	AD	Fas	↑	+	↑	+	+	?	+	+
Ib	AR	FasL								
II	AR	Caspase 10								
Phagocytic defects										
Leukocyte adhesion deficiency										
I	AR	CD18	+	+	+	+	↑Neut	BMT	–	–
II	AR	Sialyl-Lewis X	+	+	+	+	↑Neut	?	–	–
Chediak-Higashi syndrome	AR	*LYST*	+	+	+	+	+	BMT	–	–
Chronic granulomatous disease	X-linked AR	gp91, p22, p47, p67	+	+	+	+	+	IFN-γ, BMT	–	–
Mannose-binding lectin deficiency	AD	MBL	+	+	+	+	+	Abx	–	–
IFN-γ receptor deficiency	AR	IFN-γR	+	+	+	+	+	Gene transfer?	–	–
Complement deficiencies										
Complement components	AR	Complement	+	+	+	+	+	Immunization	+	–
Properdin, factors I and H	X-linked, AR	Properdin, I, H	+	+	+	+	+	?	+	–

[a]Modified from R. A. Ten, *Mayo Clin. Proc.* **73:**865–872, 1998. Abbreviations: Abx, antibiotics; AD, autosomal dominant; ADA, adenosine deaminase; AR, autosomal recessive; BMT, bone marrow transplant; BTK, Bruton's tyrosine kinase; Eos, eosinophils; FasL, Fas ligand; IFN, interferon; IL, interleukin; IVIg, intravenous immunoglobulin; MBL, mannose binding lectin; MHC, major histocompatibility complex; Neut, neutrophils; NK, natural killer cells; Plat, platelets; PNP, purine nucleoside phosphorylase; R, receptor; RAG, recombinase activating genes; WASP, Wiskott-Aldrich syndrome protein. Symbols: +, present at essentially normal levels; –, absent or decreased below normal; +/–, normal or decreased.

[b]–↑ IgM, increase in IgM and decrease in other Igs; +↓IgA or +↓IgG, decrease in IgA or IgG, respectively, but general increase in Igs; +↑IgE, general increase in Igs but much greater increase in IgE than in other Igs.

Table 18.3 Some immunodeficiency mutations in mice

Gene	Gene symbol	Chromosome	Major manifestations
Nude	*nu*	11	Thymic aplasia, hairlessness, T-cell deficiency, increased NK and macrophage activity
SCID	*scid*	16	Absence of T and B cells; defect in antigen receptor gene rearrangement; normal myeloid, NK, and macrophage function
Motheaten	*me*	6	Decreased T-cell, B-cell, NK activity; increased macrophage proliferation, granulocytic skin lesions, and pneumonitis
Dominant hemimelia	*Dh*	1	Absence of spleen; decreased IgM, IgG2, antibody responses
X-linked	*xid*	X	B-cell dysfunction; reduced IgM, IgG3, defective antibody responses
Hemolytic	*Hc*	2	Homozygotes lack C5, impaired neutrophil complement chemotaxis, increased infections
Beige granulocyte	*bg*	13	Decreased NK, T_{CTL} cells; lysosomal membrane defect; decreased chemotaxis
Steel	*Sl*	10	Loss of stem cell growth factor (c-Kit ligand), mast cell defect, impaired resistance to parasitic infections
Hairless	hr^{rh}	14	Decreased T-cell response to mitogens, reduced antibody formation, thymic lymphomas
Dwarf	*dw*	11	Decreased cortical thymocytes, primary defect in anterior pituitary
Xid	*Btk*	X	Severe B-cell deficiency; low IgM, IgG3; defective antibody response
Jak3 null	*Jak3*		B-cell development blocked, T-cell activation impaired, decreased IL-2

Anlage Defects (Reticular Dysgenesis)

The failure of development of all blood cell lines, presumably because no hematopoietic stem cells are present, is known as reticular dysgenesis. Affected fetuses lack all types of white blood cells and at autopsy have no lymphoid tissue. All have been stillbirths. The genetic defect is unknown.

Alymphocytosis

Patients with alymphocytosis have mutations in the recombinase activating genes. In SCID mice, precursor lymphocytes have active, but defective, VDJ recombinase activity. They are able to cleave the immunoglobulin genes at the appropriate sequences but are unable to correctly join the cleaved ends of the coding strands of the variable-region gene segments. Patients with alymphocytosis are unable to rearrange Ig genes or T-cell receptor genes, resulting in a failure of lymphocyte development and the absence of circulating T and B cells. However, a classical feature of this disorder is normal numbers of natural killer (NK) cells. Since NK cells do not require antigenic stimulation for development and thus may not rearrange receptors, they are not affected by defective recombinase activity.

Hyper-B Syndrome

Hyper-B syndrome is due to a congenital deficiency of the γ chain of IL-2 (X-linked form) or to a deficiency of Janus kinase 3 (Jak3, autosomal recessive form). Patients with hyper-B syndrome have normal or high numbers of B cells but have a complete absence of T cells and NK cells, because both the IL-2 receptor (IL-2R) and Jak3 are essential for development of these cells. The γ chain for the IL-2 receptor chain is also shared by the IL-4, IL-7, IL-9, or IL-15 receptor, so multiple stages in the growth of T and B cells are affected.

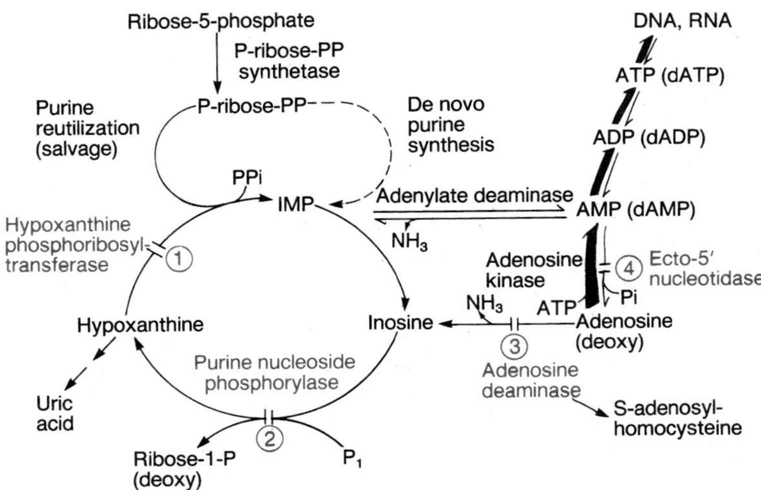

Figure 18.2 Purine metabolism and immunodeficiencies.

Purine Metabolism and Primary Immunodeficiencies

Purine interconversions are required for normal maturation of the rapidly dividing cells of the lymphoid system. Blocks in purine biosynthesis may lead to accumulation of deoxynucleosides, which are toxic to lymphocytes (Fig. 18.2). In addition to adenosine deaminase (ADA), purine nucleoside phosphorylase (PNP), and 5′ nucleotidase deficiencies (Table 18.2), there is a deficiency in hypoxanthine-guanine phosphoribosyl transferase. The immune manifestations include a T-cell deficiency, a B-cell deficiency, and a combined deficiency (Table 18.4).

T-Cell Activation Deficiencies

T-cell activation deficiencies include various disorders in which the T-cell response to antigens or mitogens is depressed or lacking because of a block at some stage of T-cell activation (see Fig. 5.7).

MHC Deficiencies

The "bare lymphocyte syndrome" is caused by a mutation in one of the genes for the major histocompatibility complex (MHC): the MHC class II mutations are in multiple transactivating regulatory genes, and the MHC class I mutation is in the gene encoding the TAP2 transporter protein. Defects in MHC expression on lymphocytes interfere with the self-recognition mechanisms required for induction of effective immune responses. Individuals with this deficiency may have normal or decreased serum Ig and antibodies and/or normal or decreased cell-mediated immunity. Severely affected individuals develop oral candidiasis, *Pneumocystis carinii* pneumonia, bacteria pneumonia, herpes, diarrhea, and wasting. Although B-cell numbers are normal, there are very few plasma cells and very low serum immunoglobulin levels in patients with clinical manifestations.

CD3, ZAP-70 Kinase, and Calcium Influx Deficiencies

Other T-cell activation defects involve defective expression of the γ or ϵ chains of the CD3 molecule or of the ZAP-70 kinase associated with the T-cell receptor, a defect of calcium influx during the T-cell activation process,

Table 18.4 Clinical symptoms and expression of diseases associated with defects in purine metabolism

Disease	Symptoms
Hypoxanthine-guanine phosphoribosyl transferase (Lesch-Nyhan syndrome) (possible B-cell immunodeficiency)	There is a marked overproduction of purines and overexcretion of uric acid. These children have severe neurological impairment and self-destructive behavior. Their lymphocytes respond poorly to stimulation with pokeweed mitogen.
Purine nucleotide phosphorylase deficiency (T-cell immunodeficiency)	Features large quantities of ribonucleosides (inosine and guanosine) as well as 2′deoxyribonucleosides (2′-deoxyinosine and 2′-deoxyguanosine) in urine, in red cells, and in lymphocytes; a loss of purines that are necessary for lymphocyte proliferation; and severe impairment of DNA synthesis. There are recurrent infection and anemia, severe lymphopenia, pronounced depression of lymphocyte responses to mitogenic and allogeneic cell stimuli, and decreased T-cell rosette formation.
Adenosine deaminase deficiency (T- and B-cell immunodeficiency)	Children have high concentrations of AMP and dAMP in erythrocytes and lymphocytes (2 to 10 times normal), and large amounts of 2′-deoxyadenosine are excreted in urine. Children may have a mild or severe disease with respiratory infections, lymphopenia, and no delayed-type hypersensitivity response to *Candida,* mumps virus, and streptokinase-streptodornase, as well as skeletal abnormalities. Their lymphocytes respond poorly to phytohemagglutinin, pokeweed mitogen, and allogeneic cells, and they fail to develop isohemagglutinins. Adenosine deaminase deficiency accounts for 15% of patients with SCID.
Nucleotidase deficiency (Omenn's syndrome)	Children have increased concentrations of toxic deoxyribonucleotides in lymphocyte subpopulations and agammaglobulinemia. There are activated circulating T cells that infiltrate organs, B-cell lymphopenia, eosinophilia, and lymphocyte depletion from lymphoid organs infiltrated with macrophages. The syndrome features erythrodermia, polyadenopathy, hepatosplenomegaly, severe infections, and failure to thrive. Such patients always die within the first year of life, unless they have a bone marrow transplant.

or abnormal binding of the transcription factor NF-AT. An abnormality in activation of T cells may result in defective production of IL-2, IL-3, IL-4, and IL-5 as a result of decreased transcription of the cytokine genes and a clinical presentation of SCID. The clinical manifestations of these abnormalities may be mild to severe infections and lesions of autoimmunity. Treatment of patients with bare lymphocyte syndrome or T-cell receptor abnormalities is bone marrow transplantation (BMT); those with calcium influx or transcription abnormalities may be effectively treated with intravenous immunoglobulin. One child of a pair of siblings who inherited mutations in the CD3-γ gene from both parents died at the age of 31 months with SCID and features of autoimmunity, whereas the brother was alive and healthy at 10 years of age. Two independent point mutations were identified in both the genes coding for the CD3-γ protein subunit of the T-cell receptor–CD3 complex; the mutations hindered but did not abolish the expression of the T-cell receptor–CD3 complex on the surface of T cells. About half of the complexes that lacked the CD3 γ chain reached the cell surface, indicating that the CD3-γ protein is not essential for expression of about half of the T-cell receptor–CD3 complexes. The expressed T-cell receptors contained α β CD3-δ and CD3-ϵ and CD3-ζ subunits. Why one sibling had severe disease and the other, with the same genetic defect, did not is not clear.

Down's Syndrome

Patients with Down's syndrome (mental retardation, abnormal brain development, and "mongoloid facies" associated with trisomy of chromosome 21) have up to 100-fold higher mortality from respiratory infections than normal. They have smaller than normal thymi, with large Hassall's corpuscles and marked depletion of thymocytes. There is also hypoplasia of the thymus-dependent zones of the spleen and lymph nodes and a selective deficiency in the response of blood T cells to bacterial and fungal antigens, although not to T-cell mitogens. There are also varied abnormalities in phagocytosis, but B-cell function is usually normal. The relationship of the thymic abnormalities to the increased mortality from respiratory infection is not clear. The pathogenesis of the immunosuppression and its relationship to the inheritance of the other abnormalities are not known.

Idiopathic $CD4^+$ Lymphocytopenia

Idiopathic $CD4^+$ lymphocytopenia is an abnormal laboratory finding without a disease. With the widespread determination of $CD4^+$ T-cell levels in the blood as a test for AIDS, individuals have been identified with low CD4 counts but without evidence of AIDS. Idiopathic $CD4^+$ lymphocytopenia includes two or more counts of $CD4^+$ T cells below 300/mm^3 of blood or a percentage of less than 20 of $CD4^+$ lymphocytes, with no evidence of HIV-1 or HIV-2 infection and no defined cause of therapy that accounts for the low level of $CD4^+$ cells.

Defects in DNA Repair

Diseases with defects in DNA repair include ataxia telangiectasia, Bloom's syndrome, Nijmegen's syndrome, and xeroderma pigmentosum. Defects in DNA repair lead to chromosomal instability and predisposition to the development of cancer because of increased sensitivity to agents that cause DNA strand breaks and mutations.

Ataxia telangiectasia is caused by a mutation of the *ATM* gene, believed to code for a tumor suppressor. The serum IgA is very low, IgG is low or normal, and IgM is usually normal. The lymphoid organs are atrophic or absent. There is also occulocutaneous telangiectasia (dilated and redundant vessels), progressive cerebellar ataxia, and increased lymphoreticular malignancies. Treatment is supportive, and patients are usually physically incapacitated by their early teens and die of lung infections or cancer before they are 30 years old. Relatives of these patients also have a higher than normal incidence of lymphomas and breast and colon cancers.

Bloom's syndrome is due to a mutation in *BLM,* a gene that encodes a protein homologous to the RecQ helicases. Patients with Bloom's syndrome are short and have photosensitive facial reactions and recurrent infections.

Nijmegen's syndrome features short stature, birdlike facies, microcephaly, and recurrent infections. The genetic defect has been mapped to 8q21, but the functional gene product is not known.

Xeroderma pigmentosum patients have an inability to repair radiation-induced DNA damage and have increased skin and mesodermal cancers. The immunodeficiency in these diseases may be controlled to some extent by intravenous immunoglobulin therapy.

These syndromes are associated with cellular immunodeficiencies.

Other T-Cell Deficiencies

Wiskott-Aldrich syndrome is an X-linked recessive combined immunodeficiency with a marked deficiency in IgM and usually depressed cellular immunity resulting in death in early infancy from infections. Serum IgA and IgG levels are usually normal, but affected males have defects in T-cell functions. There is also eczema and thrombocytopenia (low blood platelets), and bleeding may be the first manifestation of the disease. The molecular defect appears to be in a protein called the Wiskott-Aldrich syndrome protein (WASP), normally found on lymphocytes and megakaryocytes. The exact function is not clear, but WASP appears to be a component of the cytoskeleton. The absence of WASP results in decreased platelet size, loss of T-cell microvilli, and defective T-cell and platelet function. BMT may alleviate the immune deficiency, and splenectomy may alleviate the loss of platelets.

Thymic aplasia (DiGeorge's syndrome) has a deletion of chromosome 22q11, absence of the thymus, deficiency of cellular reactions, and a normal immunoglobulin-producing system. The third and fourth pharyngeal pouches fail to develop, resulting in an absent or rudimentary thymus, absent parathyroids, and aortic arch defects. Neonatal tetany occurs owing to a lack of parathyroid hormone. The level of immunodeficiency is variable. In complete DiGeorge's syndrome, T-cell levels are markedly depressed, and responses to T-cell mitogens are absent. In patients with partial DiGeorge's syndrome, which is more prevalent, there are intermediate peripheral blood lymphocyte counts and T-cell responses. Serum immunoglobulin levels are often normal. These patients are susceptible to viral and fungal infections.

Hyper-IgM syndrome, an X-linked disorder expressed by increased levels of IgM but depressed IgA and IgG, is due to a defect in isotype switching from IgM to other classes. This is associated with recurrent pyogenic infections but fortunately is very rare. The genetic defect is in signaling through CD40 on IgM-expressing B cells and through the CD40 ligand on activated T cells. The CD40 ligand gene is located on the X chromosome and is defective in patients with hyper-IgM. Without the CD40 signaling pathway, activated B cells continue to produce IgM and do not switch to other Ig classes. Eventually, it may be possible to replace the gene responsible by giving these patients a good copy of the gene.

Chronic mucocutaneous candidiasis (CMC) patients have histories of *Candida* infections associated with high antibody responses to *Candida* spp. and absent delayed skin test responses to *Candida* antigens. CMC is a genetic disorder in T-cell function, although the specific gene has not yet been identified. These patients frequently have polyendocrinopathy, suggesting autoimmune destruction of endocrine organs. As in lepromatous leprosy, these patients respond poorly to therapy unless delayed-type hypersensitivity can be demonstrated. CMC is another example of *immune deviation* in which the type of immune response determines the nature of the disease manifested, i.e., antibody is not effective; cellular immunity, particularly delayed-type hypersensitivity (DTH), is.

B-Cell Immunodeficiencies

Bruton's congenital sex-linked agammaglobulinemia (infantile sex-linked agammaglobulinemia), in which B cells are absent in peripheral blood and lymphoid organs, has an incidence of 1 in 50,000 births. Symptoms appear when transplacentally acquired maternal antibodies disappear from the circulation at the age of 5 to 6 months. Affected infants lack all three types of the major immunoglobulins but can develop reactions of the delayed type. The structure of the thymus is normal. However, there is a striking lack of tonsilar, appendiceal, and Peyer's patch lymphoid tissue, and plasma cells are absent. However, there are near-normal numbers of pre-B cells expressing Ig heavy chains in the bone marrow, indicating a block in the transition of pre-B cells to B cells, not a lack of B-cell precursors. The B cells do not respond to lymphokines that usually drive B-cell maturation. The missing gene appears to encode a protein kinase called Bruton's tyrosine kinase, related to the *src* kinase family that is required for B-cell maturation. This disease may be treated with antibiotics and gamma globulins. Treatment prolongs duration and quality of life, but early death is usual without treatment. In the future, these patients may be treated by gene transfer therapy using their own bone marrow stem cells that contain good copies of the defective gene.

Common variable immunodeficiencies are listed in Table 18.5. They are late-onset (after 4 to 5 years of age and usually later) immune deficiencies with different immune defects not associated with an identifiable cause (e.g., not related to drugs). Clinically, the immune defects may be predominantly in antibody, owing to (i) abnormalities in B-cell numbers or maturation, (ii) defects in T-helper cells or increased activity of T-suppressor cells, or (iii) secondary to autoantibodies to T or B cells. In all cases, there is a decrease in one or more immunoglobulin classes associated with variable defects in cellular immunity. These defects appear to be abnormalities in control of the immune response, a maturation arrest at the level of the germinal center B cells, or defects in transmembrane signaling.

IgA deficiencies (<5 μg/dl) are the most common deficiency, affecting about 1 in 700 people in the United States. It is usually asymptomatic, unless associated with an IgG subclass deficiency. IgA deficiencies are associated with autoantibodies to IgA, allergies, recurrent sinopulmonary infections, and autoimmune diseases. It is postulated that IgA deficiency allows intestinal transfer of environmental antigens that induce antibodies that

Table 18.5 Common variable immunodeficiency[a]

Designation	Usual phenotypic expression					Presumed nature of basic defect	Inheritance
	Serum Ig	Serum antibodies	Circulating B cells	Circulating T cells	CMI		
Common variable immunodeficiency with predominant B-cell defect	Decreased	Decreased	Near-normal numbers but abnormal proportions of subtypes	Variable	Variable	Intrinsic defect in cell differentiation of immature to mature B cells	Unknown AR, AD
Common variable immunodeficiency with predominant immunoregulatory T-cell disorder							
Deficiency of T-helper cells	Decreased	Decreased	Normal	Variable	Variable	Immunoregulatory T-cell disorder: defect in thymocyte to T-helper cell differentiation	Unknown
Presence of activated T-suppressor cells	Decreased	Decreased	Normal	Variable	Variable	Immunoregulatory T-cell disorder, cause unknown	Unknown
Common variable immunodeficiency with autoantibodies to B or T cells	Decreased	Decreased	Decreased	Decreased	Variable	Variable; no differentiation defect known	Unknown

[a]CMI, cell-mediated immunity; AR, autosomal recessive; AD, autosomal dominant.

cross-react with host antigens or that there is a common genetic defect in IgA-deficient and autoimmune individuals.

IgG subclass deficiencies are rare and sometimes occur in pairs, such as IgG2 and IgG4. In addition, IgG subclass deficiencies are not stable; a patient presenting with one subclass deficiency may develop additional deficiencies or switch to a different subclass deficiency. Selective deficiencies of IgG are usually asymptomatic but may be associated with increased infection with pneumococci, *H. influenzae,* and *Staphylococcus aureus*. Selective IgM deficiencies are very rare and are associated with autoimmune disease and increased incidence of pneumococcal pneumonia.

Antipolysaccharide antibody deficiency is found in some patients with recurrent infections who have normal serum Ig levels but are unable to produce a specific antibody response to polysaccharides of encapsulated bacteria, such as pneumococci.

Hyper-IgE syndrome features very high serum levels of IgE (>3,000 IU/ml), diminished antibody responses to specific immunizations, and pulmonary and upper respiratory infections, predominantly *S. aureus*. Also found is a high eosinophil count, a pruritic dermatitis, coarse facies, and growth retardation. There may be a mutation in the gene encoding the α chain of the IL-4 receptor. Defective gamma interferon (IFN-γ) production is also suspected, because IFN-γ turns off IgE production.

Lymphoproliferative syndromes are characterized by uncontrolled proliferation of B cells. The X-linked form is asymptomatic until males are exposed to the Epstein-Barr virus. These patients will then develop B-cell lymphomas. Three hereditary forms of autoimmune-associated lymphoproliferative syndromes have been identified, with mutations in Fas (type Ia), Fas ligand (type Ib), or capase 10 (type II) that interfere with Fas-mediated apoptosis. The result is development of B-cell lymphomas and autoimmune lesions.

Most of the hereditary *dysgammaglobulinemias* are caused by a decreased synthesis of immunoglobulins, but low levels of immunoglobulins may also be caused by increased catabolism. Increased catabolism of all immunoglobulin classes is found in *familial hypercatabolic hypoproteinemia,* of IgG in *myotonic dystrophy,* and of both immunoglobulin and lymphocytes in *intestinal lymphangiectasia*. Although these patients may have very abnormal laboratory tests, they usually do not have increased infections.

Inflammatory Defects

Defects in Inflammatory Mechanisms

Immunologically mediated defense against bacterial infections involves (i) the reactions of specific antibody with the bacteria, (ii) the activation of complement components, resulting in chemotaxis and immune phagocytosis, (iii) the ingestion of the bacteria by phagocytic cells (polymorphonuclear leukocytes or macrophages), and (iv) the destruction of the ingested bacterial by-products of the phagocytic cells. Therefore, increased susceptibility to bacterial infections may be due to a deficiency in certain complement components or an abnormality in phagocytic cells (phagocytic dysfunction), as well as to a lack of immunoglobulin antibody.

Phagocytic Dysfunction

Disorders of neutrophil or macrophage function include a lack of production (congenital neutropenia, leukemia), accessory deficiencies (complement), leukocyte adhesion deficiency, activation defects (Job's syndrome), phagocytic dysfunction, and extrinsic factors, such as drug effects (steroids) or immunoglobulin abnormalities (rheumatoid factor, IgA, or IgE). Phagocytic dysfunction occurs when phagocytic cells cannot ingest bacteria normally or can ingest but cannot kill. Such dysfunctions may be due to an abnormality in the digestive vacuole (lysosome) or to a lack of digestive enzymes in the vacuole. A summary of the steps in phagocytosis and the postulated level of phagocytic defects is illustrated in Fig. 18.3. These disorders are characterized by increased susceptibility to bacterial infections associated with the accumulation of lipochrome-laden macrophages and granulomas in the affected tissues. The granulomas are caused by a reaction to bacterial products and the debris of the dead and dying phagocytic cells. Macrophages stuffed with material that they are unable to digest accumulate in tissues. Such macrophages are able to phagocytose normally, but they process ingested materials less rapidly or less efficiently. The following are examples of phagocytic deficiencies.

Deficiency of opsonization is not a defect in the phagocytic cell itself but in opsonizing molecules, antibody and complement, or mannose-binding lectin (see below).

Leukocyte adhesion deficiency (LAD) has two forms. LAD-I is caused by a mutation in the gene encoding CD18, the common β chain of the leukocyte adhesion proteins. These include lymphocyte function-associated antigen 1 (LFA-1), the iC3b receptor (CD3), and p150,95. Each of these has a distinct α subunit but a common 95,000-Da β subunit. LFA-1 is present on lymphocytes, monocytes, and neutrophils and is critical for cell adherence-related functions. iC3b is the opsonic fragment of the third component of complement. The function of p150,95 is not known. Affected patients have an absence or deficiency of these molecules on the surface of their white cells. These receptors are required for phagocytosis and chemotaxis, and most of the clinical manifestations are the result of phagocytic defects and include recurrent bacterial infections with increased circulating neutrophils but without pus formation; the polymorphonuclear neutrophils do not respond to inflammatory stimuli. There is also a mild T-cell deficiency manifested by decreased help for B cells and lowered cytotoxic activity, presumably because of poor cell-cell adhesion. This is inherited as an autosomal recessive and exists in severe and mild forms, depending on decreased or complete lack of expression of LFA-1. There is partial compensation by increased CD2–LFA-3, and LFA-1 expression may be increased by IFN-γ. LAD-II is due to a defect in fucose metabolism that results in an absence of sialyl-Lewis X, a selectin ligand, on the surface of neutrophils. Patients with LAD-II have severe neutropenia, recurrent bacterial infections, and mental retardation.

Chediak-Higashi syndrome features a microtubular defect in *LYST,* a gene that encodes a protein important in cellular signaling. The result is a deficit in phagosome-lysosome fusion, resulting in accumulation of large abnormal lysosomes in all white cells. The defect is inherited as an autosomal recessive, and there is a partial defect in heterozygotes. Patients have recurrent infections due to decreased chemotaxis and bacterial killing, partial albinism, and a peculiar aggressive lymphoproliferative disease with diffuse organ involvement.

Chronic granulomatous disease (CGD) is caused by a deficiency in NADP oxidase activation, with a failure to develop superoxide and hydrogen peroxide and hydrogen radicals. It is estimated to affect about

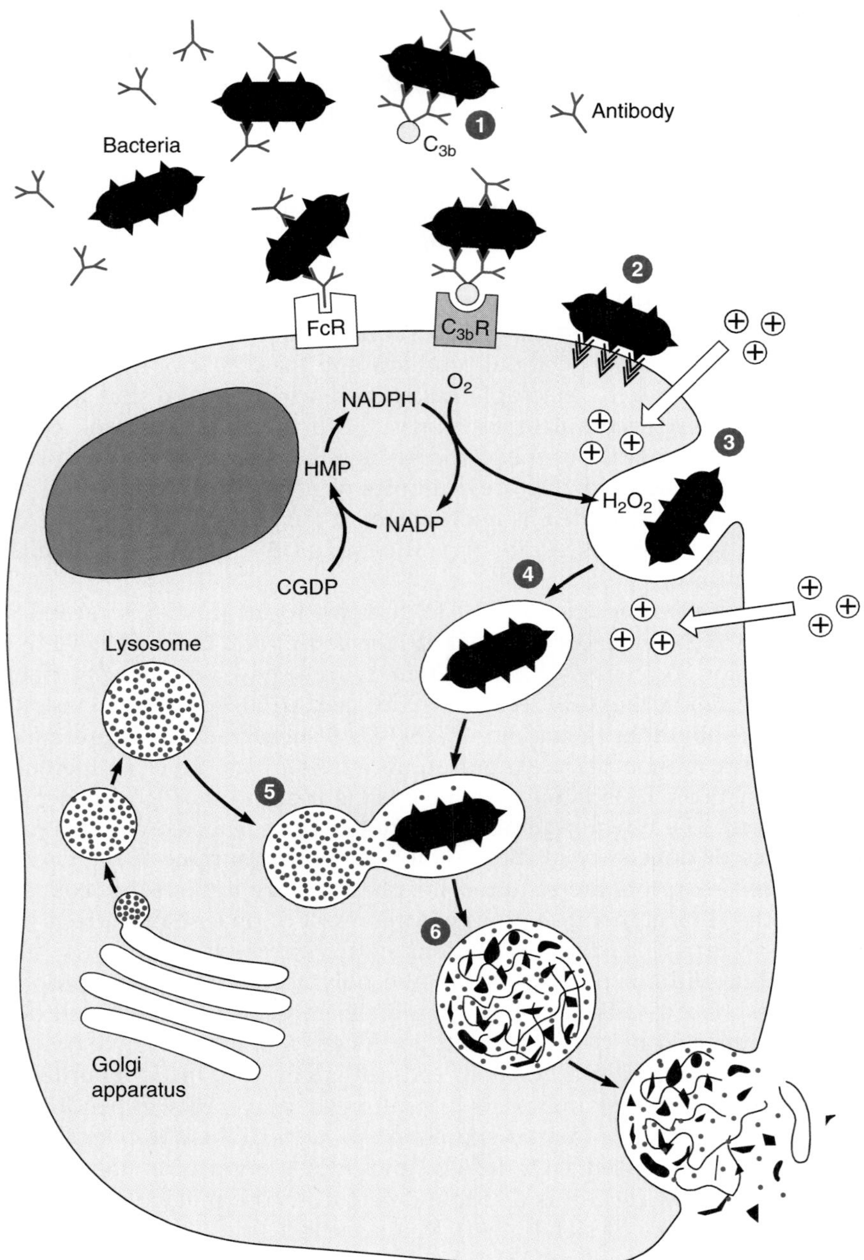

Figure 18.3 Schematic drawing of steps in phagocytosis and postulated levels of defects in phagocytic disorders. **(1)** Opsonization: aggregated Fc, C3b (defects in antibody, complement, or mannose-binding lectin). **(2)** Recognition through receptors and patching (defect in adhesion molecules). **(3)** Ingestion. Cation influx stimulates transduction of hexose monophosphate shunt and conversion of O_2 to H_2O_2 (defect in chronic granulomatous disease). **(4)** Specific granule formation. A congenital lack of granules precludes intracellular digestion. **(5)** Fusion of lysosome and phagosome to form a phagolysosome (defect in Chediak-Higashi syndrome), a microtubule defect. **(6)** Digestion of bacteria in a phagolysosome (defect in myeloperoxidase deficiency).

4,000 people worldwide. It is inherited as a defect in any one of four genes. Two-thirds of cases have the sex-linked form, affecting male children. Mothers of affected children have a partial defect. Neutrophils from patients with the X-linked form of CGD lack the enzyme cytochrome b_{558}, whereas neutrophils from patients with the autosomal recessive forms have normal levels of this enzyme. Cytochrome b_{558} is a 22,000-Da peptide that is tightly bound to a highly glycosylated 91,000-Da peptide. Patients with X-linked cytochrome b_{558}-negative CGD have defects in the gene encoding the 91,000-Da subunit of the cytochrome complex. It is believed that the 91,000-Da subunit is required to anchor the cytochrome complex in the cell membrane. The genetic basis for the cytochrome b_{558}-positive CGD is not known, but the neutrophils of these patients fail to phosphorylate a 44,000-Da membrane-associated protein found in activated neutrophils.

The functional problem in CGD is that the first line of bacterial killing, oxidative-dependent killing, fails. The neutrophil dies during the battle with the invading microorganism, leaving macrophages to deal with dead cells and the invading organisms. Macrophages (which also lack respiratory burst activity) ingest the debris and kill the microorganisms using nonoxidative defenses (e.g., lysozyme, neutral proteases, and defensins). This killing is usually successful but prolonged, leading to the formation of granulomas after each infectious episode. Marked improvement has been noted following IFN-γ treatment, but cure requires BMT.

It has been suggested that CGD might be called Jonah's syndrome. The Biblical character Jonah was phagocytized by a large multicellular organism that was unable to digest him, and he was eventually released. The enzymatic defect in CGD can be tested by the inability of isolated polymorphonuclear cells from affected individuals to kill bacteria in vitro or to reduce the dye nitroblue tetrazolium, which measures superoxide formation.

Mannose-binding lectin deficiency (MBLD) is a common disorder of the natural or innate immune system. MBL opsonizes bacteria, fungi, and some viruses and is also involved in activation of complement. A mutation in the MBL gene occurs in approximately 25% of the population of the United States. There are very low levels of MBL in homozygous mutants and intermediate levels in heterozygotes. MBLD is associated with recurrent infections, especially in the newborn after maternal antibodies have cleared.

IFN-γ receptor (IFN-γR) deficiency is caused by a mutation in the IFN-γR gene. Affected individuals have a defect in antigen presentation and increased susceptibility to atypical mycobacterial infections. Immunization with BCG may result in fatal disseminated infections.

Myeloperoxidase is responsible for the azurophilic granules in neutrophils, and its activity in inflammation causes the greenish color of pus. In the presence of hydrogen peroxide and halide, myeloperoxidase produces hypochlorous acid and chlorine, which is very toxic for bacterial cells. Hereditary *myeloperoxidase deficiency* is a relatively common (1:3,000) autosomal recessive disorder, with about one-third of patients having a total absence of myeloperoxidase and the other two-thirds having a partial absence. Fortunately, increased infection in this disorder is unusual, most likely because other microbiological mechanisms compensate for the deficiency.

Complement Deficiencies

A listing of complement deficiencies is given in Table 18.6. Activation of complement occurs upon reaction of antibody with antigen. If the antigen is an infectious agent, the complement system may activate phagocytosis (opsonization) or cause lysis of the offending agent. Thus, a deficiency in complement might be expected to be associated with an immune-deficient state. Deficiencies in a complement component are extremely rare. Most occur as autosomal recessive inherited abnormalities. Complement deficiencies are also associated with rheumatoid diseases, primarily systemic lupus erythematosus. Chronic complement consumption may also be associated with glomerulonephritis (hypocomplementemic glomerulonephritis). A deficiency in C1 inhibitor is associated with hereditary angioedema, in which massive swelling lesions of the body surface or gastrointestinal tract are believed to be caused by loss of control of early complement components C1, C4, and C2 and increased formation of anaphylatoxin, resulting in increased vascular permeability and edema. C1 inhibitor deficiency is the most commonly identified complement disorder and may be caused by insufficient production of the protein or an abnormal C1 inhibitor protein. The increased availability of reliable assays for complement components allows for screening for complement deficiencies (see below) and greater recognition of deficiencies in complement.

Table 18.6 Complement deficiencies[a]

Component	Chromosomal location	Inheritance of deficiency	Approximate no. of kindreds/patients	Clinical manifestations
C1q	1p	Autosomal recessive	14/24	Rheumatic diseases and pyogenic infections
C1r/s	12p/12p	Autosomal recessive	7/11	Rheumatic diseases
C4	6p	Autosomal recessive	17/21	Rheumatic diseases and pyogenic infections
C2	6p	Autosomal recessive	79/109	Rheumatic diseases and pyogenic infections
C3	19q13	Autosomal recessive	14/19	Pyogenic infections and rheumatic diseases
C5	9q	Autosomal recessive	17/27	Meningococcal sepsis and meningitis
C6	5q	Autosomal recessive	49/77	Meningococcal sepsis and meningitis
C7	5q	Autosomal recessive	50/73	Meningococcal sepsis and meningitis
C8	1p A, B 9q G	Autosomal recessive	52/73	Meningococcal sepsis and meningitis
C9	5p	Autosomal recessive	15/18	Meningococcal sepsis and meningitis
Factor D	?	Unknown	2/3	Meningococcal sepsis and meningitis/ sinopulmonary infections
C1 inhibitor	11q	Autosomal dominant	100s/100s	Angioedema
C4-binding protein	1q	Unknown	1/1	Behçet's disease and angioedema
DAF	1q	Unknown	2/2	Inab phenotype
Factor I	4q	Autosomal recessive	12/14	Pyogenic infections
Factor H	1q	Autosomal recessive	8/13	Hemolytic uremic syndrome
Properdin	Xp	X-linked recessive	23/70	Meningococcal sepsis and meningitis
CD59	11p	Unknown	1/1	Paroxysmal nocturnal hemoglobinuria

[a]Modified from M. Frank, *N. Engl. J. Med.* **316:**1525, 1987.

Interleukin Deficiencies

Deficiencies in IL-1 or IL-2 production may occur secondary to loss of function of macrophage (IL-1) or lymphocyte (IL-2) populations. However, the clinical significance of interleukin deficiencies has not been extensively documented. IL-2 production by blood lymphocytes appears to be depressed in burn patients and may be responsible for depressed cellular immunity in some burn patients. A simplistic explanation for the defects in B-cell maturation seen in common variable hypogammaglobulinemias could be a failure of production or response to B-cell differentiation factors, such as IL-4, IL-5, and IL-6. However, no convincing evidence for such a defect has been found.

Secondary Immunodeficiencies

Secondary immunodeficiencies may result from naturally occurring disease processes or subsequent to the administration of suppressive agents. In either case, the process operates upon an already developed immune system and, therefore, either destroys or interferes with the expression of established defense mechanisms. "Opportunistic" infection with organisms not usually pathogenic for normal individuals is a common terminal event in these patients.

Diseases affecting cellular immune reactions include Boeck's sarcoidosis, leprosy, tuberculosis, measles, diabetes, cancer, and now, most critically, AIDS. All these processes may affect lymphoid tissue directly or may secondarily alter nonspecific innate defense systems. Burn patients not only have destroyed epithelial barriers but also have a decreased ability to produce IL-2. Uremic patients have depressed cell-mediated immunity.

Multiple abnormalities have been reported in patients with diabetes. Vascular changes lead to decreased tissue perfusion, resulting in increased susceptibility to tissue damage as well as an impaired ability to mount an inflammatory response. In addition, abnormalities in glycogen metabolism depress the phagocytic and digestive capacity of neutrophils and macrophages. There may be depressed numbers of T cells in the blood, decreased responsiveness to mitogens, increased CD4/CD8 ratio, decreased IL-2 production, and decreased NK cell function, as well as decreased chemotaxis and bacterial killing by neutrophils in vitro. Some patients have low C4 levels. Although it is clear that diabetic patients have increased susceptibility to infections, there is no general agreement on why this is.

Iatrogenic Deficiencies

The mechanisms of action of the so-called immunosuppressive agents is extremely varied (Table 18.7). These agents may affect (i) the specific induction of the immune response (primary response), (ii) the expression of humoral antibody formation only, (iii) the expression of cellular immunity only, or (iv) the expression of both humoral and cellular immunity. All these agents have systemic effects on cells other than those of the lymphoid system. The damage caused by these agents in vivo is quite variable. In high doses, most cause derangements of any tissue that is metabolically active, e.g., depression of the bone marrow with subsequent loss of peripheral blood cell elements, or denudation of the lining epithelium of the gastrointestinal tract.

Table 18.7 Mechanism of action of immunosuppressive agents[a]

Agents	Mechanisms of action	Examples
Irradiation	Direct destruction of lymphoid cells, toxic for proliferating cells	Whole body, localized, extracorporeal
Steroids	Multiple, direct destruction of lymphoid cells, alterations in protein synthesis and lymphocyte circulation; anti-inflammatory	Hydrocortisone, prednisone
Alkylating agents	React chemically with nucleophilic centers of molecules, in particular DNA, RNA, and proteins; affect B-cell function more than T-cell function	Nitrogen mustard, cyclophosphamide, chlorambucil, busulfan
Purine analogs	Incorporated into DNA and RNA and interfere with nucleic acid synthesis; affect T-cell function more than B-cell function	Azathioprine, 6-mercaptopurine, thioguanine
Pyrimidine analogs	Inhibition of enzyme activity; active in RNA and DNA synthesis; affect B-cell function more than T-cell function	5-Fluorouracil, azaribine, 5-fluoro-2-deoxyuridine, cytosine arabinoside
Folic acid antagonists	Bind to dihydrofolate reductase, thereby interfering with purine, protein, and DNA synthesis	Methotrexate, amethopterin, aminopterin
Methylhydrazines	Formation of hydroxyl radicals causes changes in DNA similar to ionizing radiation	Procarbazine
Hydroxyureas	Kills DNA-synthesizing cells, block entry of cell into S phase	Hydroxyurea
Alkaloids	Block assembly of the mitotic spindle leading to metaphase arrest; also inhibit RNA and protein synthesis	Vinblastine, vincristine
Enzymes	Hydrolysis of L-asparagine to L-aspartate and ammonia	L-Asparaginase
Antibiotics	Multiple actions: (i) inhibit DNA-dependent RNA polymerase, (ii) alkylating agent, (iii) DNA binding	Mithramycin, mitomycin, actinomycin C
Antilymphocyte globulin	Alters lymphocyte circulation; lymphocytotoxic, opsonization of lymphocytes, receptor blockage	Horse, goat, rabbit, anti-human lymphocyte globulin
Cyclosporine	Blocks T-helper-cell effect, other effects?	Used to inhibit tissue graft rejection

[a]Modified from N. L. Gerber and A. D. Steinberg, *Drugs* **11**:14–35, 1976.

The effects of various drugs on the immune response are best considered in relation to the site of action during an immune response. Immunosuppressive therapy has become of paramount importance in preventing homograft rejection, especially in regard to organ transplantation, and experimental results indicate that such agents may be effective in suppressing various autoimmune reactions. These benefits are counterbalanced by the increased incidence and severity of opportunistic infections.

Infectious Diseases

Infectious diseases produce a generalized debilitation or may be associated with a selective "anergy" to the infectious agent. Anergy specifically refers to a loss of skin test DTH reaction to antigens of infectious organisms. This may represent lymphocyte sequestration or a disproportionate response of a nonprotective immune mechanism. For instance, in leprosy (see chapter 14), high antibody production (lepromatous leprosy) is associated with progressive disease, whereas high DTH and granulomatous reactivity (tuberculoid leprosy) is associated with arrested disease. The "wrong" type of immune response appears to have occurred, i.e., protection against leprosy requires cellular immunity: antibody alone is not effective. If the individual infected with leprosy produces antibody but not

DTH, protection is not effective. In our time, the most striking association of immunodeficiency with infection is in AIDS.

Full-blown *AIDS* (see chapter 19) is essentially a wasting syndrome as a result of a loss of cell-mediated immunity permitting a variety of opportunistic infections. HIV infects $CD4^+$ T cells. Although the pathogenesis of AIDS is not fully understood, the most likely hypothesis is that the causative virus directly inhibits functions of T-helper cells. The classic, but not invariable, presentation is of oral candida infection or of enlarging perianal ulcers containing herpes simplex virus (genital herpes). This is often followed by a prolonged course characterized by weight loss, fever, lymphadenopathy, multiple cutaneous nodules, and evidence of other opportunistic infections, including cytomegalovirus, *P. carinii, Mycobacterium avium-M. intracellulare,* and *Candida albicans,* as well as syphilis, tuberculosis, and gonorrhea. There is a marked depression in cellular immunity and a marked decrease in $CD4^+$ T cells in the peripheral blood ($<500/mm^3$).

Cancer (see chapter 20) causes depressed immunity in many ways. Perhaps the most significant is the general debilitation seen in terminal cancer patients. In addition, cancer patients are often treated with drastic chemotherapy or irradiation, further compromising immunity and setting the stage for opportunistic infections. Although "immunosuppressive" factors isolated from cancer tissue have been shown to suppress immune reactivity in vitro, the role of such factors in clinical immunosuppression remains poorly defined.

Selected immune effects may be seen with *leukemias* and *lymphomas,* tumors of the white blood cells and lymphoid organs (see chapter 17). In leukemia, the normal inflammatory function of the white blood cells is depressed because the neoplastic cells force out the normal population by occupying "living space." Neoplastic leukemia cells are unable to provide the same function as normal cells. Thus, the lymphocytes of chronic lymphocyte leukemia do not function properly. However, some acute lymphocytic leukemia cells may function as T-suppressor cells. The addition of small numbers of some acute lymphocytic leukemia cells to normal peripheral blood lymphocytes will inhibit lipopolysaccharide-induced Ig synthesis. In addition, autoantibodies to lymphocytes, particularly T cells, may be associated with lymphoproliferative disease and cause abnormalities in T-cell function.

Other lymphoproliferative neoplasias may affect both cellular and humoral immunity, either by occupying the bone marrow and forcing out normal products (living space) or by producing abnormalities in immune control systems. In Sézary syndrome, there is a malignant proliferation of T-helper cells. When graded numbers of Sézary cells are added to B cells, the amount of immunoglobulin synthesized as a result of lipopolysaccharide stimulation increases. However, at high T-cell/B-cell ratios, normal T cells suppress B-cell Ig synthesis; this may occur in later stages of the disease. In addition, it is not likely that Sézary cells can provide the T-cell help that is required for a specific immune response.

A number of immune abnormalities have been found in patients with tumors of plasma cells *(multiple myeloma,* or *plasmacytoma).* Most notably, these tumors produce large amounts of nonantibody monoclonal immunoglobulin. There is suppression of normal antibody responses to immunization. The primary cause of this appears to be "suppressor macrophages," which can inhibit the normal response of B cells. In addition, these patients have defects in complement and granulocyte function.

The high levels of circulating myeloma immunoglobulin increases the catabolic rate of normal immunoglobulin so that there is less functional antibody. In addition, there are large numbers of T cells with membrane-bound Fc receptors for the immunoglobulin isotope of the paraprotein being secreted by the plasma cell tumor. These isotope-specific T cells have a suppressor phenotype and can inhibit normal B-cell production of immunoglobulin of the same isotope as the myeloma protein.

Malcirculation of Lymphocytes

Lymphocytopenia (low numbers of blood lymphocytes), particularly of T cells, is frequently found in diseases such as Hodgkin's disease, Crohn's disease, hepatitis, rheumatoid arthritis, multiple sclerosis, and tuberculosis. The lymphopenia in these diseases may be due to sequestration of lymphocytes in tissues so that the numbers of lymphocytes in the blood is lower. In Hodgkin's disease, large numbers of T cells are present in the spleen; the blood lymphocytes respond poorly to T-cell mitogens, whereas the spleen lymphocytes respond normally. There also appears to be a selective sequestration of T-helper cells in the spleen. Splenectomy of patients with Hodgkin's disease may be associated with correction of the lymphopenic condition. T cells may be sequestered in the lesions of Crohn's disease, chronic hepatitis, rheumatoid arthritis, and tuberculosis. Such maldistribution of lymphocytes may lead to depressed immune responsiveness in other organ systems, such as anergy in tuberculosis and Hodgkin's disease.

Trauma

Bacterial sepsis is responsible for 75% of deaths following major thermal burns or traumatic injury. In thermal injury, there is a loss of host mechanical barriers to invading organisms, not only over the skin, but also in the lungs due to inhalation, producing a chemical tracheobronchitis with dysfunction of ciliary and alveolar macrophage function. Although conflicting results have been reported, there also appears to be an increase in "T-suppressor activity" after burns and abnormalities in chemotaxis and neutrophil function following major trauma.

Surgery is an immunosuppressive event that is intensified if the patient has an underlying disease, trauma, or complications that may contribute to suppression. The mere act of surgery violates the barriers of the body, and even with great attention to sterile procedures, the surgical patient is more likely to become infected. Surgery, as a function of its duration, complexity, and magnitude, directly influences immune reactions. On the other hand, resection of inflammatory or infected lesions, removal of tumors, or drainage of an abscess can return altered host defenses to normal. Attempts to identify immunopharmacologic treatments that might alleviate surgical immunosuppression have not been fruitful.

Chronic Fatigue Syndrome

Chronic fatigue syndrome is a complex of clinical findings with no clear pathogenesis associated with a variety of infectious agents. The major symptom is relapsing fatigue with all other chronic clinical conditions excluded. Other symptoms include low-grade fever, sore throat, lymph node pain, generalized muscle weakness and pain, generalized headaches, arthralgias, neuropsychological symptoms, and sleep disturbances. Laboratory test abnormalities include elevated antibodies to viruses, abnormal gamma globulin levels (high or low), increased serum IL-2 levels, decreased IL-2 production in vitro, increased CD4/CD8 ratio, increased or decreased NK activity, and variable antinuclear antibody levels. Infectious associations include a variety of agents. Most often implicated are Epstein-Barr virus, *Borrelia burgdorferi*, *Mycobacterium tuberculosis*, enteroviruses, and human T-cell leukemia virus type 1, but no convincing association has been established. The ability of tumor necrosis factor and IL-2 to produce symptoms similar to those of chronic fatigue syndrome has suggested that they might be responsible, but clinical testing has not found increased levels of tumor necrosis factor or IL-2.

Opportunistic Infections

The clinical manifestations of immune deficiency diseases are due to infections, often with organisms that are not usually pathogenic in a normal individual. Because many patients have immune deficiency secondary to another disease, they are exposed to organisms in the hospital and acquire the infection in the hospital. Such infections are termed *nosocomial*. A partial listing of pathogens in the immune-compromised host and the source of infection is given in Table 18.8. Most infections are acquired from the patient's own flora, but *Aspergillus* and *Zygomyces* infections are nosocomial. Some infections may be traced to application of devices, such as urinary catheters or endotracheal tubes, in particular, *Staphylococcus epidermidis* and *Corynebacterium*. Such hospital manipulations may help establish infections with host organisms by breaching of mechanical barriers.

Table 18.8 Some nosocomial pathogens in the immunocompromised host[a]

Organism	**Frequency with indicated source of infection[b]**	
	Endogenous	**Exogenous**
Bacteria		
Staphylococcus aureus	++	+
Staphylococcus epidermidis	++	0
Corynebacterium	++	0
Gram-negative rods *(Escherichia coli, Pseudomonas, Klebsiella)*	++	+
Fungi		
Candida, yeasts	++	0
Aspergillus	0	++
Zygomyces	0	++
Viruses		
Herpes simplex virus	++	0
Varicella-zoster virus	+	+
Cytomegalovirus	+	+
Parasites		
Pneumocystis carinii	++	+
Toxoplasma	++	+
Cryptosporidium	+	+

[a]Modified from L. S. Young, *Hosp. Pract.* **16:**73–84, 1981.
[b]++, high; +, low.

Evaluation of Immunodeficiency

The primary clue to the diagnosis of an immune deficiency disease is obtained by history and physical examination. The first clue to immune deficiency is the type, severity, cause, and frequency of infections in a patient. Clinical tests serve as confirmation, definition of the type and severity of the defect, and a guide for therapy. The specific diagnosis may then be confirmed by molecular testing for the specific gene loss or mutation. Also important is the presence of other factors, such as drug therapy or cancer. A summary of the laboratory evaluation of immune deficiency disease, exclusive of testing for specific genetic changes, is given in Fig. 18.4.

A patient with a history of recurrent infections must be critically examined for a potential defect in defense against infectious agents. The age, condition, and clinical and family history of the patient are vital in establishing the necessity for further laboratory work-up. Because of the complexity of findings in primary or secondary immune deficiencies, a systematic series of tests should be performed to permit adequate evaluation. Some of the tests indicated are presented below. From the type of recurrent infection, one can obtain a clue to the type of deficiency. If mainly viral or fungal, a defect in DTH (T-cell function) must be suspected. Recurrent bacterial infections indicate a defect in humoral antibody production, polymorphonuclear neutrophils, or complement. Complete white blood count and differential is an obvious first-level evaluation for major abnormalities in numbers or types of white cells in the blood. Serum immunoglobulin levels will reveal major disorders in humoral defenses. The availability of a large number of monoclonal antibodies and new methods for phenotypic analysis of lymphocyte subpopulations has made this a more practical and popular early evaluation technique; of particular importance are CD3, CD4, CD8, CD16, and CD19. Various nonimmunological factors can be tested by measuring general inflammatory indices, such as white blood count, or serum factors, such as complement or various inhibitors. Phagocytic capacity should be determined to rule out a phagocytic defect. Hu-

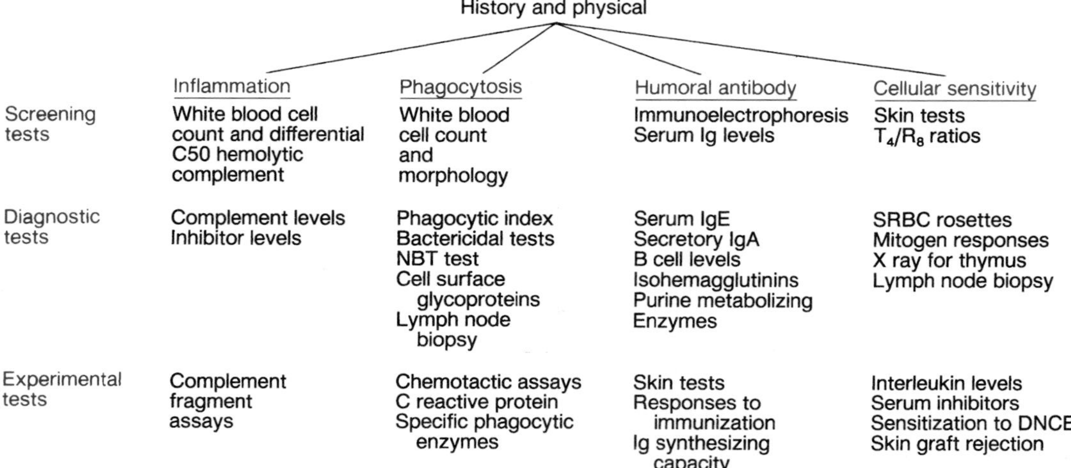

History and physical
Inflammation
Phagocytosis
Humoral antibody
Cellular sensitivity
Screening tests
White blood cell count and differential
C50 hemolytic complement
White blood cell count and morphology
Immunoelectrophoresis
Serum Ig levels
Skin tests
T_4/R_8 ratios
Diagnostic tests
Complement levels
Inhibitor levels
Phagocytic index
Bactericidal tests
NBT test
Cell surface glycoproteins
Lymph node biopsy
Serum IgE
Secretory IgA
B cell levels
Isohemagglutinins
Purine metabolizing
Enzymes
SRBC rosettes
Mitogen responses
X ray for thymus
Lymph node biopsy
Experimental tests
Complement fragment assays
Chemotactic assays
C reactive protein
Specific phagocytic enzymes
Skin tests
Responses to immunization
Ig synthesizing capacity
Interleukin levels
Serum inhibitors
Sensitization to DNCB
Skin graft rejection

Figure 18.4 Clinical laboratory evaluation of immunodeficiencies.

moral antibody capacity can be measured by determining serum immunoglobulin concentrations, by the presence of preformed antibody or the number of B lymphocytes, by the response to antigens that elicit antibody, such as immunization to diphtheria, pertussis, and tetanus or Pneumovax (pneumococcal vaccine), or by the response to specifically selected antigens such as keyhole limpet hemocyanin. Skin tests may also demonstrate anaphylactic or Arthus reactivity. Polyclonal activation of the patient's lymphocytes with lipopolysaccharide or pokeweed mitogen and the effect of cell fractionation or mixing with normal cells may be particularly revealing. Delayed reactivity can be determined by the transformation response of blood lymphocytes to mitogens such as phytohemagglutinin, pokeweed mitogen, or concanavalin A, as well as to selected specific antigens. The production of lymphocytic mediators, such as macrophage inhibitory factor or IL-2, as well as the presence of serum inhibitors of transformation, can be measured. In addition, the number of blood lymphocytes that react with monoclonal antibodies to T-cell surface markers are used to phenotype T-cell subpopulations. In vivo tests for DTH include skin tests to antigens such as the purified protein derivatives of tubercle bacilli or coccidioidin; the ability to induce contact reactivity to dinitrochlorobenzene or other haptens; skin graft rejection; X-ray examination for the thymic shadow; and, in rare cases, lymph node biopsy. From the results of a selection of these tests, one can define the nature of defect leading to recurrent or unusual infections and institute appropriate therapy. Finally, as stated above, specific testing for gene deletions, mutations, or rearrangements offer the final specific diagnosis of the genetic abnormality.

Therapy

Treatment of immune deficiency diseases may be divided into three general approaches: (i) treatment of the infectious agent by antibiotics, (ii) treatment of the underlying disease, if present, and (iii) replacement of the immune defect. In this section, replacement of the immune defect is presented in more detail.

Passive Antibody

Since immunoglobulin deficiencies are caused by the lack of antibody, some immunoglobulin deficiencies may be replaced by injections of pooled normal immunoglobulins. A number of commercially available preparations are available for intravenous administration, some containing Ig selected for reactivity with a specific infectious agent (Table 18.9). The manufacturers recommend 300 to 400 mg/kg of body weight at monthly intervals. These preparations contain about the same spectrum of specific antibodies. Preparations with low IgA should be administered to patients with combined IgG-IgA deficiencies to prevent allergic reaction to IgA. Whereas such injections give some protection, they do not provide the high levels of specific antibody that are produced in response to an infectious organism by a normal person and do not provide any cell-mediated immunity. However, some immunoglobulin preparations are made from sera containing high titers of antibodies to specific infections agents, such as hepatitis B, rabies, cytomegalovirus, and respiratory syncytial virus (Table 18.9). Passive immunoglobulin is the most effective maintenance procedure for patients with hypogammaglobulinemia, supplemented with antibiotics to cover specific infections.

Table 18.9 Commercially available licensed immunoglobulin preparations for infectious diseases

Product	Manufacturer	Isolation	Comments
Gamimmune N	Cutter Biol., Berkeley, Calif.	Cold ethanol, pH 4.0	5 or 10% in maltose; low IgG4; delivery pH, 4.0
Gammagard	Baxter Corp., Glendale, Calif.	Cold ethanol, DEAE	5% in glucose; low IgA, IgG4; delivery pH, 6.8
Sandoglobulin	Sandoz, East Rutherford, N.J.	Cold ethanol, pepsin	3 or 6% in sucrose; lyophilized; delivery pH, 6.6
BayHep B	Bayer Corp., West Haven, Conn.	Cold ethanol	15 to 18% in glycine, pH 6.4 to 7.2; contains antibodies to hepatitis B virus
BayRab	Bayer Corp.	Cold ethanol	Contains antibodies to rabies virus
BayTet	Bayer Corp.	Cold ethanol	Contains antibodies to tetanus toxin
CytoGam	Medimmune, Inc., Gaithersburg, Md.	Cold ethanol	50 mg/ml in sucrose and albumin; contains antibodies to cytomegalovirus
RespiGam	Medimmune, Inc.		Contains antibodies to respiratory syncytial virus
H-BIG	NABI, Boca Raton, Fla.	Cold ethanol	16.5% in glycine; contains antibodies to hepatitis B virus
Imogam	Pasteur Merieux Connaught, Swiftwater, Pa.	Cold ethanol	10 to 18% in glycine; contains antibodies to rabies virus

Passive Cell-Mediated Immunity

Attempts have been made to treat immunologic deficiencies of the cellular and combined cellular and immunoglobulin types by bone marrow or thymus transplantation or transfer of cell products. Such transplants must be selected carefully to correct the specific immune deficiency with a minimum potential of unwanted effects, in particular, graft-versus-host reactions. For general application, only BMT has met with consistent clinical success. Patients with only cellular deficiencies, such as DiGeorge's syndrome, have rarely been successfully treated with thymus transplants. Patients with combined immune deficiencies may be reconstituted by transfer of bone marrow cells that contain stem cells. Reconstitution of immune reactivity is due to proliferation of donor cells that repopulate the host tissue.

Thymus Transplants

Fetal thymus transplants have been reported to restore cellular immunity in a few patients with combined immune deficiencies; these people have then been maintained with passive gamma globulin to cover humoral antibody deficiency. The responding cells in patients treated with transplantation of the thymus are of donor origin, indicating the presence of T-cell precursors in the transplanted thymus. But B-cell precursors are not present, and humoral antibody production is not restored. The thymus must be selected from fetuses before the 14th week of gestation. Under these circumstances, only minimal graft-versus-host reactivity has been observed. However, thymus transplantation is not generally found to be useful in present practice.

Bone Marrow Transplantation

A growing number of hematologic diseases, including aplasias, leukemias, and lymphomas, as well as immune deficiency diseases, are being successfully treated by BMT to replace the loss of hematopoietic cells. For leukemias and lymphomas, bone marrow is used to restore the loss of hematopoietic tissue following ablative irradiation. In some forms of previously fatal leukemias and aplasia, 2-year disease-free survival exceeds 60%. BMT by intravascular infusion is much simpler to carry out than transplantation of solid organs, and since donor cells may be obtained by bone marrow aspiration, it is usually easy to find a living related donor.

In SCID, as well as many other immune deficiency diseases, it is possible to restore complete immune function by transfer of bone marrow cells. The transplantation of living immunocompetent cells to an immune-deficient recipient is possible because the recipient is unable to reject the transplanted cells. In leukemia and lymphomas, or other cancers, such as breast, in which ablative irradiation is used to treat the cancer, the patient's bone marrow is destroyed, so there are no immune-competent cells to react to the donor cells. However, if there is not close HLA matching, the transplanted immunocompetent cells may react to the recipient tissues, and death may result from a graft-versus-host reaction. The first successful BMT in a SCID infant was carried out in 1968. Since then, a number of successful transplants of bone marrow cells have been made to immune-deficient individuals with not only some spectacular successes but also some disappointing failures. Using HLA-matched sibling donors, there is about 85% successful long-term survival. Using unrelated HLA-matched donors, there is greater than 50% long-term survival, and this figure is continuing to improve. The establishment of an international marrow-donor registry has made HLA phenotypically matched marrow from unrelated donors available to patients who lack a suitable related donor. Recently, the possibility has been raised of replacing the specific genes that are missing in SCID with adenosine deaminase deficiency by transferring back to the patient his or her own bone marrow stem cells that have had the missing human gene inserted.

Even with successful "takes," BMT recipients may have cellular and humoral immunodeficiencies for months to years after transplantation. The precise reasons for this effect is not clear, but it appears that the immune system undergoes a recapitulation of ontogenesis. Immature B cells undergo differentiation processes and have low IgG levels that correlate with the incidence of pneumococcal infections after transplantation. There is also evidence of insufficient T-cell help and/or exaggerated $CD8^+$ T-cell or NK-cell suppression. Because of the frequency of immunoglobulin deficiencies after transplantation, administration of intravenous passive immunoglobulins may have beneficial effects in individual patients, and reimmunization with childhood vaccines is often recommended.

Graft-versus-host reactions. Transfer of cell populations such as bone marrow, which contain immune-competent lymphocytes, may lead to a reaction of the transferred cells to antigens of the recipient. This is called a graft-versus-host (GVH) reaction. GVH reactions occur when immune-competent cells from an allogeneic or xenogeneic donor are transferred to a recipient whose own immune responsiveness has been impaired by immunosuppression or neoplastic disease or because of immature development. Rarely, GVH reactions may occur after blood transfusions, usually in children under 18 years of age with evidence of immunosuppression. The transferred cells colonize in the recipient, recognize host tissue antigens as foreign, and react to them. The immunoreactive cells responsible for the GVH reaction are the mature T cells present in the bone marrow. Some components of the GVH reaction may include reaction of residual host cells to the grafted cells. When the lymphoid tissue of the recipient is not completely destroyed, regeneration of the host immune system in the presence of donor cells may result in a state of mutual tolerance of grafted and recipient cells. Individuals whose tissues contain cells of more than one genotype are called *chimeras*. A chimera is a fire-spouting monster of Greek mythology with a lion's head, a goat's body, and a serpent's tail. In lymphoid cell chimeras, the recipient maintains both its own and the donor lymphoid components—an interesting condition in which two separate immune and hematopoietic systems coexist.

Wasting disease. The reaction of grafted immune cells to host antigens and vice versa produces a disease known as GVH disease (GVHD), secondary disease, or wasting disease (Table 18.10). Acute GVHD usually occurs 20 to 100 days after transplantation and is fatal in 10% of the affected individuals. Acute GVHD consists of two pathologic processes: (i) infiltration of tissues, especially the skin, intestine, spleen, and liver with proliferating lymphocytes, resulting in hepatosplenomegaly, diarrhea, and a scaly contact dermatitis-like skin lesion, and (ii) loss of immune reactivity with susceptibility to opportunistic infections. The major reaction appears to be by $CD4^+$ T_{DTH} cells to class II MHC antigens on lymphoid cells, activated epithelial cells in the skin and intestine, and bile duct cells. Proliferating host cells may make a major contribution to the lymphoid hyperplasia, and it is the host's MHC class II^+ lymphopoietic tissue that bears the brunt of the attack by the transferred cells. The hyperplasia of spleen and other lymphoid organs is followed by atrophy, presumably because the grafted cells have attacked and destroyed the host's lymphoid tissue. A variety of causative factors may contribute to the severity of GVH, including effects of antineoplastic drugs or total body irradiation (for treatment of leukemias or lymphomas), medications used for treatment of GVHD, infectious complications, and antimicrobial therapies. Veno-occlusive disease of the liver occurs in up to 20% of cases. Chronic GVHD may lead to sclerodermalike skin lesions and liver lesions resembling primary biliary cirrhosis. The success of BMT depends largely on controlling the extent of the GVH reaction and preventing opportunistic infections from loss of the recipient's immune system.

Hybrid resistance. Hybrid resistance refers to the failure of inbred parental bone marrow cells to induce GVHD in lethally irradiated F_1 recipient mice. Since the F_1 hybrid immune system shares only one MHC

Table 18.10 Findings in acute and chronic graft-versus-host disease

	Findings in:	
Organ	**Acute disease**	**Chronic disease**
Skin	Erythroderma, rash, desquamation, inflammation of hair follicles and basal cells	Sclerodermalike skin atrophy, papulosquamous dermatitis dyspigmentation, alopecia
Liver	Elevated bilirubin and liver enzymes, periportal inflammation	Cholestatic disease with biliary cirrhosis
Gastrointestinal tract	Diarrhea, ileus, inflammation at base of crypts	Destruction of mucosa with intestinal strictures
Lymphoid	Delayed immunologic recovery	T- and B-cell deficiencies, opportunistic infections

haplotype with the homozygous parent, parental cells are able to recognize F_1 cells, but F_1 cells should not react against the parent homozygous cells. Thus, the parental cells should survive and produce GVHD. Parental bone marrow cells are rejected by a multistep process involving an antigen, termed Hh-1, linked to H-2D region that is only expressed in the homozygous condition. The hybrid resistance reaction involves two steps. First, a radioresistant $CD4^-$ $CD8^-$ $CD5^+$ cell in the F_1 hybrid recognizes the Hh-1 antigen and stimulates macrophages to secret IFN-α/β. The IFN activates an NK cell that specifically kills parental cells bearing Hh-1 antigens using an antibody-dependent recognition mechanism. Expression of the Hh-1 antigen is associated with the homozygous haplotype: heterozygous mice do not express this Hh-1 antigen. Since the F_1 recipients are heterozygous and the parental mice are homozygous, the radioresistant F_1 T cells are able to initiate the hybrid resistance response.

Clinical bone marrow transplantation. The objective of BMT is to replace hematopoietic stem cells. Bone marrow grafts have been used to treat patients with aplastic anemia (failure of blood cell production), SCID, or patients with cancer treated with irradiation or ablative radio- or chemotherapy. With careful follow-up, excellent results are obtained in most of the cases of aplastic anemia or immune deficiency, if an HLA-identical sibling donor is used. Similarly, bone marrow failure following accidental irradiation can be treated with BMT. Irradiation leads to failure of blood cell production and reduction in immune function.

Leukemia. In leukemias or other cancers, BMT is used to "rescue" patients following irradiation and/or chemotherapy. Irradiation or doses of chemicals sufficient to cause a potentially curative reduction in tumor cell mass frequently result in death by infection or bleeding secondary to loss of bone marrow function, i.e., loss of production of white cells and platelets. This can be circumvented by transfer of bone marrow from a healthy donor. Unless an identical twin is available, some degree of GVH reactivity seems inevitable. If possible, autologous bone marrow obtained during remission may be stored, treated with monoclonal antibodies to try to remove any residual leukemia cells, and reinfused back into the patient after ablative treatment for recurrence.

BMT following radiation and chemotherapy treatment of leukemia has had increasing success. For instance, approximately 25% of patients with acute nonlymphocytic leukemia will have long-term disease-free survival after intensive chemotherapy alone. Of the 75% who do not have long-term remission after chemotherapy, one-third will go into long-term remission after ablative therapy and BMT. Chemotherapy alone is ineffective against chronic myelogenous leukemia, but BMT after radiation leads to long-term remission in 25 to 65% of cases. The therapeutic process starts with *conditioning,* the administration of high-dose chemotherapy or irradiation or both to eliminate the malignant cell population, as well as host cells that might react against the transplanted cells. Conditioning is not required for most patients with immune deficiencies. This is followed by *transplantation* of bone marrow and *supportive care* of the patient against infection and bleeding. Support includes administration of antibiotics and transfusions of platelets and red blood cells, as well as transfusions of granulocytes in some cases.

Prevention of GVH reactions. Efforts in improving BMT have centered on ways to reduce the severity of the GVH reaction yet provide sufficient bone marrow stem cells to reconstitute the immune-deficient or irradiated recipient. In most remissions, a transient GVH reaction occurs, and the treated individual demonstrates both host and donor cells after the reaction (chimerism). Thus, there is a delicate balance between removing the alloreactive cells and preserving the stem cells. In numerous clinical trials, a variety of methods have proved to be at least partially feasible in reducing the reactivity of the donor cells to the host. Since it is the mature T cells in the marrow that are responsible for the GVH reaction, one approach has been to remove these cells. For clinical application, fresh bone marrow preparations to be used for transplantation are purged of mature T cells with anti-CD6 monoclonal antibody and complement. Another approach is to use cord blood stem cells. Cord blood has a relatively high number of stem cells and a low number of mature T cells as compared with adult bone marrow. Treatment of the recipient with drugs, such as serine protease inhibitors, to block T-cell-mediated cytotoxicity or with other immunosuppressive drugs is sometimes effective. When BMT is used for treatment of cancer, some GVH reactivity may be beneficial if directed to the cancer (graft-versus-malignancy effect). This procedure significantly reduces the severity of GVHD.

Mild GVHD is expected and is not treated. Treatment of moderate to severe acute GVHD consists of antilymphocyte preparations, cyclosporine, high-dose steroids, and azathioprine in various combinations. Infection is the most common cause of death, because immunosuppression is both a component of the disease and the effect of therapy. Abnormalities of T cells, B cells, macrophages, and neutrophils have been found, and responses to immunization with new antigens are severely impaired. The entire immune system is affected, and the cellular interactions required for induction and expression of immunity are dysfunctional. As time passes, the balance and regulation of the immune system is restored. Antibiotics are used to cover infections but may also contribute to the manifestations of GVHD. Recovery is dependent upon stem cells in the donor bone marrow repopulating the hematopoietic and lymphopoietic systems, with recapitulation of neonatal development of the immune system over a 1- to 2-year period. Early after bone marrow transfer, primitive functions such as $CD8^+$ T_{CTL}-cell-mediated cytotoxicity and suppression are predominant, and T_{DTH} and T-helper cell functions are inhibited. This stage may be necessary for the donor cells to become established.

Transplant leukemia. A particularly interesting and perplexing finding is that in a few cases of leukemia treated by whole-body irradiation and bone marrow from an HLA-matched sibling of the opposite sex, the donor's blood cells became established but subsequently became leukemic. This could be because of excessive antigenic stimulation of donor cells in a foreign environment, an abnormal homeostatic mechanism in the recipient that also applies to donor cells, fusion of donor and recipient cells resulting in transfer of donor chromosome markers to recipient leukemic cells, transmission of an agent (oncogenic virus) from host to donor cells, or the presence of an oncogenic virus in the donor cells that was not expressed in the donor. In some cases, Epstein-Barr virus has been demonstrated in the leukemic cells. Clearly, use of BMT clinically has moved from being an experimental procedure to a clinically applicable method and, if carefully done, may result in a satisfactory therapy for leukemia, lymphoma, aplastic anemia, or immune deficiency diseases.

Self-recognition. An additional factor in determining the effectiveness of stem cell transfers is the necessity of self-recognition of T and B cells in order for cooperation to occur. Unless donor and recipient are adequately HLA matched, it is possible that the T and B cells that develop from the engrafted donor stem cells may not be able to cooperate. At first glance it would seem that after transfer, a given population of stem cells from both the developing T and B cells would be of donor origin. However, in experimental systems the ability of T cells to recognize self depends not on the origin of the pre-T (stem) cell but on the thymic environment in which T-cell maturation takes place (adaptive differentiation). Thus, if type X stem cells, containing both T- and B-cell precursor potential, are engrafted into a type Y recipient, the type X pre-T cells will mature in the environment of the type Y thymus and acquire the capacity to recognize Y and not X as self. On the other hand, the type X pre-B cells will mature as type X cells. The person so reconstituted will have X type T cells that recognize Y and cannot cooperate with X type B cells.

Adoptive transfer of effector T cells. Adoptive transfer of immune-specific effector cells may provide vital defense against specific infections in T-cell-depleted patients after BMT. For example, most adult humans harbor cytomegalovirus (CMV), which is normally contained by circulating CMV-specific $CD8^+$ T cells. Loss of these cells after irradiation and bone marrow transfer releases latent CMV infections, which are responsible for up to 25% of serious complications after BMT. These infections may be held in check by transplantation of allogeneic $CD8^+$ T_{CTL} cloned cell lines expanded by in vitro culture and infused at 10^9 cells per square meter of recipient body surface. This may protect against CMV for up to 3 months, but persistent defense requires recovery of $CD4^+$ helper function in the recipient, as the donor $CD8^+$ cells must eventually be replaced by recipient $CD8^+$ cells. Such an approach has also proved effective in treatment of Epstein-Barr virus infections after BMT. The risk of GVHD after transfer of cell lines is much less than that with polyclonal T-cell populations.

Gene transfer therapy. In the last few years, the availability of retroviral techniques for transferring specific genes with high efficiency into various cell types has permitted the development of methods for specific gene replacement. The cells of choice for gene transfer therapy are stem cells, such as the hematopoietic stem cell found in bone marrow. DNA-mediated gene transfer using viruses such as adenoviruses, simian virus 40, adeno-associated viruses, or herpes simplex have not been shown to transduce or transfect hematopoietic cells effectively. Hepatocytes, endothelial cells, muscle cells, keratinocytes, and fibroblasts have all been suggested as potentially useful cells for gene transfer; however, bone marrow is considered the best means for such transfer, as it contains self-renewing stem cells and is easy and relatively safe to obtain. Such "gene transfer therapy" has been used to replace missing enzymes in SCID caused by adenosine deaminase deficiency and is now being developed for many other genetic diseases. Table 18.11 lists some of the diseases that

Table 18.11 Some diseases treated by gene transfer using bone marrow cells

Disease	Gene defect
Red cells	
β-Thalassemia	β-Globin
Lymphocytes	
ADA deficiency	Adenosine deaminase
PNP deficiency	Purine nucleotide phosphorylase
Monocytes and neutrophils	
Chronic granulomatous disease	Cytochrome *b,* β chain
Leukocyte adhesion deficiency	CD18 β subunit
Lysosomal storate diseases (mostly macrophages)	
Gaucher's disease	Glucocerebrosidase
Mucopolysaccharidosis I	α-L-Iduronidase
Niemann-Pick type B	Sphinogomyelinase
Metachromatic leukodystrophy	Arylsulfatase A

have been cured or in which symptoms have dramatically improved after bone marrow transfer of transfected cells. Use of more primitive embryonic stem cells for gene transfer of other diseases, using modified genes to correct a specific gene defect, requires more efficient methods of gene targeting. The use of genetically engineered cells for tumor therapy is discussed in chapter 20.

Liver Transplants

In one case, an allograft of fetal liver to a 3-month-old boy with SCID and ADA deficiency restored both T- and B-cell functions as well as ADA activity and clinical improvement. One year later, the child died with a fatal immune complex glomerulonephritis, which could have resulted from reaction to exogenous antigen or from a GVH reaction.

Summary

Primary immune deficiency diseases are genetically controlled developmental abnormalities in the maturation of the immune system. The type of deficiency manifested depends upon the level of maturational arrest that the abnormality affects. Secondary immune deficiencies are the result of naturally occurring diseases or administration of immunosuppressive agents that operate upon a mature immune system. The type of deficiency observed depends upon the location of the defect for the given disease or the mechanism of action of the immunosuppressive agent. Defects may occur in antibody formation, cellular immunity, accessory systems (complement, phagocytosis), or mechanical barriers or other nonspecific innate immune mechanisms. Patients with immune defects acquire pathogenic infections with organisms that are not usually pathogens in normal individuals (opportunistic infections). Replacement of the specific defect or therapy for the infection or for an underlying disease causing the immune defects may be effective. In general, BMT is effective for individuals with defects in cellular immunity, and intravenous immunoglobulin is used for patients with defects in antibody formation.

Bibliography

Mouse Models

Kerner, J. D., M. W. Appleby, R. N. Mohr, S. Chien, D. J. Rawlings, et al. 1995. Impaired expansion of mouse B cell progenitors lacking BTK. *Immunity* **3**:301–312.

Khan, W. N., F. W. Alt, R. M. Gerstein, B. A. Malynn, I. Larsson, G. Rathbun, et al. 1995. Defective B cell development and function in BTK-deficient mice. *Immunity* **3**:283–299.

Nosaka, T., J. M. A. van Deursen, R. A. Tripp, W. E. Thierfelder, B. A. Witthuhn, et al. 1995. Defective lymphoid development in mice lacking Jak3. *Science* **270**:800–802.

Rihova, B., and V. Vetvica (ed.). 1990. *Immunological Disorders in Mice.* CRC Press, Boca Raton, Fla.

Thomas, D. C., C. B. Gurniak, E. Tivol, A. H. Sharpe, and L. J. Berg. 1995. Defects in B lymphocyte maturation and T lymphocyte activation in mice lacking Jak3. *Science* **270**:794–796.

Primary Immune Deficiencies

Afzelius, B. A. 1985. The immobile-cilia syndrome: a microtubule associated defect. *Crit. Rev. Biochem.* **19**:63–87.

Allen, R. C., R. J. Armitage, M. E. Conley, H. Rosenblatt, N. A. Jenkins, N. G. Copeland, et al. 1993. CD40 ligand gene defects responsible for X-linked hyper-IgM syndrome. *Science* **259**:990–993.

Epps, R. E., M. R. Pittelkow, and W. P. Su. 1995. TORCH syndrome. *Semin. Dermatol.* **14**:179–186.

Greenberg, F. 1993. DiGeorge syndrome: an historical review of clinical and cytogenetic features. *J. Med. Genet.* **30**:803–806.

Liblau, R. S., and J.-F. Bach. 1992. Selective IgA deficiency and autoimmunity. *Int. Arch. Allergy Immunol.* **99**:16–27.

Mandell, L. A. 1990. Infections in the compromised host. *J. Int. Med. Res.* **18**:177–190.

Ochs, H. D., C. I. E. Smith, and J. M. Puck. 1998. *Primary Immunodeficiency Diseases.* Oxford University Press, New York, N.Y.

Rasio, D., M. Negrini, and C. M. Crocy. 1995. Genomic organization of the ATM locus involved in ataxia-telangiectasia. *Cancer Res.* **55**:6053–6057.

Rawlings, D. J., and O. N. Witte. 1994. Bruton's tyrosine kinase is a key regulator in B-cell development. *Immunol. Rev.* **138**:105–119.

Rieux-Laucat, F., F. Le Deist, C. Hivroz, I. A. Roberts, K. M. Debatin, A. Fischer, and J. P. de Villartay. 1995. Mutations in Fas associated with human lymphoproliferative syndrome and autoimmunity. *Science* **268**:1347–1349.

Russell, S. M., N. Tayebi, J. Nakajima, M. C. Riedy, J. L. Roberts, M. J. Aman, T. S. Migone, M. Noguchi, M. L. Markert, R. H. Buckley, et al. 1995. Mutation of Jak3 in a patient with SCID: essential role of Jak3 in lymphoid development. *Science* **270**:797–800.

Schwarz, K., G. H. Gauss, L. Ludwig, U. Pannicke, Z. Li, D. Lindner, W. Friedrich, R. A. Seger, T. E. Hansen-Hagge, S. Desiderio, M. R. Lieber, C. R. Bartram. 1996. RAG mutations in human B cell negative SCID. *Science* **274**:97–99.

Snapper, S. B., and F. R. Rosen. 1999. The Wiskott-Aldrich syndrome protein (WASP): roles in signaling and cytoskeletal organization. *Annu. Rev. Immunol.* **17**:905–929.

Steim, E. R. 1990. *Immunologic Disorders in Infants and Children,* 3rd ed. The W. B. Saunders Co., Orlando, Fla.

Strober, W., and J. C. Sneller. 1991. IgA deficiency. *Ann. Allergy* **66**:363–375.

Ten, R. M. 1998. Primary immunodeficiencies. *Mayo Clin. Proc.* **73**:865–872.

Turner, M. W. 1998. Mannose-binding lectin (MBL) in health and disease. *Immunobiology* **199:**327–339.

Ugazio, A. G., R. Maccariio, L. D. Notarangelo, and G. R. Burgio. 1990. Immunology of Down syndrome: a review. *Am. J. Med. Genet.* **7S:**204–214.

Vetrie, D., I. Vorechovsky, P. Sideras, J. Holland, A. Davies, F. Flinter, et al. 1993. The gene involved in X-linked agammaglobulinaemia is a member of the *src* family of protein-tyrosine kinases. *Nature* **361:**226–233.

Phagocytic Defects

Anderson, D. C. 1989. Leukocyte adhesion deficiency: an inherited defect in the MAC-1, LFA-1, and P150,95 glycoproteins, p. 315–323. *In* A. L. Beaudet, R. Mulligan, and I. M. Verma (ed.), *Gene Transfer and Gene Therapy.* Alan R. Liss, Inc., New York, N.Y.

Clark, R. A., H. L. Malech, J. I. Gallin, H. Nunoi, B. D. Volpp, D. W. Pearson, W. M. Nauseef, and J. T. Curnutte. 1989. Genetic variants of chronic granulomatous disease: prevalence of deficiencies of two cytosolic components of the NADPH oxidase system. *N. Engl. J. Med.* **321:**647–652.

Kume, A., and M. C. Dinaurere. 2000. Gene therapy for chronic granulomatous disease. *J. Lab. Clin. Med.* **135:**122–128.

Yang, K. D., and H. R. Hill. 1991. Neutrophil function disorders: pathophysiology, prevention and therapy. *J. Pediatr.* **119:**343–354.

Complement (see also chapter 3)

Coulton, H. R., and F. S. Rosen. 1992. Complement deficiencies. *Annu. Rev. Immunol.* **10:**809–834.

Petry, F. 1998. Molecular basis of hereditary C1q deficiency. *Immunobiology* **199:**286–294.

Sullivan, K. E. 1998. Complement deficiency and autoimmunity. *Curr. Opin. Pediatr.* **10:**600–606.

Interleukins, Lymphokines, and Monokines

Cacalano, N. A., and J. A. Johnson. 1999. Interleukin-2 signalling and inherited immunodeficiency. *Am. J. Hum. Genet.* **65:**287–293.

Spickett, G. P., and J. Farrant. 1989. The role of lymphokines in common variable hypogammaglobulinemia. *Immunol. Today* **10:**192–195.

Uribe, L., and K. I. Weinberg. 1998. X-linked SCID and other defects of cytokine pathways. *Semin. Hematol.* **35:**299–309.

Secondary Immunodeficiencies (see also chapters 19 and 20)

Baker, C. C. 1986. Immune mechanisms and host resistance in the trauma patient. *Yale J. Biol. Med.* **59:**387–393.

Gaspar, H. B., and D. Goldblatt. 1998. Immunodeficiency syndromes and recurrent infection. *Br. J. Hosp. Med.* **58:**565–568.

Jacobson, D. R., and S. Zolla-Pazner. 1986. Immune suppression and infection in multiple myeloma. *Semin. Oncol.* **13:**282–290.

Meakins, J. L. 1991. Surgeons, surgery and immunomodulation. *Arch. Surg.* **126:**494–498.

Moutschen, M. P., A. J. Scheen, and P. J. Lefebvre. 1992. Impaired immune responses in diabetes mellitus: analysis of the factors and mechanisms involved. Relevance to the increased susceptibility of diabetic patients to specific infections. *Diabet. Metab.* **18:**187–201.

Pennington, D. J., G. J. Lonergan, and E. C. Benya. 1999. Pulmonary disease in the immunocompromised child. *J. Thorac. Imaging* **14:**37–50.

Graft-versus-Host Reactions

Champlin, R., I. Khouri, S. Kornblau, J. Molldrem, and S. Giralt. 1999. Reinventing bone marrow transplantation: reducing toxicity using nonmyeloablative, preparative regimens and induction of graft-versus-malignancy. *Curr. Opin. Oncol.* **11:**87–95.

Craven, C. M., and K. Ward. 1999. Transfusion of fetal cord blood cells: an improved method of hematopoietic stem cell transplantation? *J. Reprod. Immunol.* **42:**59–77.

Exner, B. G., I. N. Acholonu, M. Bergheim, Y. M. Mueller, and S. T. Ildstad. 1999. Mixed allogeneic chimerism to induce tolerance to solid organ and cellular grafts. *Acta Haematol.* **101:**78–81.

Ferrara, J. L. M., and H. J. Deeg. 1991. Graft-versus-host disease. *N. Engl. J. Med.* **324:**667–674.

Quaranta, S., J. Shulman, A. Ahmed, Y. Shoenfeld, J. Peter, G. B. McDonald, et al. 1999. Autoantibodies in human chronic graft-versus-host disease after hematopoietic cell transplantation. *Clin. Immunol.* **91:**106–116.

Saigo, K., and R. Ryo. 1999. Therapeutic strategy for post-transfusion graft-vs.-host disease. *Int. J. Hematol.* **69:**147–151.

Bone Marrow Transplantation

Fischer, A., P. Landais, W. Friedrich, B. Gerritsen, A. Fasth, F. Porta, et al. 1994. Bone marrow transplantation (BMT) in Europe for primary immunodeficiencies other than severe combined immunodeficiency: a report for the European Group for BMT and the European Group for Immunodeficiency. *Blood* **83:**1149–1154.

Greenberg, P. D., and S. R. Riddell. 1999. Deficient cellular immunity—finding and fixing the defects. *Science* **285:**546–551.

Gross, T. G., M. Steinbuch, T. DeFor, R. S. Shapiro, P. McGlave, N. K. Ramsay, J. E. Wagner, and A. H. Filipovich. 1999. B cell lymphoproliferative disorders following hematopoietic stem cell transplantation: risk factors, treatment and outcome. *Bone Marrow Transplant.* **23:**251–258.

Locatelli, F., C. Perotti, M. Zecca, and P. Pedrazzoli. 1998. Transplantation of peripheral blood stem cells mobilized by haematopoietic growth factors in childhood. *Bone Marrow Transplant.* **22**(Suppl. 5):S51–S55.

Lockhorst, H. M., and D. Liebowitz. 1999. Adoptive T-cell therapy. *Semin. Hematol.* **36:**26–29.

Russell, N. H., A. Gratwohl, and N. Schmitz. 1998. Developments in allogeneic peripheral blood progenitor cell transplantation. *Br. J. Haematol.* **103:**594–600.

Gene Therapy

Blaese, R. M., K. W. Culver, A. D. Miller, C. S. Carter, T. Fleisher, M. Clerici, et al. 1995. T lymphocyte- directed gene therapy for ADA^- SCID: initial trial results after 4 years. *Science* **270:**475–480.

Bordignon, C., L. D. Notarangelo, N. Nobili, G. Ferrari, G. Casorati, P. Panina, et al. 1995. Gene therapy in peripheral blood lymphocytes and bone marrow for ADA^- immunodeficient patients. *Science* **270:**470–475.

Hershfield, M. S. 1998. Adenosine deaminase deficiency: clinical expression, molecular basis, and therapy. *Semin. Hematol.* **35:**291–298.

Kohn, D. B., K. I. Weinberg, J. A. Nolta, L. N. Heiss, C. Lenarsky, G. M. Crooks, et al. 1995. Engraftment of gene-modified umbilical cord blood cells in neonates with adenosine deaminase deficiency. *Nat. Med.* **1:**1017–1023.

Immunology of AIDS

19

Acquired immune deficiency syndrome (AIDS) is a secondary immune deficiency caused by infection with a human retrovirus called human immunodeficiency virus (HIV). HIV infects and kills $CD4^+$ T-helper cells. This causes a profound, irreversible immunosuppression that, without treatment, rapidly progresses from opportunistic infections to death in almost all infected individuals.

Human Immunodeficiency Virus

AIDS-Related Retroviruses

HIV belongs to the subfamily *Lentivirinae* (slow viruses) in the family of animal retroviruses (Table 19.1). In general, retroviruses cause either proliferation (transforming viruses) or destruction (cytopathic viruses) of the cells they infect. Human T-cell leukemia virus types 1 and 2 (HTLV-1 and HTLV-2) are transforming viruses. They are also called oncoviruses and cause cancers in a variety of animals. HIV is a cytopathic virus. The cytopathic viruses were first identified in animals, where they cause wasting diseases after a long interval of latent or subclinical infection. Because of the chronic course of the diseases they cause (slow diseases), this group of viruses is called "lentiviruses" or slow viruses. HIV produces a profound immunosuppression in almost every infected individual. In contrast, HTLV-1 infection produces proliferation of lymphocytes and a particular form of leukemia, adult T-cell leukemia, in a very small percentage of infected individuals. It was once proposed that HIV be called HTLV-III. However, HTLV-1 is an oncovirus, whereas HIV is a lentivirus.

There are two HIVs, HIV type 1 (HIV-1) and HIV-2. HIV-1 and HIV-2 share about 60% RNA sequence homology in some regions and 30 to 40% in other regions. HIV-1 is by far the most common cause of AIDS in the Western world. HIV-2 produces a disease similar to that caused by HIV-1 and is present in high incidence in West Africa but is being found increasing outside of Africa, in particular in India. HIV-2 is very closely related to simian immunodeficiency virus (SIV), which causes a form of AIDS with encephalitis in monkeys (macaques) that is very similar to AIDS in humans. SIVmac, the macaque form of SIV, has 75% sequence similarity to HIV-2 and 50% similarity to HIV-1. The extensive degree of genetic disparity among the new SIV isolates and between these and HIV-1 or HIV-2 isolates, as well as the lack of closely related sequences in the primate

Table 19.1 Human and animal retroviruses

Group	Examples	Comments
Oncoviruses		
Avian leukosis	Rous sarcoma virus	Contains *src*
	Avian myeloblastosis virus	Contains *myb*
	Avian erythroblastosis virus	Contains *erbA* and *erbB*
Mammalian type C	Moloney murine leukemia virus	Causes T-cell lymphoma
	Harvey murine sarcoma virus	Contains *H-ras*
	Abelson murine leukemia virus	Contains *abl*
	Feline leukemia virus	Causes T-cell lymphoma
Mammalian type B	Mouse mammary tumor virus	Causes mammary carcinoma, T-cell lymphoma
Mammalian type D	Mason-Pfizer monkey virus	Immunodeficiency (simian AIDS)
HTLV-BLV	Human T-cell leukemia virus	Causes T-cell lymphoma and neurological disease
	Bovine leukemia virus	Causes lymphosarcoma
Lentivirinae (lentiviruses)		
	Human immunodeficiency virus	Causes human AIDS
	Simian immunodeficiency virus	Causes AIDS in monkeys
	Visna/maedi virus	Causes neurologic and lung disease in sheep
	Equine infectious anemia virus	
	Caprine arthritis-encephalitis virus	
Spumavirinae ("foamy" viruses)	Many human and simian forms	Benign

genome, suggests that a family of exogenous lentiviruses has existed in African nonhuman primates for a long time. HIV-1 and HIV-2 may have started their divergence from a common ancestor in the last 30 to 50 years. Analysis of an African HIV-1 sequence from 1959 suggests that all major HIV-1 types may have evolved from a single introduction into the African population not long before 1959. Now, the primate reservoir of HIV-1 appears to be the chimpanzee *(Pan troglodytes)*, whereas that of HIV-2 is the sooty mangabey *(Cercocebus atys)*. HIV-1 appears to be more easily transmitted to humans than HIV-2 is. SIV infection has been transmitted to humans in laboratory accidents. These individuals become seropositive for SIV but as yet have not developed AIDS symptoms. At present, HIV-1 is accumulating mutations at a high rate as it spreads through the human population.

Clades

As HIV-1 spread to different parts of the world, differences among HIV-1 isolates in properties such as ability to form syncytia in vitro, surface antigens, and genetic sequences have been recognized. To date, 11 HIV-1 subtypes, or "clades," have been identified (A to J and O). Clade A is found primarily in central Africa; clade B in North America and western Europe; clade C in sub-Saharan Africa; clade D in central Africa; clade E (among heterosexuals) and clade B (among intravenous drug abusers) in Thailand; clade G in Russia; clade H in Taiwan and Africa; and clade J in Africa. O refers to "outlier" and has been found in low frequency in African countries. Clade E appears to be more efficiently spread during vaginal intercourse than clade B. Clade C contains only non-syncytium-forming virus (NSI types). Although the presence of clades originally raised the possibility of designing polyvalent vaccines, it appears that cytotoxic T cells raised against viral antigens from different clades of HIV-1 cross-react extensively.

The HIV Genome

Essential features of the genome of the virus and the structure of the virus are presented in Fig. 19.1. In general, a viral protein is cited with a capital first letter (e.g., Tat), whereas the viral gene is cited in lowercase italics *(tat)*. There are three major genetic regions: *gag, pol,* and *env. gag* codes for core structural proteins, *pol* for enzymes (polymerase) required for virus replication, and *env* for surface (envelope) proteins. The *gag, pol,* and *env* genes are common to all retroviruses and have different levels of RNA sequence homology. The term Gag originally referred to "group antigens"—the products of the *gag* region are recognized serologically as specific for different retrovirus groups. The Gag and Pol proteins are found in the inside (core) of the viral particle, whereas Env glycoproteins

Figure 19.1 The HIV genome and its products. The HIV genome, its products, and the structure of the virion are related to the proteins identified by Western blot (see Fig. 19.8). The HIV genome consists of two long terminal repeats (LTR), structural *(gag, pol,* and *env)* regions, and split segments coding for controlling factors. The *gag* region codes for internal structural proteins, including nucleic acid binding proteins (p7 and p9), the major structural protein of the nucleoid (p24), and p17, which covers the inner leaflet of the viral envelope. *pol* codes for reverse transcriptase and other enzymes that are necessary for synthesis, processing, and assembly of virion. *env* codes for the extracellular (gp120) and transmembrane (gp41) glycoproteins of the virion membrane. *vif, rev, tat,* and *nef* code for activating and controlling factors for HIV synthesis (see text).

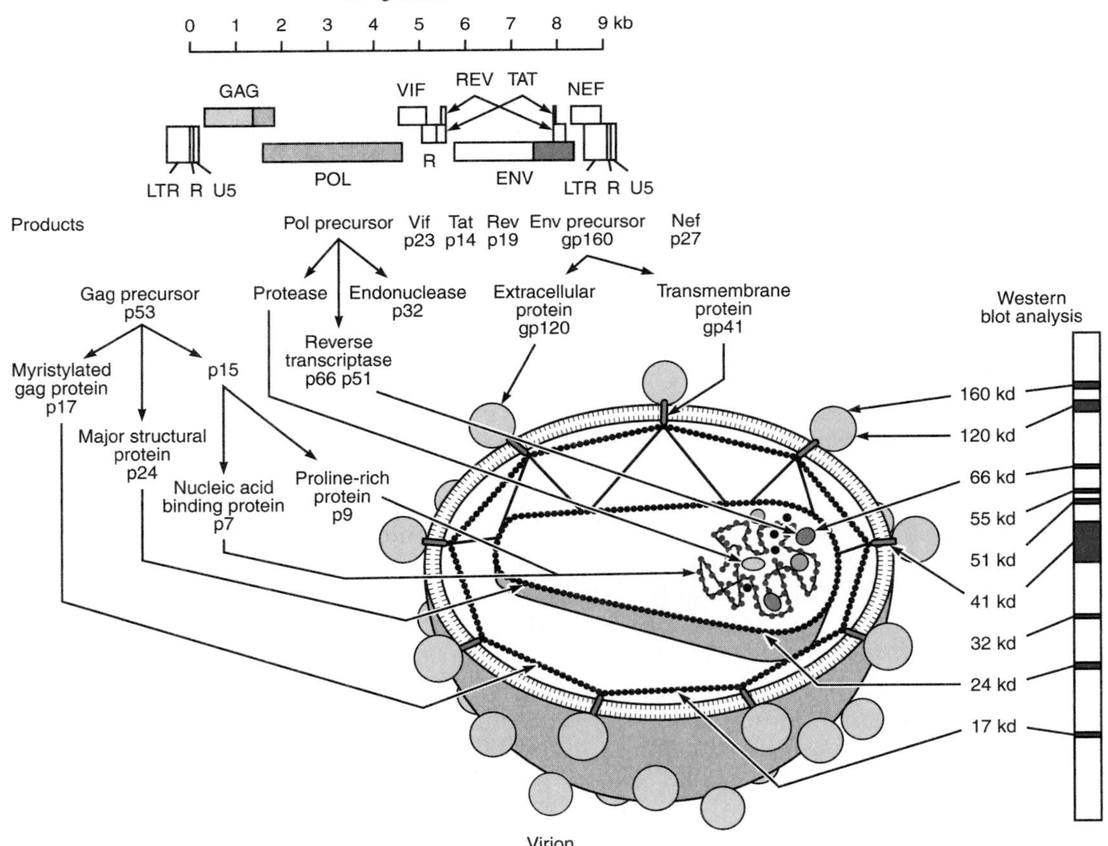

are embedded into or are on the surface of the lipid bilayer of the viral capsid.

The *gag* gene codes for a 53-kDa precursor polypeptide that is cleaved during assembly of the virus by HIV protease to form p24, p7, p9, and p17 proteins. The most abundant Gag protein, p24, is derived from the central portion of p53 and forms the core shell of the virus. p24 is strongly immunogenic during infection, and antibodies to p24 are usually the first seen. p7 and p9 are located in the RNA nucleoid and are derived from a p15 precursor that is cleaved from the carboxyl terminus of p53. p17 comes from the amino terminus of p53 and lines the inner surface of the viral envelope. It appears to serve as a scaffold for the assembly of the viral envelope.

The Pol precursor is cleaved to produce three enzymes that function at different stages of viral replication: RNA-dependent DNA polymerase (reverse transcriptase), endonuclease, and protease. The reverse transcriptase directs DNA synthesis from the genomic RNA strand during early infection. The p32 endonuclease removes the RNA in the RNA-DNA hybrid before the formation of DNA-DNA hybrids. The protease catalyzes processing events during the later stages of viral assembly, cleaving the protein precursors to allow formation of the virus.

The *env* gene codes for a glycosylated precursor of 160 kDa that is cleaved to yield the amino-terminal gp120 and the carboxy-terminal gp41. gp120 becomes located on the external surface of the viral envelope. gp41 has carboxyl-terminal hydrophobic amino acids that form the transmembrane anchor that holds the gp120 external protein by noncovalent interactions. A specific portion of the extracellular gp120 binds to the amino-terminal domains of CD4 molecules on the surface of lymphocytes and monocytes. After binding to CD4, the gp120 is cleaved off by a protease, exposing the underlying gp41. gp41 has amino-terminal residues similar to the fusogenic domain of paramyxoviruses and initiates endocytosis of the virus by fusing to the cell membrane. gp41 may serve to permit infection of cells not expressing CD4 by allowing the virus to fuse with $CD4^-$ cells. Antibodies to gp41 can block the formation of syncytia (fused infected cells in vitro) by HIV.

HIV Replication and Gene Expression

Like other retroviruses, HIV has sets of transactivators and *cis*-acting factors controlling transcription (Table 19.2). The two major products that regulate viral gene expression are Tat and Rev.

Tat

Tat acts as a highly effective transactivator of HIV long terminal repeat (LTR)-dependent transcription by increasing initiation or promoting elongation of transcripts. The two *tat* coding exons are joined by RNA splicing to produce a transcript that encodes the 14-kDa Tat protein. The Tat protein activates transcription by binding to an RNA stem-loop structure called the transactivating response element (TAR), which is located between sequences +19 and +42 in the 5′ LTR. A cellular protein kinase, Cdk9, binds to the activation domain of Tat and can phosphorylate the COOH-terminal domain of RNA polymerase II. The transactivating effects of Tat may cause proliferation of other cells, leading to the lesions of B-cell lymphoma or Kaposi's sarcoma. In addition, T-cell activation factors, such as nuclear factor κB (NF-κB) and nuclear factor of activated T cells (NFAT)

Table 19.2 HIV-activating proteins

Name	Cellular localization	Function
Tat, transactivator (p14)	Nucleus/cytoplasm	*trans*-activator of viral proteins and lymphocytes
Rev, regulator of expression (p18)	Nucleus	Expression of virion proteins
Vif, virion infectivity factor (p23)	Cytoplasm/inner membrane	Determines virus infectivity
Nef, negative factor (p27)	Cytoplasm	Accelerates endocytosis of CD4
Vpu (p16)	Cell membrane protein	Targets CD4 for proteolysis in the cell
Vpr, viral protein R (p16)	In virion	Controls viral replication
Vpx (p16)	In virion	Like Vpr, but expressed in HIV-2

react with sequences in the LTR upstream from TAR after Tat binding to form an activation complex for HIV replication (see below) associated with lymphocyte activation.

Rev

Rev is a 19-kDa protein encoded by RNA sequences which overlap those of *tat* but are in a different reading frame. Rev binds to a *cis*-acting RNA target, the *rev*-responsive region, which is a 204-nucleotide sequence (nucleotides 62 to 265) in the *env* region of HIV. Rev acts posttranscriptionally on HIV RNA transcripts and targets them for nuclear export in concert with a cellular protein called exportin 1.

Vpr

Vpr is an accessory/regulatory protein that delivers viral RNA to the nucleus, inhibits proliferation of HIV-infected cells, causing them to delay for extended periods in the G_2 phase of the cell cycle during which HIV replication takes place, then inducing apoptosis of infected T cells, allowing release of the virus particles. These effects maximize virus production during the short time that infected cells survive in vivo. Vpx is a similar protein found in HIV-2.

Nef

Nef and Vpr act to downregulate expression of cell surface molecules, such as CD4. Nef causes increased endocytosis of CD4, and Vpr targets CD4 to the endoplasmic reticulum and for proteolysis by recruitment into the ubiquitin-proteasome pathway. Downregulation of CD4 in the HIV-infected cell may enhance the ability of *env* to transit to the cell surface and assist in virus release. In addition, Nef induces production of the cytokines macrophage inflammatory proteins 1α and 1β in HIV-infected macrophages. These cytokines serve to attract and activate $CD4^+$ T cells and may contribute to transfer of infective virus from macrophages to T cells. Nef also downregulates expression of major histocompatibility complex (MHC) class I on HIV-1-infected cells and appears to protect infected cells against $CD8^+$ T-cell killing (see below).

The HIV Replicative Cycle

The HIV replicative cycle is depicted in Fig. 19.2. The mature virion forms a sphere with 72 spikes that contain the Env (gp120 and gp41) glycoproteins. The interaction between HIV and the cell surface is shown in Fig. 19.3. A region on the viral envelope gp120 first binds to a domain on CD4 on the lymphocyte surface. This interaction causes a conformational change in the gp120, resulting in binding of another domain on the virus to CCR5 or CXCR4 on the cell surface. Different HIV variants use either CCR5 (R5 variants), CXCR4 (X4 variants), or both (R5/X4 variants). X4 variants form syncytia in vitro (see below) and appear to evolve in vivo from R5 variants. Progression of latent infection to AIDS (see "Natural History of HIV Infection" below) is often associated with a switch from R5 to X4 variants in a given patient, but AIDS can clearly develop without this switch.

A further conformation change then allows a region of the gp41 on the virus to interact with a fusion domain on the cell surface. This is followed

Figure 19.2 The HIV replication cycle. HIV replicates by entering the cell, using reverse transcriptase to synthesize complementary DNA copies of virion RNA, which insert into the host genome and then are used as templates for viral RNA synthesis. The integrated DNA may remain inactive for a long time but will be activated to synthesize viral RNA when the infected cell is stimulated to proliferate by mitogens, antigens, allogeneic cells, or other viral infections through transactivating factors. The newly synthesized viral RNA is then assembled into a nucleoid in the cytoplasm, and the virion is formed during budding from the cell, where the external glycoproteins are added along with host cell membrane structures, such as MHC markers. (Modified from D. D. Ho, R. J. Pomerantz, and J. C. Kaplan, *N. Engl. J. Med.* **317:**278–286, 1987.)

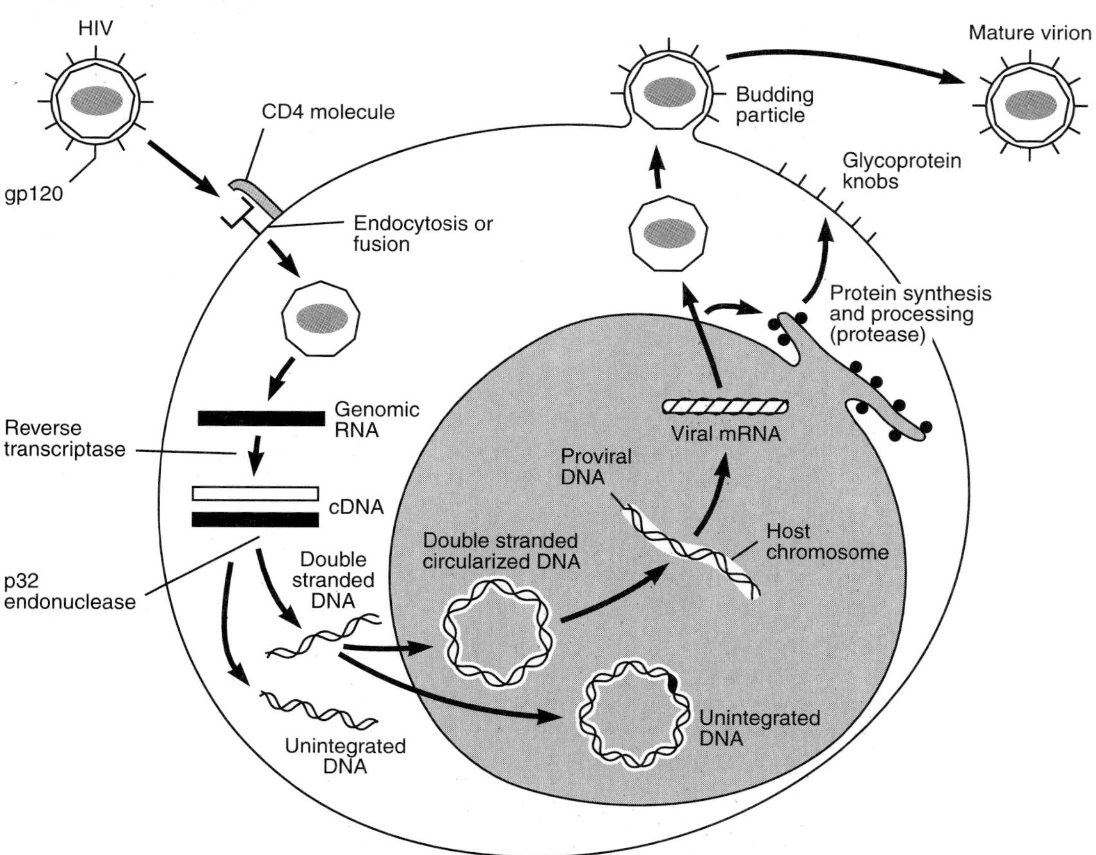

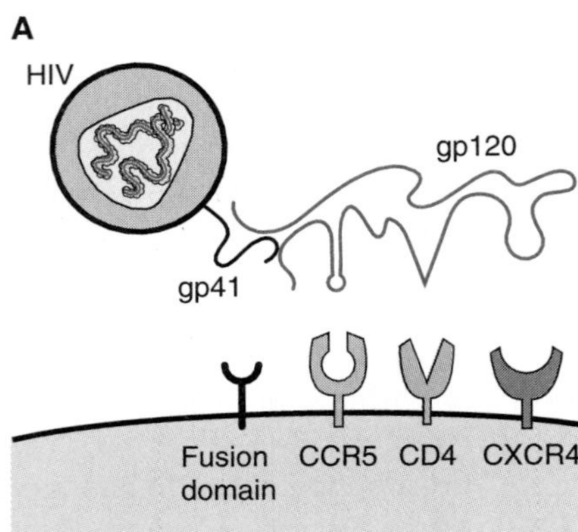

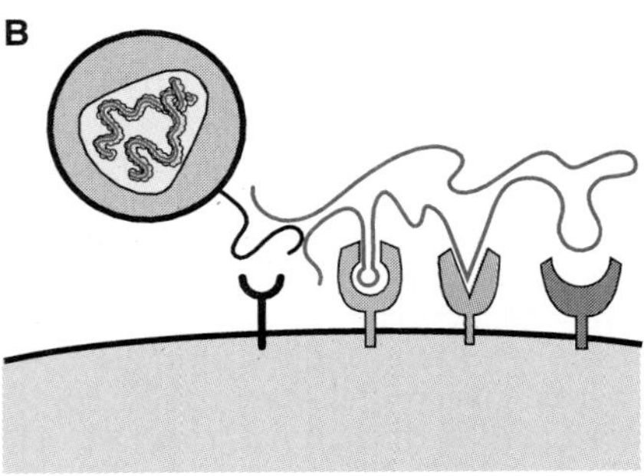

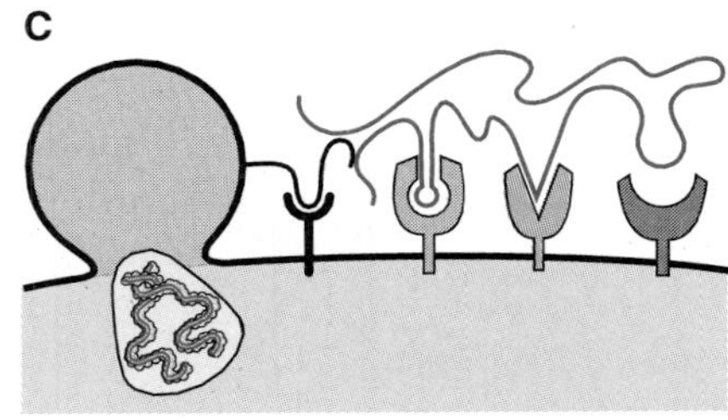

Figure 19.3 Interaction and fusion of HIV with the cell membrane. **(A)** HIV external proteins gp41 and gp120 contain domains that react with receptors on $CD4^+$ cells. **(B)** HIV first reacts with cell surface CD4 through a binding site on gp120. This is followed by conformation changes in gp41/120 that allow interaction with other cell surface receptors, such as the chemokine receptors CXCR5 and CCR5. Some strains of HIV-2 can attach directly to CD4 without chemokine receptor interaction. **(C)** This brings the viral envelope closer to the cell surface, where interaction of a domain on gp41 with a fusion domain on the cell surface results in fusion of the viral capsid with the cell surface membrane, followed by entry of the viral core into the cell cytoplasm. (Modified from J. A. Levy, *HIV and the Pathogenesis of AIDS*, 2nd ed., ASM Press, Washington, D.C., 1998.)

by fusion of the viral and cell surface membranes and release of the viral core into the cell cytoplasm. The virion is uncoated in the cytoplasm, and virion-associated reverse transcriptase produces hybrid RNA/DNA molecules. These are converted to double-stranded linear DNA molecules by HIV endonuclease. The linear HIV DNA is translocated to the nucleus of the infected cell, where covalently closed supercoiled molecules are generated, and the viral DNA is integrated into the host DNA. In the integrated proviral form, HIV may remain latent in infected cells for months or years. Activation of infected cells causes production of host cellular transcription factors that form activation complexes with Tat. This leads to the synthesis of Gag, Pol, and Env precursor polypeptides, which are then assembled into viral particles together with two copies of single-stranded genomic HIV RNA. During budding from the cell, surface proteins, such as MHC molecules, are also incorporated into the viral coat. The final maturation steps, such as cleavage of the Gag and Pol precursor proteins and other posttranslational modifications of viral proteins, occur during the budding process. Acquisition of host proteins in the viral coat produces "pseudotypes" of HIV with different host-derived surface epitopes.

Immune Evasion

A critical factor in the progression of HIV infection is the way that HIV manages to subvert or avoid immune defense mechanisms. These mechanisms will be presented in more detail throughout this chapter. During HIV infection there is continuous production of virus; billions of virions are produced every day. These, in turn, infect and kill billions of $CD4^+$ cells, which must be replaced to maintain immune function. During latency, high titers of antiviral antibodies are produced (up to 5% or more of the total immunoglobulin G [IgG] may be antiviral antibodies), and enormous numbers of $CD8^+$ T-cytotoxic cells (T_{CTL} cells) are produced. How then does the infection eventually evade the immune defense?

Immune Exhaustion

The enormous numbers of HIV virions produced may simply overwhelm the immune system. With the onset of clinical symptoms, there is a decrease in antibody titers and numbers of $CD8^+$ T_{CTL} cells. The war between the immune system and HIV infection may be viewed as a battle of attrition, with HIV eventually outproducing the ability of the immune system to make antibodies and effector cells.

Integration of HIV DNA into $CD4^+$ T Cells

In resting infected cells, HIV RNA has been reverse-transcribed into the DNA of the host cells. In this site, it is not available for reactivity to antibody or T_{CTL} cells. Activation of the dormant infected lymphocytes by immune stimulation will lead to activation of viral reproduction.

Destruction of $CD4^+$ T Cells

$CD4^+$ cells are helper cells for other immune responses and effector cells for delayed-type hypersensitivity (DTH). With the loss of these functions as a result of HIV infection, the immune response to both HIV and other infections is impaired.

Inaccessibility of HIV Surface Antigens

Antibodies that react with soluble HIV gp120 or gp40 may not react with these glycoproteins on the virion. The virion capsid is extensively glycosylated, covering up the potential reactive antigens on the virus.

Incorporation of Host Cell Antigens into the Capsid

On budding from the infected cell surface, the capsid may incorporate host cell surface molecules and in this way mask viral antigens.

Downregulation of MHC

Viral products, such as Nef, decrease expression of MHC class I on infected cells. Since $CD8^+$ cells recognize cell surface antigens complexed with MHC class I molecules, loss of MHC class I results in decreased recognition of HIV-infected cells by $CD8^+$ T_{CTL} cells.

Loss of $CD8^+$ T_{CTL} Cells

Production of $CD8^+$ T_{CTL} cells requires $CD4^+$ T-cell help. With the loss of this help, the numbers of $CD8^+$ T_{CTL} cells decrease.

Loss of Noncytotoxic $CD8^+$ Cells

Perhaps the most important effector mechanism in HIV infection is that mediated by noncytotoxic $CD8^+$ cells. Individuals with high repeated exposure to HIV, who nevertheless do not develop infection, have a strong $CD8^+$ noncytotoxic anti-HIV response. These $CD8^+$ cells inhibit HIV replication in $CD4^+$ cells, without the requirement for MHC class I recognition and without killing the infected cells. Noncytotoxic $CD8^+$ cells produce an antiviral factor (CAF) that suppresses HIV replication at the level of viral transcription by interrupting the ability of Tat or host cellular factor to interact with the HIV LTRs.

AIDS

Epidemiology

Although there is retrospective evidence that the first case of AIDS in the United States was seen in 1968, it is generally accepted that AIDS was first recognized in the United States in June 1981, when the Centers for Disease Control (CDC) published a report of five cases of *Pneumocystis carinii* and Kaposi's sarcoma in young homosexual men. One month later, 26 more cases were reported from New York and Los Angeles. By February 1983, more than 1,000 cases had been reported in the United States. At first, diagnosis and recognition of the disease depended on clinical signs and symptoms. The causative agent, HIV, was isolated from a man with lymphadenopathy in 1983 at the Pasteur Institute. With the identification of HIV and development of laboratory tests for HIV infection (see below), surveillance for AIDS became much more accurate. The incidence of AIDS in the United States essentially doubled every year from 1981 to 1993. The incidence has since slowed; almost 70,000 new cases of AIDS were reported in 1996, slightly less than a 50% increase over that reported in 1993. Now, about 40,000 new cases are expected each year. It is estimated that about 1 million persons in the United States are infected with HIV. Recently, the rate of death from AIDS has decreased because of more effective therapy, and the rate of HIV infection, estimated at about 1 in every 250 individuals, has stabilized. The estimated cost of medical care for these patients is approximately $10 billion. In the last few years, the incidence of HIV infection has soared in other countries, such as China, India, and Korea. The World Health Organization estimates that about 30 million people are infected worldwide and that 8 to 10 times this number will be infected in the coming years. As the rate of infection peaks and starts to decline in Africa, it is increasing exponentially in Asia, where it is projected that there will be up to 1.5 million new adult infections per year.

The origin of the disease AIDS is not clear. HIV appears to have surfaced in central Africa as early as 1959, but the disease was not recognized as endemic there until the late 1970s. HIV may have evolved from a monkey virus (SIV) within the last 30 to 50 years or may have existed unrecognized in isolated areas of central Africa for many years. The rapid mutation rates of the retrovirus family are consistent with either possibility. The evolutionary precursor may have been present for a long time in monkeys, and HIV may be a recent mutation transmitted to humans. On the other hand, the virus may have been present in humans for a long time in limited populations, and the present human epidemic could be a recent event.

A shift in circumstances may have allowed an avirulent HIV strain to mutate into a virulent strain. Opening up areas of endemic infection in Africa by war, tourism, and commercial trucking appears to have greatly increased the spread of HIV infection. The availability of many more susceptible hosts may have allowed more virulent strains of HIV to become established. A virulent organism requires more hosts for perpetuation, because infected individuals survive for relatively short times and are not able to pass the infection to as many other individuals as those infected with avirulent organisms. Confined to an isolated population where no carrier has numerous sex partners, a sexually transmitted organism is better off not producing illness, allowing the host to live and be mildly infective for many years. HIV-2 is now much less virulent than HIV-1. However, if allowed to spread as HIV-1 has, HIV-2 may mutate into more virulent strains.

HIV Transmission

HIV is believed to be transmitted by passage of viable infected blood lymphocytes or macrophages, such as by transfusion of infected blood, by sharing of contaminated needles by intravenous drug users, or by passage of infected lymphocytes or macrophages in semen or cervical secretions during sexual contact through contusions of breaks in the skin or mucous membranes or by direct passage of virus through the mucous membranes of the genital tract. It is estimated that only 1 in 60,000 viral particles is actually infectious. Infected mononuclear cells expressing viable virus may be able to transfer HIV more efficiently, perhaps directly to epithelial cells. However, sexual transmission is increased if the act results in trauma to the skin or mucous membranes, such as is common during anal intercourse, and transmission rates are higher if there is a coexisting genital ulcer disease, such as herpes, syphilis, or chancroid, which cause ulcerative lesions that increase the possibility of passage of infected white blood cells. Maternal-fetal transmission may occur both by transplacental transfer of infected cells from the mother to the fetus and by transmission through nursing via milk containing infected mononuclear cells. Neutralizing antibodies in milk or maternal serum may protect against transmission. Maternal immunization or aggressive chemotherapy may decrease maternal-fetal transmission. Treatment of mothers from the 36th week of pregnancy through 1 week after delivery with zidovudine (AZT) and lamivudine (3TC) reduced the risk of transmission by 50% in a large trial in Africa.

The first cells targeted for HIV infection are either $CD4^+$ lymphocytes or monocytes, in particular, follicular dendritic cells (Fig 19.4), but a wide range of cell types, including many epithelial cells, are susceptible to HIV infection. During early infection, cells of the monocytic series, including macrophages and astrocytes in the brain, dendritic follicular cells in lymph nodes, and Langerhans cells (dendritic macrophages) in the skin, have been shown to contain HIV by in situ hybridization. SIV DNA sequences have been identified in the Langerhans cells in the mucous membranes of the vaginas of monkeys infected via the vaginal route. Infected monocytes may serve as "reservoirs" for HIV and deliver HIV to the brain. In addition, infection may be passed from macrophages to $CD4^+$ lymphocytes during immune stimulation (see below) or to epithelial cells that have internalized infected monocytes. There appears to be a continuous cycle of infection from T cells to macrophages (follicular dendritic cells). Virus is

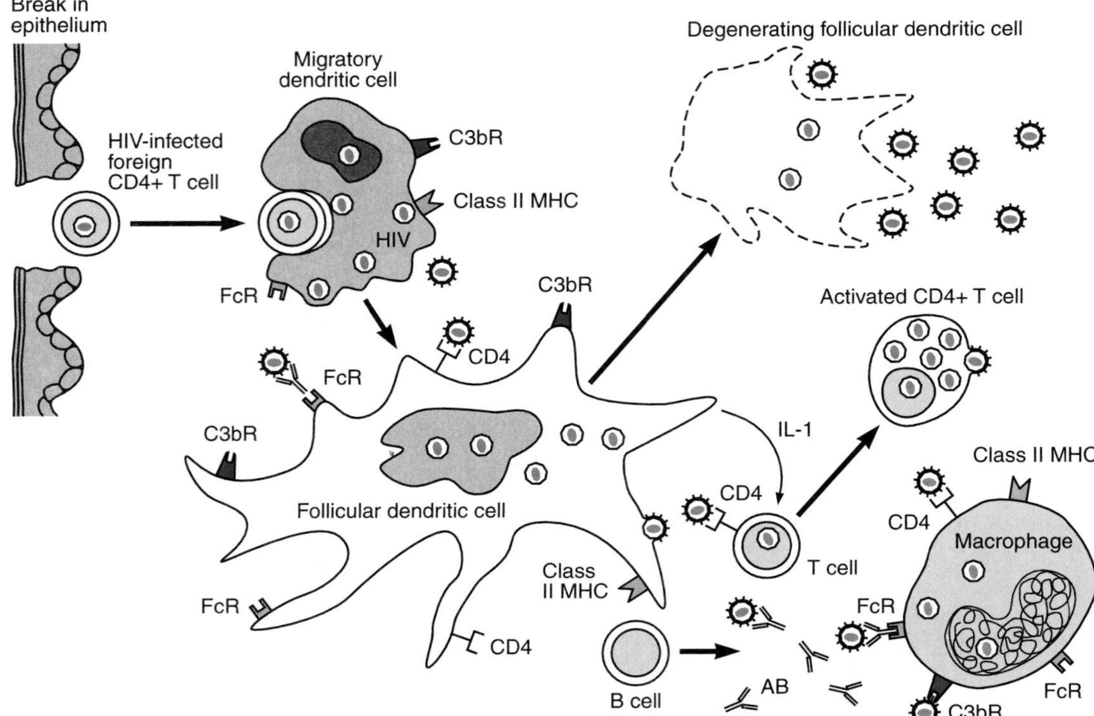

Figure 19.4 Cellular transmission of HIV infection. The most likely means of transmission of HIV infection is through HIV-infected $CD4^+$ peripheral blood lymphocytes that enter the body through breaks in the epithelial surface. The infected $CD4^+$ cells are phagocytosed by migratory dendritic cells, which localize in follicles in draining lymph nodes. The infection is passed from the DNA of the lymphocytes to the DNA of the migratory phagocytic cells. Infection may be increased by the presence of FcR, C3bR, and CD4 on the macrophages. During immune activation, the infection is passed to host $CD4^+$ T-helper cells through class II MHC-antigen receptor interactions. During this process, HIV is passed from dendritic antigen-presenting cells to $CD4^+$ T-helper cells, and stimulation of the infected T-helper cells activates virus production (see Figure 19.6). HIV infection eventually causes disintegration of the lymph node structure by destruction of $CD4^+$ T cells and degeneration of follicular dendritic cells.

passed from the infected monocytes to $CD4^+$ lymphocytes during cell contact and activation. Infected $CD4^+$ lymphocytes produce viruses and die. The released viruses are coated with IgG antibody and transported to the germinal centers, where they are picked up by dendritic macrophages after binding to Fc receptors. The level of detection of HIV infection in blood mononuclear cells does not necessarily reflect the level of infection in the lymph nodes, where the number of viruses per $CD4^+$ T cell may be much higher. In addition, many variants of HIV have now been identified that have different tropism for lymphocytes or macrophages. Monocytotrophic HIV variants produce a higher incidence of brain infection.

Natural History of HIV Infection

Although a number of variations are seen in different patients, a hypothetical course of the natural history of HIV infection is illustrated in Fig. 19.5, and stages of infection are listed in Table 19.3.

Table 19.3 Stages of HIV infection

Stage (duration)	Symptoms and laboratory findings
Acute infection (weeks)	Acute onset of fever, malaise, weakness (similar to influenza symptoms), high levels of virus in blood; serological tests negative; may be elevated $CD8^+$ cells
Asymptomatic (2–10 years)	Serum antibody to HIV antigens detected; no clinical signs or symptoms; declining numbers of $CD4^+$ cells; viral RNA may be detected in blood; may be periodic elevations of virus levels in the blood
Symptomatic (2–3 years)	Fever, weight loss, diarrhea,lymphadenopathy, fatigue, night sweats; HIV antibody, decreased $CD4^+$ T cells, leukopenia, thrombocytopenia, anemia, hypergammaglobulinemia, low mitogen response, decreased DTH skin test reaction
AIDS (<2 years)[a]	Opportunistic infections; $CD4^+$ blood lymphocytes <200/μl

[a]Length of survival after occurrence of opportunistic infections has been considerably extended by chemotherapy.

Acute Infection

Up to 60% of infected individuals experience an acute flulike illness accompanied by swollen lymph nodes and a nonpruritic rash that resolves after a few days or weeks. This most likely represents an acute infection with production of virus that is brought under control by the immune response. Those with acute symptoms generally have a poor prognosis, most likely a result of the severity of the infection. Many infected individuals do not have any symptoms immediately after infection but enter a period of inapparent infection or latency.

Asymptomatic Infection (Pre-AIDS)

There is no symptomatic evidence of disease, but the serologic test, antibody to HIV, is positive. The duration of asymptomatic infection has not yet been clearly documented, but latency may last from 2 to 10 years before progressing to symptomatic AIDS. There is evidence that those individuals who have evidence of HIV infection but respond early with antibody to p24 are less likely to progress to AIDS than those with low anti-p24 levels. In latency, HIV sequences may be detected in lymphoid tissues by using polymerase chain reaction (PCR), and there may be periodic episodes of viremia. In SIV, peripheral blood cells from animals known to be infected but having neither positive laboratory test results (including PCR) nor clinical evidence of infection are able to transfer the disease to naive animals.

Symptomatic Infection

Development of symptoms signals progression to a more severe form of the infection. Clinical manifestations include fever, weight loss, diarrhea, enlarged lymph nodes, fatigue, and night sweats. Laboratory abnormalities include decreased $CD4^+$ lymphocytes, leukopenia, thrombocytopenia, anemia, increased serum immunoglobulins, decreased response of lymphocytes to mitogen stimulation, and absence of reaction to DTH skin tests. Any combination of these manifestations or abnormalities in

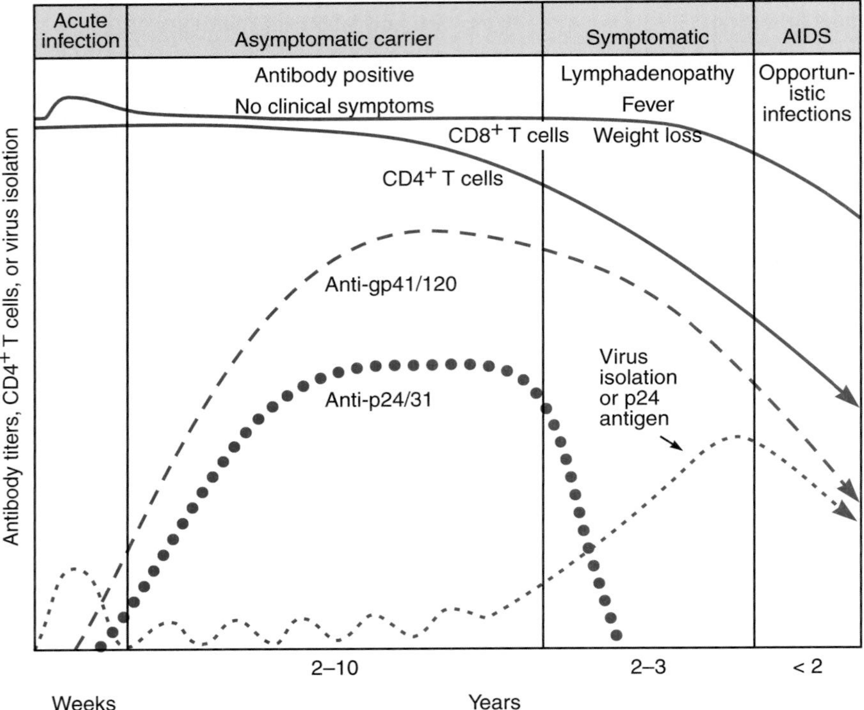

Figure 19.5 Natural history of HIV infection. The course of AIDS may begin with an acute febrile illness, during which there is systemic viral infection and a limited period of viral replication that is checked by an effective immune reaction. This is usually followed by a long latent period, followed by AIDS-related complex (ARC) and then full-blown AIDS, signaled by the diagnosis of an opportunistic infection. During the period of asymptomatic infection, HIV sequences may be detected in cells of the macrophage series in tissues by in situ hybridization, and antibody to HIV antigens, in particular anti-gp41 and anti-p24, can be detected during the asymptomatic latent period by Western blotting. Periodic cycles of HIV production at low levels may occur. Progression to ARC is signaled by development of systemic symptoms (e.g., fever, weight loss, and diarrhea), decreased numbers of $CD4^+$ cells in the blood, lymphadenopathy, appearance of HIV antigen in the blood, and falling titers of anti-p24. $CD8^+$ T cells may rise during the acute infection, then remain at stable levels until they also become depleted, but not to the same extent as $CD4^+$ cells. Once ARC is recognized, progression to symptomatic AIDS may occur in a few months or several years. (Modified from D. P. Bolognesi, *Microbiol. Sci.* **5:**236–241, 1988.)

addition to a positive serologic test for HIV is considered symptomatic infection.

AIDS

The CDC has defined a person with AIDS as any HIV-seropositive person with a $CD4^+$ cell count of $<200/mm^3$. This definition has changed estimates of the time from HIV infection to AIDS and survival time after diagnosis. Previously, AIDS was determined clinically as any time there was a manifestation of an opportunistic infection occurring on the background of other symptoms (Table 19.4). Most of these opportunistic infections are secondary to a defect in DTH. Opportunistic infections of an amazing va-

Table 19.4 Infections associated with AIDS[a]

Organism	Comment
Viruses	
Cytomegalovirus	Found in almost all AIDS patients; encephalitis, pneumonia, hepatitis, colitis, disseminated
Herpes simplex virus	Skin ulcers, persistent and recurrent
Varicella-zoster virus	Local, severe, and disseminated
Epstein-Barr virus	Aggressive B-cell lymphomas, central nervous system lymphomas, intestinal lymphomas
Papillomavirus	Invasive cervical cancer
Human herpesvirus 8	Kaposi's sarcoma
HIV	HIV encephalopathy
Bacteria	
Mycobacterium avium	Disseminated, gastrointestinal; many acid-fast organisms
Mycobacterium tuberculosis	Pulmonary adenitis
Listeria monocytogenes	Bacteremia
Salmonella	Recurrent septicemia
Variable	Recurrent pneumonia
Parasites	
Pneumocystis carinii	Pneumonia, large numbers of organisms
Toxoplasma gondii	Encephalitis, brain abscess
Cryptosporidium spp.	Gastroenteritis, diarrhea
Fungi	
Candida spp.	Oropharyngitis, esophagitis, vaginitis
Cryptococcus neoformans	Disseminated meningitis, pneumonia
Histoplasma capsulatum	Disseminated

[a]Modified and updated from D. Armstrong, J. W. Gold, J. Dryjanski, E. Whimbey, B. Polsky, C. Hawkins, A. E. Brown, E. Bernard, and T. E. Kiehn, *Ann. Intern. Med.* **103:**738–743, 1985.

riety are, in fact, responsible for most of the clinical manifestations of AIDS. More than half of AIDS patients develop *P. carinii* pneumonia, and almost all have oral candidiasis. Cytomegalovirus infection is frequently associated with clinical deterioration, and almost all AIDS patients have rapidly deteriorating courses once opportunistic infection occurs, unless aggressively treated. The prominence of opportunistic infections with organisms that are not usually pathogenic, such as *Mycobacterium avium* and *P. carinii* (in contrast to other organisms, such as staphylococci or streptococci, that are more common pathogens in immunologically normal individuals) is most likely due to the fact that AIDS patients are unable to mount an effective immune response to organisms that are held in check in normal individuals by immune responses, in particular DTH. AIDS patients have a more prominent deficit in cell-mediated immunity than in antibody production and so are more susceptible to infections normally controlled by DTH or T-cell cytotoxicity than to those controlled by humoral antibody. However, the increase in active infections with some classic pathogens in AIDS patients has led to an increase in previously declining diseases, such as syphilis and tuberculosis, in non-AIDS contacts; children of parents with AIDS and tuberculosis are at high risk for contracting tuberculosis.

Cellular Dynamics of HIV Infection

The progression of HIV infection is determined by the relationship of the rate of reproduction of virus to the production of new $CD4^+$ T cells. During latency, it is estimated that about 100 billion new viral particles are being produced every day and about 2 billion $CD4^+$ cells are dying and being regenerated every day. The immune system is unable to regenerate the incredibly large number of $CD4^+$ cells being destroyed by the HIV infection, and the number of $CD4^+$ cells gradually falls. When the level of $CD4^+$ cells falls below $200/mm^3$, the infection has progressed to AIDS. The immune system, through reactivity of $CD8^+$ cells, can hold the infection in check for prolonged periods of time. For example, in neonatal infections, the immune system is able to clear the infection during the first year of life. However, the virus is not cleared, and eventually the immune system is unable to maintain latency. There is some evidence that during active infection, HIV also causes apoptosis of $CD8^+$ T cells by reaction of gp120 from X4 variants of HIV with CXCR4 on $CD8^+$ T cells in association with the presence of tumor necrosis factor (TNF) from activated macrophages. Effective chemotherapy (see below) inhibits reproduction of the virus and allows the $CD4^+$ and $CD8^+$ cell levels to recover by expansion of the peripheral (nonthymic) T-cell population in the gastrointestinal tract. However, a reservoir of infection remains; quiescent $CD4^+$ T cells in effectively treated patients carry proviral DNA, which may be activated if therapy is discontinued or the immune system is activated.

Immune Stimulation and Activation of AIDS

The process of immune activation, which is critical for protection against infection, may, in the case of HIV infection, actually serve to activate expression of HIV and accentuate progression of inapparent infection to AIDS (Fig. 19.6). The interaction of antigen-processing dendritic macrophages with $CD4^+$ T-helper cells during induction of an immune response may serve to transmit virus from HIV-infected dendritic cells to $CD4^+$ T cells through formation of cell-cell interactions. Then, activation of the $CD4^+$ T cells by interleukins produced by macrophages, such as IL-1 and TNF, may stimulate HIV production by activated T cells. In addition to the viral activation factors mentioned above, several cellular transcription factors are also involved in regulating HIV gene expression. The HIV LTR contains binding sites for factors produced by activated T cells, such as NFAT-1, NF-κB, AP-1, SP-1, and the Tat-binding proteins, which can cause large increases in LTR-directed gene expression. These factors interact with Tat at sites on the LTR of the HIV gene, forming a "transcription complex" that stimulates high levels of transcription of the HIV gene and can result in very high levels of viral replication (Fig. 19.7).

Thus, events that lead to activation of T cells, such as stimulation of DTH by mycobacterial infections, may contribute to increased HIV production in latent individuals and to the onset of AIDS-related complex (ARC) or AIDS. In addition, other viruses, including herpesviruses (cytomegalovirus, Epstein-Barr virus, and herpes simplex virus), adenoviruses, hepatitis viruses, and HTLV-1 can transactivate the HIV LTR. Infection with these agents may not only stimulate an immune response leading to immune activation of HIV infection, but also produce cofactors that act synergistically to transactivate HIV gene transcription. The presence of these infectious agents in the patient with activated HIV destruction of $CD4^+$ T-helper cells results in impaired ability of the immune

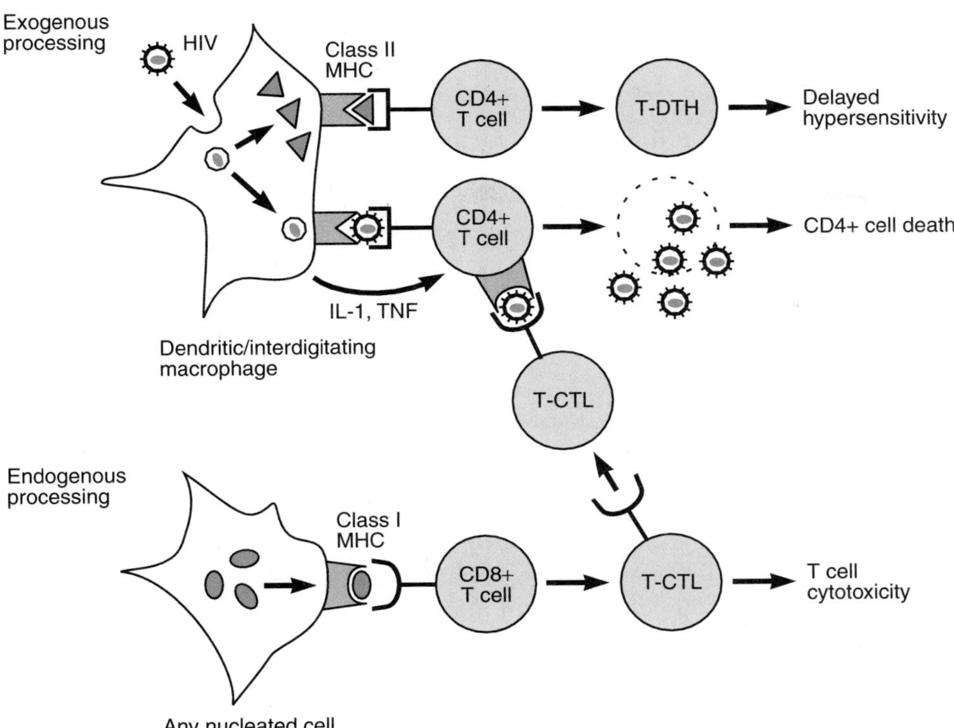

Figure 19.6 Induction of immunity and immune activation of HIV infection. HIV infects antigen-presenting macrophages. HIV antigens are presented to $CD4^+$ T-helper cells through class II MHC (exogenous processing). HIV antigens are also presented to $CD8^+$ T_{CTL} cells through class I MHC (endogenous processing). In addition, $CD4^+$ cells are infected with viable virus through class II MHC and CD4, a receptor for the gp120 surface antigen of HIV.

Figure 19.7 Activation of HIV in stimulated lymphocytes. Stimulation of proliferation of HIV-infected T cells activates production of HIV virions. Nuclear activation factors in stimulated lymphocytes (NF-κB and NFAT) form an activation complex with Tat that promotes HIV messenger RNA (mRNA) synthesis and virion assembly, leading to the death of the HIV-infected cell. The insets show the Tat binding region (TAR) and a model of the activation complex. After RNA transcripts initiate, Tat binds to nascent transcripts at TAR. After this, cellular factors are recruited (?) that enhance transcription and/or elongation of the mRNA.

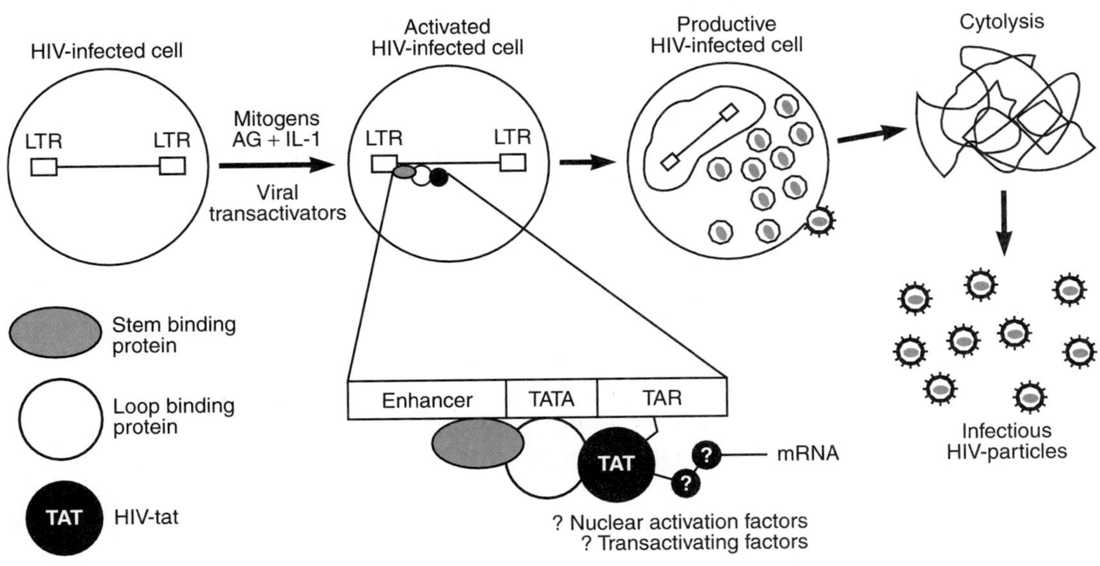

system to combat the infection, further contributing to the pathogenesis of AIDS. Finally, most AIDS patients eventually develop autoantibodies and autoreactive T_{CTL} cells that may contribute to lesions such as orchitis, thrombocytopenic purpura, demyelinating neuritis, and graft-versus-host-like lesions. The occurrence of so many different infections and inflammatory components in the AIDS picture has led some to question if AIDS is actually caused by HIV or if HIV infection is secondary to immunosuppression in multiply infected patients. Similar epidemiologic and pathogenic questions could be raised about other complex diseases. For instance, the same logic that HIV does not cause AIDS has been used to argue, disingenuously, that the tubercle bacillus does not cause tuberculosis.

Laboratory Diagnosis of HIV Infection

The laboratory diagnosis of latent AIDS has depended upon the detection of antibody to HIV in sera from infected patients, but recent advances in detecting HIV or provirus in patients may lead to more accurate and sensitive tests (Table 19.5). More than 130 tests from more than 40 commercial companies are now available for testing for antibodies to human retroviruses. The most widely applied screening test is the enzyme-linked immunosorbent assay (ELISA). This test is very sensitive and easy to do, but there is a problem with false-positive reactions. The initial reaction depends upon antibody binding to plastic beads coated with HIV antigens. Some human sera contain immunoglobulins that bind to these beads nonspecifically or to trace contaminating materials in the beads. Because the HIV antigens are prepared from human cell lines, trace contamination of human MHC antigens may account for some false-positive reactions owing to reactivity of antibodies to MHC antigens found in multiparous women or frequently transfused patients. Second-generation tests using artificially derived recombinant antigens expressed in bacterial or fungal systems or chemically synthesized peptides that are now under evaluation should eliminate these problems.

A positive ELISA is confirmed first by a repeat of the ELISA on a new sample and then by Western blotting. ELISAs for HIV antigen utilize solid-phase anti-HIV on beads or plastic wells to capture HIV antigens. Test serum is added to these plates. After incubation and washing, goat anti-human Ig will bind if there is antibody to HIV in the test serum. Enzyme-labeled anti-goat Ig is added, and the result is read spectrophotometrically after addition of substrate. The Western blot detects antibodies to HIV antigens after electrophoresis of the antigens in a polyacrylamide gel (Fig. 19.8). Although this test is much more specific than the ELISA, there has been considerable variation in its application among different laboratories. However, it is now the accepted standard for HIV diagnosis. Positive interpretation depends on the bands that appear on the nitrocellulose membrane (Table 19.6). The most important bands are p24 (the major structural protein), p31 (endonuclease), and p41 (transmembrane protein) or gp120/gp160 (extracellular protein). Approximately 0.5% of individuals tested by Western blotting will have indeterminate results. The reactivity is usually to only one or more of the HIV-1 core proteins (p17, p24, and p55) and therefore does not meet the definition of a positive specimen or a negative specimen. Approximately 1 to 5% of individuals with indeterminate test results will seroconvert within 6 months. The CDC recommendation is that "a person whose Western blot test results continue to

Table 19.5 Laboratory tests for AIDS

Screening: ELISA for antibody
Confirmation: Western blot
Others:
p24 antigen ELISA
Radioimmunoprecipitation (gp120/160)
Culture in vitro: cytopathic effect
Polymerase chain reaction
Indirect immunofluorescence
In situ hybridization
Prognosis: $CD4^+$ blood lymphocyte count

be consistently indeterminate for at least 6 months—in the absence of any known risk factors, clinical symptoms, or other findings—may be considered to be negative for antibodies to HIV-1."

Some laboratories also carry out in vitro culture assays. These are done by adding the tissue, blood, or other test material to a tissue culture line or mitogen-stimulated freshly prepared human peripheral blood mononuclear cells that will support the growth of HIV. The most useful cells are human T-cell lines transformed by HTLV-1. After several days of incubation, the cultures are assayed for the presence of HIV-produced reverse transcriptase or HIV p24 antigen. Cytopathic effects (syncytium formation and cell death) may also be used to detect HIV infection but are less reliable than the other assays.

PCR can detect extremely small amounts of HIV RNA or integrated DNA. For PCR, oligonucleotide primers containing HIV sequences are added to RNA or DNA extracted from test cells. In the presence of a thermostable DNA polymerase, multiple cycles of replication are controlled automatically to allow rapid and exponential synthesis of new DNA sequences that depend on the presence of HIV RNA or DNA in the original sample. In this way, the RNA or DNA present can be multiplied over 10

Figure 19.8 Western blot test for antibody to HIV proteins. HIV antigens are obtained from tissue culture and electrophoresed in a polyacrylamide slab gel; the separated proteins are transferred to a nitrocellulose membrane, and reaction with antibody is identified by a color reaction after incubation with the patient's serum, followed by peroxidase-labeled goat anti-human Ig. Antibodies reacting with the individual identifiable proteins can be detected. The separated antigens are transferred to a nitrocellulose membrane by electrophoretic blotting, and the blot is cut into strips that are incubated with test and control sera. During incubation, antibodies to HIV antigens will react with the antigens in the blot and can be visualized by addition of peroxidase-labeled anti-human immunoglobulin and enzymatic reaction with a colorless substrate that is converted to color. If antibody binds to the proteins on the nitrocellulose strip, a band of color will appear. In this way, antibodies to the different antigens of HIV can be identified.

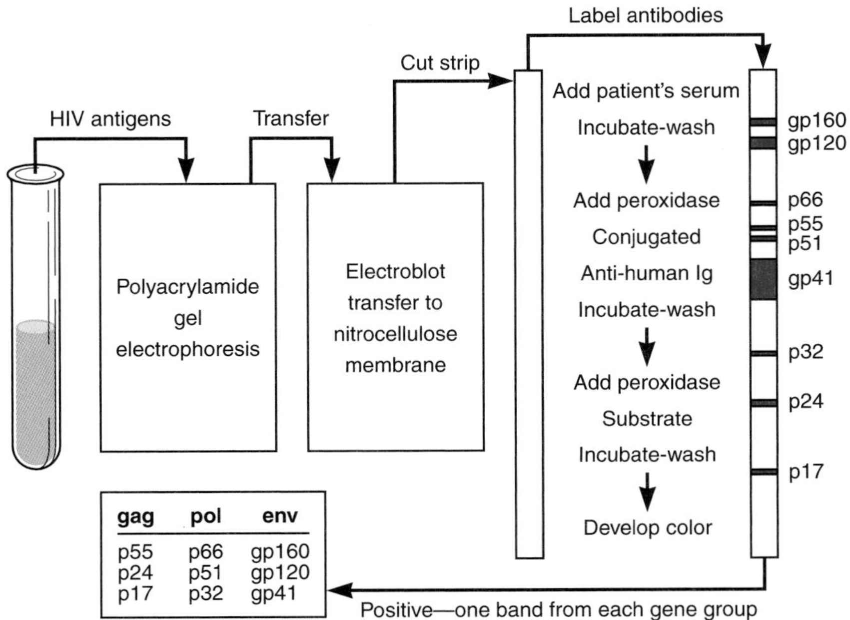

Table 19.6 Interpretive criteria for Western blot tests[a]

Organization	Criterion
American Red Cross	At least one band from each gene product region: *gag, pol,* and *env*
Association of State and Territorial Public Health Laboratories/CDC	Any two of p24, gp41, and gp120/160
Du Pont	p24 and p31 and gp41 or gp120/160

[a]*gag* region = p18, p24, p55; *pol* region = p31, p51, p66; *env* region = gp41, gp120, gp160.

million times in just a few hours. The presence of the expanded nucleotide sequences can then be detected with the appropriate complementary DNA probe. The major problem with the clinical application of PCR is the well-known high risk of false-positive results. Every laboratory with experience in PCR has had this problem at one time or another. Strict guidelines on sample preparation, PCR conditions, and positive and negative controls need to be standardized among different laboratories. When done carefully, PCR can detect HIV-1 proviral sequences directly from infected cells taken from the patient.

In situ hybridization using oligonucleotide probes for HIV sequences may be used to identify cells infected with HIV. Using this technique, HIV has been identified in macrophages and other cells in infected tissue, as well as in lymphocytes. The localization of HIV DNA sequences in dendritic cells in lymphoid follicles has led to the postulate that such cells may serve as a site for chronic "latent" HIV infection.

During 1992, reports appeared of rare cases of clinical AIDS in which no evidence of HIV infection could be detected. In a review by the CDC, 21 persons with unexplained $CD4^+$ lymphocyte depletion below 200 cells/μl but without HIV infection were identified. Five patients who developed opportunistic infections were reviewed in depth. No evidence of clustering or other findings suggesting another, yet unknown virus was found. The condition has been termed "idiopathic $CD4^+$ lymphocytopenia" (see chapter 18).

Immune Dysfunction in AIDS

There are a number of possible mechanisms of immune dysfunction in AIDS that can explain the loss of defense against infections (Table 19.7). The most direct mechanism is the infection and destruction of $CD4^+$ lymphocytes by HIV. The most consistent finding in patients with AIDS is the loss of CD4 lymphocytes. Since CD4 lymphocytes are also helper cells, the loss of this function may cause depressed cellular defenses as well as impaired antibody responses. Other suggested possibilities include the decreased production of $CD4^+$ cells, loss of specific immune responsiveness to infectious agents reflected by the loss of specific lymphocyte proliferation responses to specific antigens of infectious agents, increased T-cell suppressor activity, blocking of T-cell receptors by HIV proteins, nonspecific activation of B cells leading to nonspecific hyperglobulinemia but also to decreased specific antibody production, decreased neutrophils and loss of acute inflammatory reactivity, blocking or destruction of macrophages, as well as autoimmunity to lymphocyte antigens contributing to destruction of $CD4^+$ cells. Decreased hematopoiesis may contribute not only to lymphopenia but also to granulocytopenia, thrombocytopenia, and anemia.

Table 19.7 Immune dysfunctions in AIDS

Infection and destruction of $CD4^+$ helper cells
Interference with production of $CD4^+$ helper cells
Loss of DTH reactivity to antigens of infectious agents
Decreased number and activity of $CD8^+$ cytotoxic cells
Increased T-suppressor activity
Blocking of T-cell receptors by HIV products
Nonspecific activation of B cells leading to hyperglobulinemia and B-cell lymphomas
Decreased specific antibody formation
Decreased neutrophils
Decreased monocytes
Decreased number and function of dendritic cells
"Autoimmune" activation of Fas cell death gene
Increased expression of cell adhesion molecules (CD11/CD18)

The immune dysfunctions seen in an early symptomatic stage, ARC, point to hyperactivation and stimulation of autoimmune reactivity. This suggests some abnormality of immune regulation rather than strictly an immune deficiency through direct destruction of $CD4^+$ cells by HIV infection. These "autoimmune" dysregulatory events may lead to destruction or decreased production of $CD4^+$ cells more typical of the later stages of the disease. The immune abnormalities in early AIDS have been compared to the immunostimulatory phase of graft-versus-host reactions. It now appears that this "autoimmune" destruction of $CD4^+$ cells may be caused by activation of the Fas cell death (apoptosis) gene. HIV-infected $CD4^+$ T cells may actually be protected against cell death by blockade of the Fas gene, and AIDS may be the result of destruction of noninfected $CD4^+$ T cells after activation of Fas in these cells. According to this model, soluble gp120 is released from infected $CD4^+$ cells, reacts with CD4 on uninfected cells, and induces expression of Fas. Reaction of the Fas with FasL on T-cytotoxic cells or with soluble FasL released from activated cells causes the death of the noninfected $CD4^+$ T cell.

Another factor is the increased expression of CD11/CD18 adhesive molecules in HIV-infected lymphocytes and monocytes. The increased adhesive molecules may account for the extravascular accumulation of mononuclear cells in tissues of AIDS patients associated with lesions that are not directly related to immune deficiency, such as myositis, pulmonary dysfunction, and dementia. In any case, the most important clinical manifestations are secondary to an inability to defend against a wide variety of infectious agents that are not usually pathogenic. This secondary immune deficiency is reflected primarily in a loss of delayed-type hypersensitivity mechanisms but also in decreased antibody production.

Pathology and Clinical Staging

Staging

Clinical staging of AIDS using seropositivity, CD4/CD8 lymphocyte ratios, CD4 depletion, and degree of lymphopenia (low white blood cell count), as well as decreasing titers of antibody to p24 and loss of reactivity to DTH skin tests (Fig. 19.5), is useful in predicting when patients can be expected to develop opportunistic infections. The most useful indicators of progressing disease are a $CD4^+$ lymphocyte count below 400/mm^3, falling titer of antibody to p24, and appearance of HIV antigen in the blood. In one study, nearly all deaths occurred in individuals with <50 $CD4^+$ cells/mm^3. Lymphadenopathy appearing in the context of seropositivity is critical for defining transition from latency to early symptomatic AIDS. In fact, the term lymphadenopathy syndrome was used to emphasize this. Loss of DTH skin reactivity to standard test antigens (purified protein derivative, mumps virus, *Candida,* tetanus toxoid, and *Trichophyton*) is an independent predictor of progression to AIDS in persons with HIV infection.

Lymph Nodes

Pathologic examination of the lymph nodes reveals a progression of lesions from hyperplasia to lymphoid depletion. Early in AIDS, lymph nodes show hyperplasia of both nodular and diffuse cortex. This evolves to florid nodular hyperplasia, followed by a mixed pattern of follicular hyperplasia and follicular fragmentation. Generalized lymphocyte depletion is then seen with severe follicular atrophy. HIV proviral sequences may be detected within the follicular dendritic cells by means of radiolabeled RNA during the hyperplastic phase, but little or no HIV RNA is seen after follicular involution with advancing disease. Thus, the follicular dendritic cell may play a critical role in the cellular interactions involved in activation of HIV infection (Fig. 19.4). A number of other infectious agents, such as herpes simplex virus, cytomegalovirus, and mycoplasmas, as well as superantigen activation of T cells, have been implicated in either activation of HIV production or induction of cell death (apoptosis) in T cells. In addition, HIV may trigger a variety of autoimmune reactions, both antibody and auto-T-cytotoxicity to $CD4^+$ T cells, as a result either of shared antigen between the HIV envelope and $CD4^+$ cells or of loss of $CD8^+$ regulatory T cells.

Kaposi's Sarcoma

Kaposi's sarcoma was first described by a Hungarian physician, Moritz Kaposi, in 1872 as a nonaggressive, well-demarcated vascular neoplasm of the lower extremities of older men. A more aggressive disseminated form of the disease, which involves visceral organs as well as skin, was described as a major feature of AIDS cases described in the early 1980s. The tumor is made up of immature blood vessels and would be more appropriately called an angiosarcoma. In 1994, it was found that Kaposi's sarcoma lesions carried an associated human herpesvirus, HHV-8. HHV-8 may be found in otherwise normal individuals, and the incidence of antibodies to HHV-8 increases at the time of puberty. Thus, it appears that latent HHV-8 infection may be activated in AIDS patients, allowing proliferation of infected cells. HHV-8 encodes a constitutively active G-protein-coupled chemokine receptor that induces transformation and angiogenesis, a viral homolog of interleukin-6 (IL-6), and sequences for cyclin D as well as for a *bcl-2*-like sequence.

HIV Encephalopathy

Early in the history of the manifestations of AIDS, neurological dysfunction (AIDS encephalitis) was reported. Clinically, the affected patients manifested cognitive changes, lethargy, social withdrawal, and psychomotor retardation, with marked dementia in the late stages of the illness.

Some affected patients have severe cortical nerve cell loss associated with profound encephalopathy and encephalitis, but many symptomatic patients do not have these lesions. The now classic feature of HIV encephalitis is the development of perivascular multinucleated giant cells in the central nervous system. These cells contain virus particles and are believed to result from a process of syncytia formation of infected monocytes similar to that seen in vitro. In addition, there are nonspecific loose collections of microglial and giant cells (microglial nodules) and diffuse leukoencephalopathy (pallor of the white matter). The only cells in the central nervous system that can be readily demonstrated to contain HIV-1 are monocyte-derived: macrophages, microglial cells, or giant cells. The exact relationship between HIV encephalitis and dementia is not clear. Some people with typical HIV-1-associated dementia have no neuropathological evidence of HIV-1 encephalitis. In addition, no convincing infection of neuroectodermally derived nerve or glial cells has been demonstrated in any AIDS patient. Suggested explanations are that there is sufficient involvement of the subcortex to affect the cortex indirectly, that there are toxic proteins produced by HIV (possibly gp120), or that toxic products are released from HIV-infected macrophages (cytokines, possibly TNF-α). Some patients develop spasticity and leg weakness associated with a spongioform or vacuolar change in the lateral and dorsal columns of the spinal cord (vacuolar myelopathy). AIDS patients may also exhibit a variety of central nervous system symptoms as a result of opportunistic infections as well as lymphoma, vasculitis, and other lesions. Clearly, we have much to learn about the neuropathologic mechanisms in HIV infection.

Opportunistic Infections

At autopsy, the ravages of AIDS are revealed in multiple pathologic changes. Profound depletion of lymphoid organs and lesions caused by various opportunistic infections reflects the severe terminal immunosuppression characteristic of the disease. Prominent infections include necrotizing arteritis and intestinal ulcerations with cytomegalovirus inclusions, enlarged lymph nodes containing macrophages filled with *M. avium,* and pulmonary alveoli filled with *P. carinii.* Also notable are lymphomas, particularly in the brain, and Kaposi's sarcoma involving not only the skin but also many internal organs, such as the lung and gastrointestinal tract. As with lymphomas associated with other immunosuppressive conditions (congenital immune deficiencies, transplantation), most of the tumors are high-grade B-cell lymphomas. It is proposed that ongoing B-cell proliferation, induced by HIV (or Epstein-Barr virus), sets the stage for mutations in oncogenes or tumor suppressor genes, leading to development of monoclonal B-cell lymphomas. The brain may have infection with cytomegalovirus, *Toxoplasma, Cryptococcus,* polyomavirus, *M. avium, Aspergillus,* or other organisms, as well as demyelinating lesions such as those seen in progressive multifocal leukoencephalopathy. Finally, there is an increased incidence of cervical carcinoma as a result of infection with human papillomavirus. The most telling impression from pathologic studies is that essentially any organ of an AIDS patient may be the site of an extensive opportunistic infection.

Therapy

Theoretically, infection with a retrovirus such as HIV could be controlled by interfering with some stage of the life cycle of the virus (Fig. 19.2 and

Table 19.8). In experimental models, all of the approaches listed in Table 19.8 have been tested, but only chemotherapy using reverse transcriptase inhibitors and protease inhibitors has progressed to approved clinical use.

Binding to the Cell Surface

Binding could be inhibited by neutralizing antibodies or by the use of soluble CD4 molecules that might compete with cell surface viral receptors for CD4. The protective effect of neutralizing antibodies is not clear, as there is not a close correlation between the titer of neutralizing antibody and the course of HIV infection, either in humans or in primates immunized with HIV antigens and challenged with HIV. In addition, passive transfer of antibodies has not proved effective and may actually increase infectivity by opsonizing the virus so that it is taken up by macrophages, which then become infected. Soluble CD4 can inhibit infection of tissue culture cells by binding to the gp120 glycoprotein on HIV, which would otherwise bind to the CD4 on the T cell. However, this has not yet been shown to be effective in vivo. A genetically engineered hybrid of CD4 and IgG has been produced in which the two immunoglobulinlike domains of CD4 have been inserted in place of the Fab region of IgG. This molecule is able to bind to the gp120 of HIV and should be able to kill the virus or virus-infected cells by activation of complement or activation of antibody-dependent cell-mediated cytotoxicity. In preliminary studies, the CD4-IgG is able to kill HIV-infected cells but does not kill uninfected cells coated with gp120. Thus, CD4-IgG may be able to eliminate infected cells without contributing to AIDS pathogenesis by killing uninfected cells coated with

Table 19.8 Status of approaches to AIDS therapy

Stage of infection	Potential inhibitor(s)	Status
Binding to cell surface	Neutralizing antibody	Passive transfer not effective
	Soluble CD4	Trials under way
	Dextran sulfate	Active in vitro
Endocytosis or fusion	Antibodies to gp41 fusion domain	Under development
	Receptor CCR5, CXCR4 inhibitors	
Uncoating	Not yet identified	
DNA synthesis	Reverse transcriptase inhibitors, i.e., dideoxynucleosides (ddI)	Partially effective, used in combination with protease inhibitors
DNA circularization	Not yet identified	
Integration into host genome	Not yet identified	Integrase, drugs being developed
HIV mRNA synthesis (Tat or Rev)	Antisense oligonucleotides	Effective in vitro
	Transactivating factor analogs (ribavirin)	
	Transcription inactive retroviral vectors	Effective in vitro
Processing of viral proteins	Glycosylation inhibitors	
Viral RNA packaging	Protease inhibitors	Effective in combination with reverse transcriptase inhibitors
Budding from cell	Glycosylation inhibitors, interferons	May make symptoms worse
Directed to infected cell	Trichosanthin	Experimental trials under way
	Antiviral antibodies (anti-gp120)[a]	
	Anticell antibodies (anti-CD4)	
	Cytotoxic T cells (CD8$^+$ T_{CTL} cells)	

[a]Toxin conjugated to anti-gp120.

gp120. This molecule also has a longer half-life when passively transferred and is able to cross the placenta, allowing the possibility for use in congenital AIDS.

Inhibition of Reverse Transcriptase

The most effective therapy is directed to inhibition of reverse transcriptase (RT) using dideoxynucleosides. The most effective agent, zidovudine (3′-azido-3′-deoxythymidine, formerly azidothymidine [AZT]), is an in vitro inhibitor of RT that can also depress HIV replication in vitro. AZT has proved to be an important palliative agent in all stages of HIV infection. It may produce dramatic improvement, particularly in the neurologic status of AIDS patients with central nervous system signs and symptoms. In mildly symptomatic patients, treatment resulted in 90% event-free survival for 18 months, whereas there was 76% event-free survival in placebo-treated control subjects. Other dideoxynucleotides, such as 2′,3′-dideoxycytidine (ddC) and 2′,3′-dideoxyinosine (ddI), have also been shown to be effective. These compounds are toxic (bone marrow depression) if given for prolonged periods. Currently recommended guidelines for HIV-infected patients are based on $CD4^+$ cell count and clinical features. After diagnosis, therapy is started if CD4 count is $<400/mm^3$. Patients with higher CD4 counts are followed up every 3 to 6 months and treated if their CD4 count falls below 400.

Virus Production and Assembly

Inhibition of virus in vitro has been obtained by using four approaches: antisense oligonucleotides, which interfere with viral RNA production; guanosine analogs, such as ribavirin, which inhibit mRNA production; protease inhibitors, which interfere with later stages of virus assembly; and agents that inhibit glycosylation of viral envelope proteins. Protease inhibitors act at different stages of virus reproduction than RT inhibitors and will synergize with AZT. A third viral enzyme, integrase, is also essential for viral replication. This enzyme has been crystallized, and drugs targeted to this enzyme may also be effective in blocking HIV production.

Combination Therapy

Because the positive effects of treatment with one RT inhibitor were promising but of limited effectiveness, combination therapy using two or three drugs is now being used (Table 19.9). One of the most effective combinations is AZT and 3TC. The effective dose is well tolerated, and the improvement in $CD4^+$ cell counts and virus levels is better than that with either drug alone. In addition, this combination appears to inhibit emergence of drug resistance mutations. 3TC induces a mutation in codon 184 of the viral RT, and this mutation appears to prevent emergence of resistance to AZT by increasing the fidelity of the polymerase.

Even more effective is the combination of AZT and 3TC with a protease inhibitor. Treatment with inhibitors alone results in rapid development of resistant strains, and this effect is greatly decreased by the addition of the RT inhibitors. Such combinations have led to a substantial improvement in survival, but there are many common clinical side effects. A list of the drugs approved by the U.S. Food and Drug Administration for the treatment of AIDS is given in Table 19.9. An example of combination therapy is highly active antiretroviral therapy (HAART; ritonavir or saquinavir plus one or more nucleoside analogs). These combination therapies have

Table 19.9 Licensed drugs for therapy of HIV[a]

Type, approved brand name, and generic name	Combined with:	Times administered/ day	Side effects
RT inhibitors			
Retrovir (AZT)	ddI, ddC, 3TC, protease inhibitors	2 or 3	Anemia, agranulocytosis
Videx (ddI)	AZT, d4T, protease inhibitors	2	Pancreatitis, neuropathy
Hivid (ddC)	AZT, saquinavir	3	Pancreatitis, neuropathy
Zerit (d4T)	ddI, 3TC, nelfinavir	2	Neuropathy
Epivir (3TC)	AZT, d4T, protease inhibitors	2	Fatigue, nausea, headache
Viramune (nevirapine)	AZT, ddI	1 or 2	Transient rash
Rescriptor (delavirdine)	AZT, ddI	3	Transient rash
Protease inhibitors			
Invirase (saquinavir)	AZT, ddC	3	Nausea, diarrhea
Norvir (ritonavir)	AZT, 3TC, ddC	3	Nausea, diarrhea, numbness
Crixivan (indinavir)	AZT, 3TC, ddI	3	Kidney stones
Viracept (nelfinavir)	d4T, AZT, 3TC	3	Diarrhea

[a]Modified from M. Markowitz, *Combination Therapy for HIV Infection,* International Association of Physicians in AIDS Care, Chicago, Ill., 1997; cited by J. A. Levy, *HIV and the Pathogenesis of AIDS,* 2nd ed., p. 342, ASM Press, Washington, D.C., 1998. Abbreviations: AZT, 3′-azido-3′-deoxythymidine (zidovudine); ddI, 2′,3′-dideoxyinosine (didanosine); ddC, 2′3′-dideoxycytidine (zalcitabine); 3TC, 2′-deoxy-3′-thiothiadine (lamivudine); d4T, 2′3′-didehydro-3′-deoxythymidine (stavudine).

been very effective in increasing the production of $CD4^+$ T cells and prolonging symptom-free life for AIDS patients but are not curative.

The major reason for the failure to cure AIDS lies in the natural history of the infection and the relationship of the reproduction of the virus to the proliferation of the major host cells, $CD4^+$ T cells (see above). Therapy is effective only when the virus is reproducing in activated $CD4^+$ cells. Resting infected $CD4^+$ cells contain HIV DNA integrated into the host genome. This is not accessible to treatment. Replication-competent HIV can be obtained after activation of $CD4^+$ lymphocytes from patients who have had prolonged suppression of plasma viremia. Since aggressive treatment has serious side effects, causes a major alteration in lifestyle, and is very expensive, it is unfortunate that once started it is essentially impossible to stop. Even when the infection has been held in check, discontinuation of the therapy is inevitably associated with relapse, because the virus cannot be eradicated by this approach.

Immune Reconstitution

Attempts to reconstitute AIDS patients by transfer of immune-competent cells, thymus replacement, or immune serum have not been successful, even when there are identical twins as donor and recipient. Biological response modifiers, such as IL-2, IL-10, IL-12, and gamma interferon, as well as the drugs cyclosporin, levamisole, and thymopoietin, have also not been effective when given individually. Recently, a large clinical trial, estimated to cost $43 million, has been approved to add IL-2 to the drug therapy regimens. In small-scale studies, IL-2 has been shown to raise $CD4^+$ cell levels in patients undergoing combined chemotherapy.

Opportunistic Infections

Treatment of the opportunistic infections in AIDS patients may also be effective. For instance, acyclovir may slow the progression of cytomegalovirus, and amphotericin B is effective against cryptococcal infections. Aerosolized pentamidine has been effective in prevention of *P. carinii* pneumonia.

Animal Models

There is a critical need for the development of more useful animal models, particularly those addressing the question of therapy of, and a vaccine for, AIDS. A listing of the most relevant animal models is given in Table 19.10. Thought by many to be the most promising animal model for AIDS is SIV in macaques (SIVmac). SIVmac is carried without symptoms in African green monkeys *(Cercopithecus* spp.) and sooty mangabeys *(Cercocebus atys)* but produces an AIDS-like illness in Asian macaques *(Macaca mulatta).* SIV does not seem to inhibit the functions of lymphocytes in African green monkeys and induces a very weak immune response. Combined HIV-SIV chimeric viruses infect macaques or cynomolgus monkeys.

The course of infection with HIV in chimpanzees appears to be similar to that of latent AIDS in humans. Chimpanzees have humoral and cellular responses similar to those of humans and contain $CD4^+$ T cells, but they do not manifest AIDS-like symptoms when infected with HIV. The chimpanzee model may be used for vaccination trials to determine if a vaccine can prevent infection, but not for pathogenesis or therapy. Interestingly, the rabbit appears to have a response to HIV infection very similar to that of the chimpanzee, but even though rabbit studies would be much less expensive than studies in chimpanzees, support for the rabbit model has not been forthcoming.

Mouse models are useful for studies of pathogenesis, but not for vaccine development. Several transgenic mouse models for AIDS studies have been established. One line contains complete copies of HIV genes. After

Table 19.10 Animal models for AIDS

Species	Agent	Result	Use
Experimentally occurring			
Chimpanzees	HIV-1	Latent infection	Vaccine testing
Macaques	SIV	Wasting disease, AIDS-like	Vaccine testing, therapy, pathogenesis
Rabbits	HIV	Defective infection	Latent infection
Mice	Transgenic (complete)	AIDS-like disease	
	Transgenic *(tat)*	Kaposi's sarcoma	Pathogenesis
	SCID-human	AIDS-like disease	Therapy
	Lymphoid cell chimera		
Naturally occurring			
Sheep	Visna virus	Chronic neurodegeneration	Pathogenesis
Goats	Caprine arthritis-encephalitis virus	Chronic arthritis	Pathogenesis
Horses	Equine infectious anemia virus	Hemolytic anemia	Pathogenesis

one of the founder transgenic mice was bred with nontransgenic animals, the F_1 progeny that contained the HIV transgene developed an AIDS-like syndrome. Another transgenic mouse line containing the HIV *tat* gene develops fibroblastic tumors similar to Kaposi's sarcomas. A different mouse model has been produced by transfer of human fetal thymus, liver, and lymph node cells to SCID mice, which allows the proliferation of $CD4^+$ and $CD8^+$ human T cells as well as production of human Ig. In situ hybridization has revealed the presence of HIV-infected cells in the thymus and lymph nodes of these mice. A similar model has been produced by injection of SCID mice with human blood lymphocytes. These mice develop wasting disease and severe lymphoid atrophy, and most die 6 to 8 weeks after infection with HIV. Finally, *bg/nu/xid* mice injected with human bone marrow serve as a host system for human cells of macrophage lineage. Each of these models has great promise in the study of certain aspects of AIDS infection, but considerable care will need to be taken in extrapolating any results on pathogenesis to the human situation. An additional model used to study pathogenesis, therapy, and vaccination is the related murine leukemia virus (MuLV) infection of mice, which has some features in common with human HIV infection but is clearly different.

Vaccination against HIV Infection

Vaccines in Experimental Models

Development of an effective vaccine requires identification of a potential vaccine and design of an effective immunizing strategy. This process requires extensive testing in an experimental model. Unfortunately, none of the experimental models listed above is well suited to this type of testing. A listing of some of the putative immunogens and adjuvants is given in Table 19.11. From what is known about animal retroviruses, such as feline leukemia virus (FeLV), it should be possible to immunize against HIV infection. Although there are conflicting reports regarding effectiveness, a vaccine for FeLV has been prepared from polypeptides shed from FeLV-infected tumor cell lines. This vaccine contains the gp70/85 surface polypeptide of FeLV.

Inactivated virus. Experimental trials with chemically inactivated HIV have not provided convincing or consistent evidence of protection. Infection of chimpanzees with inactivated whole virus has resulted in some protective effects, but the vaccines have been shown to contain human antigens from the cell lines used to prepare the virus, and the response of the chimpanzees to immunization with human cells alone was also protective. Chimpanzees "vaccinated" with normal human blood cells were resistant to challenge with HIV grown in human cells. Purified HIV grown in human cell lines contain HLA antigens. These results are interpreted to show that HIV grown in human cells will acquire human antigens in the viral envelope (pseudotypes) and that an immune response in the chimpanzees to the human antigens is responsible.

Genetically modified virus. The most successful experimental vaccine is a genetically modified SIV with a deletion in the *nef* region. Monkeys vaccinated with this "weakened" form of SIV were healthy for over 3 years and had low virus levels and normal $CD4^+$ lymphocyte counts. Vaccinated monkeys were resistant to challenge with high doses of fully infectious SIV that were fatal to nonvaccinated control monkeys. Because this "immunization" is essentially inducing an infection with a low virulence form of the virus, there are many reservations that would have to be overcome before such an approach would be applicable to humans. First, it would not seem to be a good idea to intentionally infect humans with a viable virus that might cause infection, and second, if an individual is already infected with a virulent form of the virus, superinfection with a less virulent form may not provide any beneficial effect. In fact, in one study using modified SIV in rhesus monkeys, 4 of 18 monkeys developed active infections.

Hypervariable regions of gp120 appear to be the most likely candidates to provide immunogenic peptides (Fig. 19.9). This major surface molecule of HIV contains five hypervariable regions. Of these, a segment in the third region from 315 to 329 is not only the immunodominant region with which neutralizing antibody reacts but also the site of epitopes that stimulate transformation of sensitized lymphocytes as well as an active site for $CD8^+$ T-cytotoxic lymphocytes. In addition, the amphipathicity of different regions of gp120 has been analyzed to find potential amphipathic alpha-helical domains that might be selectively immunogenic for $CD8^+$ T_{CTL} cells. Three T-cell-stimulating regions are amino acid (aa) residues 428 to 443, gp120 (EnvT1); aa residues 112 to 124, gp120 (EnvT2); and aa residues 834 to 848, gp160 (EnvT4) of the Env region. Of particular interest is EnvT1, because it contains the CD4 binding site. Immunization of healthy volunteers with these peptides in alum resulted in stronger in vitro responses of T cells as measured by IL-2 production after exposure to antigen than what was found in T cells from infected patients. In fact, in naturally infected individuals, only 62% demonstrated T-cell recognition of p24, 18% recognized gp160, and 23% recognized gp120. It is possible that some of these peptides, individually or in combination, might not only provide a protective vaccine but might also stimulate T-cell responses in already infected individuals (vaccine therapy). In one study, immunization with a candidate gp160 vaccine resulted in new humoral (antibodies to different epitopes) and cellular (T-cell proliferation) responses in 19 of 30 HIV-infected individuals, and booster effects were noted on repeated immunizations. Thus, postinfection immunization is effective in increasing the immune response to HIV; it is not yet known if this has a beneficial effect on the course of infection.

One of the more effective immunization strategies in experimental models has been to immunize with recombinant viral vectors expressing HIV proteins and boosting with recombinant proteins (Table 19.12). However, this approach has produced only partial protection from infection in very small numbers of animals.

DNA vaccines have been shown to be effective in chimpanzees. An HIV-1 vaccine encoding *env, rev,* and *gag/pol* induced cellular and humoral immune responses, and the vaccinated animals were resistant to challenge infection.

Table 19.11 Possible approaches to an AIDS vaccine

Antigens
Whole inactivated HIV
Formalin
Genetically modified virus
Avirulent deletions
Alphaviruses
Recombinant DNA products
gp120
gp160
Peptides
V3 loop (gp120)
CD4 receptor (gp120)
Anti-idiotypes
Experimental
Passive antibody or sensitized T cells
DNA gene transfer
Plant-derived proteins
Carriers
For T cytotoxicity
ISCOMs
Vaccinia virus vectors
DNA transfection
For DTH
Freund's adjuvant
Muramyl dipeptide
BCG vectors

Immunization Protocols

Selection of immunization protocols for the desired type of immune response may be critical. Although there is still much to be known about the role of different immune responses in defense against AIDS, it seems likely that the most desired response is T cytotoxicity. However, there is a paradox, in that immune products may increase, as well as inhibit, the progression of HIV infection (Fig. 19.10). Immunization protocols that

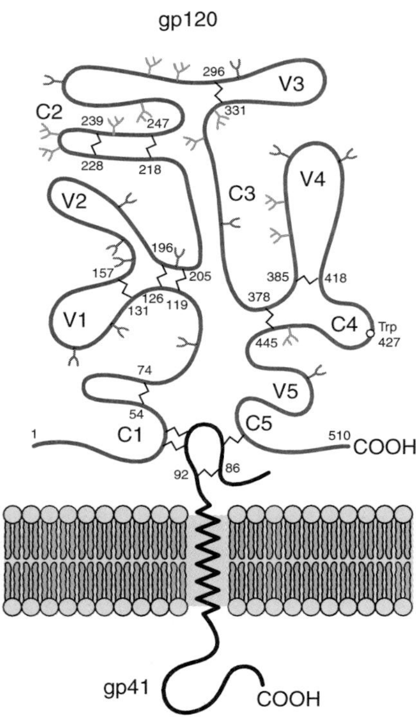

Figure 19.9 Epitope map for Env. Hypervariable regions of gp120 appear to be the most likely candidates to provide immunogenic peptides. There are five of these regions, marked V1 to V5. Of these, a segment in the third region from aa 325 to 329 (EnvT3) is not only the immunodominant region with which neutralizing antibody reacts but also the site of one of the epitopes that stimulate proliferation of reactive lymphocytes, as well as a reactive site for $CD8^+$ T-cytotoxic lymphocytes. There are three other T-cell-activating regions: aa 428 to 443 (EnvT1); aa 112 to 124 (EnvT2), and aa 834 to 848 (EnvT4). Of particular importance is EnvT1, because it also contains the CD4 binding site. Immunization of healthy volunteers with these peptides in alum induces in vitro responses measured by IL-2 production on exposure of peripheral blood lymphocytes to the peptide. (Modified from the NIH HIV epitope map and from D. F. Nixon, K. Broliden, G. Ogg, and P.-A. Broliden, *Immunology* **76:**515–534, 1992.) Gray forked symbols indicate complex-type oligosaccharides; blue-green ones represent mannose-rich oligosaccharides.

may specifically induce $CD8^+$ T_{CTL} cells include immunostimulatory complexes (ISCOMs), vaccinia virus vectors, and DNA transfection. Key to induction of T_{CTL} cells is endogenous antigen presentation by class I MHC^+ cells. Most immunization protocols involve nonliving antigens that are processed by the endosomal system (exogenous processing). This processing usually leads to production of humoral antibodies and $CD4^+$ MHC class II-restricted T-helper or T-cytotoxic cells. Organisms, such as viruses or malaria protozoa, that live within epithelial cells produce antigens that are not processed by the exogenous endosomal system (endogenous processing) and induce $CD8^+$ class I-restricted T_{CTL} cells. ISCOMs, vaccinia virus vectors, and DNA transfection are able to deliver amphipathic peptides to class I MHC molecules for endogenous antigen processing. ISCOMs are stable matrix structures produced by incorporation of protein or peptide antigens into an adjuvant glycoside. ISCOMs are processed during an immune response like an endogenous antigen in which the antigen is presented in association with class I MHC. Thus, ISCOMs could direct the immunodominant gp120 peptide to induction of an immune effector cell that will prove to be selectively protective rather than pathogenic. Vaccinia virus vectors will infect epithelial cells and present antigen endogenously, and transfection of epithelial cells with DNA that produces peptide antigens will also lead to endogenous presentation.

Problems in Vaccination against HIV

Major problems in inducing a protective immune response to HIV infection are (i) the intracellular location of the viral DNA in a provirus form, (ii) variations in the antigen expression of HIV, and (iii) stimulation of nonprotective, immunopathologic immune responses.

Table 19.12 Recombinant HIV vaccine prime-and-boost strategy

Virus	Primary immunization	Secondary immunization	Animal tested
HIV-1	Vaccinia virus gp120	rpg160	Chimpanzee
SIV	Vaccinia virus gp130	rgp130	Rhesus monkey
SIV	Vaccinia virus gp160	rgp160	Rhesus monkey
SIV	Vaccinia virus gp160	Gag	Rhesus monkey
HIV-2	Canarypox virus gp120	rgp120 or V3 peptide	Cynomolgus monkey
HIV-2	Canarypox virus gp120	rgp120	Rhesus monkey
HIV-2	Canarypox virus gp120, Gag, Pol	rgp160	Rhesus monkey

Intracellular location. Because of the intracellular location of HIV and the integration of HIV DNA into the host genome, it may not be possible to produce immunity that will prevent transmission by HIV-infected cells, because these cells may not express HIV antigens on the cell surface. Such infected cells might be able to infect the recipient's cells by direct interaction and fusion with uninfected cells, even in the presence of an immune response to the virus.

Antigenic modulation of HIV during infection. HIV is highly mutable, most likely because of inaccuracy in reverse transcriptase. This results in a single predominant virus genotype in an infected individual with multiple related minor variants of the virus in the same individual (Fig. 19.11). Most of the variants express minor differences in the gp120 membrane glycoprotein, which could be important immunologically or biologically. The "evolution" of variants could allow HIV to shift antigenicity and avoid attack by specific antibodies or change the nature of the infectivity by producing variants with different trophism for lymphocytes or monocytes and different abilities to infect the brain. Single amino acid substitutions in the V3 hypervariable region of gp120 may eliminate reactivity with specific neutralizing antibody or T_{CTL} cells. It is postulated that the slow rise in antigenic diversity of HIV during an infection results in a level of diversity that eventually cannot be controlled by the immune system. This model predicts that antigenic diversity is a major factor that drives disease progression, enabling the virus to escape from control by the immune response.

Inappropriate immune response. The effect of immunization may actually enhance immune defects in AIDS patients (Fig. 19.10). On the one hand, antibody may neutralize virus in vitro but provide aggregated Fcs that facilitate binding and uptake of virus by macrophages. Cytotoxic T cells may hold the infection in check by killing HIV-infected cells. On the other hand, specific T_{CTL} cells may mediate depletion of $CD4^+$ cells in AIDS patients. $CD4^+$ T cells are killed by gp120 *env*-specific killer cells in vitro that recognize class II MHC markers in the context of gp120 on activated $CD4^+$ T cells. Thus, immunization against gp120 may actually contribute to the immune deficiency of AIDS by activating an autoimmune mechanism that selectively kills $CD4^+$ lymphocytes. Delayed-type hypersensitivity to HIV may activate macrophages to destroy HIV in their cytoplasm, but coactivation of macrophages and infected $CD4^+$ T_{DTH} cells may result in stimulation of virus proliferation in activated $CD4^+$ infected cells.

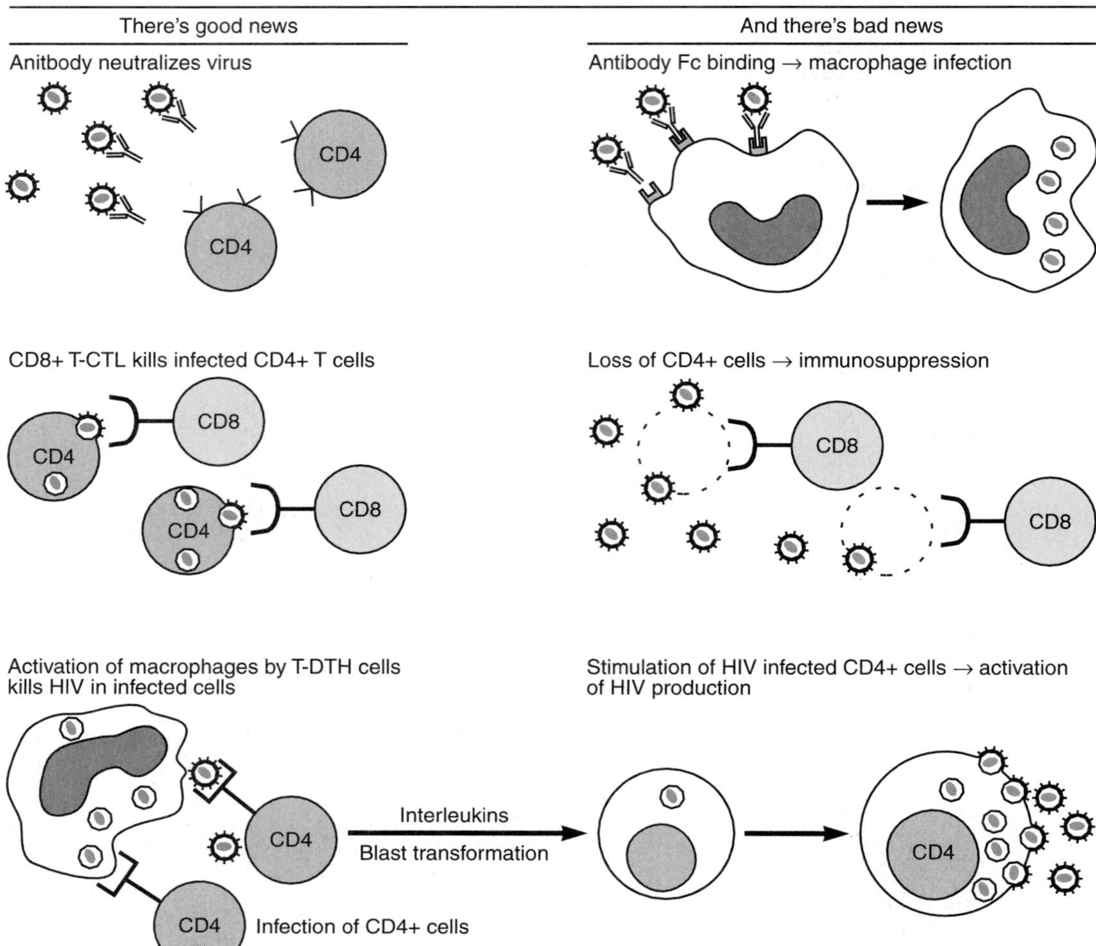

Figure 19.10 Vaccination against HIV: a paradox. Antibody to HIV may neutralize the virus (block infection) or increase infectivity by providing aggregated Fcs or binding of C3b that increases adherence and infection of macrophages. $CD8^+$ T_{CTL} cells limit infection by killing virus-infected cells but also reduce the number of CD4 T-helper cells and produce immunosuppression. DTH reactions can activate macrophages to kill intracellular viruses but also stimulate HIV production in infected cells.

Human trials. Although prevention is the ultimate goal of vaccination, realistically, human vaccine trials may be effective as therapy and not for prevention. It may not be possible to prevent HIV infection by vaccination, but the immune system may be activated to hold the infection in check. Although no experimental model has proved consistently effective in protection, the need to produce some type of human vaccine has driven stage I and II clinical trials. These have shown that vaccines can induce humoral and cellular immunity to HIV. Stage I clinical trials using recombinant gp160 (VaxSyn HIV-1) or gp120 or proteins purified from cultures of lepidopteran cells infected with recombinant baculovirus have been without serious side effects and induced antibody and some cellular responses to laboratory strains of HIV-1. Immunization with recombinant vaccinia virus/*env* vector followed by boosting with gp120 induced much higher T-cell responses in

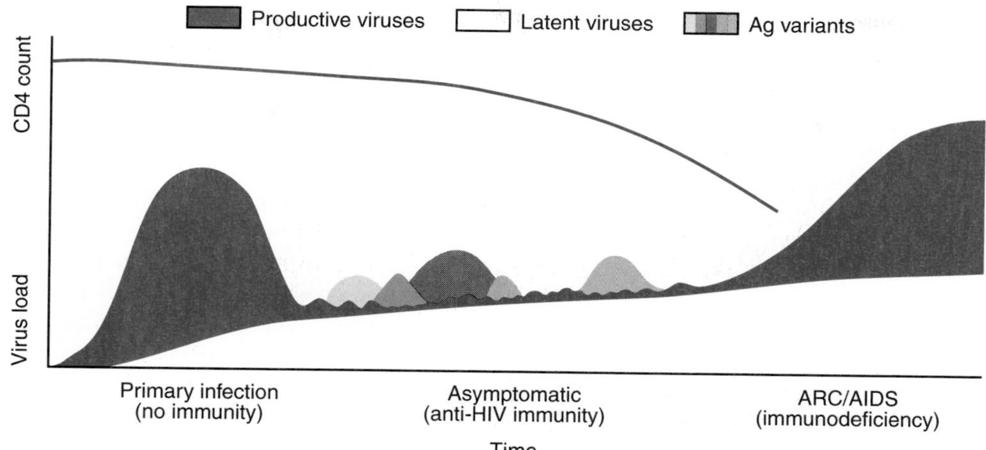

Figure 19.11 HIV vaccination and viral evolution. In natural infection, at the end of the asymptomatic stage, a wave of wild-type virus replication may occur in the absence of immunity, leading to the asymptomatic stage. Then specific immunity controls viral replication as new antigenic variants emerge. With development of ARC and AIDS, specific immunity is lost, and the viral load increases rapidly. (From P. Sonigo, M. Girard, and D. Dormont, *Immunol. Today* **11**:465, 1990.)

seronegative human volunteers than in subjects receiving either vaccine alone. In another trial, using muramyl tripeptide phosphatidylethanolamine containing glycosylated gp120, high levels of neutralizing antibodies and cellular responses were obtained. In addition, a low dose of canarypox virus expressing an envelopelike protein induced T_{CTL}-cell activity in seronegative volunteers. However, no study has yet been able to demonstrate protection against infection. In fact, some volunteers immunized with gp160- or gp120-based vaccines have subsequently become infected with HIV-1, suggesting that these vaccines are not protective even when neutralizing antibody is produced. Even so, large-scale trails of these vaccines are now being conducted in Thailand and Africa. One direction of these trials will focus on the effectiveness of active immunization on prevention of transmission of HIV from mother to child. It is predicted that at least 50% of pediatric AIDS cases may be prevented if this approach is successful.

Summary

AIDS is a secondary immunodeficiency caused by infection with a human retrovirus, HIV. The virus selectively infects and destroys $CD4^+$ T-helper lymphocytes. This results in a loss of T-cell function and a severe immunodeficiency manifested by fatal opportunistic infections by infectious agents that are not pathogenic for individuals with normal immune systems. HIV appears to infect selected cells in the macrophage lineage, such as glial cells, dendritic follicular cells, and Langerhans cells in the skin. The virus is able to persist in these cells for long periods of time and deliver the infection to $CD4^+$ T cells with immune stimulation. The surface of the virus contains molecules that bind to $CD4^+$ markers on $CD4^+$ T cells. The virus then enters the cell by fusion or endocytosis. Once in the cell, the RNA core of the virus unravels, and complementary DNA is synthesized by reverse transcriptase. The DNA enters the nucleus, where it integrates into the host DNA as a provirus. The virus may remain latent in this form for many years. Asymptomatic infection is indicated by the production of circulating antibody to HIV core (p24 or p31) and surface (gp41 or gp120) antigens. After a latent period of 2 to 10 years, disease appears in most infected individuals. However, 3 to 5% of infected people remain asymptomatic for much longer periods, indicating that survival with HIV infection may be possible. There are now individuals who are asymptomatic for over 22 years with no symptoms and normal $CD4^+$ cell counts and low viral loads. Activation of productive infection appears to result from immune stimulation, leading to activation of infected T cells by IL-1 and TNF produced by activated macrophages. This in turn leads to synthesis of activation products of T cells (NFAT and NF-κB), which form a "transcription complex" that greatly increases HIV gene transcription.

Progress of the disease is heralded by the onset of symptoms. The major features of symptomatic HIV infection are the presence of antibodies to HIV, lymphadenopathy, a decrease in the numbers of $CD4^+$ lymphocytes in the blood, and symptoms of systemic disease, including fever, diarrhea, weight loss, and night sweats. The CDC has defined AIDS as evidence of HIV infection (seropositive) associated with CD4 cell counts of $<200/mm^3$. True AIDS occurs when an opportunistic infection is diagnosed on the ARC background. Among the most important of such agents are *P. carinii,* cytomegalovirus, *M. avium,* herpes simplex virus, and *Candida albicans,* although there are many others. In addition, other infectious agents, such as *Mycobacterium tuberculosis* and *Treponema pallidum,* may be transmitted to non-HIV-infected individuals. A number of immune abnormalities occur in AIDS patients, suggesting an immune-related pathogenesis that is much more complex than simply HIV destruction of T-helper cells. These abnormalities include the production of antiantibodies and autoreactive T-killer cells leading to lymphopenia, thrombocytopenia, granulopenia, and anemia, and a stage of hyperplasia of lymphoid tissue followed by lymphoid organ depletion.

Since the spring of 1981, when a few unusual cases of *P. carinii* pneumonia and Kaposi's sarcoma among young homosexual men in New York and California were reported by the CDC, AIDS has grown to epidemic proportions and spread rapidly to the heterosexual community. Epidemiologic data indicate that the virus arose in central Africa and spread rapidly among sexually active populations, especially male homosexuals. Transmission of the infection may occur by passage of the free virus or by infected cells. Natural infection of humans occurs most often by sexual activities in which blood, semen, or vaginal fluids carrying virus or infected cells come into contact with breaks in the skin or mucous membranes, or through the use of contaminated needles or syringes by intravenous drug abusers. Transmission may also occur across the placenta from mother to fetus and actually occurs in about half of pregnancies in which the mother is infected with HIV. Effective therapy utilizes combinations of drugs that inhibit viral reverse transcriptase and protease, critical steps in HIV replication.

Attempts to produce vaccines to prevent HIV have met with little success in experimental models, as has immunotherapy. Therapy directed to restoring immune reactivity by passive transfer of cells or serum, immunostimulating agents, or interleukins has not been successful. The intracellular location of the virus, the marked variability that occurs in RNA sequences, particularly of the *env* region, during an infection, and the possibility of producing an immunopathologic effect by immunization are all factors contributing to difficulties in finding a vaccine. Clinical trials using synthetic HIV surface antigens (e.g., gp160 or gp120) demonstrate increased antibody and cellular immunity to HIV epitopes, and trials are under way to determine if immunization with envelope proteins will delay the development of AIDS in HIV-infected individuals. Animal models using macaques, chimpanzees, mice reconstituted with human cells, or transgenic mice that carry the HIV provirus, as well as rabbits infected with HIV, are being evaluated for use in vaccine and therapy trials as well as for experimental studies of pathogenesis.

AIDS is the most potentially threatening infectious disease to appear in the Western world in the 20th century. The rapid advances in immunology and molecular biology that have occurred in the last 20 years have provided an amazing armamentarium of approaches to study the virus and to learn how to modify its effects. Yet much more needs to be learned, and much more needs to be accomplished before effective therapy or vaccination will be achieved. At present, infection can be prevented by appropriate behavior to avoid transmission of the virus.

Bibliography

Highly Recommended

Levy, J. A. 1998. *HIV and the Pathogenesis of AIDS,* 2nd ed. ASM Press, Washington D.C.

General

AIDS: an International Bimonthly Journal. Gower Academic Journals, London, United Kingdom.

AIDS Research and Human Retroviruses. Mary Ann Liebert, Inc., New York, N.Y.

DeVita, V. T., S. Hellman, and S. A. Rosenberg (ed.). 1997. *AIDS: Etiology, Diagnosis, Treatment and Prevention.* Lippincott-Raven, Hagerstown, Md.

Ioachim, H. L. 1989. *Pathology of AIDS.* J. B. Lippincott Co., Philadelphia, Pa.

Neiburgs, H. E., and J. G. Bekesi. 1988. *Immune Dysfunctions in Cancer and AIDS.* Alan R. Liss, New York, N.Y.

Wormser, G. P. (ed.). 1992. *AIDS and Other Manifestations of HIV Infection,* 2nd ed. Raven Press, New York, N.Y.

Human Immunodeficiency Virus

AIDS-Related Retroviruses

Gao, F., E. Bailes, D. L. Robertson, Y. Chen, C. M. Rodenburg, et al. 1999. Origin of HIV-1 in the chimpanzee *Pan troglodytes troglodytes. Nature* **397:**436–441.

Gotch, F. 1998. Cross-clade T cell recognition of HIV-1. *Curr. Opin. Immunol.* **10:**388–392.

Korber, B., J. Theiler, and S. Wolinsky. 1998. Limitations of a molecular clock applied to considerations of the origin of HIV-1. *Science* **280:**1868–1871.

Zhu, T., B. T. Korber, A. J. Nahmias, E. Hooper, P. M. Sharp, and D. D. Ho. 1998. An African HIV-1 sequence from 1959 and implications for the origin of the epidemic. *Nature* **391:**594–597.

The HIV Genome

Wong-Staal, F. 1988. Human immunodeficiency virus: genetic structure and function. *Semin. Hematol.* **25:**189–196.

Wyatt, R., and J. Sodroski. 1999. The HIV-1 envelope glycoproteins: fusogens, antigens and immunogens. *Science* **280:**1884–1888.

HIV Replication and Gene Expression

Emerman, M., and M. H. Malin. 1998. HIV-1 regulatory/accessory genes: keys to unraveling viral host cell biology. *Science* **280:**1880–1884.

Lefevre, E. A., R. Krzysiek, E. P. Loret, P. Galanuaud, and Y. Richard. 1999. HIV-1 tat protein differentially modulates the B cell response of naive, memory, and germinal center B cells. *J. Immunol.* **163:**1119–1122.

Swingler, S., A. Mann, J. Jacque, B. Brichacek, V. G. Sasseville, et al. 1999. HIV-1 Nef mediates lymphocyte chemotaxis and activation by infected macrophages. *Nat. Med.* **5:**997–1003.

HIV Replicative Cycle

Grivel, J.-C., and L. B. Margolis. 1999. CCR5– and CXCR4–tropic HIV-1 are equally cytopathic for their T-cell targets in human lymphoid tissue. *Nat. Med.* **5:**344–346.

Kwong, P. D., R. Wyatt, J. Robinson, R. W. Sweet, J. Sodroski, and W. A. Hendrickson. 1998. Structure of an HIV gp120 envelope glycoprotein in complex with the CD4 receptor and a neutralizing human antibody. *Nature* **393:**648–659.

Tang, H., K. L. Kuhen, and F. Wong-Staal. 1999. Lentivirus replication and regulation. *Annu. Rev. Genet.* **33:**133–170.

Immune Evasion

Baker, E. 1999. CD8+ cell-derived anti-human immunodeficiency virus inhibitory factor. *J. Infect. Dis.* **179**(Suppl. 3)**:**S485–S488.

Collins, K. L., B. K. Chen, S. A. Kalams, B. D. Walker, and D. Baltimore. 1998. HIV-1 Nef protein protects infected primary cells against killing by cytotoxic T lymphocytes. *Nature* **391:**397–401.

Desrosiers, R. C. 1999. Strategies used by human immunodeficiency virus that allow persistent viral replication. *Nat. Med.* **5:**723–725.

Reitter, J. N., R. E. Means, and R. C. Desrosiers. 1998. A role for carbohydrates in immune evasion in AIDS. *Nat. Med.* **4:**679–684.

Stranford, S. A., J. Skurnick, D. Louria, D. Osmond, S.-Y. Chang, et al. 1999. Lack of infection in HIV-exposed individuals is associated with a strong CD8(+) cell noncytotoxic anti-HIV response. *Proc. Natl. Acad. Sci. USA* **96:**1030–1035.

AIDS

Epidemiology of AIDS

Garry, R. F., M. H. Witte, A. A. Gottlieb, M. Elvin-Lewis, M. S. Gottlieb, et al. 1988. Documentation of an AIDS virus infection in the United States in 1968. *JAMA* **260:**2085–2087.

Jaffe, H. W., D. J. Bergman, and R. M. Selik. 1983. Acquired immune deficiency syndrome in the United States: the first 1,000 cases. *J. Infect. Dis.* **148:**339–345.

O'Brien, T. R., J. R. George, and S. D. Holmberg. 1992. Human immunodeficiency virus type 2 infection in the United States. *JAMA* **267:**2775.

Transmission of AIDS

Cao, Y., P. Krogstad, B. T. Korber, R. A. Koup, M. Muldoon, et al. 1997. Maternal HIV-1 viral load and vertical transmission of infection: the Ariel Project for the prevention of HIV transmission from mother to infant. *Nat. Med.* **3:**549–552.

Peckham, C., and D. Gibb. 1995. Mother to child transmission of the human immunodeficiency virus. *N. Engl. J. Med.* **333:**298–302.

Stahl-Henning, C., R. M. Steinman, K. Tenner-Racz, M. Pope, N. Stolte, et al. 1999. Rapid infection of oral mucosal-associated lymphoid tissue with simian immunodeficiency virus. *Science* **285:**1261–1265.

Natural History of HIV Infection

Armstrong, D. 1987. Opportunistic infections in the acquired immune deficiency syndrome. *Semin. Hematol.* **14:**40–47.

Cameron, P. U., P. S. Freudenthal, J. M. Barker, S. Gezelter, K. Inaba, and R. M. Steinman. 1992. Dendritic cells exposed to human immunodeficiency virus type-1 transmit a vigorous cytopathic infection to CD4+ T cells. *Science* **257:**383–387.

Daar, E. S., T. Moudgil, R. D. Meyer, and D. D. Ho. 1991. Transient high levels of viremia in patients with primary human immunodeficiency virus type 1 infection. *N. Engl. J. Med.* **324:**961–964.

Meltzer, M. S., D. R. Skillman, P. J. Gomatos, D. C. Kalter, and H. E. Gendelman. 1990. Role of mononuclear phagocytes in the pathogenesis of human immunodeficiency virus infection. *Annu. Rev. Immunol.* **8:**169–194.

Sheppard, H. W., W. Lang, M. S. Ascher, E. Vittinghoff, and W. Winkelstein. 1993. The characterization of non-progressors: long-term HIV-1 infection with stable CD4+ T-cell levels. *AIDS* **7:**1159–1166.

Cellular Dynamics of HIV Infection

Brodie, S. J., D. A. Lewinson, B. K. Patterson, D. Jiyamapa, J. Keieger, et al. 1999. In vivo migration and function of transferred HIV-1 specific cytotoxic T cells. *Nat. Med.* **5:**34–41.

Finzi, D., M. Hermankova, T. Pierson, L. M. Carruth, C. Buck, et al. 1997. Identification of a reservoir for HIV-1 in patients on highly active antiretroviral therapy. *Science* **278:**1295–1300.

Herbein, G., U. Mahlknecht, F. Batliwalla, P. Gregersen, T. Pappas, et al. 1998. Apoptosis of CD8+ T cells is mediated by macrophages through interaction of HIV gp120 with chemokine receptor CXCR4. *Nature* **395:**189–194.

Mohri, H., S. Bonherffer, S. Monard, A. S. Perelson, and D. D. Ho. 1998. Rapid turnover of T lymphocytes in SIV-infected Rhesus macaques. *Science* **279:**1223–1227.

Roquews, P. A., G. Gras, F. Parnet-Mathieu, A. M. Mabondzo, C. Dollfus, et al. 1995. Clearance of HIV infection in 12 perinatally infected children: clinical, viral and immunological data. *AIDS* **9:**F19–F26.

Schmidt, J. E., M. J. Kuroda, S. Santra, V. G. Sasseville, M. A. Simon, et al. 1999. Control of viremia in simian immunodeficiency virus infection by CD8+ lymphocytes. *Science* **283:**857–860.

Immune Stimulation and Activation of AIDS

Cheynier, R., S. Gratton, M. Halloran, I. Stahmer, N. L. Letvin, and S. Wain-Hobson. 1998. Antigenic stimulation by BCG vaccine as an in vivo driving force for SIV replication and dissemination. *Nat. Med.* **4:**421–427.

Psallidopoulos, M. C., S. M. Schnittman, L. M. Thompson III, M. Baseler, A. S. Fauci, H. C. Lane, and N. P. Salzman. 1989. Integrated proviral human immunodeficiency virus type I is present in CD4+ peripheral blood lymphocytes in healthy seropositive individuals. *J. Virol.* **63:**4626–4631.

Stellrecht, K. A., K. Sperber, and B. G. T. Pogo. 1992. Activation of human immunodeficiency virus type 1 long terminal repeat by vaccinia virus. *J. Virol.* **66:**2051–2056.

Laboratory Diagnosis of HIV Infection

Centers for Disease Control. 1989. Interpretation and use of Western blot assay for serodiagnosis of human immunodeficiency virus type 1 infections. *Morb. Mortal. Wkly. Rep.* **38**(Suppl. S-7)**:**1.

Centers for Disease Control. 1992. Unexplained CD4+ T-lymphocyte depletion in persons without evident HIV infection—United States. *Morb. Mortal. Wkly. Rep.* **41:**541.

Consortium for Retrovirus Serology Standardization. 1992. Serologic diagnosis of human immunodeficiency virus infection by Western blot testing. *JAMA* **260:**674–679.

Constantine, N. T., J. D. Callahan, and D. M. Watts. 1992. *Retroviral Testing: Essentials for Quality Control and Laboratory Diagnosis.* CRC Press, Boca Raton, Fla.

Constantine, N. T., L. Zekeng, A. K. Sangare, L. Gurtler, R. Saville, H. Anhary, and C. Wild. 1997. Diagnostic challenges for rapid human immunodeficiency virus assays. Performance using HIV-1 group O, HIV-1 group M, and HIV-2 samples. *J. Hum. Virol.* **1:**45–51.

Defer, C., H. Agut, A. Garbatg-Chenon, M. Moncany, F. Morinet, D. Vignon, M. Mariotti, and J.-J. Lefrere. 1992. Multicenter quality control of polymerase chain reaction for detection of HIV DNA. *AIDS* **6:**659–663.

Stute, R. 1988. Comparison in sensitivity of 10 HIV antibody detection tests by serial dilutions of Western blot confirmed samples. *J. Virol. Methods* **20:**269–273.

Immune Dysfunction

Janossy, G., B. Autran, and F. Miedema. 1992. *Immunodeficiency in HIV Infection and AIDS.* S. Karger, Farmington, Conn.

Levy, J. A. 1993. Pathogenesis of human immunodeficiency virus infection. *Microbiol. Rev.* **57:**183–289.

Pathology and Clinical Staging

Blatt, S. P., C. W. Hendrix, C. A. Butzin, T. M. Freeman, W. W. Ward, et al. 1993. Delayed-type hypersensitivity skin testing predicts progression to AIDS in HIV-infected patients. *Ann. Intern. Med.* **119:**177–184.

Wormser, G. P. (ed.). 1992. *AIDS and Other Manifestations of HIV Infection.* Raven Press, New York, N.Y.

Therapy

Cohen, J. 1999. Cheap treatment cuts HIV transmission. *Science* **283:**916–917.

Fleury, S., R. J. de Boer, G. P. Rizzardi, K. C. Wolthers, S. A. Otto, C. C. Welborn, et al. 1998. Limited CD4+ T-cell renewal in early HIV-1 infection: effect of highly active antiretroviral therapy. *Nat. Med.* **4:**794–801.

Gulick, R. M., J. W. Mellors, D. Havlir, J. J. Eron, C. Gonzalez, et al. 1998. Simultaneous vs sequential initiation of therapy with indinavir, zidovudine, and lamivudine for HIV-1 infections: 100 week follow-up. *JAMA* **280:**35–41.

Hellerstein, M., M. B. Hanley, D. Cesar, S. Siler, C. Papageorgopoulos, E. Wieder, et al. 1999. Directly measured kinetics of circulating T lymphocytes in normal and HIV-1–infected humans. *Nat. Med.* **5:**83–89.

Wong, J. K., M. Hezareh, H. F. Gunthard, D. V. Havlir, C. C. Ignacio, C. A. Spina, and D. D. Richman. 1997. Recovery of replication-competent HIV despite prolonged suppression of plasma viremia. *Science* **278:**1291–1294.

Animal Models

Desrosiers, R. C. 1988. Simian immunodeficiency viruses. *Annu. Rev. Microbiol.* **42:**607–625.

Gardner, M. B., and P. A. Luciw. 1989. Animal models of AIDS. *FASEB J.* **3:**2593–2606.

Kock, J. A., and R. M. Ruprecht. 1992. Animal models for anti-AIDS therapy. *Antiviral Res.* **19:**81–69.

McCune, J. M., R. Namikawa, H. Kaneshima, L. D. Schultz, M. Lieberman, and I. L. Weissman. 1988. The SCID-hu mouse: murine model for the analysis of human hematolymphoid differentiation and function. *Science* **241:**1632–1639.

Morse, H. C., S. K. Chattopadhyay, M. Makino, T. N. Fredrickson, A. W. Hugin, and J. W. Hartley. 1992. Retrovirus-induced immunodeficiency in the mouse: MAIDS as a model for AIDS. *AIDS* **6:**607–621.

Schellekens, H., and M. Horzinek. 1990. *Animal Models in AIDS.* Elsevier, New York, N.Y.

Vaccination against HIV Infection

Boyer, J. D., K. E. Ugen, B. Wang, M. Agadjanyan, L. Gilbert, M. L. Bagarazzi, et al. 1997. Protection of chimpanzees from high-dose heterologous HIV-1 challenge by DNA vaccination. *Nat. Med.* **3:**526–532.

Cooney, E. L., M. J. McElrath, L. Corey, S. L. Hu, A. C. Collier, et al. 1993. Enhanced immunity to human immunodeficiency virus (HIV) envelope elicited by a combined vaccine regimen consisting of priming with a vaccinia recombinant expressing HIV envelope and boosting with gp160 protein. *Proc. Natl. Acad. Sci. USA* **90:**1882–1886.

Kennedy, R. C. 1997. DNA vaccination for HIV. *Nat. Med.* **3:**501–504.

Letvin, N. L. 1998. Progress in the development of an HIV-1 vaccine. *Science* **280:**1875–1879.

Lubeck, M. D., R. Natuk, M. Myagkikh, N. Kalyan, K. Aldrich, et al. 1997. Long-term protection of chimpanzees against high-dose HIV-1 challenge induced by immunization. *Nat. Med.* **3:**651–658.

Phoolcharoen, W. 1998. HIV/AIDS prevention in Thailand: success and challenges. *Science* **280:**1873–1874.

Tumor Immunity

20

History of Tumor Immunity

A short history of tumor immunology is presented in Table 20.1. Early pathologists noted infiltration of some cancers with lymphocytes, and William Halsted, a surgeon, reported in 1898 that tumors with lymphocytic infiltration had a better prognosis than those without such infiltration. Investigators in the early 1900s found that transplanted tumors in laboratory mice were rejected. But this rejection was based on histocompatibility differences; normal tissues were also rejected. With the development of inbred mice, it was found that most tumors would not be rejected if there were no histocompatibility differences, but there were some outstanding exceptions. Some tumors could be rejected even in the absence of a histocompatibility rejection response. Rejection of a tumor by the same animal in which the tumor arose was demonstrated in an autochthonous (primary) host by George Klein in 1960 (see below). These experimental transplantation studies established the concept of tumor-specific transplantation immunity. Although the evidence for tumor-specific transplantation antigens accumulated in experimental models, tumor-specific immunity in humans remained controversial. The history of immunotherapy of cancer is presented in more detail at the end of this chapter.

Evidence for Tumor Immunity in Humans

The evidence supporting the hypothesis that immune reactivity may control or limit the growth of human tumors is listed in Table 20.2. However, the evidence is circumstantial, and definitive proof of effective tumor immunity in humans has remained elusive.

After an extensive survey of many cases of spontaneous remission of cancer, T. C. Emerson accepted 130 cases as valid in 1964. Of these, 10% were choriocarcinomas, in which paternal antigens foreign to the maternal host are expressed. Spontaneous regressions have also been reported in about 15% of nodular lymphomas, a form of B-cell cancer that is subject to control by the immune system, and in malignant melanomas, the cancer most likely to elicit immune rejection. Thus, although spontaneous remissions do occur, they are very rare.

Regression of metastases after removal of a primary tumor is also a rare and complex phenomenon. One explanation is that removal of the

Table 20.1 A short history of tumor immunity

Year	Investigator	Discovery
1898	Halsted	Lymphocytic infiltration of breast cancer associated with good prognoses
1900	Erlich	Proposed tumor-specific immunity, similar to immunity to infection
1904	Loeb	Tumor transplantation successful in inbred Japanese waltzing mice
1906	Schone	Tumor immunity induced by fetal tissues in outbred mice
1908	Wade	Tumor grafts rejected in outbred animals; lymphocyte infiltration seen
1941	Gross	Tumor grafts rejected in partially inbred mice
1953	Foley	Tumor grafts rejected in fully inbred mice (tumor-specific immunity)
1957	Prehn	Primary tumor used to immunize syngeneic mice
1960	Klein	Tumor-specific rejection in autochthonous host (mice)

primary tumor permits an immune response to tumor antigens to become directed to metastatic lesions. However, other complex phenomena involving the biology of the tumor and host factors, such as hormonal requirements for tumor growth being altered by removal of the primary tumor, production of antiangiogenic factors that suppress growth of metastases by primary cancers, or dependence of the metastases on factors produced by the primary tumor, could be the explanation.

Reappearance of metastases after a long latent period is an example of tumor dormancy. It has been documented in experimental models that

Table 20.2 Evidence for tumor immunity in humans

Event	Comment
Spontaneous regression	Rare, usually tumors that could be controlled by developmental factors or that contain foreign antigens (e.g., paternal antigens in choriocarcinomas)
Regression of metastases after removal of primary tumor	Rare, not necessarily immune mediated
Reappearance of metastases after long latent periods	Not necessarily immune-mediated, determined by nature of the tumor
Failure of circulating cells to form metastases	Most likely not immune-mediated; circulating cells may not find supportive environment
Infiltration of tumors by mononuclear cells	Could be secondary effect; not always associated with tumor regression
High incidence of cancer in immunosuppressed, aged, or immunodeficient patients	Circumstantial evidence; usually lymphomas; may be due to loss of controlling T cells or virus infection
Depressed immune reactivity in cancer patients	Depressed immunity associated with debilitated state of patient;a secondary effect of cancer
Tumor antigens identifed by in vitro assays on human cancers	In vitro assays not reliable indication of in vivo tumor rejection
Tests for delayed-type hypersensitivity skin reaction to cancer extracts (in some cancer patients)	Significance of skin tests not clear
Immune complexes and glomerulonephritis found (in some cancer patients)	Relationship of immune complexes to tumor resistance not documented, antigens in complexes may not be to tumor antigens; antibodies to tumor antigens may aid tumor growth (enhancement)

tumor cells may exist in a quiescent state for many years. Changes in blood supply, operative trauma, or other events are associated with tumor cells escaping from the dormant state. This is sometimes related to an immunosuppressive event.

Failure of circulating tumor cells to form metastases has been well documented in both animal and human studies. During cancer surgery, large numbers of tumor cells may be released into the circulation, and yet later, metastases are not found. This can be explained by a number of nonimmune mechanisms, such as the inability of the tumor cells to escape successfully from the circulation and proliferate away from the primary site, clearing of tumor cells from the circulation by the reticuloendothelial system, or distribution of tumor cells to nonsupportive environments.

Tumor tissue is often infiltrated by large numbers of lymphocytes, perhaps because of a cellular immunologic reaction to tumor antigens. In 1898, William Halsted described perivascular infiltration by lymphocytes and hyperplasia of draining lymph nodes in patients with large breast cancers that had a relatively prolonged course without metastases, as compared with breast cancers *without* infiltrating lymphocytes. However, this generalization is not supported by more extensive data, and tumor infiltration by lymphocytes is not used as a prognostic indicator by pathologists. Lymphocytes infiltrating the base of a malignant melanoma are associated with a more favorable prognosis than melanomas in the vertical growth phase that lack a lymphocytic infiltrate. Lymphocytes that are found in tumors are known as tumor-infiltrating lymphocytes. These cells can be isolated from tumors, expanded and activated in vitro, and have been used for passive immunotherapy trials of human cancer (see below).

An increased incidence of cancer is found in patients with primary or secondary immune deficiency states. A tabulation of the occurrence of primary cancer in transplant patients during immunosuppressive therapy showed that the overall occurrence for all cancers was far greater (13 of 2,000) than in the general population (8.2 of 100,000). However, immunosuppressed individuals have a preponderance of lymphomas and skin cancers that may reflect abnormalities in control of lymphoid cell proliferation rather than suppression of immunity or susceptibility to cancer in general. A good case has been made that all cancers in immunosuppressed patients are viral or associated with UV light exposure.

Since the majority of cancers occur in patients over 65 years of age, it has been suggested that this is due to the age-associated decline in immune function. However, many important interactions of normal aging and carcinogenesis are incompletely understood. It is likely that other factors, such as the time required for the multistep process of carcinogenesis to become manifest and the effect of aging on DNA repair, are more important than the decline in immunity with aging.

Some cancer patients have decreased cell-mediated immune responses to a variety of antigens, and these patients appear to have more rapid tumor growth than cancer patients whose cell-mediated immunity is not decreased. In addition, cellular immune deficiency is more marked in patients with disseminated tumor growth or those who respond poorly to therapy. This may reflect the debilitated state of a terminal cancer patient more than a specific immune deficit, and some tumors may produce immunosuppressive products.

Some human tumors have tumor antigens detectable by in vitro assays. Several human tumor-specific antigens have been identified by these assays (see below). Although reasonable data have been obtained in various animal systems that correlate cellular immune reactivity to the ability of an animal to resist tumor challenge, the specificity of cellular tests for human tumors has been questioned. One major problem has been the finding of lymphocytes that are cytotoxic for tumor cells in normal individuals. Thus, whereas lymphocytes from cancer patients may react with certain tumor target cells, similar cells from normal persons often react just as strongly. These are called natural killer (NK) cells (see below). In addition, tumor cell lines have been used almost exclusively as target cells for human lymphocytic killer cells. These cell lines may not express the same antigenicity as the original tumor. Therefore, most of the data in which in vitro human tumor immunity was tested using cell lines is now being reinterpreted. It may be necessary to perform all such tests using primary cultures of freshly obtained tumor target cells.

A tumor-bearing patient may produce a delayed-type hypersensitivity skin reaction against a membrane extract of his or her own tumor cells, but the significance of such a reaction is difficult to evaluate. In addition, immediate (2-min) skin reactions to tumor extracts preincubated with the patient's serum (Markari test) have been reported to be an indicator of the presence of tumors, but this has not been generally accepted.

Circulating immune complexes and glomerular immune complex disease, frequently subclinical, are found in up to about 10% of cancer patients. In a few cases, the glomerular deposits of complexes have been demonstrated to contain tumor-associated antigen (carcinoembryonic antigen) or antibody to carcinoembryonic antigen. The relationship of these complexes to tumor resistance is not known, but it suggests that an antibody to a tumor "antigen" is present. Such antibodies may actually aid tumor growth.

In summary, the evidence that an immune response does occur to some human tumors and that this response may, in rare cases, be responsible for regression of inoperable primary tumors remains circumstantial. Demonstrations of effective tumor resistance in humans due to an immune response to the tumor are exceptions to the general rule.

Carcinogenesis and Tumor Immunity

If the immune system is playing a prominent role in the development of cancers, then agents that cause cancer (carcinogens) would be expected to be immunosuppressive, and immunosuppressive agents would be expected to be carcinogenic. Two potent skin carcinogens, dimethylbenzenanthracene and UV radiation, cause convincing immune suppression, whereas most others do not. Thus, although immunosuppression is not a common feature of carcinogens, it does play a role in some, such as UV radiation.

UV exposure acts not only by inducing alteration of DNA (mutations), which results in transformation of epithelial cells (inducing cancerous changes in growth behavior), but also by causing both local and systemic immune-suppressive effects. Locally, there is a marked loss of Langerhans cells in the skin and T-suppressor cell activation that blocks an immune response to the developing tumors. UV-induced tumors are highly immunogenic in syngeneic nonirradiated mice but not in the primary host, because UV irradiation suppresses the immune response in the primary animal. In addition, UV irradiation causes a transient depression of delayed-type hypersensitivity and contact dermatitis reactions to nontumor antigens, believed to be caused by release of suppressive cytokines from keratinocytes. UV irradiation thus produces both a tumor-specific and a nonspecific immunosuppression that allows strongly antigenic tumors to develop. UV-induced tumors appear to express tumor-specific antigens for T-effector cells but shared antigens for T-suppressor cells.

On the other hand, strong hepatocarcinogens, such as acetylaminofluorene and diethynitrosamine, produce little if any immunosuppression. Phorbol esters, which are promoting agents, may produce up to a 50% reduction in NK activity, but they are also mitogenic for lymphocytes. With the high interest in this aspect of carcinogenesis, it is noteworthy that there are not more published results indicating that carcinogens are immunosuppressive. Thus, it appears that carcinogens, such as UV radiation, that induce tumors with relatively strong transplantation antigens also cause immunosuppression, whereas carcinogens that do not induce transplantation antigens are not immunosuppressive.

Types of Tumor Antigens

TSTAs

Many changes in cell surface markers have been detected on tumor cells (Fig. 20.1), but the most important functionally are those identified by transplantation in laboratory animals (tumor-specific transplantation antigens [TSTAs]). These antigens may be divided into two general classes: those that are specific for a given tumor and those that are shared by two or more tumors, generally of a particular histologic type. A given tumor

Figure 20.1 Some antigenic features of tumor cells. Some antigenic changes in tumors include loss or gain of major histocompatibility complex (MHC) antigens, loss or gain of carbohydrates (CHO), appearance of virus-associated tumor antigens (TAVA), tumor-associated transplantation antigens shared by different tumors (TATA), tumor-specific transplantation antigens essentially unique for a given tumor (TSTA), and markers shared by embryonic tissues and tumors (oncodevelopmental antigens [ODA]).

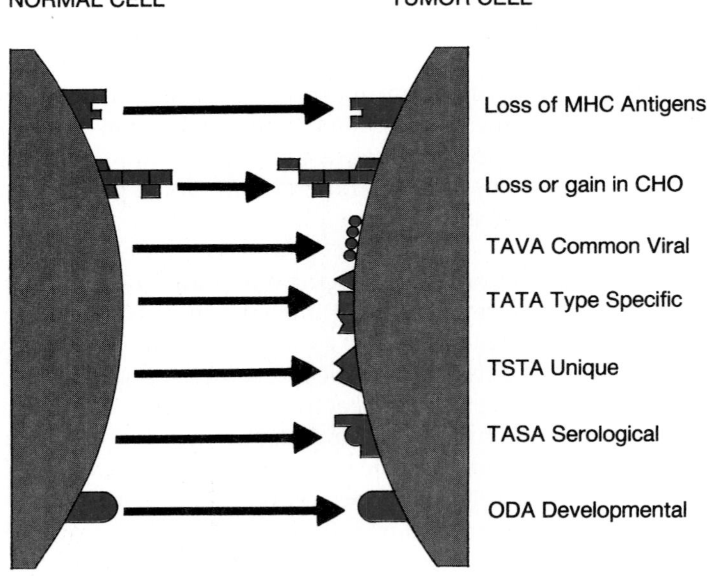

may have both unique and shared antigens. For diagnostic and therapeutic purposes in humans, antigenic specificities shared by a large number of tumors of a given class are potentially much more valuable than unique antigens; detection of a shared antigen could be used as a screening test for tumors in different persons or used for preventive immunization. On the other hand, a unique tumor-specific antigen would not be detected by a common antigen screening test and would be effective as an immunogen only in the individual with that tumor.

Skin tumors induced in mice by the carcinogen methylcholanthrene are usually antigenically different from every other skin tumor induced by methylcholanthrene. Indeed, two primary tumors induced in the same animal are antigenically distinct. This demonstration of tumor-specific antigens extends to other chemically induced tumors, including sarcomas induced by aromatic hydrocarbons, hepatomas induced by azo dyes, and mammary carcinomas induced by methylcholanthrene, as well as tumors induced by physical agents, such as implantation of cellophane films or Millipore filters.

TSTAs may be related to, but are clearly different from, histocompatibility transplantation antigens. As early as 1910, it was observed that the serum of mice that had recovered from tumors inhibited tumor growth in other mice, sometimes causing regression and an apparent cure. Attempts were made to treat cancer with immunization methods similar to those that had proved successful with infectious diseases, and promising results were obtained in laboratory animals. This raised hopes that tumor-specific immune reactions could cure cancer. However, it soon became apparent that the results obtained were not due to tumor-specific antigens but to histocompatibility antigens. In other words, normal tissue and tumor tissue from the tumor donor were rejected in a similar manner by the same recipient. Terms used to identify host-tumor relationships are the same as those used for tissue graft donor-recipient relationships (Table 20.3). Both tissue and tumor grafts will survive in autochthonous or syngeneic recipients but not in allogeneic or xenogeneic recipients.

The inability to demonstrate TSTAs led to a general loss of interest in tumor immunity between 1910 and 1940 (but see below), until the development of inbred strains of mice. In 1943, Ludwig Gross transplanted tumors (sarcomas), induced by the chemical methylcholanthrene, in inbred mice. He found that tumor nodules appeared after tumor cells were injected into the skin, grew for a few days, and then regressed. After regression, reinjection of cells from the same tumor did not produce a tumor nodule, demonstrating that the syngeneic animals that had rejected the transplanted tumor were now resistant to it. Almost 20 years later, Richmond Prehn followed up Gross's observations. Prehn tested 3-methylcholanthrene-induced sarcomas of C3H/He mouse origin. Immunization was accomplished by strangulation of the first or second

Table 20.3 Terminology of host-tumor graft relationships

Relationship	Terminology
Same individual	Autochthonous
Genetically identical (twin, inbred strain)	Syngeneic
Different individual, same species	Allogeneic
Different species	Xenogeneic

transplant generation of tumor grafts. Following tumor regression, the animals were rechallenged with living cells, and the frequency of "takes" was then compared with that in untreated controls. Resistance to challenge was noted when the mice were reinjected with the same tumor. Appropriate controls involving skin grafts and immunization with normal tissue ruled out the possibility that rejection was caused by antigens present in normal tissue and not specific for the tumor. In 1957, Prehn extended these observations by showing that tumor-specific immunity could be produced by allowing a tumor to grow and then removing it by surgical excision. Animals that had been immunized in this way could then reject the same transplantable tumor, even if greater numbers of tumor cells were injected. He also found that chemically induced tumors possessed individually specific tumor antigens; immunization of an animal to one chemically induced tumor did not protect it from growth of a different chemically induced tumor.

The Immune Response of the Primary Tumor-Bearing Host and Concomitant Immunity

The studies cited above describe immunity to transplanted tumors in syngeneic animals, but can an individual make an immune response to his or her own "autochthonous" tumor? The term autochthonous is used to indicate the relationship between a tumor and the individual in which that tumor arose (primary host). To demonstrate autochthonous tumor immunity, primary methylcholanthrene-induced sarcomas were excised from the autochthonous animal and maintained by passage in syngeneic recipients. Transplantation of the passaged tumor back to the autochthonous host resulted in rejection of the tumor 3 to 4 weeks later (Fig. 20.2). Thus, a laboratory animal may make an immune response to its own tumor, and this response may be effective in controlling the growth of the tumor (autochthonous tumor resistance). In some instances, the primary tumor-bearing animal (autochthonous host) may have an immune response that can be demonstrated by rejection upon transplantation of part of the tumor to another site or by in vitro tests, but despite this response, the primary tumor grows progressively in vivo. This is termed "concomitant immunity." Primary tumors in individuals with concomitant immunity are able to avoid immune attack that is effective if the same tumor cells are inoculated at another site.

Etiology and Immunogenicity of Tumors

The immunogenicity of a given tumor-specific antigen is related to the etiology of the tumor. Virus-induced tumors have strong antigens that are shared by other tumors caused by the same virus. Skin cancers induced by UV light demonstrate both common and tumor-specific antigens and are much more immunogenic than tumors induced by chemicals. Tumors induced by large doses of carcinogens are generally more likely to express tumor-specific transplantation antigens than tumors induced by smaller doses of carcinogens. In addition, tumors induced by "strong" carcinogens are more likely to be immunogenic than tumors induced by "weak" carcinogens (Table 20.4).

Individual tumor-specific antigens are more easily demonstrated on chemically induced tumors than on virus-induced tumors because of the presence of common viral antigens on virus-induced tumors. Spontaneous tumors of mice may lack tumor antigens or express them very weakly.

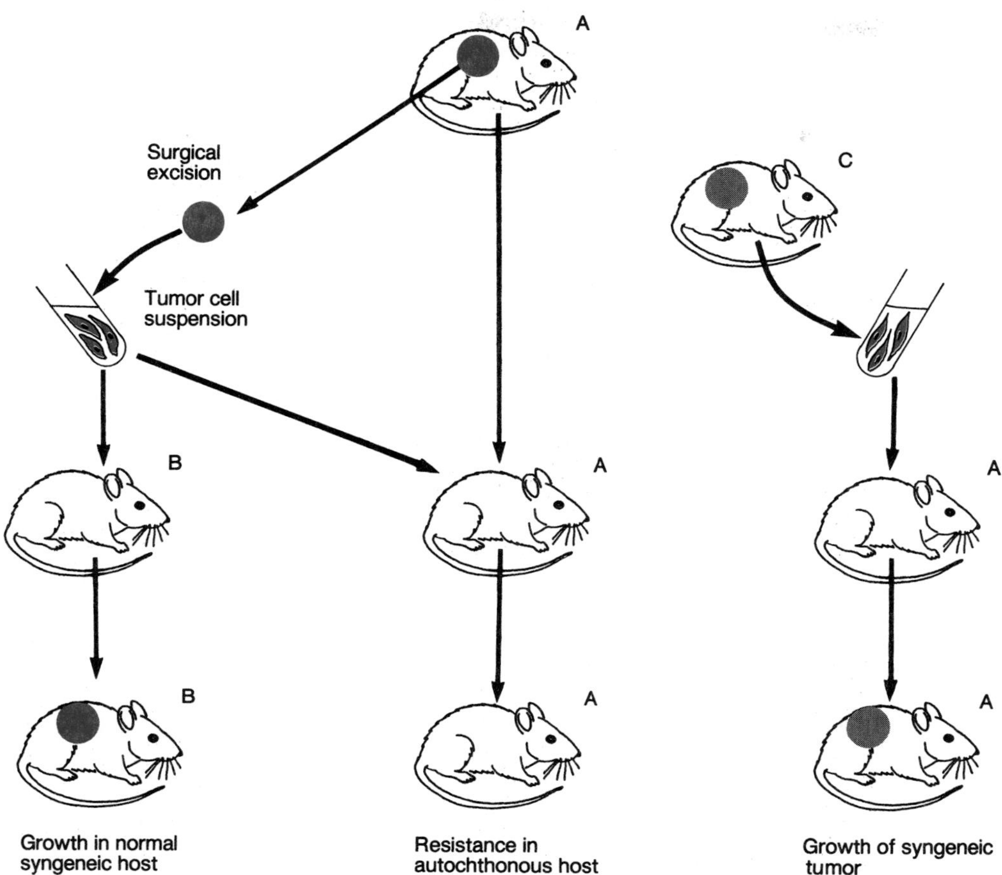

Figure 20.2 Demonstration of specific rejection of an autochthonous tumor. A chemically induced primary tumor is induced in mouse A and then removed surgically. A suspension of the tumor cells is made, and a transplantable dose of tumor cells is injected back into mouse A as well as into a normal syngeneic mouse of the same strain (B). The tumor grows in mouse B but not in the original primary tumor-bearing animal (autochthonous host). Thus, mouse A, the animal in which the tumor arose, has developed immune resistance to the growth of its own tumor. However, the tumor will grow when injected into a normal, previously unexposed recipient of the same strain (mouse B). On the other hand, a second tumor arising in another individual of the same strain (mouse C) will grow when injected into the animal in which the first tumor was produced (mouse A). Thus, the tumor resistance shown in mouse A is specific for the first tumor induced in mouse A and does not extend to other tumors (TSTA). This experiment demonstrates that an individual can develop specific immunity to an autochthonous tumor.

Some tumor antigens may be identified only serologically. Epitopes identified serologically do not necessarily induce a rejection reaction. Other tumor antigens are identified by reactivity of T cells. Specific antigens identified on human tumors are discussed below.

Virus-Induced Tumor Antigens

In contrast to chemically induced or spontaneous cancers, virus-induced tumors share common antigens. These shared antigens may be products encoded by the viral genome or cellular products not expressed in the virus itself.

Table 20.4 Immunogenicity of rat tumors[a]

Origin of tumor	Immunogenicity of: Common antigens	TSTAs	ODTAs
Virus	++++	++	+
UV radiation	++ (T_s)	++++	+
Methylcholanthrene	+	+++	+
Diaminoazobenzene	+	+	+
Acetylaminofluorene	0	+	+
Spontaneous	0	+/−	+

[a]++++ to 0, degree of immunogenicity; T_s, T-suppressor cells.

DNA Viruses

Each DNA virus induces unique nuclear and cell surface antigens. A given virus induces the expression of the same antigens regardless of the tissue origin or animal species. Although these antigens are coded for by the virus, they are distinct from virion antigens and are referred to as tumor-associated antigens. Virus-induced tumors may also express other antigens coded for by the host genome (such as TSTAs or oncodevelopmental tumor antigens [ODTAs]) as a result of host gene deregulation by the transforming event.

The association of DNA viruses with cell transformation and cancer in animals is well established and is linked to certain human tumors. For example, Epstein-Barr virus, one of the herpesviruses, is the cause of human infectious mononucleosis and is believed by many to be the etiologic agent of Burkitt's lymphoma and nasopharyngeal carcinoma. Similarly, papillomaviruses are found in human cervical carcinoma, and hepatitis B virus is found in hepatocellular carcinoma. In animals, herpesviruses have been shown to be oncogenic, as exemplified by Marek's lymphoma of chickens.

RNA Viruses

Tumors produced by RNA virus contain chromosomally integrated DNA that has been transcribed from the viral RNA by reverse transcriptase. When the oncogenic RNA viruses (oncornaviruses) infect the host cell, a double-stranded circular DNA copy of the RNA genome is synthesized and inserted into the host cell genome during cell transformation. Tumor cells induced by oncornaviruses express antigens coded for by both the viral and host genomes. These include (i) the viral envelope antigens, mostly the envelope glycoprotein; (ii) intrinsic viral proteins; and (iii) virus-induced cell surface antigens. While antibodies to viral envelope antigens will prevent infectivity, immunity against the neoplastic cell surface antigens is mainly responsible for the immunologic rejection of the malignant cell. These cell surface antigens are distinct from the viral antigens and also from the major histocompatibility antigens. The complexity of neoantigens expressed in virus-induced tumors is illustrated by the Rous sarcoma system of hamsters and human T-cell leukemia virus type 1 in humans: the antigens include virus envelope antigen, virus group-specific antigens, virus-encoded nonviral proteins, cell-encoded determinants activated by the virus, and oncodevelopmental antigens encoded by cellular genes that are activated by virus-induced transformation.

A number of retroviruses have been identified as having oncogene sequences by their ability to transfect cultured cells and effect changes in growth of the transfected cells (transformation). Human T-cell leukemia virus type 1 is a prime example. In addition, the tumors of many human cancers have been found to contain complementary DNA sequences similar to transforming oncogenes. Normal human DNA has also been found to contain such DNA sequences (proto-oncogenes), and some oncogene products may be used to estimate the prognosis of patients with cancer (see below). These oncogenes code for cellular products, particularly kinases, growth factors, or growth factor receptors, which are produced normally during development but which are also believed to contribute to the altered growth characteristics of transformed adult cells. Monoclonal antibodies (MAbs) to oncogene products of human tumors have been produced and are being used to measure the altered or overexpressed product in neoplastic tissues.

ODTAs

Oncodevelopmental antigens are found in embryonic or fetal tissues and in tumors of adults but are not present or barely detectable in normal adult tissues. ODTAs were identified by transplantation as early as 1906, when G. Schone found that tumor transplants that would kill normal mice would be rejected by mice that had been previously immunized with fetal tissue; immunization with adult tissue was ineffective. In the 1930s, humoral antibodies that cross-reacted with fetal and tumor tissue were reported. These studies were complicated by histocompatibility differences and are difficult to duplicate. General interest in ODTAs received little attention until the late 1960s, when antigens common to embryonic tissue and tumors were demonstrated in inbred strains by serologic cross-reactivity. In 1970, it was reported that lymph node cells from pregnant mice incubated in vitro with chemically induced syngeneic sarcoma cells caused death of the tumor cells. Although extensive experimental investigation of ODTAs followed, the significance of such antigens in regard to tumor immunogenicity remains undefined. The following general conclusions seem valid. Tumors and fetal tissue may share antigens that are different from TSTAs. ODTAs are not specific for a given tumor but are shared by tumors of different histologic type and even of different species of origin. Immune products that react with tumors in vitro (antibody or sensitized cells) may be generated by immunization of adults with fetal tissue or by exposure to fetal antigen during pregnancy. However, no effect of this immunization on tumor incidence or growth has been consistently demonstrated. Animals that have in vitro immune reactivity to ODTAs may have resistance to tumor challenge, demonstrate no differences from nonimmune recipients, or have increased growth of transplanted tumors. In systems that have shown oncodevelopmental transplantation antigens, immunogenicity is much more difficult to demonstrate than in the case of TSTAs or viral tumor antigens. In humans, ODTAs have been tentatively identified by in vitro tests. However, there is little or no evidence that immunization to fetal antigens protects against cancer in humans. Only one study has shown that the course of cancer differs in multiparous and nulliparous women. Previously pregnant women, after treatment for malignant melanoma, had slightly better survival rates than women with no previous pregnancies. Multiparous women have a higher incidence of carcinoma of the cervix but a lower incidence of carcinoma of the breast, but these differences are believed to be due to hormonal rather than immunological differences. ODTAs detected serologically are used as clinical "markers" of cancer (see below), but these epitopes are not involved in tumor rejection.

Mechanisms of Tumor Cell Destruction by the Immune System

In Vitro Assays of Tumor Immunity

A partial listing of the methods used to demonstrate immune reactivity to tumors in vitro is given in Table 20.5. These include almost every conceivable method of measuring the reaction of antibody or sensitized cells with antigens. Tests for humoral (circulating) antibody to tumor antigens are hampered by the difficulty in obtaining soluble antigens from tumor cells and the lack of characterization of nonviral tumor-specific antigens. Both humoral and cellular reactions are usually measured by determining some effect of immune products on tumor target cells. The most frequently used assays measure target cell lysis (such as by ^{51}Cr release) as an endpoint. In general, a positive in vitro test may or may not be an indication of an immune response that is effective against the tumor.

Cell-Mediated Tumor Immunity

Studies of these in vitro mechanisms have resulted in new insights into how immune mechanism might restrict the growth or kill tumor cells in vivo. Although humoral antibody/complement lysis of tumor cells in suspension in vitro may be demonstrated, this mechanism does not appear to act on solid tumors. The major in vivo mechanism for tumor cell killing appears to be T-cell cytotoxicity or delayed-type hypersensitivity; the contribution of NK cells or antibody-dependent cell-mediated cytotoxicity (as defined by in vitro assays) to in vivo tumor killing is not clear, but there is evidence that NK cells kill blood-borne tumor cells. Properties of cells mediating tumor immunity are listed in Table 20.6.

Table 20.5 Some in vitro assays for tumor antigens

Tests measuring:	
Human antibody	**Cell-mediated immunity**
Immunodiffusion	Effect of immune cells on targets
Antibody binding	Reduction of cell number
Fluorescence	Cytotoxicity
Radiolabeled	Vital dye uptake
Immunoperoxidase	Visual cell death
Blocking of antibody binding	^{51}Cr release
Complement-dependent killing	Inhibition of metabolism
Complement fixation	Loss of cell adherence
Complement fixation and transfer	Cytostasis
Mixed hemadsorption	Colony inhibition
Cytostasis	In vitro incubation, in vivo growth (Winn assay)
Loss of cell adherence	Effect of targets on immune cells
Blocking of cellular reactions	Mixed lymphocyte-tumor reactions
Immune adherence	Lymphokine release (IL-2, IFN-γ, etc)
ELISA (enzyme-linked immunosorbent assay)	Leukocyte adherence inhibition
Cytofluorometry	Blastogenesis (T-cell proliferation)

Table 20.6 Properties of cells mediating tumor immunity

Abbreviations	Name	Marker	Specificity	Mechanism(s)	Function	MHC restriction
T_{CTL}	Cytotoxic T cell	CD8	Specific	Lysis	Tumor rejection	Class II
T_{DTH}	Delayed-type hypersensitivity T cell	CD4	Specific	Macrophage activation	Tumor rejection	Class I
NK	Natural killer cell	NK	Nonspecific	Lysis	Tumor surveillance?	NR[a]
LAK	Lymphokine-activated killer cell	LAK	Nonspecific	Lysis	Immunotherapy?	NR
		IL-2R				
ADCC	Antibody-dependent cell-mediated cytotoxic cell	FcR	Nonspecific	Lysis	Uncertain	NR
TIL	Tumor-infiltrating lymphocyte	Mixed	Both?	Lysis and macrophage activation	Uncertain	Both
AMϕ	Activated macrophage	Monocyte	Nonspecific	Lysis and phagocytosis	Tumor rejection	NR

[a]NR, not restricted.

T-Cell-Mediated Cytolysis (T_{CTL} Cells)

T_{CTL} cells directly recognize cell surface antigens of the target cell via the T-cell receptor. One effector T cell can react with and lyse many target cells. The reaction of specific T cells with the target cell causes membrane alterations in the target cell and results in swelling of the target cell and eventual osmotic lysis. Lysis is frequently measured by the release of radiolabeled intracellular molecules (^{51}Cr release). T_{CTL} cells have Fas ligand (FasL) on their cell surface and react with Fas on tumor cells, activating the Fas-dependent cell-killing mechanism. There may also be exocytosis of granules containing perforin or granzymes from the T-killer cell that form complementlike lesions in the cell membrane of the target cell (see Fig. 12.1).

One of the first successful demonstrations of the effect of immune cells on tumor growth was accomplished by mixing effector lymphoid cells with tumor target cells in vitro, then injecting the mixture into a normal or irradiated syngeneic recipient. (Although first described by Klein, this has become known as the Winn assay [Fig. 20.3].) If growth of the transplanted tumor cells is inhibited by the in vitro pretreatment, it may be concluded that the tumor cells had been killed or damaged by the immune effector cells.

Delayed-Type Hypersensitivity (T_{DTH} Cells)

T cells responsible for delayed-type hypersensitivity reactions (T_{DTH} cells) specifically recognize antigens in tissues and are activated to release mediators that attract and activate macrophages. The activated macrophages are able to phagocytose cells and destroy them. In some animal models, this mechanism is highly effective in killing tumors in vivo, but the mechanism cannot be duplicated in vitro.

NK Cells

NK cells are large granular lymphocytes of a particular lineage with defined markers (e.g., CD16). They are operationally defined as cells present in normal individuals that are capable of cytotoxic activity against a variety of target cells. Lymphocytes from normal persons may be just as reactive against tumor cell lines as those from patients with tumors of the

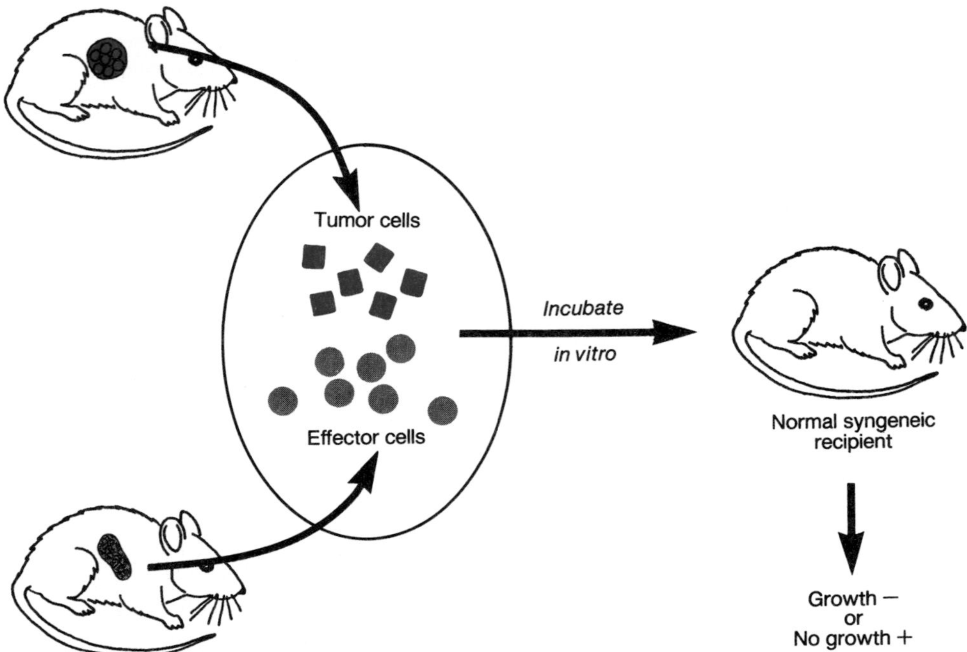

Figure 20.3 Winn assay. To determine the effect of a given cell population on the viability of tumor cells, the effector cells (lymphoid cells) are admixed in vitro with the tumor target cells, and the mixture of cells is transplanted into a normal syngeneic recipient. If growth of the tumor is inhibited in comparison to tumor cells alone or tumor cells treated with control (unsensitized) lymphoid cells, it may be concluded that the effector lymphoid cell population has adversely affected the tumor cells.

same or different histologic types. The role of NK cells in tumor surveillance in humans has recently been questioned because of the finding that a patient with a virtual lack of NK cells had problems with viral infections but did not have cancer.

LAK Cells

In 1980, Elizabeth Grimm demonstrated that incubation of "normal" mouse spleen cells or human peripheral blood lymphocytes for 3 to 4 days in vitro with interleukin-2 (IL-2) resulted in the generation of lymphokine-activated killer (LAK) cells that did not bear T-cell markers, were not major histocompatibility complex (MHC) restricted, lysed cell lines resistant to NK killing, and were effective in reducing large tumor cell masses in mice. There has been some disagreement on the nature of the precursor cell for LAK cells, but most evidence indicates that they arise from NK cells. LAK cells are being tested in clinical immunotherapy trials (see below). LAK cells are not immunologically specific, and a given population of LAK cells will lyse a number of different tumor target cell lines but not normal cells. Further stimulation of LAK cells with antibodies to the T-cell receptor (CD3, anti-TCR $\alpha\beta$) enhances release of gamma interferon (IFN-γ) from LAK, but antibodies to other T-cell surface markers do not. This suggests that LAK cells may have receptors similar to those of conventional T cells but are not necessarily of the same lineage.

ADCC

Effector cells that have surface receptors for the Fc of aggregated antibody (usually immunoglobulin G [IgG]) may react with antibody bound to target cells and cause lysis. The effector cell types are heterogeneous and include polymorphonuclear leukocytes, macrophages, and lymphocytes. The lymphocytes involved usually have no distinguishing T- or B-cell surface markers. They have been called null cells or K (killer) cells. The Fc receptor for IgG is a common feature of antibody-dependent cell-mediated cytotoxic (ADCC) effector cells. Killing requires effector-target cell interaction accomplished by the antibody binding by its antigen recognition sites to the target cell and by its Fc to the effector cell. Lysis of the target cell by ADCC follows interaction with the killer cell. The mechanism of target cell destruction is not well understood, and its in vivo significance remains unclear.

TILs

The attempt to use specific autologous cells for treatment of cancers has met with limited success. Recently, the application of tumor-infiltrating lymphocytes (TILs) or tumor-derived activated cells has been reported to have in vivo antitumor effects against both animal and human tumors. These cells are extracted from tumor tissue, treated with IL-2 in vitro, and injected back into the individual from which the tumor tissue was obtained. Cell lines with antitumor activity that have been derived from TILs are being used for passive immunotherapy (see below).

Activated Macrophages

Macrophages are activated as a result of a delayed-type hypersensitivity reaction initiated by T_{DTH} cells or by nonspecific macrophage activators such as polynucleotides. The role of macrophages as scavengers that "clean up" injured cells is well known. Macrophages may be activated and attracted to inflammatory sites by mediators released from T_{DTH} lymphocytes in vivo. However, nonspecific killing by activated macrophages has also been observed in vitro. Macrophages may be activated by a variety of agents, including mycobacteria (bacillus Calmette-Guérin [BCG]) and polynucleotides (see below). The mechanism of this type of killing involves the phagocytic activity of macrophages, through formation of oxygen radicals and activation of proteolytic enzymes.

Antibody-Mediated Tumor Immunity

Through the use of diffusion chambers (permeable to antibody and complement but not to cells), it has been demonstrated that antibody and complement may cause the death of some kinds of tumor cells. Leukemias, which exist as single cells in suspension, are sensitive to antibody both in vivo and in vitro, whereas sarcoma and carcinoma cells that form solid tumor masses are usually resistant to the effect of antibody and complement. Thus, ADCC reactions may be responsible for the death of tumor cells that grow primarily in suspension, whereas T-cell-mediated reactions are responsible for the rejection of solid tumors.

In Vivo Tumor Killing

The immune mechanism responsible for the rejection of solid tumors in laboratory animals is essentially the same as that responsible for homograft rejection. The mechanism is either T_{CTL}-cell lysis of tumor cells or T_{DTH}-cell-mediated delayed-type hypersensitivity. Studies of transplantable hepatomas in syngeneic guinea pigs have shown destruction of tumor cells in vivo by a two-step delayed-type hypersensitivity-like mechanism. Sensitized cells (T_{DTH} cells) are necessary to initiate the reaction with tumor cells, but macrophages accumulate at the site of the reaction with tumor cells and are responsible for the final tumor cell destruction. If macrophages are mixed with tumor cells, or if they are brought to the site of tumor cell inoculation by nonspecific means, tumor cell destruction is still seen. The contribution of T_{CTL} cells in this model of tumor cell rejection is not clear but may be critical for effective destruction of tumor cells in other systems.

Immunosurveillance

The Phenomenon

Does the immune system prevent cancer? If tumors have specific antigens that are recognizable by the autochthonous host, then it is possible that such antigens may stimulate an "early warning" immune reaction that will eliminate small tumors or developing cancer cells. Sir MacFarlane Burnet and Lewis Thomas independently developed the theory of immune surveillance and postulated that if it were not for the immune rejection mechanism, vertebrates would die at an early age from tumor growth. The immunosurveillance hypothesis states that potential malignant cells that develop new antigenic determinants are recognized as foreign by the immune system and are eliminated. Burnet went on to suggest that the allograft rejection mechanism prevents tumors from being contagious; if allogeneic tissue were not rejected, the tumors of one person could easily grow in another, such as occurs in nude mice.

The findings in nude mice illustrate the difficulty in using an experimental system to confirm or deny the hypothesis of immune surveillance. Nude mice do not have functional T cells, are unable to reject foreign tissue grafts, and will support the growth of allogeneic or even syngeneic tumors. In addition, the nude mouse is highly susceptible to virus-induced tumors. At first glance, these findings imply that the nude mouse proves the theory that the lack of an immune surveillance system leads to cancer. However, nude mice do not have an increased incidence of spontaneous tumors or increased susceptibility to chemical carcinogens. Therefore, at second glance, the lack of a T-cell surveillance system does not appear to result in an increase in tumor development. On the other hand, nude mice do have active NK cells, even more than most normal mice. Thus, on third glance, it is possible that immune surveillance of tumors in nude mice may depend on the NK system. However, in mice deficient in NK activity, such as mice with the beige mutation, there is no increased susceptibility to chemically induced tumors. These findings and the lack of in vivo correlation between tumor development (either high or low) and NK activity in other models leave in doubt a role for NK as a general mechanism for immune surveillance.

Immune surveillance may be weakened by natural selection mechanisms. There is a clear difference in the vigorous response to many virus-induced tumors in animals compared with little or no response to spontaneously arising human tumors. There appears to be a host selection for an immune mechanism favoring prompt rejection of virus-transformed cells along the lines of the response to other infectious agents. On the other hand, there does not seem to be strong host selection for immune resistance to spontaneous tumors, presumably because most spontaneously occurring tumors arise after the host has passed the reproductive age. Thus, immune surveillance may be effective against "strongly antigenic" tumors such as tumors caused by viruses but not against spontaneously developing tumors. In support of the above hypothesis is the observation that strongly antigenic virus-induced tumors of humans are relatively rare compared with nonantigenic spontaneous tumors, except in immunosuppressed individuals. Alternatively, cancer may result from an adaptive mechanism of a cell line against toxic cell injury, an adaptation with advantages for the cell line albeit at the expense of the whole organism.

Failure of Immunosurveillance

If progressive growth of a tumor implies breakdown of an immune surveillance mechanism, then malignancy may represent a failure of the host's tumor immune defense. There are at least 16 explanations for the failure of the immune response in the tumor-bearing host (Table 20.7).

Nonantigenic Tumors

Clearly, if a given tumor does not have an antigen that can be recognized by the autochthonous host, an immune response to the tumor will not take place. Spontaneous tumors in rodents frequently do not have demonstrable tumor antigens, and tumors induced with low doses of carcinogens are less immunogenic than those induced with higher doses. Antigenicity is not necessarily a constant feature of all tumors, and in some instances, tumor-specific antigens are undetectable even after extensive examination.

Tumor Antigens May Not Be Immunogenic in the Primary (Autochthonous) Host

The tumor may contain an antigen that is recognized in another species, such as carcinoembryonic antigen, but is not immunogenic in the tumor-bearing animal. Most serologically defined tumor antigens are not able to induce an effective immune response in the autochthonous host.

Table 20.7 Factors responsible for failure of immune surveillance of cancer

Lack of tumor antigen
Tumor antigen is not immunogenic
Immune tolerance to tumor antigen
Immune suppression
Immune enhancement
Antigenic modulation of tumor antigens
Immunoselection of nonantigenic clones
Imbalance of tumor growth and immune response
Suppressor cells for tumor immunity
Growth of tumor in privileged site
Lack of self MHC recognition
Immunostimulation
Alteration of T-cell receptor
Loss of Fas/Fas-L receptor system
Production of molecules that inactivate T cells
Lack of expression of costimulatory molecules on tumor cells

Immune Tolerance

The encounter of mature T cells with antigens may result in tolerance rather than immunity. According to a recent theory (danger signal), immunity results when inflammation and tissue destruction occurs, such as in a bacterial or viral infection. During the early growth of a cancer, there may be no "danger signal," and the putative tumor antigen induces tolerance. When the tumor gets bigger and tissue destruction occurs, the tolerant state may persist.

Immunosuppression

Increased tumor incidence has been observed in patients who have been treated with immunosuppressive drugs or who have congenital immunologic deficiency diseases. As stated above, tumors in immunosuppressed individuals frequently arise in the lymphoreticular system and do not necessarily imply a loss of immune surveillance in general but may indicate an abnormality in control of lymphoid cell proliferation. Surveys have generally concluded that while patients with solid tumors may have normal ability to form antibodies, they often have an impaired delayed cutaneous hypersensitivity. Even if impaired cellular immune mechanisms have no cause-and-effect relationship to the growth and/or development of the tumor, they have importance in respect to the problem of infectious diseases complicating cancer.

Immune Enhancement

The tumor-bearing animal may not only make an ineffective immune response, but also the immune response to the tumor may allow the tumor to grow more readily. Immune enhancement was described by N. Kaliss in 1956 as the progressive growth of normally rejected strain-specific tumors in recipients who had been pretreated with either antiserum directed against the tumor (passive enhancement) or repeated injections of antigenic material of the tumor (active enhancement). Although first seen in allogeneic systems, enhancement has been demonstrated to occur in syngeneic transplantation models with methylcholanthrene-induced sarcomas, mammary adenocarcinomas derived from mammary tumor virus-carrying mice, and possibly Moloney virus-induced lymphomas. Most of these later studies involved immunization of animals with tumor-derived materials in such a way as to induce the formation of humoral antibody but not delayed-type hypersensitivity. Transfer of tumors to such immunized recipients or to recipients injected with serum from immunized donors results in a more rapid growth than occurs in untreated tumor recipients. Growth of the tumor is enhanced in the presence of serum antibody, and such enhancement has been attributed to the presence of "blocking antibodies."

Mechanisms of enhancement in relation to the immune response may be afferent, efferent, or central. Afferent inhibition implies that the recipient did not become immunized by graft antigens because the simultaneous presence of antibody prevents antigen from becoming available to immune responsive tissues. Central inhibition would occur if the host lymphoid cells failed to be stimulated, despite being presented with the antigen in a suitable immunogenic form. Efferent inhibition would apply if the recipient became immunized but the response that resulted was ineffective against the tumor. It appears that enhancement is usually an efferent effect. In some instances, both cellular sensitivity and humoral factors are present in the autochthonous host, but the humoral factor blocks the colony-inhibiting effect of the sensitized cells (blocking factor). Although the term blocking antibody has been used to identify this factor, the antibody or immunoglobulin nature of the blocking factor has not been clearly established. It is possible that "blocking factor" is a complex of tumor antigen and antibody that inhibits the reaction of sensitized lymphocytes with antigen on the tumor cells, or, it may be free antigen. In addition, a serum factor that can decrease the effects of blocking factor has been described and is called unblocking factor. Humoral factors may also cause enhanced tumor growth, either through physiologic changes in the tumor cells or through stimulation of a substance produced by tumor cells that produces unresponsiveness in lymphoid cells.

Antigenic Modulation

Complete loss of antigenicity or a significant antigenic change with selective overgrowth of the changed variant has been demonstrated to be a mechanism of escape from immune rejection. Loss of the MHC antigens of one parental strain can be induced by passage of a tumor arising in an F_1 animal in the other parental strain, and cell surface antigens of mouse leukemic cells, the TL antigen, may disappear after treatment of the cells with antiserum to the TL antigen but reappear after removal of the antiserum. A stable subline of a Moloney tumor that is resistant to specific antiserum to the parent tumor has been produced by incubating tumor cells in cytotoxic antiserum in the presence of complement and then inoculating these samples into preimmunized mice. These observations support the concept that tumor cells under immunologic attack may be able to survive by not expressing the tumor-specific antigen to which the immune response is directed and thus thwarting immune surveillance.

Immunoselection of Nonantigenic Clones

Spontaneous tumors may produce successive clonal variants that replace each other as the tumor progresses. Each successful variant has greater autonomy and is less affected by restricting host mechanisms. Thus, by natural selection, the tumor may evolve new clones with different antigens or nonantigenic clones that are not limited by host immune response.

Imbalance of Immunity and Tumor Mass

The ability of an immune response to protect against the continued growth of a tumor depends upon the mass of the tumor that is being contained. Lloyd Old and Edward Boyse postulated that "sneaking through" of tumor cells might occur with a low number of tumor cells. In this situation, there may be insufficient antigenic stimulation to provide effective immunization until the tumor grows larger. At the higher cell number, antigenic stimulation is sufficient to provide effective immunization, which in turn prevents tumor growth. However, the presence of a large tumor mass may exhaust the supply of lymphocytes produced by the host (a form of desensitization). Most forms of immunotherapy effective in laboratory animals may be overcome by a tumor of sufficient size. Immunotherapy is effective only for relatively small tumors or in preventing growth of small numbers of injected tumor cells. On the other hand, immune rejection can destroy large tumor allografts.

Suppressor Cells

Specific suppressor cells may depress the effect of an immune response to a tumor antigen. Thus, an immune response to a tumor might result in the production of not only killer cells to the tumor but also suppressor cells that protect the tumor by inhibiting the production of T-killer cells.

Immune Privileged Site

A tumor may arise in an immunologically sheltered site, where surveillance functions play no role in antagonizing tumor development. Such a site is known to occur in the hamster cheek pouch. The hamster cheek pouch is frequently used to transplant tumors in a way that will avoid an immune reaction to the tumor. It is possible that such sites may serve as a locus for the development of primary tumors that avoid immune surveillance until the growth of the tumor cannot be reversed by the immune mechanism. However, a high incidence of tumors in similar sites in humans is not observed.

Lack of Self Recognition

It is possible that progression, a change in the growth potential of a given tumor, may be related to selection for cellular variants of a tumor with altered class I gene expression. The expression of MHC antigens, especially class I antigens, has been demonstrated to play an important role in the behavior of tumors in experimental models. In mice, some tumors having a TSTA, but lacking the self class I antigen H2K, are resistant to T-cell killing and readily grow when transplanted into normal syngeneic hosts. However, if these same tumors are transfected with DNA coding for the H2K antigen and are thereby induced to express the H2K antigen, the tumors are rendered untransplantable. For these tumors, recognition of a TSTA in combination with self class I MHC antigen may be needed either for induction or expression of tumor rejection. In other systems, resistance to macrophage and/or natural killing may be correlated with a loss of class I antigen expression. In at least one instance of a virus-transformed cell line, low class I antigen expression may be reversed by IFN treatment. In other instances, viral transfection or enhanced invasiveness of tumors is associated with increased class I antigen expression.

Skin cancers induced by UV radiation express TSTAs and are rejected upon transplantation into syngeneic hosts. Yet, UV-induced tumors grow progressively in the original UV-irradiated host. UV treatment induces suppressor components capable of specifically eliminating the T-cell response against the autochthonous tumor. This suppressor effect is not demonstrable against chemically induced tumors. Thus, alterations in self recognition may be important in the host-tumor immune relationship for some cancers. Yet, many metastatic tumors do not have demonstrable alterations in the level or nature of the class I products expressed as compared with normal tissue.

Immunostimulation

A major premise of tumor immunology is that a cell-mediated immune response to a given tumor is a beneficial reaction, that is, cell-mediated immunity, in contrast to humoral antibodies that may mediate enhancement, serves to limit or prevent tumor growth. However, Richmond Prehn has argued that, in some instances, the lymphocytic infiltrate seen in tumors is actually required for early stages of tumor growth. Under certain circumstances, immune reactions stimulate tumor target cells rather than inhibit or kill them. This result is dependent on dose. Immune cells that kill tumor target cells in vitro when added at high killer cell/target cell ratios in vitro (100:1 is commonly used) may actually increase tumor cell growth when present in smaller relative numbers in vivo. Although the specificity of immunostimulation has been questioned, it must be considered that tumors could escape immune surveillance by immunostimulation at a critical point in their development and later become resistant to the specific inhibitory effects of immune cells.

Alteration of T-Cell Receptors

T cells in tumor-bearing animals may have an altered T-cell receptor affecting the ability of $CD8^+$ cytotoxic cells to become activated after reaction with tumor antigens. The expression of the CD3γ is low, and CD3ζ is replaced by Fcϵ γ-γ, so that the T_{CTL}-cell receptor is unable to function. The role of this mechanism in humans has not been demonstrated.

Alteration of the Fas Receptor and Ligand System

T_{CTL}-cell killing of tumor cells is mediated largely by the Fas/FasL system. Cytotoxicity is initiated by reaction of FasL on T_{CTL} cells with Fas on tumor cells. Tumors may evade killing by expressing FasL, which will induce apoptosis of activated T cells. In addition, some tumors have been shown to lack Fas, and infiltration with mononuclear cells leads to release of soluble Fas, which further serves to block FasL on T_{CTL} cells. Human hepatomas that express Fas have a better prognosis than hepatomas that do not.

Production of Receptors Which Inhibit T Cells

Human cancers may express a cell surface molecule, RASC1 (receptor-binding cancer antigen expressed on SiSo cells), which is a ligand for receptors on normal lymphocytes, including T, B, and NK cells. RASC1 inhibits the proliferation of lymphocytes and causes apoptosis of activated lymphocytes.

Lack of Expression of Costimulatory Molecules on Tumor Cells

Interaction of the B7 molecule on antigen-presenting cells with its receptors CD28 and CTLA-4 on T cells provides costimulatory signals for T-cell activation (Fig. 20.4). $CD8^+$ precursors of T_{CTL} cells are also activated by costimulator signals: (i) $CD8^+$ T-cell receptor–MHC class I molecule on tumor cells, and (ii) CD28 and B7 on tumor cells. In experimental systems, transplantable tumors that express B7 are rejected in syngeneic hosts, whereas tumors that lack B7 inactivate $CD8^+$ T_{CTL}-cell precursors, allowing the tumors to grow.

Immunodiagnosis of Cancer

Pathologists recognize cancer tissue to be "less organized" and cancer cells to be "less differentiated" than normal tissue. In fact, tumors are graded histologically according to their degree of resemblance to normal tissues: well differentiated, poorly differentiated, or anaplastic (without form). Cancer markers are the biochemical or immunological counterparts of the

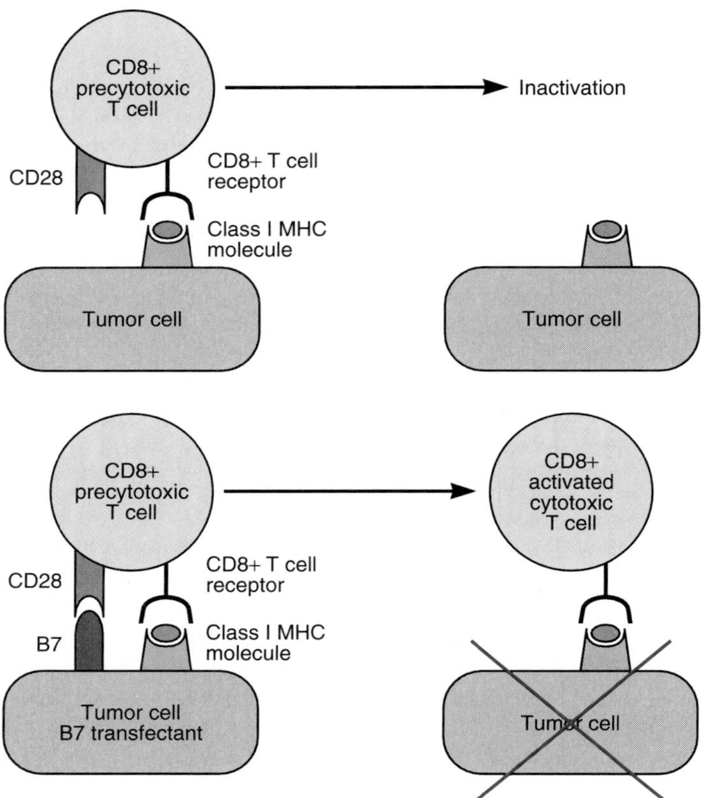

Figure 20.4 Activation of $CD8^+$ cytotoxic T cells requires two signals: T-cell receptor reacting with antigen presented by MHC class I molecule and interaction of CD28 with B7 on the tumor cell. Tumor cells that lack B7 will not activate $CD8^+$ precytotoxic cells. The same tumor cell transfected with B7 will activate T_{CTL} cells, which will kill target cells that do not express B7. Interaction of T-cell receptor with antigen on MHC class I in the absence of costimulatory signals results in inactivation of the $CD8^+$ precytotoxic cells.

morphology of the tumors. During the last 20 years, there has been a growing appreciation that the morphologic resemblance of cancer cells to embryonic or fetal cells is also reflected in the production of cellular macromolecules by cancer cells that are more typical of embryonic or fetal cells than of adult tissue (Fig. 20.5).

Many of these macromolecules are not only present in the cell or on the cell surface but are also secreted into the body fluids. Measurement of these oncodevelopmental markers by the clinical laboratory has become increasingly important in the diagnosis of cancer. In addition, antibodies to cancer markers are being used to localize tumor tissue in vivo and to treat certain selected cancers. Some clinical applications of cancer markers are listed in Table 20.8.

Various types of cancer markers are listed in Table 20.9. These are only a few examples of an increasingly recognized number of markers associated with cancer. In most, if not all, instances, cancer markers are produced normally at some time during development but are present in low or undetectable amounts in the adult (Fig. 20.5). The adult tumors that produce these oncodevelopmental markers usually originate from the

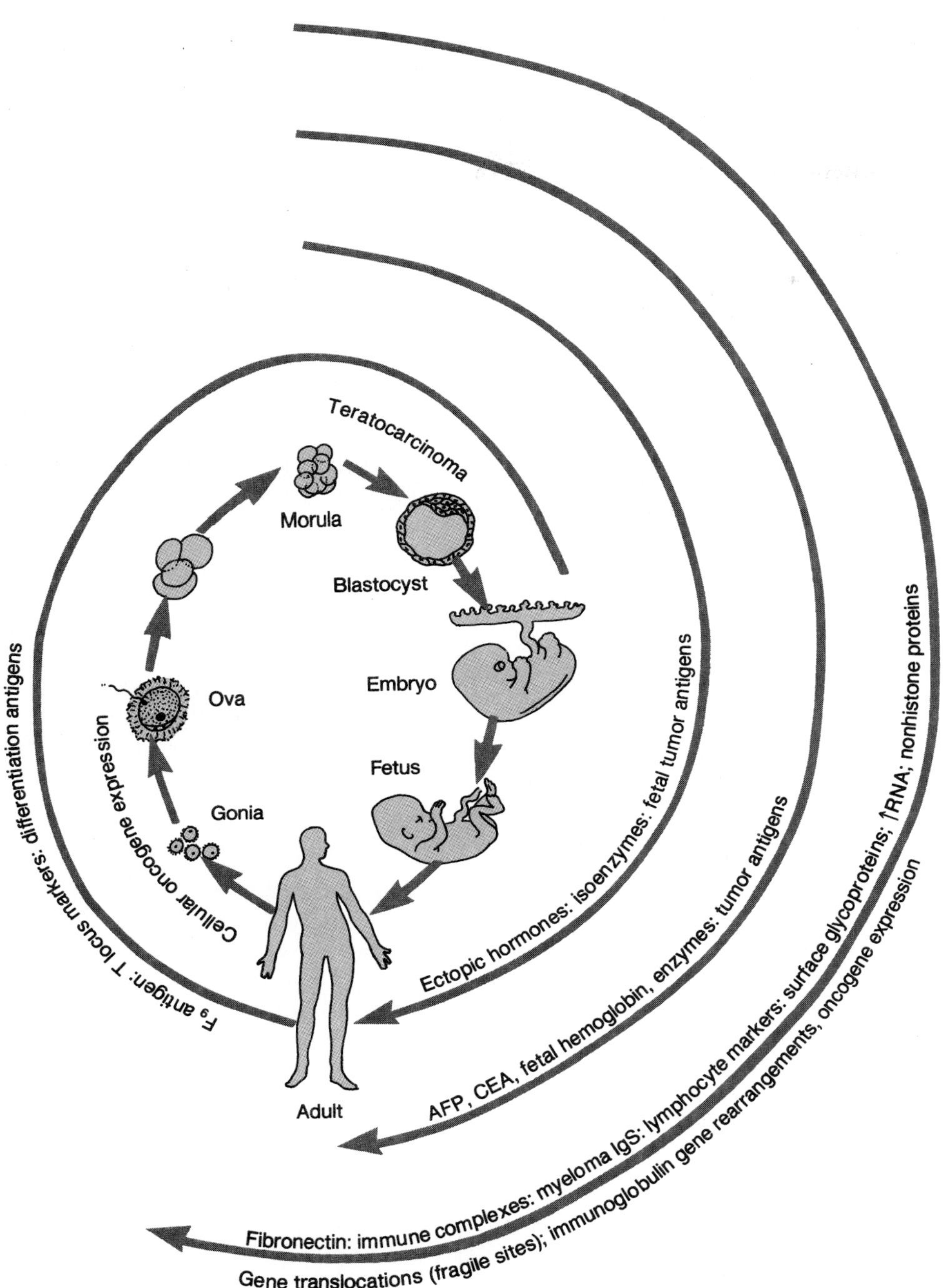

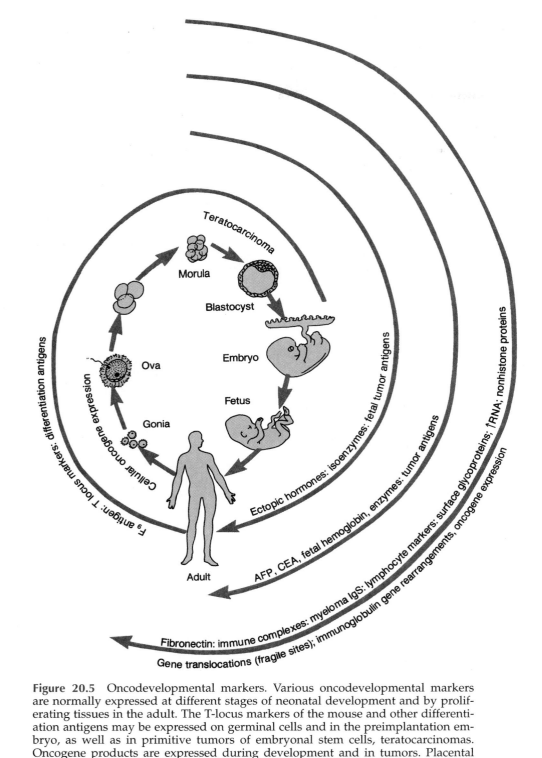

Figure 20.5 Oncodevelopmental markers. Various oncodevelopmental markers are normally expressed at different stages of neonatal development and by proliferating tissues in the adult. The T-locus markers of the mouse and other differentiation antigens may be expressed on germinal cells and in the preimplantation embryo, as well as in primitive tumors of embryonal stem cells, teratocarcinomas. Oncogene products are expressed during development and in tumors. Placental hormones, isoenzymes, and proteins may be expressed in adult tumors of testes, ovary, liver, and breast. Other markers, such as alpha-fetoprotein (AFP) and carcinoembryonic antigen (CEA), are produced normally by developing liver or colonic mucosal cells, respectively, and are frequently expressed in tumors of these tissues, i.e., hepatocellular carcinomas and adenocarcinomas of the colon, as well as in other tumors of embryologically related tissues. Immunoglobulins and lymphocyte differentiation markers (CDs) are found to be associated with lymphoproliferative tumors. Many surface glycoprotein and glycolipid carbohydrate differences recognized by monoclonal antibodies are due to the activity of glycosylating enzymes in tumors that are normally active during normal development. Gene rearrangements that occur normally during plasma cell development are used to identify clonality and B-cell origin of lymphoid tumors.

Table 20.8 Some clinical applications of cancer markers[a]

Activity or therapy	Example(s)
Activity	
Screen asymptomatic patients	Occult fecal blood
Screen high-risk patients	Complete blood count (leukemia), AFP, PSA
Confirm a suspected clinical diagnosis	CEA, PSA, lymphocyte markers (CDs)
Monitor response to therapy	CEA, AFP, PSA, myeloma protein, CHO, mucins
Therapy	
Antibody, monoclonal antibodies	CEA, AFP, anti-CDs, anti-idiotype (B cells)
Antibody–drug/toxin conjugate	Ricin, diphtheria, toxin, exotoxin A, daunomycin
Radiolabeled antibody	Iodine-131, yttrium-90

[a]Abbreviations: AFP, alpha-fetoprotein; CEA, carcinoembryonic antigen; PSA, prostate-specific antigen.

tissue that normally produces the markers during development (Table 20.10). For instance, alpha-fetoprotein (AFP) is normally produced by fetal liver and yolk sac. Tumors that arise from liver or germ cell tumors that contain yolk sac elements are the most frequent producers of AFP, and the order of frequency of other cancers correlates with embryonic lineage relationships: stomach > lung > lymphoma.

Myeloma Proteins

The first cancer marker was recognized by Dr. Henry Bence Jones in 1846. "Bence Jones protein" was identified as a urinary precipitate that occurred upon heating at pH 4 to 6 the urine of a patient with "mollities ossium," a bone disease now known as multiple myeloma. It is remarkable that it took over 100 years from the first recognition of Bence Jones protein to identify Bence Jones proteins as immunoglobulin light chains. Bence Jones proteins are produced in excess by about half of the patients with plasmacytomas. The molecular mass of the light chain (about 22 kDa) is below that excluded by the basement membrane of glomerulus of the kidney, so it appears in the urine as Bence Jones protein. It is associated with the presence of monoclonal immunoglobulins in the serum. The amount of Bence Jones protein found in urine or the amount of myeloma immunoglobulin in the serum may be used to monitor the effects of therapy;

Table 20.9 Some types of cancer markers

Type of marker	Example
Deletions of blood group markers	ABH blood group antigens
Backbone or blood group markers	Monosialoganglioside
Cell surface glycoproteins	Carcinoembryonic antigen
Secreted proteins	Alpha-fetoprotein
Enzyme alterations	Glycosyltransferases, prostate-specific antigen
Isozymes	Alkaline phosphatase
Ectopic hormones	Chorionic gonadotropin
Tumor antigens	MAGE-1, MAGE-3, gp120, etc.
Cytoskeletal elements	Epidermal tumors (cytokeratin)
Immunoglobulin gene rearrangements	B-cell tumors
Gene translocations	Lymphomas (Philadelphia chromosome, etc.)

Table 20.10 Levels of expression of oncodevelopmental markers by tumors

Marker	Normal producing tissue	Tissue(s) that is:		
		Embryogenically closely related	**Distantly related**	**From a different germ line**
Carcinoembryonic antigen	Colon	Stomach, pancreas, liver	Lung, breast	Lymphoma
Alpha-fetoprotein	Liver, yolk sac	Colon, stomach, pancreas	Lung	Lymphoma
Serotonin	"Entero-endocrine"	Adrenal, carcinoid (GI)	Oat cell, lung	Epidermal, lung
Chorionic gonadotropin	Placenta	Germinal tumor	Liver	Epidermal, lung

the amount of these proteins in a given patient closely reflects the amount of myeloma tumor mass. This general principle also applies to other secreted tumor markers, including hormones and serum enzymes.

AFP

The modern era of cancer markers began with the discovery of AFP by Garri Abelev of the Soviet Union in 1963. He identified this protein in the sera of normal fetal mice and in the sera of adult mice with hepatocellular carcinoma but not in normal adult mice. AFP is an antigenically distinct serum protein with properties similar to those of albumin. It is found in high concentrations (up to 10 mg/ml) in fetal serum and in the serum of patients with hepatocellular carcinomas or teratocarcinomas but in low concentrations (<10 ng/ml) in the serum of normal adults. Elevations up to 500 ng/ml occur frequently in association with a variety of nonmalignant diseases, such as hepatitis or cirrhosis, but elevations above this are essentially diagnostic of an AFP-producing tumor. Approximately half of the patients with hepatocellular carcinoma can be diagnosed by such an elevation. Serial determinations of AFP may be used clinically to determine the effectiveness of therapy. Failure of elevated serum AFP levels to return to normal after surgery is an indication that the tumor has not been completely removed or that metastases are present (Fig. 20.6). These patterns essentially hold true for other cancer markers found in the serum.

CEA

Carcinoembryonic antigen (CEA) is a cell surface glycoprotein that is normally produced by colonic epithelium and secreted in the intestine. In colonic and other CEA-producing cancers, alterations in the polarity of cells is associated with release of CEA in elevated levels into the blood. During development, CEA is produced by the fetal gastrointestinal tract; elevations of CEA associated with cancers in the adult reflect the developmental relationship to gastrointestinal tissue. CEA elevations also occur in association with nonmalignant diseases, so elevated serum CEA levels can be used only as an adjunct to other diagnostic procedures (Table 20.11). In patients with colorectal cancer who have elevated serum CEA, the serum levels may be used to determine the effectiveness of therapy. Unfortunately, re-elevation of CEA has not proved useful as an indication for "second-look" surgery. CEA levels in breast cancer become elevated when metastases occur, and serial CEA determinations are useful for determining effectiveness of chemotherapy, for determining prognosis, and for measuring progression of the disease.

Radiolabeled antibodies to AFP and CEA have been used to localize clandestine tumors by radioimmunescintigraphy. Labeled antibodies are

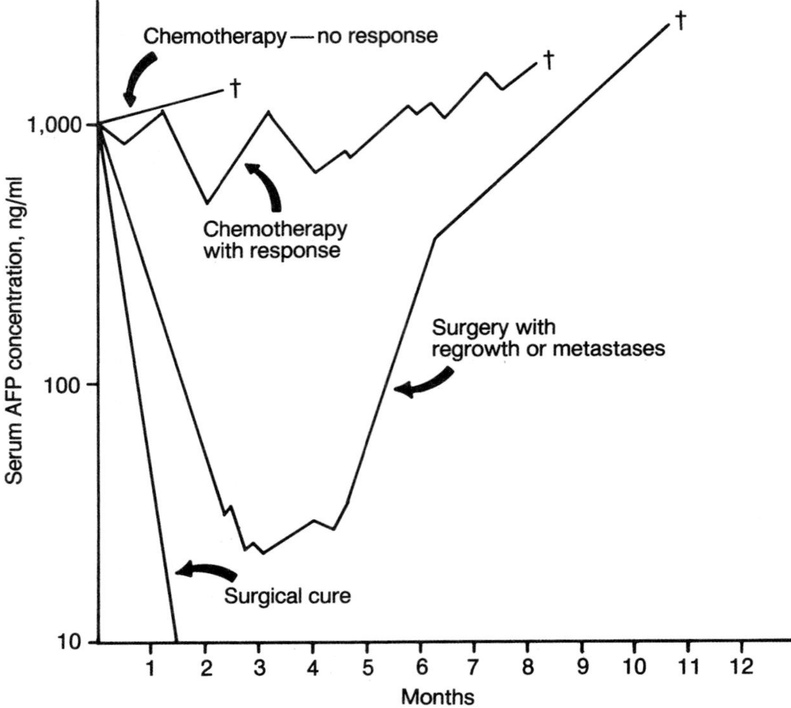

Figure 20.6 Representative changes in the concentration of AFP in serum in response to therapy. Successful treatment is reflected in a rapid fall of the serum concentration to normal. If the concentration does not fall rapidly or becomes re-elevated, tumor is still present.

injected into patients, and localization of the label in tissues is determined by scanning the body for radioactivity. Accuracy of diagnosis has been improved by application of computer analysis to the photoscans. Primary cancers have been localized in 83% of cases of colorectal cancer, and in 22% of patients, cancer sites were located that no other detection method had found.

Antibodies to CEA and AFP have also been used to treat tumors producing these markers in animals. So far, the results, even when drugs such as daunomycin have been attached to the antibodies, have been equivocal. Trials in humans are not yet interpretable as being effective.

PSA

The approval of prostate-specific antigen (PSA) for clinical use in 1985 by the U.S. Food and Drug Administration (FDA) represents the most important development in cancer markers since the early 1970s, when CEA was approved. PSA was identified by Ming Chu and his coworkers as a single-chain 34-kDa protein (serine protease) containing 7% carbohydrate that is produced by normal prostate cells and functions to help liquefy seminal fluid. It is produced in increased amounts by prostatic cancer cells. An increase in serum PSA level is now used clinically as a strong indication for prostate cancer. However, a rise in PSA may also occur with benign prostatic disease, such as prostatitis and benign prostatic hypertrophy, so elevations of PSA should be followed by careful digital rectal exam (DRE) and transrectal ultrasound (TUS). The positive predictive values for posi-

Table 20.11 CEA concentrations in human sera[a]

Type of patient	No. of patients tested	% patients with CEA concn (ng/ml) of:			
		0–2.5	2.6–5.0	5.1–10	10
Healthy subjects					
Nonsmokers	892	97	3	0	0
Smokers	620	81	15	3	1
Colorectal carcinoma	544	28	23	14	35
Pulmonary carcinoma	181	24	25	25	26
Pancreatic carcinoma	55	9	31	25	35
Gastric carcinoma	79	39	32	10	19
Breast carcinoma	125	53	20	13	14
Other carcinoma	343	51	28	12	9
Benign breast disease	115	85	11	4	0
Severe alcoholic cirrhosis	120	29	44	25	2
Active ulcerative colitis	146	69	18	8	5
Pulmonary emphysema	49	43	37	16	4

[a]Modified from V. Go, *Cancer* **37**:562–566, 1976.

tive findings are as follows: +TUS alone, 8%; +TUS+DRE, 26%; +TUS+PSA, 41%; +DRE+PSA, 58%; +TUS+DRE+PSA, 80%.

PSA is now used to monitor men over the age of 40 for development of prostatic cancer. Levels below 4 μg/liter are considered normal. Although elevations above this level may occur with benign prostatic hypertrophy, any individual with a PSA level above 4 μg/liter or with increasing levels upon serial determinations should be examined by DRE and TUR. When reaching the circulation, enzymatically active proteases, like PSA, are inactivated by complexing with protease inhibitors in the blood. The majority of PSA in the blood is in the form of a complex with the protease inhibitor, α_1-antichymotrypsin; 5 to 40% is free; and minor portions are complexed with α_1-protease inhibitor or α_2-macroglobulin. The proportion of free PSA is actually a stronger diagnostic factor than total PSA in the critical concentration range of 4 to 10 μg/liter. A low proportion of free PSA is associated with higher-grade carcinomas.

MAbs to Cancer Markers

The development of MAbs to "cancer antigens" has produced a new generation of "cancer markers." These markers include carbohydrate and mucin epitopes, as well as cytoplasmic antigens and lymphocyte differentiation markers (CDs). A comparison of newly defined markers with "classic" cancer markers is given in Table 20.12.

Routine use of a given marker for diagnosis requires a specificity of >90%. Thus, most tumor markers are not sufficiently specific for diagnosis and must be used in conjunction with other diagnostic indicators. Lower specificities are acceptable for monitoring. A marker such as tissue polypeptide antigen (TPA) may not be at all useful for the diagnosis of cancer, but if a patient who is known to have cancer has an elevated TPA, serial determinations of TPA may be useful for follow-up. The markers that are the most useful for diagnosis include AFP, human chorionic gonadotropin (hCG), PSA, TAG-72, and terminal deoxytransferase. On the other hand, many of the markers not used for diagnosis have proved

Table 20.12 Cancer markers in clinical use[a]

Marker	Nature	Minimum concn for detection	Type of cancer	Diagnosis	Prognosis	Monitoring	Sensitivity (%)	Specificity (%)
Proteins								
AFP	70-kDa glycoprotein, 4% carbohydrate	15 ng/ml	Hepatocellular germ cell (yolk sac)	+++	+	+++	60–90	60–100
CEA	200-kDa glycoprotein, up to 70% CHO	3–5 μg/ml	GI, pancreas, lung, breast, others	+	++	+++	42–96	10–90
hCG	Glycopeptide hormone	3 IU/ml	Embryonal, choriocarcinoma	++	+++	+++	60–100	40–90
Ferritin	450-kDa iron-binding protein	200 μg/μl	Liver, lung, breast leukemia	+	++	++	5–56	76–97
PSA	33-kDa glycoprotein, 7% carbohydrate	2.5 μg/ml	Prostate	+++	++	+++	33–89	89–97
Carbohydrates								
CA 19-9	Sialylated Lewis X[A]	37 U/ml	GI, pancreas, ovary	+	++	+++	33–89	82–97
CA 50	Sialylated Lewis X-1 (afucosyl form)	14 U/ml	GI, pancreas, lung	++	++	+++	40–78	80–98
TAG 72	Sialylated T antigen	4–7 U/ml	Breast, ovary, GI	+	++	++	9–72	97
CA 242	Sialylated carbohydrate coexpressed with CA 50	200 U/ml	GI, pancreas	+	++	+++	44–83	75
Mucins								
CA 15-3	Transmembrane protein	30 U/ml	Breast, ovary, lung (adenocarcinoma)	+	++	+++	88–97	30–90
CA 125	200 kDa, up to 50% carbohydrate	35 U/ml	Ovary (epidermal), endometrial	+	+	+++	40–86	86–99
DU-PAN 2	High-molecular-weight glycoprotein	400 U/ml	Pancreas, ovary, GI, lung	+	++	+++	34	86
MCA	1,000-kDa mucin peptide	11 U/ml	Breast, ovary, GI	+	++	+++	20–80	84–90

[a] +, slightly useful; ++, moderately useful; +++, very useful.

Table 20.13 CD antigens on lymphoid tumors

CD antigen	Normal expression	Indication in a tumor expression
CD3	Mature T and B cells	Good prognosis
CD4	T helper/inducer cells	Not useful
CD5	Pan-T cell	Marker for CD5$^+$ chronic lymphocytic leukemia (good prognosis)
CD8	T-suppressor/cytotoxic	Not useful
CD10	Thymocytes, pre-B cells	Common leukemia antigen
CD15	Monocytes/myeloid cells (Leu-M1)	Hodgkin's, histiocytic lymphoma
CD16	Large granular lymphocytes (FcR)	Large granular lymphocytic
CD25	Tac (IL-2 receptor)	Prognosis related to serum level
CD38	Thymocytes, pre-B cells	Poor prognosis
Ki-1	Activated T cells	Some Hodgkin's cells
Ki-67	Cell cycle marker	Prognosis related to percentage of positive cells

useful for determining prognosis (i.e., high levels at the time of diagnosis indicate poor prognosis) or for monitoring the effects of therapy.

A summary of the CDs (clusters of differentiation) useful in human lymphomas is given in Table 20.13. As discussed above, these CDs are markers found on cells of the lymphatic lineage during development and maturation. Their "overexpression" on cells of a leukemia or lymphoma represent "maturation arrest" of a clonal population of cells at a set point on the differentiation pathway of these cells.

Cell Surface Carbohydrates

Many of the "tumor markers" detected by monoclonal antibodies are oligosaccharides. Oligosaccharides on the surface of mammalian cells are attached to lipid (glycosphingolipid) or protein (glycoprotein). The lipid or protein is hydrophobic and is located in the cell membrane, whereas the oligosaccharide is hydrophilic and extends from the cell surface, where it is readily accessible for reaction with antibody.

Of the more than 100 possible monosaccharides, only 7 make up the oligosaccharides of the mammalian cell surface:

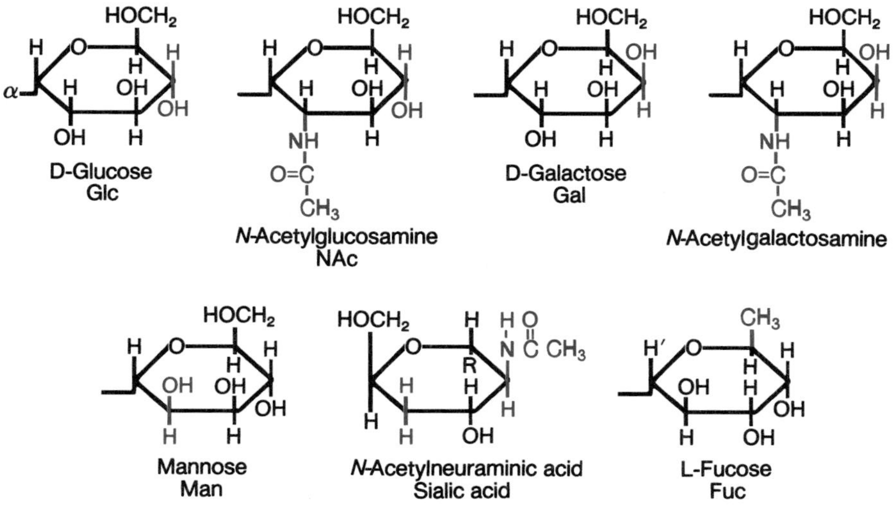

D-Glucose Glc

N-Acetylglucosamine NAc

D-Galactose Gal

N-Acetylgalactosamine

Mannose Man

N-Acetylneuraminic acid Sialic acid

L-Fucose Fuc

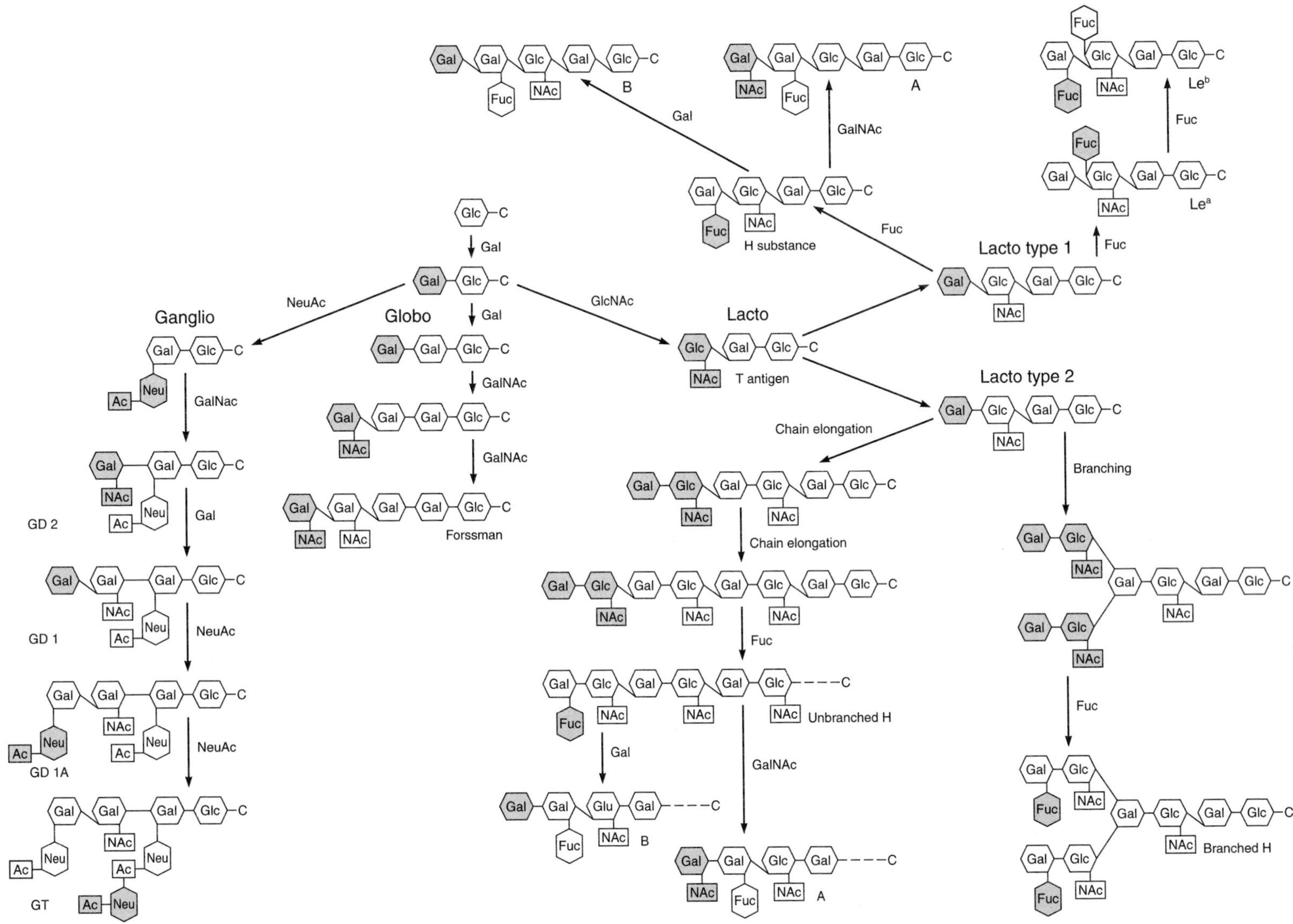

Figure 20.7 Cell surface carbohydrate structures. Cell surface carbohydrates are synthesized from a common Gal-Glu disaccharide by addition of linear or branched monosaccharides. The four major classes are ganglio, globo, lacto-type 1, and lacto-type 2. (From S. Sell, *Hum. Pathol.* **21:**1003–1019, 1990.)

Through different linkages and sequences, chains of these monosaccharides provide an enormous variety of oligosaccharide cell surface structures. The composition and linkage of these polysaccharides and oligosaccharides are not only important in determining the biological behavior of cells but also provide numerous epitopes that may be recognized by MAbs. The appearance of "new" cell surface carbohydrates on cancer cells may be due to (i) the synthesis of different oligosaccharides by tumor cells, (ii) the postsynthetic modification by glycolytic enzymes, or (iii) the "unmasking" of cell surface carbohydrates by shedding or loss of masking cell surface material. Thus, the changes found in cell surface carbohydrates in tumor cells as compared with normal cells are usually secondary to changes in activity or levels of glycosylating enzymes or glycosidases in cancer cells. Cancer carbohydrates belong to four major structural classes: ganglio, globo, lacto-type 1, and lacto-type 2 (Fig. 20.7).

The identification of MAbs to cancer-associated carbohydrates may reflect the immunogenicity of the rigid restricted structure of the oligosaccharides or the relative stability of these structures to formalin fixation. This latter feature is important because many laboratories use formalin-fixed tissues to screen for MAb activity. The major carbohydrate alterations expressed on cancer cells are shown in Fig. 20.8.

Figure 20.8 Carbohydrate structure of some major human cancer markers recognized by MAbs. The epitope designated SLEX (sialylated Lewis X, also known as SSEA or LEX) is formed by fucosylation of the type 2 lacto chain. CA 50 is formed by sialylation of the type 1 lacto chain, and CA 19–9 (Sialyl Le[al]) is formed by fucosylation of CA 50. The Forssman antigen is not found normally on human cells but may be identified on cancer cells because of an increase in expression of *N*-acetylgalactosamine transferase, producing the Forssman pentasaccharide in the globo series. OFA-2 (oncofetal antigen 2) is produced by addition of the *N*-acetygalactosamine to the core trisaccharide of the globo series; OFA-1 is produced by sialylation of OFA-2. (From S. Sell, *Hum. Pathol.* **21:**1003–1019, 1990.)

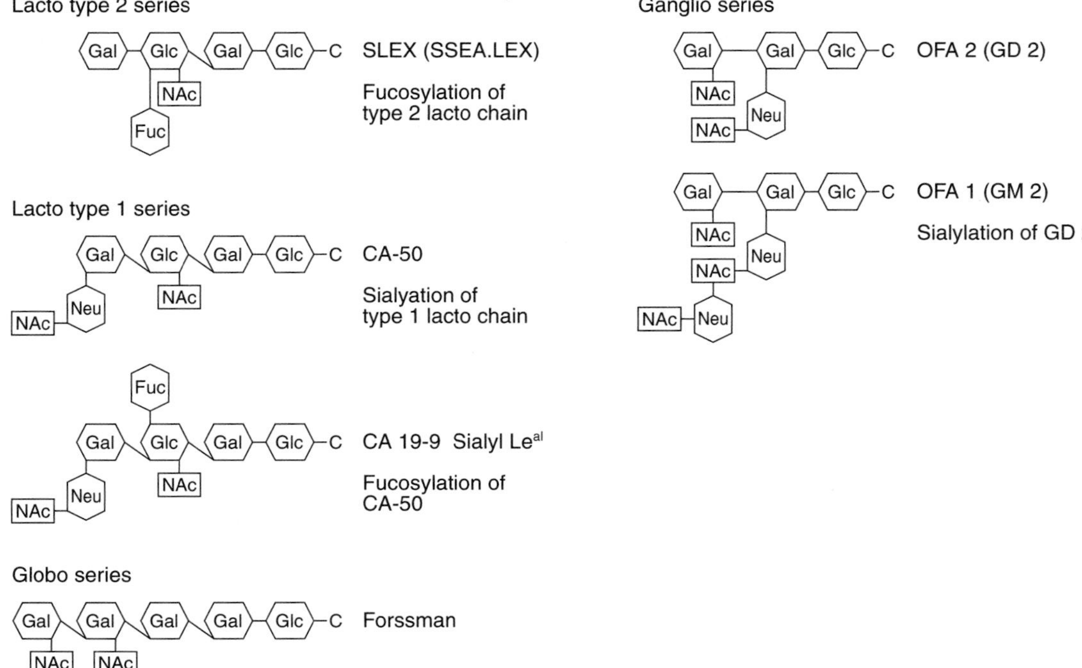

Table 20.14 Comparison of CEA, CA 19-9, CA 50, and CA 242 in patients with colorectal or pancreatic-biliary cancer

Marker	Recommended cutoff value	Colorectal cancer			Pancreatic-biliary cancer	
		Sensitivity (%)		Specificity (%)	Sensitivity (%)	Specificity (%)
		Dukes A-B	Dukes C-D			
CEA	30 ng/ml	32	71	83	39	79
CA 19-9	37 U/ml	16	44	100	76	75
CA 50	17 U/ml	26	47	97	73	67
CA 242	20 U/ml	47	59	90	68	95

A comparison of some carbohydrate epitopes defined by MAbs in the diagnosis of colorectal and pancreatic-biliary cancer is given in Table 20.14.

Mucins

MAbs that react with epitopes of mucins produced by adenocarcinomas have been made. These include CA 15-3 (episialin), CA 125, DU-PAN 2, and MCA (mucinlike cancer-associated antigen). Mucins are high-molecular-weight glycoproteins with a high carbohydrate content (about 50%) that are secreted by glandular cells into glandular lumens and protect glands from self-digestion. With an increase in the numbers of cells in an adenocarcinoma producing these mucins and alterations in the polarity of the adenocarcinoma cells, the mucins are released into the circulation. For a given adenocarcinoma, the serum levels of a mucin epitope may be used to monitor the size of an adenocarcinoma and determine prognosis. Mucin antigens may also be detected by T-cell clones reactive with human breast and pancreatic cancers.

Gangliosides

The ganglioside series specificities (Fig. 20.9) are found on malignant melanomas. GM2, GM3, GD2, and GD3 gangliosides are highly expressed on melanoma and neuroblastoma cells. Patients have been immunized with vaccines containing GM2 and have produced IgM antibodies that are cytotoxic for melanoma target cells expressing GM2. High-affinity antibodies to GD3 have been used for passive antibody therapy with little effect. GM2 is being used in tumor vaccines now undergoing clinical trials (see below).

Mixed Markers

Since some tumors may produce more than one marker, the simultaneous measurement of more than one marker often provides information leading to a more precise diagnosis or prognosis than one marker alone. For instance, differentiation of germ cell tumor types can be accomplished on the basis of elevation of serum AFP or hCG (Table 20.15).

The combined use of more than one cancer marker may greatly increase sensitivity but also may greatly decrease the specificity of detection of cancer. For instance, using placental alkaline phosphatase (PL-ALP) and CA 125 as markers for ovarian cancer, the sensitivity was 59% for CA 125 and 31% for PL-ALP, but by using both CA 125 and PL-ALP, the sensitivity was increased to 67%. On the other hand, the specificity with PL-ALP was 94% and with CA 125 was 87%, but using both, the

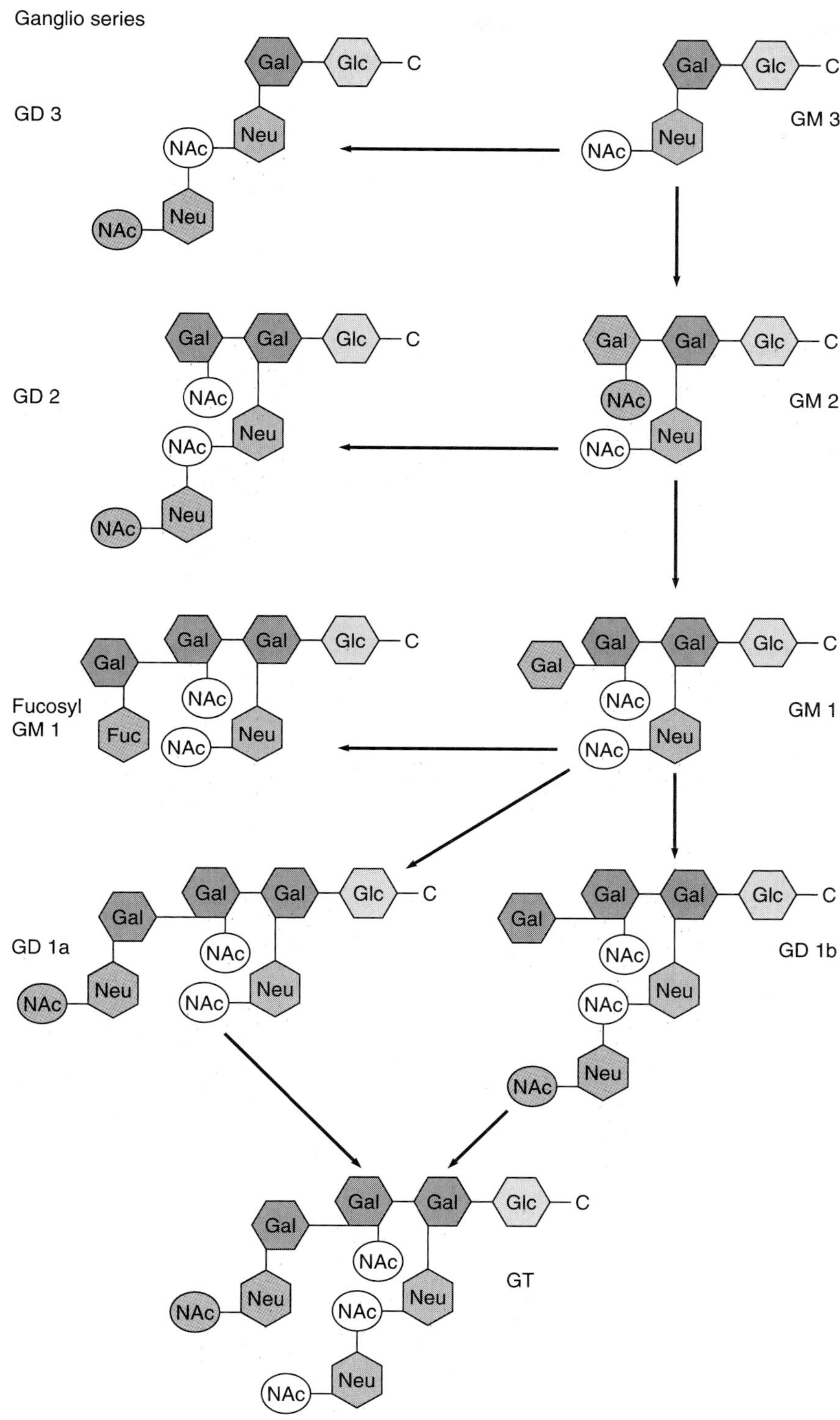

Figure 20.9 Cancer-associated ganglio chains. Monoclonal antibodies to epitopes of the ganglio series have a high specificity for the terminal sialic acid (NeuNAC) residues produced by increased sialylation of the ganglio chains. The additional monosaccharide added to produce a new epitope is indicated by slanted lines.

Table 20.15 Percentages of patients with elevated serum HCG or AFP in germ cell tumors

Type of tumor	% of patients with elevated:		
	hCG	AFP	hCG or AFP
Seminoma	10	0	10
Seminoma, metastatic	38	0	0
Embryonal	60	70	87
Choriocarcinoma	100	0	100
Yolk sac	25	75	100
Teratoma	0	0	0

specificity dropped to 82%. The application of multiple makers is fraught with many difficulties in interpretation. Setting the specificity of each cancer marker at the 95th percentile and using multiple markers greatly increases the likelihood of a false-positive diagnosis of cancer. A normal person who has 13 separate cancer marker tests has, by chance alone, a probability of 50% of being diagnosed as having cancer. It is, in fact, the potential for the overdiagnosis of cancer that has contributed largely to the limited approval for cancer marker tests by the FDA panel. The application of multiple markers for screening is now being evaluated using higher cutoff values for each marker, thus decreasing the false-positive rates.

Cytoskeletal Elements

MAbs to cytoskeletal elements have been used to identify the cellular origin of cancers by immunohistochemistry (Table 20.16). Glial fibrillary acidic protein is a major component of the intermediate filaments of astrocytes and appears to be useful for diagnosis of astrocytic neoplasms and mixed glial tumors, because it is not found in epidermal tumors, meningiomas, or other nonastrocytic brain tumors. Prekeratin, in the form of intermediate-sized filaments, is found exclusively in cells of epidermal origin and may be used immunohistochemically to identify cancer cells of epithelial origin. Neurofilament antigens are found in neuroblastomas and pheochromocytomas; vimentin is found in sarcomas and lymphomas.

Immunoglobulin Gene Rearrangements

The presence of immunoglobulin gene arrangements in lymphomas may give evidence of B-cell lineage even if the tumor cells do not produce cy-

Table 20.16 Cytoskeletal elements in cancers

Element	Normal distribution	Occurrence in cancers
Prekeratin	Epithelial cells	Epithelial cancers
Glial fibrillary acidic protein	Astrocytes	Astrocytic tumors
Neurofilaments	Neural cells	Neuroblastomas, pheochromocytomas
Vimentin	Mesenchymal cells	Sarcomas, lymphomas
Desmin	Muscle	Myosarcomas

toplasmic or surface monoclonal Ig. Immunoglobulin gene rearrangements that result in splicing out of intervening DNA sequences have been associated with maturation of B cells and the ability to produce Ig. However, some gene rearrangements are not associated with the capacity to synthesize Ig but are still believed to be characteristic of B cells. Some non-Ig-producing null cell lymphomas will demonstrate gene rearrangements, but others will not. The finding of Ig gene rearrangements in a null cell tumor indicates (i) that the cell line is monoclonal and therefore probably neoplastic and (ii) that the tumor is most likely of B-cell origin.

Oncogene Products

Since oncogene activation is associated with cancer, products of oncogenes should be useful as cancer markers. The major oncogenes and their products under study as determinants of prognosis in human cancer are listed in Table 20.17. The expression of these genes in cancer tissue has also been measured by gene amplification and messenger RNA levels. In general, the higher the expression of the oncogene, the poorer the prognosis. The identification of *ras* oncogene mutations in the DNA of stool from patients with colorectal cancers has been reported to be an effective way to detect these tumors while they are still curable by surgery. Most patients with chronic myelogenous leukemia (CML) possess the Philadelphia chromosome, which is formed by a reciprocal translocation between chromosomes 9 and 22. This exchange joins the 5′ two-thirds of the *BCR* gene on chromosome 22 to a large portion of the *ABL* gene from chromosome 9. The detection of BCR-ABL fusion proteins in the blood cells of patients with CML by Western blotting is now being used to monitor patients with acute myelogenous leukemia and CML.

Cancer Marker Summary

Cancer markers include secreted proteins, cell surface molecules, hormones, enzymes and isozymes, and cytoplasmic constituents, as well as gene rearrangements and oncogene products. Many cancer markers are identified by heteroantisera or MAbs. Cancer markers may be used for diagnosis, prognosis, or therapy. The most useful cancer markers are monoclonal Igs, AFP, PSA, and CEA. Although the clinical applications of AFP and CEA have not fulfilled all the optimistic expectations that many predicted, these markers have achieved a place in cancer diagnosis and management. Many other cancer markers have not been nearly as

Table 20.17 Oncogene products being considered as candidates for tumor markers

Oncogene	Function (product)	Change in tumor	Detection method	Types of cancers[a]
HER2/neu	Signal transduction (estrogen receptor)	Mutation	Immunohistology	Breast, prostate, GI
c-*ras*	Signal transduction (P12 tyrosine kinase)	Mutation/amplification	Immunohistology	Breast, prostate, GI, neuroblastomas
n-*myc*	Transcription regulation (P62 DNA binding protein)	Amplification	Southern blot	GI, SCLC, neuroblastomas
c-*erbB-2*	Growth factor receptor (P64 tyrosine kinase)	Amplification	Southern blot	Ovary, breast
int-2/hst-1	Fibroblast growth factor	Amplification	Southern blot	Breast, head, and neck

[a]GI, gastrointestinal; SCLC, small cell lung carcinoma.

useful, and the verdict has not yet been returned on several markers now being studied. Claims of a universal cancer marker have been made repeatedly but have not been fulfilled. However, the availability of new hybridoma and immunoassay technology, such as enzyme-linked immunosorbent assays and flow cytometry, as well as extremely sensitive computerized programs for in situ hybridization and microarray (chip) assays, may justify a new wave of excitement. Identification of cancer markers by MAbs offers an exciting opportunity not available with previous approaches. Recognition of abnormal expression of products produced normally by adult or fetal tissues appears to hold more promise in tumor diagnosis than identification of tumor-specific markers. It is possible that molecular probes for human oncogenes or gene rearrangements might become a diagnostic approach in the future. A continued search for new tumor markers is more than justified by the tremendous potential for clinical applications.

Immunotherapy of Cancer

Therapeutic Approaches

Immunotherapy of cancer is defined as any immune procedure that adversely affects the growth of an established tumor. Such immune procedures may be specific or nonspecific, active or passive (Table 20.18). Specific immunotherapy involves the use of tumor-specific antigens for targeting, whereas nonspecific therapy involves procedures that increase the activity of the effector arm of the rejection response in a manner that does not involve the recognition of a specific tumor antigen.

Clinical Trials

The possibility of successful immunotherapy of cancer has raised great excitement and led to numerous clinical trials. The phases of clinical trials and types of response to therapy are defined in Table 20.19. The introduction of a new form of immunotherapy usually generates great expectations. In the past, the enthusiasm of claims of success in the first clinical trials has been followed by the reality of limited or no beneficial effect after phase III and IV trials. For an appreciation of the extent of the work, the frustration involved, what the enormous cost and effort has achieved, and where we may be going, a selected review of the history of human immunotherapy of cancer is much more illuminating than a systematic review of essentially negative studies would be. The short historical presentation of immunotherapy presented here is essentially a synopsis of the exceptional presentation by Steven Hall in *A Commotion in the Blood: Life, Death and the Immune System* (see Bibliography).

History of Immunotherapy

Coley's Toxin

In 1890, about 1 year after being licensed to practice medicine and surgery in New York, William B. Coley was involved in the treatment of a young woman, Elizabeth Dashiell, a family friend of the Rockefellers. She had noticed a lump on her hand, which was first attributed to an infection. However, it did not respond to treatment and enlarged in size. When removed surgically, it was diagnosed by none other than famous pathologist James Ewing as a "round cell sarcoma," also known as a "Ewing's sarcoma." The

Table 20.18 Immunotherapeutic approaches to human cancer

Approach	Status
Specific	
Active	
Autologous tumor cells	Not effective
Autologous tumor extracts	Not effective
Autologous tumor lysate and BCG	Not effective
Cell line lysates and BCG	Under study
Haptenated autologous cell lysates and BCG	Not effective
Selected tumor antigens	Under study
Passive cellular	
Autologous lymphocytes	Not effective
Allogeneic lymphocytes	Some effect in bone marrow transplant recipients
Autologous stimulated lymphocytes (LAK)	Not effective
TILs	Under study
Autologous gene-modified lymphocytes	Clinical trials under way
Donor cytotoxic cell lines	Protect against cytomegalovirus infection
Transfer factor	Not effective
Immune RNA	Not effective
Passive humoral	
Xenogeneic antisera	Not effective
Monoclonal antibodies	Clinical trials under way
Anti-idiotypic antibody	Some remissions in clinical trials
Anti-CD4	Some remissions in Sézary syndrome
Bispecific antibodies	Clinical trials under way
Nonspecific	
BCG, *Cryptosporidium parvum*	Effective for superficial bladder carcinoma
Mycobacterial extracts	Experimental
Levamisole, polynucleotides	Experimental
Dinitrochlorobenzene	Limited effect in selected skin cancers
Lymphokines	
IFN-α	Hairy cell leukemia
IL-2	20% partial response in selected tumors

treatment was then amputation of the arm above the wrist, with about a 1 in 10 chance of cure. Three weeks after operation, she developed abdominal pain, multiple metastases, and died about 2 months later. This devastating case stimulated an intense and lifetime pursuit by Coley to find a way to treat cancer. He began by investigating cases of apparent regressions of incurable cancers to try to find out from these experiments of nature how the body might be able to defend itself against cancer.

In 1891, Coley searched the tenements of New York to find a cancer survivor named Fred K. Stein, whom he had identified in hospital records. When found, Stein had a large healed scar on his face but was otherwise healthy. According to hospital records, 11 years earlier, Stein had a lump the size of a hen's egg removed from his cheek by surgeon William Bull.

Table 20.19 Clinical trials: definitions

Phase or response	Definition
I	Dose toxicity titration studies to determine maximum safely tolerated dose
II	Determination of most effective antitumor activity at doses chosen from phase I trials; scheduling of dose and timing relationships for phase III
III	Comparison of treatment protocols with new agent to effects of standard therapy
IV	Application of effective new therapy protocol into general oncology practice: integration into multimodality regimens
Complete response	Disappearance of all clinical, radiological, and biochemical evidence of tumor disease; usually of limited duration
Partial response[a]	Decrease of at least 50% in the product of two perpendicular diameters of all measurable disease manifestations (usually radiological) and >50% decrease in serum concentration of a tumor marker (AFP, CEA, CA 19-9, CA 50, PSA)

[a]Partial remissions may be misevaluated because of exposure differences in X rays. Since more accurate methods (magnetic resonance imaging, ultrasound) have been applied, partial remissions can be more precisely determined and fewer reports of successful clinical trials have been reported.

Within a year, the tumor had regrown and was a grapelike mass 4 inches in diameter. After four more operations, it was deemed impossible to remove all of the tumor, which had grown around the carotid artery and infiltrated other vital structures. It was diagnosed as round cell sarcoma. One week after the fourth operation, when all appeared hopeless, Stein developed a severe infection with *Streptococcus pyogenes*. Known as erysipelas, this infection produced angry red inflammation across most of his face, as well as debilitating fever and chills. A common name for this infection was "St. Anthony's fire." During the two episodes of this infection, the open cancerous wound on his face showed remarkable healing, and the tumor masses decreased. After resolution of the infection, the tumor masses disappeared. Eleven years later, there was no evidence of residual tumor, and Stein was a healthy man with the healed surgical scar on the side of his face that Coley had first seen.

Later that year, Coley was called upon to see an immigrant from Italy, a Mr. Zola. Previously, surgery for sarcoma of the neck had revealed inoperable cancer, and physical signs indicated that Zola had lung metastases. Coley decided to treat Zola with deliberate infections with *S. pyogenes*. After several mild infections with little if any effect, the tumors began to enlarge even more rapidly. Coley decided to push his infection therapy. A large inoculum of bacteria given directly into the tumor produced a severe infection, with shaking chills and high fever, and Zola came close to dying. During this infection, there was a noticeable inflammatory reaction at the site of the tumors. Remarkably, Zola survived, and, over the next few months, his tumor masses decreased and essentially disappeared. Zola lived for at least 8 more years, apparently free of tumors, and died in Italy, where he was lost to follow-up.

After this remarkable result, from 1891 to 1893, Coley treated 12 more patients with advanced cancer by deliberate infection with *S. pyogenes*. In only four patients was he able to induce severe infections. Two of these patients died of the infection, but the two others had complete remissions; eight were reported to show some improvement but were not cured. On the basis of these clearly mixed results and fatal infections, Coley then decided to abandon active infections in favor of treatment with bacterial extracts (Coley's toxins).

Coley's toxins consisted of extracts of cultures of *S. pyogenes,* as well as *Bacillus prodigiosus,* a gram-negative bacterium. Fortuitously, *B. prodigiosus* produces endotoxin. Unknown to Coley at the time, this endotoxin acts as a superantigen and activates release of cytokines, including tumor necrosis factor (TNF), IFN, and interleukins. In 1893, John Ficken, a 13-year-old boy with inoperable metastatic cancer, was given injections of Coley's toxin directly into his tumors. This produced chills and fever, the tumors shrank, and Ficken lived to the age of 47, when he appears to have died of other causes. By 1913, Coley had treated over 500 patients with Coley's toxin, claiming significant improvement in 150. However, others were not successful, and the treatment generated great controversy. By the turn of the century, radiation had become the treatment of choice, championed by James Ewing, and Coley's toxins never became a generally accepted treatment for cancer. The controversy over Coley's toxins continued into the 1920s, with some anecdotal cases of remarkable remissions still reported in 1926. However, the lack of a consistent response, the failure of others to be able to achieve positive results, and the predominance of radiotherapy for treatment of cancer led to the eventual demise of this approach. Coley's experience with incredible early results with a few patients, followed by an inexplicable inability to duplicate these results, establishes a pattern that haunts those working in tumor immunotherapy to this day (see below).

Evaluation of Immunotherapy

Coley's experience also exemplifies how difficult it is to evaluate cancer therapy trials. The variable course of cancer as a disease makes therapeutic assessment extremely difficult. One of the major problems in the past has been the failure to include a valid control group. In addition, although the most desirable end point of any treatment is survival and quality of life, most clinical trials evaluate effectiveness in terms of complete or partial remission of tumor masses (Table 20.19). In fact, remissions may be short-lived and have little long-term effect on survival. Regardless of the means of evaluation, the effect of immunotherapy on many solid nonlymphoid tumors, following the experience of Coley, has been limited to a few individual patients and is clinically unsatisfactory in most cases. The biologic problems involved in evaluating the effects of therapy are even more complicated for immunotherapy than for chemotherapy. For instance, there are a number of mechanisms whereby an otherwise immunologically adequate individual is unable to make an effective response to a tumor (Table 20.8). It is possible that by attempting to treat cancer, the physician may actually cause the tumor to grow more rapidly, produce severe side effects or increase susceptibility to infection. The next chapter in the story is the application of nonspecific, active stimulation using BCG.

BCG

BCG is an attenuated form of tubercle bacillus used with limited success as a vaccine for tuberculosis. Large-scale epidemiology studies in Europe suggested a slight decrease in the incidence of cancer in populations immunized with BCG, compared with populations not immunized. In early

1960s, Herb Rapp and Tibor Borsos of the National Institutes of Health (NIH) demonstrated complete rejection of tumors by injection of BCG into transplanted tumors in guinea pigs and an ocular tumor of cattle. Georges Mathe, a French hematologist, claimed to be able to cure children of leukemia and of cutaneous melanoma by injection of BCG into the tumors. These results were reported widely but were never reproduced. However, an exception to the many unrewarding clinical trials that followed was the observation that BCG is one of the most effective treatments for superficial bladder cancers. For this treatment, BCG is repeatedly inoculated into the bladder lumen. This local application results in recruitment of activated lymphocytes into the bladder wall, increases interleukins in the urine, and induces systemic immunity to BCG. Long-term remission is achieved in 50% of patients, and 35% show no response. In addition, severe adverse effects are seen in about 5% of patients. Preclinical data show that these results may be improved by combining BCG with IFN-α. Another attempt at nonspecific immunostimulation involves the use of skin-sensitizing haptens, such as dinitrochlorobenzene.

DNCB

Dinitrochlorobenzene (DNCB) is a contact sensitivity hapten. It binds to proteins in the skin and induces a T_{CTL}-cell response. The T_{CTL} cells (T-killer cells) enter the epidermis and attack cells expressing the hapten, causing death of the cells and a poison ivy-type skin reaction. In the 1970s, Edmund Kline of the Roswell Park Cancer Institute treated basal cell and squamous cell skin carcinomas by painting the skin lesions with contact sensitivity haptens such as DNCB. In persons sensitized systemically to this agent, Kline found complete regression in approximately one-third of the treated lesions and partial regression of another third. Untreated lesions in patients with multiple basal cell carcinomas did not undergo regression at the time that other treated lesions were regressing. A contact sensitivity reaction occurred to the sensitizing chemical, and the tumor tissue appeared to be destroyed by the accumulation of macrophages stimulated by the reaction of sensitized lymphocytes to the DNCB. This therapy was applicable only to cutaneous tumors and had no effect on noncutaneous tumors. However, no long-term remission or significant change in survival was found. Unfortunately, others were unable to repeat Kline's results, and this interesting approach was abandoned. The next stage was the application of cytokines, including interferons and interleukins.

Interferon

Viral interference, a mysterious phenomenon discovered in the 1930s, results in protection of cells or animals against a serious viral infection, if there has been a recent previous infection with a less severe, unrelated virus. Viral interference was thought to be caused by something produced by the first virus. A breakthrough observation regarding this phenomenon occurred in 1956, in France, when Jean Lindeman found, using heat-inactivated influenza virus, that interference occurred even if the first virus did not actually infect the cell. Lindeman went to Mill Hill, in London, and teamed up with Alex Isaacs. In 1957 to 1958, they found that the interference phenomenon could be transferred from treated cells to uninfected cells by tissue culture fluid. They called the active factor interferon and later proved that interferon was produced by the cell and not by the virus. In 1961, Ion Gresser, at Harvard University, found a new interferon made by lymphocytes, IFN-γ. The original interferon was called IFN-α. In 1962, Kurt Packer and Kari Cantell, in Philadelphia, discovered that interferon could affect cell growth. In 1966, Gresser found that interferon not only inhibited virus-induced tumors (Friend leukemia virus) but also reversed growth of transplanted epithelial tumors. In the 1970s, Cantell, then in Helsinki, observed that human lymphocytes infected with Sendai virus produce relatively large amounts of IFN-γ. He set up a laboratory to produce large amounts of IFN-γ and become the world's source for clinical trials until the interferon genes were cloned in 1980.

Many clinical trials using interferons were performed in the 1970s, with initial reports of substantial remissions followed by more complete but disappointing data. At about the time IFN therapy was being discarded, an exception occurred. In 1977, a 25-year-old man with advanced hairy cell leukemia (a rare T-cell tumor), was seen by Jorge Quesada at the M. D. Anderson Cancer Center in Houston, Tex. At that time, hairy cell leukemia had no effective treatment. The patient was treated with daily doses of 3 million units of IFN-α. No side effects were observed, and within 2 weeks his blood counts improved and he went on to complete remission. By 1984, IFN-α was used to treat six other patients; all had either complete or partial remissions. IFN-α was approved by the FDA for treatment of hairy cell leukemia. Although not effective with other cancers, this positive result, after so many failures, reinvigorated the field of cytokine treatment of cancer.

IL-2

In the 1960s, it was noted that supernatants from cultures of lymphocytes stimulated with mitogens, such as phytohemagglutinin, produced "factors" that had biologic effects on other cells (conditioned medium). These factors were subsequently named for their effects on other cells; for example, MIF (migration [of macrophages] inhibitory factor), MAF (macrophage activation factor), LAF (lymphocyte activating factor), and LIF (lymphocyte migration inhibitory factor). In 1974, supernatants of phytohemagglutinin-stimulated human lymphocyte cultures used as conditioned medium to culture leukemic cells were found to contain a factor that stimulated growth of T cells. This factor was identified as LAF or T-cell growth factor. It could be produced in conditioned medium in a way that would allow massive expansion of T cells. In 1979, this factor was renamed IL-2.

In 1977, Steve Rosenberg began to build a team to study immunotherapy of cancer at NIH. He started with spleen lymphocytes from pigs inoculated with tumor cells from selected patients, and after 12 completely negative results, he began to look for another approach. Elizabeth Grimm, also then at NIH, in attempting to culture T cells with cancer cells and IL-2 in vitro to obtain a tumor-reactive T-cell line, obtained a subpopulation of cells with weak tumoricidal activity. However, these cells did not have T-cell markers. They became known as lymphokine-activated killer cells (LAKs).

Many years earlier, Karl-Eric and Ingegard Hellstrom, in Seattle, were culturing tumor cells with lymphocytes from the same patients in an attempt to identify immune cells that would inhibit growth of the tumor cells in vitro, the colony inhibition assay. They had noted that some patients with remissions appeared to have lymphocytes that would cause colony inhibition. However, this inhibition was only significant when compared with highly selected control individuals whose lymphocytes had no effect on the tumor cells in vitro. When other normal donors were used, their lymphocytes would also inhibit colony formation, even though there was no evidence that these donors had been exposed to the tumors. This effect was interpreted to be due to the presence of nonimmunized lymphocytes, so-called natural killer cells. Grimm had found that IL-2 could activate these NK cells to become more active.

In the meantime, Michael Lotze had joined Rosenberg and was attempting to use large amounts of IL-2 for immunotherapy. By 1984, 75 patients had been treated with IL-2 plus LAK with no responses. However, when the dose of IL-2 was increased to the maximum tolerated by the patients, several spectacular cures were seen. However, these patients developed severe side effects, including vascular leak syndrome, and almost died from fluid in the lung. This was so severe that some patients were sent home in a moribund state after the treatment was discontinued. Two patients given up for dead actually survived and were completely cured of their tumor. These results were hauntingly similar to those in patients treated with Coley's toxins many years earlier. In follow-up, it was noted that biopsies of their tumors showed lymphocytic infiltrate and necrosis, and over the next 3 to 4 months the tumors had disappeared!

Again, it appeared that a breakthrough had happened. By 1985, LAK/IL-2 treatment of 45 patients was reported, and a response rate of 45% was claimed. Later, with more complete studies, complete responses were reported in about 8% and partial responses in another 10% of those treated. However, severe side effects, including hypotension (capillary leak syndrome), fever, nausea, chills, vomiting, diarrhea, cutaneous erythema, anemia, and moderate to severe renal or hepatic dysfunction, as well as thyroiditis, caused most centers to discontinue this approach. IL-2 is still used in trials on otherwise hopeless cases with some remarkable responses, but use in most cancer patients is limited by the severe side effects. Perhaps more specific immune effector cells would be more effective.

TILs

For years, it was recognized that some tumors contained lymphocytes, and the general impression was that these tumors were less aggressive than tumors not containing lymphocytes. In 1983, Thomas McAllester and Alexander Knuth extracted lymphocytes infiltrating a tumor, cultured them with IL-2, and showed that they could lyse the tumor cells. These were not LAK, but T_{CTL} cells, more strongly cytotoxic and apparently specific for the tumor from which they were isolated. Rosenberg was quick to pick this up and soon reported that reinfusion of TILs back into the patient from which they came induced "substantial remission" in 8 of 9 patients with melanoma. Later, after treatment of more patients, a partial response rate of 55% was claimed. Subsequent studies revealed a much lower response rate, and again after considerable expectations, this approach was also abandoned. However, the next step, planned by Rosenberg, was to transfect TILs with cytokine genes that might increase the efficiency of TILs against tumor cells (see below). Although adoptive passive specific cellular immunotherapy has yet to be proved to be useful for tumor immunotherapy, this approach has proved valuable for treatment of one of the major complications of bone marrow transplantation.

CMV and T-Killer Adoptive Immunotherapy

About half of immunosuppressed bone marrow transplant recipients develop life-threatening infection with cytomegalovirus (CMV). Prophylactic treatment with ganciclovir is expensive ($6,000 per patient) and has severe side effects. Using just the right amounts of serum, IL-2, and antigen, it is possible to culture specific T_{CTL} cells for CMV from CMV-reactive individuals in vitro. Serum is required to keep cells alive; antigen and IL-2 provide two signals for proliferation of CMV-specific T cells. This process selects for a few specific T_{CTL} cells in billions of lymphocytes. Stimulation of T-cell clones requires repeated cycles of stimulation and growth. This difficult task was accomplished in the laboratory of Philip Greenberg in Seattle. They inject 600×10^6 cloned T_{CTL} cells for CMV beginning 4 to 5 weeks after bone marrow transplantation. (Clones are derived from marrow donor, so they are compatible with transplanted bone marrow cells.) This procedure has virtually eliminated CMV infections in bone marrow recipients (see chapter 18).

TNF

In 1957, Lloyd Old and Elizabeth Carswell discovered that a factor in the serum of mice after treatment with BCG and endotoxin produced necrosis of tumors (TNF). Another effect, independently discovered by others, is to cause wasting in animals with large cancers. This was called cachectin and was later found to be the same factor as TNF. In early treatment attempts, it was found that administration of TNF to humans produced severe systemic effects (the dark side), including high fever and poorly tolerated shock. At the maximum tolerated dose, no clear effect on tumors in humans was found.

In 1988, Ferdy Lejeune infused 10 times the maximum tolerated dose of TNF into the isolated limb of a patient bearing multiple melanoma lesions. They faded away. The systemic shock caused by the TNF that escaped into the systemic circulation had to be aggressively treated. Later, it was found that this effect was enhanced by adding low-dose IFN-γ and chemotherapy (mephalan). This became known as "triple therapy." Softball-sized tumors showed complete regression. This approach has limited applications, because essentially all patients with melanomas this size have systemic metastases and will die of these metastatic lesions. Lejeune stated, "You can cure the limb, but you can't cure the patient." Since the effectiveness of cytokines, such as IL-2, was limited by the severe and sometimes fatal side effects of the high doses required to have an effect on tumors, studies on lower doses of mixtures of cytokines were undertaken.

Cytokine Mixtures

Lower doses of toxic cytokines, such as IL-2 and TNF, given in mixtures are now being tested in other systems. For example, a commercially available preparation of natural cytokines called "leukocyte interleukin" (Cel-Sci Corp., Vienna, Va.), which includes IL-2, granulocyte-macrophage colony-stimulating factor (GM-CSF), IFN-γ, and TNF-α, is now being tested by direct injection into primary tumors. One possible mechanism of the action of these cytokines is to increase expression of CD40 on tumor cells, rending them more susceptible to T_{CTL}-cell lysis. The results of these trials were not available at the time of this writing.

IL-12

In experimental models, it was found that IL-12 activates NK cells, activates Th1 $CD4^+$ helper cells (DTH), blocks angiogenesis, and cures human tumors in nude mice. In phase I clinical trials (test for toxicity and dose level that can be given), no problems were found using a protocol in which the patients were "primed" with IL-12, then after waiting for 2 weeks given daily doses of IL-12. In 1995, in moving to phase II trials (to see if there was an effect on late-stage tumors), it was decided to omit the priming dose; of 15 patients treated, all became severely ill, and two died. The priming dose appears to be necessary to prepare patients for later daily doses. After this setback, IL-12 is now being retested after transfection of tumor cells with the IL-12 gene so they express IL-12 (see "Gene Therapy," below).

CD40 Ligand

Another approach under study is to use CD40 ligand (CD40L). T_{CTL} cells use CD40L to induce apoptosis of CD40-expressing tumor cells. In addition, CD40L upregulates expression of cytokines by different cells, including IL-6, IL-8, GM-CSF, and TNF-α by tumor cells, and IL-12 by macrophages. CD40L-transfected fibroblasts deliver an apoptotic signal to carcinoma cells. The present era of tumor immunotherapy is applying gene therapy in a number of specific and nonspecific approaches (see below). At the same time that these cellular techniques were being applied to tumor immunotherapy, antibody-directed tumor therapy was also being applied.

MAbs: Magic Bullets

In 1980, a patient with disseminated B-cell lymphoma after several remissions induced by IFN treatment suddenly became progressively debilitated and wasted and was given less than 1 year to live. In Ron Levy's laboratory at Stanford, a MAb to the Ig idiotype on the patient's B-cell tumor was made. Infusion of this MAb into the patient resulted in remarkable recovery. In 1987, after undergoing coronary bypass surgery, the patient developed the same B-cell tumor at the sites of incision for removal of leg veins used in the graft procedure. No evidence of tumor was found at other sites. Treated with low-dose irradiation, it disappeared. More than 200 patients have now been treated in this fashion, and about 10% show some remission (at a cost about $50,000 per patient). None have had the spectacular result seen in the first patient.

In 1906, Paul Ehrlich proposed antibodies, "bodies which possess a particular affinity for a certain organ," to serve as "magic bullets" to target cytotoxic agents to specific tissues. Over the next 80 years, attempts to effect this approach using conventional antibodies to cancers were not successful. With the development of hybridoma techniques, the possibility of the application of MAbs as a new specific mode of cancer therapy for treatment of human cancers became possible. Many MAbs to human tumor-associated antigens are now available and theoretically could be used to treat human cancers. Problems limiting the application of MAbs and possible approaches to circumvent these problems are listed in Table 20.20. These approaches are now being used in both experimental models with animals and in clinical trials. A recommended strategy for production, testing, and application of MAbs is given in Table 20.21. At present, MAbs are being tagged with radioisotopes, drugs, or toxins to increase their ability to kill target cells. In early studies, a conjugate of ricin A chain

Table 20.20 Problems and possible solutions to MAb immunotherapy of cancer in humans

Problem	Possible solution(s)
Tumors not antigenic in mice	Use of immune-enhancing mechanisms (adjuvants, carriers, etc.)
Tumor antigens present in normal tissue	Selection of antibodies that selectively react with tumor tissue
Presence of circulating free tumor antigen	Increasing doses of antibody to "clear" antigen
Modulation of tumor antigen	Use of mixtures (cocktails) or different antibodies sequentially
Selection of new antigens on tumor cell clones	Use of mixtures (cocktails) or different antibodies sequentially
Immune response to foreign MAb	Use of mouse-human chimeric antibodies
Lack of cytotoxic effect of MAb	Selection of cytotoxic MAbs; use of bifunctional antibodies linking effector cells to cancer cells; conjugation of cytotoxic drugs to MAbs

with an antibody that is common to melanoma cells produced only one complete response and three partial responses when tested in clinical trials on 58 patients. Other trials are too small to allow satisfactory evaluation at this time. Factors under evaluation in animal models include selection of radionucleotide or toxin, frequency of administration, regional administration, cocktails of antibodies, chimeric antibodies, use of a second antibody, and combined use with lymphokines. In addition to producing "immunoconjugates" of antibodies, strategies for directing recombinant toxins to cell surface receptors, such as the epidermal growth factor receptor, IL-2 receptor, IL-6 receptor, and ErbB-2 protein, are under investigation. Other constructions include recombinant antibodies to tumor cell antigens linked with IL-2. Now under study in clinical trials are antibodies to HER-2/neu for breast cancers, to vascular endothelial growth factor for sarcomas, and to A33 for colon cancers. A MAb to CD20 (proprietary name, Rituxin) has been approved by the FDA for treatment of non-Hodgkin's B-cell lymphoma.

"Bispecific" antibodies that contain two paratopes, one reacting with an immune cell and the other with a target cell, have been produced by chemically cross-linking a MAb that reacts with a tumor-associated antigen to an antibody that reacts with the T-cell receptor complex (CD3) or other lymphocyte activation molecules, such as CD16. These bispecific

Table 20.21 Strategy for development of MAbs for cancer immunotherapy

1. Identification of "antigen" in cancer tissue, not detectable or present in low amounts in normal tissue
2. Production of hybridoma cell line producing MAbs to tumor antigen
3. Selection of a MAb that binds and kills tumor cells in vitro but that is not toxic to normal cells
4. Isolation and characterization of MAbs
5. Demonstration of tumor binding and cytotoxic effect in vivo (nude mice with transplantable tumor)
6. Evaluation in clinical trials (phases I and II)

antibodies serve not only to bind the effector lymphocyte to the target cell but also to activate the release of lymphokines or lytic activity of the lymphocyte. Some examples are bispecific antibodies to CD2 and the epidermal growth factor receptor, FcγRIII and c-ErbB-2, CD3 and CD30 (Hodgkin's disease), and bispecific antibodies to CD3 and the tumor antigen Ep-CAM with Fc regions that activate FcγR-positive accessory cells. These bispecific antibodies are now being evaluated in phase I and II clinical trials.

Gene Therapy

Human gene therapy started in the attempt to replace the missing adenosine deaminase gene in SCIDs by transfecting it into T cells and putting the transfected T cells back into the patient (see chapter 18). The first hurdle was to obtain permission to use transfected cells in human trials. To do this, preliminary studies were designed to test the ability of transfected T cells to survive after transfer and then express the marker gene, *neo,* to make sure that transfected cells survive after transplantation and actually make the gene product. This was first attempted in 1989, when a patient with terminal malignant melanoma was injected with 200×10^6 TILs obtained from the patient's tumor after transfection with *neo*. Within about 2 weeks, the *neo* marker appeared in the patient's T cells. In 1990, the first gene therapy experiments for adenosine deaminase were done. A child's immune system appeared to be partially restored, allowing reduction of other drugs, but it remains unclear what role gene therapy actually had in the improvement (for further discussion, see chapter 18). Meanwhile, a separate protocol for gene therapy of cancer using the TNF gene and TILs was under way. By 1991, the TIL/TNF protocol had been carried out on 17 patients with no apparent effect. However, it was never determined where the transfected TILs went and how much TNF they made.

A number of gene therapy experiments have shown success at the preclinical stage. In these protocols, genes for cytokines or receptors are stably transfected into tumor or carrier cells, and growth of the transplantable tumor in syngeneic mice is determined (Table 20.22). Clinical trials in humans using gene therapy that are now planned or under way include cancer cells with insertion of genes for TNF, IL-2, HLA-B7 (for melanoma), IL-4, and IL-12.

Human Tumor Antigens

Tantalizing results using selected tumor models in animal studies (Fig. 20.2) provided evidence that it is possible to immunize an animal against its own tumor. However, many attempts to identify tumor-specific antigens or to effect growth of a tumor using autologous cells in humans have failed to achieve any success.

In 1981, Alexander Knuth in Frankfurt took cancer cells from a patient with melanoma to Thierry Boon in Brussels, who induced mutations in cancer cells with chemicals (mutagens). After irradiation, the nonviable mutated cells were injected back into the patient. (A similar approach using "mutagenized" cancer cells had been shown to produce an immune response to teratocarcinoma cells in animals.) By 1983, the patient had developed multiple metastases that no longer responded to chemotherapy. Her spleen and one kidney containing tumor were removed. In spring of 1984 a "tumor vaccine" based on the reactivity of her cloned T_{CTL} cells (see below) was given to her, and the tumor masses "melted away." The injections have been repeated every 6 months, and the tumors have not come back.

Table 20.22 Some examples of preclinical trials in mice of immune gene therapy for cancer[a]

Gene	Target cell(s)	Proposed effect(s)	Result
IL-2/3	Fibroblasts	Activate T_{CTL} cells, increase BMT proliferation	Partial response
IL-12	MC-38, adenocarcinoma	Enhance CMI	Complete regression
IL-12	Neuroblastoma	Enhance CMI	Effective vaccine, prevents growth
IL-15	MethA, sarcoma	Activate DTH	Complete rejection
IL-18	MCA205, sarcoma	Enhance DTH, increase IFN-γ	Complete rejection (with IL-12)
IFN-β	Human prostate cancer	Decrease growth, angiogenesis	Decreased growth in nude mice
IFN-γ	MCA 102, sarcoma	Enhance immunogenicity	Complete remission
CD40L	B16 melanoma	Present tumor antigen	60% complete response of transplanted tumor

[a]Abbreviations: BMT, bone marrow transplantation; CMI, cell-mediated immunity; DTH, delayed-type hypersensitivity.

Using IL-2 and lymphocyte culture techniques, Boon and colleagues cloned a T-cell line from the patient that killed her cultured tumor cells. They then made a DNA library of tumor cells and screened transfected colonies of tissue culture cells using the T-cell line. They found 1 in 13,000 colonies positive. From one colony, they identified a 9-amino-acid peptide presented by class I HLA. This peptide was called MAGE-1 and was found to be encoded by a gene present, but not expressed, in normal melanocytes. This technique of screening for tumor antigens using T_{CTL} cells has been used by the Boon laboratory and others to identify other putative "tumor antigens" (Table 20.23). Another method to identify putative tumor antigens is the SEREX technique (serological identification of antigens by recombinant expression cloning). For this procedure, sera from patients with cancer are used to screen complementary DNA expression libraries from the freshly isolated tumor.

Antigen-Targeted Adoptive Transfer Therapy

Expansion of T-cell-specific cell lines from cancer patients is now being done in an attempt to treat cancers by passive cellular transfer, as is successful for CMV infection (see above). Tumor-specific T cells are stimulated using melanoma antigens (MART-1, gp100) pulsed with peptide tetramers linked to MHC. In this process, human β_2-macroglobulin and HLA-A heavy-chain residues are linked to a tumor peptide, and tetramers are isolated. These tetramers are used to stimulate proliferation of antigen-reactive T cells in vitro. High-affinity tumor-reactive T cells may then be isolated by flow cytometry and expanded in vitro by mitogenic stimulation. In the future, these cells will be tested for adoptive immunotherapy in clinical trials.

Tumor Vaccines

Design of a tumor vaccine involves two basic questions: what antigen should be used, and how should it be delivered? Some examples of ongoing animal and human studies on tumor vaccines are given in Table 20.24.

Table 20.23 Some antigens on human tumors recognized by antibody or T-cell reactions

Antigen[a]	Tumor type	Normal tissue expression	Comments
Antibody defined			
gp100	Melanoma	Melanocytes/neuorectoderm	Combined with IL-2, modified to increase HLA-A2 binding
gp75/brown	Melanoma	Melanocytes	Melanosomal protein
Gangliosides (GM2, GD2)	Melanoma	Neuroectoderm-derived tissue	Carbohydrate antigens
Melanotransferrin	Melanoma	Melanocytes, others	Potential unique determinant
HER-2/neu	Breast	Epthelium	Estrogen receptor
p53, wild-type	Multiple	Epithelium, low	Mutant highly expressed in tumors
T, TN, SialylTn	Breast	Epithelium	Carbohydrate antigens
CD20	Non-Hodgkin's lymphoma	Lymphocytes	B-cell differentiation marker
T-cell defined			
MAGE-1,3	Melanoma, lung	Testes	Not expressed by melanocytes
Tyrosinase	Melanoma	Melanocytes	Melanosomal protein
MUC1	Pancreas, breast	Melanocytes	Non-MHC restricted
CAGE-1,2	Melanoma	Melanocytes	MHC restricted
CAGE-3	Melanoma, breast	Testes	Non-MHC restricted
Melan-A/MART-1	Melanoma	Melanocytes	Melanocytes and retina
TRP-1/2	Melanoma	Melanocytes	Melanocyte differentiation antigen
PMEL17/silver	Melanoma	Melanocytes	Melanosomal protein

[a]Antigens recognized on autologous tumor cells. BAGE is another antigen on melanomas, RAGE is an antigen on renal cell carcinoma, and mutated KIAA0205 is an antigen on bladder carcinomas.

Because of the proprietary nature of some trials and the many different approaches now being used, it is impossible to list all such studies. As can be seen in Table 20.24, a variety of approaches are being tried. In humans, most of the results are in patients with malignant melanoma using polyvalent vaccines. Other ongoing trials for melanoma include the use of the tumor antigens identified above, such as MAGE-3, MELAN-A, tyrosinase, and gp100. Other possibilities for tumor vaccines include HER-2/neu, carbohydrates such as gangliosides (GM2) and sialyl Tn, Ras mutated in the 12 position, BCR/ABL protein, p53, and idiotypes on T- and B-cell receptors.

A number of approaches have been tested to increase the immunization effect of a tumor antigen. For example, immunization with tumor cells transfected with cytokines, such as IL-12 or IFN-γ, is designed to enhance sensitization and proliferation of reactive T cells. In addition, genetically modified (transduced) whole-cell tumor vaccines using B7 (costimulator) or cytokine genes, such as GM-CSF (which promotes local antigen-presenting cell differentiation at the vaccine site) or IL-2 (which activates T-cell immunity) are also designed to increase immunogenicity. Since the cytokine does not have to be produced by the tumor cell, the cytokine effect may be obtained by admixing tumor cells with genetically transduced bystander cells or biopolymer microspheres containing cytokines. Immunogenicity of tumor antigens may be enhanced by providing MHC processing. In ongoing clinical trials, immunization with gp100 had no effect unless it was modified at the MHC anchor residue to produce higher-affinity binding to HLA-A2, combined with injections of IL-2 (41% partial response in a pilot study). In addition, preclinical animal studies using recombinant virus (vaccinia virus) and bacteria *(Salmonella* or *Listeria)* are

Table 20.24 Some techniques to induce tumor immunity (tumor vaccines)

Antigen	Adjuvant(s)	Effect(s)
Mouse (preclinical)		
MUC-1 (mucin)	"Naked" DNA Vaccinia virus-vectored DNA	Inhibition of growth of transplanted tumor
CEA	"Naked" DNA	Induction of antibody and T-cell response
CEA	Vaccinia virus vectored	Antibody, cell-mediated immunity (CMI), and inhibition of tumor growth
Modified MHC class I	Transfected tumor cells	Changes Th2- to Th1-type response
Mutated p53	Anti-idiotype (PAb240)	Resists growth of transplanted tumor cells
Wild-type p53	Complete Freund's adjuvant	Decreased chemical carcinogenesis
Anti-B cell idiotype	"Naked" DNA	Antibody-mediated inhibition of tumor
E1A peptide	Anti-CD40	Primes for T_{CTL} cells
Neu	Plasmid	Immunity to Neu-expressing tumor
ErbB-2	Linked to superantigen gene	Regression of tumor growth
ErbB-2 (breast cancer)	"Naked" DNA	Inhibits tumor growth
Tumor cells (breast)	MHC class II, B7.1 transfected	Reduces metastases, does not affect primary tumor
Myeloma cells	IL-2-IgG transfected	Tumor rejection, immunity to rechallenge
sLeX (Lewis antigen)	Anti-idiotype	Slowed tumor growth
CHO peptide mimes	QS-21 adjuvant	Slowed tumor growth
Tn (CHO) antigen	Linked to CD4 epitope	Slowed tumor growth
Human melanoma		
Polyvalent melanoma	None	At 12 years, 17% response rate; 17% complete response
	BCG	Phase III trial under way; antibody and T_{CTL}cells induced to melanoma antigens
Melanoma lysate (Melacine)	Lipid A, mycobacterial cell walls, cyclophosphamide	Phase III trial negative
Melanoma lysate	Vaccinia virus	Phase III trial negative
Polyvalent melanoma (shed culture medium)	Alum	Preliminary results positive
gp100 peptide	IL-2	Preliminary evidence of partial regression
GM2 ganglioside (melanoma)	BCG, cyclophosphamide	Trials negative
	Keyhole limpet hemocyanin (KLH) conjugation	Trials under way
Irradiated melanoma	GM-CSF transfection	Lymphocyte infiltration of tumors seen
Irradiated melanoma	IL-2-transfected cells	Induction of T_{CTL} cells, no clinical response
Melanoma antigens	Anti-idiotype (Melimmune)	Antibody and CMI induced to melanoma antigens
Human other		
PSA-liposome	BCG, GM-CSF	Induces antibody and CMI, clinical trials
Prostate peptides (ONCO-VAX)	Dendritic cells, cyclophosphosphamide	30% responders in phase II trial under way (prostate cancer)
Human papillomavirus (E6 and E7)	Peptides; DNA + cytokines	Phase I trials in cervical cancer patients
Sialyl-Tn (STn)	KLH conjugate	Antibody and CM induced to STn
CEA	Canarypox virus vectored	Induces T_{CTL} cells, safe in phase I trial
Colon cancer cell lines	DETOX, IL-1α	Some side effects in phase I trial
HER-2/neu peptides	GM-CSF	Antibody and CMI induced

under way. Another approach is to use antigen-presenting dendritic cells to reprocess tumor antigens.

Immunization must involve professional antigen-presenting cells that provide stimulation of both MHC class II-restricted $CD4^+$ (T_{DTH}) and class I-restricted $CD8^+$ (T_{CTL}) effector cells. Dendritic cells are professional antigen-presenting cells that present antigens to T cells. Isolation and tissue culture techniques have been developed that allow the generation of large numbers of dendritic cells by culturing bone marrow or blood monocytes using selected growth factors, such as GM-CSF, IL-4, TNF, and stem cell factor. Such dendritic cells may then be used to process tumor antigens in vitro, including those listed above for melanoma (tyrosinase, gp100, MART-1, MAGE, etc.) as well as other tumor antigens (prostate peptides, irradiated leukemic cells, etc.). Preclinical studies in rats and mice show that immunization with dendritic cells mixed with tumor cells or pulsed with tumor antigens leads to induction of T_{DTH}-, NK-, and T_{CTL}-cell responses and inhibition of growth or induction of cancers. Preliminary clinical trials show that autologous pulsed dendritic cells can induce T_{CTL}-cell responses to human tumors and may enhance clinical responses.

Summary

There is documented evidence in laboratory animals and circumstantial observations in humans that tumors contain specific antigens and that immune responses to these antigens occur. The identification of cancer-associated markers in the serum of affected patients has resulted in diagnostic tests for a few human tumors (hepatoma, teratocarcinomas, prostate cancer) and tests for evaluation of prognosis after treatment for many more. Immune recognition of new tumor antigens may be important in preventing growth of newly mutated cancer cells (immune surveillance). Active or passive immunity to tumor antigens may restrict the growth of an established tumor under appropriate circumstances, but a number of coexisting phenomena may interfere with this effect. Specific passive immunotherapy using MAbs and TILs and nonspecific immune stimulation using IFN, IL-2, and LAK has led to occasional spectacular results but also to many clinical failures in the face of severe side effects. More recently, new tumor antigens identified both serologically (SEREX) and by reactivity of cell lines from patients to tumors, genetically modified cells expressing these antigens, as well as a variety of adjuvants, including liposomes, cytokines, conjugates, viral vectors, BCG, and dendritic cell processing, are now being tested in clinical trials. Understanding and control of these phenomena may result in effective immunotherapy of cancer in humans.

Bibliography

History and Basic Concepts of Tumor Immunity

Challis, G. B., and H. J. Stam. 1990. The spontaneous regression of cancer. A review of cases from 1900 to 1987. *Acta Oncol.* **29:**545.

Emerson, T. C. 1964. Spontaneous regression of cancer. *Ann. N. Y. Acad. Sci.* **114:**721.

Foley, E. J. 1953. Antigenic properties of methylcholanthrene-induced tumors in mice of strain of origin. *Cancer Res.* **13:**835–837.

Gross, L. 1943. Intradermal immunization of CSH mice against a sarcoma that originated in an animal of the same line. *Cancer Res.* **3:**326–333.

Hewitt, H. B., E. R. Blake, and A. S. Walder. 1976. A critique of the evidence for active host defense against cancer, based on personal studies of 27 murine tumors of spontaneous origin. *Br. J. Cancer* **33:**241–259.

Hersy, P., D. E. Stone, G. Morgan, W. H. McCarthy, and G. W. Milton. 1977. Previous pregnancy as a protective factor against death from melanoma. *Lancet* **i:**451–452.

Kaplan, B. S., J. Klassen, and M. H. Gault. 1976. Glomerular injury in patients with neoplasia. *Annu. Rev. Med.* **27:**117–125.

Klein, G., H. O. Sjogren, E. Klein, and K. E. Hellstrom. 1960. Demonstration of resistance against methycholanthrene-induced sarcomas in the primary autochthonous host. *Cancer Res.* **20:**1561–1572.

Kripke, M. L. 1986. The immunology of skin cancer, p. 113–120. *In* M. L. Kripke and P. Frost (ed.), *M.D. Anderson Symposium on Fundamental Cancer Research,* vol. 38. *Immunology and Cancer.* University of Texas Press, Austin.

Loeb, L. 1906. Further experimental evidence into the growth of tumors. Development of sarcoma and carcinoma after the inoculation of a carcinomatous tumor of the submaxillary gland in a Japanese mouse. *Univ. Pa. Med. Bull.* **19:**113.

Penn, I. 1984. Cancer in immunosuppressed patients. *Transplant. Proc.* **16:**492–494.

Prehn, R. T., and J. M. Main. 1957. Immunity to methycholanthrene induced sarcomas. *J. Natl. Cancer Inst.* **18:**769–778.

Schone, G. 1906. Untersuchungen über Karzinomimmunität bei Mausen. *Munch. Med. Wochenschr.* **53:**2517.

Vose, B. M., and M. Moore. 1985. Human tumor infiltrating lymphocytes: a marker of host response. *Semin. Hematol.* **22:**27–40.

Types of Tumor Antigens

Chism, S. E., S. Wallis, R. C. Burton, and N. L. Warner. 1976. Analysis of murine oncofetal antigens as tumor associated transplantation antigens. *J. Immunol.* **117:**1870–1876.

Davidsohn, I., and Y. N. Louisa. 1969. Loss of isoantigens A, B, and H in carcinoma of the lung. *J. Pathol.* **57:**307–334.

Festenstein, H. 1987. The biological consequences of altered MHC expression on tumours. Br. Med. Bull. **43:**217–227.

Klein, G. 1968. Tumor specific transplantation antigens—GHA Clowes Memorial Lecture. *Cancer Res.* **28:**625–635.

Kobayashi, H., T. Kodama, and E. Gotohda. 1977. *Xenogenization of Tumor Cells.* Hokkaido University Medical Library Series, Hokkaido University, Sapporo, Japan.

Prehn, R. T. 1968. Tumor-specific antigens of nonviral tumors. *Cancer Res.* **28:**1326–1330.

Schreiber, H., P. L. Ward, D. A. Rowley, and H. J. Stauss. 1988. Unique tumor-specific antigens. *Annu. Rev. Immunol.* **6:**465–483.

In Vitro Assays of Tumor Immunity

Bloom, B. R., and P. R. Glade (ed.). 1971. *In Vitro Methods in Cell-Mediated Immunity.* Academic Press, Inc., New York, N.Y.

Tumor Enhancement and Stimulation

Kaliss, N. 1970. Dynamics of immunologic enhancement. *Transplant. Proc.* **2:**59–67.

Prehn, R. T. 1977. Immunostimulation of the lymphodependent phase of neoplastic growth. *J. Natl. Cancer Inst.* **59:**1043–1049.

Immune Surveillance

Burnet, F. M. 1970. The concept of immunological surveillance. *Prog. Exp. Tumor Res.* **13:**1–27.

Chen, L., S. Ashe, W. A. Brady, I. Hellstrom, K. E. Hellstrom, et al. 1992. Costimulation of antitumor immunity by the B7 counterreceptor for the T lymphocyte molecules CD28 and CTLA-4. *Cell* **71:**1093–1102.

Fenyo, E. M., E. Klein, G. Klein, and K. Sweich. 1968. Selection of an immunoresistant Moloney lymphoma subline with decreased concentration of tumor-specific surface antigens. *J. Natl. Cancer Inst.* **40:**69–89.

Ioachim, H. L. 1976. The stromal reaction of tumors: an expression of immune surveillance. *J. Natl. Cancer Inst.* **57:**465–475.

Nagao, M., Y. Nakajima, M. Hisanaga, N. Kayagaki, H. Kanehiro, et al. 1999. The alteration of Fas receptor and ligand system in hepatocellular carcinomas: how do hepatoma cells escape from the host immune surveillance in vivo. *Hepatology* **30:**413–421.

Nakashima, M., K. Sonoda, and T. Watanabe. 1999. Inhibition of cell growth and induction of apoptotic cell death by the human tumor-associated antigen RCAS1. *Nat. Med.* **5:**938–942.

Rygaard, J., and C. O. Poulsen. 1976. The nude mouse vs the hypothesis of immunological surveillance. *Transplant. Rev.* **48:**43–61.

Thomas, L. 1959. Discussion. *In* H. S. Lawrence (ed.), *Cellular and Humoral Aspects of the Hypersensitive State.* Harper & Row, Publishers, Inc., New York, N.Y.

Immunodiagnosis

Abelev, G. I. 1968. Production of embryonal serum α-globulin by hepatomas: review of experimental and clinical data. *Cancer Res.* **28:**1344–1350.

Bence Jones, H. 1847. Papers on chemical pathology, lecture III. *Lancet* **ii:**269–274.

Chan, D. W., and S. Sell. 1999. Tumor markers, p. 722–749. *In* C. A. Burtis and E. R. Ashwood (ed.), *Tietz Textbook of Clinical Chemistry,* 3rd ed. The W. B. Saunders Co., Philadelphia, Pa.

Gold, P., and S. O. Freedman. 1965. Specific carcinoembryonic antigens of the human digestive system. *J. Exp. Med.* **122:**467–481.

Hakomori, S.-I. 1991. Possible function of tumor-associated carbohydrate antigens. *Curr. Opin. Immunol.* **3:**646–653.

Sell, S. 2000. Tumor markers. *Sci. Med.* **7:**8–17.

Immunotherapy

Hall, S. S. 1997. *A Commotion in the Blood: Life, Death and the Immune System.* Henry Holt & Co., New York, N.Y. (A vivid exposition of the research in human tumor immunity; the discussion of human tumor immunotherapy is partially based on this book.)

BCG

Bast, R. C., Jr., B. Zbar, T. Borsos, H. J. Rapp. 1974. BCG and cancer. *N. Engl. J. Med.* **290:**1413, 1458.

Lamm, D. L. 1992. Long term results of intravesicular therapy for superficial bladder cancer. *Urol. Clin. N. Am.* **19:**573–590.

Lao, Y., X. Chen, T. M. Downs, W. C. DeWolf, and M. A. O'Donnell. 1999. INF-α 2B enhances Th1 cytokine responses in bladder cancer patients receiving *Mycobacterium bovis* bacillus Calmette-Guérin immunotherapy. *J. Immunol.* **162:** 2399–2405.

Waisbren, B. A. 1999. Update on the treatment of cancer with multiple immunotherapy. *Cancer Biother. Radiopharm.* **14:**27–30.

DNCB

Klein, E., O. A. Holterman, F. Helm, H. Milgrom, H. L. Stoll, et al. 1984. Topical therapy for cutaneous tumors. *Transplant. Proc.* **16:**507–515.

Cytokines (IFN, IL-2, TNF, IL-12, etc.)

Alexandroff, A. B., R. A. Robins, A. Murray, and K. James. 1998. Tumour immunology: false hopes—new horizons. *Immunol. Today* **19:**247–250.

Bonnem, E. M. 1991. Alpha interferon: the potential drug of adjuvant therapy: past achievements and future challenges. *Eur. J. Cancer* **27**(Suppl. 4)**:**S2–S6.

Carswell, E. A., L. J. Old, R. L. Kassel, S. Green, N. Fiore, and B. Williamson. 1975. An endotoxin-induced serum factor that causes necrosis of tumors. *Proc. Natl. Acad. Sci. USA 72:*3660–3670.

Harris, D. T., G. R. Matyas, L. G. Gomella, E. Talor, M. D. Winship, L. E. Spitler, and M. J. Mastrangelo. 1999. Immunologic approaches to the treatment of prostate cancer. *Semin. Oncol.* **26:**439–447.

Heaton, K. M., and E. A. Grimm. 1993. Cytokine combinations in immunotherapy for solid tumors: a review. *Cancer Immunol. Immunother.* **37:**213–219.

Kammula, U. S., D. E. White, and S. A. Rosenberg. 1998. Trends in the safety of high dose bolus interleukin-2 administration in patients with metastatic cancer. *Cancer* **83:**797–805.

Lissoni, P. 1997. Effects of low-dose recombinant interleukin-2 in human malignancies. *Cancer J. Sci. Am.* **3**(Suppl. 1)**:**S115–S120.

Nooijen, P. T. G. A., A. M. M. Eggermont, L. Schalkwijk, S. Henzen-Logmans, et al. 1998. Complete response of melanoma-in-transit metastasis after isolated limb perfusion with tumor necrosis factor α and melphalan without massive tumor necrosis: a clinical histopathologcal study of the delayed type reaction pattern. *Cancer Res.* **58:**4880–4997.

Rosenberg, S. A., J. C. Yang, D. E. White, and S. M. Steinberg. 1998. Durability of complete responses in patients with metastatic cancer treated with high-dose interleukin-2: identification of the antigens mediating response. *Ann. Surg.* **228:** 307–319.

Vedantham, S., H. Gamliel, and H. M. Golomb. 1992. Mechanism of interferon action in hairy cell leukemia: a model of effective cancer biotherapy. *Cancer Res.* **52:**1056–1066.

Chemokines

Rollins, E. (ed.). 1999. *Chemokines and Cancer.* Humana Press, Totowa, N.J.

Monoclonal Antibodies

Blakey, D. C. 1992. Drug targeting with monoclonal antibodies. *Rev. Oncol.* **1:**91–97.

Farah, R. A., B. Clinchy, L. Herrera, and E. X. Vitetta. 1998. The development of monoclonal antibodies for the therapy of cancer. *Crit. Rev. Eukaryot. Gene Exp.* **8:**321–356.

Reisfeld, R., and S. Sell. 1985. *Monoclonal Antibodies and Cancer Therapy.* Alan R. Liss, Inc., New York, N.Y.

Schlom, J. 1986. Basic principles and applications of monoclonal antibodies in the management of carcinomas: the Richard and Hinda Rosenthal Foundation Award Lecture. *Cancer Res.* **46:**3225–3238.

Wild, M. K., W. Strittmatter, S. Matazhku, B. Schraven, and S. C. Meuer. 1999. Tumor therapy with bispecific antibody: the targeting and triggering steps can be separated employing a CD2–based strategy. *J. Immunol.* **163:**2064–2072.

Xiang, R., H. N. Lode, T. Dreier, S. D. Gillies, and R. A. Reisfeld. 1998. Induction of persistent tumor-protective immunity in mice cured of established colon carcinoma metastases. *Cancer Res.* **58:**3918–3925.

Zeidler, R., G. Reisbach, B. Wollenberg, S. Lang, S. Shaubal, B. Schmitt, and H. Lindhofer. 1999. Simultaneous activation of T cells and accessory cells by a new class of intact bispecific antibody results in efficient tumor cell killing. *J. Immunol.* **163:**1246–1252.

Adoptive Cellular Transfer

Grimm, E. A. 1986. Human lymphokine-activated killer cells (LAK) as a potential immunotherapeutic modality. *Biochim. Biophys. Acta* **865:**267–279.

Mitchell, M. S., W. Harel, J. Kan-Mitchell, L. G. LeMay, P. Goedegebuure, et al. 1993. Active specific immunotherapy of melanoma with allogeneic cell lysates. *Ann. N. Y. Acad. Sci.* **690:**153–166.

Rosenberg, S., and M. T. Lotze. 1986. Cancer immunotherapy using interleukin 2 and interleukin 2 activated lymphocytes. *Annu. Rev. Immunol.* **4:**681–709.

Gene Therapy (some examples of active work are included)

Davidoff, A. M., S. A. Kinbrough, C. Y. Ng, S. J. Shochat, and E. F. Vanin. 1999. Neuroblastoma regression and immunity induced by transgenic expression of interleukin-12. *J. Pediatr. Surg.* **34:**902–906.

Dong, Z., G. Greene, C. Pettaway, C. P. Dinney, I. Eue, et al. 1999. Suppression of angiogenesis, tumorigenicity, and metastases by human prostate cancer cells engineered to produce interferon-β. *Cancer Res.* **59:**872–879.

Farzaneh, F., U. Trefzer, W. Sterry, and P. Walden. 1998. Gene therapy of cancer. *Immunol. Today* **19:**294–296.

Gambotto, A., T. Tuting, D. L. McVey, I. Kovesdi, H. Tahara, M. T. Lotze, and P. D. Robbins. 1999. Induction of antitumor immunity by direct intratumoral injection of a recombinant adenovirus vector expressing interleukin-12. *Cancer Gene Ther.* **6:**45–53.

Kikuchi, T., and R. G. Crystal. 1999. Anti-tumor immunity induced by in vivo adenovirus vector-mediated expression of CD40 ligand in tumor cells. *Hum. Gene Ther.* **10:**1375–1387.

Lode, H. N., R. Xiang, S. R. Duncan, A. N. Theofilopoulos, S. D. Gillis, and R. A. Reisfeld. 1999. Tumor-targeted IL-2 amplifies T cell-mediated immune response induced by gene therapy with single-chain IL-12. *Proc. Natl. Acad. Sci. USA* **96:** 8591–8596.

Osaki, T., W. Hashimoto, A. Gambotto, H. Okamura, P. D. Robbins, M. Kurimoto, M. T. Lotze, and H. Tahara. 1999. Potent antitumor effects mediated by local expression of the mature form of the interferon-gamma inducing factor, interleukin-18 (IL-18). *Gene Ther.* **6:**808–815.

Stewart, A. K., N. J. Lassam, I. C. Quirt, D. J. Bailey, L. E. Rotstein, M. Krajden, et al. 1999. Adenovector-mediated gene delivery of interleukin-2 in metastatic breast cancer and melanoma: results of a phase 1 clinical trial. *Gene Ther.* **6:**350–363.

Thompson, T. C. 1999. In situ gene therapy for prostate cancer. *Oncol. Res.* **11:**1–8.

Human Tumor Antigens

Boon, T. 1993. Tumor antigens recognized by cytolytic T lymphocytes. Present perspectives for specific immunotherapy. *Int. J. Cancer* **54:**177–180.

Bystryn, J.-C., M. Henn, J. Li, and S. Shroba. 1992. Identification of immunogenic human melanoma antigens in a polyvalent melanoma vaccine. *Cancer Res.* **52:** 5948–5953.

Lucas, S., F. Brasseur, and T. Boon. 1999. A new MAGE gene with ubiquitous expression does not code for known MAGE antigens recognized by T cells. *Cancer Res.* **59:**4100–4103.

McCarty, T. M., X. Liu, J.-Y. Sun, E. A. Peralta, D. J. Diamond, and J. D. I. Ellenhorn. 1999. Targeting p53 for adoptive T-cell immunotherapy. *Cancer Res.* **58:**2601–2605.

van der Bruggen, P., C. Traversari, P. Chomez, C. Lurquin, E. De Plaen, B. Van den Eynde, A. Knuth, and T. Boon. 1991. A gene encoding an antigen recognized by cytolytic T lymphocytes on a human melanoma. *Science* **254:**1643–1647.

Antigen-Targeted Adoptive Transfer Therapy

Lumm, L. G. 1999. T cell-based immunotherapy for cancer: a virtual reality? *CA Cancer J. Clin.* **49:**74–100.

Valmori, D., M. J. Pittet, D. Rimoldi, D. Leinard, R. Dunbar, V. Cerundolo, F. Lejeune, et al. 1999. An antigen-targeted approach to adoptive transfer therapy of cancer. *Cancer Res.* **59:**2167–2173.

Yee, C., P. A. Savage, P. P. Lee, M. K. Davis, and P. D. Greenberg. 1999. Isolation of high avidity melanoma-reactive CTL from heterogenous populations using peptide-MHC tetramers. *J. Immunol.* **162:**2227–2234.

Tumor Vaccines

Mouse (Preclinical)

Conry, R. M., A. F. Lobuglio, F. Loechel, S. E. Moore, L. A. Sumerel, et al. 1995. A carcinoembryonic antigen poly-nucleotide vaccine has in vivo antitumor activity. *Gene Ther.* **2:**59–65.

Graham, R. A., J. M. Burchell, and J. Taylor-Papadimitriou. 1996. The polymorphic epithelial mucin: potential as an immunogen for a cancer vaccine. *Cancer Immunol. Immunother.* **42:**71–80.

Hu, H.-M., W. J. Urba, and R. A. Fox. 1998. Gene-modified tumor vaccine with therapeutic potential shifts tumor-specific T cell response from a type 2 to a type 1 cytokine profile. *J. Immunol.* **161:**3033–3041.

Kieber-Emmons, T., P. Luo, J. Qui, T. Y. Chang, O. Insug, et al. 1999. Vaccination with carbohydrate peptide mimotopes promotes anti-tumor responses. *Nat. Biotechnol.* **17:**660–665.

Lo-Man, R., S. Bay, S. Vichier-Guerre, E. Deriaud, et al. 1999. A fully synthetic immunogen carrying a carcinoma-associated carbohydrate for active specific immunotherapy. *Cancer Res.* **59:**1520–1524.

Ruiz, P. J., R. Wolkowicz, A. Waisman, D. L. Hirschberg, P. Carmi, et al. 1998. Idiotypic immunization induces immunity to mutated p53 and tumor rejection. *Nat. Med.* **4:**710–712.

Saleh, M. N., D. Y. Lalisan, Jr., M. W. Pride, A. Solinger, M. S. Mayo, et al. 1998. Immunologic response to the dual murine anti-Id vaccine Melimmune-1 and Melimmune-2 in patients with high-risk melanoma without evidence of systemic disease. *J. Immunother.* **21:**379–388.

Soiffer, R., T. Lynch, M. Mihm, K. Jung, C. Rhuda, J. C. Schmollinger, F. S. Hodi, L. Leibster, et al. 1998. Vaccination with irradiated autologous melanoma cells engineered to secrete human granulocyte-macrophage colony-stimulating factor generates potent antitumor immunity in patients with metastatic melanoma. *Proc. Natl. Acad. Sci. USA* **95:**13141–13146.

Syrengelas, A. D., and R. Levy. 1998. DNA vaccination against the idiotype of a murine B cell lymphoma: mechanism of tumor protection. *J. Immunol.* **162:** 4790–4795.

Human

Disis, M. L., K. H. Grabsteni, P. R. Sleath, M. A. Cheever. 1999. Generation of immunity to the HER-2/neu oncogenic protein in patients with breast and ovarian cancer using a peptide-based vaccine. *Clin. Cancer Res.* **5:**1289–1297.

Gillespie, A. M., and R. E. Coleman. 1999. The potential of melanoma antigen expression in cancer therapy. *Cancer Treat. Rev.* **25:**219–227.

Harris, D. T., G. R. Matyas, L. G. Gomella, E. Talor, M. D. Winship, L. E. Spitler, and M. J. Mastrangelo. 1999. Immunologic approaches to the treatment of prostate cancer. *Semin. Oncol.* **26:**439–447.

Jantsheff, P., R. Herrmann, and C. Rochlitz. 1999. Cancer gene and immunotherapy; recent developments. *Med. Oncol.* **16:**78–85.

Morton, D. L., D. W. Ollila, E. C. Hsueh, R. Essner, and R. K. Gupta. 1999. Cytoreductive surgery and adjuvant immunotherapy: a new management paradigm for metastatic melanoma. *CA Cancer J. Clin.* **49:**101–116.

Pardoll, D. M. 1998. Cancer vaccines. *Nat. Med.* **4**(Suppl.)**:**525–531.

Rosenberg, S. A., J. C. Yang, D. J. Schwartzentruber, P. Hwu, et al. 1999. Impact of cytokine administration on the generation of antitumor reactivity in patients with metastatic melanoma receiving a peptide vaccine. *J. Immunol.* **163:**1690–1695.

Sandmaier, B. M., D. V. Oparin, L. A. Holmberg, M. A. Reddish, G. D. MacLean, and B. M. Longenecker. 1999. Evidence of a cellular immune response against sialyl-Tn in breast and ovarian cancer patients after high-dose chemotherapy, stem cell rescue, and immunization with Theratope Stn-KLH cancer vaccine. *J. Immunother.* **22:**54–66.

Dendritic Cells

Fernandez, N. C., A. Lozier, C. Flament, P. Ricciardi-Castagnoli, D. Bellet, M. Suter, et al. 1999. Dendritic cells directly trigger NK cell functions: cross-talk relevant in innate anti-tumor immune responses in vivo. *Nat. Med.* **5:**405–411.

Fujii, S.-I., K. Fujimoto, K. Shimizu, T. Ezaki, F. Kawano, et al. 1999. Presentation of tumor antigens by phagocytic dendritic cell clusters generated from human CD34+ hematopoietic progenitor cells: induction of autologous cytotoxic T lymphocytes against leukemic cells in acute myelogenous leukemia patients. *Cancer Res.* **59:**2150–2158.

Gong, J., D. Chen, M. Kashiwaba, and D. Kufe. 1999. Induction of antitumor activity by immunization with fusions of dendritic and carcinoma cells. *Nat. Med.* **3:**558–561.

Henry, F., O. Boisteau, L. Bretaudeay, B. Lieubeau, et al. 1999. Antigen-presenting cells that phagocytose apoptotic tumor-derived cells are potent tumor vaccines. *Cancer Res.* **59:**3329–3332.

Tjoa, B. A., A. A. Elgamal, and G. P. Murphy. 1999. Vaccine therapy for prostate cancer. *Urol. Clin. N. Am.* **26:**365–374.

Appendixes

APPENDIX 1

History of Immunopathology

A listing of the major events in the history of immunopathology (Table A1.1) and a list of winners of the Nobel Prize in physiology or medicine whose field was immunology (Table A1.2) are given in this appendix. Adaptive immunity was recognized in the ancient societies of China and Egypt. Application of this phenomenon by introduction into lesions scratched on the skin ("variolation") or by inhalation into the nasal cavity of smallpox organisms was practiced by the Chinese in about 1000 A.D., and artificial vaccination was introduced in England in 1798. In the late 1800s and early 1900s, many immune-mediated phenomena were described. The cellular immune system was emphasized by Elie Metchnikoff, and the humoral system was emphasized by Emil von Behring. Modern immunology can be said to have begun in the late 1950s with the recognition of histocompatibility antigens, identification of the structure of antibodies, and the study of immune mechanisms that cause disease. More recently, the contributions of molecular biology and genetic engineering have resulted in a breakthrough in our understanding of the molecular mechanisms of antibody diversity and the nature of the T-cell receptor, as well as how immune cells recognize and are activated by antigens.

Table A1.1 A short history of immunopathology[a]

Event or discovery	Location(s) or investigator	Date
Fever	Mesopotamia	ca. 3000 B.C.
Recognition of adaptive immunity	Egypt, China	ca. 2000 B.C.
Anatomic identification of organs	Hippocrates	ca. 400 B.C.
Acquired resistance to poisons	Mithridate Eupator, King of Pontus	ca. 80 B.C.
Four cardinal signs of inflammation	Celsus	25
"Snuff" variolation for smallpox	Sung Dynasty, China	ca. 1000
Renaissance of anatomy	Andreas Vesalius	1540
Bursa of birds described	Johann Christian Fabricius	1590
Peyer's patches	Johann Conrad Peyer	1690
Cowpox vaccination	Edward Jenner	1798
Rheumatic endocarditis	Jean-Baptiste Bouillard	1840
Tuberculous granulomas	Karl Freiherr von Rokitansky	1855
Langhans giant cells	Theodor Langhans	1868
Waldeyer's ring	Heinrich W. G. Waldeyer-Hartz	1870
Cellular pathology	Rudolf Virchow	1880
Attenuated vaccines	Louis Pasteur	1880
Phagocytosis	Elie Metchnikoff	1882
Anti-snake venom	Léon Calmette	1887
Neutralization (antitoxin)	Emil von Behring	1890
Delayed-type hypersensitivity skin test	Robert Koch	1890
Bacteriolysis (antibody and complement)	Jules Bordet	1894
Blood groups	Karl Landsteiner	1900
Side-chain theory, tumor immunity, horror autotoxicus	Paul Ehrlich	1900
Anaphylaxis	Charles Richet and Paul Portier	1902
Arthus phenomenon	Maurice Arthus	1903
Serum sickness	Clemens von Pirquet and Bela Schick	1905
Organ transplantation	Alexis Carrel	1905
Delayed-type hypersensitivity	Clemens von Pirquet	1906
Immune surveillance of cancer	Paul Ehrlich	1909
Viral cancer immunity	Peyton Rous	1910
Passive cutaneous anaphylaxis	Carl Prausnitz and Heinz Küstner	1921
Toxoid immunization	Gaston Ramou	1923
Chemical mediators of inflammation	T. Lewis	1925
Quantitative precipitin reaction	Michael Heidelberger	1935
Gamma globulin	Arne Tiselius and Elvin Kabat	1938
Yellow fever vaccine	Max Theiler	1938
Rheumatoid factor	E. Waaler	1940
Hemolytic disease of newborns (Rh)	Karl Landsteiner, Philip Levine	1941
Immunofluorescence	Albert Coons	1942
Concept of collagen disease	Peter Klemperer	1942
Immune tolerance	Peter Medawar and Macfarlane Burnet	1944
Passive transfer of cell-mediated immunity	Merrill Chase	1945
Gel diffusion antibody tests	Örjan Ouchterlony, Jacques Oudin	1946–1948
Agammaglobulinemia	Ogden Bruton	1952
Cellular transfer of transplantation immunity	Nicholas Mitchison	1953
Mechanism of immune complex disease	Frank Dixon	1956
Autoimmune thyroiditis	Ernest Witebsky and Deborah Doniach	1957
Histocompatibility antigens	George Snell and Jean Dausset	1958
Structure of antibodies	Rodney Porter and Gerald Edelman	1959
Lymphocyte recirculation	James Gowans	1959
Mitogenic activation of lymphocytes	Peter Nowell	1961
Function of the thymus	Jacques Miller and Robert Good	1961
Classification of immune mechanisms	Philip Gell and Robin Coombs	1962

Table A1.1 *(continued)*

Event or discovery	Location(s) or investigator	Date
Migration inhibitory factors	John David and John Vaughn	1962
Mixed lymphocyte reaction	Barbara Bain et al.	1963
Lymphocyte surface immunoglobulin and lymphocyte activation	Stewart Sell and Philip Gell	1964
Identification of T and B cells	Henry Claman	1966
In vitro primary immune response	Robert Mishell and Richard Dutton	1967
IgE as reaginic antibody	Kunishige Ishizaka and Teruko Ishizaka	1967
Accessory cell role in immune response	Donald Mosier	1968
Immune response genes	Baruj Benacerraf and Hugh McDevitt	1969
Tolerance in T and B cells	William Weigle and Jacques Chiller	1971
T-cell helper factors	Richard Dutton and Anneliese Schimpl	1972
Idiotype network	Niels Jerne	1974
Hybridoma (monoclonal antibodies)	Georges Kohler and Cesar Milstein	1975
Natural killer cells	Rolf Kiessling and Ron Herberman	1975
MHC class-restricted T-cell cytotoxicity	Rolf Zinkernagel and Peter Doherty	1975
Ig gene rearrangements	Susumu Tonegawa	1978
CD4 and CD8 subsets of T cells	E. L. Reinherz, P. C. Kung, and Stuart Schlossman	1979
Immunoglobulin structure	Elvin Kabat, Gerald Edelman, and Rodney Porter	1980
Antigen-specific T-cell hybridoma	John Kappler and Philippa Marrack	1981
Antigen-presenting B cells	Robert Chestnut and Howard Grey	1981
Antigen processing		
MHC class II	Emil Unanue	1982
MHC class I	Alan Townsend	1985
Lymphokine-activated killer cells	Elizabeth Grimm	1982
T-cell receptor	James Allison, Katherine Haskens, et al.	1982
Transgenic mice	Ralph Brinster and Richard Palmiter	1982
B-cell antigen presentation	Laurie Glimcher et al.	1982
Somatic generation of Ig variable regions	Susumu Tonegawa	1983
Discovery of HIV	Luc Montagnier and Robert Gallo	1983
Dendritic cell antigen processing	Ralph Steinman	1983
T-cell receptor gene	Steven Hedrick, Mark Davis, and Tak Mak	1984
Thymic maturation of $CD4^+CD8^-$ cells	Thomas Folks and Bonnie Mathieson	1984
Cell adhesion molecules	Erkki Ruoslahti and T. A. Springer	1985
MHC binds antigenic peptides	Soren Buus, Alessandro Sette, and Howard Grey	1986
Antibodies to T-cell receptor chains	John Kappler and Philippa Marrack	1988
Class I MHC antigen binding site	Pamela Bjorkman and Jack Strominger	1987
Endogenous superantigens and Vβ genes	Philippa Marrack, John Kappler, and Robson MacDonald	1988
RAG genes	David Schatz, Marjorie Oettinger, and David Baltimore	1988
Thymic selection of T-cell receptor	Hans von Boehmer	1988
Peripheral tolerance	Jacques Miller, Ronald Schwartz, and Dennis Loh	1988
Th1 and Th2 cells	Tim Mossman and Robert Coffman	1989
Igα and Igβ in membrane Ig	Walter Reth	1990
Peptide transporter proteins (TAP1 and TAP2)	John Monaco, T. Spies, and Robert DeMars	1990
Immunopathology of AIDS	David Ho, Jay Levy, Anthony Fauci, and others	1992
Molecular diagnosis of immunodeficiencies	Rebecca Buckley, H. D. Ochs, Warren Leonard, et al.	1993
Cancer antigens	Alexander Knuth and Thierry Boon	1993
Chemokines	Tom Schall, Albert Zlotnik, and S. L. Kunkel	1994
T-cell receptor–antigen interactions	Mark Davis and John Altman	1994
Role of TNF in rheumatoid arthritis	Marc Feldman et al.	1994
Signal transduction (T cells)	Paul Allen, Roger Perlmutter, and others	1995
Control of NK cell stimulation	Lewis Lanier and Wayne Yokoyama	1995
IL-15 and immune memory	Jonathan Sprent, Philippa Marrack, and John Kappler	1999

[a]Abbreviations: Ig, immunoglobulin; MHC, major histocompatibility complex; HIV, human immunodeficiency virus; AIDS, acquired immune deficiency syndrome; TNF, tumor necrosis factor; NK, natural killer; IL, interleukin.

Table A1.2 Nobel prizes in physiology or medicine awarded for research in immunology

Yr	Recipient	Country	Discovery
1901	Emil von Behring	Germany	Antitoxins in serum
1905	Robert Koch	Germany	Cellular immunity (tuberculosis)
1908	Elie Metchnikoff	Russia	Phagocytosis
	Paul Ehrlich	Germany	Antitoxins, side-chain theory
1913	Charles Richet	France	Anaphylaxis
1919	Jules Bordet	Belgium	Complement-mediated bacteriolysis
1930	Karl Landsteiner	United States	Human blood groups
1950	Philip Hench	United States	Cortisone treatment of rheumatoid diseases
	Edward Kendall	United States	Cortisone treatment of rheumatoid diseases
	Tadeus Reichstein	Switzerland	Cortisone treatment of rheumatoid diseases
1951	Max Theiler	South Africa	Yellow fever vaccine
1957	Daniel Bovet	Switzerland	Antihistamines
1960	Macfarlane Burnet	Australia	Acquired immunological tolerance
	Peter Medawar	Great Britain	Acquired immunological tolerance
1972	Gerald Edelman	United States	Chemical structure of antibodies
	Rodney Porter	Great Britain	Chemical structure of antibodies
1977	Rosalyn Yalow	United States	Radioimmunoassay for insulin
1980	George Snell	United States	Major histocompatibility complex
	Jean Dausset	France	Major histocompatibility complex
	Baruj Benacerraf	United States	Major histocompatibility complex
1984	Georges Köhler	Germany	Monoclonal antibody
	Cesar Milstein	Great Britain	Monoclonal antibody
	Niels Jerne	Denmark	Immune regulatory theories
1987	Susumu Tonegawa	Japan and United States	Immunoglobulin genes
1990	E. Donnall Thomas	United States	Bone marrow transplantation
	Joseph Murray	United States	Renal transplantation
1996	Peter C. Doherty	Australia	Specificity of T-cell-mediated killing
	Rolf M. Zinkernagel	Switzerland	Specificity of T-cell-mediated killing
1997	Stanley Prusiner	United States	Prions

Bibliography

Bibel, D. J. 1988. *Milestones in Immunology: a Historical Exploration.* Science Tech Publishers, Madison, Wis.

Boyd, W. C. 1943. *Fundamentals of Immunology.* Interscience Publishers, Inc., New York, N.Y.

Gell, P. G. H., and R. R. A. Coombs. 1963. *Clinical Aspects of Immunology.* F. A. Davis Co., Philadelphia, Pa.

Haggard, H. W. 1933. *Mystery, Magic and Medicine.* Doubleday, Doran and Co., Garden City, N.J.

Kabat, E. A. 1968. *Structural Concepts in Immunology and Immunochemistry.* Holt, Rinehart and Winston, New York, N.Y.

Landsteiner, K. 1962. *The Specificity of Serological Reactions.* Dover Pub., New York, N.Y.

Long, E. R. 1965. *A History of Pathology.* Dover Pub., New York, N.Y.

Majno, G. 1975. *The Healing Hand.* Harvard University Press, Cambridge, Mass.

Raffel, S. 1953. *Immunity, Hypersensitivity, Serology.* Appleton-Century-Crofts, Inc., New York, N.Y.

Silverstein, A. M. 1985. History of immunology: a history of theories of antibody formation. *Cell. Immunol.* **91:**263–283.

Silverstein, A. M. 1989. *A History of Immunology.* Academic Press, Inc., San Diego, Calif.

APPENDIX 2
Evolution of Immunity (Phylogeny)

Adaptation to the environment is the driving force in evolution and survival of a species. Organisms must not only accommodate to changes in temperature, pH, nutrients, oxygen, and water but also must defend against potentially fatal effects of other organisms (parasites). The most primitive defense system is the ability to recognize that something is foreign (not self). Shared domains in cell recognition molecules, in particular β2-microglobulin domains in immunoglobulins, T-cell receptors, and cell adhesion molecules, suggest that the adaptive immune response may have evolved from much older cell-cell interaction mechanisms. The following is a simplified version of the phylogenity of immunity. For a more detailed molecular presentation of the phylogeny of immune-related genes, see L. DuPasquire and M. Flajnik, Origin and evolution of the vertebrate immune system, p. 605–650, *in* W. E. Paul (ed.), *Fundamental Immunology*, 4th ed., Lippincott-Raven, Philadelphia, Pa., 1999.

Invertebrates

A simplified phylogenetic tree as related to evolution of immune functions in invertebrates is presented in Fig. A2.1.

The ability to identify foreign species and strains is present in each individual species. However, specific immunoglobulin antibody and T- and B-cell lymphocyte differentiation are later developments and are not seen in invertebrates. Protozoa are able to recognize other protozoa as different because of different enzymes in different species and can defend themselves by phagocytosis. In this process, they are able to distinguish foreign nuclei (different species) from self (same species) nuclei. The ability to recognize tissue of different species (self versus nonself) clearly exists in sponges. Identical pairs of sponges will fuse when mixed, whereas foreign pairs show a cytotoxic (necrotic) rejection response at their interface. The strength of rejection depends on the degree of genetic difference. A more rapid and extensive rejection occurs when two allogeneic (different) species are put together a second time (secondary response or immune memory). In higher organisms, this phenomenon is tested by whether or not an individual will accept a graft of tissue from another individual (graft rejection implies recognition of foreign tissue). In coral, the extent of parabiotic incompatibility suggests that each clone of coral is different.

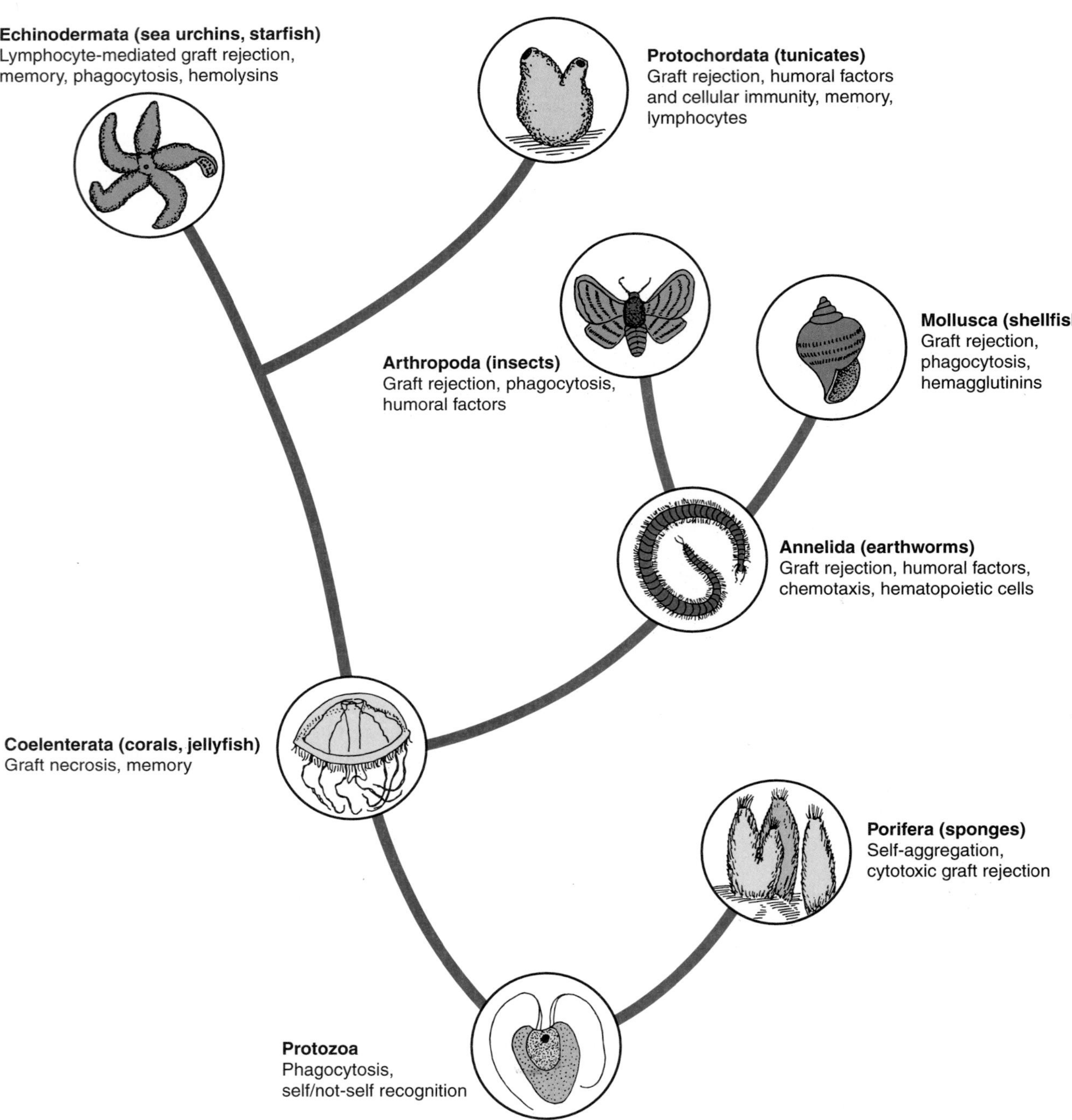

Figure A2.1 Phylogeny of immunity in invertebrates.

This principle of the uniqueness of the individual also applies to humans *(histocompatibility differences).*

White blood cell differentiation appears first in echinoderms and protochordates (for a description of white blood cells, see chapter 2). In the celomic cavity of earthworms are primitive white blood cell types that combine features of polymorphonuclear cells and lymphocytes. These cells appear to be responsible for graft rejection in these species, and some appear to respond to *mitogen* stimulation. A mitogen is a substance that stimulates cell proliferation (mitosis). Protochordates contain nodules of lymphatic cells and circulating lymphocytes that respond to stimulation. Lymphocyte-like cells also infiltrate grafts of sea urchins. Humoral factors also appear in earthworms, and hemolysins (causing lysis of red blood cells) and hemagglutinins (causing agglutination of red blood cells) are found in starfish and shellfish. However these are not immunoglobulins and are not antigen specific. Snails have at least four cell types that impede the dissemination of microbes, but the most prominent role in defense is played by mobile *hemocytes,* which have phagocytic capacities and granules (phagosomes) with properties similar to those of vertebrate granulocytes. Tunicates express both cellular and humoral immune factors, including some differentiation of lymphocytes. Immune memory, expressed as a shorter time to induce necrosis in grafts of different strains upon second exposure, is seen in coral. Some insects (arthropoda), such as cockroaches, have antibodylike proteins that have properties of specificity and memory, as well as cell-mediated ability to reject grafts from other strains of roaches. A major defense mechanism in insects is mechanical isolation (walling off) of parasites by collections (nodules) of blood cells (hemocytes), with deposition of melanin on the surface of the parasites (melanization). In general, cellular immune responses appear to precede the development of humoral responses during evolution.

Vertebrates

The phylogeny of immunity in vertebrates is illustrated in Fig. A2.2.

T and B Cells

The immune system in vertebrates is characterized by a true two-component (T- and B-cell) system, specific immunoglobulin antibody production, highly developed specific cellular immunity, and specific immune memory. Immunoglobulins first appear at the level of agnatha, although cyclostomes do not appear to have immunoglobulins. T- and B-like cells exist in teleost fishes but are not clearly defined in agnatha, although a primitive T-cell response can be demonstrated. Table A2.1 lists evolution of lymphoid organs in vertebrates (human lymphoid organs are described in chapter 3). Agnatha demonstrate diffuse lymphoid tissue in the gut but do not have other lymphoid organs. Thymus and spleen appear in fishes, and lymph nodes appear in amphibians.

Clearly defined T and B cells are first seen in amphibians, where thymectomy results in loss of cellular responses such as graft rejection, and T- and B-cell responses can be demonstrated. Reptiles have demonstrable T-regulatory cells, cells with surface immunoglobulin, and lymphoid organs that resemble those of mammals. Most amphibians do not have clear-cut graft rejection, but some amphibians have slow, chronic graft rejection reactions compared with reptiles, birds, and mammals. The evolutionary trend from slow to fast graft rejection may reflect expression of histocompatibility antigens rather than a weakness in the immune reaction.

Epithelium and Lymphoid Organs

Associations of epithelial tissue and lymphoid tissue in some lymphoid organs appear to be of critical importance in the development of the mammalian immune system. To survive on land, changes in the gill pouches

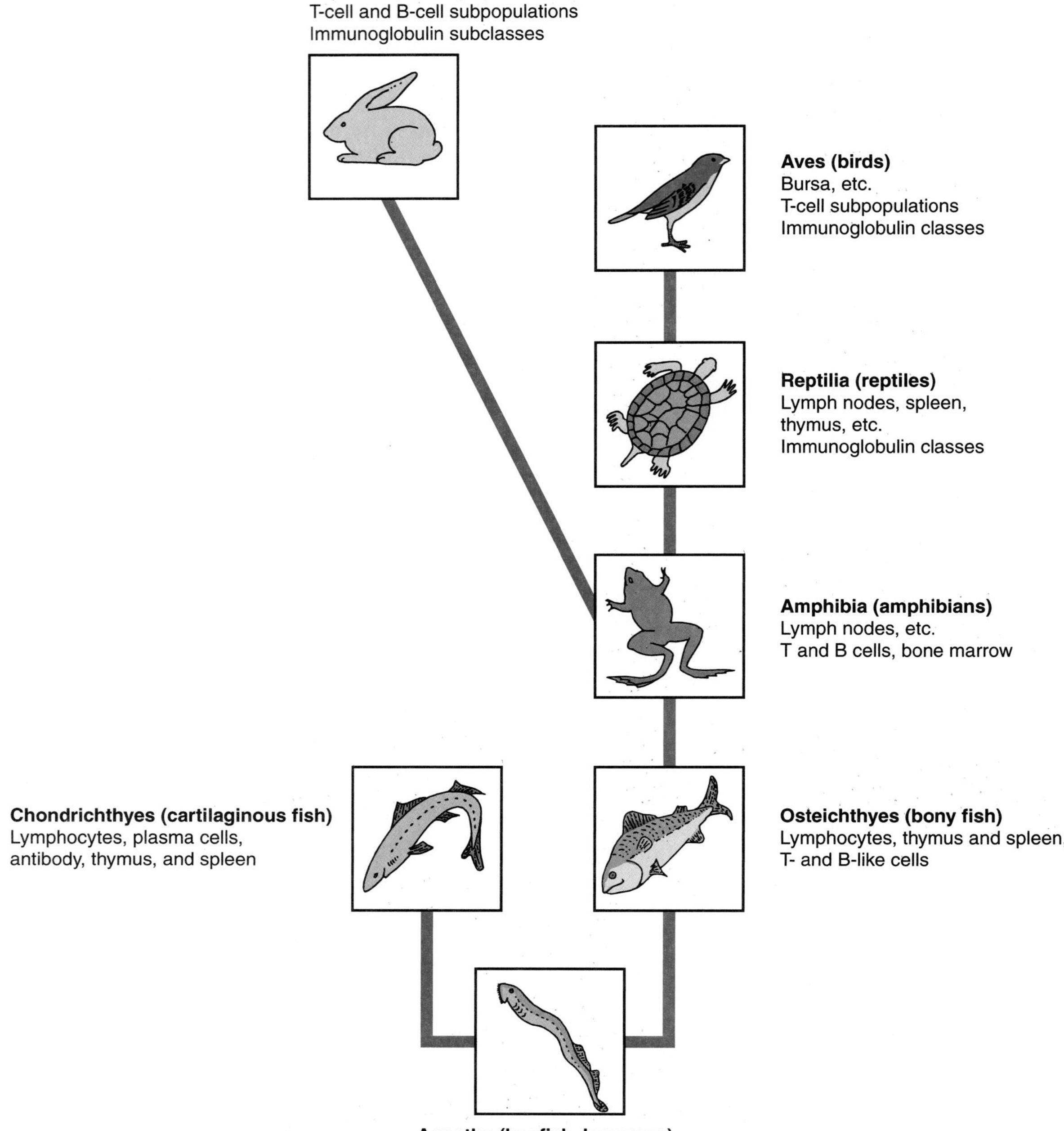

Figure A2.2 Phylogeny of immunity in vertebrates.

and cloaca bursa of amphibians had to evolve in birds and mammals. During embryogenesis of higher vertebrates, the five paired gill pouches cease absorbing oxygen and develop to supply epithelium for cervical organs. In primitive coelenterates, the celomic cavity serves not only to absorb nutrients but also to absorb oxygen. This function evolves into gills in the neck (foregut) of fishes and the hindgut of mollusks and arthropods. The five

Table A2.1 Phylogeny of the immune system from primitive fishes to mammals[a]

Class or group	Presence of: Thymus	Bone marrow	Lymph glands or nodes	Blood granulocytes and lymphocytes	Reactions to primary tissue allografts (cell-mediated immunity[b]): Moderate	Strong
Hagfish and lampreys	0	0	0	+	+	0
Sharks and rays	+	0	0	+	+	0
Bony fishes	+	+	0	+	+	+
Amphibians	+	+	+	+	+	+
Reptiles	+	+	+	+	+	0
Birds	+	+	+	+	+	+
Mammals	+	+	+	+	+	+

[a]From W. H. Hildemann, *in Frontiers in Immunogenetics,* Elsevier/North-Holland Publishing Co., New York, N.Y., 1981. +, presence of corresponding types of cells or reactivity; 0, not present or not reactive.
[b]Moderate histocompatibility barriers are found in animals representing all vertebrate classes, but strong barriers are the rule in advanced bony fishes, anuran amphibians, and most birds and mammals.

gill pouches in fish become vestigial in amphibia, but the epithelial tissue of the third pharyngeal pouch provides the stroma of the medulla of the thymus. This epithelial stroma produces thymic hormones essential for the maturation of thymocytes (see chapter 3). The hindgut gills evolve into the cloaca in turtles and further into the cloacal bursa of Fabricius of birds. The bursa of Fabricius is essential for the development of the B-cell system in birds. In mammals, there is evidence that the gastrointestinal-associated lymphoid tissue (GALT) plays an important role in the development of the B-cell system (see below).

Summary

1. Some form of recognition of self and nonself is present in the simplest animal species.
2. Cellular immunity precedes humoral immunity in evolution.
3. A bifunctional (T- and B-cell) system with developed lymphoid organs is the most recent immunological development.
4. Epithelium that evolves from the gills of fishes (i.e., pharyngeal pouches) plays a major role in the development of the lymphoid organs of mammals (thymus and GALT).

Selective pressures during evolution are believed to have resulted in the development of protective immune mechanisms. Primitive immune mechanisms may have had a number of other functions in lower organisms, such as recognition of cell surface markers required for aggregation of cell types in the early stages of development of multicellular structures (recognition of self and nonself). Immune recognition mechanisms may be variants of the cell-cell interactions that occur during embryologic development. It is likely that the immune system, as we now see it, is expanding and being modified to perform other new functions, such as regulation of neuroendocrine or hormonally expressive cells.

Bibliography

Brehelin, M. 1985. *Immunity in Invertebrates.* Springer-Verlag, New York, N.Y.

Cohen, N. 1975. Phylogeny of lymphocyte structure and function. *Am. Zool.* **15:**119–133.

Cooper, E. L. 1976. *Comparative Immunology.* Prentice-Hall, Englewood Cliffs, N.J.

Goetz, D. (ed.). 1977. *Evolution and Function of the Major Histocompatibility System.* Springer-Verlag KG, Berlin, Germany.

Good, R. A., and B. W. Papermaster. 1964. Ontogeny and phylogeny of adaptive immunity. *Adv. Immunol.* **4:**1.

Hildemann, W. H., E. A. Clark, and R. L. Raison. 1981. *Comprehensive Immunogenetics.* Elsevier/North-Holland Publishing Co., New York, N.Y.

Karp, R. D. 1990. Cell-mediated immunity in invertebrates: the enigma of the insect. *Bioscience* **40:**732.

Ohno, S. 1987. The ancestor of the adaptive immune system was the CAM system for organogenesis. *Exp. Clin. Immunogenet.* **4:**181.

van der Knapp, W. P. W., and E. S. Loker. 1990. Immune mechanisms in trematode-snail interactions. *Parasitol. Today* **6:**175.

APPENDIX 3
Cluster-of-Differentiation Molecules

Updated information on CD molecules is available through the National Library of Medicine at the PROW (Protein Resources of the Web) at http://www.ncbi.nlm.nih.gov/PROW. Tumor expression is listed for most commonly used markers, in particular those used to classify lymphoproliferative lesions.

Table A3.1 Cluster-of-differentiation molecules

CD designation	Other names	Molecular mass (kDa) and comment	Cellular expression	Family	Function(s)	Tumor expression(s)
CD1 (a, b, c, d, e)	T6, MHC-class I-like structure	43–49; β_2-microglobulin-associated	Thymocytes, dendritic cells (including Langerhans cells), B cells (CD1c), intestinal epithelium, smooth muscle, blood vessels (CD1d)	Ig superfamily (IgSF)	Presentation of nonpeptide and glycolipid antigens for T cells	Langerhans cell histiocytosis
CD2	T11, LFA-2, sheep red blood cell receptor, CD58-binding adhesion molecule	45–58	T cells, thymocytes, NK cells	Ig superfamily	Adhesion molecule (binds CD58 [LFA-3]); T-cell activation	T-cell malignancies
CD3	T3, Leu-4	Composed of three polypeptide chains: γ, 25–28; δ, 20; ϵ, 20	Thymocytes, T cells, NK1 T cells	Ig superfamily	Signal transduction as a result of antigen recognition through the T-cell receptor	T-cell malignancies
CD4	T4, Leu-3, L3T4 (mice)	55	Thymocyte subsets, class II MHC-restricted T cells; Th1 and Th2 cells, monocytes, macrophages	Ig superfamily	Coreceptor for MHC class II; signal transduction for T-cell activation; receptor for HIV-1 and HIV-2 gp120	T-cell malignancies
CD5	Leu-1, T1, Lyt1	67	Thymocytes, T cells; B-cell subset	Scavenger receptor	Modulation of TCR and BCR signaling	T- and B-cell malignancies
CD6	T12	100–130	Thymocytes; subset of T cells; some B cells	Scavenger receptor	Binds CD166; adhesion molecule binding developing thymocytes to thymic epithelial cells; costimulator for T cells?	T-cell malignancies
CD7	Leu-9, gp40	40	Subset of T cells, hematopoietic precursors	Immunoglobulin	Cytoplasmic domain binds PI-3 kinase	T-cell acute leukemia; stem cell leukemia

CD8	T8, Leu-2, Lty2	Composed of two 34-kDa chains; expressed as αα or αβ dimer	Thymocyte subsets, class I MHC-restricted cytotoxic T cells	Ig superfamily	Coreceptor for class I MHC-restricted T cells; signal transduction	T-cell malignancies/ LGL leukemia
CD9	MRP-1, p24, BA-2, J-2	24	Pre-B and immature B cells; monocytes, platelets, eosinophils, basophils	Transmembrane protein 4	Platelet aggregation, migration, and activation through FcγRIIa	
CD10	CALLA, neural endopeptidase, metalloendopep-tidase	100	Immature and some mature B cells; T-cell progenitors, bone marrow stroma	Tetraspanning membrane protein	Neural endopeptidase (enkephalinase); zinc metalloproteinase	Pre-B-cell ALLs, lymphomas
CD11a	LFA-1, α-L integrin chain	180; associates with CD18 to form LFA-1 integrin	White blood cells	Integrin α	αL subunit of integrin LFA-1 (binds to ICAM-1, -2, and -3)	
CD11b	Mac-1, CR3 (iCR3, iC3B receptor) α chain; Leu-15	165; associates with CD18 to form Mac-1 integrin	Granulocytes; monocytes, NK cells; subsets of T and B cells	Integrin α	Adhesion to extracellular matrix; phagocytosis of iC3b-coated (opsonized) particles	NGL (NK) leukemia
CD11c	αX integrin chain, p150,95; CR4 α chain; Leu M5	150; associated with CD18 to form p150,95 integrin	Monocytes granulocytes, NK cells	Integrin α	αX subunit of integrin CR4 (binds to fibrinogen)	HCL, histiocytic tumors
CD11d		125	White blood cells	Integrin α	αD subunits of integrin (binds to CD50)	
CDw12		90–120	Monocytes, granulocytes		Unknown	
CD13	My-7, aminopeptidase N, gp150	150	Myelomonocytic precursors and mature cells		Zinc metalloproteinase; role in oxidative burst?	AMLs
CD14	LPS receptor; Leu M3, Mo2	53–55	Myelomonocytic cells		Receptor for complex of LPS and LPS-binding protein; activation of monocytes	AML (M4 and 5)

continued

Table A3.1 Cluster-of-differentiation molecules *(continued)*

CD designation	Other names	Molecular mass (kDa) and comment	Cellular expression	Family	Function(s)	Tumor expression(s)
CD15	Lewis X, Lex, SSEA-I, Leu M1 (lacto-*N*-neo-fucopentose III)	Terminal trisaccharide expressed on glycolipids and many cell surface glycoproteins	Granulocytes monocytes	Blood group antigens	?Cell adherence	AMLs, Hodgkin's disease, adenocarci-nomas
CD15a	Sialyl Lewis X (sLEX), poly-*N*-acetyl lactosamine	Carbohydrate polymer	White blood cells, endothelium	Blood group antigens	Ligand for CD62E, P; cell adhesion?	Many epithelial tumors, AMLs
CD16	FcRIII, Leu II	50–80; trans-membrane	NK cells, granulocytes, macrophages	Ig superfamily	Low-affinity Fcγ receptor: ADCC, activation of NK cells	LGL leukemia
CDw17	T5A7	Carbohydrate epitope (lactosyl-ceramide)	Granulocytes, macrophages, platelets	Blood group antigens	May enhance phagocytosis of bacteria	
CD18	β chain of LFA-1 family (β_2-integrins)	95; noncovalently linked to CD11a, CD11b, or CD11c	Leukocytes	Integrin β	Associates with CD11a, b, c, and d to form integrins; adhesion and signaling during inflammation	
CD19	Leu 12, B4	95	Most B cells	Ig superfamily	Forms complex with CR2 (CD21) and TAPA-1 (CD81), coreceptor for B cells; activation or regulation of B cells through tyrosine kinases and PI-3 kinase	B-cell malignancies
CD20	Leu 16, B1, Bp35	Heterodimer: 35- and 37-kDa chains	Mature B cells; follicular dendritic cells	Tetraspanning membrane protein	Oligomers for Ca^{2+} channel; B-cell activation or regulation	B-cell malignancies
CD21	CR2; C3d receptor, Epstein-Barr virus receptor	145	Mature B cells, follicular dendritic cells, subset of immature thymocytes	Complement control protein superfamily	Receptor for C3d, Epstein-Barr virus; role in B cell activation?	B-cell malignancies

CD22	BL-CAM, Leu-14; Lyb8 in mouse	α, 130; β, 140	Mature B cells	Ig superfamily	Binds sialoconjugates; cell adhesion signaling	B-cell malignancies
CD23	FcεRIIb, B6, BLAST-2, low-affinity IgE receptor	45	Mature B cells, activated macrophages, eosinophils, FDC, platelets	C-type lectin	Low-affinity FcE receptor, induced by IL-4; regulates IgE synthesis; triggers cytokine release from monocytes	B-cell malignancies
CD24	BA-1, heat-stable antigen (HAS) in mouse	35–45	B cells, granulocytes		Not known	B-cell malignancies
CD25	TAC; p55; low-affinity IL-2 receptor	55	Activated T and B cells; activated macrophages	Complement control protein superfamily	Complexes with p70 to form high-affinity IL-2 receptor; T-cell growth	T-cell tumors, HCL
CD26	Dipeptidyl peptidase IV, adenosine deaminase binding protein	110, 120	Activated T and B cells; macrophages	Type IV transmembrane glycoprotein	Exo-serine peptidase, cleaves N-terminal X-pro of Xala dipeptides from polypeptides; costimulator for T cells	
CD27	S152, T14	Homodimer of 55-kDa chains	Medullary thymocytes, T cells; NK cells and some B cells	TNF receptor superfamily	Binds CD70; co-stimulator for T and B cells	
CD28	Tp44	Homodimer of 44-kDa chains	$CD3^+$ thymocytes, peripheral T cells, activated B cells	Ig superfamily, CD86 (B7.2)	T-cell receptor for costimulator signal 2, binds CD80 and 86	
CD29	β chain of VLA (β_1-integrins)	130; noncovalently associated with VLA α chains (CD249)	White blood cells	Integrin β	Adhesion to extracellular matrix proteins, cell-cell adhesion (see CD49)	
CD30	Ki-1 antigen, Ber-OH2 antigen	120	Activated T cells, B cells, and NK cells	TNF receptor	Binds CD30, enhances proliferation or apoptosis of T and B cells	Reed-Sternberg cells in Hodgkin's disease, lymphoma

continued

Table A3.1 Cluster-of-differentiation molecules *(continued)*

CD designation	Other names	Molecular mass (kDa) and comment	Cellular expression	Family	Function(s)	Tumor expression(s)
CD31	Platelet gplla; platelet endothelial adhesion molecule (PECAM-1)	130–140	Platelets; monocytes, granulocytes, B cells, T cell subsets, endothelial cells	Ig superfamily	Adhesion	
CD32	FCRII, FcγRII	40	Macrophages, granulocytes, B cells, eosinophils	Ig superfamily	Low-affinity Fc receptor for aggregated Ig	
CD33	MY 9; gp67	67	Monocytes, myeloid progenitor cells	Ig superfamily	Binds sialoconjugates, cytoadhesion	AMLs
CD34	MY 10; gp105–120	105–120	Precursors of hematopoietic cells; capillary endothelium	Mucin	Ligand for CD62L (L-selectin); cell-cell adhesion	Acute leukemias
CD35	Complement receptor type 1 (CR1); C3bR, C4bR, immune adherence receptor	Polymorphic; four forms are 190–280 kDa	Granulocytes, monocytes, erythrocytes, B cells, dendritic cells	Complement control protein superfamily	Binding and phagocytosis of C3b-C4b-coated particles and immune complexes	
CD36	Platelet gpIIIb, gpIV, OKM5 antigen	88–113	Monocytes, platelets, endothelial cells		Platelet adhesion, recognition, and phagocytosis of apoptotic cells	
CD37	gp40–52	Composed of two or three 40- to 52-kDa chains	B cells, some T cells, granulocytes	Tetraspanning membrane protein 4	Signal transduction, complexes with MHC class II, CD53, CD81, CD82	
CD38	T10, Leu 17	45	Plasma cells, early T and B cells, thymocytes, activated T cells		NAD glycohydrolase, augments B-cell proliferation	Multiple myeloma, follicular lymphoma
CD39	Bp50	40–78	B and T cells, granulocytes, dendritic cells		Signal transduction	
CD40	Bp50	Heterodimer of 44- and 48-kDa chains	B cells, macrophages, dendritic cells, basal epithelial cells	TNF receptor superfamily	Binds CD154, costimulatory for B cells, B-cell growth, isotype switching and	

					differentiation, cytokine reproduction by monocytes	
CD41	gpIIb, complexes with gpIIIa to form platelet fibrinogen receptor	Complex of gpIIb αβ heterodimer (125 kDa) or ββ dimer (22 kDa)	Platelets, macrophages	Integrin α	αIIβ integrin, associates with CD61 to form gpIIβ; binds RDG (fibrinogen, fibronectin, von Willebrand factor, thrombospondin), platelet aggregation and activation	AML (M7)
CD42a, b, c, d	a, gpIX; b, gpIb-α; c, gpIb-β; d, gpV	a, 23; b, 23, 135; c, 22; d, 85	Platelets, megakaryocytes	Leucine-rich repeat	Platelet adhesion, binding to von Willebrand factor	
CD43	Sialophorin, leukosialin	95–115; highly sialylated	Leukocytes (except circulating B cells)	Mucin	May be anti-adhesive for leukocyte binding	
CD44	Pgp-1; Hermes; ECMR II, H-CAM; HUTCH-1	80→100, highly glycosylated	Leukocytes, erythrocytes	Link protein	Receptor for matrix components (hyaluronate); leukocyte adhesion	
CD45	T200; leukocyte common antigen, isoforms: CD45R, CD45RA, CD45RB, CD45RC, CD45RO	Four isoforms, 180–220	All hematopoietic cells, isoforms on different cell types	Fibronectin type III	T- and B-cell signal transduction (tyrosine phosphatase)	Lymphomas
CD46	Membrane cofactor protein (MCP)	35–58	Peripheral blood lymphocytes; epithelial cells, fibroblasts	Complement control protein superfamily	Binds to C3b and C4b, leads to degradation by factor I	
CD47	Integrin-associated protein, Rh-associated protein, neurophilin, ovarian carcinoma antigen 3 (OA3)	47–52	Essentially all cells	Rh blood group?	Thrombospondin receptor, adhesion	Ovarian carcinoma

continued

Table A3.1 Cluster-of-differentiation molecules *(continued)*

CD designation	Other names	Molecular mass (kDa) and comment	Cellular expression	Family	Function(s)	Tumor expression(s)
CD48	Blast-1, HU Lym 3, CD-BCM-1 in mouse; OX-45 in rat	40–47	All white cells	Ig superfamily	Binds CD2, adhesion	
CD49a	VLA α1 chain; α_1-integrin chain	200	Activated T cells, monocytes, neuronal cells, smooth muscle	Integrin α	Associates with CD29 to form VLA-1 (β_1-integrin); adhesion to collagen, laminin-1	
CD49b	VLA α2 chain; platelet gpla	160	Platelets, monocytes, B cells, neuronal, epithelial, and endothelial cells, osteoclasts, megakaryocytes	Integrin α	Associates with CD29 to form VLA-2 (β_1-integrin); adhesion to extracellular matrix: receptor for collagen and laminin-1	
CD49c	VLA α3 chain, α-integrin chain	Dimer of 130 and 25 kDa	B cells, many adherent cells	Integrin α	Associates with CD29 to form VLA-3 (β_1-integrin); adhesion to fibronectin, laminin-5, collagen	
CD49d	VLA α4 chain, α_4-integrin chain	150	T cells, monocytes, B cells	Integrin α	Associates with CD29 to form VLA-4 (β_1-integrin); Peyer's patch homing receptor, binds to VCAM-1, fibronectin; T-cell activation	
CD49e	VLA α5 chain, α_5-integrin chain	Dimer of 135 and 25 kDa	Memory T cells, monocytes, platelets, others	Integrin α	Associates with CD29 to form VLA-5 (β_1-integrin); adhesion to fibronectin, invasin	

CD49f	Platelet gpI, VLA-6 α chain, α_6-integrin chain	Dimer of 125 and 25 kDa	T cells, monocytes, platelets, megakaryocytes, trophoblasts	Integrin α	Associates with CD29 to form α_6-integrin; binds laminin, invasin, merosine	
CD50	Intercellular adhesion molecule 3 (ICAM-3)	130	Thymocytes, T cells, B cells, monocytes, granulocytes	Immunoglobulin	Binds integrin CD11a/CD18; costimulatory molecule, regulates ICAM-1 and integrin-β adhesion	
CD51	α chain of vitronectin receptor (VNR-α)	140-kDa heterodimer, associates with CD61	Platelets, megakaryocytes	Integrin α	Associates with CD61 to form α V integrin; receptor for vitronectin, fibrinogen, von Willebrand factor (binds RGD)	
CD52	CAMPATH-1, HE5	25–29	Thymocytes, T cells, B cells, monocytes, granulocytes, spermatozoa		Unknown, target for antibodies used to remove T cells from bone marrow	
CD53	MRC OX44	35–42	Leukocytes, plasma cells	Transmembrane membrane 4	B-cell signal transduction	
CD54	Intercellular adhesion molecule 1 (ICAM-1)	75–115	Broad; many activated cells (cytokine-inducible)	Ig superfamily	Binds CD11a/CD18 integrin (LFA-1) and CD11b/18 integrin (Mac-1), receptor for rhinovirus	
CD55	Decay-accelerating factor (DAF)	55–70	Most cells	Complement control protein superfamily	Binds C3b, disassembles C3/C5 convertase; limits effects of complement	
CD56	Leu-19, neural cell adhesion molecule (NCAM)	Heterodimer of 135- and 220-kDa chains	NK cells	Ig superfamily	Neural cell adhesion molecule (NCAM)	LGL leukemia
CD57	HNK-1, Leu-7	110-kDa oligosaccharide	NK cells, monocytes, subsets of T and B cells		Oligosaccharide attached to many cell surface proteins	LGL leukemia

continued

Table A3.1 Cluster-of-differentiation molecules *(continued)*

CD designation	Other names	Molecular mass (kDa) and comment	Cellular expression	Family	Function(s)	Tumor expression(s)
CD58	LFA-3	55–70; phosphoinositol-linked	Most cells	Ig superfamily	Adhesion: ligand for CD2	
CD59	Membrane inhibitor of reactive lysis (MIRL, MACIF); IF-5Ag, H19, HRF20, P-18	18–25	Most cells	Ly-6	Binds C8 and C9, blocks assembly of membrane attack complex (MAC)	
CDw60	9-*O*-acetyl-GD3, carbohydrate component of gangliosides	Carbohydrate epitope	Subset of T cells, platelets, thymic epithelium, monocytes, many epithelial cells, fibroblasts, etc.		Possible costimulatory signal for T cells	
CD61	β_3-integrin, gpIIb/IIIa	110	Platelets, megakaryocytes, macrophages	Integrin β	Associates with CD41 (gpIIb/IIIa) or CD51 (vitronectin receptor)	
CD62E	E-selectin, ELAM-1, LECAM-2	140	Endothelial cells	C-type lectin, EGF, and CCP	Binds sialyl-Lewis X; neutrophil adhesion to endothelium (rolling)	
CD62L	L-selectin, LAM-1, LECAM-1, Leu-8, MEL-14, TQ-1	150	B cells, T cells, monocytes, NK cells	C-type lectin, EGF, and CCP	Binds CD34, GlyCAM; lymphocyte homing and rolling	
CD62P	P-selectin, PADGEM, GMP-140	140	Platelets, megakaryocytes, endothelium	C-type lectin, EGF, and CCP	Binds CD162 (PSGL-1); mediates platelet binding to endothelial cells; monocyte and leukocyte rolling	
CD63	Platelet-activating antigen, LIMP, MLA1, PTLG40, melanoma-associated antigen	53	Activated platelets; monocytes, macrophages	Transmembrane 4	Present in platelet lysosomes, translocated to cell surface upon activation?	Malignant melanoma

	(ME491), neuroglandular antigen (NGA), granulophysin					
CD64	FcRI, FcγRI	72	Monocytes, macrophages	Ig superfamily	High-affinity Fcy receptor; mediates phagocytosis, ADCC, macrophage activation	
CD65	Ceramide-dodecasaccharide, VIM-2	Carbohydrate epitope	Myeloid series	Oligosaccharide	Neutrophil activation?	Brain tumors
CD65s	Sialylated CD65, VIM-2	Carbohydrate	Granulocytes, monocytes	Oligosaccharide	Phagocytosis?	Brain tumors
CD66a	NCA-160, biliary glycophorin	180–180; phosphorylated glycoprotein	Granulocytes	Immunoglobulin	Adhesion molecule for *Neisseria gonorrhoeae, Neisseria meningitidis*	Member of CEA family
CD66b	CD67, CGM6, NCA-95	95–100	Granulocytes	Immunoglobulin	Nuetrophil adhesion and activation	Member of CEA family
CD66c	Nonspecific cross-reacting antigen, NCA, NCA-50/90	90	Neutrophils	Immunoglobulin	Neutrophil activation	Colon carcinoma
CD66d	CGM1	30	Neutrophils	Immunoglobulin	Receptor for *N. gonorrhoeae* and *N. meningitidis*	Member of CEA family
CD66e	CEA	180–200	Colonic epithelium	Immunoglobulin	Adhesion?	Colon and GI carcinomas
CD66f	Pregnancy-specific b1 glycoprotein (SP-1), pregnancy-specific protein	54–72	Fetal liver, placenta	Immunoglobulin	Role in maintenance of pregnancy?	Member of CEA family, liver cancer
CD68	KP1, gp110, macrosialin	110; intracellular protein, weak surface expression	Monocytes, macrophages, basophils, large lymphocytes	Mucin	Not known	Histiocytic lesions
CD69	Activation-inducer molecule (AIM), EA 1, MLR3, very early activation (VEA)	Homodimer of 28- to 32-kDa chains, phosphorylated glycoprotein	Activated B and T cells, macrophages, NK cells	C-type lectin	Early activation, Ca^{2+} influx?, transcription activation	
CD70	KI24, CD27 ligand	75, 95, 170	Activated T and B cells, macrophages	TNF	Binds CD27; costimulation of B and T cells	Lymphoid malignancies

continued

Table A3.1 Cluster-of-differentiation molecules *(continued)*

CD designation	Other names	Molecular mass (kDa) and comment	Cellular expression	Family	Function(s)	Tumor expression(s)
CD71	T9, transferrin receptor	190; 95-kDa homodimer	All proliferating cells		Transferrin receptor; uptake of ferrotransferrin; iron metabolism	Many tumor types
CD72	Lyb-2, Ly-19.2, Ly-32.2	42-kDa homodimer	B cells (not plasma cells)	C-type lectin	Unknown, ligand for CD5	Lymphoid malignancies
CD73	Ecto-5′-nucleotidase	69	B-cell subsets, T-cell subsets		Ecto-5′-nucleotidase, dephosphorylates nucleotides to allow nucleoside uptake	
CD74	Invariant chain, Ii, Iγ; MHC class II-specific chaperone	33, 35, 41, 43 (alternative initiation and splicing)	B cells, macrophages, monocytes, MHC class II-positive cells		Intracellular distribution of MHC class II molecules	
CD75	LN-1, sialylglycan		Mature B cells, T-cell subsets, erythrocytes	Blood group oligosaccharide	Ligand for CD22, B-cell/B-cell adhesion	Lymphoid malignancies
CD76	α2, 6-sialylated polyactosamine		Mature B cells, T-cell subsets	Blood group oligosaccharide	Not known; possible oligosaccharide, dependent on sialylation	
CD77	Globotriaocyl ceramide (Gb_3), P^k blood group		Germinal center B cells	Blood group oligosaccharide	Not known	Burkitt's lymphoma
CD79α, β	Igα, MB1 Igβ, B29	α, 40–45; β, 37	B cells	Ig superfamily	Component of B-cell antigen receptor analogous to CD3, required for cell surface expression and signal transduction	
CD80	B7 (now B7.1), BB1	60	B-cell subset	Ig superfamily	Costimulator, ligand for CD28 and CTLA-4	
CD81	Target of antiproliferative antibody (TAPA-1)	26	Lymphocytes, endothelial and epithelial cells	Transmembrane 4	Associates with CD19, CD21 to form B-cell coreceptor	

CD82	R2, 4F9, C33, IA4, KAI1	50–53	Leukocytes	Transmembrane 4	T-cell activation costimulator
CD83	HB15	43	Activated B cells, activated T cells, circulating dendritic cells (Langerhans cells)	Immunoglobulin	Not known
CDw84	GR6	73	Monocytes, platelets, circulating B cells		Now known
CD85	GR4	110	Monocytes, circulating B cells		Not known
CD86	B7.2, FUN-1, GR65	80	Monocytes, activated B cells, dendritic cells	Immunoglobulin	Ligand for CD28 and CTLA4, major costimulatory molecule
CD87	Urokinase plasminogen activator receptor (uPAR)	35–68	Granulocytes, monocytes, macrophages, activated T cells, NK cells, others	LY-6	Urokinase plasminogen activator receptor
CD88	C5aR	43	Polymorphonuclear leukocytes, macrophages, mast cells	G-protein-coupled receptor	Receptor for complement component C5a
CD89	FcαR, IgA receptor	Multiple, 45–100	Monocytes, macrophages, granulocytes, neutrophils, B-cell subsets, T-cell subsets	Immunoglobulin	IgA receptor; phagocytosis, respiraory burst
CD90	Thy-1	25–35	Hematopoietic stem cells, thymocytes, HEV endothelium	Immunoglobulin	Inhibition of stem cells?
CD91	α2-Macroglobulin receptor, low-density-lipoprotein receptor-related protein	515, 85	Monocytes, many non-hematopoietic cells	EGF, LDL receptor	α_2-Macroglobulin receptor
CDw92	GR9	70	Neutrophils, monocytes, platelets, endothelium		Not known
CD93	GR11	120	Neutrophils, monocytes, endothelium		Not known

continued

Table A3.1 Cluster-of-differentiation molecules *(continued)*

CD designation	Other names	Molecular mass (kDa) and comment	Cellular expression	Family	Function(s)	Tumor expression(s)
CD94	KP43	70	T-cell subsets ($CD8^+$ $\alpha\beta$ and $\gamma\delta$ T cells), NK cells	C-type lectin	Forms complex with NKG2-A (contains cytoplasmic immunoreceptor tyrosine-based inhibition motifs)	
CD95	Apo-1, Fas antigen	45, 90, >200	Wide variety of cell lines, in vivo distribution uncertain	TNF receptor superfamily	Binds TNF-like Fas ligand, induces apoptosis	
CD96	T-cell activation, increased late expression (TACTILE)	160	Activated T cells, NK cells	Immunoglobulin	Not known	
CD97	GR1, BL-KDD/F12	75–85	Activated T and B cells, macrophages, granulocytes	G-protein-coupled receptor	Binds CD55; may protect against complement activation	
CD98	4F2, FRP-1, RL-338 in mouse	80; heterodimer 45	T cells, B cells, NK cells, granulocytes, all human cell lines		Regulates cell activation, amino acid transporter?	
CD99	MIC2, E2	32	Peripheral blood lymphocytes, thymocytes		Not known	
CD100	GR3	150; homodimer 300	Broad expression on hematopoietic cells	Semaphorin	T-cell adhesion and activation	
CD101	BPC#4, P126, V7	120; homodimer 240	Granulocytes, macrophages, dendritic cells, activated T cells	Immunoglobulin	T-cell activation?	
CD102	ICAM-2	55–65	Vascular endothelial cells, monocytes, platelets, resting lymphocytes	Immunoglobulin	Binds CD11a/CD18 (LFA-1) but not CD11b/CD18 (Mac-1); costimulator of lymphocytes, lymphocyte recirculation	
CD103	HML-1, α_6, α_E-integrin	150, 25; dimer 175	Intraepithelial lymphocytes, 2–6% peripheral blood lymphocytes	Integrin α	Localization and activation of intraepithelial lymphocytes in intestine	

CD104	β_4-integrin chain, tumor-specific protein 180 in mouse	220	$CD4^-CD8^-$ thymocytes, epithelial cells, Schwann cells, some tumor cells, trophoblasts, endothelial cells	Integrin β	Associates with CD45f, binds to laminin
CD105	Endoglin	180; homodimer 95	Endothelial cells, bone marrow cell subset, in vitro-activated macrophages		Binds TGF-β; control of cell growth
CD106	VCAM-1, INCAM-110	100, 110	Endothelial cells	Ig superfamily	Adhesion molecule, ligand for VLA-4
CD107a	Lysosome-associated membrane protein 1 (LAMP-1)	110	Activated platelets, T cells, neutrophils, and endothelium		Lysosomal membrane protein translocated to the cell surface after activation
CD107b	LAMP-2	120	Activated platelets, T cells, neutrophils, and endothelium		Lysosomal membrane protein translocated to the cell surface after activation
CDw108	GR2, John Milton-Hagen blood group antigen	76–80	Activated T cells in spleen, some stromal cells, erythrocytes		Adhesion?
CD109	Platelet activation factor, GR56, 8A3, E123	170	Activated T cells, platelets, and endothelium		Not known
CD114	Granulocyte colony-stimulating factor receptor (GM-CSFR), HG-CSFR, CSF3R	150	Granulocytes, platelets, monocytes, endothelium, placenta	Immunoglobulin, fibronectin type III	Regulator of myeloid proliferation and differentiation
CD115	Macrophage colony stimulation factor receptor (M-CSFR), c-Fms, colony-stimulating factor 1R (CSF-1R)	150	Monocytes, macrophages	Immunoglobulin, tyrosine kinase	Macrophage colony-stimulating factor (M-CSF) receptor; macrophage proliferation

continued

Table A3.1 Cluster-of-differentiation molecules *(continued)*

CD designation	Other names	Molecular mass (kDa) and comment	Cellular expression	Family	Function(s)	Tumor expression(s)
CD116	GM-CSFRα	70–85	Monocytes, neutrophils, eosinophils, endothelium	Cytokine receptor, fibronectin type III	Granulocyte-macrophage colony-stimulating factor (GM-CSF), receptor α chain	
CD117	*c-kit,* stem cell factor (SCF)	145	Hematopoietic progenitors	Immunoglobulin, tyrosine kinase	SCF receptor, hematopoiesis	
CD118	IFN-a, βR		Broad cellular expression		IFN-β receptor	
CDw119	IFN-γR	90–100	Macrophages, monocytes, B cells, endothelium	Fibronectin type III	IFN-γ receptor	
CD120a	TNFR-I	50–60	Hematopoietic and nonhematopoietic cells, highest on epithelial cells	Tumor necrosis factor receptor I (TNFR-I)	TNF receptor (binds both TNF-α and TNF-β)	
CD120b	TNFR-II	75–85	Hematopoietic and nonhematopoietic cells, highest on myeloid cells	TNFR-II	TNF receptor, binds both TNF-α and TNF-β	
CDw121a	IL-1 receptor type I (IL-1R type I, IL-1R)	80	Thymocytes, T cells	Immunoglobulin	Type I interleukin-1 receptor (binds IL-1α and IL-1β)	
CDw121b	IL-1R type II	60–70	B cells, macrophages, monocytes	Immunoglobulin	Type II interleukin-1 receptor, binds IL-1α and IL-1β	
CD122	IL-2 receptor β chain (IL-2Rβ)	75	NK cells, resting T-cell subsets, some B-cell lines	Cytokine receptor, fibronectin type III	Takes part in IL-2 and IL-15 signaling	
CD123	IL-3 receptor α subunit (IL-3Rα)	70	Bone marrow stem cells, granulocytes, monocytes, megakaryocytes	Cytokine receptor, fibronectin type III	IL-3 receptor; hematopoietic differentiation	
CD124	IL-4R	130–150	Mature B and T cells, hematopoietic precursor cells	Cytokine receptor, fibronectin type III	IL-4 receptor; B-cell differentiation	

CD125	IL-5 receptor α chain (IL-5Rα)	55–60	Eosinophils, basophils, activated B cells	Cytokine receptor, fibronectin type III	IL-5 receptor; B-cell, eosinophil, basophil differentiation	
CD126	IL-6 receptor α subunit (IL-6Rα)	80	Activated B cells and plasma cells (strong), most leukocytes (weak), some nonhematopoietic cells	Immunoglobulin, cytokine receptor, fibronectin type III	IL-6 receptor; B-cell differentiation	
CD127	IL-7 receptor α subunit (IL-7Rα)	68–79, 90; may form homodimers	Bone marrow lymphoid precursors, pro-B cells, mature T cells, monocytes	Fibronectin type III	IL-7 receptor	
CDw128a	CXR1, IL-8 receptor A (IL-8R A)	58–67	Neutrophils, basophils, T-cell subset	G-protein-coupled receptor	IL-8 receptor	
CDw128b	CXR2, IL-8R B	58–67	Neutrophils, basophils, T-cell subset	G-protein-coupled receptor	IL-8 receptor	
CD130	IL-6Rβ, IL-IIRβ, OSMRβ, LIFRβ	130	Activated B cells and plasma cells (strong), most leukocytes (weak), endothelial cells	Immunoglobulin, cytokine receptor, fibronectin type III	Receptor for IL-6, IL-11, LIF, CNF, oncostatin M, and cardiotropin-1	Many
CDw131	Common β subunit	120–140	Early myeloid progenitor cells, immature B cells	Cytokine receptor, fibronectin type III	Receptor subunit for IL-3, GM-CSF, IL-5	
CD132	Common cytokine receptor γ chain	64, 65–70	T cells, B cells, NK cells, macrophages, neutrophils	Cytokine receptor	Subunit of IL-2, IL-4, IL-7, IL-9, and IL-15 receptors	
CD134	OX40	50	Activated T cells	TNF receptor	Adhesion molecule co-stimulator	
CD135	FMS-like tyrosine kinase 3 (flt3, FLK-2 in mice, STK-1)	130	Myelomonocytic precursors, primitive B cells	Immunoglobulin, tyrosine kinase	Growth factor receptor for early hematopoietic factors	
CDw136	Macrophage-stimulating protein receptor (msp receptor), p158-ron	180	Monocytes, epithelial cells	Tyrosine kinase	Chemotaxis, cell growth and differentiation	

continued

Table A3.1 Cluster-of-differentiation molecules *(continued)*

CD designation	Other names	Molecular mass (kDa) and comment	Cellular expression	Family	Function(s)	Tumor expression(s)
CDw137	4-1BB, induced by lymphocyte activation (ILA)	85	T cells, B cells, monocytes, and some epithelial cells	TNF receptor	Costimulator of T-cell proliferation	
CD138	Heparin sulfate proteoglycan, syndecan-1	Not known	B cells		Binding to collagen type I	
CD139		209, 228	B cells, monocytes, granulocytes, follicular dendritic cells		Not known	
CD140a, b	Platelet-derived growth factor (PDGF) receptor α and β chains	180	Stromal cells, some endothelial cells	Growth factor receptor	Receptor for PDGF	
CD141	Fetomodulin, thrombomodulin (TM)	75, 105	Vascular endothelial cells, megakaryocytes, platelets, monocytes, neutrophils	C-type lectin, EGF	Anticoagulant; binds thrombin, activates protein C	
CD142	Coagulation factor III, thromboplastin, tissue factor (TF)	45–47	Keratinocytes, epithelial cells, activated endothelial cells, and monocytes	Fibronectin type III	Major initiating factor of coagulation; binds factor VIIa and activated factors VII, IX and X	
CD143	Angiotensin-converting enzyme (ACE), peptidyl dipeptidase A	170–180	Endothelial cells, brush borders of kidney and small intestine, neuronal cells, activated macrophages, some T cells		Cleaves angiotensin II and bradykinin from precursors; regulates blood pressure	
CD144	Cadherin-5	130–135	Endothelial cells	Cadherin	Organizes adherens junctions in endothelial cells, controls vascular permeability	
CDw145		25, 90, 110	Endothelial cells		Not known	
CD146	A32, MCAM, MUC18, mel-CAM	110, 130	Endothelial cells, subpopulation of activated T cells	Immunoglobulin	Cell adhesion	

CD147	M6, neurothelin, EMMPRIN, basigin, OX-47, gp42 in mouse	55–65	Most blood cells and endothelial cells	Immunoglobulin	Cell adhesion
CD148	HPTPη, high-cell-density-enhanced PTP1, p260	240–260	Myelocytes, monocytes, dendritic cells, T cells, fibroblasts, nerve cells, platelets	Fibronectin type III, protein tyrosine phosphatase	Contact inhibition of cell growth
CDw149	MEM-133	120	White blood cells, platelets		Not known
CD150	IPO-3, signaling lymphocyte-activating protein (SLAM)	75–95	Thymocytes, activated lymphocytes, dendritic cells, endothelial cells, B cells	Immunoglobulin	B-cell costimulation
CD151	PETA-3, SFA-1	32	Platelets, megakaryocytes, immature blood cells, endothelial cells	Transmembrane 4	Adhesion molecule, associates with β_1-integrins
CD152	Cyotoxic T lymphocyte protein 4 (CTLA-4)	22	Activated CD4 T cells	Immunoglobulin	Receptor for B7.1, B7.2; negative regulator of T-cell activation
CD153	CD30 ligand (CD3OL)	38–40	Activated T cells and macrophages, neutrophils, B cells	TNF	Ligand for CD30, costimulator of T cells
CD154	CD40 ligand, T-BAM, TNF-related activation protein	30	Activated CD4 T cells	TNF receptor	Ligand for CD40, inducer of B-cell proliferation and activation
CD155	Poliovirus receptor	80–90	Monocytes, macrophages, thymocytes, CNS neurons	Immunoglobulin	Normal function not known
CD156	ADAM8, MS2 human	69	Neutrophils, monocytes		May be involved in extravasation of white cells
CD157	BP-3/IM-7, BST-1, Mo5	42–45, 50	White blood cells, lymphocyte precursors, bone marrow stroma, endothelial cells, follicular dendritic cells		ADP-ribosyl cyclase, cyclic ADP-ribose hydrolase; support for lymphocyte progenitors

continued

Table A3.1 Cluster-of-differentiation molecules *(continued)*

CD designation	Other names	Molecular mass (kDa) and comment	Cellular expression	Family	Function(s)	Tumor expression(s)
CDw158a, b	a-EB6, b-GL183, MHC class I-specific receptors	50,58	NK-cell subsets, some T cells	Immunoglobulin	Inhibits NK cytotoxicity upon interaction with HLA-c alleles	
CD161	NKR-P1A	44, 80	NK cells, subset of T cells, thymocytes	C-type lectin	Regulates NK cytotoxicity through Fc receptor on targets; induction of immature thymocyte proliferation	
CD162	PSGL-1	120; homodimer 240	Neutrophils, lymphocytes monocytes	Mucin	Ligand for CD62P, mediates leukocyte rolling	
CD163	GHI/61, M130	130	Monocytes, macrophages		Not known	
CD164	MUC-24, multi-glycosylated core protein 24	80	Epithelial cells, monocytes, bone marrow stromal cells	Mucin	Not known	
CD165	AD2, gp37	37	Thymocytes, thymic epithelial cells, monocytes, PBLs, CNS neurons, pancreatic islets, Bowman's capsule		Adhesion between thymocytes and thymic epithelial cells	
CD166	BEN, DM-GRASP, KG-Cam, neurolin, SC-1, activated leukocyte adhesion molecule (ALCAM)	100–105	Activated T cells, thymic epithelium, fibroblasts, neurons	Immunoglobulin	Ligand for CD6, integrin neurite extension	
TCRζ	T-cell receptor ζ chain	12	T cells, NK cells	ζ chain	Part of T-cell receptor activation of T cells	

APPENDIX 4
Cytokines

Cytokines are polypeptides secreted by one cell that may act on the cell that secreted it (autocrine) or on other cells nearby (paracrine) or may be released systemically and act on distant cells in other tissue sites (holocrine) to regulate the function of the target cell. These include interleukins (cytokines made by white blood cells that act on other white blood cells); growth factors, which act in hematopoiesis; interferons, which inhibit viral infections; ligands, which act on T and B cells; and factors which promote or inhibit inflammation. Activation requires interaction with a cell surface receptor in the the responding cells, and the responding cells may increase or decrease reactivity by changing the number of receptors available.

A chalone is classically defined as a cytokine that specifically decreases activity or proliferation of a cell type. The only true chalone in Table A4.1 is transforming growth factor β1.

Table A4.1 Cytokines

Cytokine	Family	Size (kDa) and form	Receptor(s)	Producer cells	Action(s)	Disease association(s)
IL-1α	Unassigned	159, monomer	CD121a (IL-RI), CD121b (IL-1RII)	Macrophages, epithelial cells	T-cell activation, macrophage activation	Fever, inflammation, RA, CLL, etc.
IL-1β	Unassigned	153, monomer	CD121a (IL-RI), CD121b (IL-1RII)	Macrophages, epithelial cells	T-cell activation, macrophage activation	Fever, inflammation, RA, CLL, etc.
IL-1RA	Unassigned	Monomer	CD121a	Monocytes, macrophages, neutrophils, hepatocytes	Binds to IL-1R, blocks action of IL-1	Weight loss, septic shock
IL-2	Hematopoietin	133, monomer	CD25 (α), CD122 (β), CD132 (γc)	T cells	T-cell proliferation	Inflammation, SLE, autoimmune disease
IL-3 (CSF)	Hematopoietin	133, monomer	CD123 (βc)	T cells, thymic epithelial cells	Stimulates hematopoiesis and differentiation	Leukemia, mastocytosis, malaria, asthma, allergy
IL-4 (BCGF-1)	Hematopoietin	129, monomer	CD124, CD132 (γc)	T cells, mast cells	B-cell activation, IgE switch, suppresses Th1 cells	Allergy, leukemia, immune deviation
IL-5 (BCGF-2)	Hematopoietin	115, homodimer	cd125 (βc)	T cells, mast cells	Eosinophil growth and differentiation	Eosinophilia, allergy, rhinitis
IL-6 (IFN-β2)	Hematopoietin	184, monomer	CD126, CD132 (γc)	T cells, macrophages, endothelial cells	T- and B-cell growth and differentiation	Fever, RA, psoriasis, myeloma, Castleman's disease
IL-7	Hematopoietin	152, monomer	CD127, CD132 (γc)	Thymic and bone marrow stroma	Growth and differentiation of T- and B-cell precursors	Pre-B-cell tumors, leukemia
IL-8	Chemokine	69–79, dimer	CXR1, 2	Monocytes, T cells, fibroblasts, etc.	Attracts and activates neutrophils	Inflammation, RA, psoriasis, neutrophilia
IL-9	Hematopoietin	125, monomer	CD132 (γc), IL-9R	T cells	Activates mast cells	Allergies, Hodgkin's disease, lymphomas
IL-10	Unassigned	160, homodimer	IL-10Rα, CRF2-4 (IL-10Rβ)	T cells, macrophages, EBV-infected cells	Suppresses macrophages	Burkitt's lymphoma
IL-11	Hematopoietin	178, monomer	IL-11R, CD130	Fibroblasts	Synergizes with IL-3 and IL-4; hematopoiesis	Megakaryocytic leukemia
IL-12	Unassigned	197 and 306, heterodimer	ILR-β1, ILR-β2	B cells, macrophages	Activates NK cells, induces differentiation of Th1 cells	Leukemia

IL-13 (P600)	Hematopoietin	132, monomer	IL-13R, CD132 (γc), CD24?	T cells	B-cell growth and differentiation; inhibits MIF production, Th1 cells	
IL-15 (TGF)	Hematopoietin	114, monomer	IL-15R, CD122 (IL-Rβ), CD132 (γc)	T cells	IL-2-like, proliferation of intestinal epithelium, T cells, and NK cells	Inflammation, leukemia
IL-16	Unassigned	130, homotetramer	CD4	T cells, mast cells, eosinophils	Attracts CD4 T cells, monocytes, and eosinophils; increases survival of IL-2-stimulated T cells	Inflammation, autoimmune diseases
IL-17 (mCTLA-8)	Unassigned	150, monomer		CD4 memory cells	Stimulates cytokine production by epithelium, endothelium, and fibroblasts	Inflammation
IL-18 (IGIF)	Unassigned	157, monomer	IL-1R-related protein (rp)	Activated macrophages, Kupffer cells	Stimulates IFN-γ production, Th1 cell differentiation	
G-CSF (granulocyte colony-stimulating factor)	Hematopoietin	174, monomer	G-CSFR	Fibroblasts, monocytes	Granulocyte proliferation and differentiation	Chronic neutropenia, leukemia
GM-CSF (granulocyte-macrophage CSF)	Hematopoietin	127, monomer	CD116, βc	Macrophages, T cells	Myelomonocytic growth and differentiation	Myelodysplasia, leukemia, osteosarcoma
OSM (oncostatin M)	Hematopoietin	196, monomer	OSMR, LIFR, CD130	T cells, macrophages	Inhibits melanoma	Kaposi's sarcoma
LIF (leukemia inhibitory factor)	Hematopoietin	179, monomer	LIFP, CD130	Fibroblasts, bone marrow stroma	IL-6-like, growth factor for embryonic stem cells	Cachexia, anemia, pancreatitis, osteoporosis
TGF-β	Unassigned	112, homo- and heterotrimers	TGF-βR	Chondrocytes, monocytes, T cells	Inhibits cell growth	Anti-inflammatory
IFN-γ	Interferon	143, homodimer	CD119, IFNGR2	T cells, NK cells	Activates macrophages, MHC expression, antigen processing, Ig class switching	Increased resistance to infections, autoimmunity, SLE, Sjögren's syndrome
IFN-α	Interferon	166, monomer	CD118, IFNAR2	White blood cells	Increased MHC class I	Antiviral immunity
IFN-β	Interferon	166, monomer	CD118, IFNAR2	Fibroblasts	Increased MHC class I	Antiviral immunity
TNF-α	TNF	157, trimer	p55, p75, CD120a, CD120b	Macrophages, NK cells, T cells	Activates endothelial cells, leukocyte adherence	Inflammation, cachexia, RA, lymphoma, septic shock, multiple sclerosis, etc.

continued

Table A4.1 Cytokines *(continued)*

Cytokine	Family	Size (kDa) and form	Receptor(s)	Producer cells	Action(s)	Disease association(s)
TNF-β (LT, lymphotoxin)	TNF	171, trimer	p55, p75, CD120a, CD120b	T cells, B cells	Cell killing, endothelial activation	Autoimmune diseases, inflammation
LT-β	TNF	Transmembrane, trimerizes with TNF-β	LT βR, HVEM	T cells, B cells	T-cell, B-cell development	Loss results in defective development of peripheral lymphoid organs
CD40 ligand (CD40L)	TNF	Trimers	CD40	T cells	B-cell activation, Ig class switching	Loss causes hyper-IgM syndrome
Fas ligand (FasL)	TNF	Trimers	CD95 (Fas)	T cells	Apoptosis, cytotoxicity	Loss leads to lymphomas, autoimmunity
CD27 ligand (CD27L)	TNF	Trimers	CD27	T cells	T-cell proliferation	
CD30 ligand (CD30L)	TNF	Trimers	CD30	T cells	T- and B-cell proliferation	Loss leads to autoimmunity
B7.1 (CD80)	Immunoglobulin	262, dimer	CD28, CTLA-4	Antigen-presenting cells	Costimulates T cells	Loss leads to increased infections
B7.2 (B70, CD86)	Immunoglobulin		CD28, CTLA-4	Antigen-presenting cells	Costimulates T cells	Loss leads to lymphoproliferation
MIF (migration inhibitory factor)	Unassigned	115, monomer		T cells, pituitary cells	Inhibits macrophage migration	Inflammation

APPENDIX 5
Clinical Immunology Tests

Immunologically based tests (Table A5.1) are used for diagnosis and determination of prognosis for many human diseases. The tests may be classified as to which diseases they are used, as follows:

Serum proteins	Immune deficiencies Inflammation Myeloma
Cell-mediated immunity	Immune deficiencies Leukemia/lymphoma Cancer (prognosis)
Tissue typing	Blood transfusion Tissue grafting
Specific antibodies	Infectious diseases Autoimmune diseases Allergic reactions (IgE)
Tumor-associated antigens	Cancer

As techniques in molecular biology become more available and reagents better characterized, many assays, such as those for specific infectious agents or for determination of prognosis in cancer, are being replaced by assays using multiplication of DNA (polymerase chain reactions) and specific complementary DNA (cDNA) probes. Immune-labeling procedures for detection of organisms in tissues are being replaced by in situ hybridization using cDNA, a method that is also being applied to detect genetic changes in cancers. It is expected that molecular hybridization will soon replace serologic methods for determination of HLA phenotypes. Flow cytometry has been used increasingly for quantitation of expression of cell surface markers detected by antibodies. In addition, many colorimetrically based assays have been automated, greatly decreasing cost and turnover time.

For more details on clinical immunologic testing, see the references in the bibliography.

Table A5.1 Some clinical immunology tests[a]

Measurement	Assay used	Disease(s)
Serum proteins; humoral immunity		
Major globulins	Serum electrophoresis	Immune deficiencies, myeloma, other protein anomalies
Serum Ig classes	Nephelometry, RID	Immune deficiencies, myeloma
Serum proteins	Isolectric focusing, immune fixation, isoelectric focusing, electrophoresis	Immune deficiencies, myeloma, immune globulin aberrations
Total complement	Hemolytic assay	Immune deficiencies, immune complex disorders
Serum complement components	Nephelometry, RID	Immune deficiencies, immune disorders
C1 esterase inhibitor	Nephelometry, inhibition of C1	Angioedema
C breakdown products	ELISA	Acute inflammation
Bence Jones protein (urine)	Precipitation/nephelometry	Myeloma
Cryoglobulins	Cold precipitation	Raynaud's phenomenon, arthralgias
Immune complexes	Raji cell binding, C1q binding, anti-Ig binding	Immune complex diseases
Cellular immunity (for cytokines, see appendix 4; for CD markers, see appendix 3)		
Total cells	Complete blood count, differential count	Infection, leukemia/immune deficiency
T cells		
Total/subpopulations	Flow cytometry	Immune deficiency, leukemia/ lymphoma, AIDS
Mitogen response	PHA, concanavalin A	Immune deficiency, leukemia/lymphoma
Interleukins	ELISA	Immune deficiency, inflammation, etc.
Cytokine production	ELISA	Immune deficiency, inflammation, etc.
T-cell receptor gene rearrangements	Flow cytometry, cDNA binding on gels	Immune deficiency, leukemia/ lymphoma
IL-2 receptors	Flow cytometry	Leukemia/lymphoma prognosis
Soluble IL-2R	ELISA	SLE, RA prognosis
ICAM-1	ELISA	Inflammation, RA, lymphoma
Neopterin (T-cell activation)	RIA	Infections, inflammation, prognosis
B cells		
Surface Ig, subpopulations and Ig class clonality	Flow cytometry	Immune deficiency, leukemia/lymphoma
Ig gene rearrangements	cDNA binding on gels	Myeloma
Monocytes/macrophages		
Subpopulations	Flow cytometry	Leukemia/lymphoma
IL-1 production	Growth of T-cell lines	Immune deficiency
Bacterial killing	Cytotoxicity in vitro	Immune deficiency
Activation	Production of oxygen radicals	Immune deficiency
Neutrophils		
Subpopulations	Flow cytometry	Myeloid leukemia
Phagocytosis	Particle uptake	Immune deficiency
Digestion	Nitroblue tetrazolium reduction	Immune deficiency
Bacterial killing	Bactericidal test in vitro	Immune deficiency
Migration	Micropore filter in vitro	Immune deficiency
Infectious diseases (microbiology)		
Bacterial	Antibody titers, PCR	Specific diagnosis
Mycobacterial	Immunofluorescence, PCR	Specific diagnosis
Parasitic	Antibody, PCR	Specific diagnosis

Table A5.1 *(continued)*

Measurement	Assay used	Disease(s)
Fungal	Antibody (ELISA), PCR, immunofluorescence, Western blot	Specific diagnosis
Viral	Antibody, immunofluorescence, PCR, ELISA, in situ hybridization, immunoblots	Specific diagnosis
Rickettsial	Antibody, PCR, immunoblots	Specific diagnosis
Chlamydial	Immunofluorescence, PCR, immunoblots	Specific diagnosis
Transfusion		
Blood group antigens	Type and cross-match	Donor selection
Platelet antigens	Flow cytometry	Donor selection
Ig allotypes	Hemagglutination inhibition	Donor selection
HIV antibody	ELISA, Western blot	Donor selection, diagnosis
HIV antigen	PCR	Donor selection, pediatric infection
Hepatitis antibody	ELISA	Donor selection, diagnosis
Hepatitis antigens	PCR (cDNA)	Donor selection, diagnosis
Fibrin split products	ELISA	Bleeding disorders
Transplantation		
HLA (A–D) antigens	Serologic cytotoxicity, PCR	Donor selection
HLA-D cellular antigens	Mixed lymphocyte reaction, PCR	Donor selection
Lymphocyte killing	Cell-mediated cytotoxicity	Rejection reaction
Antilymphocyte antibody	Serological cytotoxicity, flow cytometry	Donor activity
Allergic reactions		
Serum IgE	ELISA	Allergic predisposition
Allergen-specific IgE	RAST, immunoblot	Specific allergen
Basophil reactivity	Histamine release (fluorimetry)	Specific allergen
Skin test	Wheal and flare	Specific allergen
Schultz-Dale test	Constriction of smooth muscle in vitro	Specific allergen
Antibody-mediated diseases		
Tissue antibodies		
Acetylcholine receptor	ELISA, binding inhibition	Myasthenia gravis
Pancreatic islet cells	ELISA, IF	Type I diabetes mellitus
Basement membrane	ELISA, IF	Goodpasture's syndrome
Mitochondria	ELISA, IF	Primary biliary cirrhosis
TSH receptor	ELISA, IF	Graves' disease
Thyroglobulin	ELISA, IF, passive hemagglutination	Thyroiditis
Thyroid microsomes	IF, passive hemagglutination	Thyroid diseases
Adrenal antigens	IF	Idiopathic Addison's disease
Parathyroid antigens	IF	Idiopathic hypoparathyroidism
Striational	IF	Myasthenia gravis with thymoma
Smooth muscle antigens	IF	Chronic hepatitis, cirrhosis
Cardiac muscle	IF	Rheumatic myocarditis, bypass surgery
Gastric parietal cells	IF, ELISA for intrinsic factor	Pernicious anemia
Gliadin, reticulin, endomysin	ELISA	Gluten sensitivity
Antineutrophil cytoplasmic antibodies	RIA, IF, flow cytometry	Wegener's granulomatosis, vasculitis
Antiphospholipids	ELISA	SLE, fetal loss, PAPS
Antineurons	ELISA	SLE with CNS symptoms
Skin, basement membrane	IF	Pemphigus vulgaris
Skin, epidermal cells	IF	Bullous pemphigoid

(continued)

Table A5.1 Some clinical immunology tests *(continued)*

Measurement	Assay used	Disease(s)
Antinuclear antibodies/collagen diseases		
Anti-ssDNA	ELISA	Scleroderma, SLE, etc.
Anti-dsDNA	ELISA	SLE
Anti-Sm	ELISA, immunoblot	SLE
Anti-RNP	ELISA, immunoblot	SLE, MCTD, polymyositis, scleroderma
Antihistones	Immunodiffusion, ELISA	SLE, drug-induced SLE
Anti-Scl 70	Immunodiffusion, ELISA	Scleroderma
Anticentromere	IF	CREST syndrome
Anti-JO1	ELISA, immunodiffusion	Polymyositis, scleroderma
Anti-Pn-Ac1 (Pn-1)	ELISA, immunodiffusion	Polymyositis, scleroderma
Anti-Mi2	ELISA, immunodiffusion	Dermatomyositis
Anti-La (SS-B)	ELISA, immunodiffusion	SLE, Sjögren's syndrome
Anti-Ro (SS-A) (cytoplasm)	ELISA, immunodiffusion	SLE, Sjögren's syndrome
Rheumatoid factor	Nephelometry, latex agglutination	Rheumatoid arthritis
Cancer		
Tumor immunity (see chapter 20)		
Antitumor antibodies	ELISA, IF, cytotoxicity, cell/antigen	Reactivity to specific tumor
Cell-mediated cytotoxicity	Cell lysis (^{51}Cr release), colony inhibition in vitro	Specific and nonspecific killing
ADCC	Cell lysis	Antibody-directed cell-mediated cytotoxicity
Lymphocyte reactivity	Blast transformation, IL-2 and lymphokine production	Specific reactivity to tumors
Blocking factors	Inhibition of cell-mediated immunity	Blocking of tumor immunity
Tumor markers, serum (see chapter 20 for other markers not listed)		
Alpha-fetoprotein	ELISA	Diagnosis, prognosis
Carcinoembryonic antigen	ELISA	Prognosis
Prostate-specific antigen	ELISA	Screening, diagnosis, prognosis
Cancer carbohydrates	ELISA	Different cancers, prognosis
Cancer mucins	ELISA	Prognosis
Hormones[b]	ELISA	Differential diagnosis, prognosis
Myeloma proteins	Electrophoresis, immunofixation	Diagnosis, prognosis
Isoenzymes	Electrophoresis, immunofixation	Diagnosis
Melanoma antigen	ELISA	Diagnosis
Tumor markers, cellular		
Alpha-fetoprotein	IF or IP	Differential diagnosis
Carcinoembryonic antigen	IF or IP	Differential diagnosis
Prostate-specific antigen	IF, IP	Differential diagnosis
Pancreatic antigen	IF, IP	Differential diagnosis
Melanoma antigen	IF, IP	Differential diagnosis
Cancer carbohydrates	IF, IP	Differential diagnosis
Cancer mucins	IF, IP	Differential diagnosis
Lymphocyte markers	IF, IP	Differential diagnosis
Enzymes	Enzyme activity	Hematopoietic tumors
Molecular biologic markers		
Various oncogene products	IF, IP, blots	Prognosis
Ig gene rearrangements	cDNA binding on gels	B-cell tumors
T-cell receptor rearrangements	cDNA binding on gels	T-cell tumors

[a]AIDS, acquired immune deficiency syndrome; CD, cluster of differentiation; CNS, central nervous system; dsDNA, double-stranded DNA; ELISA, enzyme-linked immunosorbent assay; IF, immunofluorescence; Ig, immunoglobulin; IL, interleukin; IP, immunoperoxidase; MCTD, mixed connective tissue disease; PAPS, primary antiphospholipid syndrome; PCR, polymerase chain reaction; PHA, phytohemagglutinin; RA, rheumatoid arthritis; RAST, radioallergosorbent test; RIA, radioimmunoassay; RID, radial immunodiffusion; SLE, systemic lupus erythematosus; ssDNA, single-stranded DNA; TSH, thyroid-stimulating hormone.

[b]Insulin, gastrin, renin-angiotensin, growth hormone, placental hormones, thyroid hormones, cortisol, estradiol, testosterone, etc.

Bibliography

Folds, J. D., and D. E. Normansell. 1999. *Pocket Guide to Clinical Immunology.* ASM Press, Washington, D.C.

Rich, R. R., T. A. Fleisher, B. D. Schwartz, W. T. Shearer, and W. Strober (ed.). 1995. *Clinical Immunology.* The C. V. Mosby Co., St. Louis, Mo.

Rose, N. R., E. C. de Macario, J. D. Folds, H. C. Lane, and R. M. Nakamura (ed.). 1997. *Manual of Clinical Laboratory Immunology,* 5th ed. ASM Press, Washington, D.C.

APPENDIX 6
Tables of Lymphoproliferative Diseases

Lymphoproliferative lesions include benign hyperplasias (usually related to infections which are reversible when the infection is cleared) and cancerous proliferations of lymphocytes and monocytes. The basic classification of these lesions is based on morphology, as described in chapter 17. However, on the basis of morphology alone, some tumors arising from different cells may look essentially the same, particularly undifferentiated tumors. Thus, undifferentiated B-cell tumors may be made up of large lymphoblastic cells with loss of any follicular architecture, so they cannot be distinguished from T-cell tumors.

In recent years, the application of phenotypic markers, particularly cell surface markers, has been applied to provide a more precise definition of lymphoproliferative lesions. First, cancerous proliferations may be distinguished from noncancerous proliferations of lymphocytes because all the cells in a cancerous proliferation express the same markers, whereas noncancerous lesions are made up of cells expressing different markers. Second, lymphocytic and monocytic tumors may be subclassified on the basis of differentiation markers of lymphocytes and monocytic cells. In general, a cancer consists of a population of cells that arrested at a particular stage of differentiation. Differentiation markers (clusters of differentiation [CD]), or other cell markers characteristic of the stage of maturation arrest, may be used to classify lymphoproliferations more accurately than can be done by morphology alone. Tables A6.1 to A6.3 present a state-of-the-art classification, which is constantly changing as more markers are found and more clinical observations are made.

Table A6.1 Nonmalignant lymphoid hyperplasias (lymphadenopathies)

Lymphoproliferative condition	Features	Example(s)
Suppurative lymphadenitis	Draining a zone of acute infection; polymorphonuclear leukocytes early, macrophages later; basic lymph node structure intact	Tonsillitis
Postvaccinial and viral lymphadenitis	Mixed cellular response; mainly paracortical (T cells); also blast cells, giant cells	Vaccination
AIDS-related lymphadenopathy	Early polyclonal follicular (B-cell) and diffuse (T-cell) hyperplasia; later mixture of follicular hyperplasia and diffuse hypoplasia; terminally, marked lymphocyte depletion; sometimes Epstein-Barr virus-associated B-cell lymphoma	Human immunodeficiency virus
Drug-induced lymphadenopathy	Loss of normal architecture with a pleomorphic cell infiltrate: blasts, eosinophils, neutrophils, and plasma cells; history of drug exposure; also skin rash and fever	Diphenylhydantoin, mephenytoin
Sinus histiocytosis with massive lymphadenopathy	Massive cervical lymphadenopathy, fever, and leukocytosis; subcapsular and medullary sinusoids filled with proliferating histiocytes that phagocytose normal lymphocytes	Rosai-Dorfman disease
Lumphodermatitis (dermatopathic lymphadenitis)	Mixed inflammation: granulomas, histiocytosis, follicular hyperplasia, polymorphonuclear exudation	Tuberculosis, sarcoidosis, cat scratch disease, contrast media reaction
Giant lymph node hyperplasia	Hyaline vascular (i) and plasma cell (ii) varieties: (i) hyalinized blood vessels in small follicules, (ii) sheets of plasma cells in the interfollicular tissue	Castleman's disease
Infectious mononucleosis	Immature mononuclear cells in the peripheral blood; polyclonal Epstein-Barr virus-driven B-cell and reactive T-cell proliferation, fatigue, general malaise, and loss of appetite	Epstein-Barr virus infection

Table A6.2 Characterization of B-cell tumors[a]

Tumor	Phenotypic markers	Characteristics
Bone marrow origin		
CLL	Mature B-cell, sIg+, $CD5^{+}$	Mature B-cells, small lymphocytes, blood involved, indolent course
CLL (prolymphocytoid)	Like CLL, but with immature cells	>10% large (immature B) cells, accelerating course
Acute lymphocytic leukemia	Immature B cell, sIg^{+++}, $CD5^{+/-}$	Large cells, spleen prominently involved, rapid
Multiple myeloma	Cytoplasmic Ig, monoclonal Ig, rearranged Ig gene	Plasma cell tumors arise in bone marrow, usually high serum levels of monoclonal Ig, and, less often, monoclonal Ig light chain in urine
Hairy cell leukemia	sIg^{+++}, $CD5^{-}$, IL-$2R^{+}$	Splenomegaly, serum contains IL-2R
Lymph node origin		
Follicular lymphoma	sIg^{+++}, Bcl-2 rearranged, $CD5^{-}$	Atypical lymphocytes, germinal center type, prominent node and spleen involvement, variable course, usually follicular but may progess to diffuse tissue pattern
Mantle zone lymphoma	$sIgM^{+++}$, Bcl-1 rearranged, $CD5^{-}$	Usually cleaved lymphocytes, lymph node and spleen involvement, variable course, responds to chemotherapy
Burkitt's lymphoma	sIg^{++}, $CD5^{-}$, c-*myc* translocation	Small noncleaved cells, jaw mass, Epstein-Barr virus
Hodgkin's disease	Rearranged Ig genes, dendritic cell cytokines	Reed-Sternberg cells, many reactive cell types

[a]Modified from G. P. Schecter, p. 1734, *in* R. H. Rich, ed., *Clinical Immunology, Principles and Practice,* The C. V. Mosby Co., St Louis, Mo., 1996. Abbreviations: CLL, chronic lymphocytic leukemia; sIg, surface immunoglobulin; IL-2R, interleukin-2 receptor.

Table A6.3 Characterization of T-cell tumors[a]

Tumor	Phenotypic marker(s)[b]	Characteristics
Bone marrow origin		
T-cell acute lymphoblastic leukemia	Heterogeneous; most $CD1^+$, $CD4^-$, $CD8^-$ TdT^+, acid $phosphatase^+$, $CD2^-$ (ER)	Bone marrow origin; rapid course; poor response to chemotherapy as compared with B-cell tumors
T-cell chronic lymphocytic leukemia	Mature T cell ($CD4^+$, $CD5^-$, sIg^-, TdT^-, $CD1^-$, $CD3^+$), rare $CD8^+$, $CD2^+$	Very rare; most CLLs are $CD5^+$ B cells; do worse than B-cell CLL
IgG FcR^+ (T_G) lymphoproliferative disease	Large granular lymphocytes; mature T-cell phenotype; NK activity; $CD2^+$	Anemia, hypogammaglobulinemia, recurrent infections; benign course; NK-LGL is aggressive
Mycosis fungoides (MF)/Sézary syndrome (SS)	Mature Th ($CD9^-$, $CD4^+$, $CD8^-$, $CD1^-$, $CD2^+$)	Skin (MF); blood (SS); associated with dermatitis; survival varies with stage from 1 to 12 years
T-cell type of hairy cell leukemia	Mature T-cell phenotype	Usually B-cell tumor; splenomegaly
Adult T-cell leukemia/lymphoma	Mature Th ($CD9^-$, $CD4^+$, $CD8^-$, $CD1^-$, $CD2^+$) also HLA-$B5^+$ (shared with HTLV-1)	Skin, hypercalcemia, often aggressive HTLV-1-associated; Japan, Caribbean
Thymus		
Thymoma	Immature: $CD1^+$, $CD4^-$, $CD8^-$, $CD2^-$	Anterior mediastinum: usually epithelial with nonmalignant T cells; true thymic lymphoma very rare
Lymph node		
T-lymphoblastic lymphoma	Heterogeneous, most express immature thymocyte phenotype; TdT^+, sIg^-, $CD2^+$	Rare, usually in children, begins in thymus, extends to other organs and blood
T-cell non-Hodgkin's lymphoma	Mature T-cell phenotype	Rare, diffuse lymphoma, usually B-cell tumors

[a]Modified from E. A. Harden, T. J. Polker, and B. F. Haynes, *in* S. Sell and R. Reisfeld, ed., *Monoclonal Antibodies in Cancer,* Humana Press, Totowa, N.J., 1985. Abbreviations: TdT, terminal deoxynucleotidyl transferase; CLL, chronic lymphocytic leukemia; sIg, soluble immunoglobulin; NK, natural killer; LGL, lymphogranulocytic leukemia; Th, T helper; HTLV-1, human T-cell leukemia virus type 1.

[b]Many variations in phenotyic expression are seen. CD2 = ER (sheep erythrocyte receptor).

Index

Page numbers followed by *f* indicate a figure; page numbers followed by *t* indicate tabular material.

C

H

J

M

X

Z